Ambulatory Pediatric Care

Ambulatory
Pediatric Care

SECOND EDITION

Edited by
Robert A. Dershewitz, M.D., Sc.M., F.A.A.P.

Chief of Pediatrics
Harvard Community Health Plan
Braintree and Quincy Centers;
Clinical Assistant Professor of Pediatrics
Harvard Medical School;
Assistant in Pediatrics
Massachusetts General Hospital;
Courtesy Staff (Medicine)
The Children's Hospital, Boston;
Associate Pediatrician
Brigham and Women's Hospital
Boston, Massachusetts

WITH 141 CONTRIBUTORS

J. B. LIPPINCOTT COMPANY
Philadelphia

Acquisitions Editor: Charles McCormick, Jr.
Developmental Editor: Kimberley Cox
Project Editor: Mary Rose Muccie
Indexer: Victoria Boyle
Designer: Chris Laird
Production Manager: Helen Ewan
Production Coordinator: Nannette Winski
Compositor: G & S Typesetters, Inc.
Printer/Binder: Courier Book Company/Westford

2nd Edition

1 3 5 6 4 2

Library of Congress Cataloging-in-Publication Data

Ambulatory pediatric care / edited by Robert A. Dershewitz ; with
    141 contributors. — 2nd ed.
        p.   cm.
    Includes bibliographical references and index.
    ISBN 0-397-51196-5
    1. Ambulatory medical care for children.   I. Dershewitz,
Robert A.
    [DNLM: 1. Ambulatory Care.   2. Pediatrics.   WS 200
A4965]
RJ101.A42   1992
618.92—dc20
DNLM/DLC
for Library of Congress   92-13524
                                                      CIP

The authors and publisher have exerted every effort to ensure that drug
selection and dosage set forth in this text are in accord with current
recommendations and practice at the time of publication. However, in
view of ongoing research, changes in government regulations, and the
constant flow of information relating to drug therapy and drug reactions, the reader is urged to check the package insert for each drug for
any change in indications and dosage and for added warnings and precautions. This is particularly important when the recommended agent
is a new or infrequently employed drug.

To my wife, daughters, parents, and patients,
with my gratitude for your gifts of
joy, happiness, growth, and fulfillment

Contributors

Corrie T. M. Anderson, M.D.
Assistant Clinical Professor of Anesthesiology and
Pediatrics
University of California, Los Angeles
UCLA School of Medicine
Centers for the Health Sciences
Los Angeles, California

Russell S. Asnes, M.D.
Clinical Professor of Pediatrics
Colombia University
College of Physicians and Surgeons
New York, New York
Attending Pediatrician
Englewood Hospital
Englewood, New Jersey

Irving W. Bailit, M.D.
Instructor in Pediatrics
Harvard Medical School
Associate in Allergy
Children's Hospital
Boston, Massachusetts

Sophie J. Balk, M.D.
Assistant Professor of Pediatrics
Albert Einstein College of Medicine
Attending Pediatrician
Bronx Municipal Hospital Center
Bronx, New York

Victor C. Baum, M.D.
Assistant Professor of Anesthesiology and Pediatrics
UCLA School of Medicine
Attending Physician
Departments of Anesthesiology and Pediatrics
(Critical Care)

UCLA Center for Health Sciences
Los Angeles, California

Margaret L. Bauman, M.D.
Assistant Professor of Neurology
Harvard Medical School
Assistant Pediatrician and Neurologist
Massachusetts General Hospital
Boston, Massachusetts

David Bergman, M.D.
Clinical Associate Professor of Pediatrics
Stanford University School of Medicine
Stanford, California
Medical Director for Quality Management
Lucille Packard Children's Hospital
Palo Alto, California

James H. Berman, M.D.
Clinical Assistant Professor of Pediatrics
University of Chicago
Chicago, Illinois

Donald M. Berwick, M.D., MPP
Associate Professor of Pediatrics
Harvard Medical School
Associate in Pediatrics
Children's Hospital Medical Center
Pediatrician
Harvard Community Health Plan
Boston, Massachusetts

Franny Billingsley
Children's Book Buyer
57th Street Books
Chicago, IL

Herbert Boerstling, M.D.
Clinical Instructor in Pediatrics
Harvard Medical School
Pediatrician
Harvard Community Health Plan
Wellesley, Massachusetts

William P. Boger, III, M.D.
Clinical Instructor in Ophthalmology
The Children's Hospital
Harvard Medical School
Associate in Ophthalmology
Children's Hospital
Boston, Massachusetts
Active Staff
Emerson Hospital
Concord, Massachusetts

Kenneth M. Boyer, M.D.
Professor of Pediatrics and Immunology/
    Microbiology
Rush Medical College
Director, Section of Infectious Diseases, and
    Associate Chairman
Department of Pediatrics
Rush Presbyterian–St. Luke's Medical Center
Chicago, Illinois

Murray A. Braun, M.D.
Clinical Instructor in Neurology
Harvard University Medical School
Consultant, Pediatric Neurology
Harvard Community Health Plan
West Roxbury, Massachusetts

Jean R. Brodnax, M.D.
Clinical Instructor in Pediatrics
Harvard Medical School
Boston, Massachusetts
Pediatrician
Harvard Community Health Plan
Braintree, Massachusetts

David I. Bromberg, M.D.
Clinical Assistant Professor
University of Maryland Medical School
Baltimore, Maryland

Lorin M. Brown, M.D.
Instructor of Clinical Orthopedic Surgery
Northwestern University
Attending Surgeon
The Children's Memorial Hospital
Chicago, Illinois

Thomas R. Browne, M.D.
Professor of Neurology
Associate Professor of Pharmacology
Boston University School of Medicine
Boston, Massachusetts

Paul K. Bruchez, Psy.D.
Psychologist
Child Mental Health
Harvard Community Health Plan
Wellesley, Massachusetts

Hugh A. Carithers, M.D.
Clinical Professor of Pediatrics
Jacksonville Health Education Programs
Division of the Health Center
University of Florida
Jacksonville, Florida

Robert A. Catalano, M.D.
Vice President for Medical Affairs
Olean General Hospital
Olean, New York

Verne S. Caviness, Jr., M.D., Ph.D.
Joseph and Rose Kennedy Professor of Child
    Neurology and Mental Retardation
Harvard Medical School
Chief, Division of Child Neurology
Massachusetts General Hospital
Boston, Massachusetts

Tien-lan Chang, M.D.
Instructor
Harvard Medical School
Assistant in Pediatrics
Massachusetts General Hospital
Boston, Massachusetts

Paul H. Chapman, M.D.
Associate Professor of Surgery
Harvard Medical School
Chief, Pediatric Neurosurgery
Massachusetts General Hospital
Boston, Massachusetts

Evan Charney, M.D.
Professor of Pediatrics
University of Massachusetts Medical School
Chairman, Department of Pediatrics
University of Massachusetts Medical Center
Worcester, Massachusetts

Katherine Kaufer Christoffel, M.D., MPH
Professor, Pediatrics and Community Health and
      Preventive Medicine
Northwestern University School of Medicine
Director, Nutrition Evaluation Clinic
Attending Pediatrician
The Children's Memorial Hospital
Chicago, Illinois

Edward R. Christophersen, Ph.D.
Professor of Pediatrics
University of Missouri at Kansas City
School of Medicine
Chief, Behavioral Pediatrics Section
Children's Mercy Hospital
Kansas City, Missouri

William D. Cochran, M.D.
Clinical Associate Professor of Pediatrics
Harvard Medical School
Physician-in-Charge
Newborn Service
Beth Israel Hospital
Boston, Massachusetts

Herbert E. Cohn, M.D.
Clinical Instructor in Pediatrics
Harvard Medical School
Consultant in Pediatric Cardiology
Harvard Community Health Plan
Boston, Massachusetts

Edward C. Connor, M.D.
Associate Professor of Pediatrics
University of Medicine and Dentistry of New Jersey
New Jersey Medical School
Newark, New Jersey

John F. Crigler, Jr., M.D.
Associate Professor of Pediatrics
Harvard Medical School
Divisions of Endocrinology and Adolescent and
      Young Adult Medicine
The Children's Hospital
Boston, Massachusetts

Barry Dashefsky, M.D.
Associate Professor of Pediatrics
University of Pittsburgh School of Medicine
Children's Hospital of Pittsburgh
Pittsburgh, Pennsylvania

G. Robert DeLong, M.D.
Associate Professor of Pediatrics
Chief, Division of Pediatric Neurology

Duke University Medical Center
Durham, North Carolina

Robert A. Dershewitz, M.D., Sc.M.
Clinical Assistant Professor of Pediatrics
Harvard Medical School
Chief of Pediatrics
Harvard Community Health Plan
Braintree and Quincy Centers
Braintree, Massachusetts

Colette Deslandres-Leduc, M.D.
Assistant Professor in Pediatrics
Montreal Children's Hospital
McGill University
Montreal, Quebec
Canada

Thomas G. DeWitt, M.D.
Associate Professor of Pediatrics
University of Massachusetts Medical School
Director, Division of General and Community
      Pediatrics
University of Massachusetts Medical Center
Worcester, Massachusetts

Daniel P. Doody, M.D.
Assistant Professor of Surgery
Harvard Medical School
Assistant Surgeon
Massachusetts General Hospital
Boston, Massachusetts

Elizabeth C. Dooling, M.D.
Associate Professor of Neurology
Harvard Medical School
Neurologist and Associate Pediatrician
Massachusetts General Hospital
Boston, Massachusetts

Henry L. Dorkin, M.D.
Associate Professor of Pediatrics
Tufts University School of Medicine
Chief, Pediatric Pulmonology and Allergy Division
Director, Cystic Fibrosis Center
Tufts University Medical School
Boston, Massachusetts

A. Stephen Dubansky, M.D.
Assistant Professor
Division of Pediatric Hematology and Oncology
State University of New York
Health Science Center
Syracuse, New York

Paul G. Dyment, M.D.
Professor of Clinical Pediatrics
Director, Student Health Center
Tulane University
New Orleans, Louisiana

Arthur B. Elster, M.D.
Director, Department of Adolescent Medicine
American Medical Association
Chicago, Illinois

Helen M. Emery, M.D.
Associate Professor of Clinical Pediatrics
Pediatric Rheumatology and Immunology
University of California, San Francisco
Moffitt-Long Hospital
San Francisco, California

Anita Feins, M.D.
Instructor, Harvard Medical School
Pediatrician
Harvard Community Health Plan
Boston, Massachusetts

Robert P. Foglia, M.D.
Associate Professor of Surgery
Chief, Division of Pediatric Surgery
Washington University School of Medicine
Surgeon-in-Chief
St. Louis Children's Hospital
St. Louis, Missouri

Victor L. Fox, M.D.
Instructor in Pediatrics
Harvard Medical School
Assistant in Medicine
Director, Endoscopy Unit
Children's Hospital
Boston, Massachusetts

Deborah A. Frank, M.D.
Associate Professor of Pediatrics
Director, Growth and Development Program
Boston University School of Medicine
Assistant Professor of Public Health
Boston University School of Public Health
Boston, Massachusetts

Ellen M. Friedman, M.D.
Associate Professor in Otolaryngology
and Communicative Sciences
Associate Professor of Pediatrics
Chief of Service
Texas Children's Hospital
Houston, Texas

Glenn T. Furuta, M.D.
Fellow in Pediatric Gastroenterology
Harvard Medical School
Massachusetts General Hospital
Boston, Massachusetts

Charlene Gaebler-Uhing, M.D.
Fellow, General Academic Pediatrics
University of Illinois at Chicago
School of Medicine
Chicago, Illinois

Pierre Gaudreault, M.D., FRCP(C)
Clinical Associate Professor
Department of Pediatrics
University of Montreal
Director
Clinical Pharmacology and Toxicology Service
Sainte-Justine Hospital
Montreal, Quebec
Canada

Samuel P. Gotoff, M.D.
The Woman's Board Professor and Chairman
of Pediatrics
Rush Medical College
Rush-Presbyterian/St. Luke's Medical Center
Chicago, Illinois

Edward S. Gross, M.D.
Instructor in Pediatrics
Harvard Medical School
Pediatrician and Pediatric Director
Harvard Community Health Plan
West Roxbury, Massachusetts

Mohammad Haerian, M.D., MPH
Senior Psychiatrist
Service Chief, Children's Inpatient Service
The Sheppard and Enoch Pratt Hospital
Towson, Maryland
Clinical Assistant Professor of Psychiatry
Johns Hopkins University School of Medicine
Baltimore, Maryland

Roopa S. Hashimoto, M.D.
Staff Pediatrician
Nightime Pediatrics Clinic
Salt Lake City, Utah

Thomas J. Hathaway, M.D.
Clinical Instructor in Pediatrics
Harvard Medical School
Pediatrician
Harvard Community Health Plan
Braintree, Massachusetts

Peter T. Heydemann, M.D.
Director, Pediatric Neurology
Assistant Professor of Pediatrics and Neurology
Rush Medical College
Rush-Presbyterian-St. Luke's Medical Center
Chicago, Illinois

Martin I. Horowitz, M.D.
Clinical Instructor, Pediatrics
Harvard Medical School
Health Center Director
Peabody Center
Harvard Community Health Plan
Peabody, Massachusetts

Esther Jacobowitz Israel, M.D.
Assistant Professor of Pediatrics
Harvard Medical School
Associate Pediatrician
Massachusetts General Hospital
Boston, Massachusetts

Joseph J. Jankowski, M.D.
Associate Clinical Professor of Pediatrics
and Psychiatry
Tufts University School of Medicine
Director of Consultation/Liaison and Emergency
Services in Child Psychiatry
New England Medical Center
Boston, Massachusetts

Paula Kienberger Jaudes, M.D.
Associate Professor of Clinical Pediatrics
Chief, Section of Chronic Disease
University of Chicago
Pritzker School of Medicine
Associate Director
La Rabida Children's Hospital and Research Center
Chicago, Illinois

Michael S. Jellinek, M.D.
Associate Professor of Psychiatry and Pediatrics
Harvard Medical School
Chief, Child Psychiatry Service
Director, Outpatient Psychiatry
Associate Chief, Psychiatry Service
Massachusetts General Hospital
Boston, Massachusetts

David W. Johnson, M.D.
Assistant Professor
Division of Emergency Medicine,
and Clinical Pharmacology — Toxicology
The Hospital for Sick Children
Toronto, Ontario
Canada

Murray M. Kappelman, M.D.
Professor, Pediatrics and Psychiatry
Director, Division of Behavioral and
Developmental Pediatrics
University of Maryland School of Medicine
Baltimore, Maryland

Harvey P. Katz, M.D.
Associate Professor of Pediatrics
Harvard Medical School
Health Center Director
Braintree and Quincy Centers
Harvard Community Health Plan
Braintree, Massachusetts

Lucinda Lee Katz, Ph.D.
Director
The University of Chicago Laboratory Schools
Chicago, Illinois

Constance H. Keefer, M.D.
Instructor, Harvard Medical School
Director, Clinical Services
Child Development Unit
Children's Hospital
Director, Regular Nurseries
Brigham and Women's Hospital
Boston, Massachusetts

Dorothy H. Kelly, M.D.
Associate Professor of Pediatrics
Harvard Medical School
Associate Director of Pediatric Pulmonary Unit
Massachusetts General Hospital
Boston, Massachusetts

Janice D. Key, M.D.
Assistant Professor
Department of Pediatrics
Medical University of South Carolina
Children's Hospital
Charleston, South Carolina

Robert Z. Klein, M.D.
Professor, Maternal and Child Health
Dartmouth Medical School
Lebanon, New Hampshire

Ronald E. Kleinman, M.D.
Associate Professor of Pediatrics
Harvard Medical School
Associate Chief of the Children's Service
Chief, Pediatric GI and Nutrition Unit
Massachusetts General Hospital
Boston, Massachusetts

Ilana Kraus, M.D.
Chief of Pediatrics
Harvard Community Health Plan
West Roxbury Center
West Roxbury, Massachusetts

Kalpathy S. Krishnamoorthy, M.D.
Assistant Professor in Pediatrics (Neurology)
Harvard Medical School
Associate Neurologist and Pediatrician
Massachusetts General Hospital
Boston, Massachusetts

Hal Landy, M.D.
Instructor in Pediatrics
Harvard Medical School
Assistant in Endocrinology
Children's Hospital
Boston, Massachusetts

Craig B. Langman, M.D.
Associate Chair of Pediatrics
Department of Pediatrics
Northwestern University Medical School
Director, Mineral Metabolism
Children's Memorial Hospital
Chicago, Illinois

Allen Lapey, M.D.
Assistant Professor of Pediatrics
Harvard Medical School
Associate Pediatrician
Director, Cystic Fibrosis Center
Massachusetts General Hospital
Boston, Massachusetts

Laura A. Latchaw, M.D.
Assistant Professor of Surgery
Tufts University School of Medicine
New England Medical Center
The Floating Hospital for Infants and Children
Boston, Massachusetts

A. Alyssa LeBel, M.D.
Fellow, Pediatric Neurology
Massachusetts General Hospital
Boston, Massachusetts

Wayne I. Lencer, M.D.
Assistant Professor of Pediatrics
Harvard Medical School
Assistant in Medicine
The Children's Hospital
Boston, Massachusetts

Stephen J. Lerman, M.D., M.P.H.
Clinical Instructor in Pediatrics
Harvard Medical School
Chief of Pediatrics
Kenmore Center
Harvard Community Health Plan
Boston, Massachusetts

Lynne L. Levitsky, M.D.
Associate Professor of Pediatrics
Harvard Medical School
Chief, Pediatric Endocrine Unit
Massachusetts General Hospital
Boston, Massachusetts

Sonia Lewin, M.D.
Instructor in Pediatrics
Harvard Medical School
Assistant in Emergency Medicine
Massachusetts General Hospital
Boston, Massachusetts

Jacob A. Lohr, M.D.
Professor and Associate Chairman for
    Ambulatory Programs
Chief, Community Pediatric Division
Department of Pediatrics
University of North Carolina School of Medicine
Chapel Hill, North Carolina

Michael L. Macknin, M.D.
Clinical Associate Professor of Pediatrics
Pennsylvania State University
College of Medicine
Associate Professor of Pediatrics
The Ohio State University School of Medicine
Head, Section of General Pediatrics
The Cleveland Clinic Foundation
Cleveland, Ohio

William C. MacLean, Jr., M.D.
Medical Director, Pediatric Nutrition
Ross Laboratories
Clinical Professor of Pediatrics
The Ohio State University
Columbus, Ohio

M. Joan Mansfield, M.D.
Assistant Professor of Pediatrics
Harvard Medical School
Associate in Endocrinology and Adolescent
    Medicine
Children's Hospital
Boston, Massachusetts

Colin D. Marchant, M.D.
  Associate Professor of Pediatrics
  Tufts University School of Medicine
  Division of Pediatric Infectious Diseases
  New England Medical Center
  Boston, Massachusetts

John F. Marcinak, M.D.
  Assistant Professor of Pediatrics
  University of Illinois at Chicago
  Chicago, Illinois

Steven M. Marcus, M.D.
  Associate Professor of Cinical Pediatrics
  Preventive and Community Medicine
  University of Medicine and Dentistry of New Jersey
  New Jersey Medical School
  Director, Poison Control Center
  Assistant Director, Department of Pediatrics
  Newark Beth Israel Medical Center
  Newark, New Jersey

Steven M. Matloff, M.D.
  Clinical Instructor in Medicine
  Harvard Medical School
  Allergist
  Harvard Community Health Plan
  Assistant Physician
  Harvard University Health Services
  Cambridge, Massachusetts

Paul L. McCarthy, M.D.
  Professor of Pediatrics
  Yale School of Medicine
  Head, Division of General Pediatrics
  Yale — New Haven Medical Center
  New Haven, Connecticut

Michael A. McGuigan, M.D., C.M.
  Associate Professor
  University of Toronto
  Medical Director, Poison Control Centre
  The Hospital for Sick Children
  Toronto, Ontario
  Canada

Henry S. Metz, M.D.
  Professor and Chairman
  Department of Ophthalmology
  University of Rochester School of Medicine
    and Dentistry
  Strong Memorial Hospital
  Rochester, New York

Mohamad Mikati, M.D.
  Assistant Professor of Neurology
  Harvard Medical School
  Assistant in Neurology
  Children's Hospital
  Boston, Massachusetts

Michael L. Miller, M.D.
  Assistant Professor of Pediatrics
  Division of Pediatric Infectious Diseases
  University of Texas Health Science Center at San
    Antonio
  San Antonio, Texas

Anthony B. Minnefor, M.D.
  Associate Dean, Seton Hall University
  School of Graduate Medical Education
  South Orange, New Jersey
  Chief, Division of Infectious Disease
  St. Joseph Hospital and Medical Center
  Paterson, New Jersey

Jody R. Murph, M.D., M.S.
  Assistant Professor in Pediatrics
  University of Iowa College of Medicine
  Assistant Professor in Pediatrics
  Division of General Pediatrics
  University of Iowa Hospitals and Clinics
  Iowa City, Iowa

Marilyn Warren Neault, Ph.D.
  Instructor in Otology and Larnygology
  Harvard University Medical School
  Director of Audiology Services
  Children's Hospital
  Boston, Massachusetts

Leonard B. Nelson, M.D.
  Co-Director, Pediatric Ophthalmology Service
  Wills Eye Hospital
  Associate Professor of Ophthalmology and
    Pediatrics
  Jefferson Medical College
  Thomas Jefferson University
  Philadelphia, Pennsylvania

L. Gerard Niederman, M.D., M.P.H.
  Clinical Associate Professor of Pediatrics
  University of Illinois at Chicago
  Head, General and Emergency Pediatrics
  University of Illinois Hospital and Clinics,
    and Humana–Michael Reese Hospital
  Chicago, Illinois

Samuel N. Nurko, M.D.
Chief of Pediatric Gastroenterology
Hospital Infantil de Mexico Federico Gomez
Edo De
Mexico City, Mexico

Joan M. O'Connor, D.M.D.
Private Practice of Orthodontics
Winchester, Massachusetts

James M. Oleske, M.D., M.P.H.
Francois-Zavier Bagnour Professor of Pediatrics
New Jersey Medical School
Medical Director
Children's Hospital AIDS Program
Newark, New Jersey

Eileen Ouellette, M.D.
Assistant Professor of Neurology
Harvard Medical School
Assistant Neurologist
Assistant Pediatrician
Massachusetts General Hospital
Boston, Massachusetts

Amy Paller, M.D.
Associate Professor of Pediatrics and Dermatology
Northwestern University Medical School
Head, Division of Dermatology
The Children's Memorial Hospital of Chicago
Chicago, Illinois

Mark S. Pasternack, M.D.
Assistant Professor of Pediatrics
Harvard Medical School
Chief, Pediatric Infectious Disease Unit
Massachusetts General Hospital
Boston, Massachusetts

James C. Pert, M.D.
Clinical Instructor in Pediatrics
Harvard Medical School
Pediatrician
Harvard Community Health Plan
Medford, Massachusetts

Odette Pinsonneault, M.D., CSPQ, FRCS(C)
Associate Professor of Obstetrics and Gynecology
University of Sherbrooke
Centre Hospitalier Universitaire de Sherbrooke
Sherbrooke, Quebec
Canada

Orah S. Platt, M.D.
Associate Professor of Pediatrics
Harvard Medical School

Senior Associate in Medicine
   (Hematology/Oncology)
Children's Hospital
Boston, Massachusetts

Algis K. Rasymas, B.Sc.Phm., Pharm.D.
Lecturer, University of Toronto
Coordinator, Therapeutic Drug Monitoring
The Hospital for Sick Children
Toronto, Ontario
CANADA

Margaret B. Rennels, M.D.
Associate Professor of Pediatrics
Chief, Pediatric Clinical Studies Section
Center for Vaccine Development
University of Maryland School of Medicine
Baltimore, Maryland

Peter B. Rosenberger, M.D.
Assistant Professor of Neurology
Harvard Medical School
Neurologist and Associate Pediatrician
Massachusetts General Hospital
Boston, Massachusetts

Linda V. Ross, Ph.D., R.N.
Assistant Professor, Department of Pediatrics
University of Missouri–Kansas City
Assistant Professor, Department of Human
   Development
University of Kansas
Psychologist, Behavioral Pediatrics
Children's Mercy Hospital
Kansas City, Missouri

Daniel P. Ryan, M.D.
Instructor in Surgery
Harvard Medical School
Assistant Surgeon
Massachusetts General Hospital
Boston, Massachusetts

Charles F. Sanzone, M.D., Ph.D.
Assistant Professor
Boston University School of Medicine
Director of Orthopaedics
Franciscan Children's Hospital
Brighton, Massachusetts

Richard M. Sarles, M.D.
Clinical Professor of Psychiatry and Pediatrics
University of Maryland School of Medicine
Director, Division of Child and Adolescent
   Psychiatry

The Sheppard and Enoch Pratt Hospital
Towson, Maryland

Sylvia Schechner, M.D., M.P.H.
Assistant Clinical Professor
Harvard Medical School of Pediatrics
Neonatologist
Brigham and Women's Hospital
Children's Hospital
Beth Israel Hospital
Boston, Massachusetts

Edward L. Schor, M.D.
Associate Professor of Pediatrics
Tufts University School of Medicine
Staff Physician, Floating Hospital for
 Infants and Children
New England Medical Center
Boston, Massachusetts

Janet L. Schwaner, M.D.
Pediatrician
Harvard Community Health Plan
Medford, Massachusetts

Jonathan H. Schwartz, M.D.
Clinical Fellow
Harvard Medical School
Department of Psychiatry
Massachusetts General Hospital
Boston, Massachusetts

David J. Seidman, M.D.
Physician
Fairfax Hospital
Fairfax, Virginia

Bruce K. Shapiro, M.D.
Associate Professor of Pediatrics
The Johns Hopkins University School of Medicine
Director, Center for Learning and Its Disorders
The Kennedy Institute for Handicapped
 Children, Inc.
Baltimore, Maryland

Edward Sills, M.D.
Associate Professor, Pediatrics
The Johns Hopkins University School of Medicine
Director, Pediatric and Adolescent Rheumatoalogy
The Johns Hopkins Hospital
Baltimore, Maryland

Deborah E. Smith, B.M., B.Ch.
Assistant Professor of Pediatrics
Director of Adolescent Medicine

University of Virginia
University of Virginia Health Sciences Center
Charlottesville, Virginia

Howard G. Smith, M.D.
Chief of Staff
Cigna Health Plans of California
Department of Otolaryngology
Irvine Health Care Center
Irvine, California

Brook Swearingen, M.D.
Neurosurgical Service
Massachusetts General Hospital
Harvard Medical School
Boston, Massachusetts

Charles N. Swisher, M.D.
Associate Professor of Clinical Pediatrics
 and Clinical Neurology
Northwestern University School of Medicine
Acting Head, Division of Neurology
Children's Memorial Hospital
Chicago, Illinois

Katherine C. Teets Grimm, M.D.
Associate Professor, Department of Pediatrics
The Mount Sinai School of Medicine of
 the City University of New York
Chief, Division of Ambulatory Pediatrics
The Mount Sinai Medical Center
New York, New York

Kenneth H. Tellerman, M.D.
General/Behavioral/Pediatric Practitioner
Baltimore, Maryland

Milton Tenenbein, M.D., FRCPC
Associate Professor, Pediatrics, Pharmacy
 and Community Health Sciences
Faculty of Medicine
University of Manitoba
Director, Emergency Services
Children's Hospital
Director, Manitoba Poison Control Centre
Winnipeg, Manitoba
Canada

David Van Buskirk, M.D.
Associate Professor of Psychiatry
University of Vermont
Director of Child Psychiatry
Department of Psychiatry
Medical Center Hospital of Vermont
Burlington, Vermont

Ellen R. Wald, M.D.
Professor of Pediatrics
University of Pittsburgh School of Medicine
Children's Hospital of Pittsburgh
Divisions of Infectious Diseases and Ambulatory
    Care
Pittsburgh, Pennsylvania

Mark A. Ward, M.D.
Assistant Professor of Pediatrics
Rush Medical College
Rush Presbyterian–St. Luke's Medical Center
Chicago, Illinois

Anthony E. Webber, M.D.
Clinical Instructor in Orthopaedic Surgery
Harvard Medical School
Children's Hospital
Boston, Massachusetts

Marc Weissbluth, M.D.
Associate Professor of Pediatrics
Northwestern University Medical School
Active Attending
Children's Memorial Hospital
Chicago, Illinois

Harland S. Winter, M.D.
Associate Professor of Pediatrics
Harvard Medical School
Boston University
Director, Pediatric Gastroenterology and Nutrition
Boston City Hospital
Associate in Gastroenterology
Children's Hospital
Boston, Massachusetts

Raoul L. Wolf, M.D.
Associate Professor, Clinical Pediatrics
Pritzker School of Medicine

The University of Chicago
Director, Section of Allergy, Immunology, and
    Pulmonology
Wyler Children's Hospital and
    La Rabida Children's Hospital
Chicago, Illinois

Jerold C. Woodhead, M.D.
Associate Professor
Department of Pediatrics
University of Iowa College of Medicine
University of Iowa Hospitals and Clinics
Iowa City, Iowa

Basil J. Zitelli, M.D.
Associate Professor of Pediatrics
University of Pittsburgh School of Medicine
Children's Hospital of Pittsburgh
Pittsburgh, Pennsylvania

Johan Zwaan, M.D., Ph.D.
Professor of Ophthalmology, Pediatrics, Cellular,
    and Structural Biology
University of Texas Health Science Center
    at San Antonio
Staff Ophthalmologist
Medical Center Hospital
Santa Rosa Hospital
San Antonio, Texas

Robert G. Zwerdling, M.D.
Associate Professor of Pediatrics
University of Massachusetts Medical School
Director of Pediatric Pulmonology
University of Massachusetts Hospitals and Clinics
Worcester, Massachusetts

Preface

Ambulatory pediatrics is a broad and burgeoning field. Many changes have taken place in this area since the first edition of *Ambulatory Pediatric Care* was published in 1988, and this second edition reflects advances in the practice of outpatient pediatric medicine.

Ambulatory Pediatric Care is meant to be a working text, to be kept on one's desktop and used for quick information retrieval and management guidelines. Each chapter is succinct and has practical applicability to the general pediatrician. To attain an even greater "front line" clinical focus, several chapters from the first edition were either deleted or combined. Sixteen new chapters, a new section, "The Newborn," and one appendix were also added. Although this book is neither encyclopedic nor intended to replace a "standard" reference textbook, the reader will find that nearly every topic, question, or medical problem that arises in the course of office-based pediatric care is covered logically and with timely information. Many areas integral to ambulatory pediatrics, such as social issues, community pediatrics, teaching, and clinical research are not included because of space constraints, not for lack of importance.

The audience and format of *Ambulatory Pediatric Care* have remained unchanged. The book is targeted to pediatric primary care providers (pediatricians, family practitioners, nurse practitioners, and physician assistants) and students learning this discipline. Because of its focus and relatively limited size, multiple points of view, or diverse management alternatives could not always be presented. In trying to create a balance between a "glimpse" and a "treatise," a pertinent, concise approach representing accepted current practice was chosen. (For those who desire greater depth, an annotated bibliography is included at the end of each chapter.) These clinical choices reflect the diversity, challenge, and even beauty of ambulatory pediatrics.

Robert A. Dershewitz, M.D., Sc.M., F.A.A.P.

Acknowledgments

I am indebted to the contributing authors and section editors, for without their substantial efforts, this book would not have been possible. It has also been a pleasure working with the professionals at the J. B. Lippincott Company, most notably Charles McCormick, Jr. (Medical Editor), Kim Cox (Developmental Editor), and Mary Rose Muccie and Debbi Stein (Project Editors). Gert Barcella, Georgene Blight, Marianne DelConte, Lindsay Dowd, Anthony Graziano, and Lorenzo Iacovello efficiently and graciously handled the mail and faxing. So many others deserve special thanks, especially Jerold Woodhead, M.D., Wesley Brooks, PA-C, and Ina Cushman, PA-C. I am also grateful for the support given to me by the Harvard Community Health Plan. And Naomi and Dana, thank you for modulating your blasted music.

Contents

Ambulatory
Pediatric Care

1

THE OFFICE

1

Planning and Staffing an Office

Martin I. Horowitz

When a pediatrician considers establishing an office, it is assumed that he or she has already made certain decisions concerning professional and personal goals (such as joining an established or institutional practice), and about the location and style of the practice. Because it would be imprudent to proceed without forethought and research, many factors should be considered before the pediatrician decides where to locate an office. The central issues usually are desirability and compatibility with one's own lifestyle. One must consider the type of residential community, the kind of school system (an important consideration for the pediatrician with a family), the existing organizations, recreational and cultural opportunities, and other nonmedical opportunities in the area. There are, however, several disadvantages to residing in the community in which one's practice is located, such as intrusions on privacy, restrictions on involvement in local political activity for fear of offending a segment of the practice, and family members' feelings of "living in a fishbowl." These disadvantages (or advantages) often vary depending on whether the community is urban, suburban, or rural.

A good way to evaluate the community is to examine the demographics of the population, such as wealth, growth, birth rate, and age distribution (a vital consideration for a new pediatrician). It may be risky to establish a pediatric practice in an area with an aging and declining population. United States census data from the local Chamber of Commerce are usually readily available. Personal surveys may also be helpful.

A good way to learn about a community is to visit and talk to several people, including pediatricians with established practices. One must, however, evaluate whether a "potential competitor" is being open and honest or is trying to discourage the start of another pediatric practice in the community. Discussions should also be with obstetricians, whose newborn referrals would be critical, and the staff at the hospital where you would practice. Often, the hospital administrator will give a frank assessment of the need for an additional pediatrician in the community. Discussions with the clergy of one's faith and realtors for both professional and personal opportunities are recommended to further assess the community.

After choosing the appropriate community, the next step is to find a suitable site. Cost and location are prime considerations. Hospitals are often more than eager to help new physicians locate nearby and to market these new practices to the community. Hospitals may even financially assist these new practices. The major reason to consider locating near a hospital is that pediatricians situated as such have an improved quality of life because their rounds, practice, and emergency care can be more efficiently regulated. This convenience minimizes office disruption and allows the pediatrician to monitor seriously ill children with greater ease, permitting even multiple visits to the hospital each day. The location of the office must also be easily accessible to patients.

When planning an office, one should visit other practices to study their layouts. Out of courtesy, permission should first be sought. One must remember patient competition, because in many locations pediatricians are faced with an increasing number of well-trained colleagues and organized health care delivery systems, with most seeking relatively fewer patients.

The nature and style of one's practice largely determine the office design, particularly when there are special facility requirements. For example, an allergy testing area would be needed if this were to be an important part of one's practice. Will other ancillary services (e.g., x-rays, electrocardiograms) be performed? Will the office have a laboratory, and, if so, which tests (e.g., hematology, bacteriology, urinalysis) will be performed? Areas must be devoted to visual and hearing screening, an integral part of well-child care. The type of testing may be determined by office space. For example, a Titmus vision screen requires only a small area, as opposed to a 20-foot lane for Snellen eye chart testing.

One must also think of the employees one will hire and whether or not they will have specific facility requirements. Another important consideration is planning for growth. Will partners be added at a later date, and how might their needs be incorporated into the design of "expandability" of the facility to save the future expense of remodeling or relocation? The biggest error that can occur in designing an office is failing to plan for practice growth and ample file space. Present and future computer needs should also be anticipated. Computer work stations and the necessary linkage between such stations should be taken into account in the office design.

Space requirement recommendations for a pediatric office range from 1000 sq ft to 1200 sq ft per doctor. Additionally, it is recommended that parking for six to 10 cars be available per doctor. In planning the outside of one's office, the landscaping should be attractive and should include an open space design at least one half the total inner space plus the parking area. Future expansion will require at least one half of the aforementioned total space.

When planning the layout of any medical office, it is important not to underestimate the required size of the business area, hallways, and storage areas. Many medical supply houses offer the services of office designers or architects for a nominal fee (or no fee) to advise the new physician. In return, it is expected that the office furnishings be purchased from the supply house. These designers can be extremely helpful; however, the physician should know his or her budget, style, and system of practice so that overly expensive or unnecessary purchases will be avoided.

The ideal internal space of an office should be functional and free-flowing, yet tightly controlled, and there should be a balance between public (i.e., patient) and medical space. The waiting room requires about three to four chairs per doctor. This conforms well to a suggested space need for two children and two adults for each pediatric patient scheduled, because almost all of these youngsters are accompanied by one or several family members, or even friends. The waiting room should be about 40 sq ft plus 10 sq ft for each individual (adults and children included) using a room; this does not include a children's play area. The adult chairs in the waiting room should allow an adult to sit comfortably while holding an infant. Current magazines and books relating to family, child rearing, and other contemporary issues should be available in the waiting area. In addition, a bulletin board with timely articles, pictures, or patient artwork is an interesting and personal touch. Today, when marketing has become an important tool in building one's practice, it might be useful to offer personally tailored literature on pediatric health and safety issues that patients and their families can take home to read.

In a pediatric office, a special children's play area is essential. It should be furnished with solid, sturdy chairs that can be stood upon and not easily tipped over, and it should have durable and attractive toys. It is important that all toys be easy to thoroughly clean and store. A small table in this area for play, perhaps with blackboards, is also a favorite of children.

An area with a coffee pot or other appliances for staff use, where employees may take a break or eat their lunch, is a worthwhile office amenity. This area need not be large and could also allow for staff meetings. Moreover, this room could provide additional storage space. Restrooms for both staff and patients are required. A special area may be needed if smoking is permitted. Areas for drinking water and a public telephone should be considered.

The business aspects of the practice should be conducted in the receptionist/bookkeeping area. A practical guideline is for the receptionist's area to have twice the square footage as the number of patients at the busiest hour. It is suggested that in a solo practice the combined waiting room/receptionist area be between 150 sq ft and 200 sq ft. Space requirements in a group practice are dependent upon the number of people required to do bookkeeping, data entry, telephone, and reception chores. In some large offices, the billing area is placed away from the reception area to reduce noise and enhance privacy, especially when a patient's financial status is discussed. The receptionist/bookkeeping area should have enough space for at least two desks and file space for both the medical and the financial records. When designing this space, one should keep in mind both security and privacy considerations. The use of safety glass is encouraged so that the staff may see the entire waiting area.

It is suggested that an efficient office requires three examining rooms per physician. The size most commonly recommended for these rooms is approximately 8 ft by 10 ft if they are used exclusively for examination purposes. If the physician's office is combined with an examination room, then the room should be 9 ft by 13 ft. However, for many reasons, including the need for privacy and contemplation, combination rooms should be avoided wherever possible. Because it is not uncommon to have an entire family come in while a youngster is being examined, each examining room should be able to comfortably accommodate three adults and two children, as well as the patient's clothing. It is important to place the chairs in an area where the adults would be out of the way of the examiner.

If there is no combination room, each physician should have a consultation room. This room should be about 100 sq ft and should contain a desk, two or three chairs, bookcases, and a telephone. The consultation room's decor should be tasteful and appropriate. Adequate filing space is an important consideration.

All examining rooms should contain a sink and a table long enough for a large adolescent. Although some pediatricians set aside a special examining room for the adolescent patient, this may not always be possible. If a separate room is available, an adult-sized table on which pelvic examinations may be performed offers the most flexibility. Equipment and supplies in an adolescent room are generally similar to those in other examining rooms but should also include appropriate lighting, screens for privacy, and supplies necessary for gynecologic examinations. This room should be decorated in a manner appropriate for the adolescent.

Both infant and adult scales should be placed in the other examining rooms, although a third, or auxiliary room, may not be as well equipped and might be used only for brief visits. It is important to have an accurate height scale available somewhere in the office. All rooms should contain equipment for complete examinations, including an otoscope, ophthalmoscope, sphygmomanometer, hammer, syringes, bandages, rubber gloves, water-soluble gel, and immunization materials. They should also have tissues; paper goods such as gowns, table paper, and cups; and simple first aid equipment such as splints and bandages. It is essential that the supplies in these rooms be checked daily. Each examining room should be laid out identically so that the clinician knows where all the equipment is kept.

An additional room may be designed for special procedures such as suturing, blood drawing, lumbar punctures, minor surgical procedures, débridement, and so forth. This room might be equipped with an overhead operating light or at least a spotlight, as well as surgical equipment, including suture kits. Bandages and casting material can be kept here as well. The table may be an operating type, so that a child can be positioned in various ways depending on the procedure; however, the cost of such a table may be prohibitively expensive.

A laboratory and a nurse's station may be desirable in a busy practice. Many offices efficiently combine the nurse's station and laboratory into one area. The laboratory itself should be approximately 8 ft by 4 ft and should include a refrigerator, an incubator, a small sink, a microscope, an autoclave, and a centrifuge. There must be space for enough supplies to keep the laboratory well stocked.

The most common tests conducted in pediatricians' offices are hemograms, including hemoglobin and hematocrit; urinalyses; throat and urine cultures; Gram's and Wright's stains; rapid strep tests; mono spot tests; stool guaiac tests; test strips for blood glucose; and several other commercial tests (e.g., pregnancy tests). The need for these tests in the office is determined by frequency, medical necessity for rapid results, expense, and patient convenience. Because of quality assurance concerns, the federal government recently promulgated regulations that may restrict the physician's ability to run an office laboratory. One should thus be fa-

miliar with these regulations as well as license requirements and how they affect the cost and scope of tests offered in the office. The price of each laboratory test should be based on the fixed overhead costs in the use of the allotted space, the price of materials, and staff time, and it should be compared with charges for the same or similar tests in the community.

The nurse's station should have a 5-ft counter wall or base cabinets. The nurse may give allergy injections or immunizations in this area and may also answer the phone here. It is important that adequate space be provided for writing in patients' records.

Professional assistance may be useful for designing optimal soundproofing, lighting, and telecommunications, including interoffice communications. Lighting is critical, and most experts recommend 100 foot-candles of light at table height. Lighting also plays a large role in office decor and must not be addressed casually. Soundproofing and window treatments for privacy are especially important in treating adolescents.

Telecommunications planning should include the placement of telephones and the number of incoming and private outgoing lines. For efficiency, many authorities recommend a telephone in each examining room. The system should be equipped with a private intercommunication system so that the doctor may be quickly interrupted for emergencies; however, the use of this system for routine problems should be avoided.

Careful consideration must be given to the purchase of computer systems. During the last several years, computer systems have become increasingly personalized while adding more power and speed. The novice may easily become confused when seeking to purchase a system for the medical office. A list of functions for the computer to perform must first be determined (e.g., billing both one's patients and third-party carriers, payroll, access to hospital or other laboratory results, medical records, and so forth). There are many books on the market concerning computer systems. The reader is referred to Chapter 3 for a more complete discussion.

A safe milieu is necessary in any office, especially in a pediatric one. Indeed, the entire office should be a model for good safety practices. The ambience should evoke a feeling of warmth and friendliness. The office must be a pleasant environment for the pediatrician, who often spends more of his or her waking hours in the office than anywhere else, as well as for patients and staff.

The importance of having the right staff in any office cannot be overemphasized. Thus, hiring staff is one of the most important decisions a new pediatrician makes when opening an office. For example, the receptionist is usually the patient's or parent's first exposure to the office, and the climate created in this initial contact will affect how the physician–patient relationship develops. Ideally, the physician should employ as many assistants as necessary to ensure that he or she does virtually nothing in the office but practice medicine, and does that as efficiently as possible. Trained office personnel are important to ensure maximum office harmony and efficiency. Uniform staffing ratios have not been defined, and they depend mainly on variables such as style of practice, patient volume, the number of physicians and midlevel clinicians, and physician time in the office. Twenty percent of pediatric offices have one medical assistant, 27% have two, 12% have three, and 20% have four or more. It would seem wise, therefore, to start with one or two assistants and periodically evaluate one's needs. The need for receptionists, bookkeepers, and other staff will reflect personal preferences and practice requirements. Frequently, in a small office, tasks are combined and one or two assistants perform these other functions as well. The delegation of certain office tasks must be weighed against greater contact between patient and physician. However, additional staff increases productivity. Physicians with three office assistants see 50% more patients than do physicians with only one assistant. Be aware, however, that overstaffing not only is inefficient but also can lead to inadequate training.

Other ancillary personnel to consider hiring include an office manager (usually in a large and complex practice), registered or licensed practical nurse(s), physician assistant(s) or nurse practitioner(s), laboratory or x-ray technician(s), and secretarial (clerical) employees. It is prudent to have carefully written job descriptions for the positions one wishes to fill. All personnel policies should be carefully detailed. The offered salary should be competitive, have a merit plan, and should be integrated with regular cost-of-living adjustments. Fringe benefits should also be competitive.

There are many ways to find excellent staff. Usual sources include private employment agencies, other medical offices, advertisements, and appropriate vocational and technical schools and colleges. Recommendations from present staff or from families of patients already in the practice may be helpful. Written advertisements or postings should be as explicit as possible.

The options for screening applicants are varied and include an agency or a trusted employee, such as the office manager. The physician must interview the applicants if he or she is just beginning to form a staff. Some applicants can be eliminated by questioning them about their availability, salary requirements, typing skills, and background (e.g., if they have worked in a medical office before). Ascertain the academic credentials and experience of the applicant. If the initial screening is favorable, consider whether the candidate should be tested for typing or other skills needed for the job. This testing is usually done in the pediatrician's office.

The interviewing process must be carefully arranged. The same person should interview all the candidates who have passed the initial screening. In addition, the candidates should be asked to provide a list of personal references, including previous employers. The interviewer should ask open-ended questions such as: Why would you like to work in a pediatrician's office? How do you react when you must occasionally stay late at work? How do you feel about pressing people to pay their medical bills? Have you handled money for anyone before? Are you willing to be bonded? Would you like to ask me anything? The health of the applicant is important, although it is illegal to ask about health status if it is unrelated to the qualifications for the position. If any problems are uncovered, such as with the applicant's work history, these should be discussed openly.

An important aspect of hiring personnel is checking references. It is prudent to speak directly with the applicant's previous employers, usually by telephone. The most important question to ask is, "Would you hire this applicant again?" It is not necessary to ask specifically if one may speak directly with personal references because they were originally supplied by the candidate.

After this careful screening process, the top candidates should be asked to return for a second interview. If the applicants were initially screened by someone else, the physician should personally interview these top candidates and choose (with staff input) the person who will be offered the position.

Sensitivity should be shown to those not selected. A fair explanation should be given, and mention should be made that they will be considered for future openings. Frequently, one may wish to employ one of these applicants in the future.

After hiring a new employee, it is important to orient him or her to the job and its responsibilities. The job description and an office manual can make the orientation process easier. Larger offices usually offer more formal training programs, including communications, patient flow, and medical records. The idiosyncrasies of a pediatrician's office and its systems should be taught. Phone training and the office's systems training are important aspects of this program, even in a small office. The standards of excellence expected of the office personnel should be emphasized. This includes spelling, giving precise phone information, and making appointments. New employee orientation provides a good opportunity to stress the importance of patient confidentiality in the medical office. Of course, this issue should be stressed periodically to all employees, whether new or old.

The first employee usually hired is the receptionist, who in the beginning may also function as a secretary, a bookkeeper, and even as a limited medical assistant. It is important that he or she be punctual, neat, and reliable and that his or her telephone voice be pleasant, reassuring, and intelligible. One may actually test an applicant for this position by having him or her use the phone with the interviewer on the other end.

When the practice grows (or even at the beginning), a clinical assistant should be hired, if financial circumstances allow. This person prepares the exam room and the patient appropriately, obtains a basic history that includes the reason for the visit, takes the vital signs, does hearing and visual screening, and may also give injections as directed by the physician. Because these tasks increase the efficiency of the pediatrician's practice, he or she can see more patients in a given time.

Clinical assistants can be trained to give telephone advice on commonly occurring pediatric illnesses such as vomiting, diarrhea, fever control, and minor respiratory infections using written protocols as a guide. They should also be able to perform tuberculosis screening and common laboratory tests such as hematocrits and urinalyses, make appointments, accept money, give receipts, call prescriptions to a pharmacy under the direction of the pediatrician and keep a record of them, file, do secretarial work, and even remind the pediatrician of his or her outside appointments or commitments. This ability to perform several common office functions keeps the staff flexible and allows for both clinician and ancillary staff absences without total disruption of the normal office routine.

A pediatric office may run efficiently with only a receptionist/bookkeeper and a clinical assistant. As the practice grows, one may wish to expand the laboratory service, and a laboratory technician may become necessary, at least on a part-time basis. If the billing or numerous third-party forms become voluminous, the addition of a separate bookkeeper should be considered.

At some point the question, "When should I hire a registered or practical nurse versus a midlevel practitioner (i.e., a physician's assistant or nurse practitioner)?" is likely to be raised. The answer is based on both personal and fiscal considerations. The RN/LPN can augment the clinical assistant's role by developing a more extensive telephone triage system and by performing procedures (e.g., giving allergy shots) that require minimal supervision from the physician. One can often use this individual to act as an office manager in the supervision of the other staff and in the distribution of office work. The distinction between an RN and an LPN involves degree of education, the ability to perform procedures (regulated by license), and often "bedside" experience.

In situations where it may be difficult to attract an additional physician or to increase practice volume (i.e., the work is more than one pediatrician can handle but is not enough for two), a nurse practitioner or physician's assistant may be ideal. If one wishes to distinguish between the qualifications of these two midlevel clinicians, it would be worthwhile to consult the appropriate boards in your state as well as nearby academic institutions who train such clinicians. All midlevel clinicians should be able to perform routine well-child care and treat most common illnesses. He or she usually sees fewer patients in a given time period than does the pediatrician. This usually allows the midlevel clinician to do more health education or be involved with health issues such as sex education or discipline, or even the long-term management of certain chronic illnesses such as diabetes mellitus.

All new employees should be subject to a period of probation not exceeding 6 months. The employee should be aware of this probation period. The new employee should be gradually delegated increasing responsibility during the probation period. At its conclusion, the physician or his or her designee (usually the office manager or senior midlevel clinician) should conduct a formal review. The review process should be appropriate for the level of the position (e.g., a clinical review for the midlevel provider and a task-oriented review for other members of the staff).

The ability to run a successful office and be fair to the staff depends on regular staff evaluation. To do this properly, one must keep a personnel folder on each employee. The folder should include notes and the written review of the employee signed by the physician, the reviewer if not the physician, and the employee. Support and encouragement are important ingredients in keeping a happy, efficient staff.

Skilled ancillary personnel operate the office, maximize the pediatrician's patient contact by making the best use of his or her time, and serve as both facilitators and ombudsmen for the patients. Patients perceive this as personalized service and are made to feel both comfortable and welcome in the office.

ANNOTATED BIBLIOGRAPHY

Bass LW, Wolfson JH: The Style and Management of a Pediatric Practice. Pittsburgh, University of Pittsburgh Press, 1977. (Helpful guide for training ancillary personnel to fit the practice style of the clinician.)

Cotton H: Medical Practice Management, 3rd ed. Oradell, NJ, Medical Economics Books, 1985. (General guide for physicians beginning an office practice, with advice on office staff and systems. Also contains practice tips.)

Farber L (ed): Medical Economics Encyclopedia of Practice and Financial Management. Oradell, NJ, Medical Economics Books, 1988. (Exhaustive resource for all aspects of medical practice.)

Kaplan E: Practice Made Perfect—The Physician's Guide to Communicating and Marketing. Boston, Barrington Press, 1990. (Explains how to market one's practice.)

Kronhaus AK: Choosing Your Practice. New York, Springer-Verlag, 1990. (General guide to assist in choosing the kind of practice suited to the individual; helpful in decision making. Not pediatric-specific.)

Pressman RM, Siegler R: The Independent Practitioner—Practice Management for the Allied Health Professional. Homewood, IL, Dow Jones–Irwin, 1983. (Useful guide for the pediatrician integrating midlevel practitioners into the practice.)

Saltzman EJ, Shea DW: Management of Pediatric Practice. Elk Grove, IL, American Academy of Pediatrics, 1986. (Essential for the pediatrician in private practice, whether new or experienced.)

Toolos PC and Moody D: How to Choose the Right Computer for Your Medical Practice. Santa Rosa, CA, Burgess Communications, 1986. (One of a series by this company outlining the role computers might play in a medical office and how to identify the right system for a specific office setting.)

Walker M (in consultation with Trowbridge JP): Starting in Medical Practice. Oradell, NJ, Medical Economics Books, 1987. (General advice concerning beginning solo practice, legal matters, staffing, and setting up business systems.)

2

Telephone Medicine

Harvey P. Katz

The volume of medical contacts by phone can be staggering. Several hundred to 1000 phone calls per day to a busy ambulatory practice is not unusual. Approximately 60% of calls are for immediate problem care, 45% result in a same-day visit, 30% of callers receive home management advice, and 25% of calls are referred to another source. The volume of calls dictates that the doctor's telephone system must be efficient and effective. More important, our patients' and families' dependence on and trust and confidence in the telephone system are compelling reasons for it to be as high in quality as all the other components of practice. Unfortunately, it frequently is not.

There are many reasons for suboptimal service: some relate to hardware, some to systems, and some to people. The reality is that the responsibility for managing most calls needs to be delegated. Appointments have to be made, and questions must be answered about bills, insurance, illness, injury triage, and emergencies. These, and an endless array of other telephone calls, are managed, at least initially, by the office staff. If done poorly, this crucial function can "break" the practice.

The telephone encounter is highly complex. Many variables determine the outcome of each encounter. The most important factors are the degree of training in telephone medicine for physicians prior to practice; how well office personnel are trained, supervised, and evaluated by their physician employer; the operation of the various systems that are necessary for a smoothly functioning office telephone; and medicolegal constraints requiring documentation and triage. Each variable should be viewed as an opportunity to improve the quality of service and care to patients. Common patient complaints about the office telephone include being placed "on hold" too long and prematurely; encountering repeated busy signals that make it impossible to "get through" to the doctor; and rude receptionists. For physicians, calls for minor complaints after midnight and the lack of compensation for telephone time are frustrations. In a survey of Baltimore and Denver pediatricians, over two thirds of these clinicians rated the telephone as the most frustrating part of their practices. Less than half of these pediatricians incorporated specific train-

ing in telephone medicine into their practices, and very few documented any calls. Because the telephone accounts for between 15 and 25% of a pediatrician's total time, a formalized telephone training curriculum should be included in residency training programs.

TELEPHONE PERSONNEL

The personnel selected for telephone medicine responsibility represent the vital link between families and the physician. How well this responsibility is performed will have a profound influence on the quality of care, patient and physician satisfaction, and the growth and vitality of the practice. Individuals selected for the telephone responsibility must be properly recruited and oriented. They are, in effect, the image and voice of the practice. Care must be taken, however, to avoid telephone "burnout," for even the right person is at high risk for this "occupational hazard." The extent of training and required supervision depend on the degree of responsibility the physician wishes to delegate; the knowledge, experience, and motivation of the person answering the telephone; and the characteristics of the population served.

GUIDELINES FOR STAFF USING THE TELEPHONE

1. Be alert and always express interest in the caller.
2. Convey a friendly greeting with your message, and refer to patients by their names.
3. Speak clearly, distinctly, and confidently.
4. Be polite, warm, and business-like at all times.
5. Be very helpful; put yourself in the patient's position.
6. Express yourself well.
7. Talk naturally. Use a normal tone of voice and a moderate rate of speech. Avoid slang, technical language, and irrelevant, personal chitchat. Other patients are waiting. Make every effort to be efficient and relevant so you can answer the other calls quickly.
8. Answer the telephone promptly. Ringing telephones are a source of irritation to everyone. Set a goal of picking up the telephone after no more than three rings, and make every effort to meet that standard (a telephone usually rings 10 times per minute).
9. Never be argumentative. Always be helpful.
10. If you cannot provide information, offer to find someone who can. When you are overloaded, take the number and call back as soon as possible.
11. Be discreet, confidential, and sensitive to the problem. A caller may be upset and anxious for reasons that are not obvious. For example, there may have been a recent death in the family, or the parent may have been up all night with an ill child.

Those who answer the telephone in a pediatrician's office should hear themselves speaking with patients by using a tape recorder for training purposes. Staff should be reminded that their voices create an image of the practice, and they should be given on-the-job training in telephone technique.

ORGANIZATION OF A TELEPHONE-CARE SYSTEM

Both conceptually and functionally, it may be helpful to view the telephone-care system in two components:

1. Nonmedical or administrative information, including future appointments
2. Medical or problem care and same-day appointment making

All staff should be trained to schedule appointments relative to the nature of the presenting complaint and to know when a same-day or immediate appointment (within 2 weeks at most) is indicated. The person who receives a request to make an appointment for a problem must make one of three triage decisions: to schedule an appointment; to give home management advice; or to refer the call elsewhere, such as to a physician, specialist, or a local emergency room.

The management of emergency situations must be reviewed carefully. All staff must know the procedure to follow if there is a life-threatening emergency, especially when the pediatrician is not immediately available.

Other situations that may require referral to the physician for management may arise: an anxious caller, a language barrier, a complicated medical problem, or a caller who provides too little information or shows questionable competence (e.g., a babysitter or a young child).

Registered nurses, licensed practical nurses, and on-the-job trained non-nursing pediatric personnel are all capable of telephone health care management if they are properly trained and supervised. The choice of how much responsibility to delegate and which kind of personnel to use is that of the supervising physician.

DOCUMENTATION

A record should be made of all medically significant telephone encounters. Methods and formats of encounter systems differ widely. Some offices use a telephone encounter form, others use a spiral notebook. Portable, pocket-sized pads adapt nicely for after-hours use and for later placement into the patient's chart. Portable dictation equipment can be used to record after-hours telephone encounters.

The telephone encounter form may appear cumbersome; however, as the person answering the telephone becomes familiar with the format, recording of the relevant information during the conversation becomes second nature. The encounter form can be ordered with a self-sticking adhesive back so that a record of the telephone contact can be easily inserted into the patient's chart, or the encounter form can be printed on both sides for economy reasons. If the docu-

mentation is in a separate log or notebook, it should be stored for as long as possible.

There are several reasons for written documentation. Salient details of past conversations, as well as the date and name of the office staff member who received the call, can be quickly retrieved. This information is invaluable if the patient subsequently registers a complaint and medical liability is an issue. There have been several malpractice experiences that focused on telephone advice given to the patient. Risk management training as it relates to telephone medicine is essential for all staff. Also, in a group practice, it is helpful for a pediatrician to be able to review details of prior telephone instructions when the patient's regular physician is absent.

OUT-OF-OFFICE NEEDS

Rapid on-call accessibility to the pediatrician is crucial for quality of care and patient satisfaction. An answering service, where available, is literally a necessity. It increases accessibility for the pediatrician on call, and when he or she is not on call it forestalls unnecessary interruptions for the pediatrician and his or her family. Telephone calls after hours or on weekends can be managed by a direct line switch to an answering service or to a hospital switchboard if an answering service is not available. A telephone answering service should be monitored for efficiency and accuracy.

The radio paging system (beeper) enhances accessibility and should be considered a necessity. Two home telephone lines are desirable if personal and family telephone use compromises on-call accessibility. Telephone answering machines that only record messages are not appropriate for the physician on call, and many patients dislike these devices. An answering machine, however, may be useful if the message provides an emergency number and is easily understood by even a distressed parent. For example, the message may say, "Office hours are 9 A.M. to 5 P.M., Monday through Friday. In case of emergency, call _____." The use of the terminology "in case of emergency" may defer non-urgent calls until regular office hours, yet a patient who has an emergency is told how to obtain an immediate, personal response.

The use of cellular and portable telephones is increasing. They enhance availability and accessibility but also increase telephone work and stress for the pediatrician.

BASIC EQUIPMENT FOR A NEW PRACTICE

Two or three telephone lines generally are required for solo practice, but it is wise to ask the telephone company about reserving additional sequential telephone numbers for later service expansion. The placement of telephones within the office is determined by staff needs. A base unit in the appointment/reception area, an extension at the back office station, and a readily accessible, privately located telephone are minimum necessities. Telephones in examining rooms are a matter of personal taste. However, telephone calls concerning patients made in the presence of other patients may compromise patient confidentiality.

EQUIPMENT FOR THE EXPANDING PRACTICE

Three pediatricians generally require five telephone lines; five pediatricians may require eight lines. The ratio of phones per pediatrician diminishes in a large practice. If

---

Table 2-1.   Four-Step Approach to Telephone Care Training

STEP I: SURVEY OF EXISTING TELEPHONE SYSTEM

A. Objective

1. To analyze the current telephone system in a detailed, descriptive fashion, including the number of phone calls by hour and day of week. There should be a focus on predicting the busiest hours, staffing levels during these hours, and what can be done to reduce volume and smooth out peaks wherever appropriate.
2. To evaluate the telephone behavior of staff and the current training program used to prepare personnel for telephone medicine responsibility.

B. Methods

1. Use a telephone encounter form to collect important telephone data (number of calls for advice versus administrative or appointment information, total number of calls hourly and at peak times, number of referrals, and number of same-day appointments versus home management advice).
2. Personally listen to the way support staff are answering the telephone and talking to patients (with a double headset for simultaneous listening).
3. Call your office to evaluate the number of rings before the phone is answered, whether and how you were put on "hold," and how the support staff greeted you.
4. Request that a representative from the telephone company observe the telephone behavior of office personnel and the mechanics of your present system and make recommendations for improvement. This is a service that is usually free of charge.

STEP II: STUDY OF WRITTEN MATERIALS BY STAFF UNDER THE SUPERVISION OF A CLINICIAN

A. Objective

1. After studying the training material, staff should be able to obtain a relevant medical history and distinguish between:
   a. A true emergency
   b. Problems that can be safely managed at home
   c. Problems that require an appointment
2. For problems that require an appointment, staff should be able to determine when the appointment is needed:
   a. Immediately
   b. As soon as possible
   c. Same day
   d. Future appointment
3. Staff should be able to present home management advice for specific symptoms accurately, safely, and efficiently.
4. Staff should be aware of how evaluations by telephone are different from face-to-face encounters and how to avoid potential pitfalls and errors.
5. Staff should appreciate the importance of how the voice creates an image of the practice and the value of professional telephone behavior to the medical program.

B. Methods

1. Staff should read and use a reference such as *Telephone Medicine: Training and Triage. A Handbook for Primary Health Care Professionals.*

2. Mock telephone role playing should be incorporated into team meetings where one support staff plays the patient and another plays the telephone assistant. The scenarios described in the *Handbook* can be used in combination with those created by the staff from actual cases.
3. Lectures and discussions of specific disease entities and management techniques should be regular agenda items for office or team meetings.

STEP III: DIRECT OBSERVATION OF EXPERIENCED SENIOR STAFF

A. Objective

1. To reinforce techniques in history taking that improve the ability to differentiate between problems that need appointments and those that can be managed safely at home with treatment advice.
2. To learn how to schedule appointments and keep pace with heavy volume.
3. To learn how to respond to acute emergency situations.
4. To learn how to manage upset or angry patients.
5. To become fully informed about the management of administrative matters, including:
   a. Prescription refills
   b. Requests for laboratory results
   c. Referrals
   d. Health education information, such as immunization schedules

B. Methods

1. All new staff should spend approximately 24 hours, divided over a 3-month period, in direct observation of a senior staff member, listening to telephone conversations on a double headset adjusted for simultaneous listening only.

STEP IV: EVALUATION

A. Objective

1. To evaluate the telephone assistants' ability to distinguish between and manage emergency situations, problems that need appointments, and problems that can be safely managed at home with appropriate advice and follow-up.
2. To improve knowledge and skill by constructive dialogue.
3. To encourage outside reading and listening to tapes in areas recommended by the supervising clinician.

B. Methods

1. A 1-hour appointment should be made for the telephone assistant to meet with each key member of the health care team.
2. Topics (two or three each) should be divided among the health care team members and distributed in advance to the telephone assistant in preparation for the meeting.
3. Mock role playing should be incorporated into the evaluation using the audit form from the *Handbook.*
4. Live tapes of actual telephone scenarios, as well as video scripts if available, should be used as springboards for discussion.
5. Strong points should be congratulated, and further study or tapes should be assigned for those areas needing improvement.

(Katz HP. Telephone Medicine: Training and Triage. A Handbook for Primary Health Care Professionals. Philadelphia, F.A. Davis, 1991.)

requested, the telephone company will monitor the office service and provide a printout that will identify busy signals at peak periods; this is one way to know if additional lines are needed. Reserved sequential phone numbers prevent the inconvenience of having to change the office number later. As more staff members are added, more extension phones may be needed. Appointment, business office, insurance, and laboratory staff all generally require telephone access, as do the pediatricians' offices, consultation rooms, and a library or lounge.

Investigate needs thoroughly. It may be necessary to talk with a professional management consultant periodically as well as with representatives of the telephone company and some of the private telephone system vendors. Too little equipment sacrifices efficiency, and too much wastes money.

Microprocessing has revolutionized telephone equipment. Previously unknown features are now commonly available and affordable. Formerly available only by rental, these systems may now be purchased. Many other "own-your-own" systems (called interconnects) are widely available from private companies. Remember that, when purchasing equipment, the local telephone company's responsibility ends at the point of access. The decision about what to buy depends on four factors: reliability, service, features, and cost.

Some features to consider are one-direction lines, digital switching, speed dialing, call forwarding, line privacy, call paging, speakerphones, and intercom systems. Optional software may be added, such as an automatic call distribution and an electronic sequencer that holds calls sequentially and provides data, including the total number of calls, the number and duration of calls placed on hold, and the number of abandoned calls.

TRIAGE AND TRAINING

A common question parents ask is, "When should my sick child see the pediatrician?" There are no firm rules, but a child should be seen whenever parents are worried about how their sick child is acting. These decisions vary tremendously from parent to parent. An appropriate balance between the benefits and risks of home management for a particular medical situation, and sound, informed judgment are required.

Telephone decision guidelines are directed toward helping parents decide when it is safe not to bring a child to the office and what they should do and look for while the child is at home. Algorithms and guidelines also provide information for when the child should see the pediatrician. The objective of this approach is to help promote a more informed, safe decision-making process. For this purpose, a training approach for handling telephone calls is suggested (see Table 2-1). It must be emphasized that this training can be done only under careful supervision by the pediatrician. Other training tools may also be used, such as critiquing mock telephone calls, videoscripts, or live tapes. Whatever

Table 2-2. Telephone Quality of Care Checklist

1. Do you know how many phone calls your office receives daily, and what are the top six reasons for calls?	YES	NO
2. Is the average duration of employment for your office telephone staff greater than 2 years?	YES	NO
3. Have you recruited the right person for the job?	YES	NO
4. Do you have a formalized training of telephone management/triage in your office practice?	YES	NO
5. Do you have written protocols, specific guidelines, and office procedures for your staff?	YES	NO
6. Do you have written protocols for emergencies and for what to do when physicians are not in the office?	YES	NO
7. Do you document all medically significant phone calls?	YES	NO
8. Do you write smarter rather than longer?	YES	NO
9. Does your staff have a low threshold to bring patients in for an office visit?	YES	NO
10. Have you received no complaints from patients about the telephone or telephone staff in the last month?	YES	NO
11. Do you personally review telephone procedures regularly with your staff to ensure that only conditions that are appropriate for management by telephone are so managed?	YES	NO
12. Have you met with your staff in the last 2 months to talk about the telephone and to listen to their problems?	YES	NO

A "yes" to each answer is the correct response.
(Katz HP. Telephone Medicine: Training and Triage. A Handbook for Primary Health Care Health Professionals. Philadelphia, F.A. Davis, 1991.)

system is used, evaluation is critical. A practical tool to use is the Telephone Quality of Care Checklist (Table 2-2).

ANNOTATED BIBLIOGRAPHY

Kaplan S: The telephone in pediatric practice. In Moss AJ (ed): Pediatrics Update. Amsterdam, Elsevier Biomedical Press, 1983. (Comprehensive literature review of the role of the telephone in pediatric care.)

Katz HP: Quality telephone medicine: Training and triage. HMO Pract 4:137–141, 1990. (The application of a Quality Improvement approach in health care.)

Katz HP: Telephone Medicine: Training and Triage. A Handbook for Primary Health Care Professionals. Philadelphia, F.A. Davis, 1991. (Provides a comprehensive, how-to approach to office-based triage and training.)

Katz HP, Wick WR: Malpractice, meningitis, and the telephone. Pediatr Ann 20:85–89, 1991. (Case study of telephone malpractice involving telephone advice given to parents by a registered nurse in a pediatric group.)

Wood PR: Pediatric resident training in telephone management: A survey of training programs in the United States. Pediatrics 77:822–825, 1986. (Survey describing the extent of residency training in telephone medicine.)

3

The Pediatrician and the Computer

David Bergman

Over the past decade, the computer has played a prominent part in numerous aspects of the pediatrician's professional life. This has been particularly evident in hospital settings where order and results management are increasingly computerized, and in office settings where many of the financial and administrative reports are performed by computers. In the near future, pediatricians will likely be using computerized systems and decision support programs to enhance their medical decision making.

The computer has generally failed to have an impact on the one area of information management that accounts for a major part of the pediatrician's paperwork—the medical record. In other industries, computers have been used extensively to automate paper-based recording and ordering; the office-based pediatrician, however, still remains mired in a world of paper medical records, order forms, and results printouts. Three major barriers stand between the pediatrician and the computerized medical record: the inability of different computer systems to talk to each other (the lack of system integration), the need for computers to talk the same clinical language, and the lack of an interface that allows the pediatrician to use the familiar modes of writing and speaking to communicate to the computer.

SYSTEM INTEGRATION

The primary function of a medical record is to provide a repository of information that describes the nature of the medical problem, the associated diagnostic and therapeutic interventions and their justifications, and a compilation of findings and results. The sources of this information are many and include the pediatrician's office visit notes, results from laboratory tests, radiology results, and subspecialists' reports. This record must be legible and concise and must serve as both clinical and legal documentation of the care provided to the patient.

Maintaining a medical record is an arduous and time-consuming task for the pediatrician. Time–motion studies have shown that clinicians spend close to 50% of the visit time compiling and recording information into the medical record. Given the time constraints of current ambulatory practice, where the average visit ranges from 11 to 18 minutes in length, it is not surprising that the pediatrician will often forgo the time necessary to create a proper medical record in order to increase the face-to-face time with the patient. Unfortunately, this can result in a medical record that is no more than a set of key words and short phrases to later trigger expanded stores of clinical information in the clinician's mind. What results is a medical record that does not easily communicate important clinical information, provides an inadequate audit trail for quality of care measurement, and is frequently an inadequate legal document.

The potential for the computer to alleviate this situation is considerable. One of the strengths of a computerized information system is the ability to automate those functions that are currently done manually by the pediatrician (i.e., to record information derived from multiple sources into the medical record in a logical and intelligible format). The capability of a computer to accomplish this task, however, hinges on its ability to "talk" to these other sources of information. These can include the laboratory computer for lab results computerized order and results management system that places orders and tracks the results; a computerized radiology system for radiology results; digitized representations from medical imaging systems; computerized surgical and hospital discharge reports; and computerized medical records in other physicians' offices. Unfortunately, most office-based computer systems existing today do not and cannot connect to this long list of information sources; each requires that separate information be manually inputted into the computer. For the busy pediatrician, the time and cost commitment involved in typing this information into a computer eliminates most office-based systems as a viable alternative to the paper record.

Although there are few, if any, computerized medical record systems for the individual pediatric office, several large health maintenance organizations (HMOs) are actively involved in the design of integrated clinical information systems that replace the paper medical record with a clinical *work station*. A clinical work station in this context is a powerful personal computer capable of processing a large amount of information in the medical record and containing links to information systems throughout the health care organization. Through these work stations, the pediatrician is able to enter clinical information; order and review tests, procedures, and referrals; review past medical information; and have complete connectivity with his or her clinical colleagues. Although these systems are most easily implemented in highly integrated settings such as staff model HMOs, clinical information systems are currently being designed for less integrated settings such as Independent Practice Associations and multi-specialty group practices. The office-based pediatrician who is considering the purchase of an office computer should keep in mind that over the next 5 to 10 years the major impetus for computerizing clinical information will come not from single vendors selling to private pediatricians but rather from managed care organizations that have the financial incentive and the resources to integrate all the sources of information into one system. Because of the costs and resources involved in implementing a computerized medical record, it is likely that this effort will initially begin with managed care organizations and will eventually spread to individual pediatricians as part of their involvement with managed care.

TALKING THE SAME CLINICAL LANGUAGE

One of the most compelling reasons for introducing the computer into clinical practice is the power it gives the pediatrician to retrieve and organize clinical information. This quick and easy retrieval of important clinical information requires that several important assumptions be met. Terminology must be standardized. For example, to learn more about a heart murmur that sounds benign in an unfamiliar child, would the search be under "innocent," "functional," or "Still's murmur"? In order for efficient retrieval of information, everyone must use the same words to describe signs, symptoms, and diagnoses. This standardization safeguards against missing important information and prevents unnecessary tests.

Several efforts have been made to standardize nomenclature in the medical world. The best known examples are the International Classification of Disease with Clinical Modifications, 9th edition (ICD9-CM), and the Clinical Procedure Terminology, 4th edition (CPT-4). These classification systems have the advantage of widespread acceptance but often fall short of the needs of a primary care practitioner. The ICD9-CM was initially developed by pathologists and epidemiologists to ensure consistent coding of diagnoses at autopsy. Later iterations of the system have attempted to adapt more clinical medicine by incorporating symptoms as well as diseases. However, this system still falls short of the needs of the primary care practitioner who deals not with diseases but with symptoms or signs. Similarly, the CPT-4 codes are excellent for specific surgical or diagnostic procedures but do not offer a comparable level of detail for the cognitive services that constitute the majority of services offered by the primary care physician.

The issue of a universally accepted clinical nomenclature becomes even more problematic when efforts are made to standardize the description of specific symptoms and signs in the history and physical exam. For example, when the tympanic membrane is examined, is middle ear fluid or a middle ear effusion seen? It may seem that achieving this level of preciseness is unnecessary, but actually this has much clinical and research relevance. For example, if one wishes to determine the outcome of all patients who have middle ear disease, it will not be possible if patients' symptoms are described with different adjectives.

Efforts at implementing a clinical nomenclature for symptoms and signs are less well developed than are systems that describe diagnoses and procedures. The Reed Classification System has been developed in the United Kingdom and provides an excellent clinical nomenclature for primary care. The system has been validated but has not achieved widespread acceptance in other countries. Currently, the National Library of Medicine is developing a Unified Medical Language System (UMLS) that may accomplish many of these goals. The development of a valid, practical, and easy-to-use nomenclature system for primary care remains one of the top priorities for those interested in medical information systems.

In the ideal world of computerized medical records, different systems should be able to talk to each other. For example, it would be highly efficient for a pediatrician in Boston treating a patient who has just moved from San Francisco to "call up" the patient's automated medical record in San Francisco and with a keystroke have the medical record transferred into his medical record system. Similarly, for a federal regulatory agency or research institution that wants to examine the effectiveness of a given intervention for children, it would be extremely efficient to "call up" the medical records of a random sample of patients who received this intervention, store them anonymously in a data base, and analyze the clinical outcomes. This procedure could potentially save millions of dollars by avoiding expensive and time-consuming clinical studies. Information transfer between clinical data bases requires consistent protocols for communicating medical information between medical information systems. Efforts to develop and disseminate these protocols are currently ongoing, but to date no one system has been widely accepted or used.

The problem of "talking the same language" is not new to medicine. Considerable effort in the acculturation process of medical students involves translating what the student told us into our own clinical language. The prospect of automated medical information systems has forced us to formalize and continue this process. If a universally accepted clinical nomenclature can be defined, the potential benefits go beyond computerized medical records. Such systems may help us to communicate more clearly among ourselves and ultimately with our patients.

COMMUNICATING WITH YOUR COMPUTER

Time is the enemy of the busy pediatrician. The increased complexity of the patient's problems leads to increased time filling out forms or making phone calls. It is not surprising that the introduction of a new technology is not well received if it is perceived to add time to the clinician's day. This barrier remains even if the new technology enhances the quality of care, and unfortunately this scenario is often the case when computers are introduced into ambulatory care.

Clinicians readily accept the use of the computer to efficiently and effectively retrieve clinical information. This can be seen in the rapid acceptance of computer terminals that quickly retrieve laboratory results. Similarly, clinicians may be accepting of an automated order management system if it allows them to place orders with greater speed and accuracy. Problems arise, however, when attempts are made to automate clinical information in the medical record. The primary way information is placed into a computerized medical record is through a keyboard. This involves typing in the history, physical exam, assessment, and treatment plan. Pediatricians who dictate circumvent these problems; dictated clinical notes can be typed into the data base in lieu of producing a typewritten document. For the pediatrician who hand-writes his clinical notes, using a keyboard in place of a pen can be a daunting and time-consuming task. Few clinicians are willing to take the extra time to type in their notes.

Even if the typing problem was easily solved, there is yet another problem. The power of the computer to retrieve important clinical information lies in its ability to search a data base using key words and time delimiters. Consider again the example of the patient with a heart murmur who presents for urgent care. In order to query the computer for additional information about the patient's heart murmur, instructions have to be provided to direct a search of the data base for instances of heart murmur associated with this patient over a specified time interval. For this search to occur, clinical information, such as heart murmur, has to be put into an identified space or field in the data base so that it can be identified or coded for retrieval. When the pediatrician or the transcriptionist types clinical information into the computer in free text form, important clinical data are not coded and cannot be easily retrieved.

A common way for entering coded information into the computerized medical record is through the use of a checklist. A checklist contains a list of important symptoms, signs, or findings and is a means for the pediatrician to identify a patient characteristic as present or absent (normal or abnormal), not observed, or unknown. This is usually done with a keystroke or with the click of a "mouse." Ultimately, the information can be displayed as a checklist, or converted into a statement that appears to be free text but actually contains coded information. Coded clinical information can also be entered through the use of a template. This method consists of a standard paragraph such as might be used in an operative report or radiology report with blank spaces for the clinician to enter the needed clinical information. This allows for the creation of a narrative report that still contains important clinical information in a coded format. There are currently available several computerized medical record systems that use one or both of these formats for inputting clinical information.

Ideally, the pediatrician would like to avoid all contact with a keyboard. Until recently, the concept of conversing with a computer was an idea that was contemplated only in science fiction. Today, systems exist that can recognize up to 30,000 words. These systems, however, often achieve an accuracy of only 75% to 80% word recognition in "real world" situations. Over the next few years, voice input systems will become available that will allow the input of coded information into the computer by voice with use of a predefined clinical nomenclature and coding system.

A system intermediate between voice input and the keyboard is the pen interface. This interface allows the clinician to use a pen or a stylus to enter coded information by marking a checklist of symptoms and signs or by actually writing the clinical term into a predetermined field on the computer screen. These pen interface systems can be made quite small and light and may be particularly useful as "notebook" interface devices that can be used in the examining room or at the bedside. As voice input and pen interface systems become available over the next few years, the computer interface will grow to more closely resemble natural communication.

The computer has already proved itself to be a useful tool in the automation of the medical office. Many pediatricians have found it to be an invaluable tool for office administration tasks such as billing patients, making appointments, word processing, and creating spread sheets. Initial inroads into clinical application have been made by some pediatricians in the areas of bibliographic retrieval and linkages to laboratory computer systems. The further exportation of computers into the clinical arena of the medical record is clearly a goal whose time has come. Increasingly, the purchasers and payers of health care will be examining health care providers with greater scrutiny. The old medical record system of a few phrases on a piece of paper or a notecard will have to give way to a detailed accounting of the patient's problems, clinical characteristics, diagnosis, and treatment. This information will have to be represented in a format that will allow pooling of the data into data bases that can assess the impact of current treatments on medical outcomes, as well as constantly monitor the quality of care. This work is clearly more than the busy pediatrician can accomplish with paper and pen.

Although a compelling case can be made for the computer in clinical medicine, its full utilization in an ambulatory setting will have to await more complete system integration, an agreed-upon clinical language, and a computer interface that will allow rapid and easy entry and retrieval of clinical information. It is clear that these advancements are now under development and will likely be available in the near future. Until then, the pediatrician should consider computerized medical records with trepidation and with the cognizance of the limitations that currently exist.

ANNOTATED BIBLIOGRAPHY

Anderson JG, Jay SJ (eds): Use and Impact of Computers in Clinical Medicine. New York, Springer-Verlag, 1986. (Draws together a series of studies examining the impact of clinical computer systems on clinical practice and medical institutions.)

Blum BI: Clinical Information Systems. New York, Springer-Verlag, 1986. (One of the classic works outlining the essential components for an effective clinical computing system.)

Computers for the Practicing Pediatrician. Elk Grove Village, Il, American Academy of Pediatrics, 1989. (Practical, hands-on guide to purchasing computer systems for the office-based practice.)

Goldman L: Acute chest pain: emergency room evaluation. Hosp Pract 15:21–29, 1986. (One of the first examples of the marriage between decision science and computers to improve the accuracy of clinical decision making.)

International Classification of Diseases: Manual of the International Statistical Classification of Diseases, Injuries and the Causes of Death, 9th Rev. Geneva, World Health Organization, 1977. (This classification system will likely form the basis for almost all problem-based automated medical records.)

McDonald CJ, Hui SJ, Smith DM et al: Reminders to physicians from an introspective computer program. Ann Intern Med 100:130–138, 1984. (Classic study of the impact of an automated clinical reminder system on improving physician adherence to high standards of care.)

Reggia JA, Tuhrim S (eds): Computer Assisted Medical Decision Making. New York, Springer-Verlag, 1985. (Excellent collection of articles outlining the use of the computer as a decision support tool. Although some of the examples are currently out of date, the principles underlying their development remain solid.)

2

THE NEWBORN

4

Genetic Risk Factors and Screening

Janice D. Key

Genetics play an important role in general pediatrics. Genetic histories are taken at the initial well-child visit when a complete family history is obtained to help determine which diseases the child is at risk of developing, and to evaluate a child with birth defects. Birth defects are present in 2% to 4% of newborns and are the major cause of morbidity and mortality in the newborn period. This chapter presents an overview of general topics important in the prenatal and family history of the patient and of the newborn. A detailed discussion of specific genetics conditions is not included.

FAMILY HISTORY

Usually at the initial visit, regardless of the age of the patient, a complete family history is obtained, often by having the patient or parent answer a questionnaire listing numerous conditions, such as heart disease and hypertension, as well as more classic mendelian conditions, such as sickle cell disease and cystic fibrosis. In general, little information is available regarding what exact risk there is for these multifactorial conditions; however, knowledge in these areas is increasing rapidly. A family history for certain diseases may affect the decision to screen a patient (as with cholesterol screening) or may affect treatment during an acute illness (as with wheezing in a family with atopic disease).

HYPERCHOLESTEROLEMIA

Elevated cholesterol and low-density lipoprotein (LDL) cholesterol levels in childhood may be associated with adult heart disease. The molecular genetic basis for familial hypercholesterolemia has recently been discovered. A defect in the gene located on chromosome 19 coding for the LDL receptor is the cause of classic familial hypercholesterolemia. Homozygotes for this defect occur in one out of a million patients and patients are severely affected with greatly elevated LDL cholesterol, xanthomas, and very premature atherosclerotic heart disease. Heterozygotes, however, are not rare, occurring in 1 of 500 patients. Heterozygotes have an LDL cholesterol that is twice to three times normal. Typically they have myocardial infarctions in their 40s to 50s. It is estimated that 5% of all myocardial infarctions occur in these patients. A family history of myocardial infarction or heart disease at a young age may indicate a potential for this condition. The current American Academy of Pediatrics guidelines recommend cholesterol screening for these children after they are 2 years old. (See Chap. 53 for a more complete discussion on cholesterol screening.)

HYPERTENSION

Screening blood pressure in children over 3 years of age has been recommended since 1977 when the Task Force on Blood Pressure Control in Children established normal ranges for each age. Since that time it has been proved that blood pressures aggregate within families. It has also been shown that blood pressure in a child generally remains in the same percentile as the child gets older. Therefore, if one or both parents have hypertension, the child is more likely to also have hypertension and to have that hypertension persist into adulthood. Hypertension may result from many factors that are not genetic, such as the environment and psychological problems. Also, specific genetic conditions, such as neurofibromatosis, renal disease, aortic coarctation, dysautonomia, may cause hypertension. A family history of hypertension indicates that that child should be screened on routine physical exams, and it may contribute to diagnosing the etiology if hypertension is discovered. (See also Chap. 56.)

ATOPIC DISEASE

Allergic diseases are one of the most common health problems and reasons for seeking medical care. Overall, atopic disease affects 12% to 20% of the general population. While it is not a strict Mendelian condition, genetic factors are very important, as are environmental factors. Eighty percent of patients with atopic disease will have positive family histories of the disease. In evaluating population trends in IgE levels, the total IgE level has a heritability of over 50%. Children younger than 1 year old who have increased IgE levels have a greater risk of developing atopic disease in later childhood than do children with normal IgE levels. The tendency to develop an elevated IgE response to an antigen appears to have a genetic basis but requires environmental exposure to a particular antigen in order to develop an allergy.

PRENATAL HISTORY

Maternal Medical Conditions

Maternal medical conditions can influence the outcome of the pregnancy as well as the possibility that the baby will have neonatal problems or birth defects. Diabetes mellitus is a common condition that may cause an increased risk of both. The exact risk for each pregnancy depends on the classification of the mother's diabetes and her control during the pregnancy. As expected, the worse the classification and the poorer the control, the higher the risk to the baby. Transient neonatal effects seen in infants of diabetic mothers include large size at birth, hypoglycemia, hypocalcemia, and polycythemia. There is also a risk that the fetus will have birth defects, such as congenital heart disease, neural tube defects, among others.

Maternal epilepsy causes an increased risk of defects independent of anticonvulsant medication. Women who do not take an anticonvulsant have a risk of birth defects in their infants only slightly higher than that of normals, and women who take anticonvulsants have approximately a 10% overall risk. The exact risk and the specific birth defects depend on the anticonvulsant used.

Maternal infection can cause specific neonatal problems when the infection is transmitted to the fetus. The TORCH infections are the classic example. However, in other types of infections where the fetus is not directly infected there may be a teratogenic effect from the fever itself. A sustained fever of 103 to 104°F for several days can cause severe defects, the exact nature of which depends on the stage of embryogenesis. Most of the defects that have been described affect the central nervous system. Hot tubs, saunas, and any other extreme heat that may result in a rise in internal body temperature should be avoided during pregnancy.

Maternal age is related directly to some specific risks to the fetus. With advancing maternal age there is an increased risk of an autosomal aneuploidy in the fetus. Trisomy 21 is the most common autosomal aneuploidy in infants. The risk does not rise at a rapid rate until after age 35, and it rises at an even faster rate after age 40. There is no increased risk for other nonchromosomal birth defects in offspring of older healthy women.

One of the most common birth defects and the most common chromosomal abnormality is *Down syndrome,* or trisomy 21. Its patients are characterized by having specific dysmorphic features (upward slanted palpebral fissures, small ears that may be displaced downward and rotated, transverse palmar creases, clinodactyly, among others), as well as hypotonia and often feeding difficulty in the newborn period. Twenty-five percent of babies with Down syndrome will have congenital heart disease, such as ventricular septal defects, or more severe endocardial cushion defects. As they get older, they often have recurrent otitis media and usually require myringotomy tubes. Autoimmune hypothyroidism may develop at any age but should be screened for at least twice in early childhood and at any point where growth is less than expected. Children with Down syndrome are smaller than normal children and their growth should be charted with charts specific to Down syndrome. Because of the risk of atlantoaxial dislocation, children should be screened with cervical spine films at about 2 years of age and before they begin athletic participation.

TERATOGENS

Exposure to teratogens is an important aspect of the prenatal history. A positive history of exposure to a particular teratogen should be noted even if the infant appears unaffected at birth, because many subtle effects, such as learning disabilities, will become apparent only with time. More information about specific drugs can be obtained from teratology hotlines, texts, and the company that manufactures the drug. (For a discussion on environmental teratogens, see Chap. 18.)

Among anticonvulsants, Dilantin and valproic acid are proven teratogens. *Fetal hydantoin syndrome* has been well described and may include congenital heart disease, dysmorphic facial features (e.g., hypertelorism, flattened nasal bridge, epicanthal folds), hypoplastic nails, and central nervous system defects such as microcephaly and mental retardation. Of all exposed infants, about 10% will have one or more of these serious birth defects. More subtle effects not recognized at birth may include attention deficit hyperactivity disorder and learning disabilities.

Valproic acid is associated with neural tube defects as well as other birth defects. There is an increased risk of neural tube defects if the developing fetus was exposed to valproic acid during the closure of the neural tube. This risk is then increased from the baseline risk of 1/2000 to about 1/200. Other birth defects (e.g. mental retardation, congenital heart disease, and dysmorphic facial features) have been reported.

Isoretinoic acid is a recently recognized and highly publicized severe teratogen. It has a high risk of causing multiple birth defects, which may include central nervous system structural defects and mental retardation, congenital heart disease, and dysmorphic features.

Probably the most common teratogen and the most common cause of mental retardation is alcohol. *Fetal alcohol syndrome* was first recognized in the offspring of chronic alcoholics, where it affects at least one third of exposed infants. Its features include mental retardation that is usually mild, growth deficiency, congenital heart disease, joint abnormalities, and dysmorphic features (e.g., a long, flattened philtrum with a thin upper vermilion, hypertelorism, and narrow palpebral fissures). There are also common fetal alcohol features when the diagnosis of the full fetal alcohol syndrome cannot be made. These effects may include learning disabilities and attention deficit hyperactivity disorder. The amount and timing (trimester) of alcohol exposure should always be noted in a prenatal history even if there is no obvious defect at the time of birth, because it may be important several years later if the child is having difficulty in school.

An increasingly frequent problem is fetal exposure to cocaine. The abnormalities that may be caused by cocaine are becoming better recognized and include birth defects as well as long-term neurodevelopmental delays. There is an increased risk of obstetrical complications such as placental abruption. Birth defects include microcephaly, intrauterine growth failure, CNS hemorrhage, cardiac arrhythmias, and a variety of structural birth defects such as limb defects. The babies also go through a withdrawal syndrome at birth and may have neonatal complications such as necrotizing enterocolitis (NEC). (See also Chap. 5.)

PRENATAL TESTING

Ultrasound

Ultrasound is a common prenatal screening test. There are numerous indications for its use, most of which are obstetric. Ultrasound can visualize gross birth defects such as spina bifida or large ventricular septal defects, but it cannot detect smaller defects. The sensitivity of ultrasound is highly variable and depends on the quality of the machine and the experience of the operator. It presents no known risk to the fetus.

Maternal Serum Alpha-Fetoprotein

A prenatal screening test that is offered in virtually all pregnancies is maternal serum alpha-fetoprotein (MSAFP). Alpha-fetoprotein normally increases in the maternal serum with the advancing pregnancy until it reaches a peak in the second trimester. Conditions that are associated with an abnormally high MSAFP are multiple gestations, neural tube defects, ventral wall defects (e.g., omphalocele or gastroschisis), congenital nephrotic syndrome, cystic hygroma, and nonspecific problems such as intrauterine growth retardation and prematurity. A low MSAFP is associated with an increased risk of a chromosomal abnormality such as Down syndrome. The exact risk is determined by the mother's prior risk (age-related risk) and MSAFP level, and it may also be determined by the measurement of other hormonal levels. The MSAFP is a sensitive screening test for neural tube defects, but it is neither very sensitive nor specific in screening for Down syndrome. When using MSAFP alone, screening will detect only about one fifth of fetuses with Down syndrome. This may improve with the addition of other screening tests.

Amniocentesis

Amniocentesis is a prenatal test to determine the karyotype of the fetus, and it is also used for specific DNA and enzymatic testing. The most common indication is maternal age over 35. At this age, the risk of having a child with Down syndrome is about 1/350, a risk that is approximately equal to that of the procedure itself. Other indications are a previous child with a chromosomal abnormality or a couple known to be at risk for a specific condition. Amniocentesis can also be used to measure AFP and confirm a high MSAFP.

Chorionic Villus Sampling

Chorionic villus sampling (CVS) is an alternative method of collecting fetal cells for karyotyping or DNA analysis. It can be done much earlier in the pregnancy than amniocentesis (at 10 weeks rather than 16 weeks), and the results may be available in less time. Its risk is slightly greater than that of amniocentesis, but the risk seems to be decreasing as there is more experience with this technique.

EVALUATION OF THE NEWBORN

Neonatal Screening Tests

Neonatal screening tests are done to detect conditions for which there is preventative treatment and simple testing. *Phenylketonuria (PKU)* was one of the first conditions included in the neonatal screen. PKU and elevated blood phenylalanine may be caused by several different conditions. Classical PKU is an autosomal recessive condition caused by a deficiency of hepatic phenylalanine hydroxylase. It results in a very elevated phenylalanine (at least above 12 mg/dl in the newborn) that remains elevated unless the patient is treated with a low phenylalanine diet. Untreated patients have severe mental retardation and often seizures and autism. The patient will be normal if treatment is begun in the newborn period and continues throughout at least childhood. Other hyperphenylalaninemias may be detected in the screen, such as *transient hyperphenylalaninemia* which, as its name implies, requires no treatment. *Persistent mild hyperphenylalaninemia* will cause a chronically elevated phenylalanine level but will not cause mental retardation and therefore does not require treatment. Another much more serious condition is *dihydropteridine reductase deficiency,* which is autosomal recessive like PKU but causes severe neurologic deficits despite dietary treatment. Phenylketonuria may be important not only in childhood when dietary treatment is necessary but also in adolescence and adulthood because of the teratogenic effect of maternal PKU on the fetus. If not treated during pregnancy, maternal PKU may cause birth defects such as microcephaly and congenital heart disease.

The second screening test performed is usually a test for *hypothyroidism.* Although strictly speaking it is not a genetic condition, early detection and treatment will prevent mental retardation. Hypothyroidism may have various etiologies, from agenesis of the thyroid to ectopic hypoplastic thyroid. Screening is done by measuring the T_4 and, if it is low, by measuring thyroid-stimulating hormone (TSH). Hypothyroidism is found in one of 4000 to 5000 newborns. If left untreated, it will result in poor growth and mental retardation. (See also Chap. 10.)

Galactosemia may be included in neonatal screening. Elevated serum galactose may be caused by several conditions. Classical galactosemia is caused by a deficiency of galactose-1-phosphate uridyl transferase. If not treated with a galactose-free diet, failure to thrive, hepatomegaly and liver failure, and an increased risk of sepsis will occur. Long-term sequelae include mental retardation and cataracts. It is an autosomal recessive condition detected by enzyme measurement. Galactokinase deficiency may also cause an elevated galactose level, but it is different clinically from classical galactosemia. It will cause late-onset cataracts if it is left untreated. Finally, uridine diphosphogalactose-4-epimerase deficiency will cause an elevated galactose level but no clinical effects.

Other conditions that may be included in the neonatal screen vary from state to state. Sickle cell disease screening has recently been added in many states and will detect sickle cell disease, SC disease, sickle cell trait, and some other hemoglobinopathies. Many states also screen newborns for congenital adrenal hyperplasia.

Birth Defects

Approximately 2% to 4% of liveborn infants have major birth defects requiring medical attention. Many defects will be isolated in an otherwise normal child, but others will be found in conjunction with several other defects. Each newborn with a defect should be fully evaluated to 1) ascertain if other associated defects are present, 2) to ascertain if there is an overall unifying diagnosis, and 3) to inform the family of the prognosis for the child and the risk of a recurrence in future children. In addition to a careful physical examination, several approaches will be helpful in this evaluation, including analyses of each defect, a family history, and a differential diagnosis of each defect.

An analysis of each birth defect includes careful measurement to document that feature. The eyes, for example, appear close set both in hypertelorism (where there is a true increase in the distance between the orbits) and in telecanthus (where there is an increase in the distance between the two inner canthi but the orbits are normally placed).

The family history should be detailed, with particular emphasis on teratogenic exposures during pregnancy and history in the family of any related findings. An examination of the parents should also be made for detection of any similar features. For example, familial megalencephaly may be a benign trait, or a child with a cleft lip may have a parent with small pits in his or her lips, indicating an autosomal dominant condition (Van der Woude's syndrome).

After each finding is fully characterized, a differential diagnosis for each should be made using texts of birth defects as a reference source. Most of the differential can be eliminated because of essential features for each syndrome that the patient does not have. The remaining differential for each birth defect can be compared for common diagnoses. A correct diagnosis should be obtained as soon as possible for several reasons, with the most immediate one being the impact it will have in the medical management of that child. Once a particular diagnosis has been made, the patient should be further evaluated for other associated defects that have not already been diagnosed. The prognosis and treatment can then be determined.

ANNOTATED BIBLIOGRAPHY

Emery AEH, Rimoin DL (eds): Principles and Practice of Medical Genetics. New York, Churchill Livingstone, 1990. (Exhaustive text on most genetic disorders, including their biochemistry and pathophysiology when applicable. An excellent resource.)

Jones KL: Smith's Recognizable Patterns of Human Malformation, 4th ed. Philadelphia, W.B. Saunders, 1988. (Very readable, brief description with accompanying photographs of numerous dysmorphic syndromes. Last chapter contains tables of normal standards for anthropomorphic measurements and facial feature measurements. Appendix is helpful and has a differential diagnosis for many dysmorphic features and birth defects.)

McKusick VA: Mendelian Inheritance in Man, 9th ed. Baltimore, The Johns Hopkins University Press, 1990. (Computerized catalog of thousands of disorders that are proved to be or are hypothesized to be mendelianly inherited. Includes recent references for each disorder and a short discussion.)

5

Babies of Substance-Abusing Mothers

Sylvia Schechner

The epidemic of substance abuse in the United States, particularly in the urban centers, has prevailed since the 1960's. The drugs most often abused are cannabinoids, heroin, and, most recently, cocaine. The use of cocaine has spread rapidly because of the cheap, easily prepared freebased cocaine called "crack." Alcohol has always been prevalent and is one of the most common major teratogens to which the fetus is likely to be exposed.

Previous estimates of illicit drug use by pregnant woman may have been biased because sampling was mainly from urban areas with large minority groups of low socioeconomic status. In a recent study, toxicologic screening on the urine of pregnant women for alcohol, opiates, cocaine and its metabolites, and cannabinoids showed little difference between patients who used public clinics and private doctors. Positive drug screening results were also similar for white and black women in both urban and suburban areas. The overall prevalence of at least one of the above substances in the urine was 14.8%.

Drug-dependent mothers are at increased risk for hepatitis, sexually transmitted diseases, and AIDS, particularly if they engage in prostitution. About 30% of pregnant intravenous drug users are seropositive for the human immunodeficiency virus (HIV). Thus, not only are infants at risk for being addicted, they also are at risk for various infectious diseases.

Because most pediatricians will encounter infants who demonstrate neonatal withdrawal, it is important for them to be able to identify and treat these babies.

COMMONLY ABUSED DRUGS

Alcohol

Fetal alcohol syndrome was recognized in the United States in 1973, where it is estimated to occur in 1 to 3 per 1000 live births. Because of the variability in its presentation, the true incidence of this disorder is unknown. Fetal alcohol syndrome is thought to be the third most common cause of mental retardation in the United States, after Down's syndrome and neural tube defects.

This syndrome is characterized by intrauterine growth retardation, microcephaly, microphthalmia, short palpebral fissures, ptosis, a flattened nasal bridge, a long, smooth philtrum, and thin vermilion of the upper lip. There may be hypoplastic finger and toe nails, contractures of various

joints, and cardiac defects such as ventricular septal defects. Developmental delay and intellectual impairment are seen. It is often difficult to label an infant with this diagnosis in the perinatal period unless there is a strong maternal history, which is frequently denied. The clinical picture tends to become more apparent over time.

A crude dose–response relationship has been established for the amount of alcohol consumed and the likelihood of development of the fetal alcohol syndrome. The least amount of ethanol to cause this syndrome has been estimated to be two drinks per day, but usually it is not until four to six drinks per day are consumed that the subtle features become evident. No absolutely safe amount of alcohol consumption in pregnancy is known. Most of the children recognized as having fetal alcohol syndrome have been born to frankly alcoholic women who have more than eight drinks per day.

It is not known which is more harmful: binge drinking or steady consumption. Often, alcoholics will use other drugs (e.g., coffee, nicotine, and tranquilizers), which may potentiate the alcohol effects. The poor nutrition that is often present may further adversely affect fetal development.

Withdrawal symptoms of tremulousness, hypertonia, and irritability from fetal alcohol exposure may occur as soon as 6 to 12 hours after birth.

Alcohol passes freely into breast milk, but its effect on the infant is probably insignificant. Acetaldehyde, the toxic metabolite of ethanol, apparently does not pass into milk. The American Academy of Pediatrics considers maternal ethanol use compatible with breast-feeding.

Marijuana

Marijuana is the drug most frequently abused in the United States. It is inhaled through the lungs and is quickly absorbed, with a resulting high that may last 2 to 3 hours. Marijuana crosses the placenta and may result in shorter gestations and decreased fetal weight gain and length, but no decrease in head circumference. Infants born to women who smoke two or more marijuana cigarettes daily while pregnant are not at risk for developmental delay. Marijuana use during pregnancy does not appear to cause malformations. Newborns of women who smoke six or more marijuana cigarettes weekly often have tremors, startling, and altered visual response to stimuli within the first 4 days of life.

Although there have been no reported adverse effects with breast-feeding, nursing mothers should be encouraged to abstain from smoking marijuana.

Cocaine

Cocaine can be made into powder and inhaled into the nostrils (snorting), applied topically to mucous membranes, or converted into crystal chips and smoked (crack). Cocaine and its metabolites may be detected up to 24 hours later in urine and up to 60 hours later in breast milk. The neonate who has been exposed to cocaine within 2 to 3 days of delivery may have positive urine for up to 4 days after delivery.

Pregnancies complicated by cocaine use have a greater chance of spontaneously aborting, abruptions of the placenta, and fetal death, and babies are at increased risk for reduced birth weight, length, and head circumference. Possible etiologies include hypoxia secondary to decreased uterine blood flow, poor nutrition, low socioeconomic status, and a higher rate of infectious and sexually transmitted diseases.

Infants of cocaine-using mothers are at increased risk for neurologic and behavioral abnormalities, such as cerebral infarctions, tremors, irritability, and muscular rigidity. The latter three conditions are present in up to 87% of infants withdrawing from cocaine, and electroencephalograms are abnormal in almost half of these babies. The Brazelton Neonatal Behavioral Assessment Scale administered to cocaine-exposed infants at 3 days of age shows an impaired ability to react to the human voice and face and poor response to attempts at comforting. These babies have long, dull periods of wakefulness but with little spontaneous activity, and they have emotional lability. The association of cocaine with congenital malformations such as genitourinary defects, cardiac malformations, intestinal atresias, and CNS malformations is controversial. There is also disagreement regarding whether infants of cocaine users have an increased incidence of sudden infant death syndrome (SIDS).

Withdrawal from pure cocaine in the neonate rarely requires pharmacologic treatment. However, the newborn of a cocaine abuser who uses other drugs such as barbiturates, amphetamines, and alcohol can have more severe withdrawal and can require medication.

Because cocaine and its metabolites can be found in breast milk for up to 60 hours after use, it is recommended that women using this drug not breast-feed.

Heroin

In the United States, heroin use is always illicit. It is most often adulterated with various substances such as quinine, mannitol, lactose, starch, amphetamines, strychnine, and procaine and is frequently contaminated with bacteria, viruses, or fungi. Because heroin is often used with other drugs, it is difficult to isolate the effects of heroin alone on the fetus.

Heroin crosses the placenta and enters fetal tissues within 1 hour. When the mother is withdrawn from the drug, both she and the fetus will undergo simultaneous withdrawal. These symptoms usually begin during the first 24 to 48 hours of life. The incidence of neonatal withdrawal depends on the amount of daily heroin, when the mother last used the drug, and for how long she had been using it.

The withdrawal symptoms consist of a combination of any of the following: tremors, irritability, rubbing of the face and knees against the sheets, high-pitched cry, sweating, vomiting, diarrhea, hypertonia, and, rarely, seizures.

Structural defects have not been associated with prenatal exposure to heroin. However, babies have a high incidence of low birth weight and, less often, intrauterine growth retardation and prematurity. The latter may result from a higher rate of chorioamnionitis and other maternal infections in these women.

In follow-up studies of 3- to 6-year-olds born to heroin-addicted mothers, growth deficiency and occasional microcephaly have been observed. There is an increase in behavioral problems and learning disabilities, but overall intellectual functioning does not appear to be impaired.

Heroin crosses into the breast milk and may cause addiction in the infant. In addition, there is an increased risk of HIV infection in intravenous drug abusers. Therefore, breast-feeding should be discouraged in this group.

Methadone

Methadone is a synthetic opiate, and because of its ability to block the euphoric effects of heroin, it may be used in pregnancy to treat heroin addiction.

Methadone appears to partially prevent intrauterine growth deficiency in babies of mothers taking heroin. The earlier in pregnancy the mother initiates methadone therapy, the greater birth weight there will be. There is no known association between intrauterine methadone exposure and birth defects.

Withdrawal symptoms occur in 75% to 90% of exposed infants, and the severity of the symptoms correlates directly with the maternal methadone dose. Infants exposed to methadone in utero have more severe withdrawal and a higher incidence of seizures than do babies exposed to heroin. When methadone is given late in pregnancy, infants have fewer withdrawal symptoms. The onset of withdrawal is usually within the first 72 hours of life but may be delayed for up to 28 days.

Infants exposed to methadone in utero have behavioral and sleep disturbances identical to those of heroin-addicted infants: depressed interactive behavior, poor self-calming, tremors, increased tone, and less physical and emotional intimacy. Follow-up studies of these infants reveal a higher incidence of hyperactivity, learning and behavior disorders, and poor social adjustment. This may be a result of environmental factors rather than a consequence of in utero methadone exposure.

Methadone enters breast milk in concentrations approaching maternal plasma levels. No adverse effects have been reported in mothers taking 20 mg daily or less. Because of the risk of HIV infection in maternal intravenous drug abusers, it may not be prudent to encourage breast-feeding in this population.

Phencyclidine

Phencyclidine (PCP, angel dust) is an illicit drug used for its hallucinogenic effects. It can be either smoked, snorted, or taken orally. It may impair muscle coordination and result in bizarre behavior, such as hallucinations and prolonged schizophrenic-like psychosis.

The drug crosses the placenta and may be found in the urine of the newborn. The newborn is normal in most pregnancies in which the mother uses phencyclidine. There have been rare case reports of infants with symptoms of withdrawal (jitters, hypertonia, irritability, poor feeding). These babies may have significant changes in lability and consolability, but they abate by 3 months of age.

Because phencyclidine is excreted in breast milk, breastfeeding should be discouraged.

Lysergic Acid (LSD, Speed)

Because of reports that LSD (lysergic acid diethylamide) can cause chromosomal breakage in leukocytes, there is concern that it could be a teratogen. It should be noted that the reports are based on presumed ingestion of LSD; the identity and purity of what actually was taken are unknown.

Drug levels in breast milk have not been studied, and because of the lack of firm data, nursing should be discouraged.

CLINICAL PRESENTATION

A useful mnemonic for remembering the symptoms of withdrawal is presented in the following display. Withdrawal from the drugs discussed above will have at least one of the symptoms listed.

The onset of symptoms ranges from immediately after birth to 4 weeks after birth. The factors that influence the timing of withdrawal depend on the type of drug or drugs used, when before delivery it was last used, and dosage. Symptoms range from mild and transient to severe.

WORK-UP

The evaluation of an infant suspected of withdrawal should include a careful review of maternal history, the number of prenatal visits, and direct questions about drug use.

Urine specimens of the neonate should be collected for drug screening as early as possible. It is useful to obtain several samples of urine in case a repeat test is necessary. Serum glucose, electrolytes, and calcium should be obtained to rule out these abnormalities as the cause for symptoms. The clinical picture may warrant a full sepsis evaluation.

Parental consent is not necessary for urine drug screens on symptomatic infants. At our institution, we have been exercising this right when there is poor prenatal care and in cases of abruptio placentae.

Withdrawal

W =	Wakefulness
I =	Irritability, seizures
T =	Tremors, tachypnea, temperature elevation
H =	Hyperactivity, high-pitched cry
D =	Diarrhea, diaphoresis, disorganized suck
R =	Rub marks
A =	Apnea
W =	Weight loss or failure to gain weight
A =	Alkalosis secondary to vomiting
L =	Lacrimation, sneezing

Adapted from Committee on Drugs, American Academy of Pediatrics, Pediatrics 105:445, 1984.

It is important to know what the laboratory includes in its urine toxicology screen and to make sure that the suspected drug is included in the screening.

MANAGEMENT

Treatment should be primarily supportive; the infant should be swaddled tightly in its blanket and then kept in a quiet area to decrease sensory stimulation. Because of the increased caloric requirement from increased activity, crying, poor feeding, vomiting, or diarrhea, the baby may require a high-calorie formula.

A decision of whether detoxification is necessary should be based on one of several standard abstinence scoring sheets, which are widely available. These can enhance the clinical judgment of various observers who see the infant on different shifts, aid in documentation of the withdrawal signs, and chart response to medication.

PHARMACOTHERAPY

The three most common pharmacologic agents used for detoxification are tincture of opium, paregoric, and phenobarbital.

Tincture of opium contains opiate alkaloids and morphine (10 mg/ml), and when diluted 25-fold with sterile water it is equal to paregoric (0.4 mg/ml of morphine). This preparation contains less alcohol and lacks the additives of camphor, benzoic acid, anise oil, and glycerine that are found in paregoric.

The dose is .05 ml/kg, or 2 drops/kg q.4–6h. It is increased by 2 drops every 4 hours until the symptoms decrease so that scores of 8 or less on the abstinence scoring sheets are obtained. Tapering can be done by decreasing the dose 10% every day or every other day as tolerated.

Paregoric may cause habituation. It contains anhydrous morphine (0.4 mg/ml), narcotine and papaverine (antispasmodics), codeine (analgesic and narcotic), a high concentration of alcohol, camphor (a CNS stimulant), and anise oil.

The dose is .05 ml/kg, or 2 drops/kg every 4 hours, and is increased by 2 drops (.05 ml) after 4 hours if there is no improvement. Tapering is done as with tincture of opium. Paregoric is widely available, but because of its additives, it may not be as safe as the tincture of opium preparation.

Phenobarbital is effective, but the therapeutic blood level for control of withdrawal is unknown. Recommended dosage ranges from 5 to 16 mg/kg/day. Following a loading dose of 20 mg/kg, a maintenance dose of 4–6 mg/kg/day divided every 8 hours is begun.

If the patient scores less than 8 for 72 hours, the daily dose can be decreased by 10% every 24 hours.

Paregoric has been successfully used to treat withdrawal for over 70 years. It provides sufficient sedation with its antispasmodic activity to inhibit bowel motility and decrease diarrhea, and it also improves sucking ability. Its disadvantage is mainly the possible untoward side effects from its ingredients.

Phenobarbital is used because of its nonspecific central nervous system depression to control irritability and wakefulness. It has no effect on gastrointestinal irritability.

Infants who are exposed to narcotic agents respond better to paregoric or tincture of opium. Infants who have been exposed to multiple drugs in utero tend to have their withdrawal symptoms controlled better with phenobarbital.

If a single pharmacotherapeutic agent does not control withdrawal symptoms adequately, then a combination of phenobarbital and paregoric or tincture of opium may be effective.

REPORTING

In most states, the Department of Social Services must be notified when a newborn's urine screen is positive. Reporting is often done by the hospital social worker. The Department of Social Services evaluates the family situation and then decides whether discharge of the infant can be made to the home and if maternal detoxification is necessary, and it arranges ongoing follow-up for the family.

INDICATIONS FOR REFERRAL

Newborns requiring pharmacotherapy to control withdrawal symptoms are best cared for in at least a level-2 nursery. The added nursing care requirements caused by feeding difficulties, drug administration, and tapering make management difficult in a normal newborn nursery.

ANNOTATED BIBLIOGRAPHY

American Academy of Pediatrics Committee on Substance Abuse: Drug-exposed infants. Pediatrics 86:639–642, 1990. (Official statement of the AAP on the medical, social, mental health, and legal consequences for drug-exposed infants and their families.)

Chasnoff IJ, Landress HJ, Barrett ME: Prevalence of illicit-drug or alcohol use during pregnancy and discrepancies in mandatory reporting in Pinellas County, Fla. N Engl J Med 322:1202–1206, 1990. (Demonstrates that illicit drug use is common among pregnant women regardless of race and socioeconomic status.)

Finnegan LP: Neonatal Abstinence Syndrome: Current Therapy in Neonatal–Perinatal Medicine, pp 314–320. Philadelphia, B.C. Decker, Inc., 1990. (Detailed discussion of pharmacotherapeutic regimens for titrating and withdrawing therapy. Includes an abstinence scoring sheet.)

6
Special Needs of the Premature Infant

William D. Cochran

Premature infants have been going home from hospitals for over 100 years, and home-birthed "prematures" survived before that. However, premature infants have only recently been sent home weighing under 5½ lb, and even more recently some of the tiniest prematures, under 2 lb at birth, have been sent home and subsequently developed entirely normally. Unfortunately, most of these small babies have neurologic or other problems. The special needs of these premature infants and the special concerns of their parents are dealt with in this chapter. Generally, premature infants (well or with chronic problems) are assessed as ready-for-discharge when they can take all their feedings by mouth; can maintain their temperature while sleeping in a crib; no longer need an incubator; gain weight consistently (10 to 20 g/day) over a 2- to 3-day span; and have no apnea with color change. It is often helpful to explain to parents that their infant, until 40 weeks' gestation, is still prematurely born, and much of his or her fetal physiology continues.

TEMPERATURE CONTROL

Because the temperature control of premature infants under 40 weeks' gestation may not be well developed, both chilling and overheating assume greater importance than they do in full-term babies. Questions about either can most easily be assessed by the parents by taking the baby's rectal temperature; thus, this might be a technique taught before discharge. Generally, a rectal temperature between 97.5 and 100°F is within the normal range, with the lower temperature more common in the morning. A temperature below 97.5°F probably means the baby is too cold. Besides the usual sweaters and booties, hats are helpful in stabilizing a baby's low temperature.

Table 6-1.   Common Formula Supplements

MILK FORTIFIERS	PROTEIN	FAT	CARBOHYDRATE	CALORIES (per oz or ml)
HMF* (4 packets to 100 ml breast milk)	0.7 g	–	2.8 g	4/oz
Polycose	–	–	+	4/ml
MCT	–	+	–	7.6/ml
Corn Oil	–	+	–	9/ml

*HMF is a product of Mead Johnson. It can usually only be purchased through the distributor. Polycose and MCT can be purchased over the counter from a pharmacy.

NUTRITIONAL NEEDS

The nutritional needs of premature infants differ from those of full-term babies. Most "preemies" will be sent home from the hospital on a 20 cal/oz formula or, hopefully, on breast milk—or at least bottle feeding their mother's pumped breast milk. Generally, such premature infants will gain weight if they are getting 120 to 140 cal/kg/day, although occasional ones (especially those with continuing bronchopulmonary dysplasia [BPD]) may require 160 to 180 cal/kg/day because of their increased caloric needs. There are even a number of healthy premature infants who consume an inordinate amount of formula each day, "catching up" to their probable genetically set growth curve. They take as much as 200 to 220 ml/kg/day of formula at 140 to 150 cal/kg/day. As long as no obvious untoward reaction occurs, such infants may continue their large intake; their appetite will be satiated eventually. Other infants will be going home on milk fortifiers such as Polycose, Medium Chain Triglycerides (MCT), Human Milk Fortifier (HMF), or corn oil to increase their formula to 24 cal/oz or more in order to get sufficient calories without becoming overloaded with fluid. An occasional infant is discharged on 30 cal/ml formula (Table 6-1).

In most cases (the most common exception is infants with significant lingering BPD), by 5 lb of weight, if not before, the infant should be on a 20 cal/oz formula. The desired weight gain of 15 to 20 g/day is used as a rough guide. In fact, most infants will not be discharged home before they are on a 20 cal/oz formula. A reasonable guide to parents concerning frequency and timing of feedings is that seven feedings per day may be necessary for the first week or two at home in order to maintain a minimum weight gain. The infant should generally consume 2.5 oz/lb baby wt/day of formula. For premature infants, the time between feedings should not be longer in hours than their weight in pounds (e.g., a 5-lb baby should not wait more than 5 hours between any feedings), and the baby will have to make up feedings during the day, hopefully to get in the usual six or more feedings. As the baby's weight increases and the ounces per feeding increase, the number of feedings per day can be decreased.

Whether or not to give added *vitamins* is controversial.

All prepared formulas are supplemented with vitamins, but many parents (and some physicians) wonder if they are enough. Although the answer is not available, the added vitamins are probably adequate. Large doses of vitamin E are now usually no longer necessary. Fluoride supplementation (0.25 mg/day) is recommended for breast-feeding mothers, for those who live in communities where the water supply is deficient or for those who are using commercial ready-made formulas with fluoride content. Babies should have 400 U of vitamin D daily, which is already present in formula and should be supplemented to breast-fed babies.

Iron supplementation has proved beneficial. Premature infants tend to become more anemic in the first few months after birth than do full-term babies. In the nursery, it is customary to transfuse prematures in order to maintain their hematocrits around 40% until they weigh about 1500 g (3 lb 5 oz). This is usually done to help abort or treat "apnea of prematurity." After this weight is attained and no medical condition—such as continuing apnea or BPD—is present, the hematocrit is allowed to fall. It is not unusual to have it drop as low as 24%, occasionally even lower. A transfusion is not necessary if the baby continues to do well and the reticulocyte count rises to greater than 1%. However, because of the known poor iron stores of premature infants, it is recommended that iron supplementation (2 to 3 mg/kg/day) be started 8 to 12 weeks after the last transfusion is done in the hospital.

THEOPHYLLINE AND APNEA MONITORING

Theophylline and apnea monitoring are controversial and highly charged subjects (see Chap. 162). Parents are desperate for good advice, but, depending on the expert, that advice varies. At present, it is recommended that parents know of the conflicting recommendations, and the physician should tell them his or her opinion. The author's opinion is that monitoring is for their peace of mind only, because pneumograms in premature infants have no predictive value regarding subsequent sudden infant death syndrome (SIDS). However, whatever informed decision the parents make, they should be supported.

An occasional premature infant is sent home still on theophylline for apnea or for its potentially beneficial effect on residual BPD. It is generally true that some infants will have a tendency for continuing central apnea and therefore will need theophylline up to their 34th or even 35th week of gestation. However, many other prematures have proved that they had no need for it as early as the 30th week of gestation. If they are taking theophylline when discharged, it is usually given three to four times/day. To achieve a desired serum level of around 12, the dose is approximately 9 to 12 mg/kg/day. With 2 weeks at home of continuing apnea-free behavior (and the infant being now at least 36 weeks' gestation), the general consensus is to allow the infant to "outgrow" the dose (i.e., continuing the same dose in the face of the usual weight gain). The medication can be discontinued either around 40 weeks' gestation or when the serum theophylline level drops to less than 6.

IMMUNIZATION

Immunization of premature infants has been shown to be worthwhile. It may even be started for some of the smaller ones still in the hospital growing for discharge. The current advice is to start immunizations at the routine time (around 2 months of actual age) and at the normal dosage level. Fewer severe reactions seem to occur among premature infants, although their immune response is almost equal to that of normal full-term infants. (See Chap. 14.)

SPECIAL PHYSICAL PARAMETERS

Special physical parameters of prematures are noteworthy. For instance, almost all normally growing prematures have a head circumference (HC) that grows at a considerably faster rate than the infant's height or even weight. In fact, the sagittal suture may be split to a small degree for some time. Most small prematures will have had a cranial ultrasound in their first week of life. A normal result is reassuring that such a rapidly growing head is normal. This extra-rapid growth will usually slow down as the higher percentiles are reached. As long as the percentile of HC is not over 50% higher than the weight or it remains under 95%, expectant care is reasonable, especially in the presence of normal neurologic behavior. Declining growth parameters should also be investigated. (See Chap. 188.)

Because of changing signs and findings, the neurologic examination of all "normal" term infants as well as prematures may be difficult to interpret. Many prematures have an increased incidence of diplegia (with its tiptoe posture and hyperactive knee jerk); therefore, one may look for it—and then find it! Then one must decide whether to inform the parents of such a worrisome finding or monitor it to see if it persists, worsens, or decreases. The author strongly advocates only monitoring, especially if it is an otherwise isolated neurologic finding. If, on the other hand, there are such additional findings as continued fisting of the hands, excessive spitting or vomiting, or a marked "setting

sun sign," then further investigation should be carried out and referral to subspecialists considered.

Non-neurologic physical findings of prematures that one should be aware of are hernias, more flattened heads (mostly from positioning the baby on its back), and the characteristic high forehead that often persists for about a year.

Special attention must be paid to the premature infant's ability to see and hear, and whether these two senses are working and developing properly. Many physicians advise that otologic and ophthalmologic consultation or tests be routinely performed. The author believes that this can be done on an individual basis. An involved parent instructed to watch and observe carefully can usually see responses to visual or auditory stimuli in his or her child. The pediatrician should ask about such responses at routine well-child visits. If there is any question, further investigation is warranted.

COUNSELING

Counseling parents of a premature infant is especially important, and they will most likely need and should get special instructions, special help, extra "routine" visits, and extra time per visit. A premature birth often shatters the parents' expectation that their baby is perfect; it causes worries about cerebral palsy, mental retardation, and other defects. Thus, the parents of a premature (especially the mother) feel guilty ("that she had a premature delivery") and often become ambivalent about the increased care involved and the increased needs of such an infant. Parents often do not know how to deal with this problem. In addition to consideration and understanding on the part of the physician (allowing the parents time to ask all their questions), a worthwhile suggestion is to encourage parents of prematures to form a group, or at least talk to another set of parents of a premature. The discussion of similar problems with parents of other premature babies is generally beneficial.

Early infant stimulation programs are becoming more available, and prematures (and their parents) profit by entering them. Lastly, a wealth of literature is becoming available, and one should encourage parents to use it at the level of their need.

ANNOTATED BIBLIOGRAPHY

Goldson E: Bronchopulmonary dysplasia. Pediatr Ann 19(1):13–18, 1990. (Good review of BPD.)

Harrison H: The Premature Baby Book. New York, St. Martin's Press, 1983. (Excellent, practical book written for parents.)

Koops BL, Abman SH, Accurso FS: Outpatient management and follow-up of bronchopulmonary dysplasia. Clin Perinatol 11(1):101–122, 1984. (Useful reference for those who follow BPDer's after hospital discharge.)

Ronnholm KAR, Siimes MA: Hemoglobin concentration depends on protein intake in small preterm infants fed human milk. Arch Dis

Child 60:99–104, 1985. (Evidence that, at least when solely receiving breast milk, premature infants are more anemic by 12 weeks of age than they are when fed a protein-fortified formula.)

Southall DP, Richards JM, de Swiet M et al: Identification of infants destined to die unexpectedly during infancy: Evaluation of predictive importance of prolonged apnoea and disorders of cardiac rhythm or conduction. Br Med J 286:1092–1096, 1983. (This study of more than 2000 prematures, as well as subsequent data, supports findings that the pneumogram fails to predict SIDS.)

7

Families With Multiple Births

James Pert

The primary care provider is frequently involved with a family having a multiple birth—most often twins, but not uncommonly triplets. There are many aspects of the pregnancy, the neonatal course, and well-child care that are specific to multiples. A pediatrician will better meet the needs of these special families if he or she is aware of them. (For simplicity, this chapter will refer to all multiples as twins, unless otherwise specified.)

The incidence of twinning is the sum of the incidence of monozygotic (single ovum, or identical) twins and dizygotic (double ovum, or fraternal) twins. Monozygotic twins have an incidence of about 3 to 5/1000 births, a rate fairly constant across race and environment. The incidence of dizygotic twins ranges from 4 to 50/1000 births. Many factors contribute to this variation, such as increasing maternal age, parity (distinct from age), genetic predisposition, use of fertility agents, and serum gonadotropin levels. The highest incidence of twinning occurs in black Africans, and the lowest incidence occurs in Asians, with Japanese women having a rate of about 6/1000 births. North American white women have an incidence of about 10/1000 births. If twinning occurs with a frequency of $1/X$ in a given population, triplets will occur with a frequency of 1 in X^2, and quadruplets will occur in 1 in X^3. Having had twins once increases the chances of having another set from roughly 1/100 to 1/20.

It is not possible in the delivery room to definitively prove, on the basis of placental findings, that twins are identical. In monozygotic twins, an abnormal division (i.e., separation) of one embryo into two can occur at different times and can lead to varied placental findings. If separation occurs less than 72 hours after fertilization, there can be separate amnions and chorions. If separation occurs between 4 and 8 days after fertilization, there will be a diamnionic, monochorionic placenta; if separation occurs after 8 days, there will be a monoamnionic, monochorionic placenta; and if separation occurs after 13 days, the result is conjoined twins, occurring in 1/1500 twin pregnancies. While it is not possible initially to define twins as identical, twins of different sex are always fraternal. Paradoxically, disparity in birth weights increases the possibility of identical twinning. Anastomosis of the separate placentas leading to twin-to-twin transfusion (greater than 5 g/dl difference between infants) is more common in identical twins.

GOALS OF THE PRENATAL VISIT

Because most pregnancies of multiples are diagnosed prior to delivery (largely as a result of prenatal ultrasound), there is an opportunity for a prenatal visit with the pediatrician. These are best scheduled early in the third trimester, because 50% of twin deliveries occur before 37 weeks of gestation.

For families expecting twins, conception may have been a difficult issue. Conception may have been delayed voluntarily or because of fertility problems. In either case, the expecting couple may have great expectations and concerns, which potentiate the risk for creating vulnerable (i.e., at-risk) children. Discussion about the pregnancy, its timing, and the meaning for the expecting couple should help normalize their expectations.

Prenatal risks should be mentioned at some point during the prenatal visit. Twin pregnancies constitute 1% of all pregnancies but up to 10% of prenatal deaths, most due to lower birth weight. Twin pregnancy has an increased likelihood of caesarean delivery. If problems are anticipated, mothers are often referred to a tertiary obstetrical center for delivery. There is an increased chance for the twins to be admitted into a neonatal intensive care unit. The mechanism for such care in the pediatrician's delivery system should be reviewed. Couples expecting twins should be encouraged to visit the hospital where delivery is anticipated.

Having just one child can be a challenge for most new parents. Having twins creates considerably more stress on families. Mothers of twins are more tired, depressed, and anxious in the first months following delivery than are mothers of single births. It is very important for parents to hear the pediatrician state explicitly that having twins is different and harder than having children one at a time, for this acknowledgment will help parents maintain their self-esteem and energy.

Among the most useful advice for the family with twins is the suggestion to contact the National Mothers of Twins group. Most areas have a local chapter. This resource provides information, economic benefits through the sale of twin equipment and clothes, and psychological comfort to families of twins.

Publications are a second valuable resource. For example, *Twin's Magazine* usually contains many educational articles in each issue, and lay books such as *Having Twins,* by Elizabeth Noble, are very helpful.

Families with twins should also be encouraged to take advantage of other resources. Depending on their economic situation, each family may consider hiring a nanny or an au pair, a cleaning service, and so forth. If a family member has offered assistance, this should rarely be refused.

WELL CHILD VISITS

When scheduling visits for families with twins, extra time should be allowed. Even when both twins are healthy and developmentally normal, a well-child visit should take at least 45 minutes. Both parents are encouraged to attend. If this is not possible, advise the family to bring along another adult (e.g., grandparent, friend, babysitter) in order to allow the parent to focus on the exam rather than on the co-twin competing for attention, who will often disrupt the visit.

The pediatrician is wise to avoid scheduling appointments early in the session. It takes longer for a family of twins to travel anywhere, including getting to the doctor's office. Chronic lateness should usually be interpreted not negatively but simply as a consequence of increased strain on the family system presented by the twins.

Development does not progress at a steady rate for all infants and children. Rather, there are periods of growth followed by plateaus along each major path of development. A family of twins may achieve some respite in coping with daily life during the periods of consolidation. It is useful to anticipate that during periods of increased change (such as when infants become physically mobile, typically between 8 and 10 months) there will be an increase in stress, frequently resulting in marital discord.

The timing and content of well-child visits should occur at the customary times for singletons. (See Chap. 13, "The Well-Child Visit.") As with any individual child, visits may need to be more frequent if the children have special needs or the parents have specific issues to discuss.

Anticipatory guidance should be provided at each routine well-child visit. Safety issues need particular attention because parents of twins will be more tired and distracted by the other twin, and therefore less attentive. Moreover, and particularly for twins 15 to 48 months old, twins can cooperate in pursuing trouble more effectively than can singletons.

SPECIAL CONSIDERATIONS

Breast-Feeding

Breast-feeding should be encouraged as the major method of feeding twin infants, but exclusive breast-feeding is only rarely accomplished because feeding only one infant can take up to 8 hours a day. Most mothers are not able to breast-feed both infants simultaneously, so time demands become prohibitive. Some mothers will need permission to supplement the breast-feeding with formula. Using formula does not threaten milk production because two infants demand full volume even with partial feedings. An additional advantage of supplemental feeding is the increased involvement for the father in feeding. This enables the mother to rest while the father can enjoy feeding his children.

Sleeping

A common issue for parents of multiple births is fatigue. All parents of newborns become sleep deprived, but the demands of twins are particularly exhausting. During the period from birth to 4 months of age, families will do better if both infants are on similar hourly schedules. This optimizes the chance for parental naps and sleep. This manipulation of an infant's schedule is counter to the typical advice of promoting "on demand" feeding and sleeping, but during this period the expedient goal is similar rhythms in both infants. Many twin families report success with the following advice: Starting at the point when both twins are sleeping and the first twin awakens spontaneously, the first infant is nursed while the second is allowed to continue sleeping. When the first is finished, the second is awakened, fed, changed, and so forth. If twins can continue this pattern, parents have a better chance for coping and sleeping. Infants who deviate from this pattern may devastate the coping strategies of some parents.

Identical Versus Fraternal

Families will be asked repeatedly if the twins are identical or fraternal. As stated earlier, this will usually not be known at delivery. As the twins pass through infancy into early childhood, individuals outside the family may have progressive trouble telling the twins apart, even though the parents do not. If the twins are identical, the parenting goals become different. The definition of "self" for each individual twin is complicated when they are identical. Parental ability to identify differences in growth and development as well as to expect such differences is fostered by fraternal twinning. Strategies that promote the theme of "related but separate" are successful. Developmental patterns of fraternal versus identical twins have been of historical scientific interest and controversy for decades.

Developmental Risks of Twinning

Twins have a distinct pattern of language development, which is delayed compared to that of their singleton peers. The specific reasons for language delay may be related to reduced interaction with their parents or increased interaction between the twins, with each encouraging and responding to the other despite their language errors. However, the existence of a twin's special language should not delay pursuit of speech and language evaluations. A useful suggestion for fostering language acquisition is alternating placement of the twins in daycare or preschool to promote one-to-one interaction between each twin and their parents and to encourage separate peer interactions.

ANNOTATED BIBLIOGRAPHY

Hay DA: Update of Wilson's "A Study of Twins, with Special Reference to Heredity as a Factor of Determining Differences in Environment." Hum Biol 61(5–6):660–665, 1989. Wayne State University Press, 1990. (Review of the historical perspective of different developmental patterns in fraternal and identical twins.)

Hay DA et al: Speech and language development in preschool twins. Acta Genet Med Gemellol (Roma) 36:213–223, 1987. (Places speech delay in twins into a broader learning perspective.)

Hollenbach K, Hichok D: Epidemiology and diagnosis of twin gestation. Clin Obstet Gynecol 33(1): 1990. (Part of a lucid series giving an obstetrical perspective on multiple births.)

Niermeyer S: Clin Obstet Gynecol 33(1):88–101, 1990. (Statistics on perinatal risk of twins; also has excellent bibliography.)

Noble E: Having Twins: A Parents Guide to Pregnancy, Birth and Early Childhood. Boston, Houghton Mifflin, 1980. (Considered the "standard" lay press book, it covers a range of topics of practical importance to parents.)

Robin M, Jesse D, Tourette C: Forms of family reorganization following the birth of twins. Acta Genet Med Gemellol (Roma) 40:53–61, 1991. (Excellent review of the impact of twins on families.)

8

Breast-Feeding

Katherine C. Teets Grimm

Women have breast-fed since the beginning of time. Breast-feeding is a subject that is often made needlessly complicated. As a result, many women who are breast-feeding for the first time are anxious as to whether they can be "successful" at it. Most women can be, but some may require much counseling because it is a skill that may not "come naturally." Many books have been written about breast-feeding, including several books specifically for the medical profession: these books should be referred to for more detail.

ADVANTAGES

The advantages of breast-feeding include the following:

- *Promotion of maternal–infant bonding:* Breast-feeding encourages not only eye-to-eye contact but also close body contact and touch. Such closeness fosters the bonding process.
- *Excellent nutrition with good digestibility:* Breast milk contains all the essential nutrients required for good growth, with the possible exception of vitamin D. It is high in fat and lactose and low in casein and sodium. The low casein promotes good digestibility. The stools of breast-fed infants tend to be soft and easier to evacuate than those of formula-fed infants.
- *Allergen free:* The proteins of breast milk are species-specific and are therefore nonallergenic. Occasionally, foreign proteins that the mother ingests, such as from cow's milk, pass through the breast milk and sensitize the infant. "Colic" in a breast-fed baby can sometimes be relieved by the elimination of cow's milk products from the mother's diet.
- *Soluble and cellular immune protection:* This includes secretory IgA as well as other immunoglobulins, macrophages, lymphocytes, other cellular elements, chemotactic factors, and antibacterial factors. There is a lower incidence of enteric and respiratory infections in breast-fed infants. Of interest, the predominant intestinal flora in breast-fed infants is the nonpathogenic *Lactobacillus bifus.* In contrast, the intestinal flora of bottle-fed babies is entero-bacteria.
- *Convenience:* The nursing mother does not need to prepare bottles of formula or get up in the middle of the night to heat a bottle. If she wears proper clothing, she can easily feed the baby anytime and in any place without any preparation.
- *Low cost:* The nursing mother requires an additional 500 calories and 20 g of protein a day. The cost for these additional calories is a few dollars a week. The cost for formula will depend on whether the mother buys ready-to-feed, concentrate, or powdered formula, singly or by the case. Using any formula is considerably more expensive than breast-feeding.

DISADVANTAGES

A woman who is trying to decide whether or not to breast-feed should know that breast-fed babies tend to feed more frequently. It is also difficult to breast-feed exclusively if the mother returns to work. Working mothers, however, can easily breast-feed part-time and formula-feed part-time.

CONTRAINDICATIONS

The contraindications include the baby with an inborn error of metabolism (e.g., phenylketonuria [PKU], galactosemia) who requires a special formula, the baby born to a mother who has a highly contagious disease such as AIDS, and the baby born to a mother who is taking certain medications (see Appendix 1).

BREAST-FEEDING MANAGEMENT
PREGNANCY

The topic of breast-feeding is best introduced during the third trimester. The pediatrician can discuss feeding during the prenatal visit. The advantages and disadvantages have already been mentioned. A woman who does not find breast-feeding appealing should be supported in her decision. A woman who desires to breast-feed should be counseled on what to expect in the immediate postpartum period (e.g., colostrum, breast engorgement) and how to prepare her nipples. Although there is controversy about the need for nipple preparation in women with normal nipples, women with flat or inverted nipples will benefit from preparation. Preparation includes avoiding soap to the breast area to allow for the build-up of body lipids, rubbing the nipples with a wet washcloth ten times a day, and pulling at the nipple (Hoffman maneuver) ten times a day. (For more detail, one of the breast-feeding manuals listed in the bibliography should be consulted.)

Postpartum Care

The mother needs to be instructed in the proper mechanics of breast-feeding; for example, the whole areola goes into the baby's mouth, and the nares should not be obstructed by the breast. The baby should feed at least every 3 hours unless the mother is sick or utterly exhausted. At first, nursing should be for 3 to 5 minutes on each side and gradually increased to 10 or 15 minutes on each side. The mother should alternate which breast is offered first. The mother may want to try several positions, such as lying down and sitting up. These changes in position may decrease breast soreness. In addition, the mother needs to know how to break the suction of the baby's sucking by gently inserting her finger into the baby's mouth. The mother should also expect a loose, watery stooling pattern.

The mother needs to know that colostrum is present before the milk comes in. The baby does not require extra fluid supplementation because he or she is born with an excess of body fluid. If water is offered, it should be *after* each feed.

The mother should be aware that at about the third postpartum day she will experience engorgement that can be quite painful. This may be more of a problem for primiparas, because it takes longer for their milk to come in than it does for multiparas. The best treatment is frequent feeding. The engorgement is sometimes so tense that pumping some milk prior to breast-feeding may be necessary for the baby to insert the areola and nipple properly into his or her mouth. The use of hot pads before feeding may also relieve discomfort.

If the mother develops sore nipples, she should limit the time the baby breast-feeds on each nipple. She should try different positions and should air-dry her nipples, taking care to avoid breast pads that retain heat and moisture. She may find using a breast shield helpful if her nipples are very sore.

Because the mother's milk often does not come in until after she is discharged from the hospital, she will need a great deal of support. This help can be given by the physician or the postpartum floor nurse, by telephone, or by a visiting nurse.

Discharge Instructions

These instructions should be simple and brief. Ideally, the mother should feed the baby on demand but generally not more often than every 1½ to 2 hours. It is common for a baby to feed 8 to 12 times in 24 hours. Frequent short feeds are preferable to prolonged infrequent feeds. The mother should drink approximately 64 oz of fluids per day, be well rested, and take her prenatal vitamins with iron. Her major occupation will be to feed the baby. If the baby has six wet diapers a day without water supplementation, she should feel confident that the baby is getting enough breast milk. The mother need not avoid certain foods unless she observes consistent increased fussiness in the baby in association with the mother ingesting such foods. Foods commonly incriminated are garlic, onions, cabbage, chocolate, and great quantities of caffeine. Excessive colic has been attributed occasionally to the baby developing an allergy to cow's milk proteins, which can be excreted in the mother's milk. The mother should not take any medications without first talking to her physician. She may drink small amounts of alcohol; in fact, a glass of sherry or wine may be beneficial in the late afternoon if she is having let-down reflex problems.

The mother's clothing should be comfortable. A brassiere is not essential, although she may find that it gives her support. A tight brassiere, however, should be avoided.

The mother and father need to be counseled that the father has a major role even if the baby is exclusively breast-fed. The baby still needs much holding and cuddling, which the father can do. Furthermore, the father may wish to give the baby his or her regular bath, which can be a special time together. The father can also feed the baby a bottle of expressed milk or a bottle of water on a daily basis. This allows the mother to have a rest and also introduces the baby to a bottle.

Two-Week Check

This is an important visit because most mothers need to be reassured that their babies are getting enough milk. If the baby has gained weight, the mother will be reassured and encouraged. If breast-feeding is going well, the physician may recommend a periodic relief bottle or regular breast pumping so that the mother has milk stored for those times when she will be away from the baby. The baby should take 400 U of vitamin D daily. Some pediatricians also prescribe iron and fluoride supplementation.

COMMON PROBLEMS ENCOUNTERED WITH BREAST-FEEDING
Poor Let-Down (Milk Ejection Reflex)

The let-down is characterized by tingling or fullness in the breast. The milk will often spray from the nipple in a stream. Let-down is often precipitated by seeing the baby, hearing the baby cry, or the baby's sucking. When the let-down is active, one may hear a gulping sound when the baby is sucking. A poor let-down is characterized by the absence of these findings. The best way to condition the let-down is to have the mother relax prior to feeding, drink plenty of liquids, and rest.

Poor Weight Gain

Poor weight gain is usually caused by infrequent feeds (e.g., less than seven times a day) or an inadequate let-down. Infrequent feeds are easy to rectify. Some babies are quite placid in spite of inadequate caloric intake and need to be awakened during the day to be fed every 2 to 3 hours. If the weight is of concern, the mother can also give one or two supplementary bottles while she is increasing feeds. She should offer these relief bottles during the most stressful part of the day.

Mastitis

Infection in the breast is often characterized by fever, local redness, and soreness. It is usually precipitated by infrequent feeds. Treatment consists of rest, hot compresses, frequent feeds, and an antibiotic such as dicloxacillin or a cephalosporin.

Cracked Nipples

A sore nipple may result in a cracked or fissured nipple if the sore nipple problem is not immediately addressed. Once the nipple is cracked, the mother should use a nursing position that places the point of stress away from the fissure. She should begin each feeding on the uninvolved breast. Applying expressed milk to the fissure and allowing it to dry has been shown to be effective. Ointments should be avoided. The baby should be fed frequently but briefly. Occasionally the fissures bleed and can result in the baby vomiting blood or having dark stools.

Jaundice From Breast-Feeding

This generally occurs with the onset of the milk coming in and peaks at about 10 to 14 days of age. All other causes of jaundice should be excluded. If the bilirubin level gets dangerously high, the mother should stop breast-feeding for 12 to 48 hours. If the etiology of the jaundice is the milk, the bilirubin level will fall, even as much as 2 mg/dl in 12 hours. Breast-feeding can then be reinstituted. Generally, the bilirubin does not rise to its previous high point. The mother should pump her breasts during the observation period so that breast-feeding is not compromised when reinstituted.

OTHER CONSIDERATIONS

Working Mother

The mother who goes back to work can usually continue breast-feeding without problems. The milk supply adjusts itself to the demand. If the mother is working at least 8 hours a day, it is sometimes prudent to pump the breasts once during her work day in order to stay comfortable and maintain a good milk supply. Each woman is different in what is required to maintain a supply. Some women can work for a long time without pumping and without compromising the supply. Others have a supply that is more responsive to decreased feeds. A woman will rarely "dry up" because she has returned to work.

Logistics of Nursing Twins

A mother of twins can produce a large milk supply so that she can adequately breast-feed both babies. It is customary for the mother to breast-feed twins simultaneously; in so doing, she is breast-feeding by using a modified demand approach. Thus, if one twin wakes up and is hungry, she may awaken the other twin in order to feed him or her as well. The mother of twins who breast-feeds may be more likely to get mastitis, and she should be aware of the early symptoms. (See Chap. 7.)

Weaning

Weaning is an individual decision. Some women stop when the baby is young, and others wait until the baby is a toddler. The physician should avoid making judgments as to the "right" time. The physician should, however, advise slow weaning if possible, which involves cutting back on one feeding a day every few days. Slow weaning makes the woman's physiologic adjustment less painful.

Breast Pumps and Storage of Milk

Hand expression is superior if the mother can learn the technique. Generally, the nurse on the postpartum floor will be able to teach it. Several pumps are available if the mother is unable to express by hand. The pump that works best will depend on the woman. It is good if the woman can borrow a pump from a friend before she decides which pump to purchase. Another alternative is to rent an electric pump.

Milk should be stored in clean containers and immediately refrigerated or frozen. If refrigerated, it will stay good for 48 hours. If frozen at 0°F, it will keep for months.

ANNOTATED BIBLIOGRAPHY

Eiger US, Olds S: The Complete Book of Breast-Feeding. New York, Workman Publishing Co., 1992. (Excellent guide for the breast-feeding mother.)

Goldfarb J, Tibbetts E: Breastfeeding Handbook: A Practical Reference for Physicians, Nurses, and Other Health Professionals, rev. ed. Hillside, NJ, Enslow Publishers, 1989. (Excellent handbook for health care professionals. Contains a number of summary tables, some of which can be copied for patient use. There are also useful appendices on resources for professionals and mothers and on breast pump suppliers.)

Lawrence RA: Breastfeeding, a Guide for the Medical Profession, 3rd ed. St. Louis, CV Mosby, 1989. (Written expressly for health professionals with many diagrams and illustrations.)

9

Circumcision

Robert A. Dershewitz

The ritual of circumcision is thought to be at least 15,000 years old. It is still performed by many religions, including Judaism and Islam. Circumcision is the most frequent operation on American males but is much less frequently done in other Western countries.

Until the middle of this century, circumcision was considered standard of care in the United States, with more than 90% of newborn males being circumcised. Then the pendulum swung and the practice was discouraged by the medical profession. As late as 1983, both the American Academy of Pediatrics and the American College of Obstetrics and Gynecology declared that there was no valid indication for circumcision in the newborn. By 1987, the percentage of newborns circumcised had decreased to 61%. Now, as fewer babies are being routinely circumcised, new evidence has emerged showing that circumcision protects male babies from urinary tract infections. Thus, the debate of whether to circumcise newborns has been rekindled, and issues of risk/benefit and cost-effectiveness are being reexamined.

There are both contraindications for performing a circumcision and indications for doing a circumcision (but these are not commonly present in the newborn). The one major exception is ritual circumcision, which is performed for nonmedical reasons. Premature or unstable newborns should not be circumcised.

THE ARGUMENTS FOR CIRCUMCISION

Data are now convincing that uncircumcised males have a significantly greater risk of having urinary tract infections (UTIs) than do circumcised babies. In 1982, Ginsburg and McCracken published a study showing that 95% of infant boys who developed UTIs were uncircumcised. Subsequently, Wiswell and Geschke (1989) reported a tenfold increase in the number of UTIs in uncircumcised males, and Herzog (1989) also confirmed that noncircumcision was a highly significant risk factor for UTIs. Circumcision is thought to prevent uropathogenic bacterial colonization. Because they have fewer UTIs, circumcised newborns have significantly fewer episodes of bacteremia than do uncircumcised newborns.

Another major benefit of circumcision is the decreased risk of balanitis (inflammation of the glans), and it virtually eliminates the possibilities of posthitis (inflammation of the foreskin), phimosis (a 4%-10% risk in uncircumcised males), and paraphimosis. Avoidance of these infections reduces the need for a therapeutic circumcision later in life, which has been reported to occur in as many as one out of seven uncircumcised males. This estimate may be lower depending on the definition of what constitutes an absolute indication for performing a therapeutic circumcision (e.g., one versus recurrent episodes of balanitis) and what constitutes a relative indication (e.g., the number of episodes of posthitis). Moreover, avoiding a therapeutic circumcision in later life spares general anesthesia and psychological stress, which may be an even bigger concern.

Circumcision greatly reduces the risk of penile cancer. How this protection occurs is unclear, but it may be related to less accumulation of smegma, which is believed to be a carcinogen. Either data are lacking or beliefs have been disproved that circumcision protects against prostatic and cervical cancer, enhances sexual functioning, and improves genital hygiene. The relationship of circumcision to sexually transmitted diseases is inconclusive. It may be that circumcision protects against genital herpes. Lastly, preliminary data suggest that circumcision decreases the transmission of group B streptococcus and reduces the chance of infection with the HIV virus after heterosexual exposure.

THE ARGUMENTS AGAINST CIRCUMCISION

The major complications of circumcision are infection and hemorrhage, which occur in up to 0.6% of cases. Most infections are minor, but some may be life-threatening, such as necrotizing fasciitis, staphylococcal scalded skin syndrome, Fournier's gangrene, generalized sepsis, and meningitis. In addition to major skin loss, there may be dehiscence of the penile skin. Bleeding may occur as a complication of either a well-performed or poorly performed circumcision, or because of an underlying, unknown bleeding disorder (e.g., hemophilia). Mortality is estimated to occur in 2 out of 1 million cases.

There is no doubt that the newborn experiences pain with circumcision. Discomfort, as manifested by behavioral changes, usually resolves within 24 hours. A dorsal penile nerve block appears to reduce the pain response but may cause a hematoma and local skin necrosis.

Circumcising a newborn who has contraindications to the procedure (e.g., genitourinary anomalies) is a frequently encountered problem. In one report, 36% of boys with hypospadias were inadvertently circumcised, and thus the opportunity for using the foreskin for surgical repair was lost.

Other major complications occur infrequently: penile amputation, urethrocutaneous fistulas, and skin bridges (which result in penile curvature and painful erection). Minor, relatively common complications include adhesions, skin irritation, and needing to revise the circumcision because of poor technique. Meatitis may occur as a complication of circumcision, but there is no evidence that it results in meatal stenosis. Penile lymphedema and urinary retention (from a tight circular bandage) may also occur. It remains unresolved if a foreskin enhances penile sensitivity during sexual intercourse.

Finally, cost should be considered. With an estimated current 1.25 million circumcisions performed annually in the United States, the cumulative health care cost for this procedure is enormous.

METHODS OF CIRCUMCISION

There are many methods of circumcision. All share the same goal: to remove enough shaft skin and inner preputial epithelium to have the glans uncovered. By doing so, phimosis and paraphimosis will not be possible. All methods require adherence to the same principles: asepsis; adequate, but not excessive, excision; hemostasis; and cosmesis. Each method is equally safe and gives equally good results when performed by experienced operators.

The clamp methods (Mogen clamp, Gomco clamp, and Plastibell) are most commonly used in the newborn. In skilled hands, the freehand excision method should be equally acceptable. The reader is encouraged to consult textbooks for detailed descriptions of these easily learned and performed surgical techniques.

PATIENT EDUCATION

It is unproved that retraction of the foreskin for cleaning prevents balanitis and other foreskin problems. Indeed, the natural history of the uncircumcised foreskin is that only 4% are retractable at birth. Half are able to be fully retractable by 1 year of age, 80% by 2 years of age, 96% by the time boys enter school, and almost 100% by 17 years of age. Manual retraction does not expedite retractability. Thus, advice for caring for the foreskin is simple: no special care is necessary. Once the prepuce has separated from the glans, that body part should be cleaned no differently from any other body part.

Care to the penis after circumcision is equally simple and primarily consists of watching for bleeding and signs of infection. A good precaution is to observe the baby for bleeding for at least 1 hour after the circumcision. Direct pressure is often adequate to stop oozing. If a Gomco or Mogen clamp is used, a petroleum jelly or antibiotic ointment gauze is wrapped around the penis for a few days until healing is well under way. If a Plastibell is used, the foreskin with plastic rim usually falls off in 5 to 8 days. No special care is required, and the baby can be bathed as if he were not circumcised. Parents should be told to notify their doctor if the plastic rim does not fall off in 8 days or slips onto the shaft of the penis.

RECOMMENDATIONS

Should newborn boys be circumcised? If it is performed for religious or ritualistic reasons, no discussion is required, for the decision has already been made. This is not the case, however, with the majority of boys. The latest statement issued on this subject by the American Academy of Pediatrics modified their previous position of strongly discouraging the routine practice of circumcision. Their current posture is *not* to make a recommendation for or against circumcision but rather to explain the risks and benefits of circumcision to parents, and to let *them* make their informed decision. Many parents will not find this "official" recommendation entirely satisfactory, for they prefer more directed advice. It is the author's belief that the weight of medical evidence now favors routine circumcision because it appears to prevent (1) fairly commonly encountered conditions in newborns that are potentially life-threatening (e.g., UTIs); (2) less common serious conditions (e.g., penile cancer); (3) commonly encountered medically minor, but potentially psychologically scarring, conditions (e.g., balanitis, posthitis); and because (4) it is a low-risk procedure.

At this time, however, benefit/risk ratios have not been firmly established, and each clinician will need to individually decide the more prudent course to recommend.

ANNOTATED BIBLIOGRAPHY

Anderson GF: Circumcision. Pediatr Ann 13:205–213, 1989. (Excellent table describing surgical techniques for circumcision)

Kaplan GW: Complications of circumcision. Urol Clin North Am 10:543–549, 1983. (Detailed discussion of all that can go wrong with circumcision)

Poland RL: The question of routine neonatal circumcision. N Engl J Med 322:1312–1315, 1990. (Well-presented discussion of why circumcision should not be considered medically necessary)

Report of the Task Force on Circumcision. Pediatrics 84:388–391, 1989. (The current official stance of the AAP)

Schoen EJ: The status of circumcision of newborns. N Engl J Med 322:1308–1312, 1990. (Well-reasoned presentation explaining why the author favors circumcision)

Wiswell TE, Geschke DW: Risks from circumcision during the first month of life compared with those for uncircumcised boys. Pediatrics 83:1011–1015, 1989. (Study of 136,086 boys showing that UTIs and bacteremia are significantly greater in uncircumcised males and that complications from circumcision are uncommon)

10

Neonatal Screening for Thyroid Disease

Robert Z. Klein

The importance of neonatal screening for hypothyroidism has been firmly established. It allows the diagnosis of infantile hypothyroidism before there are sufficient physical signs to suggest a clinical diagnosis. The resultant early treatment prevents the brain damage so common after clinically diagnosed infantile hypothyroidism. Intelligence quotients of the patients are normal. Most of the relatively few children who have gone through the eighth grade in school have demonstrated no neuropsychologic or learning problems.

In addition to primary, permanent, infantile hypothyroidism, the following conditions may be diagnosed as a result of neonatal screening: transient hypothyroidism, permanent or transient compensated thyroid disease (indicated by consistently elevated thyrotropin [TSH] and normal thyroxine [T4] concentrations), hypothyroidism secondary to hypopituitarism, which in turn may be secondary to hypothalamic dysfunction, hypothyroxinemia due to thyroid-binding globulin (TBG) deficiency, and transient hypothyroxinemia due to interference in T4 binding.

SCREENING PROCEDURES AND NEONATAL THYROID PHYSIOLOGY

The ideal screening method measures the concentrations of both TSH and T4 in the filter paper blood samples obtained at 3 to 5 days of age. At present, assaying for both T4 and TSH in all neonates is too expensive, so either TSH or T4 is measured alone and the second hormone is measured only when the first is abnormal. Thus, whenever the T4 is 2 standard deviations or more below the normal mean, or the TSH is similarly above the normal mean, the alternate hormone is also measured on the same filter paper blood specimen. In New England, a T4 of 77 nmol/L (6 μg/dl) and a TSH of 20 mU/L have been taken as convenient approximations of 2 standard deviations below and above their respective means. In North America, screening is usually done by measuring T4 first, whereas TSH is the primary measure in the rest of the world. There are advantages and disadvantages to both methods without either being clearly superior. No matter what method is used, some patients cannot be diagnosed in the neonatal period because their circulating concentrations of both T4 and TSH are normal for weeks or months.

The changing normal values for thyroid-related hormones and binding globulins based on age are presented in Table 10-1. The former are necessary to understand the bases for diagnosis suggested by screening, and the latter are critical for proper treatment of the patient with permanent infantile hypothyroidism. The infant's T4 concentration at birth is higher than that of his mother, even though maternal T4 concentrations are higher than those of nonpregnant adults because of the increase in TBG stimulated by the increased estrogen concentrations of pregnancy. The neonate also has a TBG concentration higher than that of older children and adults, but this increase is too slight to account for the elevated T4 concentrations. As would therefore be expected, the free T4 concentrations are also significantly elevated in the first weeks of life. The magnitude of the TSH surge precludes the use of primary TSH screening in the first 48 hours of life.

Table 10-1. Circulating Concentrations of Thyroid Related Factors

AGE	T4 nmol/L	FT4 pmol/L (ng/dl)	T3 nmol/L (ng/dl)	TSH mU/L	TBG mg/L
Fetus @ 33 wks	116 (9)		0.45 (30)	12	
Birth	154 ± 44 (SD) (12 ± 3)		0.8 ± 0.3 (55 ± 20)	1–20	32 ± 13
1 hour				90–160	
1 day	193 ± 39 (15 ± 3)		4.5 ± 2.2 (300 ± 150)	17 ± 3	
3–7 days	142 ± 32 (11 ± 2.5)	33 ± 11 (2.6 ± 0.9)	3 ± 1.5 (200 ± 100)	12 ± 4	26 ± 8
1 month	140 ± 25 (10.9 ± 1.9)	23 ± 6 (1.8 ± 0.5)	2.3 ± 0.8 (153 ± 53)	2.5 ± 3	24 ± 7
1 year	122 ± 26 (9.5 ± 2)		2.1 ± 0.45 (140 ± 30)		
Adolescent and adult	103 ± 22 (8 ± 1.7)	17 ± 3.2 (1.3 ± 0.25)	2.1 ± 0.53 (140 ± 35)	2 ± 1.5	21 ± 2.5

CATEGORIES OF RESULTS OF SCREENING

1. A presumptive diagnosis of hypothyroidism, permanent or transient, is made when the screening T4 concentration is low and the TSH concentration is high.
2. A presumptive diagnosis of compensated thyroid disease is made when the concentration of TSH is high and the T4 is in the normal range in a primary TSH program.
3. If the screening T4 concentration is low but the TSH concentration is not increased, further testing is required before even a presumptive diagnosis can be made. The first tests to be done are the measurement of TBG and then the measurement of free T4. Because most screening laboratories are not yet capable of these measurements on filter paper blood samples, further discussion will be presented in the section on confirmatory diagnostic measures.

Caveat

These distinctions are oversimplified. The physician must remember that clinical hypothyroidism can develop in infants whose screening T4 and TSH concentrations had been normal. The progressively deteriorating hypofunction of the thyroid gland postnatally has been well documented. More commonly, infants are discovered who had low T4 concentrations with normal TSH concentrations on screening. The TSH may require as much as 1 to 3 months to reach diagnostic elevations. It is not known whether such patients have low screening free T4 concentrations. Furthermore, the filter paper screening methods are less precise than the diagnostic serum methods, and borderline values have to be reassessed frequently. Premature infants introduce further problems of interpretation.

CONFIRMATORY DIAGNOSTIC MEASURES

1. *After screening values suggestive of hypothyroidism*

   Confirmation of the diagnosis of permanent hypothyroidism is made by finding a serum TSH concentration over 40 mU/L or values over 20 mU/L in two serum specimens with T4 concentrations below 77 mmol/L (6 μg/dl). Repeat determinations are advised before diagnosis and treatment when the first serum TSH is between 20 and 40 mU/L because 80% to 85% of patients with such hormonal concentrations are eventually found to have transient disease. Conversely, the TSH concentration of 50% of patients with transient hypothyroidism is over 40 mU/L. Some patients with transient hypothyroidism will not be able to be differentiated from those with permanent hypothyroidism in the first months of life. They will require treatment with 1-thyroxine to avoid the risk of delaying treatment in a patient with permanent hypothyroidism. In New England, only about 3% of patients treated for permanent hypothy-

roidism for more than a month or two eventually were proved to have transient disease.

If the serum TSH concentration is elevated but the T4 concentration is normal, the patient has compensated thyroid disease.

If the serum concentrations of both T4 and TSH are normal, a diagnosis of transient hypothyroidism can be made with one reservation. The diagnosis is not certain if the screening TSH was between 20 and 40 μU/ml on blood obtained in the first 48 hours of life because it is conceivable that the TSH concentration might merely have represented slow clearance of the hormone following the neonatal surge. Indeed, for this reason, many European workers will not accept a diagnosis of transient hypothyroidism unless an elevated TSH concentration is found in the serum as well as in the screening blood.

2. *After screening values suggestive of compensated thyroid disease*

   Confirmation of compensated thyroid disease is made when the serum TSH is high but the T4 is normal. This condition, too, may be transient. Transiency is diagnosed when the serum TSH becomes normal and is suggested when the serum TSH is significantly less than the screening concentration. Compensated thyroid disease may also continue with the same degree of dysfunction or may progress to hypothyroidism during or after infancy. Patients developing hypothyroidism after the age of 3 years have never been shown to be at risk of brain damage. Because they obviously have significant amounts of remaining functioning thyroid tissue, once a transient condition has been excluded, patients with compensated thyroid disease are usually treated with thyroxine to prevent the development of a goiter.

3. *After screening values demonstrating isolated hypothyroxinemia*

   The most commonly identified cause of a consistently low T4 concentration with a normal TSH concentration is TBG deficiency. This is tested for first by a direct assay of TBG concentration. A few screening laboratories are able to perform this assay on the original filter paper specimen, but more often this is done after the confirmatory serum specimen shows this combination of hormonal values. In either event, if the concentration of binding globulin is low, nothing further needs to be done for the child. The family is reassured that this condition is benign. If the TBG assay is normal, an assay of free T4 should be performed. Once again, a few screening laboratories can do this on the filter paper screening blood specimen. If the free T4 concentration is normal, interference with protein binding of T4 is suggested. This is a transient condition, although it frequently persists for months but rarely for over a year. Again, there is no evidence that this has any clinical significance.

If the free T4 is low in the screening specimen or thereafter, and the TSH still is not increased in the serum specimen, an attempt to confirm the diagnosis of congenital hypopituitarism must be made at once because neonatal hypopituitarism is often fatal.

This form of hypopituitarism is suggested clinically by hypoglycemic attacks, a history of low maternal estriol concentrations, diabetes insipidus, micropenis, small testes, and the following frequently associated conditions: septo-optic dysplasia, holoprosencephaly, single central incisor, postaxial polydactyly sometimes with imperforate anus or cardiac lesions, and micro- or macrocephaly. The classically described hypopituitarism is associated with breach and traumatic deliveries and becomes clinically manifest after the middle of the first year of life, although there may be low screening concentrations of T4 and TSH. Diagnosis of these patients is less urgent. In either case, the diagnosis is made by standard means such as demonstrating failure of adrenocorticotropic hormone (ACTH) or cortisol concentrations to increase in response to clinical hypoglycemia or metyrapone administration, or failure of serum growth hormone concentration to rise after spontaneous hypoglycemia or administration of pharmacologic agents such as L-dopa and glucagon. The induction of hypoglycemia with insulin administration is dangerous in these patients. If the pituitary hypofunction is primary, the patient will not respond to thyrotropin-releasing hormone with a rise in serum TSH concentration or a rise in growth hormone following administration of growth hormone releasing factor.

FEATURES OTHER THAN HORMONAL CONCENTRATIONS SUGGESTING TRANSIENCY OF HYPOTHYROIDISM

A diagnosis of transient hypothyroidism or transient compensated thyroid disease is clearly suggested when it becomes known that an infant's mother was treated during pregnancy with iodides for asthma or with antithyroid drugs (thiourea derivatives or less frequently ^{131}I) or had autoimmune thyroid disease with circulating antithyroid antibodies. A family history of pseudohypoparathyroidism or hypocalcemic seizures also strongly suggests transiency of hypothyroidism because the thyroid dysfunction associated with this condition frequently manifests itself with low T4 and elevated TSH concentrations on screening and confirmatory tests. The infants do not develop clinical signs of hypothyroidism, but the TSH concentration may remain mildly elevated throughout adult life.

Whereas 66% to 75% of patients with permanent hypothyroidism are females, 65% of those with transient hypothyroidism are males. By itself, however, gender is not of great value in suggesting which patient may have transient hypothyroidism.

Sixty-five percent of patients with transient hypothyroidism not associated with maternal disease or treatment are premature infants. The incidence of prematurity among infants with permanent hypothyroidism is 6%, the same as in the total neonatal population. Premature infants are more susceptible to both iodine deficiency and iodine excess, and both cause transient hypothyroidism.

The incidence of transient hypothyroidism is highest in areas of iodine deficiency, so the incidence in Europe with pockets of marginal iodine intake or frank deficiency is 1:8000 births. In New England, 1:19,000 neonates were recognized to have transient hypothyroidism. The actual incidence is higher than this because blood specimens are not repeatedly obtained from small preterm infants. Lavish bathing of neonates with povidone iodine as well as administration of iodinated dyes in x-ray contrast studies have been shown to increase the incidence of transient hypothyroidism.

MANAGEMENT OF INFANTILE HYPOTHYROIDISM

The goal of treatment of infantile hypothyroidism is to prevent brain damage and to assure normal physical growth and development. Between 20% and 25% of patients treated as a result of screening are not at risk of brain damage. Most of these have compensated thyroid disease and would develop clinical hypothyroidism only after the period in which the developing brain is vulnerable to thyroid hypofunction, or they never would develop clinical hypothyroidism. As stated earlier, some patients with transient hypothyroidism are also treated because if they were determined to have permanent disease, delaying treatment could be fatal. Thus, one in 4500 to 5000 neonates is treated for hypothyroidism, but only one in 6000 is actually at risk of brain damage from hypothyroidism. In Europe, one neonate in 3000 is treated for hypothyroidism. About 50% of them have been shown to have either transient hypothyroidism or compensated thyroid disease.

Treatment should begin in patients with low screening T4 concentrations and TSH concentrations over 40 mU/L before results of confirmatory serum assays are known. It seems safe to wait for the confirmatory results before treating the remaining patients. Because the experience antedating neonatal screening suggested that delay in treatment had a deleterious effect, the first dictum is that at least those with the more severe thyroid hypofunction should be treated as soon as possible.

There is no consensus on whether to do thyroid imaging with ^{123}I at the time of diagnosis. The question is whether being able to give genetic counselling to the parents of the roughly 20% of hypothyroid patients with dyshormonogenesis outweighs the risk of administering 10 to 15μC of the radioactive iodine to 2- to 4-week-old infants. If the parents do not intend to have more children, the decision is easy. If genetic counselling of the patient with dyshormonogenesis is desired, the imaging can be done many years later when presumably the unknown risk would be lower. Improving methods of ultrasound imaging give promise that this question will become moot.

Treatment is initiated with 1-thyroxine by mouth in a dose of 10 to 12 μg/kg of body weight. Then the dose is altered to maintain the serum concentration of thyroxine between 130 and 190 nmol/l (10–15 μg/dl) in the first year and over 130 nmol/l (10 μg/dl) thereafter.

The maintenance of these concentrations requires frequent serum T4 and TSH assays. With improved assay methods, the measurement of free T4 will probably replace that of total T4 because free T4 is the active moiety of serum thyroxine, but this is unlikely to alter management guidelines substantively. The infant should be examined and blood specimens for hormonal analyses obtained 2 and 4 weeks after initiating therapy, 2 weeks after any change in dosage, routinely at monthly intervals until the child is 1 year old, and then bimonthly until the age of 3 years. Thereafter, assays should be made three to four times per year.

Careful monitoring is necessary because it has been shown that infants with serum T4 concentrations of less than 103 nmol/l (8 μg/dl) for significant periods in the first year of life had lower IQs than did patients whose serum T4 concentrations remained in the desired range. This inadequate treatment still permitted normal physical growth and development.

The average doses of thyroxine found to maintain serum T4 concentrations in the upper half of the normal range are as follows:

An initial dose of 10 μg/kg of weight at the start of treatment is continued until the child weighs 6 kg.

From 6 to 10 kg, 6 μg/kg of current weight
From 10 to 20 kg, 60 μg plus 2 μg for each kg above 10
Over 20 kg, 80 μg plus 1 μg for each kg above 20

If the patient is receiving much less than the average dose and still has T4 concentrations in the desired range, transiency of disease should be considered unless it is known that the patient has ectopic gland or goiter. If the child is receiving significantly larger doses, it is worth making sure that he or she is actually ingesting the prescribed doses. Similarly, failure of serum T4 to reach 116 to 130 nmol/l (9–10 μg/dl) 2 weeks after initiation of treatment raises the possibility of inadequate prescription or compliance. Failure of the TSH concentration to decrease to below 20 mU/L within 6 weeks of treatment need not be due to improper dose or failure of compliance because 10% to 15% of patients will have slightly elevated TSH concentrations for as long as a year unless serum T4 concentrations are raised to 193 to 219 nmol/L (15–17 μg/dl). Such failure, however, or any subsequent elevation of TSH even with normal T4 concentrations, should serve to alert the physician that the child may not be receiving adequate thyroxine regularly and both dose and compliance should be checked. Transient elevations of T4 concentrations well above the normal range have not had discernible adverse effects. To make compliance easier and anxiety less, suggest to parents that they set out a week's supply of pills each Sunday so that they can make sure they have not missed a dose. Parents can then give a missed dose with the next day's dose. This also lessens anxiety if the infant vomits and cannot take the thyroxine for a day or two. There is no evidence that slightly elevated TSH concentrations with T4 concentrations consistently in the desired range is associated with any harm. On the other hand, raising serum T4 levels to suppress TSH concentrations to normal offers a greater margin of safety in treatment. With the newer sensitive TSH assays, concentrations below the normal range give ample early warning of overtreatment. If the physician suspects noncompliance (e.g., suspects that the infant might have been inadequately treated until just before his appointment so that T4 was normal but TSH was elevated), the parents should be carefully reeducated and the baby tested again in 2 weeks. If the TSH is then normal on the same dose, the suspicion of poor compliance is strengthened.

As the children pass beyond the age of risk of permanent brain damage from hypothyroidism, compliance and its monitoring become increasingly problematic. At age 14, surprise checks of hormonal concentrations revealed significantly inadequate treatment in 50% of the patients in New England, although measurements in their doctor's offices showed only 3% to 4% noncompliance.

INDICATIONS FOR REFERRAL

The patient with neonatal hypopituitarism should be seen in consultation immediately by a pediatric endocrinologist. Consultation is also advisable when the distinction between permanent and transient hypothyroidism is difficult. It is not necessary in the classical case of infantile hypothyroidism diagnosed as a result of neonatal screening, provided that the following conditions are met:

1. The primary physician has access to a certified laboratory for hormonal monitoring.
2. He is willing to spend the time required for educating the parents about the disease and the importance of adequate treatment, and for genetic counselling in cases of dyshormonogenesis.
3. He, in addition to monitoring the clinical course, must be willing to obtain the specimens for frequent monitoring of hormonal values.

Consultation, however, can help increase the chance of adequate compliance by reinforcing the education, genetic counselling, and reassurance provided shortly before by the primary physician. Consultation becomes a necessity when hormonal concentrations deviate from the desired range and the physician cannot determine the cause on reexamination 2 weeks later.

PROGNOSIS

The ultimate IQ of infants whose hypothyroidism is diagnosed as a result of neonatal screening but before a clinical diagnosis is possible, and who are adequately treated, is unaffected by their hypothyroidism. Their mean IQ and distribution of IQs are normal. It is possible that the prognosis may not be as good for the rare patient whose intrauterine thyroid hypofunction was severe enough for a long enough time that the infant was born with the obvious classical stigmata of hypothyroidism. These patients (less than 1% of patients with infantile hypothyroidism) are too few to resolve the question of prognosis. The patients who are less than optimally treated do have lower IQs than other patients, but their IQs are in the normal range of distribution. In the New England study, the hypothyroid children did fully as well as their euthyroid siblings through the eighth grade in school.

ANNOTATED BIBLIOGRAPHY

Delange F (ed): Research in Congenital Hypothyroidism. New York, Plenum Press, 1989. (Reports of the international conference on thyroid screening—Brussels, May 1988.)

Ilicki A, Larsson A: Psychomotor development of children with congenital hypothyroidism diagnosed by neonatal screening. Acta Paediatr Scand 77:142, 1988. (Excellent results from a meticulous Swedish study.)

Klein RZ: Infantile hypothyroidism then and now: The results of neonatal screening. Curr Probl Pediatr 15:1, 1985. (Complete review of infantile hypothyroidism.)

New England Congenital Hypothyroidism Collaborative. Elementary school performance of children with congenital hypothyroidism. Pediatrics 116:27, 1990. (Largest cohort followed longest. Through third grade, did as well as sibling and classmate controls. No difference in IQs. Similar results in small group through the eighth grade unpublished as yet.)

3

The Well Child

11

Normal Growth and Development: An Overview

Constance H. Keefer

Pediatricians have a broad responsibility to promote normal growth and development and to monitor their progress, both in the community and in the office.

IN THE COMMUNITY

Since the inception of the American Academy of Pediatrics in the 1930s, pediatricians have been respected for keeping the interests of their patients above their own; the community both implicitly and explicitly gives authority for pediatricians to speak and act on behalf of children. One of the best ways pediatricians can use that authority to advocate for children is to offer thoughtful analysis of objective data to schools, hospitals, agencies, and legislatures.

Many studies have demonstrated that schools, hospitals, and daycare can have an impact on the development and behavior of children. For example, Michael Rutter has shown that the characteristics of schools (e.g., class size, teacher attitude and skill) do make a difference in the rates of behavior problems and the level of academic achievement among students. Jerome Kagan and others have demonstrated that excellent daycare (e.g., high staff–child ratio, trained staff) does not jeopardize the developmental outcome of children as compared to home-reared peers.

Closer to the pediatricians' medical domain, we know that hospitalization may lead to behavioral disturbances in children, but that these disturbances can be reduced by pre-hospital preparation and in-hospital attention to the psychosocial needs of the children and their parents. (See Chap. 27, "Preparation for Hospitalization.") In the newborn period, giving mothers a sense of control and having a personal support person for them during labor and delivery improves their later interactions with their infants. Allowing contact between mother and infant soon after birth improves the quality of the mother–infant interaction in later infancy and may even protect against parenting failures such as child abuse and neglect. It is now known that a deprived interactional setting not only jeopardizes an infant's developmental performance but actually disturbs brain development ("hard wiring" or structure on which later developmental skills will depend).

Pediatricians, by informing themselves of studies like these and bringing this information to bear on the conditions in schools, daycare, and hospitals in their communities, can help to prevent problems of behavior and development.

This communication process must be reciprocal; in addition to being an advocate for the child in the community, the pediatrician must be ready to listen to concerns from both professional and family observers. Teachers and parents often have a more complete, even if less sophisticated, assessment of a child than can be gleaned by a pediatrician in a short (15- or 20-minute) visit occurring every few months or years.

Pediatricians should also inform themselves about community or referral services available to families who have a child with a developmental problem. Not knowing what to do or to whom to turn if a developmental problem is discovered only compounds pediatricians' natural reluctance to find anything wrong with a child's development. When referred by their parents, children with cerebral palsy are seen in specialty clinics at an average age of 8 months; when referred by pediatricians, the average age is 16 months. Thus, simply knowing the phone number of an early intervention program helps to overcome this obstacle to timely referral.

IN THE OFFICE

The overriding responsibility of the pediatrician is awareness, or an encompassing attention to the following four areas: the roles and concerns of the parents; the usefulness of the timing of well-child visits; the importance of perspective; and the content and processes of behavioral development.

Parental Roles and Concerns

A child's adequacy as determined by physical growth, motor skills, and social, language, and cognitive development is as important to the parents as the child's survival. Deviations or disturbances in any of these areas produce a serious blow to a parent's sense of competence and confidence, and parents will be alert to even subtle changes in this direction. Studies of the detection of both language and motor delays have demonstrated that parental concern can be as reliable an indicator as the standard screening instruments.

One must always weigh and balance reliance on the parent as a partner in the diagnostic and therapeutic work, and assessment of the parent as an important part of the child's environment and, therefore, as a potential part of the problem. The pediatrician who says, "I'm only placating the parents" should seriously reexamine the situation to better address the needs of the parents. Nonorganic failure-to-thrive exemplifies the inextricability of parent and child needs and issues, of both psychological and somatic origins. Even in organic failure-to-thrive, the parents' competence and motivation are called into question, at least by themselves if not by others, and this invariably affects the child.

Timing of Well-Child Visits

While immunizations and screening procedures determine the timing of most well-child visits, they do coincide with many of the developmental and behavioral issues that create normal crises in the life of a family with young children. Table 11-1 presents both normal and non-normal critical *junctures* in which preventive intervention is particularly important. A pediatrician who uses the well-child visit to address these issues, even without actually diagnosing or solving them, can positively influence the later parent–child interaction. As economic pressures on medical practices increase, pediatricians must be able to articulate what they are doing in well-child visits and to defend the preventive, early diagnostic, and, therefore, cost-effective value of those visits. The American Academy of Pediatrics' Guidelines for Health Supervision are excellent in their coverage of these developmental opportunities for intervention.

Changing Perspective

When the pediatrician deals with behavior and development, his or her perspective must transcend the framework

Table 11-1. Normal and Non-normal Developmental Crises

NORMAL CRISES	NON-NORMAL CRISES
Pregnancy	Miscarriage
Birth or adoption	Birth of premature, defective, or stillborn infant
Intensity and lack of boundaries of infancy	
Aggression and autonomy of the toddler	Diagnosis of a significant illness or handicap
Developmental milestones that change the parent–child relationship	Divorce
	Family stress, without support
Regression prior to developmental progress	Abuse or neglect
Adjustment to daycare	
Transition to school	
Preparation for a well-child visit	

of traditional medicine in two ways. First, an understanding of the cultural determinants of child-rearing practices and infant behavioral development is essential to pediatric care when a patient population is ethnically diverse, and it greatly enhances that care even when the patients are culturally homogeneous. Culture can be defined as a shared system of practices, along with the beliefs and values that support those practices. In this sense, even a nuclear family functions like a culture. Helping parents to discover their own, often hidden, beliefs and values is useful in solving developmental and behavioral problems, as well as in communicating around illness. The meaning of a child's physical symptoms has a cultural dimension for parents, and a medical explanation may not satisfy them if it does not address the concerns arising out of their own theories.

Much of child-rearing advice derives from the pediatrician's own personal background or culture, often without his or her awareness. In our continuing reeducation of ourselves, recognition of those cultural and personal biases must be a goal.

The second change in perspective necessary for the practice of developmental pediatrics in primary care involves replacing the action, authority, and answer-giving of the medical model with an approach that includes negotiation with the parent, problem-solving, and tolerance of a high degree of uncertainty.

Content and Processes of a Developmental Model

Although the path of physical growth is usually uncomplicated and orderly, variations do exist and may be difficult to distinguish from pathology. Plotting height, weight, and, until age 2, head circumference on standard curves provides an objective assessment of the adequacy of growth. Parents

Growth Guidelines

WEIGHT

Birth weight is regained by the 14th day.

During the first 3 months, the average gain is about 1 kg/month (about ½ to 1 oz/day).

Birth weight doubles at about 4 months, triples at 12 months, quadruples at 24 months.

By the sixth month, the average gain per month is 0.5 kg.

During the second year, the average gain per month is 0.25 kg.

After age 2, the average annual increment is 2.3 kg (5 lb) until the adolescent growth spurt.

HEIGHT

Average birth length is 50 cm (20 in)

By the end of the first year, birth length increases by 50%.

Birth length doubles by 4 years.

Birth length triples by 13 years.

Average annual growth is 5 cm (2 in) or better per year.

can understand visually the concept of following a particular percentile curve as opposed to achieving a particular height or weight. Convenient "rules of thumb" for remembering growth norms are listed in the following display, "Growth Guidelines."

When pathologic deviations of growth occur, they may reflect a range of problems (e.g., stress in the family, an extreme temperamental difficulty in the child, or an endocrine, metabolic, or gastrointestinal disease). This "red flag" is an extremely important diagnostic and surveillance tool for the pediatrician.

A model of behavioral development must explain not just the content but also the processes of change. Most theories of child development invoke the concept of stages, which imply uneven development, with short periods of rapid change followed by plateaus or longer periods in which change is not so obvious.

A paradoxical phenomenon accompanying staged development is regression. In periods prior to a major advance, in moving from one plateau to another (e.g., crawling to walking), one often sees regression, or disorganization, either in the skill area involved or in other supportive functional areas, such as state regulation or dependency. These periods of disorganization are often easier for parents to tolerate when the clinician explains them as fueling the next, more mature, stage of development.

A similar phenomenon, occurring when new skills are being acquired, is that of the suppression of activity in one area in favor of the new skill being practiced (e.g., the child at 13 months who stops talking during a few weeks of intense practice in pulling to stand or taking first steps).

Motivation, or the child's own desire to be skillful, to

create, or to act on his or her own sense of what might be possible, is a powerful force in development. This encourages the child to seek out and use whatever the environment has to offer rather than merely sitting and waiting for the environment to act on him or her. The concepts of mastery and coping, drawn from the work of Lois Murphy and her colleagues, enlarge on this process of self-motivation and are helpful in understanding behaviors of children in new and challenging situations.

In addition to these processes, a developmental model indicates content areas in which change will occur. A standard categorization of these changing skills includes gross/fine motor, perceptive/adaptive, cognitive, language, social/peer relations, and bodily control functions. Keeping these categories in mind while taking an interim history on a patient, and referring to a few milestones (the "tip of the iceberg" items as outlined on the Denver Developmental Screen), greatly enhances the pediatrician's care of developing children. Details of specific milestones of development are presented in Chapter 37.

A temperamental/constitutional model is drawn largely from the work of Chess and Thomas and is second only to the developmental model in importance to the pediatrician's involvement in this area. Together, these two models (one addressing what children do, the other addressing how they do it) form a matrix from which the pediatrician (and parent) can more fully understand developmental and behavioral phenomena.

Temperament, or the child's style of behavior, that has some permanence over time, often explains apparent deviations in development and is an essential area to assess when behavior is a problem. The nine temperamental dimensions provide a nonjudgmental way to describe the child's behavior and interactive style, often reclassifying a difficult situation in which the child is "bad" to a situation wherein the child has a particular set of strengths and weaknesses. For parents who are burdened by the belief that they are the sole determiners of their child's future, the concept of the child himself or herself having a role in his or her own development can be freeing and confirming, enabling the parents to more fully enjoy the child and their parenting role.

Table 11-2 lists some standard developmental tests and the areas that each assesses. Even if these tests are not used in a formal way, knowledge of them makes working on developmental issues possible in a time-limited setting. For example, a full Brazelton assessment is rarely needed on a newborn, but knowledge of the categories of behavior and how they are manifested in the scale is most helpful in sorting out questions of subtle deviation from normal behavior or development in the first 3 months of life. Similarly, when a parent of a 10-month-old describes new night wakening, the following should be explored: the child's stage of attachment, stage of motor development, and temperament, and the meaning to the parents of the cry and their beliefs about their responsibility to the child.

Table 11-2. Assessing Development

ASSESSMENT	FUNCTIONS STUDIED
Dubowitz Assessment of Gestational Age	Gestational age
Brazelton Neonatal Behavioral Assessment Scale	Newborn behavior of motor, state-control, and sensory orientation Newborn neurologic function
Carey Temperament Questionnaire	Temperamental style of behaving
Denver II,* PEER,† and PEEX‡	Fine and gross motor, perceptual, cognitive, language, and social skills
Anna Freud's Lines of Development	Development of play, body functions, and social relations
Hunt and Uzgiris' Cognitive Scales	Development of thought
Margaret Mahler's Stages of Attachment	Development of attachment to others and sense of identity

*Denver II
†Pediatric Examination of Preschool Readiness
‡Pediatric Early Elementary Examination

Another common example is a 5-year-old's difficulty adjusting to school. To identify the proper locus of difficulty and to help the parents focus their efforts on understanding and managing the situation, the following should be considered: parental factors, such as maternal depression; factors directly related to the child, such as school readiness skills, temperament (especially adaptability), coping style, and level of development from self- to other-centered activities or in bodily function; and interactional factors, such as the "fit" with a particular teacher or a particular educational philosophy. Often, just mentioning these areas and helping parents to start to explore them solves the problem, even without a formal analysis.

Pediatricians have used their close and frequent contacts with families to great advantage in the detection and prevention of medical problems. In this chapter, ways in which pediatricians can broaden this relationship to also manage problems of behavioral development have been outlined. In drawing on information from theories and research in developmental psychology, and turning an interactive ear to parents and community resources, pediatricians can create a more relevant practice for their patients and a more exciting and rewarding one for themselves.

ANNOTATED BIBLIOGRAPHY

Brazelton TB: Toddlers and Parents. New York, Delacorte, 1974. (Realistic description of autonomy in the second and third years of life, with helpful suggestions for management of the negative behavior.)

Dixon SD, Stein MT (eds): Encounters with Children: Pediatric Behavior and Development. Chicago, Year Book Medical Publishers, 1987. (Practical, well-organized guidelines for developmentally based primary care pediatric practice: what to do at each well-child visit, prenatal to late adolescent; well supported with scientific information and references.)

Erikson E: Identity and the life cycle. In Klein GS (ed): Psychological Issues, vol 1. New York, International Universities Press, 1959. (Defines eight stages of psychosocial development, five of which apply from birth through adolescence. The integration of biological, psychological, and social forces and their impact on development, and the relationship of emerging stage to previous stages are particularly helpful.)

Fraiberg S: The Magic Years. New York, Charles Scribner and Sons, 1959. (Childhood blossoms before your eyes as the psychological issues of development from 2 years to 5 years are described in realistic and practical detail.)

Hunt JM, Uzgiris I: Assessment in Infancy. Urbana, IL, University of Illinois Press, 1976. (A systematic and detailed look at cognitive development from birth through 2 years, based on the work of Piaget. Particularly helpful when language is delayed or when physical problems make an accurate assessment of intelligence difficult.)

Levine MD, Carey WB, Crocker AC, Gross RT (eds): Developmental–Behavioral Pediatrics, 2nd ed., Philadelphia, WB Saunders, 1992. (Comprehensive text; chapters on developmental stages, management of common behavior problems, and developmental assessment techniques especially usable by a general pediatrician.)

Mahler M: The Psychological Birth of the Human Infant. New York, Basic Books, 1975. (Detailed look at the stages of development of attachment in the first 2 years of life.)

Murphy LB: The Widening World of Childhood: Paths Toward Mastery. New York, Basic Books, 1962. (Rich clinical examples of coping and mastery and their influence on the child's negotiation of new situations and new stages of development.)

12

Nutrition and Nutritional Status: An Overview

William C. MacLean, Jr.

Parents are increasingly concerned about nutrition, both as it affects their children's immediate growth and development and as it affects later health. Misinformation abounds, and most parents have no means of distinguishing reliable information. Pediatricians have a major role to play in guiding parents through the changing nutritional needs of their children and in inculcating sound nutritional practices that will persist throughout life. To do so requires a basic understanding of nutrient requirements, how they are estimated and how they can be met at different ages, and an appreciation of what a good diet can and cannot be expected to accomplish.

NUTRIENT REQUIREMENTS AND DIETARY ALLOWANCES

The requirement for any nutrient is related to the age, size, growth rate, and gender of the individual. It represents the amount needed to replace obligatory losses (e.g., fecal, urinary, integumentary) and to support synthesis of new tissue. Requirements of specific nutrients at different ages are known with variable degrees of precision. For example, the protein requirement of the growing low-birth-weight infant is still subject to debate, whereas the iron requirement of the adolescent is known with greater certainty.

Recommended Dietary Allowances* (RDAs) are published periodically and are an attempt to translate estimates of requirements of nutrients into the safe and adequate amounts that should be consumed as part of a normal diet to meet the requirements. Recommended daily allowances are determined with groups of people (populations) rather than individuals in mind. Consequently, RDAs virtually always exceed a given individual's requirements. The RDA for all nutrients except energy (calories) is defined as the amount needed to meet the needs of "nearly all healthy individuals" (i.e., at least 97% of the population). (The RDA for energy is given as an average figure assuming light to moderate physical activity.) The RDAs are useful in assessing nutrient intakes of population groups but are less useful in evaluating the diet of an individual because they do not define individual requirements or optimal intakes. They also make no attempt to describe adequate intakes during illness. Because of the way RDAs are defined, most normal children can and will consume less than the RDA for many nutrients yet remain nutritionally healthy. However, the lower the intake relative to the RDA and the longer low intake persists, the greater is the risk of nutrient deficiency.

The dietary choices that provide appropriate amounts of nutrients broaden progressively as an infant develops the capacity to tolerate solid foods. In the typical American family, parents frequently express concern that children may not be eating enough. Parents seem especially preoccupied with protein and vitamins. In fact, most nutrients are consumed in excess; the only serious concern for undernutrition in most children is iron.

Widely divergent diets are capable of meeting a child's nutritional needs. The concept of "a proper diet" must be broadly interpreted in the cultural and social context of the family. Most parents and pediatricians would do well to recognize that as long as the child is growing normally and maintaining a normal hemoglobin concentration, the diet is most likely adequate.

Infancy

The normal infant will gain approximately 165 grams (about 6 oz) per week for the first 6 months of life. Based on data from the National Center for Health Statistics (NCHS), birth weight is expected to double by about 4 months of age and to triple by about 12 months of age. The normal diet of the infant (human milk) is low in protein (about 6% of calories) and high in fat (about 52% of calories), specifically saturated fat and cholesterol. Mineral intakes of the full-term breast-fed infant are relatively low but are sufficient to meet requirements. Infant formula provides slightly more protein (9% of calories) than does human milk. The distribution of protein, fat, and carbohydrate in standard infant formulas approximates that found in human milk. Both human milk (possibly with vitamin D supplementation) and infant formula are sufficient to meet the full-term infant's nutrient needs for at least the first 4 to 6 months.

Solid foods are generally withheld for the first 4 to 6 months. This delay stems less from concerns about the digestibility of solids than from concerns that the infant's head control and oromotor coordination are not sufficiently developed before that age to allow the infant to participate appropriately in the feeding process. As long as the protrusion reflex persists, the infant given solids will essentially need to be force-fed. Although a specific weight is often suggested as the guideline for timing the introduction of solid foods, developmental readiness is more important and a better criterion. The possible exception to this is the breast-fed infant whose growth rate has begun to falter after lactation is well established. Some infants may outgrow their milk supply as early as 3 months of age. In these instances, earlier introduction of solids may be considered, although it may be preferable to supplement with formula.

In the United States, the order in which solid foods are usually introduced into the diet is based primarily on tradition. Typically, cereals are begun first, followed by fruits, vegetables, and meats. This order is not followed in many countries, and departures from it are of no particular nutritional concern. A good case could be made for starting meats initially in breast-fed infants to provide additional protein and iron, both of which reach low levels in human milk as lactation continues. Nevertheless, most mothers in the United States probably expect cereal to be their infant's first solid food, and there is no compelling reason to try to change this. High-protein cereals specifically should be avoided, however; they supply more protein than needed and consequently increase the renal solute load. Initial baby foods are purées. The term *junior food* usually implies a

---

*The Recommended *Dietary* Allowances of the Food and Nutrition Board, National Research Council, of the National Academy of Sciences, should not be confused with the United States Recommended *Daily* Allowances (USRDAs) of the Food and Drug Administration. Although derived from the RDAs, the USRDAs group children under 4 years together and children 4 years and over and adults together. These USRDAs are the values used for consumer labeling of nutrient contents of food products and are the "goals" some parents try to meet. Proposed changes in labeling regulations may soon replace the US-RDAs with a new system.

coarser texture or the presence of small chunks of fruit, vegetable, or meat in the product. (Some junior foods, applesauce for example, may be the same purée in a larger jar.) The age at which the infant will accept these coarser foods is highly variable. It is wise to obtain product information from the major manufacturers because the contents of protein and energy (and other nutrients) vary among food groups and among corresponding products of different manufacturers.

The older infant, 8 to 10 months of age, is usually ready for a cup. Some infants can be weaned directly to a cup at an earlier age; some prefer a bottle even at mealtime beyond this age. There seems no reason to force the issue either way. Older infants should not be put to bed with a bottle because of the danger of nursing-bottle caries. At the same age, finger foods can be introduced. Care should be taken not to offer chunks of food (e.g., cheese or small hot dogs) that can easily be aspirated.

Breast-feeding with appropriate supplementation after 4 to 6 months is desirable for at least the first year of life. When breast-feeding is declined or is stopped earlier, iron-fortified infant formula provides the most appropriate alternative. (The Committee on Nutrition of the American Academy of Pediatrics recommends that "low-iron" formulas not be used.) Most experts now agree that no cow's milk of any kind should be introduced until the child is at least 1 year of age. An analysis of dietary data from the Second National Health and Nutrition Examinations Survey (NHANES II) indicates that mothers who introduce cow's milk at an early age are also more likely to introduce table foods inappropriately. Their infants tend to be fed excessive amounts of protein and sodium and inadequate amounts of iron. Low-fat milks should never be introduced in the first year of life because of the potential for inadequate energy intake and essential fatty acid deficiency, particularly when skim milk is fed.

Toddler and Older Child

The nutrition of the toddler is characterized by a decrease in appetite and the emergence of iron deficiency as a nutritional concern. Growth rate slows toward the end of the first year of life. During the second year, the child will gain only 50 grams (1.7 oz) per week, about 30% of the rate early in infancy. Appetite decreases in parallel. Parents need anticipatory guidance to alert them to this change. The major goal is to prevent mealtimes from becoming periods of daily conflict and coaxing.

Two- to five-year-olds have been shown to vary their meal-to-meal energy intake by more than 30%, in contrast to a day-to-day variability of only 10%. A meal with high calorie intake is generally followed by a meal with low calorie intake, and vice versa, thus demonstrating that children are capable of regulating their own calorie intake. The child's appetite should be respected, and parents should be urged to be less concerned about undernutrition and more concerned with the risk of establishing a life-long pattern of overconsumption.

There is a valid concern about emerging iron deficiency between 9 and 18 months of age. Most full-term infants are born with adequate iron stores. Depending on the diet consumed during the first year, iron stores are drawn upon to meet iron needs. As the diet shifts from iron-fortified foods (e.g., infant formula, infant cereals) to whole cow's milk and table foods, iron intake decreases. Iron deficiency becomes clinically apparent when the stores are exhausted and the intake continues to be suboptimal. This occurs most commonly between 9 and 18 months of age.

Because the low-birth-weight infant and breast-fed infant are at particular risk of iron deficiency, careful attention must be paid to the iron content of the diet of these two groups of infants. The low-birth-weight infant is born without adequate iron stores. Iron supplementation is delayed in some infants. The requirement for dietary iron is higher in these infants throughout the first year of life and probably well into the second year. The breast-fed infant receives small amounts of iron in human milk (≤ 0.5 mg/L). The low concentration of iron in human milk is largely offset by high bioavailability. The addition of solid foods to the diet of the breast-fed infant, however, adversely affects iron absorption. Breast-fed infants probably rely to a large extent on their iron stores to meet iron needs during the second six months of life.

Concern about iron deficiency has been heightened recently. A number of studies have shown that iron deficiency anemia in infancy is associated with developmental delay. Two follow-up studies of these infants have now suggested that these deficits persist long-term and may be permanent. At 5 years of age, the mean IQ of children who had been anemic and iron deficient (and whose anemia had been promptly corrected) was six to eight points lower than that of infants who had never been anemic. These differences could not be explained on the basis of other variables measured, such as socioeconomic status.

There is a transition from the diet of infancy to an adult diet during the toddler years. Eating habits that may persist throughout life are established. The introduction of table foods is accompanied by a marked increase in salt intake in most households. Fiber intake also increases. Depending on the family, there may be a shift toward lower fat intake and from saturated to polyunsaturated fats. Extreme modifications of the diet of young children in an attempt to prevent later development of diseases such as atherosclerosis, cancer, or hypertension are not warranted. For example, authorities advise against any significant changes in the high-fat diet of the infant before the age of 2 years. The low-fat diet (<35% of dietary energy from fat) recommended for adults as part of a prudent diet to reduce serum lipid concentrations implies increased intake of complex carbohydrates. Foods meeting this goal are bulkier in the stomach (i.e., they tend to be more filling and they are often less digestible). It becomes difficult for many young children to meet energy needs on such a diet.

There are generally few nutritional concerns between the ages of 2 or 3 years and the onset of adolescence. Growth rate is modest, and nutrient requirements are easily met by most diets. Strong food preferences and dislikes are established during this time. The child develops progressively more control, direct or indirect, over what is eaten.

Adolescence

During no time other than infancy are growth rates as fast or nutrient requirements as high as during the pubertal growth spurt. Rapid linear growth imposes particularly high requirements for energy, protein, calcium, and phosphorus. Iron requirements are high in both sexes. Muscle mass and hemoglobin mass increase, especially in boys. Once the growth spurt is complete, however, the need for iron in the male decreases. Because of menstruation, the iron requirement for females remains high (about twice that of the male) throughout adolescence and beyond.

Meeting the iron requirements of adolescent girls can be difficult. Iron intake relates directly to energy intake. The typical American diet provides about 5.5 to 6.0 mg iron per 1000 kcal. Adolescent boys tend to eat "everything in sight." Studies of body image suggest that most teenage boys would like to be bigger and more muscular than they are. Adolescent girls, on the other hand, tend to feel they are overweight. They are often weight watchers. Their attempts to limit calorie intake effectively reduce iron intake during a period of high iron requirement. This situation is not unique to the teenaged girl and often persists into adulthood. Screening for iron deficiency in adolescent girls is an important part of their medical care.

Adolescents participating in athletics require careful nutritional monitoring. Strenuous exercise imposes nutritional stresses during a period of rapid growth. Certain sports, such as wrestling, may foster attempts to lose weight, which is undesirable at this time. Athletes may espouse inappropriate dietary regimens that promise improved performance. Excessive training, as in long-distance running, may induce amenorrhea in girls and has been associated with iron deficiency anemia, the exact cause of which is unknown.

"Junk food" and teenagers seem inseparably linked. The appropriate role of "junk food" in the diet is hotly debated. Much of this debate derives from the lack of any reasonable definition of what "junk food" truly is. (One man's hamburger is another man's junk food.) Fast food seems to have become synonymous with junk food, an unfortunate link. Fast foods often parallel what is served at home and can be quite nutritious. A quarter-pound hamburger, an order of French fries, and a chocolate shake provide the growing adolescent male with about 33% of the RDA for energy, 70% of that for protein, and more than 35% of the RDAs of calcium, phosphorus, and iron. Similarly, pizza comes as close to being well balanced as most single-dish items can. In recent years, the variety of foods offered at fast food restaurants has increased substantially. Parental concerns often center on the fear that the diet will be deficient in some nutrient, but this is rarely a problem except for iron, as noted previously. A valid nutritional concern of fast food is its potential for high intakes of sodium and fat and, in some instances, low intakes of vitamin A. "Junk foods" do have a place in the teenager's diet. Parents have little control over this in any case and should direct their nutritional concerns to what is available at home for snacks and to what is served at mealtimes.

ASSESSMENT OF NUTRITIONAL STATUS

The main use of screening of nutritional status in office-based pediatric practice is the early detection of illness or inappropriate dietary patterns. The assessment of nutritional status in the well child is essentially the assessment of growth. Iron nutriture is also a concern at the end of infancy and during adolescence. Chronic illnesses can have devastating effects on nutritional status. There is a high prevalence of malnutrition and of specific nutrient deficiencies in those conditions. More complex situations will not be discussed here.

The assessment of growth involves three steps: (1) accurate measurement of length, weight, and head circumference, (2) careful plotting of *serial* measurements on appropriate growth charts, and (3) correct interpretation of the data. The measurement of weight is done accurately in most offices. Nevertheless, it is important to standardize scales periodically with known reference weights and to weigh children consistently with minimal clothing. Measurement of length is often not done, and when it is, it is frequently done poorly. Recumbent length should be measured for children less than 2 years of age, and standing height (stature) should be measured for those over 3 years of age. Either measurement may be used for the 2- to 3-year-old child, depending on the child's cooperation, provided that it is plotted on the appropriate growth chart (recumbent length 0 to 36 months, standing height 2 to 18 years). Good equipment for measuring recumbent length and standing height is as important as any equipment in the office. The height bar attached to most scales, for example, is unacceptable. Errors of several centimeters in height are easily made. Differences of this magnitude can change the percentile ranking of a 4-year-old child from the 25th percentile to approximately the 10th percentile or *vice versa* (both directions can be a problem).

A single value for stature or weight is of little value except when a child is already obviously under- or overnourished. Serial measurements of weight, length or height, and, in younger children, head circumference, should be plotted on standard growth charts (NCHS reference data). Because growth charts are a statistical representation of the growth of a population of children, the place on the chart of a single child cannot be equated with health or illness. For example, we instinctively worry more about the 4-year-old child whose height falls at the 10th percentile and whose weight falls at the 5th percentile than we do about a child of similar age with height and weight at the 50th and 25th percentiles, respectively. Height for both children, however, is within the normal range, and both have a weight-for-height at approximately the same percentile within the normal range. On the other hand, if one of these children had a rapid decrease in percentile rank, concern about undernutrition or disease would be warranted.

A different problem arises in the interpretation of adolescent growth data. The commonly used growth charts mask the growth spurt because the pubertal growth spurt occurs in different children at widely different ages. Children with early growth spurts appear to accelerate on the chart and then appear to fall back. The reverse is true of children whose growth spurt occurs later. In some instances, charts that permit the plotting of growth velocity (increments), rather than height or weight attained, may be useful.

There are two patterns of growth, aside from frank cessation of increases in weight and stature, that should alert the pediatrician to impending problems: continuing linear growth with stable weight, and proportionately slow growth in both stature and weight. The child whose length (height) continues to increase, perhaps more slowly, while weight gain ceases or weight loss ensues will become *wasted*, a state characterized by low weight-for-height. The child who grows slowly in both stature and weight is termed *stunted*. Wasting (acute nutritional insult) may be superimposed on stunting (chronic nutritional insult) in some instances. Both wasting and stunting can be associated with marginal nutrient intakes, mild to moderate malabsorption, or chronic illness. (See also Chap. 188, "Failure to Thrive.")

Measurement of triceps or subscapular skinfold (fatfold) thickness can be useful in assessing body fatness. Inexpensive plastic calipers and good reference data (percentile charts) are available for these measurements. Skinfold measurements are likely to prove useful in separating the overweight child from the overfat child and in following fat loss in an obese child who is growing. In the latter situation, frank weight loss may be undesirable. Slower weight gain with normal linear growth can be used to achieve fat loss, which is most easily monitored by skinfold measurements. Such measurements should be reserved for specific children and need not be routine.

Screening for specific nutrient deficiencies is rarely required in the office situation. Protein status should be assessed in children with either wasting or stunting. This is most easily accomplished by measurement of serum total protein and albumin concentrations. Proteins with shorter half-lives (e.g., prealbumin) are more sensitive indicators, especially of response to recovery, but they are not needed routinely. Low serum albumin concentration is rarely the result of low protein intake in the United States but may point to pathologic conditions in which protein requirements are elevated or protein is being malabsorbed or lost. Screening for iron deficiency is routine in most offices, usually by measuring hematocrit or hemoglobin concentration. If anemia is detected, a therapeutic trial of iron may be preferred over extensive laboratory testing in office practice. Screening for other specific nutrients should be done on an individual basis. For example, children who are raised as vegetarians are known to have low intakes of vitamins D and B_{12}; thus, the screening of vitamin D and B_{12} status is indicated (see Chap. 15). Consultation with someone knowledgeable in laboratory diagnosis of nutrient deficiencies is advisable, because the plasma concentration of many nutrients is less indicative of body stores than are other indirect measures related to metabolic functions of the nutrient.

ANNOTATED BIBLIOGRAPHY

Birch LL, Johnson SL, Andresen G, Peters JC, Schulte MC: The variability of young children's energy intake. N Engl J Med 324: 232–235, 1991. (Authors' conclusion: " . . . the successful feeding of children is best accomplished by providing them with a variety of healthful foods and allowing them to eat what they wish.")

Dallman PR: Progress in the prevention of iron deficiency in infants. Acta Paediatr Scand (Suppl) 365:28–37, 1990. (Good overview of iron nutrition in infancy.)

Dietz WH Jr., Gortmaker SL: Do we fatten our children at the television set? Obesity and television viewing in children and adolescents. Pediatrics 75:807–812, 1985. (The answer is . . . yes.)

Harper AE: Dietary goals—A skeptical view. Am J Clin Nutr 31:310–321, 1978. (A respected nutritionist suggests we may be expecting too much from dietary modification.)

Jung E, Czajka-Nasius DM: Birth weight doubling and tripling times: An updated look at the effects of birth weight, sex, race and type of feeding. Am J Clin Nutr 42:182–189, 1985. (Reality for many infants differs from the NCHS growth charts.)

Lozoff B, Brittenham GM, Wolfe AW et al: Iron deficiency anemia and iron therapy effects on infant developmental test performance. Pediatrics 79:981–995, 1987. (Treatment of iron deficiency anemia may not reverse the behavioral effects, as demonstrated by this 5-year follow-up. See Pediatr Res 25:16A, 1989.)

MacLean WC Jr., Graham GG: Vegetarianism in children. Am J Dis Child 134:513–519, 1980. (A review of nutritional and non-nutritional effects of being raised a vegetarian.)

Montalto MB, Benson JD, Martinez GA: Nutrient intakes of formula-fed infants and infants fed cow's milk. Pediatrics 75:343–351, 1985. (Differences in nutrient intakes were due not only to different concentrations of nutrients in each of the milk feedings but also to the different amounts and types of solid foods fed the two groups of infants.)

Moore WM, Roche AF: Pediatric Anthropometry, 2nd ed. Columbus, OH, Ross Laboratories, 1983. (Details how to perform anthropometric measurements properly and provides guidelines for interpretation of values obtained.)

Walter T, De Andraca I, Chadud P, Perales CG: Iron deficiency anemia: Adverse effects on infant psychomotor development. Pediatrics 84:7–17, 1989. (Findings nearly identical to those of Lozoff et al. in a different study population. Five-year follow-up also shows persistent effects. See Pediatr Res 28:295, 1990.)

13

The Well-Child Visit

Katherine C. Teets Grimm

The prenatal visit and subsequent well-child visits provide the physician with an excellent opportunity to acquaint himself or herself with the child and his or her family, to develop a data base on the child, and to practice preventive pediatrics. Such visits are helpful when the physician treats the same child for an acute illness. Knowledge of what the child is like when he or she is well, and knowledge of the family, their ability to cope with illness, their judgment during crises, and their compliance with past medical regimens, helps the physician to determine how sick the child is and what the treatment plan should be.

SOME GOALS OF THE WELL-CHILD VISIT

In addition to the variable agenda that parents bring to each visit, the physician should determine his or her goals for each well-child encounter. Such goals guide the provider's content of the visit. Examples of goals might, and indeed often, include the following:

- To establish a relationship of trust and open communication with the patient and his family
- To gain an understanding of the child's cultural, ethnic, religious, and socioeconomic background (Do culturally influenced ideas strongly affect how the family deals with illness?)
- To observe and inquire about the child's relationship to his parents and to other family members and to know the attitudes and expectations that they have toward each other (Is the child considered to be a "bad" child? Is the child a "vulnerable" child? Is the child the only reason why the parents are still together? Do the parents have realistic expectations given the child's developmental level?)
- To detect stresses that affect the family and anxieties that the family or the child is experiencing (Does the mother feel overwhelmed or incompetent with her child care responsibilities? Are there financial pressures?)
- To inquire about the child's environment (Are there environmental hazards such as lead-based paint in the child's home or in the babysitter's home? Is either parent involved in an occupation that might bring hazardous materials into the home? Have proper precautions been taken in the home and the babysitter's home to prevent accidents?)
- To determine the risk for genetically transmitted diseases (For example, is there a history of early cardiovascular disease?)
- To detect early developmental and behavioral problems and to monitor their remediation
- To detect early disease processes by an interview, a physical examination, and screening tests
- To provide health maintenance (e.g., immunizations)
- To provide appropriate counseling and anticipatory guidance
- To communicate to the family that the physician is there to help and provide support

GENERAL PRINCIPLES OF THE WELL-CHILD VISIT

Frequency of the Visits

The American Academy of Pediatrics (AAP) recommends a *minimum* of five health supervision visits from birth to 2 years of age, three visits from 2 to 6 years of age, and four visits from 6 to 18 years of age. The AAP also recommends that the frequency of the visits be increased for the following situations:

a. First-born, adopted, and foster children
b. Parents with a particular need for education and guidance
c. Disadvantaged social or economic environment
d. The presence or possibility of perinatal disorders, congenital defects, or familial disease
e. Acquired illness or previously identified disease or problems

It is apparent that each child and family must be treated individually and that the number of visits should be adjusted accordingly.

Organization of the Visits

The average initial well-child visit during which a complete family history is obtained will generally take at least 30 minutes. The typical follow-up well-child visit will normally take 15 to 30 minutes. The physician frequently faces the dilemma of how to provide full services to a family and yet conserve time. The counseling and anticipatory guidance portion of the visit are often too limited. Several suggestions on how to deal with this dilemma follow:

- For the initial visit, parents can fill out a data base form while waiting for the child to be examined by the physician.
- If more intensive counseling is necessary, a separate visit with the family should be arranged.
- The physician or his nursing assistant can hold periodic parent–group conferences during which topics of com-

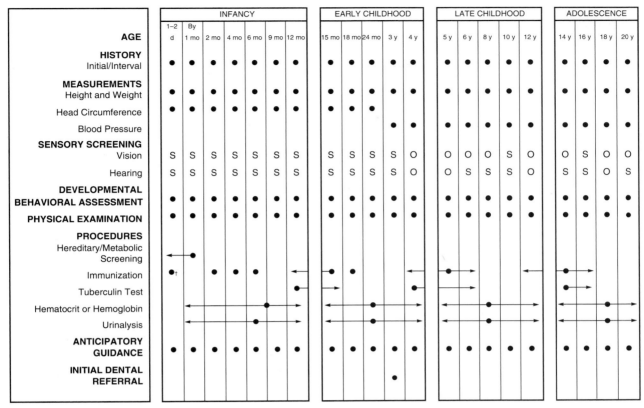

Key: ● = To be performed; S = subjective, by history; O = objective, by standard testing method; † = the first dose of hepatitis B vaccine should be given by the second day of life, the second dose at 1-2 mo of age, and the third dose between 6 and 8 mo.

Figure 13-1. Guidelines for health supervision (modified). (From the American Academy of Pediatrics, July 1991)

mon concern are discussed. The topics conducive to group discussion include: the advantages and potential side effects of vaccines, toilet training, sleep disorders, feeding problems, discipline, and limit setting.

- The physician can use written patient education materials, either commercially or personally formulated, to reinforce guidance provided during the counseling and anticipatory guidance portion of the well-child visit. The physician can also give the parent materials to read *in preparation* for the next well-child visit.
- The physician can use audiovisual materials appropriate for both the child and the parent in the waiting room. Many excellent materials are available.
- The physician can use a nursing assistant to do exit interviewing with the child and family to ensure that all the instructions are clear and to do further teaching.

Content of the Visits

Interview. The physician should gain a sense of how the child and the family are doing. Are there any stresses? What activities do the parents enjoy doing with the child? Is parenting an overall positive experience? Do the parents have

time by themselves? What are the overall supports? The physician should also ask a sufficient number of open-ended questions in order to unearth "hidden complaints." For example, "Is there anything that you are worried or concerned about today?" "Is there anything else that you would like to discuss?" "Do you have any other questions?" The initial interview should explore the family history, the perinatal history, hospitalizations, accidents, medications, allergies, dietary history, growth and development, habits, behavioral problems, discipline, living conditions, environmental hazards, and a review of systems. Subsequent interviews build on this initial base. Once the child has started to talk, the physician should interview the child as well as the parent. When the child is in early puberty, the physician should interview not only the patient alone but also the patient and parent together.

Physical Examination. The physical examination should be *complete* and should include the appropriate measurements (Fig. 13-1) and *developmental assessment*. With younger children, it is good to initiate the examination by observation and then to proceed with the least threatening part of the examination. The physician can do much of the respiratory and neurologic examination by observation and then proceed to examine the chest and abdomen. It is sometimes wise to begin the examination with the child in the mother's lap and to solicit the child's involvement as much as possible. An examination of the child's doll or teddy bear often helps to dispel anxiety. An older child should be allowed to undress and dress in privacy and to use a gown. Children who are in puberty should be examined without the parent in the room unless the patient wishes otherwise. Female patients who are being examined by a male physician may prefer to have the mother stay in the examining room.

Preventive Care and Periodic Health Screening. The content of the well-child visit at various ages, as recommended by the AAP, is described in Figure 13-1.

Counseling and Anticipatory Guidance. A well-child visit is incomplete without adequate time spent on this topic. In fact, this subject is generally considered the cornerstone of the visit. Specific guidelines for counseling and anticipatory guidance follow.

SPECIFIC GUIDELINES FOR THE WELL-CHILD VISIT AT DIFFERENT AGES

In 1988, the American Academy of Pediatrics issued *Guidelines for Health Supervision*. This manual addresses in good detail the interview, developmental assessment, physical examination, preventive care, and anticipatory guidance for each well-child visit. More abbreviated comments for each well-child visit follow, along with a collection of common parental questions with suggested answers that the physician can give.

Prenatal Visit

During this visit, the parents and the physician become acquainted, and the parents decide if they want to have this physician for their expected child. Practice arrangements and philosophy of care should be discussed. Concerns and questions should be solicited from the parents. Generally, feeding should be discussed (breast-feeding versus bottle-feeding versus both). Some anticipatory guidance, such as the need for a car seat, circumcision if the baby is a boy (see Chap. 9, "Circumcision"), and help for the mother should be provided. Appropriate patient education pamphlets might be given.

Newborn Visit

This is a time of euphoria, exhaustion, and sometimes postpartum blues. A complete physical examination with close follow-up to detect problems early is important. Parents need to be informed of all procedures and tests, including "nonconsequential" ones. Most families, but especially first-time parents, need repeated reassurance and encour-

agement. Feeding is discussed, particularly with breast-feeding mothers who may need help, especially with the mechanics (see Chap. 8, "Breast-Feeding"). Arrangements after discharge should be addressed. The first dose of hepatitis B vaccine should be given by the second day of life (see Chap. 14).

2- to 4-Week Visit

At this visit, various concerns are usually raised by the parents, but they are most often reassured that everything is fine. This is especially important for the breast-feeding mother who may fear that her child is not gaining weight properly. In addition to the interview and the physical examination, common topics to discuss include the parent's exhaustion and how to deal with it, the reactions of siblings to the new baby and how to handle them, the baby's sleep and feeding patterns, and what to do when the baby is fussy. Safety advice should include the use of car seats on *all* trips and avoiding articles in the crib, such as pillows, floppy bumpers, and toys, which could result in accidental suffocation. The physician might prescribe vitamins A, D, and C with fluoride and iron for the baby who is being exclusively breast-fed and fluoride for the formula-fed baby who receives no fluoridated water. In children discharged early from the hospital, repeat metabolic screening may be indicated. The second hepatitis B vaccine may also be given at 1 month.

2-Month Visit

By this visit, the family is generally more adjusted to the new baby. If the mother is returning to work, child care arrangements need to be discussed. Remind the parents that the babysitter's home needs to be accident-proofed as well as their own. Development is assessed: Is there a social smile? Does the child regard the parent's face? Does the child respond to sound? Does the child coo? Immunizations are normally initiated with oral polio-virus vaccine (OPV); diphtheria, pertussis, and tetanus (DTP); and a conjugate *Haemophilus influenzae* type b (Hib) vaccine (e.g., Hib-TITER™). The second hepatitis B vaccine should also be given if it was not already administered the previous month. Anticipatory guidance includes safety advice such as not leaving the child on the bed unattended and not drinking a hot beverage while holding the baby. Parents need to be encouraged to start having time "alone." Guidance concerning choosing a babysitter, even if the mother is not returning to work, should be given.

4-Month Visit

By this visit, the baby is generally more responsive to his environment and is happy most of the time. The infant often sleeps through the night; if not, the parents are often concerned and ask what to do (see Chap. 30, "Sleep Disturbances"). There are also questions about the addition of solids to the diet. Depending on the philosophy of the physician, solids are slowly introduced at this age or their addition is deferred until 5 or 6 months of age (see Chap. 12, "Nutrition and Nutritional Status: An Overview"). If the baby is being fed with formula, it should be iron-fortified. Development is assessed: Does the baby laugh or squeal? Does the baby follow objects around the room? Is the baby alert to the human voice? Does the baby hold his head high when put on his stomach? Does the baby try to roll over? Anticipatory guidance should reinforce previous counseling on the necessity of car seats and other pertinent aspects of home safety (see Chap. 19, "Injury Prevention").

Parents may want suggestions on how to play with their baby. Several excellent books are available on this subject (Eden, 1980). DTP, OPV, and conjugate Hib vaccines are given.

6-Month Visit

A baby at this age is normally highly engaging and a joy. If the parent shows signs of ambivalence, the physician should carefully explore the stresses in the parent's life and determine if supportive intervention, perhaps by a social worker or by an infant stimulation program, is indicated. The parent may simply need more time alone. Development is assessed: Does the baby babble (use vowel sounds)? Is the baby happy most of the time? Does the baby roll over, sit with or without support, pick up toys, transfer toys? Has the baby started showing anxiety toward strangers?

Anticipatory guidance includes a discussion of the need for iron-fortified foods and fluoride in the diet. The parent should avoid using the bottle as a pacifier and should not put the child to bed with the bottle because it might predispose to "milk caries." Safety instructions are reinforced. Teething and footwear might also be discussed. DTP No. 3 and OPV No. 3 (optional) are given, and, depending on the type used, a conjugate Hib vaccine may also be given. If the child was premature, a complete blood count (CBC) should be done. The third hepatitis B vaccine may be given at this visit or at any time before 18 months of age.

9-Month Visit

By this visit, the child will probably show great gains in motor skills. Generally, children are sitting by themselves, picking up small objects, and playing well with toys. It is common for children this age to pull to a stand and crawl; some are cruising or walking. The child is entering his "dangerous" developmental stage. The parent needs to understand that a child will not comprehend dangers at this age and for at least the next 12 months, and thus all hazardous or breakable items should be inaccessible. When this is not possible, rooms should be cordoned off by gates or locks, and closets that contain hazards should be locked. These precautions also make parenting much easier. Language and social interactions are considerably more im-

portant developmental milestones to assess than are motor skills. Is the child babbling with monosyllables and polysyllables? Does the child respond to his name, "No," or "Where is mama"? Does the child enjoy interactive games? If the child's babbling is decreasing rather than increasing, a hearing evaluation is necessary. Anticipatory guidance will include counseling on "accident-proofing" the home, such as the need for window gates for windows on the second floor and higher, and the avoidance of foods that could be aspirated. A *tuberculin test* may be administered at this or the 12-month visit and a *hemoglobin/hematocrit* may be checked at this visit (or at the next one). A sickle cell screening test is also done when indicated.

12-Month Visit

Babies at this age are usually highly social and interested in exploring their environments. Their motor skills make them adept at getting around. They are also developing strong likes and dislikes. Some parents find this developmental stage exciting, and others find it highly stressful. Difficulty may arise because parents are no longer completely in control; they are at a loss to manage an active toddler who gets into "trouble" and who does not respond to the word "No." Such parents need kind, supportive intervention. Developmental achievements that should be noted are language and communication: Does the child say one to three meaningful words or sounds? Does he or she point to what he needs? Anticipatory guidance may address nutrition, accident prevention, and parent–child interactions: Should the baby be switched to whole cow's milk? Should the bottle be stopped? The telephone number of a poison control center should be readily available. What should the parent do about stranger and separation anxiety? The parent should try to spend at least 10 minutes each day reading, playing games, and cuddling with the infant. The parent should also start praising the child for desired behavior. Lead screening is recommended. In communities where measles is a problem, the first MMR (measles, mumps, rubella) vaccine is given at this visit.

15-Month Visit

The 15-month-old is usually walking well and on the verge of rapid language acquisition. He or she usually uses much jargon and many gestures. The toddler can often understand simple commands such as "Go and get your book," and is usually more proficient at receptive, rather than expressive, language. The child may also be adept at self-feeding with his or her fingers and with a spoon. He or she may know one or two body parts. Anticipatory guidance might include phasing out the bottle and pacifier by 18 months, avoiding a bottle in bed, and reinforcing safety-proofing the home, including a reminder of the dangers of dangling cords, electrical sockets, plastic bags, unattended water, and small objects that could be aspirated. The child's readiness for bowel training at 18 or 24 months can be discussed. The topic of discipline can also be raised. The measles–mumps–rubella (MMR) immunization is generally given at this visit, if it was not given at 12 months of age, along with the conjugate Hib vaccine booster (see Chap. 14, "Childhood Immunizations").

18-Month Visit

The 18-month-old child is entering the "problem-solving" stage of development. He or she can make rapid intellectual advances if given the proper stimulation. The child can often say four to ten words and frequently more and can usually express two or more wants. Motor skills are more refined: the child may walk up the stairs with one hand held and may kick and throw a ball. He or she will also tend to have a low frustration threshold and may sometimes behave negatively. He or she is unlikely to share, and when he or she plays with other children, it will probably not be interactive play. Parents who are aware that this is normal development will better be able to cope when their child "misbehaves." Parents should avoid situations in which temper tantrums may be embarrassing and a major source of frustration. For example, taking a child this age to a grocery store or a restaurant is a gamble. Parents also need to know that even though their child seems to understand much more, he or she still cannot fully understand danger and is still at high risk of ingesting something poisonous or otherwise harmful, such as a small object. The house must therefore continue to be safety-proofed. The physician might also reassure the parents that toilet training can (and, indeed, often should) be deferred, and that they should have fun with the child. The value of play groups for both the child and the mother might be mentioned. The first DTP and OPV boosters are given at this visit (if it was not already given at 15 months). If the child is at increased risk of lead exposure, lead screening is repeated.

24-Month Visit

At 2 years of age, some of the child's negative behavior may decrease. However, the child will have good days and bad days. Language should be well established, with a vocabulary of more than 50 words and some two-word phrases. Words may include some pronouns and will be intelligible to parents. A hearing and speech evaluation should be considered if language has not developed to this degree. Anticipatory guidance should reemphasize accident prevention. Also, it is a good idea to discuss the importance of routines, such as a regular bedtime preceded by reading a story, prayers, and so forth. Toilet training is another topic. If the child is not yet toilet trained, which is common at this age, the parents should not feel frustrated. An explanation about physiologic readiness is helpful. Parents should continue to try to praise the child for good behavior, and they should be good role models. Children at this age are great imitators, and they are beginning to develop attitudes and habits. If the child is toilet trained, a urinalysis may be appropriate at this visit. Some pediatricians will also do a tympanogram and repeat a hematocrit/hemoglobin, tuberculin test, and lead screen.

3-Year Visit

The 3-year-old is no longer a toddler. He or she is very communicative, thoroughly enjoys being with other children, and is skilled at pretend play. The 3-year-old can also be defiant at times, which may be a source of frustration. Because of the child's communicative abilities, the parents may have greater expectations than what is developmentally appropriate. Parents should observe and then try to avoid situations that are most likely to cause the child to decompensate. For example, fatigue is a common precipitant of misbehavior. Parents also need to learn the importance of setting realistic limits and avoiding overindulgence. Limit setting, however, must be balanced by praise for good behavior and by a good deal of love, affection, and "special" times together. Injuries continue to be problematic and continue to need emphasis. Because of the problem of sexual molestation, the child needs to be taught about "good touch"/ "bad touch" and the rights that he or she has in as sensitive a manner as possible. Several children's books, including coloring books, can help in this educational endeavor. The topic of nursery school or play groups should be raised again. At this age, the child usually has his or her first dental visit and has vision and hearing screening. If the child's speech is not intelligible to nonfamily members, a speech referral should be considered. The physician should also take the child's blood pressure, do a blood count if indicated, repeat a lead level screen and administer a tuberculin test if at risk, and obtain a urine culture (if the patient is a girl).

4-Year Visit

A 4-year-old is generally self-sufficient. Motor skills are such that the child can walk up and down stairs alternating feet, hop, jump forward, and ride a tricycle well. Fine motor skills enable the child to cut and paste, begin drawing a person with face and arms or face and legs, and copy a cross, circle, and possibly a square. The child can dress and undress with supervision. Parents can begin giving the child more responsibilities, such as setting and clearing the table. They should remember to give praise when deserved. The parent and child can jointly get involved with special projects, such as going together to the museum or to a movie. If there are other siblings in the house, some of these special projects should be done alone with the child if possible. At this visit, a dental screening is advised and, if indicated, a blood count and vision screening done, a tuberculin administered, and lead screening may be repeated. Between 4 and 6 years of age, the second and last DTP and OPV boosters are administered.

5-Year Visit

The 5-year-old is generally in kindergarten or preschool. The child's development should include such tasks as naming four or five colors, knowing his or her age, defining at least one word, and drawing a person with head, body, arms, and legs. If the child is in school, the physician should seek feedback on how the child is progressing and, if there are problems, evaluate the situation more thoroughly. Because there is great variability in development from one child to another, sometimes school "readiness" and placement need to be addressed (see Chap. 38, "School Readiness"). Educational consultants can assist in this task. Parents should again be counseled about safety; the need for the child to know his or her name, telephone, and address; how to approach strangers (and *vice versa*); and discipline. The child at this age will have sexual curiosities. Parents need to answer questions at the child's level and not answer more than what the child actually asks. If parents feel uncomfortable about a particular question, they can defer an answer until the child is older and better able to understand. Pejorative explanations and accusations of "dirtiness" must be avoided. Screening procedures vary from one physician to another, but they may include a tuberculin test, a blood count, urinalysis, vision, and audiometry. A MMR booster is given either at this age or when the child is in the sixth or seventh grade. The child should be advised to have a dental check-up.

6-Year Visit

The 6-year-old may be in the first grade. The issues that relate to school readiness in the 5-year-old are also important for the 6-year-old. In terms of developmental achievements, the 6-year-old may be able to ride a bicycle, tie his or her shoelaces, count to ten, print his or her first name and numbers up to ten, know right from left, and draw a person with six parts, including clothes. The physician should inquire about the child's social interactions with family and peers. Good health habits need to be reinforced, such as avoiding junk food, eating a balanced diet, the need for adequate exercise and sleep, and good dental care. The importance of special times with the parents, the use of appropriate praise, and the importance of responsibilities in the home are reiterated. If the physician sees that the child needs adult role models other than those available at home and in school, he or she can recommend a good after-school program or other programs such as the Big Brother Program.

8-Year Visit

The 8-year-old is generally in third grade and is beginning to read reasonably well. He or she can also tell time, take care of him- or herself and his or her belongings, and participate more fully in household activities and chores. The physician should ask about school—attitudes, academic performance, and social interaction. Good health habits are again discussed, including a low-fat diet and sufficient exercise. Accident prevention, especially the use of bicycle helmets, should be stressed.

Television viewing should be included in the discussion. Television viewing should be limited, and the child should not be allowed to watch violent or sexually provocative programs. Parents should have fair rules in the house and should try to avoid being too harsh. Praise and affection are still important and will continue to be so as long as the child lives at home. The parents should become involved in the school, and they should actively seek feedback from the teacher for means by which they can help their child. Any academic problems should be vigorously addressed. Office screening tests done at this visit are variable, but they may include a tuberculin test, vision screening, and cholesterol screening. Dental screening should be done at least yearly.

10-Year Visit

A 10-year-old is usually sophisticated. Some 10-year-old girls are pubertal. It is wise to do a substantial portion of the interview with the child as well as with the parent. If the physician senses tension, it is prudent to speak to the child and parent separately. The physician should get a sense for how the child is doing in general, what sorts of things they like to do, how they are progressing at school, what kind of feelings they have, whether they have friends, and what activities they do together. Health habits and safety issues should be discussed. The physician should explore the level of communication between the parents and the child. If there is not open, supportive communication, then counseling is indicated. Screening procedures done at this visit may include a blood count, urinalysis, vision screening, audiometry, and a tuberculin test. Special attention should be given at this visit and subsequent ones to scoliosis screening.

12-Year Visit

This young adolescent should be seen not only alone but also with the parents, and he or she should be asked questions similar to those asked of the 10-year-old. The physician should also explore sexuality issues and drug or alcohol experimentation. Because these are delicate subjects, and because it may take several visits before the teenager can trust the physician, the physician might say to the patient, "I'm going to ask you some questions about your personal life and your social life, and if you would rather not answer them, that's okay. The reason I'm asking them is so that I can be of help to you, and I will not tell your parents what you say to me unless you give me permission." (See also Chap. 16, "Sexuality Education.") The physician should also explore school issues, hobbies, the family life-style, and the level of communication between the patient and his or her family. Guidance should be given on good health habits, safety, and issues related to rapid physical and sexual changes. Discussion about safe sex should be included if it is appropriate. Parents need to be reminded to respect the patient's privacy, to have rules in the home but not overly harsh ones, to continue to have special times together, and to foster open communication. Parents may also need counseling on "danger signs" to look for in terms of drug and alcohol abuse and depression. At this visit, a tuberculin test may be done and, if not done previously, an MMR booster is given.

14-Year Visit

Children in this age range are still variable in terms of development and maturity. Some behave like prepubescent children and others behave like adults. Despite these differences in behavior, most teenagers at this age are somewhat insecure about relationships with others. They are also concerned about their body images, and they are strongly influenced by peer pressure. Such issues are important for the physician to discuss alone with the patient, and the physician should reassure him or her that these feelings are normal and that they will pass with time. Parents need to be aware that "acting out" behavior is often a reflection of underlying insecurity, and they should deal with unacceptable behavior not only with consistent rules but also with love, affection, time, and sympathetic listening. A response of anger tends only to increase the schism that frequently develops between parents and teenagers. When they are upset, parents should remind themselves of the basic worth of their teenager as a human being. Parents should also strive to be excellent role models, and they should not have double standards. The physician should ask about school, likes, dislikes, performance, extracurricular activities, hobbies, and drug, alcohol, and tobacco use. Whenever possible, the physician should try to encourage and praise the teenager. Either at this visit or the next one, girls should be instructed in breast self-examination and boys in testicular self-examination. Teenage girls should be advised to take a multivitamin with iron on a daily basis with juice in order to avoid iron deficiency. Screening tests done at this visit might include a blood count, vision screen, tuberculin test, and rubella titer. A tetanus and diphtheria (Td) booster should be given if 10 years have elapsed since the last DTP. Female adolescents should be referred for gynecologic care if the primary physician does not provide it.

16-Year Visit

All teenagers should be in puberty by this age. Once again, it is good to interview the parents and the teenager separately. The physician should specifically discuss with the teenager alone sexuality issues, including birth control, because this is often an area of conflict. The physician should also gently introduce the topic of sexual abuse/incest. One

way to approach this subject is to ask, "Has anyone, including a relative, ever touched you anywhere on your body when you did not want this to occur?" Many issues previously raised should be raised again. It is also appropriate for the physician to discuss plans after high school graduation. Office screening tests are the same as for the 14-year-old, except for rubella titer and Td booster.

18-Year Visit

The 18-year-old is legally an adult. He or she can now vote, enlist in the military, and drive. The process of emotional maturation, however, will continue for many years. The patient continues to require understanding, support, and encouragement from family, friends, and physician. The physician should discuss many of the previous issues: school, work, home situation, social outlets, sexuality, and habits, including drugs or alcohol. A discussion on communication (and, if necessary, how to improve it) and on future plans and aspirations should be held. The patient needs to be counseled concerning good ongoing health maintenance, including gynecologic care. If the patient is being seen by a pediatrician and will be transferred to an internist, this transition should be discussed and made as smoothly and as easily as possible.

COMMON PROBLEMS ENCOUNTERED BY THE PARENT OF AN INFANT

Crying

In infants less than 3 months old, it is normal for the child to cry 1 to 3 hours a day. Infants will usually cry for physiologic reasons such as hunger, tiredness, excessive gas, wet or dirty diapers, and loneliness. The crying usually stops when the needs are met. It is common for a baby to have a "fussy" period, which often occurs in the evening. If the baby is not responsive to the usual comforting measures, the physician should make sure there are no underlying causes, such as milk intolerance. (For a more extensive discussion on crying and colic, see Chap. 211.)

Colic

Many physicians do not like the term "colic" because of the connotations it has for many parents. Colic basically refers to paroxysms of irritability. These paroxysms occur in healthy, well-fed infants, and they are often associated with the infant drawing up his legs as though in pain, often for more than 3 hours a day. Classically, colic begins at about 2 weeks of age and lasts until about 16 weeks of age. It is frequently worse in the evening, and it is often attributed to an immature digestive system.

Colic is frustrating to manage. Various therapies have been used, with none being consistently successful. Some modalities that have been used are:

- Picking up the infant and carrying him or her around
- Rocking the infant; exposing the infant to other motion such as car rides
- Using small doses of antacids or antiflatulents such as si-methicone, which is available in a formulation for infants
- Removing all dairy products from the mother's diet if she is breast-feeding on the chance that the child has a milk allergy
- Changing formula from cow's milk to soy or a more hypoallergenic formula, also on the chance that the child has a milk allergy

In the past, many physicians used antispasmodics combined with barbiturates, but these are generally no longer used because of side effects and possible overdosage.

Parents with a "colicky" baby need a great deal of support and empathy. Because a screaming child can be a major stress, they should be encouraged to have some time by themselves if at all possible. They should also be reminded that the condition is only temporary.

Sleep

It is normal for a baby to awaken at night for the first few months of life. Some babies develop a pattern of sleeping during the day and keeping awake most of the night. Parents can slowly reverse this pattern of sleep by awakening the child earlier and earlier during lengthy daytime naps. Putting the baby in his or her crib while still awake frequently promotes sleeping through the night because the child learns to settle him or herself. (See Chap. 30 for a more detailed discussion on sleep disturbances.)

As the child gets older, parents can also develop routines that will promote good sleep habits, such as the following:

- A regular bedtime
- Avoiding excessive stimulation to the child while the child is sleeping (e.g., the room should be dark, there should be little noise, the child should sleep alone)
- Not responding to the first cry. Occasionally, children will cry in their sleep and then stop.

Diet

Every physician has his or her own style of giving dietary advice. Some guidelines, however, are generally accepted. Breast milk or formula should be the major source of nutrition for the first 5 to 6 months of life. If the mother is breast-feeding exclusively, the child should receive a vitamin D (400 U) and fluoride (0.25 mg) supplementation daily. If the child is given formula, an iron-fortified formula should be used, and a fluoride supplementation should be given unless the formula is reconstituted with fluoridated water. When the child is drinking more than 32 oz of formula a day, many physicians will start the child on cereal and then add fruits or vegetables, one at a time. Meats are generally introduced into the diet at 6 to 8 months of age. Parents may use a mill to grind table foods, but they should avoid foods with added salt or simple sugars.(See Chap. 12, "Nutrition and Nutritional Status: An Overview.")

COMMON PROBLEMS ENCOUNTERED BY THE PARENT OF THE TODDLER

Sleep

It is normal for a child to have periodic wakening during the night. If a child awakens and cries or calls for the parent, the child should be reassured of his or her parent's presence and love. The parent should make sure the child is not sick, and then leave the room. The parent should not stimulate the child further by playing with or feeding him or her. After being comforted, the child may cry him- or herself to sleep. When the child realizes that nighttime is sleeping time for both him- or herself and his or her parents, nighttime awakening will lessen (see Chap. 30, "Sleep Disturbances").

Tantrums, Including Breath-Holding Spells

During a tantrum, the parent should make sure the child is safe and then ignore the act. When the child is not having a tantrum, the parent should be generous with love and attention (see Chap. 212, "Breath-Holding Spells").

Behavior and Discipline

As a child's verbal skills progress, many parents overestimate their toddler's ability to control his or her behavior. Thus, the "terrible twos" evolve. Some hints to decrease the stress include the following:

- Decrease the number of temptations to which the toddler is exposed. If the toddler continually hears the word "No" from his or her parents, he or she will learn how to say "No" very well; furthermore, if the toddler continually has his or her hand slapped, he or she will learn how to hit very well. Examples of temptations are leaving breakable items in easy reach of the toddler or taking the toddler to the grocery store.
- Try to anticipate misbehavior on the part of the toddler and distract him or her before it happens (Brenner, 1988).

Toilet Training

Toilet training requires patience on the part of the parent. It is common even for a precocious child not to be toilet trained until 3 years of age, but it happens sooner or later. Toilet training should be viewed as any other developmental task, as a skill for the child to acquire, such as walking or climbing the stairs, rather than as a task for parents to accomplish.

Most children are not ready to be introduced to the potty

or toilet until they are 24 months old. At that time, the parent may choose to purchase a small potty that the child can play with, sit on, or have his or her doll sit on. When the child expresses a need to urinate, the child should be put on the potty. The child should not be coerced to sit on the potty if he shows no interest whatsoever, nor should the child be overly praised for success on the potty; praise should be consistent with praise given for other accomplishments.

Some authorities advocate gradually guiding a child to the use of the potty starting at age 2. During the first week, the child is brought to sit on the potty fully clothed for as long as he likes. During the second week, he or she sits on the potty without a diaper, and, as before, he or she is not coerced. No attempt is made to catch urine. During the third or fourth week, the child is brought to the potty after wetting his or her diaper. The dirty diaper is placed in the potty to show the child where the urine or stool eventually should go. Subsequent to these introductory weeks, the child is periodically put on the potty and encouraged to urinate or defecate. In the case of boys, it is advisable to teach them to urinate standing up. They can learn this by watching their fathers.

Diet

Most children will demonstrate a decreased appetite at some time (often at around 2 years of age), and this frustrates almost every parent. The physician can reassure the parents by showing them their child's normal growth curve. The physician should encourage the parent to feed the child the wholesome foods that he or she likes. Most young children like cheese, pasta, juice, and fruit (see Chap. 31, "Common Feeding Problems in Young Children").

Preparing for the New Sibling and Sibling Rivalry

Preparing a child for a new sibling may help decrease some of the trauma of the arrival of the new sibling. Because a toddler and preschooler both have a distorted sense of time, it is probably appropriate to begin the process when the mother is in her last trimester and "showing." Parents will have different ways to introduce the topic. They may want to use one or more of the excellent books written for children who are expecting a new brother or sister or who already have one. The parents should generally make the child feel a part of the team that is expecting the new baby, and they should emphasize to the older child how important he or she is in their lives. Many hospitals now also have a special tour of the delivery room and postpartum floor for children prior to their mothers' deliveries. Most hospitals also allow sibling visitation after delivery. Such programs allow the older sibling to understand his or her mother's absence from the home and to see "his" or "her" baby very early on. Some sibling "bonding" may even occur. In spite of these measures, the older child may still regress in his or her behavior. Parents should try to tolerate this regression

and not pay much attention to it. Other ways to help the older child cope are:

- Parents should remove the child from the baby should he or she strike out against the baby. The parents should also allow the child to hold and cuddle the baby under close supervision when the older child is in a nonaggressive mood.
- The parents should take turns spending special times with the older child.
- The older child should be made to feel important in his or her new role as the older sibling. Parents can solicit the older child's opinion, such as, "Why do you think the baby is crying? What do you think we can do?" Parents can also ask the older child to help with some small tasks.
- Parents should make a concerted effort not to show favoritism.

Biting, Kicking, and Sharing

Biting and kicking are behaviors that are common between the ages of 15 months and 36 months. Frequently, they are signs that social demands, such as sharing and waiting a turn, are being placed on a child who is not mature enough to handle these demands.

Parents need to be advised that biting is a "normal" response to a stressful situation. They should try to provide play situations that are less stressful (e.g., ones that do not require ongoing sharing). They should try to anticipate biting and redirect the child's attention or have him or her bite on something inanimate, such as a wet washrag. They should *not* bite back.

With regard to sharing and interactive play, parents need to be aware that this does not occur easily until the child is about 3 years old. If the child has a temper tantrum about sharing, it is best to remove the child or the object from the situation.

COMMON PROBLEMS ENCOUNTERED BY THE PARENT OF THE PRESCHOOLER

Diet

The problem is the same as for the toddler, if not worse, and the same principles of management apply. If the child has totally eliminated all calcium-containing foods from his or her diet, the physician might recommend chewable calcium tablets, such as Tums, in sufficient quantity to provide 800 mg of elemental calcium a day. A children's multivitamin that contains vitamin D should also be given once daily. Otherwise, dietary sources of calcium other than milk should be encouraged, such as cheese or yogurt.

Behavior and Discipline

The "terrible twos" are sometimes replaced by the "defiant threes." One can often reason with children this age and make "deals." Occasionally, "time out" is required for misbehavior. "Time out" can mean sitting on a chair in the corner for a few minutes until the child has gained control of himself. Corporal punishment should be reserved for the most serious offenses. Frequent spankings become meaningless and just convey to the child that hitting is okay. Parents should also try to evaluate underlying causes for misbehavior and make appropriate interventions. For example, is the child misbehaving because he or she is tired, or bored, or because he or she needs more time with his parents?

Lying and Stealing

Preschoolers have big imaginations, and they have difficulty distinguishing between truth and nontruth, their own possessions and those belonging to others. Parents of preschoolers who "lie" or "steal" should not be harsh with them; they should instead correct the child gently and be good role models.

School

Children at about 2½ or 3 years of age become highly social and enjoy interactive play. Parents should be encouraged to provide their child with opportunities to interact with other children of the same age. This can be done in nursery school or in play groups supervised by parents.

Nightmares or Night Terrors

Nightmares occur commonly in children. A child with a nightmare wakes up fully; he or she is anxious and has excellent recall of the bad dream. Nightmares are generally infrequent and require no intervention except reassurance and affection from the parents. Occasionally, however, nightmares will be frequent, in which case they may indicate some stress in the child's life. The content of the bad dream may be a clue.

Nightmares should be distinguished from *night terrors.* Night terrors occur in 5% or less of children and are characterized by a child who is out of control but still "asleep." There is no recall of the event on the child's part. Night terrors are generally infrequent and require no therapy. In those rare cases in which they are frequent, a more thorough social, psychiatric, and sleep evaluation is appropriate with an option for pharmacologic therapy.

Imaginary Playmates

Approximately 10% to 30% of children between the ages of 3 and 5 years have imaginary companions. It is more common in first-born children and in girls. Parents need to know that this play is normal, and they should not be worried about it. Rarely, a child may be so involved in his imaginary world that he appears to have difficulty distinguishing the

real from the unreal. In such a situation, the parents should encourage more activities with real persons and less time alone.

Fears

Children in this age group have an active imagination and a fertile fantasy life. Typical fears include fear of the dark, fear of monsters, and fears of animals and scary noises. There is also the fear of losing the primary caregiver. Reassurance by parents is critical. Avoiding scary television shows may also be helpful. The child should not be criticized or punished because of his or her fears. (Schachter's book [1988] is helpful for more specific guidance.)

COMMON PROBLEMS ENCOUNTERED BY THE PARENT OF THE SCHOOL-AGED CHILD

School Problems

It is good to gain some assessment of how a child is doing the first few years in school. If a problem becomes apparent, active intervention is required. This may include a conference with the child's teacher, perhaps a psychometric evaluation, and, if a learning disability is suspected, an evaluation by a learning disability consultant or clinic (see Chap. 40, "Learning Disabilities," for a more complete discussion).

Crying

Some school-aged children cry easily. This reflects their sensitivity. They should not be criticized and called "crybaby" but rather told that it is okay for even boys and adults to cry. If the child is embarrassed about crying easily, the parents and physician can offer suggestions on how he or she can control his or her emotions.

Lying and Stealing

When these activities occur in the child aged 6 and older, the physician and parents should carefully look for reasons for this behavior. Does the child feel too much pressure so that he or she is forced into lying? Is the child fearful that the punishment will be too harsh? Is the child needy? Is the child being strongly influenced by a group of friends?

Parents should show love and attention while setting limits. Parents must also set good examples by being truthful and honest. Children who lie or steal should be corrected, and, where appropriate, the misdeed should be rectified without undue embarrassment and humiliation.

Fears

Fears continue in this age group. Some are more reality-based (e.g., fear of being robbed). There continues to be the fear of losing a parent. As children get older, there is a tendency for adults to belittle the fearful child. Parental support and understanding are essential. As the child gets older, the parents can help the child face the fears with logic and thereby give him or her power over the fears.

The Difficult Child

There are some children whose temperament makes them difficult to raise. They are often hyperactive, moody children with poor impulse control. How well they do depends in part on their families and whether their personalities "fit" well with other family members. These children need a lot of love, affection, and structure with consistent limit setting. They sometimes need psychological or psychiatric assessment and occasionally medication. (Parents will find useful advice on the difficult child in Turecki, 1985.)

COMMON PROBLEMS ENCOUNTERED BY THE ADOLESCENT

Drugs

In our present society, it is almost impossible for a teenager to escape exposure to drugs. It is important for both the physician and parent to recognize the danger signs. An excellent review on the subject is given in an article by Comerci, and the warning signs that he enumerates are quoted *verbatim*:

1. Poor school performance and attendance
2. Mood swings more pronounced than those usually experienced by teenagers
3. Recent change from age-appropriate "acceptable" friends to older, unacceptable associates
4. Increased interest in the drug culture, manifested by possession of drug literature, paraphernalia, and clothing such as belt buckles and T-shirts with a drug theme
5. A change to sloppy dress and poor grooming and hygiene
6. A rebellious and paranoid flavor to all interpersonal relationships with adults, siblings, and authority figures

Immediate intervention is indicated if a physician feels that a patient has a high potential for drug abuse or has already started experimentation. This will include counseling of both the teenager and the parents and may include referral to a drug treatment program. It is not uncommon for the parents of a drug-using teenager to be overindulgent, permissive, and uninvolved in the teenager's life. These issues need to be included in any counseling program (see Chap. 45, "Street Drugs").

Suicide

Suicide is of epidemic proportions in the 15-to 24-year-old age range. Individuals who attempt suicide often feel an overwhelming sense of hopelessness and loneliness, and they feel that their lives are not worth anything. These individuals frequently have such high expectations for themselves that they are almost "destined" to feel like chronic failures. Physicians and parents need to be sensitive to these personality traits and should intervene when such traits are seen. Healthy, open communication between the parents or another adult role model and the teenager is critical in detecting early signs and in preventing suicide (see Chap. 36, "Depression and Suicide").

Pregnancy

Many teenagers are sexually active. By the age of 15 to 19, 50% of women in metropolitan areas have had sexual intercourse. It is important for the physician to develop a trusting relationship with the teenage girl and to frankly ask her in private what her sexual activities are. Birth control may be indicated (see Chap. 42, "Pregnancy Prevention").

Some teens may wish to abstain from sex but are under peer pressure to behave like the rest of the group. The physician can help "empower" the teen who wishes to abstain, through encouragement and highlighting activities that the teen may wish to focus his or her energy on, such as sports, arts, jobs, and so forth (see Chaps. 52 and 200).

Sexually Transmitted Diseases, Including AIDS

Many teenagers who experiment with sex are not fully cognizant of the hazards involved. Safe sex (i.e., abstention or the use of a condom with spermicide) is critical. Compliance is more likely if the teen truly believes that one can contract a serious sexually transmitted disease, including AIDS, with just one sexual encounter.

ANNOTATED BIBLIOGRAPHY

American Academy of Pediatrics: Guidelines for Health Supervision. Elk Grove Village, IL, 1988. (Expanded presentation of guidelines for conducting well-child care.)

American Academy of Pediatrics: Report of the Committee on Infectious Diseases. Elk Grove Village, IL, 1991. (Comprehensive reference book that covers all aspects of immunizations, recommendations for care of children in special circumstances [e.g., daycare, isolation, and sexually transmitted diseases], summaries of infectious diseases, and information on antimicrobials and antimicrobial prophylaxis.)

Brenner B: Love and Discipline. New York, Ballantine, 1988. (Excellent book on the topic of discipline.)

Canter L, Canter M: Assertive Discipline for Parents: A Pioneer Step-by-Step Approach to Solving Everyday Behavior Problems. New York, Harper and Row, 1988. (An excellent, easy-to-read guide on how to decrease the arguing that occurs in the home of the school-aged child.)

Comerci GD: Recognizing the five stages of substance abuse. Contemp Pediatr 12:57–66, 1985.

Eden AN: Positive Parenting. New York, Signet, 1982. (Useful paperback for parents of children up to the age of 3 years. Each chapter addresses a specific age range and includes information on growth and development, nutrition, exercise and play, safety, toys, and other practical topics.)

Farber R: Solve Your Child's Sleep Problems. New York, Simon and Schuster, 1986. (A handy guide for parents on sleep problems.)

Fraiberg S: The Magic Years. New York, Charles Scribner's Sons, 1959. (A wonderful analysis of the emotional development of children from newborn to 6 years of age. Provides good insight into early childhood behavior. Appropriate for parents and health care providers.)

Illingsworth RS: The Development of the Infant and Young Child: Normal and Abnormal, 9th ed. London, Churchill Livingstone, 1987. (A lengthy book that addresses most issues related to the normal child. Its chapter on development and the evaluation of development is noteworthy.)

Schachter R, McCauley CS: When Your Child Is Afraid. New York, Simon and Schuster, 1988. (A book for parents, and also useful to physicians, that outlines by age normal fears and phobias, with concrete advice on what to do.)

Schmitt B: Your Child's Health. New York, Bantam, 1987. (A frequent columnist on behavioral problems, Schmitt provides sage advice to parents on all aspects of child health, including a large section on illnesses and when to call the physician.)

Turecki S, Tonner L: The Difficult Child. New York, Bantam, 1985. (A practical guide for parents on raising the difficult child.)

14

Childhood Immunizations

Margaret B. Rennels

This chapter contains summaries of immunization recommendations from the Immunizations Practices Advisory Committee (ACIP) of the Public Health Service, and the Committee on Infectious Diseases of the American Academy of Pediatrics. The reader is urged to refer to the bibliograpy at the end of the chapter for greater elaboration of the immunization recommendations.

Vaccine development is an active field in which there are continual additions and refinements to the arsenal of vaccines. There has also been improvement in delivery of vaccines to most segments of the population. Virtually all children entering school have received the recommended immunizations as a result of the enactment of laws in all 50 states requiring documentation of immunity as a condition of first entry into school. Enhanced efforts are required, however, to reach preschool children in "poverty pockets," such as in some of our inner cities; in some areas, only 50% of 2-year-olds have received measles vaccination. It is the responsibility of all physicians providing health care to children to improve immunization levels in the United States.

GENERAL ISSUES

Informed Consent

Parents should be told of the benefits and risks of each of the vaccines their child is to receive. The National Childhood Vaccine Injury Act of 1986 requires that the Secretary of the Department of Health and Human Services develop and distribute standard benefit and risk statements for vaccines. Another requirement of the National Childhood Vaccine Injury Act is that health care providers note in the child's permanent record the following information concerning vaccinations: (1) date of administration, (2) manufacturer and lot number, and (3) name, address, and title of the person administering the vaccine.

Vaccine Adverse Event Reporting System (VAERS)

There is now a uniform reporting system and form through which health care providers are required to report the following events occurring after vaccination: (1) *DTP, P, DTP/IPV combined*—anaphylaxis or anaphylactic shock within 24 hours; encephalopathy (or encephalitis) within 7 days; shock–collapse or hypotonic–hyporesponsive collapse within 7 days; residual seizure disorder. (2) *MMR and combinations; DT, Td, or T*—anaphylaxis or anaphylactic shock within 24 hours; encephalopathy (or encephalitis) within 15 days for MMR and combination and within 7 days for DT, Td, or T; residual seizures. (3) *OPV*—paralytic poliomyelitis in a nonimmunodeficient recipient within 30 days, in an immunodeficient recipient within 6 months, in a vaccine-associated community case with no time limit. (4) *IPV*—anaphylaxis or anaphylactic shock within 24 hours. In addition to these events, any occurrence thought to be vaccine related or any event listed in the manufacturer's package insert as a contraindication to further vaccinations should be reported to the Department of Health and Human Services on the VAERS form. Submission of a report does not necessarily constitute a claim that the vaccine caused the adverse event. The number to call for information and forms is 800-822-7967.

Logistics of Injection

Refer to the vaccine package insert for the route of immunization and the dose of vaccine. Each vaccine should be given by a separate syringe and needle at a separate site. Preferable sites for intramuscular and subcutaneous injections are the anterolateral thigh of infants, and the deltoid of older children, adolescents, and adults. A 22- or 23-gauge needle ⅞ inches or longer is appropriate for intramuscular injections. For subcutaneous or intradermal injections, a 25-gauge needle ⅝ to ¾ inches long is used. After insertion of the needle, draw back on the plunger; if blood appears in the syringe, remove and change the needle and use a new site.

Scheduling

Immunizations should not be delayed for mild illness with low-grade fever, such as upper respiratory infections. Routine physical examination and temperature measurement are not prerequisites for vaccinating children who are in apparent good health. Refer to the following sections for precautions and contraindications for the administration of individual vaccines. If a child's immunization status cannot be determined, he should be considered susceptible and vaccinated. Most of the widely administered vaccines can be given simultaneously, safely, and effectively (Tables 14-1 and 14-2). A lapse in the routine schedule of immunizations does not interfere with the immune response; it is unnecessary to reinstitute or repeat doses. Reduced doses or multiple small doses are not recommended because they may not induce an adequate immune response.

Misconceptions Concerning Contraindications to Vaccination

Conditions most often *inappropriately* regarded as routine contraindications include the following:

1. Reaction to a previous dose of DTP vaccine that involved only soreness, redness, or swelling in the immediate vicinity of the vaccination site or a temperature of <105°F (40.5°C).
2. Mild acute illness with low-grade fever or mild diarrheal illness in an otherwise well child.
3. Current antimicrobial therapy or the convalescent phase of illnesses.
4. Prematurity. The appropriate age for initiating immunizations in the prematurely born infant is the usual chronologic age. Vaccine doses should not be reduced for preterm infants.
5. Pregnancy of mother or other household contact.
6. Recent exposure to an infectious disease.
7. Breast-feeding. The only vaccine virus that has been isolated from breast milk is the rubella vaccine virus. There is no good evidence that breast milk from women immunized against rubella is harmful to infants.
8. A history of nonspecific allergies or relatives with allergies.
9. Allergy to penicillin or to any other antibiotic, except anaphylactic reactions to neomycin (e.g., found in MMR) or streptomycin (e.g., found in OPV). None of the vaccines licensed in the United States contain penicillin.
10. Allergies to duck meat or duck feathers. No vaccine available in the United States is produced in substrates containing duck antigens.
11. Family history of convulsions in persons considered for pertussis or measles vaccination.

(Text continues on p. 58)

Table 14-1.   Recommended Schedule for Immunization of Healthy U.S. Children with DTP, OPV, and MMR
(See Table 14-5 for *H. influenzae* Type b Conjugate Vaccine Schedule and Table 14-7 for hepatitis B vaccine schedule)

RECOMMENDED AGE	IMMUNIZATIONS	COMMENTS
2 mo.	DTP, OPV	*H. influenzae* b vaccination begun at 2 mo.; see separate schedule. DTP and OPV can be initiated as early as 4 wk. after birth in areas of high endemicity or outbreaks
4 mo.	DTP, OPV	2-mo. interval (minimum of 6 wk.) desired for OPV
6 mo.	DTP	
15 mo.	MMR	Tuberculin testing may be done at same visit
15–18 mo.	DTP, OPV	Should be given 6 to 12 mo. after the third dose. May be given simultaneously with MMR at 15 mo.
4–6 yr.	DTP, OPV, MMR	At or before school entry. Second MMR given here or at 11–12 yr.
11–12 yr.	MMR	At entry to middle school or junior high school unless second MMR given previously
14–16 yr.	Td	Repeat every 10 yr. throughout life

(Adapted from Report of the Committeee on Infectious Diseases. 1991 Red Book, 22nd ed., p. 17. Evanston, IL, 1991.)

Table 14-2. Recommended Immunization Schedules for U.S. Children Not Immunized in the First Year of Life

RECOMMENDED TIME/AGE	IMMUNIZATIONS*	COMMENTS
Younger than 7 years First visit	DTP, OPV, MMR	MMR if child ≥15 mo. old; tuberculin testing may be done at same visit
	HbCV*†	For children aged <60 mo., can be given simultaneously with DTP and other vaccines (at separate sites)‡
Interval after first visit‡ 2 mo.	DTP, OPV (HbCV)	Second dose of HbCV is indicated only in children whose first dose was received when younger than 15 mo.
4 mo.	DTP	Third dose of OPV is not indicated in U.S.
10–16 mo.	DTP, OPV	OPV is not given if third dose was given earlier
4–6 yr. (at or before school entry)	DTP, OPV (MMR)§	DTP not necessary if fourth dose was given after fourth birthday. OPV not necessary if third dose given after fourth birthday. Second MMR may be given here or at 11–12 yr.
11–12 yr.	(MMR)§	Second MMR at entry to middle or junior high school unless given previously
10 yr. later	Td	Repeat every 10 yr. throughout life
7 years and older‖¶ First visit	Td, OPV, MMR	
Interval after first visit 2 mo.	Td, OPV	
8–14 mo.	Td, OPV	
11–12 yr.	MMR§	
10 yr. later	Td	Repeat every 10 yr. throughout life

*HbCV = *Haemophilus influenzae* type b conjugate vaccine.

†As of June 1991, two HbCVs (HbOC and PRP-OMP) have been approved for use in children less than 15 months of age (see *H. influenzae* immunization).

‡The initial three doses of DTP can be given at 1–2-month intervals; hence, for the child in whom immunization is initiated at age 15 months or older, one visit could be eliminated by giving DTP, OPV, and MMR at the first visit; DTP and HbCV at the second visit (1 month later); and DTP and OPV at the third visit (2 mo. after the first visit). Subsequent doses of DTP and OPV 10 to 16 months after the first visit are still indicated. HbCV, MMR, DTP, and OPV can be given simultaneously at separate sites if failure of the person to return for future immunizations is a concern.

§The second MMR may be given either at first entry to school or at entry to middle or junior high school.

‖If person is ≥18 years old, routine polio virus vaccination is not indicated in the U.S.

¶Minimal interval between doses of MMR is 1 month.

(Adapted from Report of the Committee on Infections Disease, 1991 Red Book, 22nd ed., p. 18. Evanston, IL, 1991.)

12. Family history of sudden infant death syndrome in children considered for DTP vaccination.
13. Family history of an adverse event, unrelated to immunosuppression, following vaccination.

SPECIAL CIRCUMSTANCES

Premature Infants

Immunization of clinically stable premature infants with full doses of vaccine should begin at 2 months of chronologic age. Data suggest an adequate immune response and no increase in adverse reactions at that time. Oral polio vaccine (OPV) should not be administered to hospitalized infants because of the possibility of transmission of the vaccine virus to an immunosuppressed patient. Inactivated polio virus vaccine (IPV) may be given while the infant is in the hospital, followed by OPV after discharge.

Immunosuppression

No live vaccines should be given to individuals with congenital immunodeficiency diseases or those on immunosuppressive therapy; household contacts of these individuals should also not receive OPV. Topical steroid therapy should not contraindicate immunization unless systemic immunosuppressive levels are achieved. Children infected with human immunodeficiency virus (HIV) and their household contacts should be given IPV, not OPV. Because wild measles virus infection can be very severe in individuals with HIV infection, the measles, mumps, rubella (MMR) vaccine should be given to HIV-infected children.

Immunoglobulin

The MMR vaccine generally should not be given within 3 months of receipt of an immunoglobulin preparation because immunoglobulins may interfere with the replication of the vaccine viruses and the immune response. If it is necessary to give immunoglobulin within 14 days of immunization with MMR, the vaccination should be repeated in 3 months. The immune response to OPV is not inhibited by immune globulin administration.

DIPHTHERIA (D), TETANUS (T), PERTUSSIS (P) VACCINES

The whole-cell DTP vaccines currently licensed in the U.S. as of July 1992 consist of formaldehyde-inactivated diphtheria and tetanus toxins (toxoids) combined with a suspension of inactivated *Bordetella pertussis* cells. This vaccine is given intramuscularly; subcutaneous administration can result in marked local reactions and therefore is not recommended. Vaccine-induced immunity to pertussis is now known to wane after vaccination; pertussis infections in previously immunized individuals are generally mild, however.

Vaccine Use

The recommended schedules of vaccinations are shown in Tables 14-1, 14-2, 14-5, and 14-7. Between *6 weeks and 6 years of age,* children should receive a primary series of four immunizations with DTP; the first begins at 6 to 8 weeks of age. The first three doses are given at 4- to 8-week intervals, and the fourth is administered 6 to 12 months after the third, usually at 15 to 18 months of age. This fourth dose can be given concurrently with other vaccines. A booster DTP is then given at age 4 to 6 years, before school entry; this booster is unnecessary if the fourth DTP was given after the fourth birthday. An acellular pertussis vaccine combined with diphtheria and tetanus (ACEL-IMUNE by Lederle-Praxis) has recently been licensed in the United States for use as the fourth and fifth immunizations. Although the acellular pertussis vaccine is probably less reactogenic than whole-cell DTP vaccines, contraindications to whole-cell DTP apply to ACEL-IMUNE. If pertussis is prevalent in an area, DTP can be initiated at 4 weeks of age. *After 7 years of age,* the dose of diphtheria vaccine is lowered, and a routine pertussis immunization is not routinely given because side effects may be more common in older children. Individuals in whom vaccination is initiated after age 7 years should receive a primary series of three doses of Td; the second dose is given 4 to 8 weeks after the first, and the third dose is given 6 to 12 months after the second. Booster doses of Td are recommended every 10 years.

Prophylactic administration of an antipyretic at the time of vaccination and then every 4 to 6 hours will reduce the incidence of postvaccination fever and may be particularly beneficial for children at risk for seizures with fever.

Special Circumstances

When pertussis vaccination is contraindicated for a child under 7 years of age (see "Precautions and Contraindications," below), the DT combination is substituted for DTP. If immunization is begun with DT and it is subsequently determined that the child can be safely given pertussis immunization, DTP is then given to complete the recommended pertussis immunization schedule. The total number of doses of D and T should not exceed six before the fourth birthday. Because infections with diphtheria or tetanus may not confer protection, vaccination should still be performed following these infections. Pertussis infection is generally followed by lifelong immunity; children who have had disease that was confirmed by culture to be due to *B. pertussis* need not receive further pertussis immunization.

Tetanus prophylaxis for wounds varies depending upon the nature of the wound and the person's immunization history. Patients with minor, uncontaminated wounds who have already received a primary series of three tetanus immunizations require only a booster if the last tetanus shot was given over 10 years ago. If the patient with a clean, minor wound has not received the primary series, or if the vaccination history is unknown, a tetanus booster should be administered. The management of more serious wounds (such as those contaminated with dirt, feces, or saliva; puncture wounds; and those with devitalized tissue) is as follows: (1) If the patient has received three tetanus immunizations in the past, a booster should be given if more than 5 years have elapsed since the last dose. (2) A person whose primary series was incomplete or whose immunization history is unclear should be given both a tetanus booster and a tetanus immune globulin (250–500 U intramuscularly) by separate syringes at separate sites. Individuals with AIDS who sustain tetanus-prone wounds should be given tetanus immune globulin regardless of their immunization status. In all of the above situations, DTP (DT if pertussis vaccine is contraindicated) is preferred to tetanus toxoid alone for children under 7 years of age, and Td is preferred to tetanus toxoid alone in those older than 7 years.

Side effects and adverse reactions are listed in Table 14-3. Local reactions consisting of erythema, induration, and tenderness at the injection site occur commonly following immunization with DTP. Occasionally a nodule and rarely an abscess will form at the injection site. Frequently seen mild-to-moderate systemic reactions are transient mild-to-moderate fever, drowsiness, fretfulness, anorexia, vomiting, and crying. These symptoms are significantly more common following immunization with DTP than they are with DT. Although children who have experienced those reactions are more likely than other children to experience them again, subsequent doses of DTP should be given. More serious systemic events occur infrequently; these include fever ≥ 104.9°F (40.5°C) persistent inconsolable crying (≥3 hours), unusual high-pitched crying, collapse or shocklike state (hypotonic–hyporesponsive episode), and seizures. No permanent sequelae have been documented as

Table 14-3. Adverse Events Occurring Within 48 Hours of DTP Immunizations

EVENT	RATE (%) PER DOSE
Local redness	37
Local swelling	41
Local pain	51
Fever ≥38°C (100.4°F)	47
Drowsiness	32
Fretfulness	53
Anorexia	21
Vomiting	6
Persistent crying ≥3 hr.	1
High-pitched, unusual cry	0.1
Convulsions	0.06
Hypotonic, hyporesponsive episode	0.06

(Adapted from Cody CL, Baraff LJ, Cherry JD, Marcy SM, Manclark CR. Nature and rates of adverse reactions associated with DTP and DT immunizations in infants and children. Pediatrics 68:650–660, 1981.)

occurring after these reactions. Alleged reactions, including encephalopathy and permanent brain damage, occurring in temporal association with DTP vaccination have been thought to be very rarely due to the pertussis vaccine. After a reanalysis of past data, the American Academy of Pediatrics Committee on Infectious Diseases and others have concluded that whole-cell pertussis vaccine has not been proved to be a cause of brain damage.

Anaphylactic reactions following DTP immunization are exceedingly rare. Transient urticarial rashes are sometimes seen postvaccination. Unless the rash occurs within minutes of vaccination, it is unlikely to be an anaphylactic reaction and thus does not contraindicate further doses of vaccine.

Precautions and Contraindications

Before each dose of DTP, the parent or guardian should be asked about adverse reactions following the preceding DTP. Further immunization with pertussis vaccine is usually contraindicated if any of the following have occurred after receipt of DTP or P: immediate, severe allergic reaction; fever ≥104.9°F (40.5°C) within 48 hours and unexplained by another cause; persistent, inconsolable crying for ≥3 hours or unusual high-pitched crying occurring within 48 hours; convulsion (febrile or afebrile) within 3 days; encephalopathy or severe acute neurologic illness within 7 days; or collapse or shocklike state (hypotonic–hyporesponsive episode) within 48 hours. Pertussis immunization should be withheld when a child has a neurologic disorder that is progressive, unstable, or evolving (e.g., uncontrolled epilepsy, infantile spasms, or progressive encephalopathy) because further immunizations may coincide with or even exacerbate symptoms. Children who have experienced seizures (febrile or afebrile) have an increased risk of postimmunization convulsions. If the child has experienced a recent seizure, it is prudent to defer immunization until a progressive neurologic disorder has been excluded. Children with a neurologic condition that is stable, corrected, or controlled, such as well-controlled seizures or cerebral palsy, may be vaccinated. Infants for whom the decision has been made to defer pertussis immunization should not be given DT in the first year of life. At the first birthday, the decision of whether or not to give pertussis immunization should be made and either DT or DTP immunizations initiated. The reasons for withholding immunizations during the first year are: (1) a child is unlikely to sustain a tetanus-prone wound before he is ambulatory and (2) one should not give more than six DT immunizations prior to 4 years of age. Children with a family history of seizures have a higher risk of convulsion after pertussis vaccination; however, a family history of seizures is not a contraindication to pertussis vaccination. The parents of children at increased risk of seizure postvaccination should be informed and advised about fever control and measures to take should the child have a convulsion.

POLIOVIRUS VACCINES

Formulations

Oral polio vaccine (OPV) and inactivated polio vaccine (IPV) are licensed in the United States; both contain all three strains of poliovirus. The OPV vaccine consists of live attenuated poliovirus and is given by mouth, whereas IPV is killed virus that is administered subcutaneously. A highly immunogenic enhanced-potency IPV was licensed in 1988. OPV is currently recommended as the vaccine of choice for primary immunization of immunocompetent children in the United States. Advantages of OPV over IPV are that it is simple to administer; it induces intestinal immunity; it is excreted in stool, which results in immunization of some contacts; and it has virtually eliminated disease in the United States. The disadvantage of OPV is that there is a rare association with paralytic disease in vaccine recipients or their contacts. Parents should be informed of the option of IPV and the benefits and risks of both vaccines.

Vaccine Use

The OPV vaccine is generally given as a primary series of three doses integrated with DTP (at 2, 4, and 18 months of age). The third dose can be given anytime between 12 and 24 months of age and can be given with DTP, MMR, and *Haemophilus influenzae* vaccines. A booster dose of OPV is then given before school entry, at 4 to 6 years of age. In high-risk areas, an additional dose of OPV is given at 6 months of age (Table 14-1). For children who were not immunized in infancy, two doses of OPV should be given 6 to 8 months apart, a third dose 6 to 12 months later, and a booster at school entry (Table 14-2). The schedule for IPV administration is essentially the same as that for OPV administration. The first two doses are given at 4- to 8-week intervals, and a third dose is given 6 to 12 months later, with a booster at school entry. When IPV vaccination is initiated in infancy, it is generally given concomitantly with DTP doses 1, 2, 4, and 5.

Because OPV is shed in the stools, inadequately immu-nized adult contacts have a very small risk of developing OPV-associated paralytic disease. Parents should be informed of this very small risk and should be advised to take precautions when handling the infant's stools. If prompt immunization of the child can be assured, unimmunized adult contacts may be given a series of IPV prior to administering OPV to the child. *Under no circumstances should OPV be administered to immunosuppressed individuals or if there is an immunosuppressed household contact.* Immunosuppressed persons are those with HIV infection, immunodeficiency diseases, altered immune states, and immunosuppressive therapy, including radiation therapy. If OPV is given inadvertently to a household contact of a person who is immunosuppressed, the two should avoid close contact for 2 months.

Adverse Reactions

The IPV vaccine contains trace amounts of streptomycin and neomycin; individuals allergic to these antibiotics may experience a hypersensitivity reaction. There is a rare occurrence of paralytic poliomyelitis associated with OPV administration, as discussed above.

HAEMOPHILUS INFLUENZAE TYPE B CONJUGATE VACCINES

H. influenzae type b conjugate vaccines (HbCVs) consist of the capsular polysaccharide polyribosylribitol phosphate (PRP) conjugated to a protein carrier. This conjugation converts PRP from a T-cell–independent antigen to a T-cell–dependent antigen, which (1) results in the stimulation of antibody levels higher than those found in PRP alone, (2) renders it immunogenic in young infants, and (3) results in anamnestic or booster responses upon revaccination. HbCVs produced by different manufacturers are dissimilar because the protein carriers and methods of conjugation are different. As a result of this biochemical variability, the vaccines are immunologically different and the schedule of vaccination is unique to each.

Table 14-4. *H. influenzae* Type b Conjugate Vaccines

MANUFACTURER	ABBREVIATION	TRADE NAME	CARRIER PROTEIN	LICENSED BY THE FDA (AS OF FEB. 92)
Connaught Laboratories	PRP-D	ProHIBit®	Diphtheria toxoid	For children ≥ 15 months of age
Praxis Biologics, Inc. (Distributed by Lederle Laboratories)	HbOC	HibTITER™	CRM197 (a non-toxic mutant diphtheria toxin)	For infants & children ≥ 2 months of age
Merck Sharp & Dohme	PRP-OMP	PedvaxHIB™	OMP (an outer membrane protein complex of *Neisseria meningitidus*)	For infants & children ≥ 2 months of age
Pasteur Merieux Vaccins	PRP-T	—	Tetanus toxoid	Not licensed

(From Committee on Infectious Diseases, American Academy of Pediatrics. *Haemophilus influenzae* Type b Conjugate Vaccines: Recommendations for Immunization of Infants and Children 2 Months of Age and Older: Update. 1991.)

Table 14-5. Summary of Recommended Regimens for Use of *H. influenzae*
Type b Vaccines

AGE IMMUNIZATION INITIATED (MONTHS)	VACCINE PRODUCT USED AT INITIATION	TOTAL NUMBER OF DOSES TO BE CURRENTLY ADMINIS- TERED	RECOMMENDED VACCINE REGIMENS (SEE TEXT)
2–6	HbOC	4	a. Initial 3 doses at 2-month intervals b. Fourth dose at 15 months of age* c. HbOC for doses 1–3 d. HbOC, PRP-OMP, or PRP-D for dose 4*
	PRP-OMP	3	a. Initial 2 doses at 2-month intervals b. Third dose at 12 months of age c. PRP-OMP for all three doses†
7–11	HbOC	3	a. Initial 2 doses at 2-month intervals b. Third dose at 15–18 months of age* c. HbOC, for doses 1–2 d. HbOC, PRP-OMP, or PRP-D for dose 3*
	PRP-OMP	3	1. Initial 2 doses at 2-month intervals b. Third dose at 15–18 months of age* c. PRP-OMP for doses 1–2 d. PRP-OMP, PRP-D, or HbOC for dose 3*
12–14	HbOC	2	a. 2–3-month interval between doses b. If the second dose is given at or after 15 months, HbOC, PRP-OMP, or PRP-D may be given*
	PRP-OMP	2	a. 2–3-month interval between doses b. If the second dose is given at or after 15 months, PRP-OMP, PRP-D, or HbOC may be given*
15–59	HbOC PRP-OMP PRP-D	1	HbOC, PRP-OMP, or PRP-D†
60 and older‡	HbOC PRP-OMP PRP-D	1	HbOC, PRP-OMP, or PRP-D

*The American Academy of Pediatrics considers that safety and efficacy are likely to be equivalent for PRP-OMP, PRP-D, and HbOC for use in children 15 months of age or older.

†If the third dose is inadvertently delayed until the child is 15 months of age or older, the Academy considers that the safety and efficacy are likely to be equivalent for PRP-OMP, PRP-D, and HbOC for this third dose.

‡Only for children with chronic illness known to be associated with an increased risk for *H. influenzae* type b disease (see text).

(Adapted from Committee on Infectious Diseases, American Academy of Pediatrics. *Haemophilus influenzae* Type b Conjugate Vaccines: Recommendations for Immunizations of Infants and Children 2 Months of Age and Older: Update. 1991.)

Vaccine Use

Four HbCVs have been extensively studied in young infants; three are licensed for use in the United States at this time, and it is anticipated that the fourth will soon be licensed (Table 14-4). Two are licensed to be given beginning at 2 months of age (HbOC and PRP-OMP). The third (PRP-D) is licensed for use only in children 15 months of age and over because it is poorly immunogenic in young infants and because protection conferred in infancy has been inconsistent. Any of the three licensed vaccines can be used for immunization after 15 months regardless of the type of vaccine given previously.

Infants should be immunized with a conjugate vaccine beginning at 2 months of age or as soon as possible thereafter (Table 14-5). Routine immunization of infants under 7 months of age should consist of either three doses of HbOC separated by 2-month intervals and a third dose at 15 months, or two doses of PRP-OMP given at 2-month intervals and a third dose at 12 months. Until it has been established that HbOC and PRP-OMP are interchangeable, it is recommended that for children under 15 months of age all of the immunizations be with the same vaccine. Recommendations for the immunization of children who were not vaccinated in early infancy are outlined in Table 14-6. Children 7 to 11 months of age should be given two doses of either PRP-OMP or HbOC separated by 2 months, with a third dose of any licensed conjugate vaccine between

Table 14-6. Recommended Doses and Schedules of Currently Licensed Hepatitis B Vaccines*

	VACCINE			
	Recombivax HB		Engerix-B	
GROUP	Dose (μg)	(ml)	Dose (μg)	(ml)
Infants of HBsAg-negative mothers and children <11 years	2.5	(0.25)	10	(0.5)
Infants of HBsAg-positive mothers. Prevention of perinatal infection	5	(0.05)	10	(0.5)
Children and adolescents 11–19 years	5	(0.5)	20	(1.0)
Adults ≥20 years	10	(1.0)	20	(1.0)
Dialysis patients and other immunocompromised persons	40	(1.0)[†]	40	(2.0)[‡]

*See Table 14-7 for dose schedule.
[†]Special formulation for dialysis patients.
[‡]Four-dose schedule recommended at 0, 1, 2, and 12 months.
(From Centers for Disease Control. Protection against viral hepatitis: Recommendations of the Immunization Practices Advisory Committee. MMWR 40(RR-13):13; Nov. 1991.)

15 and 18 months of age. Immunization of children 12 to 14 months old should consist of two doses of PRP-OMP or HbOC separated by 2 months. Unimmunized children between 15 and 60 months of age may be given one dose of any licensed HbCV vaccine.

Special Circumstances

Unimmunized children over 5 years of age with an illness that puts them at increased risk of *H. influenzae* type b infections, such as sickle cell disease or asplenia, should receive one dose of a conjugate vaccine. If possible, children with Hodgkin's disease should be immunized 2 or more weeks prior to the induction of chemotherapy. There are no known contraindications to giving conjugate vaccine at the same time as pneumococcal and meningococcal vaccine.

Unimmunized children less than 24 months of age who develop invasive *H. influenzae* type b infection should be immunized upon convalescence, because an adequate antibody response may not have been stimulated by the infection. At this point in time, rifampin prophylaxis is still recommended for appropriate contacts exposed to an individual with invasive *H. influenzae* type b disease regardless of the vaccination status of the individual.

The HbCV vaccine may be given at the same time as OPV (or IPV), DTP, or MMR. If at the 15-month visit a choice has to be made to give either MMR or HbCV, it is recommended that priority be given to MMR and that the child be brought back for the HbCV. Studies are currently under way to evaluate the immunogenicity and safety of giving HbCV mixed in the same syringe with DTP. At this point, the vaccines are to be given by separate syringes at different sites.

Side effects and adverse reactions are uncommon and consist of low-grade fever and mild local reactions.

MEASLES, MUMPS, RUBELLA VACCINES

Vaccines consisting of live, attenuated strains of the measles, mumps, rubella virus were licensed in the United States in the 1960s. Measles infection reached an all-time low in 1983 when 1497 cases were reported, which represented a decrease of more than 95% from the prevaccine era when virtually all children were infected by age 15. There has been a progressive increase in measles since then, with 27,672 cases reported in 1990. Outbreaks of mumps also are occurring in colleges, and congenital rubella infections may be increasing.

The two age groups primarily affected in the current measles resurgence are unimmunized preschool children and immunized adolescents and young adults. Outbreaks among the latter appear to be a consequence of the small percentage of individuals who do not respond to a single vaccination; some degree of waning vaccine-induced immunity may also play a role. In 1989, a two-dose schedule of measles, mumps, rubella (MMR) vaccine was introduced to eliminate this small pool of susceptibles, and thus the opportunity for outbreaks in this older age group. Increased attention also must be directed at improving immunization levels of preschool children, particularly poor, inner-city children.

Vaccine Use

Measles, mumps, and rubella vaccines are available as individual vaccines and combined as MMR. All of the preparations must be stored at 2 to 8°C and protected from light. The combined MMR is the preparation of choice for all routine childhood vaccination programs, and a dose of 0.5 ml is given subcutaneously. Because the optimal seroresponse to measles vaccination may not occur until 15 months of age, it is recommended that the first MMR routinely be given at that age. The age of first vaccination may be lowered to 12 months in areas with continuing measles activity. In outbreak situations, monovalent measles vaccine (MMR if monovalent is unavailable) may be given to infants as young as 6 months. Children vaccinated prior to 12 months of age should be considered unvaccinated and should receive two further MMR immunizations. The Advisory Committee on Immunization Practices (ACIP) of the Public Health Service has recommended that the second dose be given at age 4 to 6 years. The reason for choosing that age is simply that it is practical; all states have laws in force requiring compliance with immunizations for school entry. Children who have not received MMR at school entry may be vaccinated, allowed to begin school, and revaccinated 1 month later. The disadvantage of this policy is that it will require several years before it will lower the incidence of measles among adolescents. Primarily for this reason, the Committee on Infectious Diseases of the American Academy of Pediatrics (AAP) has recommended that the second dose be administered at 11 to 12 years of age. Vaccination at 11 to 12 years also offers the theoretical advantage of boosting antibody closer to the period of probable need. In some areas, local public health regulations may dictate practice. Until all young adults have received two doses, a second dose of vaccine is recommended upon college entry for those who have had only one previous vaccination. Children who have had physician-documented measles or laboratory evidence of measles immunity are considered immune and need not be revaccinated.

Early measles vaccines that may have resulted in inadequate immunity were inactivated vaccines (available between 1963 and 1967 in the United States) and further attenuated vaccines given with immune globulin. Two doses of MMR, separated by 1 month or more, should be given to individuals known to have received these vaccines, those who received a vaccine of unknown type between 1963 and 1967, and those who received a vaccine of unknown type with immune globulin.

Side Effects and Adverse Reactions

Five to fifteen percent of recipients of the measles vaccine may develop a fever ≥103°F beginning 5 to 12 days after vaccination and usually lasting several days. Transient rashes are also reported in approximately 5% of vaccinees. Children with a personal or family history of convulsions may have a slightly increased risk of seizures after measles vaccination. Parents should be advised of this fact and should treat fever aggressively. A person who previously received the killed measles vaccine has a small risk of ex-

periencing an extensive local reaction and prolonged fever following receipt of the live measles vaccine. It is the consensus of both the ACIP and AAP that this risk of revaccination is outweighed by the risk of severe atypical measles that individuals who received the killed measles vaccine may develop when exposed to the wild measles virus. Adverse reactions attributable to the rubella vaccine include low-grade fever, rash, and lymphadenopathy 5 to 12 days postvaccination, and transient joint pain 1 to 3 weeks after vaccination in a small percentage of recipients (≤3%). The joint pain is usually in small peripheral joints and is more frequent in previously unvaccinated postpubertal females. Transient peripheral neuritic complaints such as paresthesia and pain in the arms and legs have been reported rarely following rubella vaccination. Reports of illnesses following mumps vaccination have primarily been episodes of parotitis and low-grade fever.

Precautions and Contraindications

The MMR vaccine, or any of its components, should not be given to *pregnant* women or those considering becoming pregnant within 3 months of vaccination because of the theoretical risk of infection of the fetus. The recommended precaution in immunizing female adolescents is to simply ask them if they are pregnant, exclude those who are, and explain the theoretical risks to the others. Pregnant women immunized with rubella vaccine who are known to have been susceptible at the time of vaccination should be reported to the Division of Immunization, Centers for Disease Control. Because rubella vaccine during pregnancy has not been documented to result in congenital defects, it is not ordinarily an indication to interrupt pregnancy.

Persons with a history of *anaphylactic reactions* either to neomycin or after egg ingestion should be vaccinated only with extreme caution. Individuals who have recently received *antibody-containing blood products* (immune globulin, whole blood) should have MMR deferred for 3 months because passively acquired antibodies might interfere with the immune response to the vaccine. *Skin testing for tuberculosis* is not a prerequisite for measles vaccination; however, vaccination may suppress the reaction to tuberculin skin tests. If tuberculosis testing is to be done, it should be performed the day of vaccination or 4 to 6 weeks after immunization.

Significantly *immunocompromised* individuals, with the exception of those with HIV infection, should not be given MMR; this includes persons with immune-deficiency diseases, leukemia, lymphoma, and generalized malignancy, and those undergoing therapy with alkylating agents, antimetabolites, radiation, or large doses of corticosteroids. The administration of vaccine is not contraindicated by the following: patients with leukemia in remission who have not received chemotherapy for at least 3 months; short-term (<2 weeks), low- to moderate-dose systemic corticosteroid therapy; topical steroid therapy; long-term alternate-day treatment with low to moderate doses of short-acting systemic steroids; and intra-articular, bursal, or tendon injection of corticosteroids. Because the vaccine virus strains in MMR are not transmitted from one individual to another, contacts of immunocompromised persons may be vaccinated with MMR. The MMR vaccine is also recommended for patients with HIV infection, symptomatic or asymptomatic, because of the severity of wild measles infection in these individuals. Regardless of the vaccination status, symptomatic HIV-infected patients who are exposed to measles should receive IG prophylaxis.

HEPATITIS B VACCINE

There are two hepatitis B vaccines currently licensed in the United States. The original plasma-derived vaccine consisting of a suspension of inactivated, alum-absorbed, 22-nm HBsAg particles (Heptavax-B) is no longer being produced in the United States. The two vaccines in current production (Recombivax-HB and ENERGIX-B) are both produced by yeast (*Saccharomyces cerevisiae*), into which the gene governing the production of HBsAg has been inserted.

Vaccine Use

The dose of vaccine varies by manufacturer and by age and immune status of the recipient (Tables 14-6 and 14-7). All hepatitis B vaccines are inactivated products, and there is no evidence of interference with other vaccines administered at the same time but it should not be mixed in the same syringe with other vaccines. Also, passively acquired antibody to hepatitis B will not interfere with vaccine-induced immunity.

Both hepatitis vaccines are effective, but the duration of immunity is unknown. It is not recommended to routinely measure antibody levels except for babies born to HBsAg-positive women. These babies should have their serologic status measured at 9 months, and if the child is negative for both anti-HBsAg and HBsAg, a fourth dose of vaccine is recommended.

Universal hepatitis B immunization of infants is now recommended in the United States; vaccinations should be given in accordance to the schedule in Table 14-7. The alternative regimen of having the first dose at 1 to 2 months of age is acceptable only if the mother is HBsAg-negative. Three other points are emphasized for infants born to HBsAg-positive women. They should: (1) receive a larger dose of vaccine than babies born to HBsAg-negative mothers (see Table 14-6); (2) receive one dose of HBIG as soon after birth as possible; and (3) receive their second dose at 1 month and third dose at 6 months of age. If the mother's HBsAg status is unknown at the time of delivery, she should be considered to be HBsAg-positive until her serologic status is determined. Thus, the infant should be vaccinated within 12 hours of birth and be given HBIG shortly after birth.

Table 14-7. Recommended Routine Hepatitis B Immunization Schedule

MATERNAL HBsAg STATUS	DOSE	AGE
Negative*	1	1–2 d
	2	1–2 mo
	3	6–18 mo
Positive†	1†	0–12 h
	2	1 mo
	3	6 mo

*Alternative schedule: dose one at 1–2 mo of age, dose 2 at 4 mo, and dose 3 at 6–18 mo.
†Administered with HBIG.
Adapted from AAP News, February 1992.

High-Risk Groups

Groups recommended for routine vaccination are those at increased risk for hepatitis B infection, including the following:

1. Health-care workers with significant exposure to blood.
2. Susceptible clients and staff of residential institutions for the developmentally disabled. Clients discharged from residential institutions into community settings should be screened for HBsAg so that appropriate prophylaxis of contacts may be undertaken. Vaccination of staff and clients in day-care programs for the developmentally disabled should be strongly encouraged if an HBsAg-positive classmate behaves aggressively or has medical problems that increse the risk of exposure to his blood or serous secretions.
3. Hemodialysis patients
4. Sexually active homosexual and bisexual males
5. Users of illicit injectable drugs
6. Hemophiliacs and other patients who receive clotting-factor concentrates
7. Household and sexual contacts of hepatitis B carriers. Adoptees from countries of high HBV endemicity (Africa, Asia) should be screened for HBsAg.
8. Heterosexual persons with multiple sexual partners in the last 6 months or with recently acquired sexually transmitted diseases
9. Travelers to highly endemic areas who plan to stay for more than 6 months or have intimate contact with the local population

The AAP also recommends that adolescents receive universal immunization when resources permit.

Postexposure prophylaxis for hepatitis B should be provided in the following situations: perinatal exposure of an infant born to an HBsAg-positive mother; an infant less than 12 months of age exposed to a primary caregiver who has acute hepatitis B; percutaneous or permucosal exposure to HBsAg-positive blood; and sexual exposure to an HBsAg-positive person. The reader is referred to Chapter 110,

"Hepatitis," for a discussion of prophylaxis of percutaneous and sexual exposures.

Side Effects and Adverse Reactions

Soreness at the injection site is the most common side effect. Hypersensitivity to yeast or the preservative, thimerosal, has been reported.

VACCINATIONS FOR SELECTED POPULATIONS

Several vaccines that are not part of the routine childhood immunization program are required for children with certain chronic medical conditions. Indications for and details of administration of pneumococcal, meningococcal, and influenza vaccines are listed in Table 14-8.

FUTURE

We are in an era of rapid evolution of childhood immunizations as new and improved vaccines become available.

These are exciting advances, but they necessitate that pediatric providers remain updated on changing recommendations. Two infections for which there are ongoing intensive vaccine development efforts are varicella and rotavirus. It is anticipated that varicella vaccine will be licensed for use in normal children in the near future.

BIBLIOGRAPHY

Centers for Disease Control. General recommendations on immunization: Recommendations of the Immunization Practices Advisory Committee (ACIP). MMWR 38(38):205–227, 1989.

Centers for Disease Control: *Haemophilus* b conjugate vaccines for prevention of *Haemophilus influenzae* type b disease among infants and children two months of age and older: Recommendations of the Immunization Practices Advisory Committee (ACIP). MMWR 40(RR-1):1–7, 1991.

Centers for Disease Control. Measles prevention: Recommendations of the Immunization Practices Advisory Committee (ACIP). MMWR 38(S-9):1–18, 1989.

Table 14-8.   Miscellaneous Vaccinations for Selected Populations

VACCINE	FORMULATION	TARGET POPULATION	USAGE*
Pneumococcal	23 valent polysaccharide vaccine	Children ≥ 2 yr. with sickle cell disease, anatomic or functional asplenia, nephrotic syndrome or chronic renal failure, CSF leaks, conditions associated with immunosuppression (including HIV infection)	0.5 ml SQ or IM
Meningoccocal	Quadrivalent A, C, Y, W-135 polysaccharide vaccine	Children ≥ 2 yr. with anatomic or functional asplenia or terminal C' component deficiencies	0.5 ml SQ
Influenza	Killed influenza strains, generally 2A and 1B strains	Children with chronic pulmonary diseases, hemodynamically significant cardiac disease, hemoglobinopathy, immunosuppression, long-term aspirin, significant renal or metabolic diseases Vaccination also recommended for providers of care to, and household contacts of, high-risk individuals	*6–35 mo.*[†] 0.25 ml of split virus, 2 doses separated by ≥ 4 weeks *3–8 yr.*[†] 0.5 ml of split virus, 2 doses separated by ≥ 4 weeks *9–12 yr.* 0.5 ml of split virus, 1 dose *≥ 12 yr.* 0.5 ml of whole or split virus, 1 dose

*Check package insert for recommended dose and route.

[†]Two doses are recommended for children <9 years of age who are receiving influenza vaccine for the first time (based upon recommendations for 1990–1991). If vaccine strains have not changed, one dose yearly thereafter.

Centers for Disease Control. Meningococcal vaccines: Recommendations of the Immunization Practices Advisory Committee (ACIP). MMWR 34(18):255–259, 1985.

Centers for Disease Control. Mumps prevention: Recommendations of the Immunization Practices Advisory Committee (ACIP). MMWR 38(22):388-400, 1989.

Centers for Disease Control. Pneumococcal polysaccharide vaccine: Recommendations of the Immunization Practices Advisory Committee (ACIP). MMWR 38(5):64–76, 1989.

Centers for Disease Control. Prevention and control of influenzae: Recommendations of the Immunization Practices Advisory Committee (ACIP). MMWR 39(RR-7):1–15, 1990.

Centers for Disease Control. Rubella prevention: Recommendations of the Immunization Practices Advisory Committee (ACIP). MMWR 39(RR-15):1–18, 1990.

Centers for Disease Control. Vaccine adverse event reporting system— United States. MMWR 39(41):730–733, 1990.

Centers for Disease Control. Hepatitis B virus: A comprehensive strategy for eliminating transmission in the United States through universal childhood vaccinations. MMWR 40(RR-13):1–19, 1991.

Committee on Infectious Diseases of the American Academy of Pediatrics. *Haemophilus influenzae* type b conjugate vaccines: Recommendation for immunization of infants and children 2 months of age and older: Update. 1991.

Committee on Infectious Diseases of the American Academy of Pediatrics. Measles: Reassessment of the current immunization policy. Pediatrics 84(6):1110–1113, 1989.

Report of the Committee on Infectious Diseases of the American Academy of Pediatrics. Red Book, 22nd ed. Elk Grove Village, IL, American Academy of Pediatrics, 1991.

15

Vegetarianism

Katherine Kaufer Christoffel

All pediatricians are likely to have some patients who are vegetarians. The number of vegetarian children in a practice may be substantial in some areas because of clustering of families who share ethnic origins, religion, or beliefs that promote vegetarianism. The practicing pediatrician needs to be familiar with various types of vegetarian diets and their dietary strengths and weaknesses to be able to evaluate possible advantages or disadvantages of a particular diet for a particular patient, and when to enlist a dietitian's help in dietary assessment.

The pediatrician may become aware from several indications that a child is on a vegetarian diet. The parent may sometimes volunteer the information. More often, the pediatrician learns of the atypical diet while taking a dietary history to assess a problem that may be related to diet, such as iron-deficiency anemia. It is preferable to know about a child's diet before problems arise so that likely problems can be anticipated; thus, a brief dietary history should be a routine part of office practice. Anticipatory guidance concerning the composition of the diet can then be tailored to prevent or minimize growth disturbances and dietary deficiencies. (See Chapter 12, "Nutrition and Nutritional Status: An Overview.")

MOTIVATIONS OF VEGETARIAN FAMILIES

Vegetarian diets may be less expensive than omnivorous diets, but economics is not a common reason for the adoption of a vegetarian diet. The diet is chosen most often because the mother or father believes that the family will benefit from it, in terms of either health or spirituality. Because a family's motives are likely to affect specific food choices, it is essential that the reasons be identified and understood by the pediatrician (Table 15-1).

TYPES OF VEGETARIANISM

Parents may mean different things when they classify themselves as vegetarians. Therefore, it is necessary to make inquiries regarding which specific food categories they avoid. Although many intermediate types of vegetarian diets exist, there are four common ones. *Ovolactovegetarians* consume eggs and milk as well as vegetable foods; they are the largest group of vegetarians worldwide and within the United States. *Ovovegetarians* consume eggs and vegetable foods, but they avoid milk. *Lactovegetarians* consume milk and vegetable foods, but they avoid eggs. *Vegans* eat only foods of vegetable origin, avoiding both milk and eggs as well as flesh foods. In addition, a large and possibly growing number of Americans may be described as *semivegetarians*. They eat flesh foods sparingly (often only fish and fowl) and thus they have a diet that in many ways resembles that of ovolactovegetarians. Followers of *macrobiotic* diets restrict their diets in various ways and to varying degrees. Some macrobiotic diets are comparable to omnivorous American diets; others are severely restricted vegan diets.

Individuals who adopt vegetarianism may lack familiarity with traditional ways of maximizing the nutritional value of vegetarian meals by combining foods with complementary nutrients. An assessment of the adequacy of a family's vegetarian diet therefore requires information about meal planning as well as about categories of foods used and avoided. Particular attention should be given to the protein content of meals, which may be low in vegan diets if the family does not use ample soy products and does not follow the principles of protein complementarity (which assure appropriate balance of the eight essential amino acids).

VEGETARIANISM AT DIFFERENT AGES

Dietary needs vary with a child's growth and activity. Consequently, the likely positive and negative effects of vege-

Table 15-1. Motivations for Vegetarianism

MOTIVE	ANTICIPATED BENEFIT
Health/Nutrition	
Lower calories	Less obesity, hypertension
Lower fat (especially saturated)	Less atherosclerosis
Less pesticides/hormones	Less cancer
More fiber/bulk	Less constipation, cancer
Spiritual	
Religious tenets	Obedience/conformity/ blessedness
Respect animal life	Ecologic awareness
Economic	
Lower family food costs	Budget stretching
Lower world food costs	Famine relief
Food Preference	Enjoying meals more
Cultural/Social	Following familiar or favored customs

tarian diets on children vary at different stages of development.

During *prenatal* life, fetal well-being depends mainly on maternal nutritional status. The physician's usual attentiveness is warranted to assure that the mother consumes the necessary calories, calcium, and iron. Extra attention is required to assure that vegetarian mothers receive adequate vitamin B_{12} and vitamin D, because mothers deficient in these vitamins put their infants at risk of abnormal postnatal growth and development. The motives of some individuals in following vegetarianism also favor the use of megavitamins or other unusual nutritional supplements. The possibility of toxicity or of a postnatal withdrawal state must be explored if a pregnant mother uses any such supplements.

In *infancy,* nutrition depends on breast milk or infant formula. Breast milk fatty acid composition reflects the mother's (vegetarian or omnivorous) diet; total fat content may rarely be reduced if the mother's diet is severely limited.

If a vegetarian mother is deficient in a nutrient (e.g., vitamin B_{12} in a vegan mother), her newborn baby may also suffer from a deficiency. Most nutritional considerations for infants of well-nourished vegetarian mothers are not different from those for other infants, but some are unique. As in prenatal life, if a nursing mother takes megadoses of vitamins or other atypical nutritional supplements, the possibility of risk to the infant must be considered, as it would be for a prescribed medication. Some vegetarian mothers prefer to prepare their own formulas, usually based on soybeans or almonds, with added oils, vitamins, or other ingredients. The nutritional adequacy of such formulas varies and must be specifically assessed if deficiencies and toxicities are to be avoided. Vegetarian infants who are fed the usual commercial formulas do not have any special dietary problems.

During *childhood,* vegetarian diets can readily meet the child's needs if properly balanced or appropriately supplemented. Children who grow up in vegetarian households become accustomed to the family diet, just as other children do. However, unless they live in a self-contained vegetarian community, children from vegetarian families face the social/cultural conflicts that arise for all children whose families differ from the mainstream culture. The degree of conflict faced by vegetarian children is likely to be proportional to the degree to which the families are atypical (i.e., least for semivegetarians and most for vegan macrobiotics). The pediatrician can help children and parents find ways to deal with these conflicts that respect both the values that underlie the choice of the vegetarian diet and also the child's inevitable drive to conform to societal norms. Such conflicts are predictably accentuated during *adolescence.* At the same time, nutritional requirements increase (e.g., for calories, protein, calcium, and iron). The adolescent's physical and emotional needs must be assessed and the diet evaluated and adjusted if necessary to meet those needs.

Although it is possible to become (or remain) obese on a vegetarian diet, individuals on vegetarian diets are generally leaner than those on omnivorous diets. This may sometimes be an advantage; thus, the pediatrician may suggest that some families with obese children explore vegetarian ways of eating.

Although nutrient deficiencies do occur, particularly on severely restricted diets, the benefits of sound life-long vegetarian nutrition for most adherents are substantial. When compared to their omnivorous counterparts, *adult* vegetarians tend to be leaner and to have lower cholesterol and blood pressure levels, a lower incidence of gallstones, less constipation, and less diabetes. There is also evidence of lower rates of diverticulosis, colon cancer, and osteoporosis.

Internationally, lower levels of food intake from animal sources are associated with reduced mortality from coronary heart disease and breast cancer, and possibly also from colon cancer.

AREAS TO MONITOR

Because vegetarian diets are often defined by food avoidances, monitoring of vegetarian children for dietary deficiencies and growth disturbances should be even more thorough than similar monitoring of omnivorous children (Table 15-2). There is good evidence that vegetarian diets have no adverse effect on intelligence; thus, special monitoring of this aspect of child development is not required.

Growth

Vegetarian children are generally lighter and leaner than their omnivorous peers.

Linear growth of vegetarian children may be slower than that of omnivorous children, particularly after weaning. Growth velocity, however, is generally not impaired unless

Table 15-2.   Most Likely Dietary Deficiencies

DIET	CALORIES	PROTEIN	ZINC	CALCIUM	VITAMIN D	VITAMIN B₁₂	IRON
Semivegetarian			X				
Ovolactovegetarian			X				
Lactovegetarian			X				†
Ovovegetarian			X	X	X	*	X
Vegan	X	X	X	X	X	X	†
Macrobiotic‡	?	?	?	?	?	?	?

*Vitamin B₁₂ is in the yolk; a deficiency is possible if the yolk is discarded or rarely eaten.
†Iron in egg yolk iṣ poorly absorbed.
‡Depends on the degree of dietary restriction.

dietary restrictions are severe. As for any child, if growth is poor, the diet must be examined for adequacy.

Table 15-3 shows the most common vegetarian dietary patterns and their consequences and makes it clear that the effects of a child's diet are difficult to predict. However, certain areas warrant monitoring.

Caloric intake may be inadequate if the diet is excessively rich in vegetable bulk, which can induce early satiety. Caloric deficiency is also possible if there is a marked avoidance of dietary fat.

Protein intake may be low as a result of the quantity or quality of dietary protein. Compared to the proteins in meat, milk, and egg white, all other proteins are less than completely usable by the human body. This occurs because in order for protein to be fully used, the essential amino acids must occur in a fixed ratio, and all vegetable proteins are relatively lacking in one or another of those amino acids.

However, because the nature and degree of these amino acid "deficiencies" vary, different vegetable proteins can be combined in a meal so that they complement each other. This protein complementarity is embodied in many traditional food combinations (e.g., beans and rice) and is both readily learned and used.

Soy protein appears to be the most complete and usable vegetable protein. For adults and older children, protein complementarity is effective if foods are consumed at successive meals; closer consumption (together or a few hours apart) may be most effective for young children.

Inadequate *calcium* intake can contribute to rickets, with associated growth arrest. In most diets, calcium is primarily obtained from milk and milk products. Other foods also contain calcium, but (with the exception of soybean products) generally in small amounts. Common nonanimal sources of calcium are listed in Table 15-4. Even though

Table 15-3.   Common Consequences of Dietary Variations Seen in Vegetarianism*

	DIETARY PATTERN	NUTRITIONAL EFFECT	HEALTH EFFECT†
Reduced	Animal food	↓ Vitamin B₁₂ intake	Anemia, neuropathy
		↓ Zinc intake	Hypogeusia, slow growth
		↓ Total protein intake	Usually none
		↓ Saturated fat intake	Reduced cardiovascular
		↓ Cholesterol intake	disease (CVD)
	Calcium	↑ Zinc, calcium absorption	None or reduced osteoporosis
	Fortified milk	↓ Vitamin D intake	Rickets
	Fat	↓ Calories	Reduced obesity‡
Increased	Legumes	↑ Fiber intake	(See below)
		↑ Zinc intake	Usually none
	Whole grains	↑ B vitamin intake	(See below)
		↑ Zinc intake	Usually none
	Soy protein	↓ Iron Absorption	Anemia possible
		↓ Saturated fat	Reduced CVD
	Carotene	↑ Vitamin A repletion	Reduced cancer
	Vitamin C (ascorbic acid)	↑ Iron absorption	Anemia avoided
	Fiber, phytates	↓ Mineral absorption	Anemia
		↓ Protein absorption	Usually none
		↓ Calorie intake	Reduced obesity‡
		↓ GI transit time	Reduced constipation
			Reduced colon cancer

*Type and degree of dietary variations differ from family to family.
†Proved or strongly suspected.
‡In infants, can result in difficulty meeting caloric requirements.

Table 15-4. Nonanimal Sources of Minerals*

CALCIUM	ZINC	IRON
Soybean products: tofu, formula/milk	Beans	Beans
	Whole grains	Whole grains
Some green vegetables: mustard greens, broccoli	Some green vegetables	Most green and yellow vegetables
Other: blackstrap molasses, medicinal supplements		Some dried fruits: prunes, peaches
		Other: black-strap molasses

*Absorption may be poor in the presence of high levels of phytates.

increased dietary calcium results in increased calcium absorption, growing children on vegetarian milk-free diets (like those on milk-free diets for other reasons) are likely to require calcium supplements to assure adequate intake, unless they are on calcium-fortified formulas.

Vitamin D deficiency may occur, either alone or with calcium deficiency, resulting in rickets. It is most likely in a child who is dark-skinned and breast-fed by a mother who was herself vitamin D depleted during pregnancy. Because most vitamin D metabolites in breast milk are inactive, the absence of rickets in breast-fed infants generally depends on prenatal repletion, exposure to the sun, or dietary or medicinal supplementation. Supplementation is mandatory for dark-skinned babies who are born in winter and who are breast-fed by vegan mothers who did not take vitamin D supplements during pregnancy. In other situations, the need for supplementation can be assessed by a review of maternal diet before and during pregnancy and a review of the child's sun exposure and diet after 6 months of age.

Vitamin B_{12} is present in flesh foods, the aqueous portion of milk, and egg yolks. Reports of vitamin B_{12} in sea vegetables and cultured soy products (e.g., tempeh) have proved to be misleading.

Vegan and most ovovegetarian diets thus require supplementation with this vitamin. Vitamin B_{12} deficiency in a nursing vegan mother can cause a deficiency in her baby, with resulting reversible slowing in growth and development, and in hematologic and biochemical problem.

Zinc, which is most plentiful in foods of animal origin, has a positive effect on appetite and growth of muscle. Zinc balance may sometimes be adversely affected by dietary excess of phytic acid, a substance present in fibrous plants (e.g., green leafy vegetables) that forms unabsorbed phytates with several minerals. The possibility of a zinc deficiency should be considered when growth is deficient and associated with a poor appetite, a marginal dietary intake of zinc, or a diet rich in phytate-containing foods. A trial of zinc supplementation (5 mg/day) may be beneficial and is benign. Some nonanimal sources of dietary zinc are listed in Table 15-4.

Laboratory Tests

If a child on any diet is severely malnourished, as evidenced by wasting or growth arrest, anthropometric and laboratory measurements are indicated. The most frequent nutrient deficiencies are listed in Table 15-2. The lab values that are most often depressed are albumin, prealbumin, ionized calcium, phosphorus, vitamin D metabolites, and ferritin.

Although vegetarianism does not predispose to iron-deficiency anemia, the most common laboratory abnormality in vegetarian children is microcytic anemia due to iron deficiency, just as it is in omnivorous children. Evaluation and treatment of microcytic anemia are the same as for an omnivorous child except that meat consumption cannot be relied on as a means of iron repletion. Anemia may sometimes be macrocytic because of vitamin B_{12} deficiency in vegan children (or nursing infants of unsupplemented vegan mothers); folate is plentiful in vegetarian diets (because of inclusion of foliage) and is not a likely cause of macrocytosis in this context.

Although heme iron (in meat) is much more available than nonheme iron (in vegetables), iron deficiency is not a common consequence of vegetarianism. This is probably due to the coincidence of several dietary and metabolic factors that promote iron homeostasis: nonheme iron absorption is increased by simultaneous consumption of ascorbic acid, which is generally plentiful in vegetarian meals; iron absorption is increased by increased need; and nonheme iron is ample in many vegetable foods. Despite these facts, severe dietary restriction (as in some macrobiotic diets) or huge phytic acid intakes can result in iron deficiency. Recommendations to avoid excess phytate intake and to have a vitamin C–rich food in most meals are practical and readily followed.

If a child has rickets, it is prudent to rule out renal, liver, and parathyroid pathology by means of a careful history and physical examination, and with appropriate laboratory tests. The possibility of other etiologies (e.g., familial hypophosphatemic rickets, vitamin D dependency) should be further explored if the child fails to respond to the usual therapy for vitamin D deficiency.

PRINCIPLES AND PRACTICALITIES IN MANAGING THE VEGETARIAN CHILD

It is essential that the pediatrician develop and convey the same attitude of respect for vegetarian parents as for omnivorous parents. It should be explicitly acknowledged that the physician recognizes that parents adhere to a vegetarian diet with the intention of improving their children's lives. This positive posture not only reflects reality but is also an essential basis for effective recommendations concerning necessary dietary changes. The physician who displays ignorance—or, worse, contempt—for vegetarianism will be ineffective in assessing or modifying the diet and growth of a vegetarian child.

Many pediatricians do not have the experience or interest necessary to assess and manage the most unusual or restricted vegetarian diets. In such instances, it is most appropriate to work with a dietitian or to refer the patient to a pediatrician with special expertise (as one might for a child on a special diet because of a metabolic error).

ANNOTATED BIBLIOGRAPHY

Dwyer JT. Health aspects of vegetarian diets. Am J Clin Nutr 48:712–738, 1988. (A thorough review of the literature concerning adult health effects. Many articles in this issue discuss other aspects of vegetarian nutrition.)

Ewald EB. Recipes for a Small Planet: The Art and Science of High Protein Vegetarian Cookery. New York, Ballantine Books, 1973. (Sequel to *Diet for a Small Planet,* with usable recipes exemplifying protein complementarity.)

Jacobs C, Dwyer JT. Vegetarian children: Appropriate and inappropriate diets. Am J Clin Nutr 48:811–818, 1988. (Thorough review of the literature concerning children: through 1986.)

Lappé FM. Diet for a Small Planet. New York, Ballantine Books, 1971. (Essential background concerning recent growth of interest in vegetarianism, with excellent figures.)

Nutritional aspects of vegetarianism, health foods and fad diets. In American Academy of Pediatrics: Pediatric Nutrition Handbook, Chap. 33. Elk Grove Village, IL, American Academy of Pediatrics, 1985. (Includes specific information on megavitamin toxicity.)

O'Connell JM, Dibley MJ, Sierra J et al. Growth of vegetarian children: The Farm study. Pediatrics 84:475–481, 1989. (Anthropometric data on 404 children aged 4 months to 10 years living in a collective community. Deficits decreased with increasing age. By age 10, deficits were 0.1–0.3 S.D., 0.7 cm, and 1.1 kg.)

Robertson L, Flinders C, Godfrey B. Laurel's Kitchen: A Handbook for Vegetarian Cookery and Nutrition. Petaluma, CA, Nilgiri Press, 1976. (Nutrition text-cum-cookbook. Highly readable, usable recipes, and fine tables of nutrient contents.)

Sabaté J, Lindsted KD, Harris RD, Johnston PK. Anthropometric parameters of school children with different life-styles. Am J Dis Child 144:1159–1163, 1990. (Two-year longitudinal study of 2272 Seventh Day Adventist children—mostly ovolactovegetarian—aged 6–18 years; the children were about 1 kg lighter than public school peers but of comparable height.)

16

Sexuality Education

Edward L. Schor

Sexuality is central to the personality and daily life of every individual. It has its beginning in the intimacy and love of the mother–child relationship, and it is developed through the child's continuing interaction with his culture and society, especially as these are represented and interpreted by his

or her family. Sexual development, like other aspects of child development, is a continuing process, susceptible to errant experience that can lead to a poor self-image and aberrant sexuality and sexual behavior. It is an area of preventive pediatrics in which the pediatrician can play a valuable role as an educator of children and their parents and as a facilitator of open and honest communication between them.

Pediatricians are uniquely able to follow a child's development over an extended period of time. Sexuality is an integral part of that development. By making sexuality education a regular part of child health care, pediatricians are able to legitimize it as an aspect of child development that should be considered and discussed. The primary goal of sexuality education is to enhance normal social and psychological development, including developing a positive self-image and the capacity for intimate, mutually supportive, and satisfying relationships. Successful sexuality education may also help to prevent sexual abuse, teenage and unwanted pregnancies, sexually transmitted diseases, and adult sexual dysfunction.

Pediatricians who omit sexuality education from their child care visits convey a strong message to the parents that such topics are uncomfortable or off-limits. Parents who avoid discussing these topics with their children give a similar message. However, although pediatricians should consciously include sexuality education as a normal and comfortable part of their interactions with parents and children, a certain amount of discretion is advisable. All families have boundaries beyond which some topics or conversations become uncomfortable, if not taboo. On one hand, pediatricians should not restrict their entry into the family's value system to the extent that normal sexual development is not discussed. On the other hand, the pediatrician must sufficiently assess the family's boundaries so that he or she does not offend them, thus limiting his or her effectiveness as an educator and child advocate.

The biologic determinants of sexuality begin at conception when the genetic gender of the child is determined. On the basis of gender, the child (boy or girl) begins to be exposed to differential societal expectations. The child, influenced by attitudes about his or her sex role, begins to actively identify with others of his or her own gender. Learning gender identity, whether by a boy or a girl, occurs by 3 years of age. The child develops the foundation for his or her gender role by perceiving differences in social roles based on gender and by valuing things that are like himself. Gender identity is a fixed characteristic. On the other hand, gender roles, masculine or feminine, may be transcended, and children and adults are able to base their behavior on personally meaningful experiences, interests, and abilities.

PRENATAL STAGE

Many of the topics routinely discussed during a prenatal pediatric visit are issues of sexuality. The decision to breast-feed is partly a decision in favor of maximum intimacy between mother and child. It also provokes questions about the intended role of the father in the care of the child and thus addresses aspects of sexuality and gender roles of both parents. Circumcision is a decision linked to the child's body image and sexuality. Even the choice of names for the child and their connotation to the parents and others have implications for the child's sexual development. By creating an atmosphere that encourages discussion of sexual matters, the pediatrician is modeling for the parents how to help their child feel safe to ask questions, show concerns, and express feelings. These parenting skills are fundamental to normal, healthy development, sexual and otherwise.

NEWBORN STAGE

Sexuality education occurs as the newborn examination is performed in the presence of the parents. As in every subsequent examination of the child, examination of the genitalia should be included as a matter of course. During the first examination, the pediatrician should, using the correct terminology, comment on the genital anatomy. Penile and clitoral erections, the former reported to occur as early as the second trimester, or vaginal secretions and bleeding should be discussed, as should the presence of breast tissue. The contribution that nestling, suckling, rocking, and other such behaviors make to the child's sense of intimacy and trust should be discussed and encouraged.

INFANCY

During infancy, children begin to learn that it is pleasant to be touched. If holding is absent or associated with unpleasant feelings, the infant may fail to learn pleasure and to be comfortable with physical contact. Infants will normally find and explore their genitals and will take pleasure in touching themselves. Masturbation is natural and inevitable, and infants appear to be capable of having an orgasm. Parental reactions to children touching their genitals will influence the formation of attitudes associated with self-pleasure and with genital parts of the body. The pediatrician may inquire whether the infant has developed the motor skills and sense of his or her own body necessary to play with his genitals. Sexuality is normalized when placed in such a developmental context.

TODDLER STAGE

The development of expressive language, which progresses rapidly between 18 and 36 months, is a period of extensive sexual learning. The child names body parts and learns of their functions along with the affect attached to the words. Toilet training also occurs during this stage. Children find pleasure in urinating or having a bowel movement, and thus toilet training, including exploring their feces, urine, or the toilet bowl, is a part of discovering their bodies. Parents' reactions to these explorations can influence children's attitudes toward bodily functions.

Children now begin to engage in mutual exploration, usually with siblings and peers, although they take careful note of their parents' anatomy and behavior. They question the reason for genitalia and other mysteries such as their umbilicus. Social sexual issues begin to arise within families. Much early parent–child communication deals with sexuality, because many of the child's first interests are with his or her own body parts and functions. Parents will find it necessary to address questions about nudity and when clothing is necessary, separate sleeping areas, and sexual privacy for themselves.

PRESCHOOL STAGE

Active psychosexual development occurs at this stage. The child now becomes aware of the physical boundaries between "me" and "somebody else." The child should learn that his or her body belongs to him- or herself. A child who has a positive view of his or her own physical anatomy and control of his or her own body is less likely to be an object of sexual misuse. Parents need to learn to listen to their children, especially if the child tells them that something happened that made him or her feel uncomfortable.

Although children need to understand when to say "No" and to respect their bodies, it is also important for them to understand that sexual behavior can and should be good. Children need experiences that reinforce a positive self-image. Sexual development includes a period of experimentation and exploration. Sex play, cuddling, touching, kissing, and playing "doctor" or "mommy and daddy" are normal. They are ways of acting out situations to test their ideas of how things happen, to discover how things look, and to learn what feels good. This may be seen as a form of sexual rehearsal play that will help them develop a sense of sexual competence. Children are also likely to be intensely attached to the parent of the opposite sex during this stage of development. They may harbor jealous feelings toward the same-sex parent. This is an affirmation of their own gender identity and an unconscious testing of their sex role.

Instead of asking for labels, children ask questions about body functions. They are not able to understand the concept of procreation; they believe that babies have always existed somewhere. Thus, the question "Where do babies come from?" is a quite literal one. Children, as they get a little older, begin to attribute babies to some cause, although their thinking is "magical" and filled with illogical connections. Their questions may then be mechanistic, such as, "How are babies made?" "How does it feel to be born?" or "Can I watch you and daddy make a baby?"

The innocent, naive, and embarrassing questions and behavior of children between 3 and 5 years should be handled graciously and respectfully. Parents should be encouraged to address such situations not as good or bad, right or wrong, but rather as appropriate or inappropriate depending on the time, place, or person. Masturbation, for example, may be permissible at home or in the car, but not in public—the place is inappropriate. Similarly, being naked with your family might be permissible, whereas with a friend's family it may be frowned on—the situation or persons are inappropriate. Although a child's behaviors and questions at this age may be embarrassing for the parents, sexual topics do not have the same emotional significance for children. The quality of this dialogue, the ability of the parent to allow the child to broach any subject without fear of judgment or censorship, can establish future patterns of sharing and relating to others.

Parents can also be guided to recognize the sexuality in the everyday life of their child. Much sexual learning can take place gradually, informally, and incidentally. Parents should take advantage of family events such as pregnancies, weddings, and birthdays to discuss sexual topics. Picture books offer examples of gender roles; discussions about family relationships can be introduced by looking at photo albums; and reproduction can be discussed when dealing with pets.

ELEMENTARY SCHOOL STAGE

When a child starts going to school, he is exposed to a world in which new information and attitudes abound and rewards are given for understanding how things work. At this age, children offer explanations, albeit less than convincing, for phenomena that seem technically feasible, and they ascribe will and purpose to all things in nature. Thus, their questions about sex and reproduction increase as they try to find reason in conflicting "facts"; as a part of their developing sexuality, they are fascinated by what they perceive as deviant, such as twins or profanity. Their interest in the fantastic and bizarre extends to their choice of toys, games, and television viewing. Parents should be encouraged to actively participate in the selection of these activities.

By 8 or 9 years of age, most of the basic facts of sexual life may have been learned, but children will not yet be able to weave them into a consistent whole with which they are comfortable. Consequently, they begin showing embarrassment when discussing sexual topics such as pregnancy and childbirth, and they may be reluctant to ask questions that might clarify their misconceptions. "Dirty jokes" appear at this time and reflect both their confusion and reluctance; such behaviors test the receptivity of their parents to discuss these topics.

During this and subsequent stages, the sexuality of single parents is a topic that pediatricians are increasingly required to address. There are no easy answers to parents'

questions, and, as always, their values and circumstances must be respected. As is true for couples, single parents need to honestly confront their own sexuality and be clear on how they wish to convey their values to their children. Divorced parents may have different sexual values; they may need to agree to disagree. Parents should be reassured that the formation of normal gender identity and roles seems to take place without the presence of a same-sex parent and under various child-rearing conditions.

Later during this stage, the pediatrician can begin to see the child alone for part of the examination, offering this option directly to the child. In this way, the pediatrician acknowledges that an advance in maturation of the child has occurred, and he or she introduces the concept of responsibility for one's own body and health. The communication between the parents and the child should be observed; it is the key to a good family relationship and to healthy psychosocial development. When communication is not adequate—when open discussions do not occur; when children's opinions are not solicited before judgments are made; or when their decisions are not respected—intervention in the office or referral for brief counseling is appropriate.

The wide variation in the age of onset of puberty makes the timing of pubertal counseling difficult to determine. Because an examination of the genitalia should occur at each well-child visit, the pediatrician will be able to identify the first changes of secondary sexual characteristic development—testicular enlargement in boys and breast buds in girls. By or at this time, discussion of secondary sexual characteristic changes should begin, including genital and breast development and gynecomastia, linear growth, voice changes, muscular development, hair pattern differences, and menstruation.

Controversy exists concerning the role of the parents, schools, and physician in sexuality education. Most would agree that the family's values should be respected. This question has led to a hesitancy on the part of many school systems to incorporate sexuality education into their curricula. The pediatrician should ascertain what the parents' values are with regard to sexuality, and he or she should offer pubertal counseling congruent with them. It should be emphasized that this is an integral part of health care. It is useful to include the parents in the process of sexuality education. This reduces their anxiety about what is being discussed and increases the potential for continued discussion in the home.

Puberty

The physical changes associated with puberty are major factors in self-image, and they are managed best by the young adolescent whose self-esteem, comfort with his or her body, and ability to communicate with significant others are well developed. Previous sexuality education should have prepared him for the more visible changes. Other changes may be more problematic. Young adolescents are concerned with how they appear to others and how they feel about themselves. Their principal concern is with normality, and thus with peer acceptance. Conventional role conformity is evident in their spoken beliefs, their dress, and their behavior. Their development is described by their ability to form intimate, interpersonal relationships outside of their families as they move toward families they may form in the future. Their behavior displays a stepwise progression of sexual behavior from kissing to intercourse.

In some ways, pubertal sexuality is undifferentiated; this can lead to concerns about both homosexuality and "adequacy" for heterosexual roles. Other topics of interest at this age and later in adolescence include menstruation, masturbation, intercourse, birth control, pregnancy, and venereal diseases. Theses subjects invoke a considerable number of questions. The pediatrician should encourage the adolescent to raise questions of his own rather than depend entirely on a planned teaching agenda.

When the pediatrician perceives that he or she will be the primary source of sexuality education for a young adolescent, an increase in the usual number of health maintenance visits is necessary to allow adequate opportunity for discussions. During each visit, most of the time should be spent with the adolescent alone. Privacy and confidentiality are important for adolescents, especially when sexual histories are taken; homosexuality, sexual activity, or an ignorance of sexual knowledge may be revealed. Parents and other adults who enjoy teenagers' confidence are those who respect their privacy, who do not expect to be told everything, and who do not push for more information than they are offered. Another reason for seeing the adolescent alone is to encourage a sense of responsibility for him- or herself that hopefully will also extend to others. The physical examination of young adolescents should be performed in a way that helps them learn about their changing bodies and that reinforces a sense of normality. Some pediatricians find it useful to guide adolescents through a self-Tanner staging. It is also a time to consider teaching breast and testicular self-examinations.

Adolescence

Whereas early adolescence is a time to experience changes, mid-adolescence is a time to manage and incorporate them into a functional life-style. Teenagers are physiologically ready for sexual activity before adulthood, before our society makes it possible for them to cope with its consequences. Sexuality should be cast in the context of relationships, a framework that is usually welcomed by adolescents and their parents.

The pediatrician can initiate a discussion about sex by taking a sexual history as a part of the general history. Aspects of physical and physiologic maturation can be explored as appropriate to the age of the adolescent. Questions may be asked about sexual feelings, concerns, and, perhaps with more difficulty, behaviors. Finally, the issues of responsibilities and consequences can be addressed. Such discussions can help adolescents explore sexuality and sexual life-styles that serve to increase their sense of self-mastery and good decision making. The pediatrician should support and encourage good communication between parents and their children throughout the span of sexuality education. Teenagers who believe that they are basically good and competent people and that they are loved and respected will be better able to cope with the pressures their sexuality creates and to develop loving and lasting relationships.

PATIENT EDUCATION

The education of patients and parents in sexuality requires a combination of teaching (e.g., providing facts) and counseling (e.g., providing emotional support and reassurance). It also requires that the pediatrician first assess his or her own beliefs, values, and experiences regarding sexuality. Thus prepared, he or she will be better able to engage in effective and empathetic communication and will more likely succeed as an educator.

When introducing education regarding sensitive topics such as sexuality, it is essential to understand the family's value system and to map out its boundaries. Similarly, the knowledge that patients and their families already possess should be assessed and used as a foundation for discussion. Problem-based learning with active participation of the patient is most effective. Concerns and questions expressed by the parent or child should be used to direct the educational process. The pediatrician should also be sensitive to unspoken messages and indirect questions, and he or she should tactfully address these covert communications. The number of issues discussed during any single visit and the amount of factual material presented should be limited. Sequential visits allow the organized presentation of information and provide the opportunity for reinforcement of previous discussions. During patient education, it is essential to evaluate as the process occurs. The pediatrician should not assume that what is being presented is being understood.

The practice of pediatrics naturally lends itself to the inclusion of the family in the educational process. This is an important advantage. Family involvement allows a more complete understanding of what knowledge, attitudes, and behaviors form the context for the sexual development of the child. During childhood and early adolescence, the parents are the primary participants in sexuality education, because they can either apply advice being offered by the pediatrician or undermine its message to the child. Parents should be made to feel competent as educators themselves, because the most successful sexuality education occurs when the parent–child communication is good. Finally, the role of the pediatrician as a health educator should extend beyond the patient and his or her family. Pediatricians can become more effective in promoting child health care by participating in educational programs in schools and communities.

ANNOTATED BIBLIOGRAPHY

Bartlett EE. Effective approaches to patient education for the busy pediatrician. Pediatrics 74(Suppl):920–923, 1984. (Brief, but one of the few practical references on health education for pediatricians.)

Bernstein AC. How children learn about sex and birth. Psychology Today, pp 73–78, Jan. 1976. (Succinct and interesting article outlining children's understanding of sexuality based on a Piagetian formulation.)

Calderone MS, Johnson EW. The Family Book About Sexuality. New York, Harper & Row, 1981. (Comprehensive, well-illustrated book that promotes open discussion within the family of all aspects of sexuality.)

Litt IF, Martin JA. Development of sexuality and its problems. In Levine M, Carey WB, Crocker AC, Gross RT (eds): Developmental–Behavioral Pediatrics, pp 633–649. Philadelphia, WB Saunders, 1983. (Useful chapter that provides an overview of several theories and concepts about childhood sexuality. Discusses sexuality during adolescence in detail.)

Parcel GS, Finkelstein JW. Adolescent sexuality. In Buchanan N (ed): Pediatric Issues for General Practitioners. Sydney, Australia, ADIS Health Science Press, 1987. (Excellent chapter on adolescent sexual development covering most of the important considerations for pediatricians providing sexuality education for this age group.)

Planned Parenthood. How to Talk with Your Child About Sexuality. Garden City, NY, Doubleday, 1986. (One of the best sexuality education resources for parents and professionals; provides sound advice and information on promoting effective parent–child communication.)

Rutter M. Psychosexual development. In Rutter M (ed): Scientific Foundations of Developmental Psychiatry, pp 322–339. London, Heinemann Medical Books, 1980. (Thorough, scholarly review of biologic and psychosocial aspects of the development of sexuality.)

17

Sports Medicine and Physical Fitness

Paul G. Dyment

The subject of pediatric sports medicine has long been considered the domain of the orthopedic surgeon alone, but most sports injuries are minor and can be handled by a primary-care physician. A physician who has an interest in preventive medicine has an important role in sports medi-

cine—performing preparticipation examinations and working to make athletics safe as well as enjoyable.

This chapter focuses on three areas of common concern to the primary-care physician interested in sports medicine: how to make the preparticipation physical examination worthwhile, the team physician's responsibilities, and the problem of physical fitness in children and youth.

PREPARTICIPATION PHYSICAL EXAMINATION

Sports preparticipation physical examinations are common reasons for adolescents to visit their doctors. The physician may see them only at these visits because half of the high-school athletes undergoing such examinations will have no other contact with a physician during that year. The number of such examinations performed annually in the United States is striking. Seven million high-school students are involved in interscholastic sports, and most state high-school athletic associations still require an annual physical examination. In the experience of most physicians, such examinations are not very productive in detecting conditions that might affect athletic participation, and the effectiveness of sports preparticipation examinations as usually performed is arguable. Most adolescents are generally healthy, and the mere fact that they are trying out for a sport further diminishes the likelihood of their having a significant disease. The fact that only 1% of such patients have a disqualifying condition revealed by the traditional examination underscores why this type of examination is widely believed to be not very cost-effective.

If, however, the physician is aware that *most sports injuries are reinjuries* and thus focuses the physical examination on the musculoskeletal system, abnormalities will be detected in 10% of patients. Most of these abnormalities will be easily treated musculoskeletal conditions, such as tight hamstring muscles, patellofemoral syndrome (chondromalacia patellae), and ligamentous ankle instabilities that generally require only some rehabilitative exercises with the use of training equipment available in most schools. Such a musculoskeletal examination is good practice and also makes the physical examination much more productive and therefore more interesting.

The sports preparticipation examination can occur during a "locker-room" type of mass screening, but this is not ideal. It is much better to incorporate this examination into the health maintenance examination in a physician's office where preventive health care and counseling, some of it sport-specific, can be offered.

Purposes

A sports preparticipation physical examination has three purposes. The first is to detect physical abnormalities that could predispose the athlete to injury or death or that could affect the athlete's ability to compete effectively. The second purpose is to evaluate the size and maturity of young adolescent athletes in order to counsel whether collision or contact sports with their peer group would be safe. During early puberty, a boy's athletic abilities are directly related to his degree of sexual maturity (i.e., his Tanner stage). Ideally, competition should be between boys of similar degrees of physical maturity. The third purpose is to identify residual disabilities from previous injuries, because this will allow the physician to recommend rehabilitative exercises that will decrease the probability of a reinjury.

Frequency

Most schools insist on an annual examination, presumably because of a vague belief that this will be legally advantageous to the school in case of litigation over an injury, or it may be because the physical educator believes that annual examinations represent optimal medical practice. Most specialists in adolescent medicine believe that all adolescents should undergo a comprehensive health maintenance examination each year, at which time anticipatory guidance (e.g., regarding sports participation) can be given. The school should require an interval history before each sports season so that illnesses or injuries that have occurred since the last examination can be discussed and decisions made as to whether an athlete needs another physical examination.

Laboratory Tests

A determination of the hemoglobin or hematocrit and a urinalysis are not considered essential for this kind of examination. In one study of 701 children undergoing a sports physical examination, 40 had abnormal urinary protein on screening, but *none* were found to have any significant abnormality after further work-up. Iron-deficiency anemia has to be severe before the body's compensatory mechanisms, such as increased stroke volume and heart rate, fail to maintain appropriate oxygen flow to the tissues. However, iron depletion that is not severe enough to cause anemia may limit endurance and ability to exercise, and it is certainly much more common than frank anemia. Because serum assays of ferritin or iron are expensive, it is recommended that they be obtained only on highly competitive state, national, and world-class female athletes and on male distance runners, many of whom can be shown to be hypoferremic.

Medical History

In addition to the usual questions asked during a medical review of systems, the athlete should be asked the following six questions:

1. Have any members of your family under age 50 had a "heart attack" or "heart problem"?
2. Have you ever been told you have a heart murmur, high blood pressure, an extra heart beat, or a heart abnormality?
3. Do you have to stop while running around a quarter-mile track twice?
4. Are you taking any medications?
5. Have you ever "passed out" while exercising or been "knocked out"?
6. Have you ever had any illness, condition, or injury that:
   a. required you to go to the hospital either as a patient overnight or in the emergency room or for x-rays?
   b. required an operation?
   c. lasted longer than a week?
   d. caused you to miss a game or practice?
   e. was caused by allergies (e.g., hay fever, hives, asthma, or medicine)?

Examination

If this examination takes place in the physician's office in the context of a health maintenance examination, then a complete physical examination should be performed. In the mass-screening form, it is acceptable to concentrate on examining the chest, abdomen, inguinal canals in the male, and the musculoskeletal system. Even then the examination should be sport-specific; thus, swimmers would also have their tympanic membranes examined and wrestlers would have their levels of body fat determined by use of skinfold calipers so that advice can be given on how to "make weight" in a medically sound manner.

Cardiopulmonary. Most sudden, unexpected deaths in adolescent athletes are from abnormalities of the heart, and few of them would have had their abnormality detected even during a carefully performed physical examination. The aberrant left coronary artery syndrome has been associated with sudden death in young persons. Although there is no heart murmur, in most instances they have had a history of fainting during exercise. Idiopathic hypertrophic subaortic stenosis (IHSS), although uncommon, is a potentially lethal defect associated with exercise. It may be associated with an apical systolic murmur that increases when the patient performs a Valsalva maneuver, and there may be a hyperdynamic left ventricular impulse. The stigmata of Marfan's syndrome should be looked for, because sudden death from a ruptured aortic aneurysm can follow vigorous activity. Particular attention should be paid to blood pressure, even though mild forms of hypertension are not a reason for disqualification from sports (in fact, exercise generally lowers the blood pressure), and levels greater than 140/90 in adolescents need repeated determinations before a decision is made that hypertension is present.

Abdomen and Genitalia. The athlete should be supine while a careful palpation for intra-abdominal masses and hepatosplenomegaly is performed. Males should then have their testicles palpated and inguinal canals examined, and at least males playing contact sports should have their Tanner pubic hair staging assessed.

Table 17-1. 2-Minute Orthopedic Examination

INSTRUCTIONS	OBSERVATION
Stand facing the examiner.	Acromioclavicular joints, general habitus
Look at the ceiling, floor, over both shoulders; touch ears to shoulders.	Cervical spine motion
Shrug shoulders (examiner resists).	Trapezius strength
Abduct shoulders 90° (examiner resists at 90°).	Deltoid strength
Do a full external rotation of arms.	Shoulder motion
Flex and extend elbows.	Elbow motion
Arms at sides, elbows 90° flexed; pronate and supinate wrists.	Elbow and wrist motion
Spread your fingers; make a fist.	Hand or finger motion and deformities
Tighten (contract) quadriceps; relax quadriceps.	Symmetry and knee effusion; ankle effusion
"Duck walk" four steps (away from examiner with buttocks on heels).	Hip, knee, and ankle motion
Keep back to the examiner.	Shoulder symmetry, scoliosis
Keep knees straight, touch toes.	Scoliosis, hip motion, hamstring tightness
Raise up on toes, raise heels.	Calf symmetry, leg strength

(Reproduced with permission from Sports Medicine Committee. Sports Medicine: Health Care for Young Athletes, 2nd ed. Elk Grove Village, IL, American Academy of Pediatrics, 1991.)

Musculoskeletal. This component of the examination can be performed in less than 2 minutes, and the emphasis should be on detecting the residua of previous injuries so that the athlete can undergo rehabilitative exercises that may prevent a reinjury. The athlete, wearing only underwear, should stand in front of the examiner, and the physician should call out the commands listed in Table 17-1. The physician should look for the listed abnormalities. After the history, this is the most productive part of the entire examination.

Disqualification

The American Academy of Pediatrics (AAP) has published a list of qualifying conditions for sports participation. This guide has replaced the now-obsolete recommendations of the American Medical Association, which were last revised by them in 1976. The AAP guidelines first divide sports by their degree of contact and strenuousness (Table 17-2) and then makes a recommendation regarding participation in these groups based upon the medical condition (Table 17-3).

SCHOOL TEAM PHYSICIAN

A physician is often asked to be the school's team doctor for the team in which his or her child is a member. If the physician agrees, then he or she cannot merely sit in the stands waiting to be called in case of an injury. The physician should agree to do the job only if a total team-physician program is instituted. The physician should also obtain in writing the school's agreement to this program with its recognition that the team physician has the ultimate authority

Table 17-2. Classification of Sports

COLLISION	LIMITED CONTACT/IMPACT	NONCONTACT STRENUOUS	MODERATELY STRENUOUS	NONSTRENUOUS
Boxing	Baseball	Aerobic dancing	Badminton	Archery
Field hockey	Basketball	Crew	Curling	Golf
Football	Bicycling	Fencing	Table tennis	Riflery
Ice hockey	Diving	Field*		
Lacrosse	Equestrian	Running		
Martial arts	Gymnastics	Skiing (cross-country)		
Rodeo	Raquetball	Swimming		
Wrestling	Skating (ice and roller)	Tennis		
Soccer	Skiing (downhill, cross-country, and water)	Track		
	Softball	Weight-lifting		
	Squash, handball			
	Volleyball			

*Field events: Jumping events such as pole vaulting and high jump are "limited-contact" sports.

Table 17-3.   Qualifying Conditions for Competitive Sports Participation

CONDITIONS	COLLISION	LIMITED CONTACT	NONCONTACT STRENUOUS	MODERATELY STRENUOUS	NONSTRENUOUS
Atlanto-axial **Instability**	No	No	Yes (no butterfly, breast stroke, or diving starts in swimming)	Yes	Yes
Acute Illness	Need individual assessment (*i.e.,* contagious to others, risk of worsening illness, and so forth)				
Cardiovascular Carditis	No	No	No	No	No
Hypertension Mild Moderate Severe	Yes Needs individual assessment Needs individual assessment	Yes	Yes	Yes	Yes Yes Yes
Congenital heart disease	Patients with mild forms of congenital heart disease can be allowed a full range of physical activities. Patients with moderate or severe forms of cardiac disease, or who are postoperative, should be evaluated by a cardiologist before athletic participation.				
Eyes Absence or loss of function of one eye	The availability of ASTM-approved eye guards may allow the competitor to compete in most sports, but this must be judged on an individual basis.				
Detached retina	Consult opthalmologist				
Hernia Inguinal	Yes	Yes	Yes	Yes	Yes
Kidney Absence of one	No	Yes	Yes	Yes	Yes
Liver Enlarged	No	No	Yes	Yes	Yes
Neurologic History of previous serious head or spine trauma, repeated concussions, or craniotomy	Needs more assessment		Yes	Yes	Yes
Convulsive disorder Well controlled Poorly controlled	Yes No	Yes No	Yes Yes (no swimming or weight-lifting)	Yes Yes	Yes Yes (no archery or riflery)
Ovary Absence of one	Yes	Yes	Yes	Yes	Yes
Respiratory Pulmonary insufficiency	May be allowed to compete if oxygenation remains satisfactory during a graded stress test				Yes
Asthma	Yes	Yes	Yes	Yes	Yes
Skin Boils, impetigo, scabies, herpes	No wrestling, martial arts, gymnastics with mats, or skin-to-skin contact until not contagious		Yes	Yes	Yes
Spleen Enlarged	No	No	No	Yes	Yes
Testicle Absence or undescended	Yes Certain sports will require protective cup	Yes	Yes	Yes	Yes

("No" = Should not participate)

to keep a player off the field. The tasks and responsibilities of the team physician include the following:

1. Know the general factors that contribute to injuries: conditioning, coaching techniques, rules, equipment.
2. Educate self, parents, coaches, and students as to the risk factors of the involved sport and what procedures are needed to reduce these risks.
3. Evaluate the playing surface and the equipment for dangerous conditions.
4. Evaluate all injuries and establish a system for the management and follow-up of these problems.
5. Evaluate the conditioning and training procedures for safety factors.
6. Establish criteria for disqualification from participation in competitive sports and for returning to competition after an illness or injury.
7. Review all histories and physical examinations done by other physicians. Re-evaluate the student or contact the physician if any questions arise from this review, and do the examination if no primary physician is available.
8. Establish a record system for all injuries.
9. Establish rehabilitation procedures for injuries.
10. Establish a transportation and referral system for all serious injuries.
11. Learn the rules of the sport and evaluate the official's adherence to enforcing the rules that pertain to player safety.
12. Observe the techniques used by the coaches in teaching the sport, and advise them of those techniques that contribute to injuries or excessive stress.

The question of compensation for the team physician is complicated by the fact that some state "good Samaritan" statutes protecting physicians from medical liability when responding to emergencies specifically include the rendering of care at school athletic events, but this protection ceases if a fee is rendered for the service. This discussion is generally moot, however, because schools rarely have any funds available for this service, and the physician should accept the fact that this care will be a service to the community.

PHYSICAL FITNESS

Concepts about what constitutes physical fitness have changed markedly during the past 30 years. Initially, physical educators interpreted fitness to be the motor components important to athletic performance (i.e., muscle strength, power, speed, and agility). However, during the past 15 years, the emphasis has changed to one promoting overall health and life-long physical activity. The components of health-related physical fitness are now believed to be: muscle strength and endurance, cardiorespiratory endurance, flexibility, and body composition (i.e., percent body fat).

Health Benefits of Physical Activity

Certain physical activities such as repeated sustained aerobic exercise can increase cardiovascular endurance, improve abnormal blood lipids, and moderate hypertension, and they have even been shown to improve the behavior of incarcerated delinquent boys. Even more modest amounts of physical activity can be associated with important health benefits. Regular exercise can reduce anxiety, increase self-esteem, promote weight loss, and improve the affect of patients with depression, and it is associated with a longer life. Finally, if muscle strength is increased, the risk of musculoskeletal injuries during a physical activity can be reduced because joint supports are strengthened. A recent text published by the American Academy of Orthopedic Surgeons for athletic trainers (see Bibliography) is an excellent source of information about conditioning exercises for the physician with little or no previous knowledge of this subject.

It is widely believed that children and adolescents in the United States are less physically fit than "before." However, the only comparative studies that have been done have shown little change in fitness levels of children and youth since 1968, with the sole exception of the body composition component, which has shown increasing amounts of body fat. There are several problems in interpreting fitness studies, including the fact that children's abilities to perform several of the test components, such as the 50-yard dash, are primarily genetically determined and, at least in prepubertal children, can be improved only slightly by training.

Until they are 10 to 12 years of age, most children are sufficiently active just responding to the normal childhood drive for play. With the onset of adolescence, tremendous *decreases in physical activity* are observed in most youth. By midpuberty, most American adolescents are quite sedentary and will likely continue that life-style into adulthood. As Table 17-4 indicates, both physical inactivity and obesity are risk factors for the development of coronary heart disease (CHD).

There are four major CHD risk factors—hypertension, elevated blood lipids, cigarette smoking, and physical inactivity, and each by itself just about doubles the risk of CHD. All four have similar relative risks, but the largest group consists of those who are physically inactive (59% of

Table 17-4.   Coronary Heart Disease Risk Factors

ALTERABLE	UNALTERABLE
Hypertension	Age
Elevated blood lipids	Male sex
Smoking cigarettes	Heredity
Diabetes	
Physical Inactivity	
Obesity	

American adults), followed by those who smoke a pack or more of cigarettes a day (18%), those who have a systolic blood pressure over 150 mm Hg (10%), and those with a serum cholesterol over 268 mg/dl (10%). Therefore, increasing the level of physical activity in the entire adult population will have a far greater impact on lowering the overall level of CHD than will improving any of the other three risk factors.

How Much Physical Activity?

Less than 8% of American adults perform regular amounts of aerobic exercise (an activity requiring at least 60% of maximum cardiorespiratory capacity for at least 20 minutes three times a week). This amount of exercise can be shown to alter blood lipids favorably (both increasing the high-density lipoprotein cholesterol level and decreasing the low-density lipoprotein cholesterol level) and has been shown to prevent or delay recurrences of myocardial infarctions. But less strenuous physical activity is also effective in decreasing the frequency and mortality of CHD. One study of Harvard alumni showed that moderate life-long exercise could add 2 years to a man's life. A large study in Dallas showed that just by walking 2 miles in under 30 minutes three times a week, or 2 miles under 45 minutes five times a week, a man can decrease by three times (and women by two times) his risk of dying from CHD during the follow-up period of that study (which averaged 8 years). It is now clearly established that moderate amounts of regular exercise can prolong life.

Role of the Physician

During health maintenance visits beginning at about age 5, questions about physical activity should be raised. When the child becomes an adolescent, these questions need to be asked in more depth, and the physician should be more assertive in recommending physical activity. *Any* form of exercise will do, the more fun the better, and the necessity of aerobic exercise should be downplayed, because most aerobic activities (e.g., running, swimming laps) are not very enjoyable and are therefore unlikely to become a sustained part of a person's lifestyle.

Because patients view their doctors as role models, physicians should also be reasonably fit and not overweight. They should adhere to a physical activity regimen recommended to their adolescent patients and will thus give the message "If a busy doctor can do it, so can you."

ANNOTATED BIBLIOGRAPHY

American Academy of Orthopedic Surgeons. Athletic Training and Sports Medicine. Chicago, IL, American Academy of Orthopedic Surgeons, 1984. (Covers the important and practical aspects of caring for and preventing soft-tissue injuries, including taping, elastic bandaging, recognition of injuries, and rehabilitative exercises.)

Borms J. The child and exercise. J Sports Sci 4:3–20, 1986. (Reviews the effects of physical training on body size, the relationships between both aerobic and anaerobic exercise and physical development, the effects of strength training on the growing body, and the influence of maturation on athletic abilities.)

Committee on Sports Medicine. Sports Medicine: Health Care for Young Athletes, 2nd ed. Elk Grove Village, IL, American Academy of Pediatrics, 1991. (Covers the entire field of pediatric sports medicine. Directed toward the primary care physician.)

Dyment PG (ed). Sports and the Adolescent. Philadelphia, Hanley & Belfus, 1991. (Thirteen chapters covering the major topics in primary-care sports medicine.)

Goldberg B, Saraniti A, Wiltman P et al. Preparticipation sports assessment—An objective evaluation. Pediatrics 66:736–745, 1980. (One half of the high-school athletes in this series had no other contact with a physician during the school year. Only about 1% of those undergoing the traditional medical examination had physical abnormalities detected that might affect safety or performance.)

Thompson TR, Andrish JT, Bergfeld JA. A prospective study of preparticipation sports examinations of 2670 young athletes: Method and results. Cleve Clin Q 49:225–233, 1982. (Study of adolescents focusing on examination of the musculoskeletal system; 10% had abnormalities detected, usually residua of previous injuries.)

4

ENVIRONMENTAL INFLUENCES ON CHILDREN

18

Environmental Concerns

Sophie J. Balk

Pediatricians and parents are becoming more aware that there are increasing numbers of environmental toxins that affect children's health. New information is accumulating rapidly about well-known hazards such as lead and environmental tobacco smoke. In addition, many other toxic substances, such as radon, asbestos, pesticides, and arts and crafts hazards, may affect children's well-being. Pediatricians should become familiar with environmental health issues to properly evaluate symptoms and to provide accurate information when responding to parents' questions. It is equally important for the clinician to ask about possible exposure to toxins during well-child and well-adolescent visits. This chapter will review important environmental hazards, give examples of questions to be asked to elicit exposure, and give suggestions for abatement of risks.

BASIC PRINCIPLES

A few basic principles should be remembered when considering children's environmental exposures. In many cases, children may be more susceptible to environmental toxins than adults. Their exposures may be greater because of their normal curiosity and mouthing behavior, because they have a breathing zone closer to the ground, and because of their rapid growth and differentiation, which may enhance toxicity at the cellular level. Toxins may be stored in biologic sanctuaries such as adipose tissue and bone. Because of a long life span, children are at risk for long-term and multiple exposures.

Toxins can have both acute and chronic health effects. The acute effects are often caused by exposure to products of combustion, such as environmental tobacco smoke or wood smoke. The effects of chronic exposure to most toxins are often uncertain or difficult to establish, although exposure to some substances, such as radon and asbestos, has been linked to specific diseases in adults.

Standards set by regulatory and scientific agencies may not guarantee safety for children. Standards reflect the best current estimates of levels of risk and thus may change as data accumulate. The change in the standard for lead poisoning best exemplifies this principle. The Centers for Disease Control (CDC), which set the blood lead level for diagnosing lead poisoning at 25 μg/dl in 1985, lowered this definition in 1991 based on evidence reporting neurobehavioral and cognitive deficits above 10 μg/dl, a blood level that was recently considered "safe."

INDOOR AIR POLLUTION

Because most infants and young children spend about 90% of their time indoors, indoor air pollution is an important concern. Children are more susceptible to air pollution than are adults. Because children breathe faster and have a larger oxygen requirement per unit weight, they inhale more air pollutants. Children have narrower airways, so irritation caused by air pollution may result in substantial obstruction. Children exposed to high levels of air pollutants appear to have a higher risk of long-term lung damage.

The most pervasive indoor air pollutant is *environmental tobacco smoke* (ETS). Over 40% of children in the United States are exposed to ETS from parental smoking. ETS contains more than 4700 different compounds, including carbon monoxide, polycyclic aromatic hydrocarbons (such as benzo[*a*]pyrene, a carcinogen), respirable particles, and cyanide. Sidestream smoke, which comes from the smoldering end of the cigarette, is more dangerous than the mainstream smoke exhaled by the smoker because the lower combustion temperature of sidestream smoke leaves behind more carcinogenic hydrocarbons and respirable particles.

Prenatal exposure to ETS adversely affects birth weight. Postnatal effects include impairment of lung growth by as much as 5% to 10%; increased incidence of upper respiratory infections, such as croup, and lower respiratory infections, such as bronchiolitis and bronchitis; and exacerbation of reactive airway disease. Pediatric exposure to ETS has been correlated with chronic middle ear effusion. It has also been linked to exposed children developing lung cancer as adults.

Questions about ETS exposure should be part of the routine history, whether or not the child has respiratory symptoms, and should be part of the investigation of recurrent respiratory infections, reactive airway disease, and recurrent middle ear infections. These include: Do the parents smoke? If so, how much and where? Do babysitters or regular visitors to the home smoke? Is the child exposed to smoke outside the home? Is smoking allowed in the car?

Parents who smoke should be encouraged to stop. Local chapters of the American Cancer Society and the American Heart Association have information about smoke cessation programs that may be made available in the pediatrician's office. Parents who do not stop smoking should be advised to smoke outside, not in the house. Visitors who smoke may be told, "The doctor says smoking is bad for my child," and that smoking is not allowed anywhere in the house. Eliminating ashtrays reinforces this message. (Smoking should also not be permitted by office staff members!)

Smoke emitted from *wood stoves and fireplaces* is another important source of indoor air pollution in colder areas. Although a certain amount of smoke release is inevitable, this is markedly increased when the stove or fireplace is not cleaned regularly or drafted properly. Symptoms of respiratory irritation, including persistent cough and wheeze, may result when children are exposed to nitrogen dioxide, hydrocarbons, and respirable particles. Infants and preschoolers confined to "tight" wood-heated homes during the winter are most at risk. When a child has recurrent respiratory symptoms, the pediatrician should determine whether the family heats with wood, how often the stove or fireplace is used, whether much smoke escapes when the door is opened, and if the stove pipe and chimney are regularly cleaned. If the family has an alternative heating source, a "wood elimination trial" may be suggested. Other suggestions include improving ventilation and ensuring that stoves and chimneys are cleaned regularly.

Nitrogen dioxide emanating from *gas stoves* may be a source of respiratory irritation. This is particularly true when there is no ventilation hood, when there is a pilot light, when children spend many hours in the kitchen, and when the stove is used as a source of supplemental heat before and after the heating season. Abatement measures include using a ventilation hood, improving ventilation in general, and switching to an electric stove.

Formaldehyde is a respiratory irritant found in many products, particularly those in mobile homes. Formaldehyde volatilizes from particle board, wood paneling, plywood, carpet adhesive, and urea formaldehyde foam insulation (UFFI). It is also found in certain permanent-press fabrics and cosmetics. Emission of formaldehyde from a product decreases with time.

Adverse health effects include upper respiratory and eye irritation, dry skin or dermatitis, headache, nausea, and general malaise. Formaldehyde may precipitate bronchospasm in asthmatics. Exposure during childhood is also of concern because formaldehyde is a probable human carcinogen.

If symptoms of irritation exist and a source of formaldehyde is present, a formaldehyde level may be obtained from local health departments or from a private laboratory. If the level is greater than 0.1 part per million (ppm), children should be removed from the source, if possible. Other abatement measures include improving ventilation and painting with vapor barrier paint.

OUTDOOR AIR POLLUTION

Outdoor air pollution is a complex mixture that comes from auto emissions, industrial emissions, power plants, and incinerators. Pollutants include sulfur dioxide, the oxides of nitrogen, volatile organic compounds, particulates, and ozone. Ozone is a highly reactive gas formed mainly by the action of sunlight on mixtures of nitrogen oxides and volatile organic compounds. When inhaled, ozone produces inflammation and irritability of the airways, dyspnea, cough, and chest tightness. In addition, ozone produces nonrespiratory symptoms such as nausea, headache, and malaise.

Current levels of air pollutants can injure children's lungs. In addition to ozone, particulates and acidic air pollutants produce respiratory symptoms and decrease pulmonary function in children. Dose–response studies have demonstrated changes in lung function in adults and children exercising for 1 to 2 hours at ozone concentrations well below the current standard of 0.12 ppm. Adverse changes in pulmonary function of children exposed to ozone and other air pollutants may be long-lasting.

The Clean Air Act of 1970 and its revisions (last revision, November 1990) have improved outdoor air quality by establishing outdoor air standards and enforcing compliance with them. Ambient concentrations of certain air pollutants, such as sulfur dioxide and particulates, have decreased over time. Major components of this bill include curtailing emissions of 189 toxic chemicals, many of which are carcinogenic; reducing coal-fired utility emissions of sulfur dioxide, a respiratory irritant and a component of acid rain; and curbing motor vehicle emissions. Critics of the bill are concerned that its standards are not stringent enough and the Environmental Protection Agency (EPA) gives states up to

15 years to enforce the standards. The federal ambient air standard for ozone (0.12 ppm) has not changed and leaves no margin of safety for children.

Pediatricians should counsel parents and patients at special risk, such as asthmatics and children with cystic fibrosis, to be aware of air quality. Susceptible children exposed to excessive air pollution may need to restrict activity while pollution levels are high.

ASBESTOS

Asbestos is a naturally occurring fiber that was widely used in schools, homes, and buildings between the 1940s and 1970s. Because of its strengthening, insulating, and fireproofing qualities, asbestos was used in a large number of products, including pipe coverings, thermal and acoustic insulation, and roofing and flooring products.

Asbestos is a known human carcinogen. Asbestos products in good condition do not usually pose a health risk, but when they become worn and friable, a large number of fibers may be released into the air and inhaled.

There are no acute health risks associated with asbestos exposure. Adults who work with asbestos are at risk for asbestosis and bronchogenic carcinoma in a dose–response relationship. Mesothelioma may occur following transient exposure to asbestos after a latency period of up to 40 years. The main concern about children's exposure to asbestos, therefore, is the possibility of developing mesothelioma later in life.

In 1986, the EPA estimated that 35,000 of the nation's schools contained friable asbestos, with 15 million school children and 1.4 million adult staff members at risk. In 1986, Congress passed the Asbestos Hazard Emergency Response Act (AHERA), which mandated inspection of all public and private elementary and secondary schools and required abatement of any hazardous situation.

There is little information about asbestos in homes. Asbestos may pose a danger to children if it is deteriorating, or when it is exposed and handled, as may happen when the home is renovated. In contrast to the situation in schools, asbestos in homes is not regulated by any governmental agency. It is therefore up to the individual homeowner to determine if the home has asbestos and whether or not it poses a health risk.

Parents should be asked if there is asbestos in the home, what condition it is in, and whether children come into contact with asbestos-containing materials. Only certified contractors should make recommendations about testing for and abating asbestos, because careless removal may release fibers into the air. Questions may be referred to the EPA's Regional Asbestos Coordinator, to state health departments, and to two EPA publications, the *Asbestos Fact Book* may be ordered by EPA's Asbestos Ombudsman Hotline (800-368-5888) and *Asbestos in the Home* may be ordered by calling the TSCA hotline (202-554-1404).

RADON

Radon, a naturally occurring, colorless, odorless gas, is a radioactive decay product of uranium. Radon and its decay products have long been known to increase the risk of lung cancer in uranium miners. More recently, radon has been recognized as a problem in many United States homes. Radon represents the most significant nonmedical radiation exposure to the general population. Approximately 13,000 lung cancer deaths per year may be attributed to exposure to radon in homes.

Radon decays into short-lived "daughters" or "progeny," which are responsible for most of radon's adverse health effects. When progeny become attached to particulates, they are inhaled into the respiratory tract but are not dispersed throughout the body because of rapid radioactive decay. This decay exposes bronchial stem cells to alpha radiation, which penetrates to no more than 70 μm. Thus, cancers produced by radon are limited to the lung. Smoking, which creates more particulate matter in the air, increases this exposure. Although the relationship between radon and cigarette smoking is not precisely known, it is thought to be nearly multiplicative.

Radon emanates primarily from rock and soil but may also be found in water, building materials, and natural gas. Radon diffuses through rocks and soil and is pulled into a home through cracks in the foundation and other entry points. The construction of "tight" homes can result in increased radon concentrations.

Radon is measured in *picocuries per liter* (pCi/L). This unit is generally used to express levels in homes. The average indoor radon concentration is 1.5 pCi/L. Five to ten percent of single family homes exceed 4 pCi/L, the lowest level at which EPA suggests taking action to decrease exposure. Some homes have extremely high levels, exceeding what is permitted in uranium mines. Although radon levels tend to cluster in similar geographic areas, there may be great variability from home to home. Thus, a measurement must be taken to determine the radon level in any one home. Activated charcoal detectors measure radon levels over 3 to 7 days. They are useful in determining high levels quickly but may miss fluctuations. Alpha track detectors, used over a period of months, give more accurate measurements.

Radon, like asbestos, poses no immediate health risk. The risk to children of developing lung cancer as adults is not precisely known. It is plausible, however, to presume that exposure during childhood may have greater effects than exposure during adulthood. This is based on evidence from Japanese atomic bomb survivors: those exposed before 20 years of age had higher relative risks of radiation-induced cancers than did those exposed later in life.

Despite uncertainties, parents and pediatricians should be aware that exposure to high levels of radon over long periods of time poses a risk of lung cancer to their children and to themselves. Information about radon levels in the community can be obtained from local health departments or environmental health authorities. Testing should be recommended in high-risk areas and when there is parental concern. Parents should consult the regional office of the EPA for a current list of reliable testing firms. Cigarette smoking should be discouraged. Parents may be referred to two EPA booklets, *A Citizen's Guide to Radon* and *Consumer's Guide to Radon Reduction,* Public Information Center, 401 M St. SW, Washington, DC 20460). Additionally, parents may call their state environment agency's radon office or the federal EPA's 24-hour hotline: 1-800-SOS-RADON.

LEAD

Lead poisoning is discussed in detail in Chapter 21. Because virtually all United States children are considered at risk for lead poisoning, CDC suggested that every United States preschool-aged child be screened. At highest risk are: children ages 6 to 72 months (especially <36 months) who live in, or are frequent visitors to, deteriorated housing built before 1950; children living in housing built before 1950 with planned or ongoing renovation or remodeling; children who are siblings, housemates, or playmates of children with known lead poisoning; children whose parents or other household members participate in a lead-related occupation or hobby; and children who live near active lead smelters, battery recycling plants, or other industries likely to result in atmospheric lead release.

If the pediatrician does not adopt universal screening, questions that will identify those children at highest risk must be incorporated into the well-child history. These include questions about the location of the home near lead industry, condition of the paint in the home, and occupations of the adults in the home.

PESTICIDES

Pesticides are substances designed to be toxic to living things. They are not, of course, intended to affect human beings, but many do. Approximately 1500 active ingredients are used in the 34,000 pesticide preparations. Legal requirements for pesticide registration by the EPA do not guarantee their safety, because most have not been tested adequately for carcinogenicity, teratogenicity, or mutagenicity. The law regulates only the active ingredients in pesticides, with no requirement that "inert" ingredients be listed on the product label. In addition, even banned pesticides may return as residues on imported food (the "circle of poison").

Pesticides may also cause long-term health hazards. This subject is complex and has not been adequately investigated, so long-term effects are difficult to determine for most exposures.

Children may be exposed to pesticides through ingestion, inhalation, and dermal absorption. In addition to acute ingestion, children take in pesticide residues remaining on foods. Awareness of this issue was heightened because of Alar (daminozide), a suspected carcinogen widely used on apples and other fruit in the 1980s. Although Alar was withdrawn from the market in 1989, concern remains about children's exposure to other residues whose long-term health effects are unknown.

Lawn care products are another source of children's exposure to pesticides. Exposure to the herbicide 2, 4-D (2, 4-dichlorophenoxyacetic acid), an active ingredient in many herbicides, has been associated with a sixfold increase in lymphomas and soft-tissue sarcomas in farmers with long-term exposure to the product. Common fungicides (e.g., maneb, zineb, mancozeb) are metabolized to ethylenethiourea (ETU), which has been shown to cause birth defects, cancer, and thyroid disorders in rats and mice.

Because these pesticides are readily absorbed dermally, they may be more hazardous to children because of children's increased surface area, increased permeability of skin, and increased skin contact with lawn areas. Young children are also at risk through the respiratory route because their breathing zone places them closer to the ground.

The application of insect repellents directly onto children's skin may also place them at risk. The most effective topical insect repellent is "deet" (N-N-diethyl-m-toluamide) which repels a variety of mosquitoes, chiggers, ticks, fleas, and biting flies. Deet is absorbed through the skin and into the systemic circulation. If used, deet should be applied to clothing of infants and young children rather than directly on the skin. Toxic encephalopathy has been reported in infants and children following prolonged application of high concentrations. Allergic skin reactions have also been reported, and ingestion of deet can be fatal.

To avoid acute poisoning, all pesticides should be locked and out of children's reach. Pesticides should never be transferred from their original containers. Parents concerned about pesticide residues on foods should encourage their children to consume a wide variety of fruits and vegetables and encourage their supermarket to stock organically grown produce.

Parents using a lawn care company should find out if the company is certified, what chemicals are used, and whether warnings will be posted. The company should provide customers with fact sheets about their chemicals. Pediatricians should urge parents to consider the risks of using lawn pesticides versus the benefits of a weed-free lawn.

ARTS AND CRAFTS HAZARDS

Art supplies used by children may be hazardous. Children may come into contact with heavy metals (lead, arsenic, cadmium in pigments, glazes, enamels, and solders), solvents (in paints, inks, thinners, and paint removers), dusts (silica and asbestos in clays, talcs, and glazes), and pesticides (used to prolong shelf life). Toxins may be encountered in stained-glass making, ceramics, air-brush painting, jewelry making, woodworking, and model building, to name a few. Lead in artists' paints is legally exempt from other bans on lead in paint, and it is also present in many glazes and solders.

Some children are at higher risk than others. Visually impaired children who work close to an art project may breathe in toxic fumes. Physically handicapped or mentally retarded children who are clumsy or cannot follow safety precautions are more likely to contaminate their skin with toxic materials, inhale toxic vapors, or put toxins into their mouths. Emotionally disturbed children may abuse art materials and endanger themselves or others. Children with asthma may be adversely affected by irritating vapors. Children need not be directly involved in hazardous activities but may be exposed merely by being present in a dangerous work area.

Federal labeling laws provide little guidance in determining the safety of children's art supplies. Until recently, only acute hazards were regulated under the Federal Hazardous Substances Act (FHSA). The "Labelling of Hazardous Materials Act," effective November 1990, required that guidelines be established to determine whether art materials present chronic hazards, such as carcinogenicity, neurotoxicity, and reproductive/developmental toxicity, but did not include other chronic effects such as those on the heart, liver, or other organs.

The Arts and Crafts Materials Institute (ACMI), an industry-supported organization, has sponsored a voluntary standard for children's art materials for over 40 years. The ACMI's Approved Product (AP) and Certified Product (CP) labels have reassured parents and teachers as to the safety of children's art products. However, independent audits suggest that despite the "AP" or "CP" label, caution is still advisable because some products contain small quantities of heavy metals, and other products, such as oil paints, require potentially toxic solvents for clean-up. The California List of Approved Children's Art Materials, previously considered the safest, has not been updated in several years and can no longer be relied on. Despite labeling deficiencies, parents and teachers should choose a product with a label over one without one. The AP/CP seal gives some reassurance that the product was reviewed by a toxicologist. Activities involving the use of sprays, dusts, and solvents should be avoided.

Parents involved in potentially dangerous arts and crafts activities in the home should confine their work to one area. They should wear disposable clothing and an approved respirator. The area should be well ventilated. Children should never be allowed to play in an area where there are toxic arts and crafts materials.

WORK-RELATED HAZARDS

Parents exposed to toxic substances at work may bring these home on their clothes and shoes, on their lunch boxes and tool kits, and in the car. A well-documented example of a "brought-home" toxin is lead carried home by parents who work in areas such as lead smelting, bridge repair, battery recycling, demolition, and rehabilitation of houses. Asbestosis has been documented in the adult children of shipyard workers, and elevated urinary mercury levels have been found in children of mercury thermometer plant workers.

A review of the literature suggested a relationship between certain types of childhood cancer (particularly leukemia and lymphomas) and parental occupation.

Because of these risks, an occupational history should be obtained. Family members employed in high-risk industries should leave contaminated clothes at work and should have them sent out to the laundry instead of washing them at home.

Children themselves, particularly teenagers, may also be employed. Employment may offer economic opportunity, development of new skills and responsibilities, and heightening of self-esteem. On the other hand, employment may place the adolescent at risk for school problems, limit time for interaction with peers and for social activities, and expose him or her to possible injury, illness, and toxins.

The Fair Labor Standards Act (FLSA) provides a broad framework for the regulation of child labor (defined as paid employment of children under 16). The FLSA prohibits children under 16 from working during school hours and sets maximum permitted numbers of hours worked per day and per week. Any person under 18 is prohibited from working in any hazardous nonagricultural occupation. This includes operating meat processing machinery, delicatessen slicers, and supermarket box-crushers. In addition, no one under 18 may work in logging, mining, brick and tile manufacture, excavating, or roofing as a helper on a vehicle or on power-driven machinery. Restrictions in agriculture are much less stringent. Most administration of the FLSA occurs at the state level. The maximum permissible hours worked varies by state.

The adolescent history should include questions about whether the patient is employed, the nature of the job, how many hours are worked, and whether the work endangers the patient in some way or interferes with normal development.

Pediatricians should also be aware that a substantial number of children are employed illegally and that child labor in this country appears to be increasing. This includes children working in fields recently sprayed with pesticides, children who do industrial work after school, and younger adolescents who work on prohibited machinery in factories, bakeries, and butcher shops.

ANNOTATED BIBLIOGRAPHY

American Academy of Pediatrics Committee on Environmental Hazards: Asbestos exposure in schools. Pediatrics 79:301–305, 1987. (Although this article was written before the AHERA legislation, it gives information about risks of disease to children and about evaluation and abatement of asbestos in schools.)

American Academy of Pediatrics Committee on Environmental Hazards: Radon exposure: A risk to children. Pediatrics 83:799–802, 1989. (Summarizes chemistry of radon, sources, and probable risks of radon exposure to children.)

Babin A, Peltz P, Rossol M: Children's Art Supplies Can Be Toxic. Center for Safety in the Arts, New York, NY, 1989. (Good reference for evaluating art supplies and labeling laws; gives a list of safe alternatives.)

Natural Resources Defense Council: Intolerable Risk: Pesticides in Our Children's Food. February 27, 1989. (First detailed analysis of children's exposures to pesticides in foods.)

Office on Smoking and Health: The Health Consequences of Involuntary Smoking: A Report of the Surgeon General. Rockville, MD, United States Public Health Service, 1986.

Pollack SH, Landrigan PJ, Mallino DL: Child labor in 1990. Annu Rev Public Health 11:359–375, 1990. (Reviews current knowledge about extent and hazards of child labor and discusses options for prevention of morbidity.)

19

Injury Prevention

Robert A. Dershewitz

On the basis of mortality and morbidity data, injury control (formerly called, and often used interchangeably with, "accident prevention") is the most important topic in pediatrics. About half of all deaths in children are caused by injuries, and 20% of all hospitalizations for children result from injuries. Motor vehicle–related injuries account for 47% of unintentional injury deaths, followed by drowning (9.2%), fires and burns (7.2%), falls (1.4%), and firearms (1.27%). After injuries from motor vehicles, homicide and suicide are the second (13%) and third (10%) leading causes of pediatric injury death. Each year, approximately 16 million children receive medical care for injuries, and over 30,000 children become permanently disabled. The cost of injuries to children exceeds 7.5 billion dollars annually. Governmental regulations and legislation have proved beneficial in reducing childhood injuries. Health education is not as effective because altering behavior is considerably more difficult.

The educational impact may be improved by limiting the content of the education, explaining its relevance, repeating the message, and having the recommendations practical and easy to implement. Most importantly, the message must be targeted to the group being taught and must be appropriate to the developmental level of the child.

There are several programs to aid the practitioner in providing safety counseling. The one most widely used is The Injury Prevention Program (TIPP) sponsored by the American Academy of Pediatrics. The injury categories listed in Table 19-1 constitute the minimum injury prevention topics that should be discussed at each visit. Pediatricians should be especially tuned into high-risk situations. Injuries have a greater likelihood of occurring at times of stress, such as moves, so counseling at these times may be particularly effective. The injury repeater may be the clue to a dysfunctional child or family and would thus warrant special attention.

AUTOMOTIVE SAFETY

Fortunately, cars are increasingly being equipped with air bags and automatic occupant restraints. These passive measures will probably have a greater impact than will counseling. The focus of education must be on parents consistently using infant car restraints. This message should start at either the prenatal or newborn hospital visit. Ideally, infants should ride semi-reclined and backward-facing in the back seat of the car. Parents must read the manufacturer's directions to ensure that the car seat is used properly. At 17 to 20 lbs, the baby is too large to remain in an infant carrier and will need to use a toddler seat, which should face forward. When the child reaches 40 to 44 lbs, he or she may use either an approved booster seat or a seat belt (which is not as safe as a booster seat). The shoulder harness should not be worn if it goes across the child's face or across the front of his or her throat. Also remind parents that all car doors should be locked.

The premature infant can safety ride in a semi-reclined position, but an adult should always monitor the baby in case the head falls forward, which may compromise the airway. All new car seats meeting current safety standards provide adequate protection. Although a convertible car seat is more expensive than an infant carrier, it is cheaper in the long run because there is no need to purchase a second car seat. Parents must not mistake the flimsy infant seats, which are not intended to be used in cars, with car seats.

The most unsafe place for a child in a car is on an adult's lap in the front seat. With an abrupt stop, the child is thrown against the dashboard, followed by the adult's body, which crushes the child and adds further injury. The outside of vehicles is even more dangerous. Nevertheless, many children ride in the back of pick-up trucks where there is a much greater risk for ejection and more severe injuries.

Parents should set an example themselves by wearing seat belts and be adamant about their child riding in a car seat. Bring toys in the car for the child to play with, if necessary. Reward the child for good behavior.

There are a variety of adaptations of car seats or commercially available special, safe car restraint systems for children unable to use standard child safety seats or safety belts. These may include children with very low birth weight, spina bifida, leg or hip casts, cerebral palsy, or ventilator

Table 19-1. Age-Appropriate Safety Counseling Topics

VISIT	TIPP* (MINIMAL TOPICS TO COVER)	OTHER RELEVANT TOPICS
Prenatal/hospital	Infant car seat† Smoke Detector Crib safety	
2–4 wk.	Falls	Car seats
2 mo.	Burns—hot liquids	
4 mo.	Choking	Toy safety
6 mo.	Poisonings Burns—hot surfaces	Poisonous plants Safety-proofing
9 mo.	Water safety Toddler car seat	Aspiration
12 mo.	Reinforce poisonings, falls, and burns	
15 mo.	Same as at 12 mo.	Guns Cuts
18 mo.	Same as at 12 mo.	Reinforce appropriateness of toys
24 mo.	Playgrounds Tricycles Pedestrian safety	Yard safety
3 yr.	Reinforce car, falls, and burns	Reinforce appropriateness of toys How to approach strange animals
4 yr.		Fire prevention Fire drills
5 yr.	Bicycle safety Pedestrian safety	
6 yr.	Fire safety	Sledding safety
8 yr.	Water safety	
10 yr.	Sports safety	
Adolescents		Car safety Risk taking Firearms Power tools (e.g., lawn mowers) Sports injuries

*The Injury Prevention Program, revised, 1989.
†Car safety counseling at every well-child visit.

dependency. (More information may be obtained by contacting the Automotive Safety for Children Program at the James Whitcomb Riley Hospital for Children, Indianapolis, IN 46202.)

PEDESTRIAN INJURIES

Pedestrian deaths account for approximately one fourth of all motor vehicle deaths. Most of the 1800 child pedestrian fatalities each year occur while the child is crossing a street. The seriousness of this danger is underscored by the fact that pedestrian injuries have the highest death-to-injury ratio of any type of motor vehicle–related injury. Thus, parents must be warned to exercise proper caution and supervision when children play outside. Children should not be allowed to play near or in traffic, and parents must teach their children how (and where) to cross streets.

BURNS

Hot Liquids

About 75% of all burns to children are scalds, and most occur in the kitchen. About 9400 young children are hospitalized annually in the United States for scald burns. Infants are often scalded when sitting on the lap of a person drinking a hot beverage. Coffeepots and teapots should not be left on the table, and pot handles should face the back of the stove. Parents should be advised to buy a cool mist vaporizer rather than a steam vaporizer. As both an energy-saving and injury-prevention measure, the home water thermostats should be set no higher than 125°F.

Hot Surfaces

Most hazards in this category are obvious. Some, such as hair dryers, are not. Young children should not be allowed to play near hot ovens and barbecues. Wire screens around fireplaces prevent children (especially hair and clothing) from catching fire. Sleepwear should be flame-resistant or retardant, and children should not be allowed to play with toys that can burn them. Guards should be placed in front of heaters, and parents should be cautioned to unplug an iron when not in use. The insertion of outlet covers in unused outlets and removing or taping extension cords to the plug prevent many electrical burns.

FIRE PREVENTION AND DRILLS

One out of every 17 homes in the United States has a fire, and house fires cause about 80% of all deaths related to fires and burns. Smoke detectors have the greatest potential for saving lives from fires, and all three types (heat, photoelectric, and ionization) are effective. Parents must be encouraged to install them and must be reminded to check the battery monthly. Matches and lighters must not be accessible, and parents ought to be warned, especially if a grandparent lives at home, never to smoke in bed. Each household should conduct periodic fire drills and have a clearly delineated escape plan in the event of a fire. It is a good idea to have an "ABC"-rated fire extinguisher in the kitchen. For any fire larger than a small, self-contained stovetop fire, the house should be left immediately and the fire department called from a neighbor's house.

FALLS

Falls are the fifth leading cause of death in children and result in enormous morbidity. Infants should never be left unattended on an elevated surface such as a changing table or bed, and the crib railing must be up. Gates on staircases should be used when children first learn to walk. This will also prevent falls from walkers, an occurrence resulting in about 24,000 emergency room visits per year in the United States. Window sills and bunk beds must be forbidden play areas. In 1987, 25,000 children under 15 years of age received emergency room care for bunk bed–related injuries. Until children are older, screens and window locks should be used to limit how high windows may be raised. Situations that greatly increase the likelihood of falls, such as overwaxing floors, storing objects on stairs, using scatter rugs, and leaving spills on floors, should be avoided. During the toddler years, sharp-edged coffee tables should be moved from the center of the living room or even removed from the room.

Each year, a staggering number of children require medical attention from falls involving playground equipment. Forty to fifty percent occur at home; the remainder occur at parks or school playgrounds. Falls from swings, slides, playhouses, and monkey bars are most common, and the head, neck, and face are most frequently injured. Preventive measures that should be emphasized include: having all equipment in good working order and encouraging parents to teach their children to minimize risk-taking behavior. If the gross motor activity is developmentally too advanced for the child, either the child should be supervised more closely or that activity should be prevented. Skateboards and trampolines are highly dangerous. Children should be discouraged from playing with the former and banned from the latter. The trampoline often is the cause of spinal cord injuries.

GUNS

Gunshot wounds to children are increasing dramatically, in part because of gang-related homicide. One half to three fourths of homes in the United States have guns, and unintentional shootings are a major cause of death in children. A little more than half of these fatalities occur at home. Guns other than firearms, such as BB guns, pellet guns, spring-operated guns, and air guns, are widely marketed as toys, so many mistakenly think they are harmless. Any type of gun is a dangerous weapon capable of, and often producing, severe injuries such as blindness. Prevention is straightforward: all firearms should be locked up, and children should not be allowed to play with *any* type of gun; better yet, guns should not be kept in homes where there are children.

CHOKING

Choking is the most common cause of indoor death in young children and may occur from either food or nonfood items. Parents should be taught proper first-aid for a choking child.

Because hot dogs, nuts, grapes, and raisins are the foods most commonly aspirated, they should not be fed to infants. Furthermore, toddlers should not be allowed to run with food in their mouth or to chew gum. Small objects are also commonly aspirated, particularly balloons, pacifiers, and jacks; thus, they should be kept away from young children.

TOY SAFETY

Children need to play with toys, but they also need toys that are safe and age-appropriate to minimize the risk of injuries. Worn and broken toys are likely to be dangerous. Darts, trampolines, and BB guns are dangerous at any age. Objects not intended to be used as toys, such as abandoned refrigerators, may also be dangerous because children may suffocate in them. Even "cuddly" toys may be lethal. For example, a stuffed animal with small parts that an infant can easily pull off are highly dangerous because the small parts might be aspirated. Pacifiers that are not of single-piece construction are also dangerous because of their potential for aspiration.

POISONS

Toddlers are at greatest risk of accidental ingestions. Largely as a result of legislative measures, the rate of poison fatalities has declined, yet poisonings remain a major pediatric problem. Safety-proofing should usually start when the child is 6 months old, before the crawling stage. The most dangerous household items are cleaning agents, especially furniture polish and products containing caustic agents. Therefore, they should all be stored high in cabinets with locks. Medicines must be kept in locked cabinets or boxes, and parents should be reminded that pocketbooks containing medications should not be within reach of youngsters. Substances found commonly in most households, such as insecticides and alcohol, should also be inaccessible to children.

Syrup of ipecac should be in each home where there is a young child, with the telephone number of the poison control center written on the label or conspicuously posted by the phone. Parents must be instructed never to give ipecac to their child without medical authorization because inducing vomiting is contraindicated for certain types of ingestions.

Five to 10% of calls to poison control centers involve plant ingestions. Most households have plants, and it is unrealistic to expect parents to know the names of the over 700 plants that have been identified as poisonous. It is, however, realistic to ask parents to know the names of *their* house plants. Regional poison control centers are sources of useful information (see also Chapter 177).

WATER SAFETY

Drowning is the second leading cause of death in children between 5 and 14 years of age. Most drownings occur when children are poorly supervised in pools and bathtubs. Boating injuries are another major cause of drowning. Infants can drown in unusual ways at home (e.g., pail immersions and toilet bowls). Supervision is the key to prevention. Other parental responsibilities include teaching their children to swim, teaching them proper conduct around water, and following other water safety precautions (e.g., having life preservers on boats). Those with swimming pools should have "isolated fencing" that completely surrounds the pool, thereby separating the pool from the house and the rest of the yard.

LACERATIONS

Most cuts occurring in children are relatively minor but account for thousands of emergency room visits each year. Kitchen knives and scissors may cause serious cuts. The most dangerous type of cut results from falls through non-safety glass (e.g., patio doors). The glass may break into razor-sharp pieces, producing severe lacerations. Children should be told not to play near glass. If high-risk glass doors cannot be replaced by safety glass, easily visible decals must be placed on them. Many children are cut in their yards, so parents should remove dangerous objects such as broken glass. Bushes with thorns should also be avoided.

BICYCLE AND TRICYCLE SAFETY

There are approximately 1 million bicycle injuries each year, with injuries peaking between the ages of 5 and 14 years. More than 600 children die annually in this age group, most by colliding with an automobile. Injuries from tricycles usually occur at an earlier age. While resultant mortality is uncommon with tricycles, serious injury may occur. Children should not ride a bicycle until developmentally ready, and they should not be permitted to ride in the street until they demonstrate competence in understanding and following traffic rules, such as riding in the direction of traffic, using hand signals, and otherwise demonstrating good judgment. This generally does not occur before age 8, and in many children it occurs years later. Children must never ride at dusk or when it is dark, and they should always wear protective helmets. Because it is risky to have passengers on bikes, children should never ride double.

OTHER SPORTS-RELATED INJURIES

The risk of sports injury varies according to the recreational activity. In Massachusetts, 1 out of every 14 adolescents becomes hospitalized each year for a sports injury. While the number of deaths is relatively low, sports injuries result in a large number of emergency room visits and hospitalizations. In addition to those recreational activities already discussed, all sports, but most notably football, basketball, skateboarding, hockey, gymnastics, and sledding have their own inherent dangers. There is a need to have coaches and other supervisory personnel better trained, because with proper knowledge, many injuries could be either avoided or minimized. It is likely that in the near future coaches will need to be certified in basic principles of sports medicine. Indeed, we should advocate for this.

All-terrain vehicles are particularly dangerous. Legislation has helped in restricting their availability but has not outlawed all models.

ANIMALS

Each year, nearly 1 million children are bitten by animals, many of whom are domestic pets. Children must be taught how to interact with and approach animals. Pets, especially if accustomed to a household without children, may become jealous and therefore must prove themselves safe to be around children. Instruct children to avoid strange animals and not to tease or hit animals. Also caution children not to awaken or take food away from an animal, feed strange dogs, or be licked by a strange dog.

ADOLESCENT CONCERNS

Adolescents are at particular risk for vehicle-related injuries. The risk of injuries is increased if the adolescent (1) is a novice driver, (2) has a tendency for risk-taking behavior (especially males), or (3) experiments with drugs and alcohol. Motorcycles are even more dangerous. Mile for mile, the death rate from motorcycles is 15 times greater than that from cars. For each year an adolescent rides a motorcycle, he has a 2% chance of being killed or seriously injured. Helmets greatly reduce the severity of injury, but unfortunately many riders choose not to wear them.

THE PEDIATRICIAN AS ADVOCATE

Although potentially time-consuming, advocating safety practices outside the office (e.g., in the political arena) can be enormously beneficial and worthwhile. As an example, the enactment of the child car safety restraint law by all 50 states was in large measure due to practitioners who convinced elected officials that such legislation was in the public interest. Depending on one's time commitment and interest, there are different levels of involvement, ranging from telephoning legislators, to writing letters, to testifying for the passage of safety standards. In addition, if dangerous toys or situations are noted (e.g., unsafe playgrounds), the pediatrician has an ethical responsibility to try to correct the situation, such as notifying the toy manufacturer or school officials.

ANNOTATED BIBLIOGRAPHY

American Journal of Diseases of Children. Vol. 144, June 1990. (Entire issue devoted to childhood injuries. Chapters on injury facts, policy, educational intervention, and the many different types of injuries.)

Baker SP, O'Neill B, Karpf RS: The Injury Fact Book. Lexington, MA, Lexington Books, 1984. (All the facts you would ever want to know about injuries.)

Moriarty RW: Poisonous plants. Drug Therapy July 1978, pp 101–109. (Summarizes the experience of one poison control center and presents a concise compilation of clinically relevant information regarding poisonous plants.)

Stout JD, Bull MJ, Stroup KB: Safe transportation for children with disabilities. Am J Occup Ther 43:31–36, 1989. (Excellent overview of safe transportation for children unable to use conventional car restraints.)

TIPP—The Injury Prevention Program. Elk Grove Village, IL, American Academy of Pediatrics, 1989. (Updated and expanded from the first 1983 program. Fulfills its goal of helping the practitioner efficiently deliver age-appropriate safety advice.)

20
Child Abuse
Paula Kienberger Jaudes

Child abuse and neglect have existed throughout the history of man. Both are written about in the Old and the New Testament. Child abuse and neglect (e.g., infanticide) were a means of population control by the ancient Greeks and other societies in which the child was considered the property of the parents and had no rights of his or her own. In more recent times, Charles Dickens depicted the problem of child abuse as it existed in England during the Industrial Revolution. Scattered reports in the medical literature described abuse, but it was not until 1962 that Dr. Henry Kempe first described and named the *battered child syndrome.*

Child abuse and neglect are major pediatric problems in the twentieth century. In the United States, it is estimated that over 1000 children die annually after battery or gross neglect. Over 1 million children are maltreated by their parents each year, and more than 200,000 children are sexually abused annually.

On the average, the practicing physician will see four to six child abuse patients each year. Child abuse and neglect exist across social, racial, geographic, and economic boundaries. The spectrum of child abuse is broad and includes physical abuse, sexual abuse, and emotional abuse. Forms of neglect include medical, supervisional, educational, physical, and failure to thrive. The physician must be aware of all these manifestations.

ABUSE

The key to the diagnosis of child abuse is the examining physician's *suspicion.* The physician must have an open mind concerning the potential of abuse in every pediatric patient. Clues that may arouse suspicion begin with the case history of an injured child. The following clues are helpful for the diagnosis of child abuse:

1. The parent's or caretaker's story does not explain the child's injuries. An important aspect that should be considered is normal child development (e.g., a 5-month-old infant cannot climb into a tub of hot water).
2. The story told by the parent or caretaker may be inconsistent or contradictory. Does the story change? Does one parent give one explanation and the other parent give another? What does the child say?
3. There is an unnecessarily long time interval between the injury and seeking of medical treatment.
4. The parent's reaction to the seriousness of the injury is inappropriate.
5. The parent's interaction with the child is inappropriate.

In addition to the history, the physical examination of the child helps the physician to determine whether to suspect abuse. The physical examination should begin with observation of the child. Is the child afraid, withdrawn, and does he or she have a frozen stare? The whole body should be examined, with documentation of injuries and the stages of their resolution. Injuries on several areas of the body, in various stages of healing, indicate physical abuse.

Physical Abuse

Bruises. The skin is the most common site where physical abuse is diagnosed. Therefore, it is important to examine the skin of the entire body. The physician must distinguish between inflicted and accidental trauma. Accidental injuries usually occur on the knees, shins, and elbows. Suspicion of abuse should be aroused by signs of trauma on the face, buttocks, neck, back, genitalia, and chest.

The shape of the lesion is also important. An electric extension cord is perhaps the most common "weapon" used on a child. An extension cord, rope, or belt, when folded back on itself, can leave a characteristic loop mark on the body. These objects may also leave linear marks. A hand slap can leave red linear marks the size of the hand on any part of the body. A human bite causes a crescent-shaped crushing injury. One can distinguish between a child's bite and an adult's bite by the size of the arch. A dog's bite characteristically causes a puncture, rip, or tear injury. If a child has been tied down, a linear circumferential burn or abrasion is usually seen around the wrists or ankles. Pinpricks cause petechiae, usually found on the palms and soles.

In documenting bruises and correlating them with the patient's history, the physician needs to estimate the age of the skin lesion. A bruise is initially red to purple. Within the first week, the color changes to dark purple, and during the second week, to yellow. By the third to fourth week, the bruise has usually resolved.

Burns. Approximately 10% of all injuries inflicted on children are burns, including cigarette burns and immersion burns. A cigarette burn initially leaves a characteristic circular ulcerative lesion that may resemble bullous impetigo or an infected insect bite. On a pigmented child, it may leave a hypopigmented circular lesion after healing has occurred. Typically, inflicted cigarette burns are found on the hands, feet, or buttocks. If a child has been burned by another object (e.g., if the child has been placed on a radiator, hot plate, or iron), the burn will resemble the outline of the object. These types of burns, however, could be accidental. Thus, a history is important to help distinguish accidental from inflicted burns. Splash burns are commonly accidental burns. Typically, such a burn is unilateral and is not well defined, and there are satellite burn lesions that are caused by the splashes. On the other hand, an immersion burn is an inflicted injury, in many cases as a form of pun-

ishment related to issues of toilet training. The child is dunked into hot water, with the buttocks and perineum making contact with the water first. The burn leaves characteristic water level marks around the buttocks and feet where these were immersed.

Fractures. In the diagnosis of accidental versus inflicted fractures, the location and the type of fracture are important. Accidental rib fractures are rare in children; they are found most often in adolescents who participate in contact sports. Rib fractures are usually caused by a fist, foot, or blunt object that strikes the front or back of the chest. Skull fractures can be caused accidentally; however, a thorough history and physical examination should be obtained in cases of skull fractures so that the possibility of abuse can be explored. A spiral fracture is caused by the twisting of a bone. Children who are not ambulatory and thus do not bear weight are unlikely to have this type of fracture occur by accident. A metaphyseal chip fracture is the result of the wrenching, forcing, or pulling of an extremity. Blunt trauma to a bone may cause subperiosteal hemorrhage, with subsequent periosteal thickening and elevation. Beginning calcification and remodeling of the bone will be seen on radiographs approximately 7 to 10 days after the trauma has been inflicted. The presence of multiple fractures of the same or various ages should be considered a sign of abuse, unless the clinical history provides another explanation for the pattern of the fractures.

Visceral Trauma. When visceral trauma is inflicted deliberately, there is often no visible evidence of injury except for bruises on the abdomen. Forceful blows to the abdomen may cause a ruptured viscus, tears of organs, and hematomas. Any abdominal structure may be damaged. The child may have a distended abdomen as well as bowel obstruction, coma, shock, or death.

Central Nervous System Trauma. Physical abuse is recognized as a leading cause of subdural hematomas in infants. The whiplash shaken infant syndrome is caused by severe shaking of an infant, usually under 1 year of age, which may cause subdural hematomas, cerebral injury, and retinal hemorrhages. The child may be lethargic or in a coma, with bruising around the arms or the chest in a pattern that fits the offender's hands. Infants who have been shaken usually do not have skull fractures or signs of scalp injury. Accidents such as a fall from a couch or a bed rarely cause serious bleeding in the brain. Therefore, all children with major head trauma, including epidural, subdural, and subarachnoid hematomas and depressed skull fractures, should be investigated for abuse.

Poisoning. Accidental poisonings are common in children under 3 years of age. Intentional poisoning is difficult to prove but should be considered if the child is over 3 years of age. Substances that have been identified in cases of intentional poisoning include tranquilizers, hypnotics, alcohol, diuretics, and all forms of street drugs. Small children have been poisoned by having water withheld and by being fed salt.

Münchausen Syndrome by Proxy. Münchausen syndrome by proxy is characterized by parents (most often the mother) giving a fictitious history and lying about symptoms in their children, causing the children to undergo multiple hospitalizations with unnecessary diagnostic and therapeutic procedures. Parents may actually poison the child in order to cause symptoms of disease or to manipulate signs and symptoms that simulate disease.

Sexual Abuse

Sexual abuse is probably the least reported and most underdiagnosed of all types of child abuse. A conservative estimate is that one in ten children will be exposed to this form of abuse. Kempe defined sexual abuse as "involvement of dependent, developmentally immature children and adolescents in sexual activities that they do not fully comprehend, or are unable to give informed consent, and that violate the social taboos of family roles." Sexual abuse of children includes incest, sexual assaults, and exposure to sexual assaults. Incest is best defined as any sexual relation or activity between various combinations of "legal relatives," including step-parents. Sexual assaults include rape, molestation, fondling of the genitalia or of the anal or oral region, fellatio, cunnilingus, and sodomy. Sexual abuse also includes exhibitionism and having the child present during the sexual acts of others.

Sex offenders are predominantly male. In approximately 90% of the cases involving a child, the child knows the offender (e.g., he is a family member, a neighbor, or someone at school). The average age of girls who are abused is 10 years old, and the average age of boys is 7 years old.

When a child reports being abused, this is not only a cry for help but also an act of courage. Children do not fabricate stories about detailed sexual activities. Thus, sexual accusations by a preadolescent child should be believed. It happens only rarely that a disturbed adolescent lies about being sexually abused. Children describing sexual encounters will use language appropriate to their developmental stage. Visual aids such as special coloring books or dolls can help a child tell his story. Above all, children should be given the benefit of the doubt about sexual abuse even if their account contradicts an adult's statements.

In all cases of suspected child sexual abuse, as in other types of abuse, the pediatrician should have a high index of suspicion. If a child does not report an incident directly, there are indirect ways of detecting that sexual abuse has occurred. Any genital injuries, irritations, or discharge may indicate sexual abuse, and all sexually transmitted diseases should be considered possible evidence of such abuse. These diseases include *Neisseria gonorrhoeae,* syphilis, *Trichomonas vaginalis,* condyloma acuminatum, *Chlamydia trachomatis,* and herpes simplex type II.

Common childhood problems, although nonspecific, could indicate sexual abuse at home. These problems include difficulty with friends, failure at school, isolation from peers, enuresis, and encopresis. Certain changes in behavior have been associated with sexual abuse. Examples are the sudden appearance of symptoms such as night terrors, fear states, clinging behavior, sudden school phobias, anxiety, depression, and insomnia. In adolescents, one may see acting-out behavior, teenage pregnancy, running away from home, drug abuse, suicide attempts, sexual acting out, or fear of any sexual activity.

If there is a suspicion of sexual abuse, a complete physical examination should be done. An examination of the genital area should be performed last. The skin should be examined closely for the presence of injuries such as abrasions, excoriations, bruises, or suction petechiae on the breasts or the body. Edema or laceration of the frenulum of the lips may be identified. The abdomen should be examined for tenderness or the presence of masses. In the male, signs of genital or anal trauma should be noted, and the presence or absence of urethral discharge should be determined. For prepubescent girls, a careful inspection should be done of the labia, vagina, hymen, anus, and adjacent skin. In pubescent girls, special attention should be given to signs of pregnancy, such as increased uterine size or bluish discoloration of the cervix.

In many cases, the findings on physical examination will be normal even though there is a history of sexual abuse. Younger pediatric patients usually show few physical signs because they are often victims of fondling only. Furthermore, the sexual assault often happens weeks, months, or years before it is mentioned by the child. The longer the time between the sexual assault and its revelation, the less likely that pertinent positive physical signs of sexual abuse will be discovered. The child should be believed, however, even if there are no abnormal findings on physical examination.

Emotional Abuse

Emotional abuse is the parental act of chronic denigration of a child. Continual verbal attacks deprive a child of love, security, and the feeling of being wanted. Emotional abuse whittles away at a child's spirit and self-esteem. This is probably the most common form of child abuse, the least often reported, and the most difficult to document.

NEGLECT

Child neglect is the type of maltreatment reported most frequently to state agencies, and it causes the greatest morbidity in children. There usually is a pattern of neglect with more than one type of neglect occurring.

In all forms of neglect, the pediatrician's role is to intervene and to be an advocate for the child. The physician, using his or her best judgment, must decide whether the neglect is hindering the growth and development of the child. Intervention may initially take the form of social service involvement but may at times require the state's child protective services.

Medical

Medical neglect includes refusing or denying treatment for serious acute illnesses such as meningitis. It also includes not treating life-threatening chronic disorders such as diabetes mellitus or asthma when appropriate treatment is known and available. Withholding treatment such as bracing, physical therapy, occupational therapy, and speech therapy for disabling or handicapping chronic diseases, such as cerebral palsy, or for potentially fatal illnesses, such as cancer, for which there is an accepted medical treatment, is also considered medical neglect.

One cannot hold all parents responsible for meeting the optimal standards recommended by the American Academy of Pediatrics for well-baby care. However, at a minimum, the child should have received immunizations (unless contrary to religious beliefs) and should have seen a physician within the first 5 years of life.

Supervisional

Supervisional neglect is expressed in morbidity and mortality of children as a result of accidents. For the first 3 to 4 years of a child's life, his or her environment needs to be controlled. Leaving a child at home alone without supervision can result in serious injuries and poisonings, many of which could have been prevented if the child were better supervised by an adult.

Emotional

Emotional neglect is the lack of a loving relationship between the parents and the child. Children who are emotionally deprived are usually withdrawn and listless, and many have developmental delays. It is difficult to define the minimum responsibilities of a parent with regard to love. There are parents who are mentally ill or mentally limited and who are thus incapable of assuming the role of parents. Whatever the reason for this deficient relationship, when the child's growth and development are adversely affected, the case is one of emotional neglect.

Educational

Educational neglect of school-aged children is defined as more than 25 days of school absenteeism in the year. The child or adolescent is often made to stay at home to babysit younger siblings. All children should attend school by 7 years of age. Children with special needs, such as disabilities, should be in school by 3 years of age, as provided by federal law.

Physical

Physical neglect is the lack of provision of adequate food, clothing, and shelter. Abandonment, when a parent cannot or will not take care of a child, is the ultimate form of physical neglect. Typically, the child is left with a member of the family or a baby-sitter, and the parent does not return.

Failure to Thrive

Failure to thrive (FTT) is the failure of an infant to properly grow and develop. Every child needs both adequate nutrition and "love" in order to grow and develop normally. Children who do not thrive are usually less than 2 years old. The first evidence of failure to thrive is usually a subnormal weight gain. The absence of physical clues is often indicative of "nonorganic" FTT (see Chap. 188).

OTHER FORMS OF MALTREATMENT

Fetal neglect is considered a form of maltreatment. This occurs when a baby is born showing signs of alcohol or drug withdrawal from maternal substance abuse. In all states, the suspicion of denial of reasonable medical care to a defective newborn may be reported to the Child Protection Agency. Another form of maltreatment is exploitation of a child, including forced exposure to drugs, alcohol, and pornography, as well as child labor.

EVALUATION AND TREATMENT

When the physician suspects child abuse or neglect, he or she must report this suspicion to the state Child Protection Agency and may also refer the child to a local hospital that has a child abuse team. Many victims of suspected child abuse or neglect may initially be admitted to the hospital. The hospital assumes the responsibility for protecting the child, following up on the reported problem and providing social service support for the child and his family. A hospital admission also allows time for a medical and social evaluation and affords an opportunity for in-depth planning for the future welfare of the child. If a parent refuses admission or threatens to remove the child from the hospital, the physician may need to take protective custody.

During hospitalization, the staff should record the child's history and the results of a physical examination, with specific attention to a description of all lesions on the child's body, including their color, type, location, and shape. Clinical photographs should be taken if the child is injured or malnourished. Parental consent is not required for these photographs. Clotting studies should be performed if bruises are present. A skeletal survey should be done on children who have signs of trauma, particularly children who are less than 3 years old. Exact documentation of growth and development is necessary, particularly if a child appears malnourished or deprived.

If there is suspicion that a child has been sexually abused, a Gram's stain of any discharge from the vagina, urethra, or anus should be done. Specimens from the cervix (in adolescents), vagina (introitus), urethra, anus, and throat should be cultured for *N. gonorrhoeae* and *C. trachomatis*. Other tests that are indicated include a serologic test for syphilis, a pregnancy test in postmenarcheal females, and a urinalysis to look for trichomonads. The state's forensic collecting kit should be used if a sexual assault has occurred within the previous 72 hours. Potentially evidential specimens should be obtained, including samples of clothing, diapers, pubic hair, scrapings of blood, and so forth, as indicated.

THE PHYSICIAN AND THE ABUSER

The most important role for the physician is that of advocate for the child. Physicians must report cases of suspected abuse or neglect to the appropriate state agency. In some cases, the identity of the abuser may be unknown or uncertain, because children may be cared for by numerous people. The physician has a moral obligation to inform the parents or caretakers of his or her concerns and to tell them that he or she is required by law to notify the state's Child Protection Agency of these concerns. This requirement may make the physician's interaction with the parent(s)/caretaker(s) difficult because these cases arouse a great deal of emotion in those involved. It is best to be honest with the parents/caretakers without being judgmental or angry. The physician should also take time to describe the process that will unfold (e.g., the involvement of the child protection service worker).

Parents and caretakers who abuse or neglect their children come in all colors, from all socioeconomic groups, and from all ethnic and religious affiliations. The bases of child abuse and neglect are many and varied; they range from the temporary stress of unemployment, to being raised in a dysfunctional family, to severe mental illness. Similarly, abusive parents/caretakers may require access to a broad range of services, such as counseling, parenting skills training, proper housing, job training, and psychiatric services. At times, because of the severity of the abuse, the severity of the parent's psychopathology, or the condition of the child, out-of-home placement may be necessary. However, the overall goal is to preserve the family unit.

CHILD PROTECTION AND LEGAL SYSTEMS

In all 50 states, if a physician *suspects* that a child has been abused or neglected, the physician is required to notify the state's Child Protection Agency. After making the report, the physician is protected by law from being sued by the alleged abusive parents. In some states, if a physician fails to report a possible case of child abuse or neglect, he or she could be jailed, lose his or her medical license, or become liable to a malpractice suit.

Once the report has been made, the Child Protection Agency has the responsibility for investigating the case. The state case worker will talk with the physician and other medical personnel and with the family, neighbors, and the child. The case worker decides whether the allegation of abuse or neglect has credence and whether to take the case to juvenile court.

In juvenile court (or family court, in some jurisdictions), the judge rules on child abuse on the basis of "preponderance of evidence" and makes decisions concerning custody issues. If the child abuse has consisted of homicide, extreme battery, or sexual abuse, the case may also be adjudicated in criminal court. In criminal court, the judgment is based on evidence "beyond a reasonable doubt" against the alleged perpetrator.

If the physician must go to court to testify, he or she should be subpoenaed. Preparation for the court appearance includes gathering the medical evidence, including a copy of the medical records, laboratory reports, radiographs, and photographs. The physician can make notes from the records and may refer to these while on the witness stand. The physician will usually be questioned by three attorneys: the prosecutor (Assistant State's Attorney), the defense attorney for the parents, and the guardian *ad litem* (for the child). The judge ultimately makes a decision in the best interest of the child. The decision is based on the testimony at the court hearing, especially the important input by the physician.

The physician's responsibility for the patient continues past reporting and possibly testifying in court. The physician should have concerns about placement of that child (i.e., whether the placement should be with the natural parents or in a foster home). The overall goal is a permanent and supportive environment for the child. Continued follow-up with the pediatrician is essential to ensure the optimal growth and development of the child.

ANNOTATED BIBLIOGRAPHY

American Medical Association: Diagnostic and treatment guidelines concerning child abuse and neglect. Council on Scientific Affairs report. JAMA 254(6):796-800, 1985. (Reference for treatment guidelines.)

Child abuse. Pediatr Clin North Am 37(4):791–1011, 1990. (Excellent medical reference.)

Committee on Child Abuse and Neglect, American Academy of Pediatrics: Guidelines for the evaluation of sexual abuse of children. Pediatrics 97(2):254-260, 1991. (Reference for sexual abuse.)

Ellerstein NS (ed): Child Abuse and Neglect, A Medical Reference. New York, John Wiley & Sons, 1981. (Excellent medical reference.)

Kempe CH, Silverman FN, Steele BN et al: The battered child syndrome. JAMA 181:17, 1962. (The original article describing the syndrome.)

Leake HC, Smith DJ: Preparing for and testifying in a child abuse hearing. Clin Pediatr (Phila) 16(11):1057–1063, 1977. (Guidelines for the pediatrician in preparing for court.)

Sarles RM: Sexual abuse and rape. Pediatr Rev 93–98, 1982. (Review of the diagnosis and management of sexual abuse.)

21

Lead Poisoning

Steven M. Marcus

Interest in lead as a poison dates back many centuries. Over the last 40 years, renewed concern has developed in lead poisoning as both an industrial and an environmental problem. The realization that childhood lead poisoning may have lasting effects on child development has kindled increasing interest. Adults and adolescents may be exposed to lead through their hobbies or occupations. Stained-glass workers, sport shooters, automobile restorers, and workers in over 900 occupations are at potential risk of developing lead poisoning. Children may be subjected to exposure through close contact with parents who have such occupations or hobbies.

Children usually develop lead poisoning by ingesting lead-containing substances, principally lead-based paint. A significant portion of the housing stock was painted at least once with lead-based paint. When this paint peels or flakes, it becomes an inviting hazard for a toddler, who tends to test his or her environment with his or her mouth. The lead in paint may further become part of household dust. The normal hand-to-mouth activities of toddlers and small children represent a significant risk of increased lead absorption.

Definition: The United States Centers for Disease Control (CDC) statement, "Preventing Lead Poisoning in Young Children," released in October 1991, established a lead level of 10 μg/dl as the lower level at which ill effects of lead are identifiable. It thus defined a national goal to reduce children's blood lead levels below this value.

Because lead is so ubiquitous in our society, virtually all children are at risk for lead poisoning. It is not surprising, therefore, that the CDC suggested universal screening of all children 6 months to 6 years of age. The CDC estimates that over 3 million U.S. children younger than 6 years of age have lead levels over 15 μg/dl.

Children living in inner-city residences appear particularly prone to develop lead poisoning, with a significantly increased incidence in the black population. Also, gentrification of inner-city dwellings by affluent people who burn or otherwise remove layers of lead-laden paint may expose entire families to excessive amounts of lead. Another major source is from lead in old pipes and soldering.

The greatest number of cases and the severest cases of lead poisoning appear to occur from late spring to early fall. This apparent seasonal variation is not well understood.

PATHOPHYSIOLOGY

Lead is a protean poison; it has been shown to disturb the cellular metabolism of almost every tissue and organ in the body. Perhaps its best known effect is on the heme synthesis pathway. This produces an anemia that mimics iron deficiency anemia with a rise in heme precursors, particularly erythrocyte protoporphyrin (EP), also known as free erythrocyte protoporphyrin (FEP) or zinc protoporphyrin (ZPP). This interference with heme synthesis also disrupts the cytochrome system, the major oxidative enzyme system of every cell in the body.

Of serious concern is the effect of lead on the central nervous system (CNS), particularly on the developing brain of the child. Lead has been reported to produce a syndrome that ranges in severity from no defects, to learning disabilities, to frank seizures, and to retardation. Lead has been implicated in the etiology of various chronic diseases such as hypertension, renal disease, and gout.

CLINICAL PRESENTATION

Most patients with lead poisoning present with little or no overt symptomatology. Among common symptoms referable to the gastrointestinal tract are vomiting, abdominal pain, constipation, and loss of appetite. Common CNS symptoms include projectile vomiting, lethargy, irritability, and lack of attention span; there may be arrest or regression in developmental stages. There may also be overt signs of peripheral neuropathy, such as hypoesthesias and paresthesias. In adolescents or adults, a lack of, or decrease in, libido is common, as are affective disorders. It is imperative that careful occupational and environmental histories be obtained in any patient presenting with complaints such as these, especially during the summer months. Often symptoms are not appreciated until treatment for lead poisoning reverses behavioral effects that were believed to be unrelated to the lead. These symptoms often recur when lead levels again increase, sometimes even after re-equilibration.

LABORATORY TESTS

Although the FEP has proven to be a valuable screening tool for lead levels above 25 μg/dl, it is not as useful for levels set at 10 μg/dl. Thus, the standard screening test is now the whole blood lead level.

The laboratory evaluation of a patient for lead poisoning is relatively simple. Reliability of the lead testing is very important. Techniques are available for capillary sampling for lead screening, but careful attention to avoid contamination is imperative. A laboratory must be chosen that is excellent in performing lead determinations, e.g., cooperates and performs well in standardized proficiency studies.

An elevated capillary lead level must be confirmed by a venous lead level before any intervention is attempted. Lead levels above 70 μg/dl by the capillary method must be confirmed by venipuncture as emergencies whereas levels above 10 can be prioritized depending on the level.

Hemoglobin (Hgb), hematocrit (Hct), or mean corpuscular volume (MCV) should not be used as the only screen for lead poisoning because mild to moderate degrees of lead poisoning may exist in small children in the absence of these hematologic abnormalities.

A peripheral smear may reveal a hypochromic microcytic anemia. Hypochromic microcytic anemia, in adolescence, indicates a need for further evaluation. If such an adolescent is occupationally exposed to lead, then he or she should be considered to have lead poisoning until proved otherwise. Iron deficiency anemia is not uncommon in menstruating females. Basophilic stippling of the red blood cells occurs in marked chronic lead poisoning. Basophilic stippling also occurs in certain hemoglobinopathies, but it is of a different character and can be differentiated by a good technologist or hematologist. Urinalysis may reveal the presence of glucose or protein secondary to the renal tubular dysfunction caused by lead. Radiographs may reveal the presence of radiopaque foreign material in the gastrointestinal tract in children who ingest lead-containing substances. Furthermore, growth arrest lines in the distal metaphyses of growing bones may be seen in individuals with chronic lead poisoning.

Screening venous lead levels between 10 and 14 μg/dl should be repeated in 3 months, along with an FEP (and perhaps a serum iron, TIBC, and ferritin). A level between 15 and 19 μg/dl should also be repeated in 3 months and the child begun on iron therapy. In addition, sources of lead should be explored and the parents educated regarding dust control and the importance of high iron and calcium in the diet to decrease lead absorption. A lead between 20 and 24 μg/dl should be repeated in 1 month, again with the child on iron and the same advice given. A home inspection should also be considered. Depending on the symptoms, children with levels between 25 to 45 μg/dl should have either chelation therapy or a mobilization test. This may be done at a lead clinic or outpatient setting. All asymptomatic children with lead levels over 45 μg/dl should promptly receive chelation therapy.

The CaNa$_2$ EDTA (ethylenediaminetetraacetic acid) mobilization test may be useful in determining which patients will excrete significant quantities of lead in response to chelation therapy. This test is not advised if lead levels are elevated above 45 μg/dl. Recent experimentation conducted in rodents suggests that the mobilized lead from bone is transferred to brain tissue during the first 24 hours after CaNa$_2$ EDTA administration. The mobilization test may thus pose a danger to a child's brain, and its use should be carefully considered. Delaying therapy to wait for the results of a mobilization test is not indicated. Children with lead levels between 25 μg/dl and 45 μg/dl who are symptomatic

should be placed on chelation therapy without any further evaluation. Children with blood lead levels between 25 μg/dl and 45 μg/dl who are asymptomatic and who have no laboratory signs of biologic damage from lead may benefit from a mobilization test in an attempt to determine if chelation therapy will successfully lower the body burden of lead. After the patient empties his or her bladder, a dose of 50 mg/kg of CaNa$_2$ EDTA is administered either intravenously (over a 1-hour period) or intramuscularly. All urine produced during the next 24 hours is collected in a lead-free container and is analyzed for total lead excretion. This test must be performed and interpreted with an awareness of the difficulties inherent in collecting 24-hour urine specimens. Lead excretion over 24 hours in excess of 1 μg of lead for 1 mg of CaNa$_2$ EDTA administered is an indication for a full course of chelation. Some studies suggest that an 8-hour collection in children is adequate. A modification is then made: A urine excretion greater than 0.5 μg Pb/mg CaNa$_2$ EDTA suggests a good result from, and hence indication for, full chelation.

Although not currently widely available, noninvasive x-ray fluorescence to measure bone lead deposit has been suggested by some as an effective measure of total body lead burden. Preliminary research suggests a close correlation between bone lead level and urinary lead excretion after CaNa$_2$ EDTA mobilization. Such indirect evidence of total body burden may prove to be an effective indication of need for chelation in the future.

TREATMENT

Treatment of patients with lead poisoning depends on the presence or absence of symptoms and the degree of lead burden. Patients should be removed from their lead-contaminated environment. Patients who are symptomatic should have chelation therapy initiated as soon as possible. Asymptomatic children with positive CaNa$_2$ EDTA mobilization tests will probably benefit from chelation therapy. Because data concerning the long-term effects of lead poisoning on development pertain to the effects of lead levels and not FEP levels, it is the lead level that determines the need for therapy.

Available lead chelation therapy regimens include BAL + CaNa$_2$ EDTA, EDTA alone, d-penicillamine, and dimercaptosuccinic acid (DMSA). Animal data suggest that of the chelators available, only dimercaprol (BAL) crosses the blood–brain barrier in any appreciable concentration. Patients presenting with lead encephalopathy should, therefore, be treated with an initial dose of BAL followed by both BAL and CaNa$_2$ EDTA. BAL is not water soluble and must be administered intramuscularly in a dose of 3 to 4.5 mg/kg per dose administered every 4 hours. Its administration carries with it a significant risk of local problems such as sterile abscesses, febrile responses, and hepatic inflammation.

Nonencephalopathic patients with lead levels above 80 μg/dl require large amounts of a chelator. Administration of sufficient amounts of either BAL or CaNa$_2$ EDTA alone in such circumstances is limited by their inherent toxicity. Concurrent administration of both CaNa$_2$ EDTA and BAL is thus recommended in such cases.

CaNa$_2$ EDTA is a water-soluble chelator that is essentially nonmetabolized. CaNa$_2$ EDTA can be used alone when patients have no signs or symptoms of CNS involvement or when lead levels are below 80 μg/dl. When used intravenously, it has been shown to have few toxic effects. Five hundred milligrams of CaNa$_2$ EDTA is added to 1000 ml of IV solution and is administered at a rate of 50 mg/kg/day. Incorporation of EDTA into a continuous intravenous (IV) infusion appears to decrease the incidence of renal toxicity and hence is preferable to bolus injection.

When CaNa$_2$ EDTA is used intramuscularly, side effects such as local irritation at the injection site and renal impairment have been common. Pain at the injection site may require that either lidocaine or procaine be incorporated into the injection solution. Creatinine phosphokinase (CPK) levels may be elevated because of the large amount of tissue damage caused by the injection. CaNa$_2$ EDTA may also produce significant renal impairment; thus, the urine must be carefully monitored.

Some physicians use intramuscular (IM) EDTA in outpatient chelation when lead levels are relatively low. Considering the need to separate children from lead sources and considering the toxicity found with IM EDTA, this technique should be restricted to selected patients (e.g., for whom hospitalization is not possible). Oral EDTA is contraindicated because it increases lead absorption from the gastrointestinal (GI) tract.

It is unclear whether CaNa$_2$ EDTA itself is harmful to the kidney or whether it is the chelated lead that causes damage. The lead–EDTA complex is water soluble and stable at physiologic pH; however, free lead may be released in the acid environment of the renal tubule. There may be justification for the alkalinization of the urine to protect against the effects of the lead–EDTA complex on the renal tubule.

D-penicillamine is an orally effective chelating agent. Although shown to be an effective chelator of lead, it has never been approved by the Food and Drug Administration (FDA) for such use. However, it is used commonly in a dose of 20 to 40 mg/kg/day and appears to produce a prompt plumburesis. D-penicillamine should be used only in the chronic phase of treatment; there is no role for it in the acute treatment of lead poisoning, especially when encephalopathy is present. It should also not be given to patients with penicillin allergy.

Dimercaptosuccinic acid (DMSA), an oral BAL analogue, was approved by the FDA in January 1991 for treating children with lead levels over 45 μg/dl. The medication, although foul-smelling and -tasting, is well tolerated by children. When used in a protocol of 10 mg/kg/dose q8h for 5 days followed by 10 mg/kg/dose q12h for an additional 14 days, DMSA has produced a dramatic reduction of blood lead levels and an increase in urinary lead excretions. Side effects have included gastric distress (primarily flatus), and transient liver transaminitis. One adult treated with DMSA may have suffered a potentially life-threatening febrile event.

Lead-poisoned children should never be allowed to return to their environment until it is proven to be free of lead. Lead abatement must only be performed by experts. All patients chelated should be retested no later than 2 weeks after completion of therapy. The lead levels of many patients treated for lead poisoning may "rebound" because of the re-equilibration of lead from bone and soft tissue or from re-exposure. If lead levels rise too high, chelation may have to be repeated.

Whether treatment after the lead level has reached the highly toxic range is effective in reversing or preventing long-term effects is still unclear. Until this point is settled, it is the physician's responsibility to attempt to keep lead levels within the low, acceptable ranges.

All children with lead poisoning warrant nutritional counseling. A diet rich in calcium, protein, and iron is beneficial, whereas excess salt and fat should be avoided. A correlation has been found between dust lead content, dust-control measures, and lead poisoning. Thus, attention must be paid to careful housekeeping. Measures such as wet-mopping and moist dusting must be implemented.

Close follow-up, removal of sources of lead, and early chelation are imperative.

CHELATING REGIMENS

Several chelating regimens accepted for treatment of lead poisoning are outlined below. They were developed by the New Jersey Lead Consortium as an adaptation of the CDC guidelines and have been used to successfully treat over 12,000 children.

1. Dual chelation therapy: BAL–EDTA combination.

Dosages:

BAL = 18 mg/kg/day (375 mg/m^2/day); a dosage range of 3 to 4.5 mg/kg/dose q4h is acceptable. Divide daily dose into six parts, give q4h.

CaNa$_2$ EDTA = 50 mg/kg/day (1000 mg/m^2/day); a dosage range of 40 to 50 mg/kg/day is acceptable. See (3) below for specifics concerning EDTA administration.

Schedule:

Divide total daily BAL dosage into six doses. Give an initial dose of BAL alone (3 to 4.5 mg/kg/dose q4h) by deep IM injection. Four hours later and continuing q4h thereafter, BAL and EDTA are given simultaneously. BAL is given by deep IM injection. EDTA is given at the same time q4h at a separate IM site, or it may be given intravenously. See (3) for specifics concerning EDTA administration. The usual course of treatment is 5 days.

Note:
On completion of this course, further chelation should be considered, as outlined under chelating regimens (3) and (4). Alternatively, further chelation therapy may be withheld until results of post-chelation rebound Pb values are available. Based on laboratory studies and the patient's medical and social condition, a regimen for further chelation therapy can be selected.

2. Modified dual therapy: BAL–EDTA combination for 3 days followed by EDTA alone for 2 days.

Dosages:
BAL: As described under (1), dual chelation therapy.
EDTA: See (3) for specifics of EDTA administration.
Schedule:
For the first 3 days of chelation, proceed as described under (1), dual chelation therapy. Beginning with day 4 when EDTA is given alone, the total daily dosage of 50 mg/kg/day may be divided into two to four portions, as best suits the patient's circumstances, to be given IM q12h or q6h, respectively, or it may be given by continuous IV infusion. Again, various schedules for giving EDTA are acceptable: q4h, q6h, q8h, q12h, or once daily.
Note:
On completion of this course, further chelation should be considered, as outlined in chelation regimens (3) and (4). Alternatively, further chelation therapy may be withheld until results of post-chelation rebound Pb values are available. Based on laboratory studies and the patient's medical and social conditions, a regimen for further chelation therapy can be selected.

3. EDTA alone.

Dosage:
50 mg/kg/day (1000 mg/m^2/day); a dosage range of 40 to 50 mg/kg/day is acceptable either as IV (preferably as a continuous slow drip) or as a divided IM dose.
Schedule:
a. Inpatient chelation — calculate the dose at 100 ml/kg/24 hr of this solution that will give the recommended EDTA dose of 50 mg/kg/day. Alternatively, 1.0 g (5 ml) of EDTA in 250 to 500 ml of 5% D/W (dextrose in water) or isotonic saline can be administered slowly by IV drip (in not less than 1 hour). Two such courses per day for 3 to 5 days can be administered.
b. Ambulatory chelation — a single dose of 50 mg/kg/day is given by deep IM injection for 5 consecutive days. Because it is irritating to veins and may produce thrombophlebitis, IV bolus should be avoided. Calculate the dose at 100 ml/kg/24 hr of this solution that will give the recommended EDTA dose of 50 mg/kg/day. Alternatively, 1.0 g (5 ml) of EDTA in 250 to 500 ml of 5% D/W or isotonic saline can be administered

slowly by IV drip (in not less than 1 hour). Two such courses per day for 3 to 5 days can be administered.

4. Penicillamine.

Dosage:
30 mg/kg/day. Maximum dose = 750 mg/day. Usual course of therapy is 1 to 3 months.
Schedule:
Daily dose may be administered in one to three doses. Give on an empty stomach, at least ½ hour before feeding. Contents of capsule may be emptied into a small amount of fruit sauce, fruit slush, or chilled fruit juice.
Note:
This drug has not been approved for use in treating lead poisoning. Penicillamine should be used in compliance with approved FDA policy.

5. Dimercaptosuccinic acid.

Dosage:
20–30 mg/kg/day. Usual course of therapy is 19 days.
Schedule:
10 mg/kg/dose q8h administered for 5 days; 10 mg/kg/dose q12h administered for the next 14 days.
Note:
This drug is approved for use in children with lead levels of over 45 μg/dl. Significant side effects have been reported. Careful monitoring of hemoglobin, white count, platelets and liver function studies are suggested. A fixed drug eruption may force discontinuation of therapy.

ANNOTATED BIBLIOGRAPHY

Agency for Toxic Substances and Disease Registry: The Nature and Extent of Lead Poisoning in Children in the United States: A Report to Congress. Atlanta, U.S. Department of Health & Human Services, 1988. (The definitive guide regarding childhood lead poisoning.)

Centers for Disease Control: Preventing Lead Poisoning in Young Children. Atlanta, US Government Printing Office, 1991. (Guidelines for the prevention and treatment of childhood lead poisoning as set forth by the U.S. Centers for Disease Control.)

Needleman HL, Gunnoe C, Leviton A, et al: Deficits in psychologic and classroom performance of children with elevated dentine lead levels. N Engl J Med 300:689, 1979.

Needleman HL, Schell A, Bellinger D, et al: The long-term effects of exposure to low doses of lead in childhood—An 11 year follow-up report. N Engl J Med 322:83, 1990. (The classic report and follow-up study of a group of children with "subclinical" lead poisoning and the effects on their social performance; findings emphasize the need for aggressive case finding and therapy.)

Shannon MW, Graef JW. Lead intoxication in infancy. Pediatrics 89:87–90, 1992. (Reviews 370 cases of lead poisoning. Fourteen percent occurred in children less than 12 months old and their causes differed from those in older children. The authors recommend that children first be screened at 6 months of age.)

5

BEHAVIORAL PEDIATRICS

22

Patient Education in Primary Care

Edward R. Christophersen

Primary health care providers have the major responsibility for educating patients about risks to their health and well-being. Although many providers have been motivated for such a mission, the optimal way for teaching health education has not been developed. Health education requires more than the simple provision of information, but the time factor is an important practical constraint. The fact that the pediatrician does not have much time to include a process (health education) that he or she knows little about and that has not been effective in the past underscores the difficulty of achieving success. There are several areas in which the effectiveness of patient education can substantially affect the outcome with the patient. A discussion follows on the primary educational opportunities for the primary provider with recommendations on how to maximize the effectiveness of each.

PRENATAL COUNSELING

Most hospitals with obstetric services offer prenatal classes. Information that needs to be conveyed to all expectant couples (e.g., normal infant behavior and development and automobile and home safety practices) can be included in these classes with little additional effort. With a group format, much more information can be covered during a 1-hour class than could be covered by a pediatrician during a one-on-one prenatal visit. The pediatric staff should also be able to work with the nursing staff who teach the prenatal classes to include certain information without the pediatrician having to give lectures.

Office-based prenatal counseling, although recommended by many individuals over the years, cannot replace group prenatal classes because the pediatrician does not have the time to cover all of the material necessary during each prenatal visit. Rather, an individual prenatal visit, after a couple has attended the group prenatal class, can be used to answer the couple's personal questions and to discuss concerns on breast-feeding, working mothers, and so forth.

ANTICIPATORY GUIDANCE

After numerous investigators demonstrated that brief "educational" encounters are of little practical value, several models that hold more promise were proposed for the delivery of well-child care. One innovative approach is group well-child care. Using this format, the provider meets with four to six mother–child dyads together for one full hour, instead of meeting with them individually. This approach has several advantages. The groups allow the pediatrician to spend significantly more time with each family, averaging 45 minutes per visit compared to about 15 minutes with traditional one-on-one care. The mothers in the groups learn from each other, and they are comforted to learn that other mothers also have similar questions regarding their children. Pediatricians who run the groups commonly report that they learn from the groups because they have the opportunity to observe the mothers interacting with their children over a longer time, and they are able to observe the mothers in a larger social situation where it is possible to make objective comparisons between the mother–child dyads.

Well-child visits provide the most "natural" opportunity to conduct well-child groups. The physical examination portion of the appointment is usually conducted at the beginning or end of the group appointment, so that the examinations do not interrupt or interfere with the groups. Lastly, convening "special" groups, such as providing parents with information about parenting, may be highly successful.

When the effect of group care on home safety practices (e.g., safe hot water heater settings and smoke detector installations) was evaluated, the well-child groups demonstrated the effectiveness of their counseling. Success was attributed to more time for interaction between the health care provider and the family.

Several things should be considered by the pediatrician who prefers one-on-one well-child care or who is unable to offer group well-child care. An important point is that a provider needs adequate time if he or she is to be an effective communicator. Recipients of health care recommendations need to be made aware of the seriousness or importance of an issue; to believe that they can follow their pediatrician's recommendations successfully; and to have time to consider the issue and to make up their minds. In addition, families should be given realistic appraisals of how both compliance and noncompliance with the provider's recommendations will affect them. As a practical application for child passenger safety, addressing both the positive and negative aspects of accident prevention is superior to either approach by itself.

An equally important consideration is the amount of effort that a health education strategy takes for parents to implement. The less amount of effort required by the parent, the more likely the parent is to follow the pediatrician's suggestions. Parents, for example, are more likely to insert plastic outlet covers than to install child safety latches on kitchen cabinet doors.

Another important factor in health education efforts is the distinction between active and passive approaches. Active approaches require varying amounts of effort on the part of the parent. Passive approaches, in contrast, require little or no effort. For example, traditionally, seat belts have involved an active approach: they have required that the driver exert effort every time he or she enters the vehicle. With a passive approach to seat belts, the seat belt is drawn around the driver when he shuts his door; no effort is required from the driver.

ACUTE CARE REGIMENS

It is well known that large numbers of patients/families do not follow their physicians' recommendations. In one study in a pediatric outpatient clinic, over 50% of patients stopped taking penicillin by the third day of a 10-day regimen; 71% stopped by the sixth day; and by the ninth day 82% of the patients were not taking their medication.

Several areas need to be addressed by the physician in order to maximize patient compliance.

Parent/Patient Education

Patient or parental understanding and recall can be increased by more efficient presentation of medical information. Whenever possible, patients should be provided with instructions and advice at the start of the information to be presented. The provider should stress how important it is that the patient follow the regimen exactly. He or she should use short, easily understood sentences and should provide concrete examples whenever possible. In one study on compliance for acute otitis media, the control group received their instructions in the standard way, with the physician telling the patient what to do; the experimental group received a written copy of the physician's recommendations and had a monitoring sheet on which they were to keep track of the medications and when they were given. The control group had 49% compliance compared with 82% compliance by the experimental group.

Increased Follow-Up

To reduce the possibility of poor compliance over time, the pediatrician can have nurses or office personnel telephone parents after the first few days of therapy and encourage them to continue the prescribed course of medications. This telephone contact should carefully avoid putting parents on the defensive. During the phone call, parents can be asked how their child is feeling and if they have any questions. Within this context of inquiring about the child's progress, the parents can then be encouraged to continue therapy even though their child is asymptomatic. It can be mentioned to parents that most people have a tendency to stop therapy when they or their children are feeling better. Parents should then be given a brief rationale about why it is important to continue therapy. The total time for this follow-up call can usually be limited to 2 or 3 minutes unless the parent has additional questions.

Physician–Patient Interaction

Data show that patient satisfaction and compliance may be related to patterns of physician–patient interaction. For example, noncompliance has been found to be related to unmet expectations of mothers who brought their children to pediatricians. Generally, the pediatrician should make sure that he or she finds out what the parents' concerns and expectations are, and then he or she should provide information about both the diagnosis and the cause of the illness. A friendly, conversational attitude, coupled with a lack of medical jargon, may also improve compliance.

CHRONIC DISEASE REGIMENS

Two important characteristics that distinguish chronic care regimens from acute care regimens are that the chronic care regimens are typically much more complex and they must be carried on for a longer time. Compliance may be facilitated by the following steps.

Regimen Checklist

A written list of the recommendations that the physician usually makes, with a space to check off those that apply in a particular instance, may make it easier for the parents to follow the physician's recommendation. The parents then have a written reminder that they can take with them when they leave the office. It is difficult for parents to follow a complex regimen without some kind of written reminder. Similarly, there are some regimen components that parents have little knowledge of and that require more guidance from the physician. For example, when parents are advised to increase the fiber in their child's diet because of constipation, a list of dietary suggestions should be provided because many parents do not know which foods are high in natural fibers.

Rehearsal

When the physician recommends a complex set of procedures for the parents to follow, those elements that can easily be rehearsed in the office should be. Whether a parent is instructed to give a diabetic child an insulin injection, provide postural drainage exercises for a child with cystic fibrosis, or monitor exercises for a child with rheumatoid arthritis, asking the parent to practice the procedures in the office and rehearsing with them while in the presence of the office nurse can help substantially with complex regimens.

Gradual Implementation

The physician should be aware of "information overload." Parents can assimilate only limited information at any one time. The regimen components can be introduced in a step-by-step fashion as the parent masters prior steps in a sequence of components ordered in terms of difficulty and necessity. Although there is a temptation to tell the parent everything during one visit, this is often the most difficult style for parents. For example, the parents of a newly diagnosed diabetic can be instructed and given the opportunity to rehearse giving the insulin injections. The next day, for an inpatient, the parents can be instructed in and allowed to rehearse the procedures for measuring their child's blood glucose levels.

Tailoring of Regimens

Tailoring refers to the practice of adapting the regimen to the personal habits and routines of a patient and his family. If possible, medications can be prescribed at times when well-established habits occur, such as when the patient eats, takes vitamins, or brushes his or her teeth. For example, parents of children with cystic fibrosis may do postural drainage exercises while their child is watching a favorite television show. Pediatricians can decide how to tailor regimens by inquiring about the daily routines of a particular patient and discussing with parents convenient times to conduct regimen components. The time that a physician spends tailoring a regimen may have long-range benefits because

the patient may continue to comply with the treatment regimen without further effort by the physician.

Increased Supervision

Increased supervision in the form of more frequent follow-up appointments may also improve compliance. By giving more frequent, shorter appointments, the physician can better monitor the patient's progress and attend to compliance problems. For example, selected diabetic patients may be asked to return to the endocrine clinic to have their Hgb A_1c checked at monthly intervals. When the result of the assay is available, a nurse calls the patient/parents to give them feedback about the patient's current degree of metabolic control. Each visit may be brief, but the cumulative effect of visits may further convince patients and their parents that the physician is concerned and ready to help. A telephone call may be substituted for a clinic visit to decrease the cost to parents and to take up less of the physician's time.

WHY IMPROVE HEALTH EDUCATION EFFORTS?

Compliance failures are costly from a therapeutic and an economic standpoint. An obvious consequence of noncompliance with medical regimens is that patients fail to receive the benefits of effective therapies and thereby may adversely affect their health. Incomplete antibiotic therapy, for example, may result in a greater probability of recurrent infections. Abrupt discontinuation of medications such as prednisone can result in life-threatening side effects. The accumulation of unused medications in the home can increase the probability of accidental poisoning of young children. Physicians may also inadvertently conclude that a particular treatment was ineffective when in fact an adequate trial of that treatment was not conducted because the patient did not adhere to the treatment regimen. The cost-effectiveness of medical care is also affected by patient compliance. Money is spent on unused medications, and parents may incur the expense of additional diagnostic and treatment procedures that may not have been necessary with optimal patient compliance. Poor compliance can also lead to more frequent hospitalization, which results in increased costs to parents. The cost of hospitalization is indirectly passed on to other families in the form of increased insurance premiums.

Most physicians report increased satisfaction with their practices when they are not constantly confronted with the frustration of patient noncompliance. The routine use of strategies to improve patient compliance may well result in increased satisfaction for both the physician and the patient.

ANNOTATED BIBLIOGRAPHY

Finney JW, Friman PC, Rapoff MA, Christophersen ER: Improving compliance with antibiotic regimens for otitis media: Randomized clinical trial in a pediatric clinic. Am J Dis Child 139:89–95,

1985. (Results of a carefully controlled study of medical compliance with pediatric patients; methodology and results may be useful to primary providers interested in medical compliance.)

Osborn LM: Group well-child care. Clin Perinatol 12(2):355–365, 1985. (Concise discussion of some of the features of group well-child care that make it so appealing to some pediatricians. Dr. Osborn, a practicing pediatrician, was one of the first advocates of group well-child care.)

Rapoff MA, Christophersen ER: Improving compliance in pediatric practice. Pediatr Clin North Am 29(2):339–357, 1982. (Discussion of factors that have an impact on patient compliance, with recommendations on how to improve compliance.)

Varni JW, Christophersen ER: Behavioral treatment in pediatrics. Curr Probl Pediatr 20(11):639–704, 1990. (In-depth discussion of a wide variety of behavioral treatments that can be incorporated into primary care.)

23

The Working Mother

Linda V. Ross and Edward R. Christophersen

An increased number of women joined the work force in the 1980s, and a large percentage of these women are combining careers with motherhood. Among mothers of children less than age 18, 35% work outside the home and 45% of those working mothers have children of preschool age. Of the many reasons why women have chosen to combine careers with motherhood, the most important one is economic necessity. Because it is becoming increasingly more difficult for a family to sustain a comfortable lifestyle on the earnings of one family member, women are continuing to work after their children are born. The combination of a career with motherhood poses several problems for families as well as society. The problems include the provision of adequate child care for children of all ages from infancy through adolescence; the possible detrimental effects on the health and development of children due to the mother working; and the possible detrimental effects on the marital relationship due to the mother working. Solutions to these problems could have substantial economic and emotional impact on the family and society.

The primary health care provider is in a unique position to assess, evaluate, and intervene with the family. Ideally, the question of child care should be raised with expectant parents during the prenatal period. Many parents, however, will not have reached a decision about the mother working outside the home until after the child is born. If the provider knew the family prior to the time the mother goes to work, he or she may know of preexisting problems that might complicate the child's adjustment to the mother's employment. For example, if the mother is seeking employment to avoid dealing with her child's behavioral problems, the provider should provide consultation or referral in order to ameliorate the behavioral problems and should counsel the mother to choose employment for more valid reasons, such as economic need or personal satisfaction.

Pediatricians can help parents select the type of child care that will be best suited to the child and the family. The provider can give anticipatory guidance that may prevent or diminish possible deleterious effects of the mother working outside the home. Day care can affect a child's development both positively and negatively. Most studies indicate that no differences in intellectual or social development occur between day care–reared children and home-reared children. Hopefully, as more infants and preschoolers experience day care, further research will be done to determine the positive and negative effects on child development. Pediatricians must, of course, be sensitive to when they are counseling parents from fact versus a personal bias.

The provider must make a distinction between the deleterious effects of maternal employment and preexisting problems that are unrelated to the mother's working status. The primary health care provider who has had ongoing contact with families has an advantage in making this decision. Families who have made good adjustments to previous changes are more likely to adjust well to the mother working outside the home. On the other hand, those families who have had difficulty coping with crises are more likely to manifest behavioral or emotional problems.

Divorce is one of the possible problems complicating the family's adjustment to the mother working outside the home. Divorce and parental separation may be the cause of the mother seeking employment and may contribute to the presenting problems (see Chap. 24, "Divorce and Single Parents"). Other problems that may complicate the family's adjustment to maternal employment include parental conflict over the mother's decision to pursue a career outside the home and parental feelings of anxiety and guilt when both parents decide to work. Such problems can create behavioral or emotional disturbances in the children.

ASSESSING THE IMPACT OF EMPLOYMENT

The American Academy of Pediatrics (AAP) published a statement on the mother working outside the home that included a discussion of questions that may be asked by the mother (American Academy of Pediatrics, 1984). The questions and the AAP's answers follow:

1. Is working harmful to the child? Answers will depend on whether a safe, caring environment is provided for the child and whether the mother is satisfied with her work, her family support, and her ability to nurture her children at the end of each workday.
2. How does a mother evaluate a substitute care-giving situation? Answers should include information about the care-giver, safety, sanitation, and nutrition.

3. What are some of the possible negative effects on children when mothers work outside the home? Answers to this question must include an evaluation of the quality of the child care and care-givers and the mother's energy available for optimal parenting.
4. When is it acceptable to return to work after the birth of a child? Answers will be determined on the basis of the mother's physical health, the infant's physical health, practical and financial considerations, the development of a satisfactory mother–infant relationship, family support, and adequate child-care arrangements.
5. What kinds of reactions can be expected in the mother and other family members if the mother works outside the home? Answers will be most helpful if the provider is aware of the frequent feelings of loss, inadequacy, and guilt experienced by mothers who work. Pointing out positive effects of quality day care and suggesting ways for the mother to spend quality time with her children may decrease the intensity of such negative feelings.
6. Are there special factors that the mother should keep in mind before going to work? The provider can supply answers to this question by recommending that the mother have a frank discussion with other family members about the change in her status and about the necessity of sharing child-care and housework responsibilities.

After a mother has been working for some time, the health care provider can assess the effects of maternal employment on the child's development by taking a complete family history, plotting physical growth, administering developmental tests, and making behavioral observations (see Chap. 24 for a discussion on screening procedures). Problems detected during the assessment should help alert the provider to the possible need for referral.

FINDING QUALITY CHILD CARE

Good child care can be identified in many ways, such as through community referral services, referrals from friends or other health care professionals, university child development departments, or local parenting centers or classes. The mother needs to decide whether she wants family day care, live-in help, a babysitter in the home, a day-care center, or a nursery school program. The advantages and disadvantages of each of these types of child care are summarized in Table 23-1. Once the parents have decided on the type of care they prefer, they should screen the facility or person by telephone for obvious positive or negative features and then visit or interview several facilities or persons. Adequate time should be allotted, and the child should accompany the mother to the final choices so that the mother can see her child's reaction to the environment and the care-giver's response to her child. The environment should be clean, cheerful, and safe, and the care-giver should be caring, patient, and responsive to the children in his or her care. Other concerns should be staff turnover, individualized attention,

stimulating activities and equipment, and an appropriate adult:child ratio for the age level (e.g., 1:3 for infants and 1:4 or 5 for older children). Once the child is being cared for in a day-care facility or by a care-giver in the home, the mother should telephone regularly and drop in unannounced occasionally. If the facility or care-giver objects to unannounced drop-ins, the mother should reconsider her choice. Proximity to the work place may allow the mother to spend occasional lunch hours with her child. On-site day-care facilities at places of employment are increasing in the 1990s and are an obvious benefit of employment. Periodic conferences should be scheduled between the care-givers and the mother to monitor the child's adjustment and progress. The mother should listen attentively to her child during quiet times when he or she is likely to express feelings and concerns about the child-care situation.

PRINCIPLES OF MANAGEMENT

The focus of family management by the primary health care provider should be on the prevention of possible deleterious effects on the entire family of the mother working outside the home. If the provider possesses optimal skills in counseling and developmental and behavioral assessment, he or she will be able to advise families more effectively about the possible results of maternal employment. Familiarity with the children prior to maternal employment can alert the provider to factors that may interfere with a satisfactory adjustment to changes for the child, such as child care outside the home, maternal absence, or increased household responsibilities. Preexisting problems may complicate the management of the family and may dictate referral to specialists.

INDICATIONS FOR REFERRAL

The primary health care provider should refer families in which there are significant psychological, behavioral, or developmental problems to appropriate specialists. Indicators of the need for referral include evidence that a child is consistently failing to reach developmental milestones; repeated reports by child-care providers that the child has a behavioral problem; multiple complaints from the parents about their child's behavior at home; or symptoms of serious childhood adjustment problems, such as depression or delinquency.

If a child is repeatedly treated for infectious diseases, the provider should investigate the health practices and sanitation of the child-care facility. It may be necessary to notify public health authorities if many cases of infectious disease are encountered from one particular day-care center.

Primary health care providers must be familiar with available community resources to which families can be referred, such as government agencies, community support groups, and child advocacy committees. In many metropolitan areas, organizations such as the United Way publish

Table 23-1. Advantages and Disadvantages of Different Types of Day Care

TYPE OF CARE	ADVANTAGES	DISADVANTAGES
Family day care	Some licensed Most have children of their own One caring adult Least costly: on sliding scale May have flexible hours	Licensing focuses on environment, not social, psychological factors Illness of family child; day-care child Taking child out in bad weather Less convenient if more than one child
Live-in help	No early-morning hassles Child's illness less problem Often also does housekeeping More flexible hours Good for more than one child More control as employer	Costly Family gives up some privacy Hidden expenses (food, utilities) Often deal with personal problems of employee Difficult to find good help Turnover Fewer children for stimulation
Babysitter in home	Often also does housekeeping Child illness less problem Good for more than one child More control as employer	Transportation difficulties Difficult to find good help Hidden expenses (food, utilities) Fewer children for stimulation
Day-care center	Child has experience with other children; socialization Planned activies spread through day Long hours, seldom closed Continuity of program Sometimes offers special services	No provision for illness Taking young child out of home in bad weather Long day in nonhome environment
Nursery school program	Geared toward cognitive development Child has experience with other children Sometimes offers special services	No provision for illness More costly than day care Taking young child out of home in bad weather May not have summer or vacation arrangements

(Adapted from Ashery RS, Basen MM, The Parents with Careers Workbook, Washington, DC, Acropolis Books Ltd, 1983.)

directories, such as *Where to Turn,* that list most of the service agencies with specific information on the types of referrals and the ways to refer.

MANAGEMENT

The health care professional should provide specific guidance to mothers in order to facilitate the best adjustment for the working mother and her children. The type of guidance varies with the ages of the children involved.

Infant

Mothers should be allowed and encouraged to take paid maternity leave of 4 to 6 months, and paternity leave should be granted to fathers to establish their role in caring for their infants. The United States is the only developed nation that does not have a statutory maternity leave policy. Many health care providers recommend a minimum of 6 months' maternity leave for mothers of both natural and adopted infants. Federal legislation to this effect has recently been proposed.

Working mothers should establish daily quality time with their infants to maintain a good mother–infant relationship. *Quality time* is defined as time when the mother and child are engaged in promoting the child's intellectual, social, or emotional development and when the mother is developing a warm, accepting, attitude toward the child's feelings and behaviors. Working mothers should be encouraged to set priorities for how they will spend their time at home. It is essential that the mother establish the relationships with her infant and her husband as higher priorities than household tasks such as cleaning and laundry. Dividing household tasks with the father, finding outside help, or decreasing expectations for neatness may allow the mother to have more time with her infant.

Preschool Child

The mother of the preschool child may be concerned about such tasks as language development, toilet training, and peer associations. Language may be stimulated in a high-quality child-care environment, but mothers should still be encouraged to talk, listen, and read to their children during their time together. Toilet training can be accomplished easily by looking for readiness characteristics, such as following two- or three-step directions, finger and hand coordination in removing and replacing clothing, and ability to stay dry for several hours. Peer associations may be enhanced in child-care settings, but the mother may also invite her child's friends to the home so that she can monitor her child's social skills.

The quality of the time a mother spends with her child continues to be important at this age. Mothers should also be advised to encourage their children to engage in play by themselves by rewarding brief periods of appropriate play.

School-Aged Child

Although the school-aged child may be in school most of the time the mother is working, she should be encouraged to find child care before and after school. The health care provider should discourage "latch-key" arrangements that expose the child to many risks during unsupervised times. The provider can recommend various community programs that may be available, such as the public school system, church facilities, and YMCAs. For older children who must at times be unsupervised, the mother can be advised to teach her child about fire safety, emergency numbers, stranger avoidance, neighborhood contacts, simple first aid, and routine telephone check-ins with the mother. There is evidence that substance abuse is increased in unsupervised school-aged and adolescent children.

Adolescent

The adolescent usually does not require day care unless he has a handicap; however, the adolescent continues to need the mother's quality time. Quality time can include setting aside a designated time each evening during which the adolescent does his homework and the parents work on budgets, correspondence, or other paperwork. Telephone calls, television, and visitors should be discouraged or prohibited during the designated time. In this way, the parents can serve as role models for the adolescent who is developing work habits for adulthood. Delegation and sharing of appropriate household tasks can also encourage increased respon-

sibility in the adolescent. Regularly scheduled family nights can provide focused quality time.

ANNOTATED BIBLIOGRAPHY

American Academy of Pediatrics: The mother working outside the home. Pediatrics 73:874–875, 1984. (Official statement of the AAP that may be used as a handout for working mothers.)

Ashery RS, Basen MM: The Parents with Careers Workbook. Washington, DC, Acropolis Books Ltd, 1983. (Excellent practical workbook for parents; covers child care, home management, and parent and career issues.)

Forehand RL, McMahon RJ: Helping the Noncompliant Child: A Clinician's Guide to Parent Training. New York, Guilford Press, 1981. (For professionals; describes strategies for training parents in child management.)

Hurwitz ES, Gunn WJ, Pinsky PF, Schonberger LB: Risk of respiratory illness associated with day-care attendance: A nationwide study. Pediatrics 87:62–69, 1991. (Reports results of a national study of day-care risk of illness in children 6 weeks to 59 months old; they have a significantly increased risk of respiratory illness.)

Lerner JV: When both parents work: Effects on the development of children. Children Are Different: Behavioral Development Monograph Series (No. 12). Columbus, OH, Ross Laboratories, 1985. (Many useful suggestions for parents and professionals when both parents work.)

Rivara FP, DiGuiseppi C, Thompson RS, Calonge N: Risk of injury to children less than 5 years of age in day care versus home care settings. Pediatrics 84:1011–1016, 1989. (Children are not at greater risk for injury in day care than they are in home care.)

Zigler E, Muenchow S: Infant day care and infant-care leaves. Am Psychol 38:91–94, 1983. (Reviews the current status of infant day care.)

24
Divorce and Single Parents

Linda V. Ross

It is currently estimated that 33% of children under the age of 18 (1 million per year) in the United States experience their parents' divorce. The divorce rate in the United States is the highest in the world, with approximately 40% of current marriages of young adults ending in divorce. Children will live an average of 6 years in a single-parent home created by marital disruption. Although there are differences of opinion, there is strong evidence that divorce can have negative effects on a child's cognitive, emotional, and social development.

Mechanisms by which the negative effects on child development can occur include a lowered socioeconomic status, the loss of a father or mother in the home, conflict in parent–child relationships, loss of external social support systems, stress- and crisis-related problems, and disruption in the nuclear family, including possible separation from siblings. Some of the negative effects of divorce on children include a lowered self-esteem, increased aggression or delinquency (particularly in boys), depression, feelings of guilt and responsibility for the divorce, fear of abandonment by the custodial parent, fantasies of reuniting the divorced parents, regression in toilet training and other developmental tasks, academic difficulties, and social withdrawal. Factors related to a child's adjustment to parental divorce include age, sex, predivorce cognitive and emotional functioning, parental adjustment, parental communication about child rearing, extent of environmental changes required, cultural and family beliefs, and social support available within and outside the family. In general, a young male child whose parents do not adjust well to the divorce and remain in conflict over child rearing and who is required to move away from his home or social support has the poorest prognosis for a healthy adjustment to his parents' divorce. On the other hand, the most important variable related to satisfactory adjustment to divorce among children seems to be a positive relationship with the custodial parent. Individual differences, including the child's cognitive and behavioral abilities, mediated by family variables are important in describing why children react differently to the stress of parental divorce.

PRESENTATION

Parents may present to the primary health care provider with specific questions or problems regarding a pending divorce. More often, however, the provider will become aware of a pending or recent divorce when the custodial parent comes with nonspecific questions or recurrent problems and does not tell the physician of the divorce. Billing problems are often the reason the family health care provider learns that there has been a change in marital status. Other presenting problems often encountered include regression in toilet training, bedtime problems, temper tantrums, and frequent minor illnesses. Occasionally, the noncustodial parent will call the physician for information regarding the physical or mental health of his or her child.

DIFFERENTIAL DIAGNOSIS

In determining the effects of divorce on children, the primary health care provider needs to rule out preexisting conditions that might impede a healthy adjustment. Children who have been exposed to a long-term marital conflict may have already developed behavior patterns that require professional intervention. Temper tantrums, bedtime problems, and noncompliance with parental instructions can become exaggerated at the time of divorce when the level of stress is elevated. In general, the child who has a history of maladjustment preceding the divorce is more likely to respond with long-lasting emotional disturbance following the divorce. These problems need to be anticipated, because early and timely counseling may minimize long-term problems.

WORK-UP

Plotting the child's weight and height on a standard growth chart allows the pediatrician to reassure the mother that the child's growth is normal. Several scales and screening tests that have been developed to help the primary care physician assess the effects of divorce on the child are summarized in Table 24-1. Most physicians, however, perform only the Denver Developmental Screening Test (DDST) in their offices, choosing to refer to psychologists for further testing. Problems detected in the screening procedures should alert the provider to the need for referral.

The primary health care provider should determine what stresses the children of the divorcing couple will be or have been exposed to. Questions regarding economic changes, living arrangements, who will be the custodial parent, non-

Table 24-1. Screening Tests to Assess the Effects of Divorce on Children

NAME	KIND	TIME	AGE	REFERENCE
Achenbach Child Behavior Checklist	Behavioral	30–45 min	4–5 yr 6–11 yr 12–16 yr	Achenbach and Edelbrock (1981)
ANSER	Developmental Health	Varies	School-age	Levine (1983)
Denver Developmental Screening Test	Developmental	15–25 min	Birth–6 yr	Frankenburg (1983)
Eyberg Child Behavior Inventory	Behavioral	10–20 min	2–12 yr	Robinson, Eyberg, and Ross (1980)
Home Screening Questionnaire	Home environment	15 min	Birth–3 yr 3–6 yr	Frankenburg (1983)
Denver Prescreening Developmental Questionnaire	Developmental	5 min	3 mo–6 yr	Frankenburg (1983)

custodial parent visitation, school and day-care arrangements, disciplinary decisions, extended family support, and other forms of social support need to be addressed at the first opportunity. The answers to these questions will help the provider identify areas in which the family is in need of counseling. The provider should have available resources such as written handouts, books written for lay people, a list of local mental health professionals well versed in divorce counseling, and a list of community workshops for divorced families to which families can be referred. The physician can attempt to keep the noncustodial parent involved in the child's health maintenance by suggesting conferences in the office and periodic telephone calls regarding the child's health status.

PRINCIPLES OF MANAGEMENT

Knowledge of normal child development and skill in educating and counseling parents and children are prerequisites for the provider who intends to help families adjust to divorce. Management will be determined by the stresses experienced and the predivorce status of the child and his parents. In general, if the custodial parent is able to make a satisfactory pre- and postdivorce adjustment and maintain a positive relationship with the child, the prognosis for the child is good.

The physician can convey directly to the child a compassionate recognition of his feelings, fears, and concerns. Such acknowledgment may diminish the child's sense of loneliness and the lack of adult support. Parental and child adjustment can be improved when both parents and children are involved in support groups aimed at developing problem-solving skills.

The primary health care provider may sometimes be involved in child custody decisions. Several studies have investigated variables affecting decisions about child custody. Laws vary from state to state. Important issues include joint, shared, or one-parent custody; the best interests of the child; and the acceptance of psychological or physician investigations. Some considerations in the custody decisions are: to determine which parent is most likely to foster visitation and respect for the other parent; to maintain continuity of child contact with friends, relatives, neighbors, and school; to provide productive support, guidance, and discipline; to maintain emotional and environmental security; to be aware of resources available for parent support; and to demonstrate flexibility and adaptability with regard to the current situation and the future. The provider is encouraged to maintain the role of advocate for the child rather than to take sides with either parent. In this role, the professional will be able to provide care and advice to either parent and to the child without being biased by considerations concerning fault in the divorce proceedings. Divorce mediation is a recent trend in deciding child custody disputes and may be recommended by the primary health care provider.

INDICATIONS FOR REFERRAL

Most acute responses to a divorce, such as anger, fear, depression, and guilt, are considered normal and usually begin to resolve during the first year following a divorce. However, continued exposure to adversity with multiple stresses may lead to developmental disruptions requiring special intervention. Some indications for referral include persistent antisocial behavior; academic failure; symptoms of depression such as insomnia, appetite disturbance, or weight loss; and coercive parent–child interactions. Results of the aforementioned screening procedures will alert the provider to the need for referral.

MANAGEMENT

Management of children and their families following a divorce will depend on the age of the child, the custodial arrangements, and the adjustments of the parents and children. The following discussion centers on common issues relating to divorce and children.

Telling the Children About Divorce

What and how to tell the children are questions often asked by parents contemplating divorce. Some authorities suggest that each child in the family be told separately with both parents present to answer questions, whereas others recommend that siblings be told together. The children should be told that the parents will be living apart and will no longer be married. They should be told what the living arrangements will be and how often they will see the absent parent. Children should not be asked their opinions about where they are going to live or whether their parents should get a divorce. In the case of older adolescents, their opinions on living arrangements may be taken into consideration in legal decisions, but the parents should not expect their children to make the decisions. Questions of loyalty and abandonment are problematic for children of all ages.

Financial arrangements often result in changes such as a new residence, the mother returning to work, the necessity for day care or after-school programs, and depleted resources for extra activities such as club memberships and dance lessons. Parents need to be aware of the effects of such environmental changes on their children and must reassure them that they will continue to be cared for and provided for despite the changes in economic resources.

Visitation

It is important that the child visit with the noncustodial parent as often as possible unless that parent has been abusive or is a substance abuser. Details of visitation such as scheduling, picking up and delivering children, vacations, grandparent visits, a child's refusal to visit, and debriefing following the visitation should be worked out by the parents, with professional assistance if necessary. The absence of the noncustodial parent (most often the father, although recently more fathers are receiving custody of their children) can have various effects, such as fears that he has abandoned the child or has had a mishap. The father–child interaction is often very different postseparation. In some cases, the relationship between absent fathers and their children improves after divorce. This relationship can be fostered by including the fathers in decisions about their children's health, education, discipline, and general child rearing. The frequent availability of the father is associated with positive adjustment, especially in boys. "Bribes" in the form of excessive gifts, trips, or weekend outings should be discouraged because they introduce unrealistic expectations and place additional stress on the other parent.

Discipline

Discipline of children following divorce may be difficult for various reasons. A mother who has returned to work may have added household responsibilities as well as job responsibilities with less time to devote to her children. Thus, children may experience the loss of both mother and father immediately following a divorce. Disruption of the parenting routine is one factor leading to adjustment problems in children of divorcing parents. It is important for the child's adjustment that home stability be restored as quickly as possible. Concrete types of discipline, such as a brief time-out period, are recommended because the use of lectures and frequent reprimands may lower the self-esteem of a child already at risk. Older children may benefit from the need for greater self-sufficiency in a single-parent family if the mother does not make excessive or inappropriate demands for emotional sustenance. It is important to monitor children frequently and praise appropriate behaviors. Physical touch is one of the best ways of communicating love, acceptance, and understanding to children of all ages.

One common practice that should be discouraged is that of having the child sleep with the custodial parent after the separation or divorce. Because it is unpleasant to remedy this situation once it has occurred, the professional can provide anticipatory guidance to the parent to prevent the habit from developing. Related to sleeping with the parent is the tendency to have a child replace the absent parent symbolically. Forewarning the parent of this possibility may avert the problem. The same advice may prevent the parent from identifying the child with the absent parent of the same sex.

Feelings

Children may have feelings of guilt about having caused the divorce. They may also feel that they can cause their parents to reunite if they behave in certain ways. It is important that parents be aware of their children's tendencies to feel responsible and not contribute to such fantasies. Parents should not involve the children in their own disputes, nor should they use the children as their confidants.

Children will have feelings of anger, fear, sadness, hurt, and loneliness. It is important that parents recognize these feelings as normal reactions to the loss of the family unit and the noncustodial parent. Such feelings are not indicative of parental incompetency. However, if ignored, such feelings may persist and lead to maladaptive responses such as antisocial behavior, depression, or academic failure. In the case of maladaptive responses, the parent should be encouraged to seek professional help for the entire family.

Step-Families

The number of children living in step-families is growing. Over 70% of divorced men and women remarry, creating a step-family when children are involved. Some problems that step-parents may face include hostile step-child behaviors; complications with the spouse's ex-husband or -wife; who makes decisions regarding discipline and other child-rearing questions; visitation; and attachment or lack thereof. Some characteristics of step-sibling relationships are that they are instantaneous; they lack a shared family history; they bring into the new family a common experience of loss in their original families; there are conflicting loyalties; there may be shifts in sibling position roles and functions; and there is an abrupt change in family size. The primary care provider may provide anticipatory guidance to parents who are about to become step-parents and direct them to books and community resources to help the family adjustment process.

ANNOTATED BIBLIOGRAPHY

Achenbach TM, Edelbrock CS: Behavioral problems and competencies reported by parents of normal and disturbed children aged four through sixteen. Monogr Soc Res Child Dev 46 (1, Serial No. 188), 1981. (Complete discussion of the Achenbach Child Behavior Checklist is presented with data from studies using the scale.)

Einstein E: The Stepfamily: Living, Loving and Learning. Boston, Shambhala Publications, 1982. (Excellent book to recommend to parents contemplating remarriage or who have already created a step-family. Discusses topics such as dating, remarriage, family traditions, noncustodial parents, step-sibling relationships, and signs of trouble.)

Frankenburg WK: Developmental assessment. In Levine MD, Carey WB, Crocker AC, Gross RT (eds): Developmental–Behavioral Pediatrics, pp 927–937. Philadelphia, WB Saunders, 1983. (Presents a two-stage developmental screening procedure that may be useful to the pediatrician assessing the effects of divorce on preschool children.)

Howell RJ, Toepke KE: Summary of the child custody laws for the fifty states. Am J Family Therapy 12(2):56–60, 1984. (Summarizes state custody laws and discusses problems often encountered.)

Levine MD: The developmental assessment of the school age child. In Levine MD, Carey WB, Crocker AC, Gross RT (eds): Developmental–Behavioral Pediatrics, pp 938–947. Philadelphia, WB Saunders, 1983. (Presents the ANSER screening instrument, which may be useful to the pediatrician assessing the effects of divorce on school-aged children.)

Robinson EA, Eyberg SM, Ross AW: The standardization of an inventory of child conduct problems. J Clin Child Psychol 2:22–29, 1980. (Discusses the Eyberg Child Behavior Inventory, which may be useful to the pediatrician assessing behavioral effects of divorce on children.)

Teyber E: Helping Your Children with Divorce: A Compassionate Guide for Parents. New York, Pocket Books, 1985. (Written for parents who are preparing their children for divorce. Discusses topics such as common fears, symptoms of depression, custody and visitation, and common childhood fantasies about reconciliation.)

25

Working with Difficult Parents

Kenneth H. Tellerman

Pediatric practitioners continuously deal with parents who appear angry, anxious, or depressed. Stressed parents may also be noncompliant with appointments and medications. Alternatively, they may repeatedly express seemingly trivial concerns (the "hidden agenda") or contact the practitioner at unusual hours. The practitioner's sense that "something is wrong" may also serve as an early warning of parental stress. Stress may surface from a child's acute or chronic illness, or from ongoing psychosocial problems within the family. Parental stress may be heightened if the physician is perceived as nonresponsive. Practitioners may develop negative feelings toward some patients, and the recognition that these feelings are present may prevent a breakdown in effective communication.

Several components of intervention are required for the primary care physician to deal effectively with these "difficult" parents.

1. Acknowledge parental concerns.
2. Explore parental concerns.
3. Help resolve parental concerns.

All of these approaches may be integrated into one session for acute problems. In fact, many of these principles can be used to allay parental stress during routine telephone encounters. For more complex problems, however, these approaches may need to be adapted over a longer time frame.

ACKNOWLEDGING PARENTAL CONCERNS

When dealing with parents experiencing emotional turmoil, it is important for the physician to convey to parents the message that their feelings and concerns have been recognized. Several effective communication techniques can be used to convey this message.

Pacing

The physician may wish to "pace" body language and statements to those of the parent in order to establish rapport. If the parent is anxious and frenetic, the physician may wish to respond in an animated fashion. If the parent is weepy and depressed, the physician may wish to approach the parent in a soft, gentle manner.

Reflective Statements

Reflective statements indicate feelings that parents have verbally or nonverbally expressed, and they convey to parents the message that the physician is aware of their emotional state.

Examples
"You seem really upset."
"It sounds like you are pretty angry."
"I noticed tears in your eyes while you were speaking."

Empathic Statements

Empathic statements are supportive statements that convey to parents the message that the physician is aware that the situation is difficult for them.

Examples
"It must be frightening to you when your daughter's fever gets that high."
"You must be exhausted after staying up all night."
"This must be very difficult for you."

Active Listening

Active listening is the technique of identifying and reiterating the feelings and concerns inherent in seemingly neutral statements made by the parent ("listening between the lines").

Examples
Parent: "This is the third ear infection he has had in 3 months."
Practitioner: "You are upset because he has had so many ear infections in a short amount of time."
Parent: "Every doctor I see tells me something different."
Practitioner: "You are frustrated because you have been given so much different advice."

Using the Parent's Sensory Representational System

People often communicate in a sensory (i.e., visual, tactile, or auditory) modality. Rapport with the parent may be potentiated by using the same sensory modality.

Examples

Parent: "I just can't *picture* going through another night like last night."
Practitioner: "I can *see* that last night's experience with your child was quite distressing for you."
Parent: "Sometimes I *feel* like I am being *pulled* in a hundred directions."
Practitioner: "I have a *feeling* that you are right."

All of these approaches convey to parents the message that the physician is sensitive to their duress. Once the physician has established this groundwork, the next step is to explore the nature of their difficulty.

EXPLORING PARENTAL CONCERNS

Direct Approach

The direct approach is best for many parents for getting to the root of the problem. Examples of direct questions include: "Can you tell me what you are concerned about?" "Why did you bring your daughter to the office today?" "What worried you about her?" "Why did that worry you?" It is also prudent to ask what the parent hopes will be accomplished as a result of the visit. The parent's expectations may influence the intervention. If the parent's expectations are unrealistic, it is important to explain why his or her expectations cannot be met.

Indirect ("Third-Person") Approach

When dealing with reserved or less articulate parents, one may use the "third-person" approach, whereby the suspected concerns of the parents are verbalized by the practitioner. This approach allows issues to become apparent that parents might not themselves raise.

Examples

"Some parents are concerned that high fevers can seriously harm their infant. Do you have such concerns?"
"When some parents have experienced a death or illness in their family, they are concerned that their child may die. I wonder if you have such concerns about your child?"

Additional techniques can be used to further delineate parental concerns as the interaction proceeds.

Clarification

When clarification techniques are used, the parent is required to elaborate on unclear points.

Examples

"I am not sure I understand what you mean by that."
"You seem upset. I wonder what is bothering you?"
"You have become quiet. I wonder what you are thinking about?"
"I saw a tear in your eye. Can you tell me what upset you?"

Summarizing Techniques

Summarizing techniques allow the physician to recapitulate what the parent has said in order to validate the accuracy of the assessment.

Example

"Let me see if I understand what you are saying . . . you had a niece who died of meningitis, so whenever your baby gets a high fever, you become worried that she has meningitis as well."

Once parental concerns have been acknowledged and delineated, the final aspect of the interaction should direct the parents toward a resolution of their concerns.

RESOLVING PARENTAL CONCERNS

An effective intervention has occurred when the parent leaves with the hope of a productive change and feels in better control of the problem. This objective can be achieved in several ways.

Viewing the Problem from a New Perspective

Implicit in the concerns of most parents experiencing duress is the fear of a "bad outcome" to the problem. A key point of intervention is to accept with the parent the fact that although the situation is bad, *the problem is not as bad as it seems* (providing, of course, that this is the case), and to help the parent view the problem from a new perspective. A classic example is related by the psychotherapist Milton Erikson. He allayed his 3-year-old son's anxiety following a laceration by getting the child to defocus on how many sutures he would require and to reflect instead on whether he would require "as many sutures" as his older siblings had received for their lacerations.

For the parent distressed by infantile colic, one might accept with the parent the fact that the infant appears to be in discomfort (the situation is bad) but that colic *will not* harm the infant (the situation is not as bad as it seems), and that, indeed, crying for some infants is a developmentally healthy mode of tension release (new perspective on an old problem.)

For the parent overwhelmed by a hyperactive child, one might accept with the parent the fact that raising a hyperactive child is a difficult endeavor (the problem is bad). One might proceed to help the parent identify his child's strengths and positive features (the problem is not as bad as it seems). In addition, one might help the overwrought parent recognize how the hyperactive child's scattered attention also presents the child with unique and creative ways of viewing the world (a new perspective for the parent to consider).

Conveying an Expectation of Improvement

In addition to helping parents gain a new perspective on a problem, it is helpful to convey to the parent (if the prognosis is not dismal) that the situation is capable of improving. The suggestion that the situation is promising for positive change can be a powerful intervention. The implicit message to convey is that "things will get better." If, for example, the parent is overwhelmed by a child with colic, the physician can convey to the parent the fact that colic is self-limited and that an improvement can soon be expected. For an acutely ill child, it is helpful to give the parent a time range over which to expect improvement. For the child with an ongoing behavioral disorder, one might review the child's strengths and assure the parent that, with work, the child is capable of improving his behavior. In the case of chronic problems, the practitioner may aim for a series of small successes (rather than sweeping changes) as a means of sustaining parental hope.

Helping Parents to Regain Control

Problems and concerns can often become magnified to the point of overwhelming a parent. The physician can help parents regain a sense of control over their problems with the following methods.

Setting a Realistic Plan of Action. The most important aspect of this intervention is to convey to parents the fact that they have choices. The physician may actively engage parents in problem-solving strategies by having them review all of their options, review the advantages and disadvantages of each option, and select a realistic plan of action. This plan should be as specific as possible, regardless of whether it is a treatment regimen for acute gastroenteritis or a "time-out" strategy for a child with behavioral problems. It is helpful to anticipate what problems may occur despite the plan and how the parent should deal with such problems. For some parents, it is helpful to have them recount the plan to ascertain whether they understand it. If the physician lets a parent leave with "something to do" about the problem, the parent's stress can be markedly alleviated.

Ongoing Availability of the Practitioner. A parent's sense of control can be enhanced when he is assured of ongoing physician availability and that resolution of the problem is viewed as a cooperative venture. It is important to the parent that the physician can be reached if a problem arises.

Positive Feedback. Parents' sense of control can be enhanced by bolstering their confidence. It is helpful to convey to parents the fact that their physician feels they are competent and capable of handling the problem, by saying, for example, "I know that this has been difficult, but you are doing an excellent job," or "I know that you are a caring parent."

WHEN TO MAKE A REFERRAL

If a parent's or child's problem seems extreme, or if the problem is refractory to the aforementioned primary intervention, it is prudent to refer the family to another colleague or in some cases to a mental health consultant (see Chap. 26 for further discussion on mental health referrals).

ANNOTATED BIBLIOGRAPHY

King M, Novik L, Citrenbaum C: Irresistible Communication. Philadelphia, WB Saunders, 1983. (Excellent and unique book on psychosocial communication techniques for medical professionals.)

Korsch B, Freeman B, Negrete VF: Practical implications of doctor-patient interaction analysis for pediatric practice. Am J Dis Child 121:110, 1971. (Summary of practical guidelines for effective communication with parents based on Korsch's classic work on communication with parents.)

Poole SR: The "overanxious" patient. Clin Pediatr 19:557, 1980. (Helpful guidelines for working with anxious parents.)

Quill T: Recognizing and adjusting to barriers in doctor-patient communication. Ann Intern Med 111:51, 1989. (Summarizes helpful approaches to recognizing and overcoming communication barriers between physicians and patients.)

Schulman J: The management of the irate parent. J Pediatr 77:338, 1970. (Good practical guidelines for working with difficult parents.)

Wender E: Interviewing, 2nd ed. In Levine M, Carry WB, Crocker AC, Gross RT (eds): Developmental-Behavioral Pediatrics. Philadelphia, WB Saunders, 1992. (Good overview of methods of conducting a pediatric psychosocial interview.)

26

The Constant Complainer

Kenneth H. Tellerman

The pediatrician frequently encounters children who experience recurrent pain. Abdominal pain, headaches, and limb pains are the most common recurrent pains in childhood. The evaluation and treatment of pain are described in Chapter 186. In this chapter, an approach is given to the "constant complainer" (i.e., the child whose pain does not have a discernible etiology [*functional pain*]) and to the child whose pain is of organic etiology but with a psychogenic component.

ASSESSMENT

When a child presents with recurrent pain, the practitioner must perform a thorough history and physical examination to assess for organic etiology. Such an approach also conveys to the child's family the fact that their concerns have been taken seriously, thus establishing the basis for potential psychosocial intervention.

Organically induced pain is indicated by pain that is constant, well-localized, or awakens the child from sleep. In the case of recurrent abdominal pain, for example, the presence of constitutional signs or symptoms such as fever, arthritis, vomiting, bloody stools, jaundice, rash, growth arrest, pain associated with meals, or weight loss is a serious indication for organic illness. The approach to the child with pain *and* constitutional or organic signs has an orientation markedly different (i.e., sense of time urgency and aggressive laboratory investigations) from that of the child with pain alone. A careful history can gather evidence of psychogenic factors and can prevent the performance of unnecessary diagnostic procedures. Of course, establishing an organic etiology of pain does not preclude the presence of significant psychosocial stressors that may exacerbate the child's organic condition. Ample time should be allotted to conduct a thorough interview.

During the assessment, the practitioner should explore the following factors:

Timing

- When do the pains occur? Pains that occur on mornings prior to school may be psychogenic. Do the pains occur during weekends or during pleasurable activities?
- Are there precipitating stressors? Do the pains occur after disagreements with family members or peers? Do the pains occur prior to anxiety-provoking events such as school examinations or athletic activities? The parents or child may be instructed to maintain a daily diary for a short time, documenting the nature of the pain, the times of occurrence, and the events or thoughts that are associated with the onset of pain.
- Does the child miss school frequently? School absenteeism is frequently an indication of underlying psychosocial issues. The child's teacher may provide valuable insight (see Chap. 39, "School Refusal").

Personality and Family Climate

- What is the child's personality like? Recurrent pains may occur in a child who is anxious or depressed. Is the child high-strung, uptight, overly dramatic, or an overachiever? Is the child withdrawn, or does he or she display a sleep or appetite disturbance consistent with depression? It may be revealing to conduct part of the interview with the child alone.
- What is the family "climate"? Is the family experiencing potent stressors such as financial difficulties, marital discord, death, or chronic illness? How do parents respond to the child's pain? Are family members preoccupied with pain? Are there other family members ("models") experiencing recurrent pain? The possibility of sexual abuse within the family should not be overlooked.

Secondary Gain

- Secondary gain may be viewed along several parameters. Recurrent pain symptoms may be reinforced by a secondary gain that the child receives. Parents may also attain a secondary gain from the child's symptoms. Such parents may inadvertently reinforce their child's recurrent complaints.
- *Nurturance issues:* Do the child's symptoms elicit caring and nurturant responses from family members? Do the parents inadvertently reinforce the child's symptoms in order to maintain a "care-giving" role?
- *Separation issues:* Are the child's symptoms a component of separation anxiety, and do they serve to maintain proximity with parents? Do the parents inadvertently reinforce the symptoms in order to prevent separation? In the "vulnerable child" syndrome, there is parental difficulty with separation, overprotectiveness, and bodily overconcerns. Children at risk include those who experienced a serious illness from which the parent believed the child would die, those who represent for the parent a significant person from the past who died prematurely, and those whose mothers have had a threatened miscarriage, a spontaneous abortion, or a stillbirth.
- *Control issues:* Does the child use the symptom as a means of gaining control over parents (e.g., "Give me what I want or I will get ill.")? Do the parents inadvertently reinforce the child's symptoms as a means of maintaining control over the child (e.g., "You are too sick to go out and play.")? For some children, high parental expectations of achievement (e.g., academic or athletic) may lead to recurrent pain symptoms as a means of reacting to or thwarting parental control.
- *Attention seeking:* Does the child use the symptom to gain attention, or does the child use the symptom to avoid negative attentions (e.g., missing school in order to avoid embarrassment due to scholastic underachievement)? Do the parents inadvertently reinforce the child's symptom in order to gain attention from peers or medical personnel? For some parents, office visits meet their need for attention.
- *Marital discord:* Parents in conflict may inadvertently reinforce their child's pain symptoms. This frequently occurs when parents either become overly preoccupied with their child's symptoms in order to avoid dealing with their own conflict or use their child's symptoms as a means of extending their own conflict. Such parents may have conflicting attitudes about their child's symptoms and use the child as a fulcrum rather than confronting the more relevant sources of their marital conflict.

MANAGEMENT

If the assessment suggests that the recurrent pains are of psychogenic etiology, several effective primary care approaches are available.

Relating Findings

It is important to acknowledge with the family that the child's pain is real, regardless of whether it is organically or psychogenically induced. The pediatrician should be careful not to convey the message that the child is "making it up" or that the pain is simply "in the child's head." By asking both parents and child what they think is causing the pain, an opportunity is provided to dispel any anxiety-provoking fears and fantasies. With less articulate families, the pediatrician may wish to use the "third-person" technique to raise hidden concerns. For example, the pediatrician might state, "It sounds like you are quite concerned about your son's chest pains. Many families fear that chest pain is a sign of a serious heart condition. I wonder if you are concerned that your son has heart disease?"

When the family's concerns have been addressed, the pediatrician can often reassure the parents that although the problem seems bad, it is not as bad as they thought. The pediatrician might address the family by saying, "I have listened to your son's medical complaints and I have examined him thoroughly, and I do not believe that your son is displaying signs of a serious illness." He might proceed to say, "It seems like your son has been under a lot of stress. You have talked about problems at home and at school. Sometimes pains such as your son is experiencing can be worsened by stress."

It is helpful to leave open the possibility of a physical disorder if the signs and symptoms change. The pediatrician might add, "I would like to continue to monitor these pain episodes, and if they change, we may need to consider a further evaluation. For now, I think it would be helpful to examine the stress-related issues going on in your son's life."

The practitioner can be helpful in delineating precipitating stressors and developing a problem-solving strategy with the family to reduce stress. He might help the family evaluate their options, review the advantages and disadvantages of each option, and select a plan of action. Strategies might be as simple as finding an after-school tutor for a child with an academic difficulty or planning constructive time with busy parents of a child who is seeking attention. Identifying and systematically eliminating sources of secondary gain are often effective strategies. In addition, numerous studies have demonstrated the benefits of teaching self-relaxation techniques to children as a means of empowering them with a sense of control over their symptoms, thereby allowing them to reduce stress and pain.

Vulnerable Child

Children with recurrent pain symptoms frequently have overprotective parents. In addition, such parents are often overly involved with the child's symptoms, overly anxious, and overindulgent. Unresolved fears of separation often exist, and many of these children meet the criteria for the "vulnerable child syndrome." Overinvolvement between family members and overprotectiveness are characteristic features of "psychosomatogenic families." Recurrent pain symptoms are commonly an outgrowth of psychosocial dy-

namics in such families. In families with overprotective and overly indulgent parents, some of the goals of intervention are to diminish the overextended parent's preoccupation with the child's symptoms and to encourage the family to foster age-appropriate behaviors. This will often lead to improvement in the child's pain symptoms.

Ways of improving an inappropriate relationship between overprotective parents and the symptomatic child include the following: (1) Encouraging the family to allow the child to engage in age-appropriate activities outside of the home, such as Scouts, church groups, and athletic activities. (2) Returning the child to school if absenteeism is an issue. Strict criteria should be set for when a child may remain home or be sent home from school (e.g., fever, vomiting). (3) Encouraging the parents and child to spend "positive time" together engaged in activities that are enjoyable and not focused on pain. Parents should be counseled to de-focus on the child's pain symptoms, and they should be advised not to inquire about the child's pain or remind the child of his symptoms. Parents need to become aware of how they respond to their child's symptoms and how their response may foster the child's symptoms. (4) Helping a less involved parent spend more time with the child and encouraging an overly involved parent to pursue alternative interests. (5) Encouraging parents to diminish overly indulgent behaviors. Some parents may need specific advice on limit setting and may be helped by using such behavioral approaches as "time out." Overly indulgent parents may need to be advised to relegate age-appropriate responsibilities to the child, such as participation in household chores.

If the parent–child relationship can be redirected toward a more appropriate interaction, the practitioner will frequently witness regression of the child's symptoms. It is important to remember that many families may require several sessions of counseling before a productive change is noted. Also, many of the aforementioned approaches can be individually introduced over the course of several counseling sessions.

MENTAL HEALTH REFERRAL

Mental health referral should be considered if the patient's symptoms are refractory to primary care intervention; if the parents are experiencing significant marital discord; or if the parent(s) or child is displaying severely disturbed behavior.

The recommendation for referral may be greatly facilitated if the family has been advised early on of the possibility that there is a psychogenic overlay to the pain. It is often more palatable to the family to convey the message that the child's symptoms may be stress-related rather than caused by an emotional problem. For example, the pediatrician might state, "It appears that your child is experiencing a number of stressful occurrences in his life. Pain can sometimes be influenced by stress factors. There is no clear indication of a serious physical illness causing the pain, but we should stay alert for changes in the nature of your son's symptoms. At this point, I believe that counseling will help your family examine and deal with some of the factors that are contributing to your son's recurrent pain."

Referrals should be made to a specific consultant, with a message clearly conveyed that the practitioner will remain available. Recommendations for referral to a mental health consultant should be stated firmly, and the practitioner should avoid being apologetic about making such a referral. Some families may require time to process the recommendation, and the practitioner should be sensitive to this need.

ANNOTATED BIBLIOGRAPHY

Allmond B, Buckman W, Gofman HF: Psychosomatic conditions. In Allmond B, Buckman W, Gofman HF: The Family Is the Patient: An Approach to Behavioral Pediatrics for the Clinician. St. Louis, CV Mosby, 1979. (Excellent chapter with practical guidelines for the pediatric practitioner on working with psychosomatic families.)

Coleman W: Recurrent abdominal pain. Pediatr Rev 8:143, 1986. (Excellent discussion with focus on integrating medical and psychosocial factors.)

Green M: Sources of pain. In Levine M, Carey WB, Crocker AC, Gross RT (eds): Developmental-Behavioral Pediatrics, 2nd ed. Philadelphia, WB Saunders, 1992. (Good review of the evaluation of children with recurrent pain, with a focus on psychosocial issues.)

Green M: Vulnerable child syndrome and its variants. Pediatr Rev 8:75,1986. (Excellent review and update on the identification of "the vulnerable child" syndrome.)

Minuchin S: Families and Family Therapy. Cambridge, Harvard University Press, 1974. (Presents a family therapy model of psychosomatic illness.)

Olness K: Recurrent headaches in children: Diagnosis and treatment. Pediatr Rev 8:307, 1987. (Excellent review; includes discussion of self-relaxation techniques.)

Schecter N: Recurrent pains in children: An overview and an approach. Pediatr Clin North Am 31:949, 1984. (Comprehensive review.)

27

Preparing the Child for Hospitalization

Thomas J. Hathaway

Admission to the hospital for medical or surgical treatment can be a terrifying and disruptive experience for a child and his family. It can awaken or heighten fears of separation, pain, disfigurement, loss of loved ones or self, and loss of control or autonomy. These well-documented negative repercussions of hospitalization can persist long after the admission.

Prehospitalization preparation can both reduce the negative impact of hospitalization and improve a family's adaptation to their child's illness and medical management. Studies of the effects of prehospitalization preparation show reduced levels of stress in parents and child, improved cooperation, improved posthospital adjustment, lower anxiety, decreased fear, and fewer behavioral problems. However, the full beneficial impact to a child or family is dependent on a number of variables that can and should be assessed prior to hospitalization or treatment.

ASSESSMENT

The clinician should assess the need for prehospital preparation in each child and family for whom hospitalization is planned. An understanding of the family's support mechanisms and coping styles, the family's comprehension of proposed treatment, and the child's developmental stage is necessary to determine the amount and kind of preparation needed. If family supports or coping strategies are limited, this opportunity to intervene or access help for the family may be critical to the success of the hospital treatment or posthospital adjustment. The family's cultural and socioeconomic background, primary language, education, parenting experience, and other potential barriers to communication should be recognized and managed.

The need for preparation can be assessed by open-ended questions to parents such as, "What do you know about this illness or condition?" "What do you know about this test or treatment?" "What is the likelihood of success?" "What are the risks?" "What have you told your child?" "What do you plan to tell him or her?" "What do you expect your child's reaction to be?" "How has your child coped in the past with separation, strangers, unfamiliar routines, pain, confinement, and medical encounters?"

The older child can be asked similar questions to assess his level of preparation prior to hospitalization. It may be helpful to de-personalize the questions to the child by asking about others' feelings, reactions, or fears concerning the illness, treatment, or hospitalization rather than asking direct questions of the child.

When the child and family are known to the pediatrician, the child's past experience with office visits, medical tests, or treatments can be of help in determining the child's preparation needs.

The extent, type, and timing of preparation will also vary depending on the child's age and developmental level; therefore, the pediatrician should keep in mind the common developmental themes or issues for each age group. Separation, stranger anxiety, autonomy, and mastery are a few of the relevant developmental issues that have an impact on adjustment to hospitalization.

In addition to assessing the family's and child's preparation needs, the clinician should be familiar with local hospital and community resources as well as hospital policies and procedures that may have an important impact on the child's course of treatment. Rooming-in policy, visiting hours, child life programs, play and educational facilities, nursing care policies, and medical staff routines and coverage should be discussed with the family.

The clinician should also be knowledgeable about the availability of child life specialists, mental health professionals, and social service supports and should have established lines of referral and communication to these providers.

MANAGEMENT

Prehospitalization preparation should begin once a decision to admit a child to the hospital has been made. For elective admissions, this preparation begins with explanations to the parent and child of why admission and treatment are needed and what to expect during the hospital stay. The youngest age for which preparation is beneficial has not been established. If a child is old enough to understand language, he or she should receive some preparation for what will be happening to him.

Guidelines for preparation suggested by Thompson and Stanford (1981) include:

1. Both children and parents should be included in the preparation process.
2. Information should be provided to children at a level commensurate with their cognitive abilities.
3. Emphasis should be placed on the sensations a child is likely to experience.
4. Parents and children should be encouraged to express their emotions throughout the process.
5. The process should result in the development of a trusting relationship between the family and those doing the preparation.
6. Parents and children should receive support throughout the stressful points of hospitalization from a figure in whom such trust is placed.

Preparation varies according to the cognitive abilities and developmental issues of the child's age group. The pediatrician can provide insight and anticipatory guidance to the parents on what reactions and issues may be expected. For a practical approach to preparation for the various age groups, the reader is referred to the book by Petrillo and Sanger, *Emotional Care of Hospitalized Children*. Several points are highlighted:

Infants and Toddlers

Separation anxiety is expected. Encourage rooming-in for parents, parental involvement in care, and transitional objects or toys from home. Stranger anxiety is also common. Parents and staff should be made aware that these reactions are normal.

Children this age may not understand explanations about the body and how it works. Use of a doll to teach or explain and to depersonalize teaching is recommended. Allow older toddlers to touch and play with appropriate equipment.

Fantasies about illness or treatment as punishment and feelings of guilt over illness are common and should be discussed during teaching.

Parents and care-givers need to be honest about pain and discomfort to the child (this is true for all ages).

This age has a limited time concept. Preparation should be one day before planned hospitalization. Explain times in terms of routines that are familiar to the child (e.g., after lunch or nap).

Preschool and Early School-Age

Separation fears and fear of the medical staff are possible concerns. Rooming-in should be encouraged; however, parents should also be encouraged to leave for periods of time if the situation allows.

Children this age can understand simple explanations of anatomy. Use dolls or drawings to explain and teach. Allow play with appropriate equipment.

Be aware of "magical thinking" in this age group. Correct fantasies around guilt or blame for illness.

Discuss the limits of treatment. Inform the child of what will and what will not be done (e.g., what parts of the body will not be touched or treated).

Use, and encourage parents to use, neutral words in discussing treatment (e.g., "opening" for incision rather than "cut"). Keep in mind that anything said can be misconstrued, especially conversations between adults within earshot of the child.

Time concepts are evolving. Preparation should be within the week of admission. Some experts recommend one day per year of age as the optimal number of days between preparation and admission.

School-Age

Separation anxiety is not as common in this group as it is in younger children. However, separation from parents, siblings, and peers may be problematic. Regular visiting by family and friends should be encouraged. Rooming-in may or may not be necessary depending on the child, the family, and the nature of the illness or treatment.

Mastery of skills, experiences, and self-esteem become increasingly important issues. Encourage self-care, continued school work, and play when appropriate.

School-age children have a developing capability for understanding explanations, anatomy, and physiology. However, be sure to explore misconceptions as to causation or nature of treatment. The use of a doll for teaching may or may not be accepted by the child. Use simple drawings and appropriate equipment for teaching.

Adolescents

Independence and development of identity become increasingly important during adolescence. The adolescent should be informed of and involved in treatment planning and decision making.

Body image and appearance are usually paramount. The effects of illness or treatment on appearance and function should be discussed.

The adolescent's understanding of his illness or treatment should not be taken for granted. Many adolescents will have misconceptions about anatomy and physiology that may go unrecognized unless they are discussed.

The issue of confidentiality should also be discussed with the adolescent.

For nonelective admissions, there is usually little time to plan prehospitalization preparation. In these circumstances, the aforementioned guidelines should be kept in mind and age-appropriate explanations given. Patient and family education and support should begin as soon as time and circumstances permit.

INDICATION FOR REFERRAL

The admission of a child to the hospital should be preceded by timely and appropriate preparation and support. This process begins with the admitting physician but is also the responsibility of the parents and office or hospital staff. In many hospitals and communities, child life specialists provide thorough prehospital preparation and support to children and their families.

The clinician may choose to use a child life specialist or other professional trained in children's emotional support in order to prepare the child and family for hospitalization. This person should also have experience or knowledge of the reasons for hospitalization and the type of procedures, tests, or treatments expected in order to accurately prepare and inform the family. All staff dealing with children should have a recognition of the child's and family's special emotional needs and adjustment during hospitalization. In addition to working with families, the child life specialist may also serve to inform and apprise staff of a child's or family's needs before and during hospitalization.

Parents have an obvious role in preparing their child for hospitalization. However, they usually do not have the medical background or experience necessary to fully prepare the child for the hospital experience. With guidance from their family physician, a child life specialist, or other experienced person, parents can have a greater impact on the preparation of the child. There are numerous resources, including books, pamphlets, and videos, that can be used at home to help the family with this preparation. Several organizations devoted to the needs of children publish newsletters, journals, catalogs, and bibliographies of relevant material. Several recommended books are listed in Appendix D. The reader is referred to the following bibliography to obtain complete listings of available materials in this area.

ANNOTATED BIBLIOGRAPHY

American Academy of Pediatrics, Committee on Hospital Care: Hospital Care of Children and Youth. Elk Grove Village, IL, American Academy of Pediatrics, 1986. (Covers many aspects of hospital care, including admission process and child life programs.)

Campione P: Play and Preparation: An Annotated Bibliography. Bethesda, MD, Association for the Care of Children's Health, 1988.

Petrillo M, Sanger S: Emotional Care of Hospitalized Children, 2nd ed. Philadelphia, JB Lippincott, 1980. (Comprehensive treatment of the subject; practical and useful guidelines, including preparation techniques for specific procedures. See especially pp. 209–233.)

Redburn L: Books for Children and Teenagers About Hospitalization, Illness, and Disabling Conditions. Bethesda, MD, Association for the Care of Children's Health, 1987. (An annotated bibliography.)

Thompson RH, Stanford G: Child Life in Hospitals: Theory and Practice. Springfield, IL, Charles C Thomas, 1981. (Thorough discussion of the theory and practice of child life in hospitals. Intended primarily for students of child life, but useful for all professionals dealing with hospitalized children.)

ORGANIZATIONS

Association for the Care of Children's Health
7910 Woodmont Ave., Suite 300
Bethesda, MD 20814
(Publishes and distributes a large number of relevant books, brochures, films, and videos, and a quarterly journal. Catalog available.)

Family Communications, Inc. (Mr. Rogers)
4802 Fifth Ave.
Pittsburgh, PA 15213
(Publishes and produces a number of resources for family growth, including books, pamphlets, and videos relating to the hospital experience. Catalog available.)

Pediatric Projects, Inc.
P.O. Box 57155
Tarzana, CA 91357
(Publishes a guide to medical toys and books for children to help them understand health care, illness, disability, and hospitalization.)

28
Children in Foster Care

Edward L. Schor

Most children who enter foster care do so because their parents are unwilling or unable to provide for their physical and emotional needs. They come most often from single-parent households, where poverty, lack of formal education, and absence of social support lead to inadequate and inappropriate child care. The vast majority of the children have experienced physical or sexual abuse or neglect. Substance-exposed infants whose mothers received inadequate prenatal care are entering foster care at increased rates. HIV-positive infants frequently are placed in foster care. Previous health care of older children is likely to have been fragmented. As a consequence, children in foster care are likely to have unrecognized or untreated chronic disorders, a high rate of emotional problems, and impaired school performance.

The foster care system is managed by child welfare agencies. These agencies are usually branches of larger public or private social service departments, which, in general, operate with severely limited resources. As the first step in the process of placing a child in foster care, social workers determine a family's need for social services such as counseling, public housing, and so forth. Should the application of these resources fail to, or appear unlikely to, improve a home situation deemed detrimental to a child's well-being, the social worker may recommend the removal of the child from his or her home. The purpose of this removal is to assist the family to remediate the circumstances that prevent adequate child rearing so that the child may be returned to the care of his family. If unsuccessful, the agency may recommend that the parents' rights to the child be terminated, thus freeing the child for adoption. Court-imposed separation of children from parents is a decision intended to be based on the best needs of the child. The burden of responsibility for reconstitution of the family is placed on the parents. A child so removed may be placed in the home of a relative or a foster family, in a group home, or in an institution under the supervision of a staff of child-care workers. Where a child is placed is determined by his or her needs and the availability of various settings. Most children are placed in foster home care, but placement with the extended family is increasingly sought as a first option. The child's caseworker is then responsible for helping the biologic family prepare for the return of their child, supervising the care provided by the foster parent, and assuring that the child's health and educational needs are being met. Limited specialized services and drug treatment for parents may impede the effectiveness of the caseworker's efforts. Additionally, an individual social worker may have several dozen or more children in his or her case load and therefore may be unable to meet all of his or her responsibilities.

Good foster homes, able to provide the appropriate mix of structure and nurturance to distressed children, are in short supply. Despite this shortage, agencies do their best to exclude prospective foster parents who are emotionally unsuited for the demands to be placed on them. While efforts are being made to upgrade the recruitment, training, and support of foster parents, foster parents ordinarily receive limited training prior to receiving children, and they receive scanty continuing education. They receive an allowance from the state for each child in their care; the rate of support barely covers the cost of providing shelter, food, and clothes for the child, and it does not presume to be a salary for professional child care. Medical care is paid for by Medicaid programs. Foster parenting, therefore, is essentially a voluntary program heavily dependent on the good intentions and intuitive abilities of altruistic lay people.

PRESENTATION

Children in foster care may present for medical care at several points during the chronology of their foster care placement. Because most children in care come to public attention through reports of abuse or neglect, pediatricians may first become involved in the emergency assessment of these children. This encounter may present the only opportunity for a physician to obtain a detailed and accurate history of the child. An increasing number of children of substance-abusing parents are identified in the neonatal period as being at risk for subsequent neglect. The subject of child abuse is discussed in detail in Chapter 20.

Because the care of children in foster care is time-consuming and reimbursement is poor, agencies have difficulty identifying physicians willing to provide ongoing care for these children. The absence of an organized system of medical care for children in foster care or a system of universal health coverage for mothers and children makes the pediatrician's role more difficult. The lack of a documented intake pediatric history, the turnover of caseworkers, the movement of the child from one foster home to another, and the too-frequent exclusion of biologic parents from child-care decisions once a child has been placed in a foster home may cause the continuing care of a child to be based on an insubstantial data base. These same constraints interfere with the completion of referrals for specialized care and with effective communication among all individuals involved in the ongoing care of the child.

The physical health problems of children in foster care do not differ substantially from those of other children from similar socioeconomic backgrounds. However, their previous lack of comprehensive health care, the family disorganization and abuse they experienced, and, ironically, the separation from their families inherent in foster care placement lead to a considerably increased rate of chronic medical conditions, educational problems, and, most notably, emotional disturbances. In addition, because a large proportion of the children who enter foster care are adolescents, health problems of this age group are seen with greater frequency than they are in the usual pediatric practice.

Short stature is twice as common in children in foster care as in the general population. They also have a higher rate of auditory and uncorrected visual acuity deficits. Dermatologic, allergic, and orthodontic problems, dental caries, and musculoskeletal deformities are also common chronic disorders. These children appear to have a higher rate of developmental disabilities and consequent educational failures. Comprehensive investigation and management of these disorders is time-consuming and requires an organized system of follow-up and consultation. Whether because of their disorganized lives or because of superimposed physical and emotional problems, children in foster care are also likely to be behind their expected grade level in school. No data are available on the incidence of specific learning disabilities in these children, although it seems to be increased. The number of substance-exposed infants entering care may further increase the rate of educational and behavioral disorders.

The most important health problems of children in foster care, which some investigators have found to be almost universal, are emotional disorders. Over one third of children in foster care have moderate to severe emotional problems, and another third have evident, although less severe, disabilities.

The spectrum of emotional disorders is wide and is related to the age, personality, and experience of the child. For a brief interval after their initial placement or subsequent replacement, evidence of emotional disturbance may subside and the foster parents may then experience a "honeymoon" of good behavior by the foster child. This phase passes rapidly, and existing mental health problems reemerge. Infants and young children will often fail to thrive, or they will have sleeping and eating disorders. Preschool and early school-aged children will have problems of discipline, toileting, and "hyperactivity." Older children and adolescents often present with exaggerations of usual adolescent behaviors, testing the limits of acceptable social behavior through truancy, delinquency, substance abuse, destructive and violent activities, and sexual experimentation. Psychosomatic symptoms such as headache and recurrent abdominal pain are common. The pediatrician, however, should not be lulled into a false sense of security by the absence of these more overt signs. Depression is common among children in dependent care, and withdrawal and social isolation strongly suggest emotional disability. These signs are accentuated during times of uncertainty and stress.

The underlying insecurity of children in foster care is often aggravated when foster parents, having been pushed to the limit of their tolerance or parental abilities and not receiving sufficient professional support, threaten the child with his or her single greatest fear—removal from their home—in an effort to control the child's behavior. This tactic is usually ineffective and may precipitate behavior requiring removal. Occasionally, physical or sexual abuse of foster children occurs in foster homes, and this possibility should be considered by the pediatrician when a child's behavior deteriorates.

The frequency and severity of emotional problems are strongly related to the child's sense of security and permanence in his life. Children whose placement conveys a sense of permanence and security fare better. These children may have exacerbations of psychobehavioral disturbances when they have contact with their natural parents and are thus reminded of the precariousness of their life's circumstances.

Unfortunately, these visitations are often too infrequent and occur as isolated, unnatural contacts in unfamiliar settings under the watchful eye of a caseworker. This surreal experience, connected as it is to decisions of reuniting the family, compounds the stress on both the child and the parent.

WORK-UP

History

The health evaluation of children in foster care extends beyond the physical, emotional, and educational problems that may be present; it must also allow for cognizance of the child's legal status and communication with the multiple people responsible for the child. Previous health care records should be requested, and the child, caseworker, foster parent, and natural parent should all be sources of information. Others, such as relatives and school teachers, can help in developing a complete picture of the child's life and problems. Much can be learned by interviewing these individuals separately, although having the opportunity to watch their interactions can be helpful in understanding the stresses in the child's life and the nature of the supports available to him.

Central to the health and well-being of a child in foster care is his placement status. The pediatrician should learn the details of the child's foster care history (e.g., the age and circumstances under which the child came into foster care). Because many of these children have had a succession of caseworkers and have lived in several foster homes, the number of replacements and the circumstances that led to them should be determined. Children often feel unjustifiably responsible for their being in foster care and for whatever alterations in their placement that subsequently befall them. In the process of developing relationships with these children, it is helpful to understand their feelings and perceptions about being in foster care. The pediatrician should ascertain whether there are plans for a child to return home and, if so, when and under what circumstances, or whether the child is free to be adopted, and what progress is being made in this regard. Long-term nonrelative foster care should be avoided if possible because of its inherent insecurity.

Natural parents, although absent, are central to the lives of children living in foster care settings. The pediatrician should learn the frequency and nature of children's contact with their parents. In their absence, natural parents become fantasy figures imbued with various attributes. A complete understanding of the foster child's sense of self requires that information about his parents be obtained. One should also obtain information about the child's natural siblings. Siblings are often separated, and little effort may be made by agencies to assure meaningful contact between them.

A description of the child's life within the foster home

should be obtained. This inquiry takes the form of the usual family social history, with the following modifications: physical accommodations and sleeping arrangements should be noted, as should other issues, such as chores and allowance, that relate to the integration of the child into the home. The foster parents' previous experience in that role, as well as with children of their own, should be explored. The composition of the foster family and the child's perceptions of the entrance or exit of other children placed in that home should be elicited. It is important to know the types of rewards and punishments being provided by foster parents, because behavior that often appears to foster parents and caseworkers as intolerable can be understood and remediated by altering the approach to discipline.

A complete school history is essential because school problems are frequent among children in foster care. Unfortunately, caseworkers and foster parents often have less communication with the child's school than would be optimal; thus, early signs of learning problems and school failure may not be noticed. Careful inquiry may provide clues to difficulties in the school setting and may prompt the pediatrician to contact school personnel directly. Disparate reports between classroom and home behavior warrant further investigation.

Physical Examination

The physical examination should be comprehensive. Areas in which positive findings are likely should receive particularly careful evaluation. These include growth parameters, vision and hearing, dental examination, and musculoskeletal and neurologic assessment. Young children should be screened with a standardized developmental assessment. Additionally, adolescents should have an assessment of maturation, an assessment of fitness for sports, and breast, gynecologic, and genital examinations.

PRINCIPLES OF TREATMENT

If the child's emotional, physical, or educational problems are treated as though they are separable from the foster child's life circumstances, the results will be unsuccessful. By being a sympathetic, objective advocate for the child, the physician can be a source of support, advice, and stability in the child's otherwise precarious world. His or her knowledge and skills offer the opportunity to recognize and address problems, both emotional and physical, that would otherwise handicap the child's future development. He or she can also educate and influence the other adults who share responsibility for the child's welfare so that their decisions are consistently in the child's best interest.

Medical care of dependent children cannot occur in isolation from the other professional services directed toward the child and his or her natural and foster families. Unlike serving as a primary care provider for the average child, pediatricians caring for children in foster care can expect to routinely invest much time acting as an advocate for the child and as a coordinator of an array of services involving the child's health, education, and welfare. The pediatrician must be cautious to avoid a situation in which the child and those responsible for his or her day-to-day care are lost in an unintegrated mixture of specialists' opinions that do not take account of the child's unique circumstances. The pediatrician may also find himself or herself in conflict with social service agencies, schools, or the judiciary, and he or she should not hesitate to lobby for the child in these arenas. It is unfortunately not unusual that the best interests of the child are subverted by conflicting interests and bureaucratic obstacles.

INDICATIONS FOR REFERRAL

The nature and frequency of the health problems of children in foster care that are identified by pediatricians make referral or consultation a customary part of their care. The frequency of referral to other medical specialists depends partly on the constraints and capabilities of the primary physician. Many of the chronic medical problems will require the input of a subspecialist. Educational problems demand the coordinated services of psychologists and educators. At least 20% of these children have emotional problems serious enough to warrant referral for ongoing psychotherapy. On occasion, the input of lawyers will be helpful in buttressing the advocacy role of the primary care pediatrician.

TREATMENT AND MANAGEMENT

The practices in which children in foster care are seen should be organized to accommodate their special needs. Appointment systems should allow sufficient time for the comprehensive care these children require. Counseling services and family planning should ideally be integrated into the primary care setting. Because of the nature of the health problems of dependent children and the transient nature of their living situations, a great deal of patient education is necessary; this is particularly important with regard to the self-management of chronic illnesses and in the area of sex education. Problems identified by the primary care pediatrician that require subspecialty consultation should be promptly referred and should then be integrated into the child's ongoing health care plan. The anticipation of a return to his or her natural parents should not delay appropriate medical assessment and care because, as a rule, these plans are rarely implemented in a timely fashion.

The system of record keeping employed by social service agencies will vary but ordinarily is not adequate. Pediatricians should keep careful office records of children in foster care because it is likely that the child's care will be transferred at some point to another physician, or that information will be requested by the agencies or the courts. It is also recommended that these children, through their foster parents, retain an abbreviated medical record that travels with them through their various placements and their return home. The American Academy of Pediatrics has made available such a record.

In his or her role as a child advocate, the pediatrician caring for dependent children may wish to participate in the broader, community-based aspects of foster care. Within the office, he or she may identify and recruit families whom he or she believes would be effective foster parents. He or she may participate as a member of a citizens' review board that monitors the planning that agencies do on behalf of children under their care. Finally, he or she may work, independently or through professional organizations, with local social services agencies. In this capacity, the pediatrician may participate in continuing education programs for agency staff and foster parents, or may help develop standards and procedures for health care for dependent children in the community.

The final arena in which pediatricians may deal with children in foster care is when these children leave foster care. Children may return to their natural home, in which case an organized transfer of medical responsibility should be initiated. They may also leave foster care at their legal age of majority to enter the adult world. Alternatively, they may be freed for adoption. This latter course is often a complicated process requiring the termination of parental rights by the courts. In general, well-formulated plans should provide children in foster care with a sense of permanency. When children in care are eligible for adoption, the pediatrician may be asked to support the adoption application of the child's foster parents. This determination should be based on knowledge of the foster parent–child relationship and on established principles of parent–child attachment.

Many children remain in foster care even though they are legally eligible for adoption. These are the "hard to place" children who are older and who have emotional, cognitive, or physical handicaps. Prospective adoptive parents are often reluctant to assume the additional burden these children may present and prefer to parent young, healthy infants. In order to facilitate adoption of children with special needs, Congress has enacted legislation allowing their medical care to continue to be financed by the federal Medicaid program after they leave foster care. The philosophy of adoption agencies is that prospective adoptive families exist for each of these children. Pediatricians should encourage families to consider adopting children from foster care in those situations in which such a process would be in the best interest of the child and the family.

ANNOTATED BIBLIOGRAPHY

Fanshel D, Shinn EB: Children in Foster Care: A Longitudinal Investigation. New York, Columbia University Press, 1978. (The major prospective study of children in foster care, which is concerned with issues of placement and how children fare developmentally during long-term separation from their parents.)

Goldstein J, Freud A, Solnit AJ: Before the Best Interests of the Child. New York, Free Press, 1979. (Considers the legal and psychological aspects of the child–parent relationships and the intrusion of the State into what should be a vigilantly protected area.)

Goldstein J, Freud A, Solnit AJ: Beyond the Best Interests of the Child. New York, Free Press, 1973. (Application of principles of child psychology to legal decisions regarding child placement in adoption, foster care, and divorce; required reading.)

Knitzer J, Allen ML: Children Without Homes. Washington, DC, Children's Defense Fund, 1978. (Compilation of valuable data on foster children and the foster care system; not specifically focusing on health issues.)

Schor EL: Foster care. Pediatr Rev 10:209–216, 1989. (Review of the foster care system and health issues of children in care.)

Schor EL: The foster care system and health status of foster children. Pediatrics 69:521–528, 1982. (Review of the history of foster care and of data describing the health problems of foster children.)

29
Death in the Family
Edward R. Christophersen

Much of the literature on grieving has been characterized by a lack of scientific rigor, an absence of data, and a dependence on clinical examples. This chapter provides a discussion of normal grieving or "uncomplicated bereavement," major depressive episodes, and suggestions for helping parents and children cope with grief.

The Diagnostic and Statistical Manual of Mental Disorders, published by the American Psychiatric Association, begins its discussion of "uncomplicated bereavement" with the following statement:

This category can be used when a focus of attention or treatment is a normal reaction to the death of a loved one. A full depressive syndrome frequently is a normal reaction to such a loss, with feelings of depression and such associated symptoms as poor appetite, weight loss, and insomnia. However, morbid preoccupation with worthlessness, prolonged and marked functional impairment, and marked psychomotor retardation are uncommon and suggest that the bereavement is complicated by the development of a Major Depression.

In Uncomplicated Bereavement, guilt, if present, is chiefly about things done or not done at the time of the death by the survivor; thoughts of death are usually limited to the individual's thinking that he or she would be better off dead or that he or she should have died with the person who died. The individual with Uncomplicated Bereavement generally regards the feeling of depressed mood as "normal," although he or she may seek professional help for relief of such associated symptoms as insomnia and anorexia.

The task for the primary health care provider is to discriminate between families who are experiencing a normal grief process and those who display significant pathology requiring a referral to an appropriate mental health practitioner. Unfortunately, in much of the published literature on grieving, the authors never state whether they are dealing with normal grief reactions or the reactions of individuals who present with significant psychopathology.

PRESENTATION

In those instances in which a family member, perhaps a child, has been hospitalized, up to the time of his death, the close family members seldom maintain a normal lifestyle. Parents who sleep in chairs in their children's hospital rooms, or on sofas in the waiting room outside of a pediatric intensive care unit, cannot be expected to look, act, or feel normal. The use of hospital restrooms, showers, and bathtubs, and changing clothes much less frequently than usual, exacerbate the acute stress. A parent, under these circumstances, will not get much quality sleep. He or she may also exhibit less affect and may have a decreased appetite. Thus, some of the reactions that are interpreted solely as grieving may very well be a result of the combined effect of the loss and a reaction to the severe disruption in lifestyle.

It is important to know about any preexisting pathology in a family who is grieving, because families with significant psychopathology cannot be expected to behave or adjust in the same manner as well-adjusted families. Primary health care providers have a major advantage in that most of the families they follow have been known to them for years, and they usually know which families have had adjustment problems. If a family is known to have had serious emotional problems prior to a death in the family, the provider should consider referring the family to a mental health practitioner for management immediately after a death or, in some cases, during the critical illness period. The preexisting condition, coupled with the death in the family, may create a condition that is simply beyond the time constraints and the training of a primary provider. The urgency or eventual need for counseling is much reduced in a well-adjusted family. In the absence of prior experience with the family, the decision becomes much more difficult, because the provider must then draw judgments from a history obtained while the family is under significant stress. It is highly desirable to spend time with the family, to listen, to provide emotional support, to help them cope, and to discover emerging or preexisting problems.

DIFFERENTIAL DIAGNOSIS

Probably the most frequently encountered differential diagnosis for the provider to make is between uncomplicated bereavement and a major depressive episode. The *Diagnostic and Statistical Manual of Mental Disorders* states that:

The essential feature (of a major depressive episode) is either a dysphoric mood, usually depression, or loss of interest or pleasure in all or almost all usual activities and pastimes. This disturbance is prominent, relatively persistent, and associated with other symptoms of a depressive syndrome. These symptoms include appetite disturbance, change in weight, sleep disturbance, psychomotor agitation or retardation, decreased energy, feelings of worthlessness or guilt, difficulty concentrating or thinking, and thoughts of death or suicide or suicide attempts.

Uncomplicated Bereavement is distinguished from a major depressive episode and is not considered a mental disorder even when associated with the full depressive syndrome. However, if bereavement is unduly severe or prolonged, the diagnosis may be changed to Major Depression.

WORK-UP

History

Primary health care providers are often the first resource that families turn to when they experience a death. To emphasize this point, it should be restated that the major advantage that the primary provider has is prior experience with the family. If the provider has seen how a family reacted to a prior serious illness or hospitalization, or to another kind of stress such as a job layoff, then he or she has a good baseline with which to compare the family's functioning shortly after a death in the family and to anticipate problems. A brief office interview, or a phone conversation, may be sufficient to decide if the family needs a referral. If the family members are very sad but there is no reason to suspect any prior history of emotional problems, then the practitioner may assume, for the present time, that the family will eventually be able to adjust. Some practitioners may want to administer a depression inventory (e.g., Beck) to one or both of the parents in order to assist in making a judgment regarding the need for a referral. However, the administration of any such inventory would be best left until at least several weeks after the death in order to give the family members time to deal with their grief. If, after several weeks, they are not functioning better, a referral may be indicated.

INDICATIONS FOR REFERRAL

In most cases, the primary provider is in the best position to offer advice and support to parents and children who have experienced a loss. Unfortunately, relatively few mental health professionals have much experience with medical disorders.

If there has been a history of significant adjustment problems, if the family either requests a referral for "counseling" or presents with enough symptoms, then the family probably should be referred to a mental health practitioner for assessment and treatment. The provider should not hesitate to inquire about the training and expertise of a professional prior to referring a family to him or her, because mental health professionals (even those who practice at tertiary care centers) are not always adept at dealing with grief reactions.

TREATMENT AND MANAGEMENT

Treatment Considerations with Parents. In most families, there will be only normal grief. Few people are competent at grieving. The provider may want to make several suggestions to families who either have a child in critical condition or have already lost a child as a result of an accident or illness.

Maintenance of Routines. Many people become accustomed to a routine, and when these individuals have a family member in the hospital, or there is a death in their family, their routine is drastically changed. It is also difficult to ascertain whether changes in the family members' habits are due directly to the emotional trauma of the illness or death or to the fact that the individuals' routines have been so drastically altered. Parents should try to return to their normal schedule, and although doing so may be difficult, they will usually report that they feel much better. Other survivors should resume their daily schedules as soon as it is practical, with no more than 2 weeks' time lapsing between the death and returning to work. The primary provider may have to deal with support people who think that the individual is going back to work too soon.

Physical Conditioning. Several studies suggest that physical exercise can help substantially in preventing or reducing clinical depression. This is particularly true in individuals who were on active exercise programs up until the time of a disease or trauma. We have frequently recommended that parents go for long walks around the Medical Center in order to get some exercise. Parents who have trouble sleeping during a child's hospitalization will often be able to cope better if they exercise and if they sleep in their own beds. The combination of exercise and a good night's sleep may also improve their appetite. Hence, the parent who exercises, eats, and sleeps well will begin to feel better.

Emotional Support for the Grieving. Most of the comments that people make to someone who is grieving are of little help and may be tasteless. Physical contact of a gentle, supporting nature is superior to anything that can be said. Holding a parent's hand without saying a word can often be more comforting than nervously babbling on. Encourage family members to express their support with physical contact—physical contact often says what we want to say but can't find the words to express.

Support Groups. Some families appreciate going to a support group and sharing their feelings with others who are in a similar situation. Other families will never attend a support group for any reason. Support groups are an individual type of experience. The provider has to know a family before making decisions about emotional support. This knowledge of a family usually comes about prior to a crisis, but if it is not available, then the provider will need to spend time with the family prior to deciding whether to refer the family to such a group.

Treatment Considerations with Children. Children usually need much less time than do adults to discuss a death: they do much better if they resume a routine as soon as possible. Rather than one or two lengthy discussions about death, children may want to discuss it briefly, and episodi-

cally, over a period of months or longer. How the child wants the format of the discussions should be respected. Naturally occurring discussion, rather than programmed marathons, will be much better received by the child and will be easier for the parent to cope with. Parents should be discouraged from lying to their children. Grandma is not asleep, nor is her state anything like sleeping. Children learn the meaning of words like "death" only by having them used in a correct and meaningful context. Death should neither be glorified nor made worse than it really is. A death should certainly not be used as a warning to a surviving sibling to improve his behavior.

Egocentricity of Children. Children may appear to act inappropriately by asking for some of the toys from a deceased sibling, but they do not understand or appreciate that their parents cannot deal with the death, much less face the task of deciding what to do with a deceased child's belongings. They may also make inappropriate remarks about a sibling, saying that they are "glad he's gone," or that they "sure won't miss him!" The parents need to decide as soon as possible if they want to tolerate such behavior. If they do not, then they will have to resume limit setting.

Discipline and Limit Setting. Families typically get very lax in their discipline and limit setting following a death in the family. The enforcement of house rules, as soon as possible after a death, will help toward restoring normality in a household. Results are often dramatic. There are few, if any, situations that warrant the suspension of usual and customary family rules.

Some parents allow their children to sleep with them after a death in the family. Typically, this practice stems from the fact that the parents do not feel like arguing with the children. However, once the parents allow this habit to be well established, it takes a good deal of effort to break it. It is usually better not to allow the bad habit to start. Some well-intentioned professionals will actually recommend that families begin bad habits (such as encouraging the children to sleep with the surviving parent), with the implication that doing so will somehow make a death easier to cope with. There is no support for such a recommendation in the literature.

No matter who is responsible for the children's caregiving during the time around a death, children need to continue with their lives. They may want to, and should be allowed to, engage in normal recreational activities. The need to do so, in children, represents a very good coping mechanism that should not be circumvented by a well-intentioned adult. A few "hot laps" around a go-cart track may do more for a child than hours of verbal discussion. Such recreational activities are also excellent therapy for the adults who accompany the children.

Obnoxious Child. Typically, a child who is obnoxious during a wake or a funeral was obnoxious before the death. The fact that his parents are preoccupied with a death exacerbates a preexisting condition. A child whose behavior was unremarkable before a death in the family and who suddenly develops a behavior problem is easy to manage. The child can be placed with a babysitter who is unrelated to the family and who is unaffected by the death. The behavior will usually show a dramatic improvement if the babysitter engages in regular activities and places limits on the child. If the child's behavior shows improvement, then the main reason for the acting-out behavior was probably that the family acted in a very different manner with him during their grieving. Because the child has the rest of his life to learn to deal with the loss, there is no hurry. Acquaintances who do not know the family well will often offer to "help in any way they can." These are excellent people to use as babysitters. They will feel as though they are doing something to help the family, and the child is removed from a setting that is obviously not beneficial to him. Just because a child knew someone before he died does not mean that the child is going to experience a profound sense of loss. If a child acts as though the death did not have a real impact, it is probably better to leave him alone than to assume that he needs to "learn to cope with his grief." The adults may be projecting their sense of loss, rather than evaluating the child's feelings correctly.

Dealing with a Child's Guilt. When parents are concerned about their child feeling guilty about a death, they need to ask themselves whether they said anything to encourage that guilt. It is not unusual for a parent to say things under stress that have an entirely different meaning to a child. The fact that thousands of families lose loved ones every day and their children continue without significant disturbances is sufficient evidence that children will ordinarily do very well in time. Most children who are verbally fluent (beyond about 4 or 5 years of age) are entitled to a brief, accurate explanation of how the family member died and to have their questions answered at that time. During this discussion, the parents (or other relative) can state specifically what caused the family member's death and that there was probably nothing more that anyone in the family could have done. If the same question (about guilt) arises continuously, it means either that the child really does feel guilty or that he is getting a lot of attention from bringing up guilt. Many parents will deny that a child would use guilt just to get attention. If the physician suspects that the behavior is meant to attract attention, it is better to mention this possibility and then drop the subject, having planted a seed that the parents will probably think about and may very well admit to later. One method for separating attention-getting behavior from honest questions about a death is to provide many opportunities for such discussions when no apparent secondary gain can be made. For example, a discussion at bedtime about a death may be used by a child as a reason to stay up later, whereas the same discussion at lunch the next day would not.

The Funeral. Most experts agree that children should attend funerals for members of their families. They should be involved in the funeral activities; however, as mentioned above, if the immediate family members are emotionally distraught, it is a good idea to identify a more distant individual to chaperone the child(ren). A child should be allowed to choose whether or not he wants to spend time with a deceased family member. Some children can carry on a perfectly lucid conversation with a deceased sibling, much to the amazement of the adults in the family.

ANNOTATED BIBLIOGRAPHY

American Psychiatric Association: Diagnostic and Statistical Manual of Mental Disorders, III-R. New York, American Psychiatric Association, 1987. (Definitive source on psychiatric diagnoses; no other source is more highly recognized.)

Beck AT, Rush AJ, Shaw BF, Emery G: Cognitive Therapy of Depression. New York, Guilford Press, 1979. (Good review of the literature on depression. Includes a depression inventory that can be administered conveniently in the office.)

Miles MS: The Grief of Parents When a Child Dies. Oak Brook, IL, Compassionate Friends, 1978. (This brief booklet, available for less than $2.00 per copy, is appropriate for distribution to parents and family members. It deals nicely with topics that will be faced by grieving parents and is short enough that parents will probably read it.)

30

Sleep Disturbances

Marc Weissbluth

Falling asleep, staying asleep at night, and napping are best considered active processes that develop when there is a harmonious synchronization between parental behaviors and the young child's developing sleep/wake rhythms. Disturbances in this process interfere with the evolution of healthy sleep patterns in the older child. Sleep patterns change as the child grows, and many sleep problems in older children originate in early-onset sleep disturbances. This chapter will therefore focus on infancy and early childhood in order to help prevent, recognize, and manage sleep disorders from the perspective of an office-based pediatrician. Child psychiatrists, psychologists, and neurologists often have different views of sleep disturbances.

PRESENTATION

The major complaint of parents whose child does not sleep well is that the child has difficulty falling asleep or staying asleep. For children under 12 to 16 weeks of age, the complaint may simply reflect parents' misperceptions. They do not appreciate the natural irregularity of sleep/wake cycles at this early age. Night sleep becomes organized after 6 weeks of age, and day sleep becomes regularized after 12 to 16 weeks. After the first few months, parents of children who do not sleep well may continue to complain of abnormal sleep schedules, frequent or prolonged awakenings at night, brief durations of night or day sleep, increased resistance to falling asleep, and an apparent failure to fall asleep except in the parent's arms or in the parent's bed; of note is the infrequent complaint of the harmful effects of sleep deprivation. They may or may not perceive that the trend of mood changes toward increasing reflex irritability, fussiness, peevishness, or crying is the direct result of disturbed sleep. Other parents will notice and complain of the increased fretfulness, excitability, and wakefulness, but they do not attribute this behavior to sleep deprivation. Such parents may incorrectly assume that both the disturbed sleep and daytime restlessness are caused by teething pain or that they have a "hyper" baby.

During the remainder of the first year of life, parents may further complain that their child cannot sleep without a pacifier, which is always dropping out, that their child rolls over away from his preferred sleeping position and cannot roll back, that their child pulls himself to standing but cannot get down by himself to sleep, or that their child awakens too early in the morning.

After the first birthday, the parents might complain that their child is climbing out of his or her crib or bed and wants to stay up to play with them or get into their bed to sleep with them. Another issue that parents often worry about after 1 year is whether the child should take only one nap instead of two. Parents of 2- to 4-year-old children often wonder if these behaviors might be related to fears of darkness, death, or abandonment, or if they might be associated with other stresses such as toilet training or the arrival of a new baby in the family.

Parents of preschool and school-age children might describe their child's disturbed sleep in terms of his or her being an "owl" or a "night" person because he or she likes to stay up late watching television, reading, or listening to music. Decreasing school performance, low self-esteem, or depression may be associated with long-standing impaired sleep quality in these older children.

DIFFERENTIAL DIAGNOSIS

The diagnosis of disturbed sleep rests on the determination of whether the child's sleep pattern is age-appropriate for the particular child. Norms are available for all age groups; however, the range of normal sleep patterns for any age is wide.

Changes of mood or performance may represent a combination of chronic fatigue and the accumulation of "nervous energy" due to the expected physiologic response to the chronic sleep loss. Thus, the adolescent might have features of depression, whereas the much younger child might have features of hyperactivity. Extreme temper tantrums or noncompliant behavior might be the sign of an overly tired toddler. "Sleep inertia" occurs upon awakening when lingering sleepiness creates a foggy, groggy, or painful sensation. Young children with disturbed sleep may suffer from severe sleep inertia, which may cause them to cry inconsolably upon awakening from their naps. Therefore, the differential diagnosis of common behavioral or emotional problems at any age should include a consideration of whether disturbed sleep is an associated feature. Often in the younger child but less so in the adolescent, a determination of which came first, the disturbed sleep or the disturbed behavior, allows the pediatrician to decide which is the primary problem and which is a complication.

Medical problems causing disturbed sleep include allergies, large adenoids or tonsils, and birth defects causing partial or complete airway obstruction during sleep. Children with these problems present with snoring, mouth breathing, sweating, or restlessness during sleep, frequent awakenings, and, in long-standing or severe cases, bed-wetting and hyperactivity.

It is important to distinguish persistent or chronic snoring from transient mouth breathing caused by a seasonal allergy or by a sequence of overlapping viral upper respiratory infections during the winter. Airway obstruction during sleep causes poor-quality sleep and results in excessive daytime sleepiness that interferes with development or academic performance. When the nocturnal breathing problem is corrected, these children sleep better and dramatically improve their mood and performance.

In many other children it is unclear whether the sleep disturbance reflects a problem within the child or represents problems between the parents. An example of a common sleep problem within the child is the postcolic baby who has learned to expect a parent's soothing attention to help him or her fall asleep. Examples of problems between parents or within the family presenting as a childhood sleep disturbance include marital discord, maternal ambivalence about breast-feeding, maternal guilt about working outside the home, life-styles that view sleep schedules as too inconvenient or artificially restrictive, and parental difficulties in allowing their baby to develop independence. For example, when there is marital discord, the nonsleeping child who clings to the mother at night provides solace to the unloved or unappreciated wife. There may be too much commotion in the family bed, thus contributing to the sleep disturbance; at the same time, this helps parents avoid issues of sexuality, intimacy, or further children. Although a parent may complain that the child is not sleeping, it may serve a useful function or reflect a long-standing problem within the family.

Thus, the three major areas to consider when a child does not sleep well are (1) innocent parental errors involving inconsistency, irregularity, or oversolicitousness, (2) a child's difficulty in breathing during sleep, and (3) family problems creating and maintaining a sleep disturbance for the child. These three types of problems may coexist. Less common medical problems should also be considered, such as severe anemia, acquired hypothyroidism causing excessive daytime sleepiness, or impaired mood and school performance associated with psychiatric or neurologic problems.

WORK-UP

It is useful to have a detailed written report that includes night sleep durations, night sleep schedule, and the frequency and duration of night wakings. The schedule and duration of naps, the time required to put a child to sleep at naps and at night, the parents' behaviors when the child does not fall asleep at naptime and bedtime, and the parents' behaviors when the child awakens at night are also important.

Inquire about snoring, mouth breathing when asleep or mouth breathing when awake, and cessation of breathing while sleeping. Parents can tape breathing sounds during sleep. Questions should also be asked about disagreements between parents regarding sleep, the parents' work schedules, child-care routines, the marriage, and time away from the children. Two issues often confuse parents: (1) distinguishing the child's need to sleep at night and day versus the child's wanting to enjoy more of his parents' company, and (2) encouraging the development of the healthy capacity to experience being alone versus thwarting independence out of fear that the child will feel abandoned. These areas should be explicitly discussed because they might not spontaneously surface. Other issues to consider are: Is one parent an insomniac searching for nighttime company? Does the mother view naps as a waste of time, depriving the child of time from being in mom-and-tot groups, or does she view nap time as restricting her social activities?

The onset of disturbed sleep often begins with naturally occurring disruptive events such as vacation trips, moves, or frequent common illnesses. Hospitalizations, severe illnesses, death of a family member, or changes in school may also be precipitating events.

The work-up for a child with suspected respiratory deficits during sleep might include endolateral radiography of the neck to determine airway patency, a formal sleep study to evaluate the quality of breathing during sleep, an allergy work-up, or a referral to an otolaryngologist.

PRINCIPLES OF MANAGEMENT

The major principle of management is to educate parents that sleep patterns are a health habit that they can encourage or discourage. Just as with other health habits such as tooth brushing and hand washing, there may be times when the child does not want to cooperate. It is hard not to give in to the demands of the child when everyone is tired. However, when the parents understand that sleeping well directly helps the child become more relaxed, calmer, more attentive, and better able to learn, then they are more motivated to establish healthy sleep habits.

Several hours may be required for counseling. If the physician or family cannot accept this time commitment, the child's sleep problem will likely continue. Counseling is time-consuming because it must address issues of parental mismanagement and parental guilt. Because crying bothers parents so much, they have to be repeatedly told, "We are letting your child learn to sleep better; we are letting him cry, but we are not making him cry in the sense of hurting him." This attitude of tough love is hard for many parents to accept. The written sleep diary may be invaluable in helping the parents cope; parents can see that, compared to the baseline, improvement has occurred. The observed improvement also helps support them in being firm without fear of creating a resentful or angry child.

The behavioral approach to helping the child sleep better should be delayed if there is a suspicion that the child has an abnormal breathing pattern during sleep. When there is a partial or complete airway obstruction during sleep, the night wakings or light sleep states represent protective arousals that prevent asphyxiation. After the airway obstruction is reversed, it is possible that long-standing unhealthy sleep patterns persist because they have become habitual or a part of the family's life-style. When the child is no longer having nocturnal respiratory problems, his or her sleep habits can be changed by reducing parental reinforcing behaviors.

INDICATIONS FOR REFERRAL

A fatigued family may readily accept only those suggestions that do not add further stresses to their frayed relationships. If it is thought that the chronicity or severity of the sleeping problem has seriously disturbed family members, or if the parents are in substantial disagreement about how the problem evolved or how to solve it, a referral should be made to an expert in pediatric sleep disorders. Alternatively, neurologists, psychologists, psychiatrists, and pediatricians who have developed skills in dealing with pediatric sleep problems may be consulted; they are usually affiliated with academic hospitals for children.

TREATMENT AND MANAGEMENT

Much has been written about young children who do not sleep well because of prenatal factors, mild obstetric problems in the newborn period, constitutional features such as low sensory threshold, colic during the first few months, and food allergies. However, the most common cause of disturbed sleep in infants and toddlers is parental mismanagement. There is unanimity in published reports that when parents change their behaviors and ignore protest crying from their child, the child's sleep habits do change. It has been amply documented, and bears restatement, that there is no psychological or emotional harm to the child when the parents do not respond at those times when the child needs to sleep.

The focus of treatment is not to impose a rigid arbitrary sleep schedule but rather to develop an orderly routine that reasonably synchronizes care-taking activities with the child's circadian sleep/wake rhythms and, most important, that ensures that the child's sleep habits meet his needs. The question that should be answered as treatment proceeds is not how many hours the child should sleep but rather if the child's behavior indicates that he or she is well rested.

When the child is between 4 and 15 months of age, parents should expect him or her to begin sleep between 7 PM and 9 PM and to awaken between 5 AM and 7 AM. Many children awaken once around midnight for a brief feeding, and they and their parents immediately return to sleep. A midmorning nap and an early afternoon nap are typically at least 1 hour. Parents usually spend about 20 minutes soothing their child to sleep at naps and at bedtimes.

If parents stop attending to all but one night waking, put the child down awake or asleep after the predetermined soothing period, and maintain this schedule, protest crying will rapidly disappear. Parents usually prefer a fade procedure whereby they gradually reduce their soothing efforts, but they often begin to observe that they are somewhat inconsistent. The inconsistency reflects the fact that their exhaustion overrides their patience in maintaining a planned withdrawal of parental attentiveness. Nevertheless, some improvement is usually observed, and many parents now have the courage to try an extinguishing procedure.

After 15 months, children usually take only one nap, but now parents may observe an increasing resistance to napping or going to bed at night. The child may soon start to climb out of the crib as he or she becomes more independent and curious.

Parents who firmly and calmly maintain healthy sleep habits and gently place the child back in the crib silently whenever he or she gets out teach the child that certain behaviors are unacceptable. Silence and an emotionless attitude help reduce the social rewards that reinforce night waking. Consistency in doing the same behaviors or rituals at sleep times and reasonable regularity when the child is tired help establish structured sleep habits. It is important to remind parents that they can establish a programmed routine regarding sleep but that they cannot force the child to sleep. Once a routine is established, however, the child will usually then sleep.

After about 2 years of age, parents should add positive reinforcing efforts to reward cooperation in maintaining a healthy sleep pattern. Rewards might include keeping the door open wider, a brighter night light, extra time playing with a parent, extra amounts of favorite foods, toys, stars on a chart, or snacks.

The exact management strategy should be tailored to each family. For all families, it is essential that parents keep a sleep log or diary before and during the treatment process. The diary should be examined to determine sleep schedules and specific parent behaviors. Parents often fail to note that intervals of wakefulness are too long, and the result is overstimulation leading to a failure to easily fall asleep or stay asleep. Thus, the diary helps improve and adjust the treatment plan to meet the specific sleep needs and the family's routines. The parents are rewarded with a better behaved, rested child.

ANNOTATED BIBLIOGRAPHY

Dinges DF, Broughton RJ: Sleep and Alertness. Chronobiological, Behavioral, and Medical Aspects of Napping. New York, Raven Press, 1989. (Discusses naps and "sleep inertia".)

Guilleminault C, Winkle R, Korobkin R, Simmons B: Children and nocturnal snoring. Evaluation of the effects of sleep related respiratory resistive load and daytime functioning. Eur J Pediatr 139: 165–171, 1982. (Respiratory deficits cause *reversible* sleep disturbances, excessive daytime sleepiness, and impaired school functioning.)

Richman N, Douglas J, Hunt H et al: Behavioral methods in the treatment of sleep disorders—a pilot study. J Child Psychol Psychiatry 26:581–590, 1985. (Parents do not cause more anxiety in their children when they give them less attention at night.)

Weissbluth M: Crybabies. New York, Berkley Books, 1989. (Second half of the book discusses fade procedures and extinguishing procedures to promote healthy sleep.)

Weissbluth M: Healthy Sleep Habits, Happy Child. New York, Fawcett Columbine, 1987. (Age-specific guidelines to prevent and correct sleep disturbances.)

Weissbluth M: Modification of sleep schedule with reduction of night waking. A case report. Sleep 5:262–266, 1982. (Presents age-specific normal data for sleep schedules.)

Weissbluth M, David AT, Poncher J: Night waking in 4 to 8 month old infants. J Pediatr 104:477–480, 1984. (Most night waking is due to postcolic sleep problems or partial airway obstruction.)

Weissbluth M, David AT, Poncher J, Reiff J: Signs of airway obstruction during sleep and behavioral, developmental, and academic problems. J Dev Behav Pediatr 4:119–124, 1983. (How sleep deficits harm the child.)

31

Common Feeding Problems in Young Children

David I. Bromberg

Few areas cause as much parental concern and consternation as those involving feeding and nutrition in infancy and childhood. Parents enter the feeding relationship with their children with a set of experiences and expectations. On the basis of these, they make decisions about nutrition and feeding practices for their families. Many parents, for example, have grown up hearing about the starving children in Europe (Asia, Africa, or Appalachia may be substituted), or they may be members of the "Clean Plate Club." These parents, therefore, feel it is important for their children to finish a serving presented to them. Similarly, parents have been presented with nutritional "truths" about the role of milk or red meat in a diet and they plan their children's diets based on these often erroneous "truths." Infants and children bring to the dinner table a set of nutritional and caloric needs as well as certain emotional and developmental requirements. These needs may be in direct conflict with parental expectations, which then results in family conflict and behavioral difficulties. The pediatrician is in an important position to educate and counsel about these differing viewpoints and to resolve many common feeding problems.

Between one quarter and two thirds of middle-class parents of 2-, 3-, and 4-year-olds have concerns over eating behaviors. These eating problems are a frequent cause of parent–child conflict. Similarly, over one third of mothers of preschool children who were interviewed expressed concerns about their children eating a limited variety of food and dawdling over their meals. Over 20% of the mothers voiced concern that their children ate too few fruits, vegetables, and meat and too many sweets.

DEVELOPMENTAL ISSUES

Three major developmental areas—(1) temperamental factors, (2) neuromaturational factors, and (3) psychosocial/emotional factors—have an impact on eating behavior and feeding problems. Infants clearly differ from one another in their ability to adjust to new situations and in the intensity with which this adjustment occurs. These factors may affect the ease of introduction of new foods and textures. Differences in biologic regularity affect the ease of meal scheduling and the ability to deviate from schedule. Once some infants start a task (e.g., eating breakfast), they stay on the task easily, whereas others are distractible and have a short attention span varying from eating to playing to crying.

New feeding behaviors often require increasing neurologic skills or the disappearance of primitive reflexes. The ability of self-feeding necessitates increasing eye–hand coordination and a *fine pincer grasp*. Until the infant develops these abilities at 9 to 12 months, he or she will be unable to feed himself. Should these milestones be delayed, the ability to self-feed will correspondingly be altered. The *extrusion reflex,* present from birth until about 4 months, causes an infant to expel solids placed in his or her mouth. This expulsion may be viewed by parents as a refusal to feed if solids and the spoon are introduced before this primitive reflex has disappeared.

Psychosocial factors also play a significant role. As the infant approaches his or her first birthday, he or she has increasing autonomy needs. This is often reflected in the infant's "need" to feed him- or herself and the desire to not allow his or her mother near him or her with a spoon. At this same time, the infant begins to develop the concept of object permanence, which is partly learned by repetitive games (e.g., peek-a-boo). The game is fun for parents when played with toys or faces, but it may become less fun when played with food thrown from the high chair. When the child is almost 2 years of age and autonomy needs increase, he or she often becomes selective in his choice of food. The child often decides at each meal what he chooses to like or reject at that time. Children develop increasing social awareness and social skills around the preschool age. Increasing chattiness at the dinner table about the day's events may result in a decreased food intake. The child's desire to use a knife and fork may cause increased frustration at mealtime.

COMMON PROBLEMS

The most frequently voiced concern about eating behavior is that children do not eat enough or that they eat too limited a variety of foods. In early infancy, nursing mothers may fear that they are not providing enough milk for their babies. They may misinterpret infant cues and misread crying after eating as hunger or lack of satisfaction with a meal. In preschoolers, aged 3 to 5, the growth velocity dramatically decreases, with a concomitant decrease in caloric needs and appetite. Parents will report that their 3-year-old does not eat enough to sustain his activity level. Parents may resort to harsh threats or ineffective cajoling in an attempt to encourage intake. The result may be tense, conflicted mealtimes with deteriorating behavior by the child.

Parents also express concern about their children's nutritional balance. This may be reported as a youngster's refusal to eat green vegetables or what a mother might consider inadequate milk intake. Many of these concerns stem from nutritional myths or misinformation. For example, parents, not recognizing the protein content of peanut butter, may have concerns about protein intake when their child eats peanut butter but little meat. Occasionally, the concerns center on a lack of variation in the diet or difficulty in getting a child to try new foods. Concerns about nutritional balance may be warranted and should be investigated by the practitioner. Serious nutritional deficiencies may result, especially when families are committed to faddish or unusual diets. (See also Chap. 15, "Vegetarianism.")

Mealtime behaviors and table manners are frequently a source of conflict in families. Typical complaints at mealtime include dawdling over meals, messiness, gulping down food, sitting with poor posture, playing with food, or an unhappy mood. Parental expectations and the family's mealtime routine play a large role in the genesis of these problems. For example, large portions and the need to finish everything on the plate may encourage dawdling and playing with food.

Spitting and vomiting are common problems in infancy and often cause parents grave concern. The spitting commonly presents as "wet burps" of 5 to 10 ml of regurgitated stomach contents shortly after a feeding. Inadequate weight gain, hematemesis or hematochezia, aspiration pneumonitis, or marked irritability with regurgitation indicates a more significant form of gastroesophageal reflux. Spitting in infancy is usually self-limited and largely disappears by 9 months. Intermittent vomiting may continue in some children throughout childhood. These children often present with a history of vomiting unaccompanied by nausea. They may vomit daily or several times a month. The vomiting does not appear to be under voluntary control. A careful history with a search for a relationship to dietary, emotional, or environmental factors should be undertaken, although frequently no relationship is found. This process, too, is self-limited, and in the presence of adequate growth, reassurance may be the only necessary intervention. (See also Chap. 102, "Gastroesophageal Reflux.")

Rumination and *cyclic vomiting* are more uncommon and represent a more serious pathology. Rumination is a voluntary self-induced vomiting usually occurring in infancy. The reverse peristaltic wave is triggered by oral movements and occasionally self-gagging. Rumination is thought to represent a self-stimulating behavior and can seriously interfere with adequate nutrition and normal growth. Serious disturbance of the mother–infant relationship is thought to exist. Treatment involves addressing the underlying social and emotional causes and using behavioral techniques to gain control of the vomiting. Cyclic vomiting is a disorder characterized by recurrent bouts of vomiting not caused by organic conditions. Each of these episodes may be sustained and can result in acute dehydration. Psychopathology is thought to play an important role, and psychiatric treatment is indicated. Colic, overeating and overweight, and failure to thrive are discussed in separate chapters.

DIFFERENTIAL DIAGNOSIS AND WORK-UP

Feeding problems are frequently uncovered during routine health screenings. Open-ended questions about mealtime and nutrition can be helpful in eliciting parental concerns. Once parents have expressed worry about feeding or nutrition, a detailed dietary and feeding history should be obtained. The pediatrician should have a clear picture of what mealtime is like. What are the typical portion sizes and what is the expectation that they will be finished? Are there frequent distractions such as television and telephone calls? How long does a typical meal last? Is the youngster required to eat the entire meal? Are there special mealtime rules, such as finishing dinner before dessert? A detailed 3-day food diary recording of what was served at each meal and how much the child ate can be helpful.

In performing a thorough physical examination, the physician should be looking for both underlying physical abnormalities and consequences of poor nutrition. In most of the feeding problems discussed, the etiology lies in difficulties in the parent–child interaction. As such, the examination of these youngsters is frequently unremarkable. However, the therapeutic implications of a normal physical examination in reassuring concerned parents cannot be overstated. A careful neurologic examination with a search for a central nervous system dysfunction is warranted in infants who experience difficulties in the transition to solid food and who demonstrate persistent or excessive extrusion reflexes past 4 months of age. In the presence of persistent vomiting, careful consideration should be given to the possibility of increased intracranial pressure, intermittent intussusception, malrotation, and volvulus. These diagnostic possibilities can usually be excluded on the basis of sustained good growth, a negative history, and a normal physical examination.

The most helpful diagnostic study in the evaluation and management of feeding problems is the meticulous use of the growth chart. Repetitive charting of height and weight over time compared to established norms is the most sensitive indicator of the significance of a feeding problem. A feeding problem exists (e.g., undereating, too many sweets, not enough vegetables, dawdling at dinner, and so forth) when it is viewed as such by parents. However, a feeding problem in the presence of a consistent weight gain and an appropriate weight for height may be managed very differently from one in which weight has substantially fallen off the curve. Educational and counseling interventions may suffice in the first situation, whereas more intensive counseling and behavioral treatments may be necessary in the latter case.

TREATMENT

When children are allowed to make their own choices regarding food, they tend to select a calorically and nutritionally balanced diet. In most families who complain of feeding problems, the children are adequately nourished and are growing well. The difficulties frequently stem from misconceptions about nutrition or family traditions that are in conflict with the developmental needs of the child. The approach to management should be reassurance and education. Reassurance should begin with a confirmation of health and nutritional status and a review of the growth record. The physician can then demonstrate the developmental level of the child and balance it against the parental expectations. A 1-year-old cannot be expected to eat in a carpeted dining room and keep all his or her food off the floor. A 4-year-old may not be able to sit civilly through a dinner involving several courses. Once this is recognized, the parent and pediatrician can develop alternative eating strategies.

When pickiness or poor intake is the concern, especially if accompanied by inadequate growth or poor nutritional balance, several behavioral interventions can improve and change the diet, such as reinforcement, portion control, and modeling techniques. Behavior modification strategies can also be helpful in improving mealtime behavior. The physician can help the parent identify desired behaviors that are positively reinforced as well as undesirable behaviors that are punished (e.g., with a time-out period). A discussion of specific mealtime routines with parents can also be useful. This discussion might include setting appropriate time limits for eating, determining appropriate portion sizes, creating a calm atmosphere, and including children in the dinner conversation.

Nutritional interventions can be helpful in alleviating feeding difficulties. Nutritionally equivalent substitutes can be found for nonpreferred foods. Preferred foods can be embellished with supplemental calories if inadequate calories are the problem. Vitamin supplements can be used when specific inadequacies are suspected. Although often requested by parents, no tonics are available to increase appetite.

INDICATIONS FOR REFERRAL

Most feeding problems are appropriately handled by the pediatrician in the primary care office. Through the use of pediatric diagnostic and counseling skills, most common problems (especially in infants and children with normal growth) can be resolved to the parent's satisfaction and the youngster's benefit. However, assistance from other professionals in developing a comprehensive management plan may occasionally be valuable. This is especially true in the presence of growth retardation or a nutritional deficiency. Dietitians can be especially helpful in assessing nutritional adequacy and in planning nutritional interventions. The pediatrician and dietitian can work together as an effective team in treating common feeding problems.

Attitudes about eating are often deeply ingrained, and even with excellent education and counseling, parents may be resistant to change. When the physician is faced with a lack of progress with a significant feeding problem or if a parent is dissatisfied with the outcome of treatment, referral to a mental health resource is indicated. Child psychiatrists, child psychologists, and feeding disorder teams (often including psychiatrists, psychologists, developmentalists, and dietitians) would all be appropriate referral sources. Psychiatric referral is also indicated for most cases of rumination and cyclic vomiting. Consultation with a gastroenterologist may be indicated when significant vomiting is a component of the problem. In selected cases, referral to a failure-to-thrive clinic would be indicated.

ANNOTATED BIBLIOGRAPHY

Birch LL et al: The variability of young children's energy intake. N Engl J Med 324:232–235, 1991. (Left to their own devices, children choose adequate diets.)

Chamberlain RW: Management of preschool behavior problems. Pediatr Clin North Am 21:33, 1974. (Overview of behavioral concerns in the preschool age group and a pediatric approach to counseling.)

Dunn J: Feeding and sleeping. In Rutter M (ed): Scientific Foundations of Developmental Psychiatry, pp 119–128. Baltimore, MD, University Park Press, 1981. (Interesting review of the biologic and psychological factors influencing feeding patterns and their relationship to the development of feeding problems.)

Eppwright ES: Eating behavior of preschool children. J Nutr Educ 1:16, 1969. (Reviews food amounts, food types, and eating behavior in preschoolers.)

Finney JW: Preventing common feeding problems in infants and young children. Pediatr Clin North Am 33:775, 1986. (Review of the behavior modification techniques available for use in the amelioration of feeding problems. Good examples of parent education material about issues of feeding and mealtime behavior are included.)

Fraiberg SH: The Magic Years, pp 72–76. New York, Charles Scribner's, 1959. (Delightful review of child development from an analytic perspective. Feeding issues are presented as they would be perceived by a toddler.)

Ilg FL, Ames LB: Child Behavior, pp 69–83. New York, Harper & Row, 1955. (Classic review of eating behavior from a developmental perspective. Discusses several specific problems and makes management recommendations.)

Satter E: The feeding relationship: Problems and interventions. J Pediatr 117:S181, 1990. (An interactional analysis of the feeding relationship between parents and infants. Offers several interventions through which the practitioner can obviate the development of long-term problems.)

32

Speech Disorders

Jonathan Schwartz

Normal children develop speech at widely varying rates. Many parents attach a great deal of importance to this milestone and may be very anxious about their child's speech development.

Because of the central role of speech in social, intellectual, and emotional development, pediatricians should be familiar with the components of speech so that they are comfortable assessing speech development, especially when a problem is suspected.

Speech disorders may result either from a problem in the acquisition or comprehension of language or from a problem in producing sounds. The presence of intact hearing is crucial to the development of normal speech.

The distinction between psychological and neurologic causes of speech disorders may be difficult to make. Several psychosocial factors may adversely affect the quantity or quality of a child's speech. In most cases, the pediatrician can narrow the differential diagnosis considerably by taking a careful history, conducting a thorough physical examination, and assessing the child's speech.

DEFINITIONS

Disorders of speech can be divided into those of sound production and those of language production. Disorders of sound production include articulation disorders (*dysarthria*), voice disorders (*dysphonia*), and fluency disorders (*dysrhythmia*). Dysarthria refers to the incorrect enunciation of distinct syllables and words; dysphonia implies a loss of voice, usually due to hoarseness; and dysrhythmias are disorders in the rhythm or fluency of speech.

Disorders of language production include both delays in the onset of speech and abnormalities in the understanding and production of formal spoken language.

CLINICAL PRESENTATION AND DIFFERENTIAL DIAGNOSIS

Disorders of Language Production

Significant *delay* in the development of speech may be caused by intellectual retardation, hearing loss, psychosocial deprivation, autism, or developmental aphasia.

Intellectual retardation is the most common cause of delayed speech acquisition. The more severe the retardation, the slower is the acquisition of communicative speech. A high proportion of intellectually retarded children also have other problems that may contribute to delayed speech development. Psychosocial deprivation and hearing loss are both more common among intellectually retarded children than they are among children of normal intelligence. Therefore, it should not be assumed that intellectual retardation is the sole cause of delayed speech development.

Hearing loss is a common cause of delayed speech acquisition. Although screening tests to detect early hearing loss have been increasingly utilized, many children who are referred to speech clinics at 3 or 4 years of age are found for the first time to have impaired hearing. Many children with retarded speech development have a history of recurrent or chronic otitis media, or a perforated eardrum. Cerumen accumulation, leading to decreased hearing acuity, is also more common in children with intellectual retardation.

Psychosocial deprivation may occur in families who place little emphasis on verbal stimulation. Typically, there is minimal verbal communication among family members. Children who grow up in such families may exhibit speech that is immature with respect to articulation, vocabulary, sentence length, and grammar, as well as a delay in the onset of speech.

Infantile autism is a rare cause of failure to develop speech. Babbling is often delayed, echolalia (repeating of the last few words said) is prolonged, and 50% of these children may not acquire communicative speech if they are left untreated. In addition to the delay in onset, the speech of an autistic child tends to be formal and is delivered in monotonous flat tones. These children also misuse pronouns—for example, using "he" or "it" instead of "I." The autistic child may occasionally appear to develop speech normally at first, only to regress before 3 years of age. The cause of autism is unknown.

Developmental aphasia has been increasingly appreciated as a cause of speech delay. There is a delay in the maturation of the central neurologic process required to produce speech. This term is generally reserved for those children who have no words by the age of 18 months or no phrases by 30 months despite normal intelligence, good emotional relationships, adequate hearing, and normal articulation skills. There is usually no difficulty in the comprehension of spoken language. A family history of late speech acquisition without sequelae is often found. Consultation with a speech pathologist should be sought when difficulty in speech comprehension (developmental receptive aphasia) is suspected or when there is no evidence of word sound acquisition by the expected age.

Disorders of Sound Production

Dysarthria should be suspected when a child's speech is difficult to understand even though the quantity and loudness are normal. Children normally may omit consonants or substitute incorrect consonants up to 5 years of age. When dysarthria persists beyond this age, the pediatrician should suspect the presence of a diagnosable cause of dysarthria. The most common causes are either neurologic abnormalities or local structural abnormalities affecting the mechanics of speech production. Neurologic abnormalities, such as upper motor neuron lesions, may be suggested by an early history of difficulty with sucking or swallowing.

The child may be observed to have abnormal muscle tone, especially of the palatal and pharyngeal muscles, and poor coordination of muscle groups used during speech. These difficulties are accentuated when the child is asked to increase the speed of his speech. Local abnormalities include cleft palate, malocclusion resulting from abnormalities of the upper or lower jaw, or an excessively large jaw. Dysarthria may also result from hearing loss.

Stuttering is a frequent concern of parents who notice that their child begins to repeat words or hesitates before starting a word. Between the ages of 2 and 4, when children are rapidly acquiring new vocabulary and grammar, a certain amount of dysrhythmia (including hesitations, repetitions, and prolongations) is normal. This dysrhythmia is symptomatically similar to stuttering. The diagnosis of stuttering should be made only if the dysrhythmia persists into the school years. Stuttering is more common in boys than girls. When a child continues to struggle with the rhythm of his speech, secondary symptoms may begin to develop, especially when negative attention is focused on his speech efforts. These symptoms, which are attempts to avoid the embarrassment of stuttering, include various facial movements, such as grimacing and blinking, and actual avoidance of situations that require the child to speak.

Dysphonia usually presents as hoarseness and affects girls more often than boys. The quality and loudness of the child's voice often fluctuate in pitch and volume from hour to hour. There is frequently a history of recurrent laryngitis, and an examination of the pharynx often reveals signs of inflamed nodules on the vocal cords.

Elective mutism is apparently the only disorder of speech with a strictly functional cause. These children usually speak freely and normally at home but do not speak at all in certain other settings, such as at school. This disorder can persist for months or years. Such children usually manifest other symptoms of poor adjustment, such as poor peer relations or overdependence on their parents. The child's developmental milestones and intelligence are usually normal. No neurologic abnormality can be identified.

WORK-UP

History

It is important to take a careful medical history, including a history of the pregnancy and prenatal course, as well as a psychosocial history. Neurologic insults, such as perinatal anoxia or pseudobulbar palsy, should be ruled out, although they rarely cause disorders of speech. Prematurity and significant illness during the neonatal period may increase the likelihood of abnormal milestones and suggest that a speech disorder is only a part of the clinical picture. A history of middle ear disease should always be noted.

The psychosocial history should include a family history, especially a history of speech development and speech disorders among family members. Stuttering is more common among family members of stutterers than it is in the general population. The child's emotional and social development should be evaluated. Children who are delayed in their speech development are usually anxious and shy in social settings, whereas an autistic child shows little emotional response. An intellectually retarded child will usually be immature in his social and emotional responses. The child who has an elective mutism may be anxious and shy or unreactive in social situations.

The child's home life and relationships with family members should be reviewed, and an evaluation should be made of the extent to which the child is stimulated and encouraged to develop speech and language skills.

Examination

First, the presence of intact bilateral hearing should be determined. The child's speech should be assessed with respect to both the timing and the normality of the speech itself. High-frequency sounds (phonemes) such as "s" or "sh" will often be distorted or omitted in the hearing-impaired child. The pediatrician will find it useful to assess three separate aspects of the child's speech—his understanding of language, his ability to articulate properly with a normal rhythm, and the production of his own language. These can usually be evaluated in the office by noting the child's responses to particular questions or commands. Table 32-1 provides a guide to normal milestones of speech acquisition.

Table 32-1.   Milestones of Speech Acquisition

AGE	SPEECH ACQUISITION
Birth–1 mo	Mainly involuntary distress responses (e.g., crying)
2–3 mo	Produces consonants; voluntary nondistress responses
7–10 mo	Reduplicated monosyllables (e.g., ma-ma); babbling
11–18 mo	Two-word combinations
36 mo	Simple sentences with subject, verb, and object

PRINCIPLES OF MANAGEMENT

The management of speech disorders is aimed at correcting any underlying anatomic defects, such as a cleft palate, or creating an environment that will promote the development of normal speech. Parents may benefit from instruction in techniques for stimulating their child's speech by certain sound or word games. Some parents should be encouraged to place their child in day programs that will provide increased stimulation for the child's speech. A professional program of speech therapy should be undertaken when a child's speech is deviant or delayed for reasons other than inadequate stimulation; in some cases, even children with inadequate stimulation should be evaluated by a speech therapist. The earlier this step is taken, the more likely it is that the child will develop normal or communicative speech. The age at which a child should be referred for evaluation depends on the clinical finding; for example, a child who has acquired no spoken language by 20 months should be referred to a speech pathologist once all the medical and surgically treatable conditions have been ruled out. "Stuttering" speech, however, is a normal finding in the preschool child, and the parents of preschool children who are dysrhythmic should be gently reassured that such errors are within the range of normal but may well become a more serious problem if the child is made to feel ashamed of his mistakes. It is best either to ignore the mistakes or to be gently encouraging.

INDICATIONS FOR REFERRAL

A child should be referred for a surgical consultation when a structural abnormality may be impairing speech. A neurologic consultation may be helpful if a neurologic cause for delayed or defective speech is suspected. Psychological testing should be requested when intellectual retardation is suspected, regardless of the patient's age. The patient should be referred for psychotherapy when elective mutism is diagnosed or when a child's speech disorder is accompanied by anxiety or depression, which may often be the case for patients who stutter. Supportive counseling may also be helpful for parents of these children, particularly when parental distress is upsetting to the child or complicates his treatment. Speech therapy should be obtained for the child whose stuttering persists into the school years.

The pediatrician should have a low threshold for referring patients with delayed or deviant speech for a specialized evaluation by a speech pathologist. Speech pathologists are best able to distinguish between normal variations in speech and problems that warrant treatment. The advantages of early intervention far outweigh the possible inconvenience of enrolling in a specialized evaluation and treatment program.

Because children with speech and language disorders are at higher risk than others for psychological problems such as anxiety and depression, the pediatrician who is following these children should evaluate the need for referral to a psychiatrist or psychologist.

ANNOTATED BIBLIOGRAPHY

Bax M, Hart H: Assessment of speech and language development in the young child. Pediatrics 66(3):350–354, 1980. (Guide to the evaluation of speech in preschool children.)

Beitchman J, Hood J: Psychiatric risk in children with speech and language disorders. J Abnorm Child Psychol 18(3):283–296, 1990. (Discussion of psychiatric sequelae in children with speech disorders.)

Eisenson J: Is Your Child's Speech Normal? Reading, MA, Addison-Wesley, 1976. (Parents' guide to understanding speech development.)

Hubatch L, Johnson C: Early language abilities of high-risk infants. J Speech Hear Disord 50:195–207, 1985. (Discussion of language delay in children with a history of prematurity and respiratory distress.)

Morley ME: Development and Disorders of Speech in Childhood. Baltimore, Williams & Wilkins, 1972. (Thorough and authoritative text.)

Rutter M, Martin EJ: The Child with Delayed Speech. Philadelphia, JB Lippincott, 1972. (Nontechnical and readable chapters on the causes, evaluation, and management of speech disorders.)

33

Enuresis

David I. Bromberg

Enuresis is a common, complex problem of childhood. The clinician treating enuresis is faced with a confusing array of etiologic considerations and an abundance of treatment possibilities. Because it is essentially a benign, self-limited disorder, there is a tendency to downplay or ignore this condition. There may, however, be significant psychosocial morbidity associated with enuresis that the primary care physician may be able to prevent.

Enuresis is usually defined as the involuntary passage of urine, more frequently than once a month, in children over the age of 5. It is *primary* if it always existed without periods of dryness, or *secondary* if a youngster was consistently dry for at least 6 months before wetting again. Enuresis is termed *nocturnal* when the wetting occurs at night (bed-wetting) and *diurnal* when wetting occurs during the day. Most enuretics are primary (70%–75%) and nocturnal.

Estimates of the prevalence of enuresis vary widely from 9% to 22% of 6-year-old males and 5% to 18% of 6-year-old females. The male-to-female ratio ranges from 1.5:1 to 2:1. Enuresis decreases with increasing age; approximately 10% to 15% of an enuretic cohort exhibit a spontaneous "cure" in a given year. By age 11, the prevalence is estimated to be between 7% and 10%, and by age 18 it is less than 3%.

The prevalence of enuresis increases with lower socioeconomic class and is higher among black youngsters, both male and female, even when controlling for socioeconomic level. Many other etiologic factors must be considered for an understanding of the clinical entity of enuresis. These can be divided into developmental, biologic, and psychological factors.

DEVELOPMENTAL FACTORS

The ability to control urinary flow involves several component tasks that are generally mastered at different ages. Between 1 and 2 years of age, children become aware of micturition. It is generally not until age 3, however, that most children can consistently postpone micturition. Children are closer to age 4 before they can voluntarily urinate on command and are often 5 to 6 years old before they can withhold urination with any degree of bladder distention.

BIOLOGIC FACTORS

Over three quarters of children whose parents both had a history of enuresis will be enuretic. The specific mode of inheritance remains elusive. Further support for biologic factors comes from the association of other biologic variables in children with enuresis. These variables include a lower mean bone age, a later sexual maturation, and a lower average height.

Children with enuresis have a reduced functional bladder capacity; as a result, they void more frequently during the day and can hold only a reduced bladder volume at night. Bladder volume appears to be functionally, but not anatomically, reduced.

Enuresis has also been conceptualized as representing a disorder of arousal from sleep or as a sleep disorder. Parents frequently describe their enuretic children as being extremely sound sleepers. Several studies, including some that used sleep polygraphy, have failed to demonstrate this relationship. Thus, the role of sleep abnormalities in enuresis remains unproved.

Recent evidence has suggested that enuretic adolescents have not developed diurnal variation in vasopressin release. In one study, normal youngsters exhibited a doubling of vasopressin release between 8:00 PM and 8:00 AM, while the enuretic group showed no similar overnight increase. The antidiuretic effects of vasopressin would normally reduce overnight urine production.

PSYCHOLOGICAL AND PSYCHOSOCIAL FACTORS

The relationship between enuresis and psychological antecedents and sequelae has received a great deal of attention and remains largely unresolved. Enuresis is not primarily a psychiatric disease. Large population studies, most notably those of Rutter on the Isle of Wight, demonstrate that although the incidence of psychiatric illness is higher in populations of enuretic children, most children with enuresis do not have a significant psychiatric disease. The prevalence of enuresis and an attendant of emotional disturbance is higher in girls than in boys; is higher in youngsters with secondary enuresis; and is higher in youngsters with diurnal enuresis. Emotional stress can precipitate secondary enuresis, and early stress factors (family disruption, separations from mother, and multiple hospitalizations) may be important in the development of primary enuresis.

Secondary psychological effects of enuresis may develop. Enuresis often engenders feelings of shame and low self-esteem in affected children. Additionally, having an enuretic child is stressful to many families.

PRESENTATION

The clinician may become aware of a patient's enuresis under several different circumstances. The complaint of enuresis may accompany several other physical or behavioral complaints, or it may be the chief complaint of a visit. Enuretic children are generally anxious about the possibility of wetting while at camp and may want to discuss their problem at a precamp physical examination. Enuresis will often be discovered during health screening at routine well-child visits.

Each of these different presentations dictates a slightly different evaluation and treatment approach. Gearing the evaluation and treatment to the degree of the family's concern and to associated findings is important. The child who presents with secondary enuresis in addition to social withdrawal and school refusal should have a thorough psychosocial and psychological evaluation. Similarly, the youngster who has secondary enuresis, polyphagia, and polydipsia should be carefully evaluated for diabetes mellitus. The

5-year-old who has primary enuresis may require only educational counseling, reassurance, and a follow-up plan.

DIFFERENTIAL DIAGNOSIS

The most important differential feature in evaluating enuresis is its primary or secondary nature. For the child with secondary enuresis, greater emphasis should be placed on evaluating recent psychosocial and emotional factors.

Most children with enuresis, both primary and secondary, have a functional problem in the absence of organic pathology. It has been estimated that only 1% to 3% of all enuretic children have organic disease. Urinary tract infection is the most common organic problem and should be considered especially in the girl with secondary enuresis. Other urinary tract abnormalities are unlikely to present as enuresis. Disorders that greatly increase urinary output may result in enuresis, and, especially in the child with secondary enuresis, consideration should be given to the diagnosis of diabetes insipidus, diabetes mellitus, and sickle cell disease. Drugs that have a diuretic effect, either as a primary action or as a side effect, may cause enuresis. Consideration should also be given to any neurologic condition that may alter the innervation to the bladder, such as meningomyelocele.

WORK-UP

History

The management of enuresis begins with a careful history obtained in a supportive fashion. The history should begin with a definition of the problem as primary or secondary and a notation of nocturnal and diurnal features. Careful documentation of the degree and frequency of wetting is essential in establishing a baseline from which to gauge the results of treatment. Frequently, the family has tried several interventions before presenting the problem to the physician. These methods should be discussed, and their effectiveness should be determined.

In view of the multifactorial etiologies of enuresis, the data base should include developmental, biologic, and psychosocial information. Any associated developmental delays should be documented. The family history will frequently reveal a close relative with a history of enuresis. This knowledge is supportive to the youngster who often feels isolated with this problem. In secondary enuresis, the recognition of recent psychosocial stresses may help the family understand the child's symptom. A history of toilet training, including the family's perception of the ease with which it was accomplished, may be useful.

In order to develop an appropriate treatment strategy, it is essential for the clinician to understand the impact of enuresis on the child and on the family. Has being enuretic kept the child from participating in peer or family activities (e.g., sleep-overs, camp experiences, or family visits)? Has extra laundry from an enuretic child been a stress on the family? Are the parents angry or frustrated with the child and the problem? Are the parents in agreement regarding their approach to wetting?

Physical Examination

The physical examination should focus on possible urinary tract abnormalities and neurologic dysfunction. Subtle neurologic differences may be associated with developmental delays. More definitive neurologic findings may suggest a pervasive neurologic problem that causes a neurogenic bladder. Abnormalities of the external genitalia may be associated with other urinary tract abnormalities. Although the physical examination will usually be entirely normal, a thorough examination is an essential part of an evaluation of enuresis and provides the necessary reassurance to the child and the family that the child appears to be anatomically and medically healthy.

Laboratory Tests

A complete urinalysis and a clean-caught urine culture are a necessary part of the evaluation. A urinary tract infection may result in enuresis and may not be suggested by either the history or physical examination. Other laboratory studies should be obtained only if indicated by the history or physical examination. There is no indication for routine radiographic studies unless the history suggests an abnormality of the urinary tract.

TREATMENT

General Considerations

Bed-wetters frequently are ashamed of their wetting and have feelings of low self-esteem and poor self-worth. Enuresis may significantly interfere with age-appropriate peer activities. Thus, treatment strategies for enuresis should have as a primary goal the prevention or alleviation of psychosocial morbidity. Optimism should be maintained because of both the spontaneous resolution in enuresis and the successful treatment interventions available. Helping a youngster get control of his bed-wetting and succeed at mastering it can provide him with an important boost in self-esteem.

In describing their enuretic youngsters, parents will often talk of the child's easy acceptance of the symptom and his nonchalance about wetting the bed. In actuality, most enuretic children are anxious to stop bed-wetting. Rather than asking children if they are sad or embarrassed about wetting, assume that they are, and then begin to educate them about the problem by teaching the multifactorial nature of enuresis. One method of informing a 7-year-old child of the prevalence of enuresis is to tell him that three or four of his classmates also wet their beds. The understanding that bed-wetting "runs in the family" and that it

represents a difference in nervous system development may also be helpful. An explanation should then follow as to why we think children wet their beds. The goal is to explain bed-wetting in a nonjudgmental way that removes blame from both the child and the parents.

Latency-aged children (6- to 12-year-olds) are confronted with the developmental challenge of being industrious (i.e., being faced with a job and accomplishing it). Overcoming bed-wetting may be presented as a challenge to the child, thereby giving him responsibility for the symptom as well as the satisfaction of mastering it once it is overcome. Parental participation is needed in most of the treatment protocols; however, the choice of whether or not to begin treatment and the responsibility for following through with the program can be the youngster's.

"Home" remedies that are often tried to control enuresis include limiting fluids after dinner time, taking the child to the bathroom when the parents go to bed ("lifting"), limiting carbonated beverages or milk in the diet, and rewarding a period of dry nights. The success rate with most of these interventions is low. If these methods are working, they need not be discouraged; however, there is little reason to promote them as a primary treatment.

Behavior Modification

Many children can consciously control their enuresis. This is evidenced by their ability to achieve a limited period of dryness in order to obtain a desired reward (e.g., bicycle, doll). In the absence of a systematic program to alter their wetting behavior, however, there is a high recidivism with this approach. Helping parents structure a standard behavior modification program may yield better results. The program should be discussed with the child before it is started and should have the desired goal of dry nights. This heightened awareness of trying to stay dry may increase the child's rate of success. Positive reinforcement of a dry bed in the morning should include social praise and perhaps a visual reinforcer (a sticker on a calender). The youngster may then be challenged to increase his run of dry nights and may be further rewarded for achieving specified goals (e.g., 4 nights of staying dry in a week). Negative reinforcement, such as social disapproval and punishment, should be avoided. The success rate with this type of system has been estimated at about 25%, although no firm figures are available. This method is particularly appropriate for the younger child (between the ages of 5 and 7) in the family who wants to try some intervention.

Urine alarms offer a more formalized behavioral intervention and yield a much higher success rate. The alarms involve an apparatus that is either worn by the child or located in the bed. When the child wets, an electrical circuit is completed and either a buzzer sounds or a bell rings. When the alarm sounds, the child goes to the bathroom and finishes urinating. He then returns to bed, changes into dry nightclothes, and resets the alarm. This method can be explained to the child and his family as an attempt to teach the child to respond to the stimulus of a full bladder. Motivation by the child and at least one parent is essential. It should be emphasized that the alarm is not a punishment for wetting. Dry nights are recorded and socially reinforced. The newer alarms (e.g., Wet-Stop from Palco Laboratories, Scotts Valley, CA) are miniaturized, more reliable, and more sensitive to small amounts of urine. Success rates of up to 70% with the newer alarms have been documented. Relapse rates range from 10% to 15%. The alarms provide an excellent intervention for the motivated youngster over the age of 7.

A third behavioral approach described as dry-bed training has been reported by Azrin and associates. This technique involves a practice phase whereby the youngster practices going to the bathroom. During the following night, intensive training occurs whereby the child is awakened every hour and is encouraged to urinate. On awakening, dryness is reinforced; wetness elicits cleanliness training, and the child changes his bed and his clothes and practices going to the bathroom. Subsequent training involves other protocols using nighttime awakening, positive reinforcement, cleanliness training, and practice sessions. The program is complex and demanding, especially in the initial phases. Success rates of up to 85% have been reported. Some of the techniques of dry-bed training (e.g., positive practice, cleanliness training) can be used in combination with urine alarms.

Bladder-Stretching Exercises

Decreased functional bladder capacity has been demonstrated in enuretic children. Based on this finding, exercises to increase bladder capacity have been recommended for the treatment of enuresis. Children are instructed to try to avoid urinating for as long as possible during the day. Their progress is monitored by recording voiding volumes on a daily basis. Normal bladder volume can be estimated in ounces as the age in years plus 2. They are encouraged to increase the average volume of their voidings. A 35% cure rate using bladder exercise techniques has been demonstrated.

Pharmacotherapy

Imipramine (Tofranil) has an antienuretic effect. The mechanism of action is unclear and has been postulated to result from an anticholinergic effect, an antidepressant effect, or an alteration in sleep cycle. In doses of 25 to 75 mg ½ to 1 hour before bedtime, 40% to 70% of enuretic children will be dry. The response to imipramine is rapid and occurs usually in the first week of treatment. The drug is usually continued for 3 months and then is gradually tapered. The remission rate is high; up to 50% of responders will again wet once the drug is discontinued. An extensive list of toxic effects of imipramine paired with a low therapeutic index in children discourages the use of this drug for treatment of enuresis.

Intranasal vasopressin analogues can be very effective in treating enuresis. Protocols begin with 20 μg of intranasal desmopressin (DDAVP), one spray in each nostril, increasing to 40 μg at bedtime. Improvement rates of up to 65% occur, but relapses on discontinuing therapy are common. Longer treatment protocols are being developed. Hypertension and heart disease are contraindications to desmopressin use. Side effects with intranasal desmopressin are rare. Cost is a major consideration, with desmopressin therapy costing up to $90 per month.

Treatment modalities should be used in combination. For an older youngster with primary nocturnal enuresis and urinary frequency, combining an enuresis alarm with bladder stretching is appropriate. Drugs may be used adjunctively as part of a treatment plan or for special occasions when dryness may be important, such as camp or a sleep-over.

INDICATIONS FOR REFERRAL

Functional enuresis should be managed by the primary care provider in an ambulatory setting. Historical or physical findings that suggest an abnormality of the urinary tract may require further diagnostic studies. A urinary tract abnormality (e.g., obstructive uropathy, reflux, or congenital abnormalities) warrants a referral to a urologist. A urology referral in the absence of strong supportive evidence of an abnormality may be harmful both in subjecting the child to possible unnecessary procedures and in suggesting the likelihood of organic problems. There is a similar danger in psychiatric referral in otherwise uncomplicated enuresis. Psychiatric referral is warranted when enuresis is accompanied by a serious secondary individual pathology or family pathology or when there are serious accompanying pathologic behaviors. The combination of symptoms of enuresis, fire-setting, and cruelty to animals is of particular concern and suggests significant psychopathology.

ANNOTATED BIBLIOGRAPHY

Azrin NH, Sneed TJ, Foxx RM: Dry-bed training: Rapid elimination of childhood enuresis. Behav Res Ther 12:147, 1974. (Complete review of the behavioral dry-bed training technique.)

Brazelton TB: Is enuresis preventable? Clin Dev Med 48/49:281, 1973. (Explores the possible connection between enuresis and toilet training.)

Gross RT, Dornbusch SM: Enuresis. In Levine MD, Carey WB, Crocker AC, Gross RT (eds): Developmental-Behavioral Pediatrics, 2nd ed. Philadelphia, WB Saunders, 1992. (Clear overview of enuresis with an in-depth look at the clinical associations of enuresis demonstrated by the National Health Examination Survey.)

Norgaard JP, Rittig S, Djurhuus JC: Nocturnal enuresis: An approach to treatment based on pathogenesis. J Pediatr 114:705, 1989. (Reviews data suggesting failure of diurnal variation in vasopressin release as an etiologic factor in enuresis; also looks at treatment with desmopressin.)

Rutter M, Yule W, Graham P: Enuresis and behavioral defiance: Some epidemiological considerations. Clin Dev Med 48/49:137, 1973. (Interesting epidemiologic analysis of data from the Isle of Wight that examines the connection between enuresis and psychopathology.)

Schmidt BD: Nocturnal enuresis: Finding the treatment that fits the child. Contemp Pediatr 7:70, 1990. (Excellent analysis of treatment options presenting a rational approach to the age-appropriate treatment of enuresis; includes parent handouts that the author uses in his practice.)

Shaffer D: The association between enuresis and emotional disorder: A review of the literature. Clin Dev Med 48/49:118, 1973. (Insightful and well-organized review of a complicated subject.)

Shaffer D: The development of bladder control. In Rutter M (ed): Scientific Foundations of Developmental Psychiatry, pp 129–137. Baltimore, University Park Press, 1981. (Careful look at the developmental issues in the etiology of enuresis; epidemiologic factors and other etiologic theories are also reviewed.)

Starfield B, Mellitis EE: Increase in functional bladder capacity and improvements in enuresis. J Pediatr 72:483, 1968. (Presents an intervention for increasing functional bladder capacity and the implications for a group of enuretic children.)

34

Encopresis

Paul K. Bruchez

Encopresis in a pediatric outpatient setting is a common problem and may be resistant to standard pediatric or mental health intervention. The incidence of all encopresis is as high as 3% of a pediatric clinic population. It requires a sensitivity both to the stigma of the symptom and to the apparent inertia toward its resolution.

Encopresis is defined as "repeated voluntary or involuntary passage of stool into places not appropriate for that purpose in the individual's own sociocultural setting." (*Diagnostic and Statistical Manual of Mental Disorders, III-R*). It is classified as primary when a child has never achieved bowel control and as secondary when a child has previously achieved regular control but has discontinued that behavior.

PSYCHOLOGICAL MECHANISMS

Encopresis has been viewed as a classic conversion symptom with the child attempting to maintain infantile pleasure of withholding and then rebelling. It often presents as a symptom of childhood stress. Studies indicate that in as many as one half of the cases, the onset of secondary encopresis is associated with beginning school, adjustment difficulties in school, separation from the mother, or birth of a sibling. School transitions (from grade to grade or from primary to secondary) and the onset of a marital separation or divorce are also frequent precedents and contributory factors. The stress-induced presentation of encopresis, when addressed early by parental education, support, and guidance, responds well and quickly. It is the family system with the more ingrained control struggle or possible covertly expressed rebellion that is more difficult to treat and requires a more prolonged and close interdisciplinary approach.

DIFFERENTIAL DIAGNOSIS

In establishing the diagnosis of functional encopresis, the following organic causes of encopresis, which may manifest as fecal soiling without retention, must be considered: diarrheal disorders causing accidental incontinence, diseases of the central nervous system, and sensory or motor deficits in the anorectal or pelvic floor muscles. The following causes of chronic retention with or without soiling should also be ruled out: Hirschsprung's disease, intestinal pseudo-obstruction syndrome, hypothyroidism, hypercalcemia, chronic codeine or phenothiazine use, disorder of the intestinal smooth muscle, and anal/rectal stenosis or fissure.

WORK-UP

The work-up must include a complete developmental and social history. A thorough physical examination including a careful inspection of the anus, a rectal examination, and a neurologic examination should be performed. A urinalysis and urine culture should be ordered for all girls because a urinary tract infection is a frequent concomitant condition in encopretic girls. When palpation cannot establish the presence of retained stool, a plain-view roentgenogram of the abdomen can detect retained stool. A rectal biopsy should be considered only if there are signs that suggest an aganglionic megacolon. Some experts recommend that a rectal biopsy not be performed unless the symptoms have not improved after long-term optimal medical management. The yield from biopsy is low even in such instances.

TREATMENT

The initial education of the family and the patient can go far to promote the resolution of encopresis. If, as is frequently the case, the encopresis is the result of chronic constipation, a complete bowel clean-out is recommended to try to return the patient's lost physical sensations and muscle tone needed for normal, routine defecation. Thus, it is important to first establish a nonimpacted colon. Levine's widely accepted regime for the initial outpatient treatment of moderate to severe stool retention recommends three to four cycles of the following: one to two Fleet enemas on the first day, Dulco-lax suppositories b.i.d. on the second day, and one Dulco-lax tablet on the third day. Mild retention may be treated by a stool softener daily for up to 14 days. If the stool retention is severe, or if the above regimen fails, hospitalization with saline enemas may be necessary to achieve initial catharsis.

Further discussion of the treatment of encopretic children may be divided into the three categories of mild, moderate, and severe encopresis. Each category has a clear presentation and a matched intervention. The importance of a nonimpacted colon before beginning any intervention must be emphasized.

Often the best treatment for encopresis is treatment at arm's length. Too often, the parent, the child-care provider, and sometimes the health care provider move too quickly as though to indicate that this is an awful problem and one for which the other party—parent, care-giver, or health care provider—has the solution. This is simply not true. It is a stance that may ultimately undercut the message we want to give: that this is the patient's body and the patient's problem. Thus, the patient will be the one to resolve it. Health professionals will play a brief but important consultative role in getting the child back firmly in control.

Most often, the encopresis is a transient reaction to either a physical event such as a dehydrating illness resulting in painfully hard stool or a developmental regression for a psychosocial reason. Simply confirming the common occurrence of such a problem and addressing the issue at arm's length without overmanagement empowers the child. It confirms the desired self-view that he or she can and should manage his or her body and that stooling will shortly get back on track. The primary alliance for the physician is with the child in this matter.

Mild Encopresis

These children can talk openly about their accidents. They can wonder about its causes and freely problem solve with their health care provider. These patients are in the best position to benefit from brief substantive intervention. Their diets should be addressed and, if necessary, improved. The child should be on a high-fiber, high-clear-fluid diet. Often this change, along with coached observation for the child to attend and respond to bodily cues of flatus, fullness, and anal pressure, is sufficient to begin the child's return to a nonencopretic pattern.

All categories of encopretic children can benefit from projected fantasy rehearsal of how they would excuse themselves from certain situations (play or school) to use the bathroom. It is often important for these children to know where they can go to use the bathroom at friends' houses, at school, and at other sites in their lives. These role-playing rehearsals can be assigned to the parents if they are agreeable and supportive. Encouraging the use of humor in this endeavor can often make it enjoyable.

Moderate Encopresis

This group of children is comprised of those patients who have enlarged, distended colons due to a long history of retaining large quantities of stool. Unlike the mild group, they profess to have lost the sensations and sensory feedback allowing them to tune in to their body. They are distinguished from the "severe" group in that these patients recognize and accept the soiling as a problem, and they are motivated to solve it.

This group requires an aggressive and thorough cleanout. It is recommended that they be put on a maintenance dose of oral laxative such as mineral oil, malt extract, or senna.

If mineral oil is chosen, multivitamins should be taken to prevent a fat-soluble vitamin deficiency. Dietary requirements of increased high-fiber foods and increased clear fluids are also important.

Severe Encopresis

The most difficult category of encopresis to treat consists of those children who have never experienced the physical sensations associated with the need to defecate and are seemingly uninterested in solving the problem.

These children are in need of establishing a clear bowel, supportive dietary habits, ongoing oral laxative maintenance, behavior management, and often conjoint psychiatric intervention. It is these children who have the poorest prognosis.

The behavioral management aspect of the intervention package is critical for the moderate and severe category patients. It can also be added to the intervention of the more slowly resolving mild encopresis patients.

Perhaps the best form of behavior management is to enlist the child and the parent to note two easily observable behaviors: bowel movements in the toilet and clean, unsoiled pants. The literature contains some elaborate systems for management that are often intensive and intrusive for both the patient and parent.

When needing to add a behavioral approach, I ask the less-involved and often less-aggravated parent (if there are two) to serve as the monitor. I give the child the task of informing the parent of the bowel movement in the toilet. One a day is sufficient for a check or a star. Clean pants are more difficult to achieve. I make this point as a way to present a challenge to the child. This establishes clean pants as an accomplishment of a higher order. The child must maintain clean pants for the entire day to receive a star. Children will sometimes hide their soiled pants. If this is the case, the pants could be numbered and checked in and out. Stars or checks should be translatable into some form of reward. While objects can be used as a reward, I find that a social or recreational event with child and family is a more potent reward; the event provides a wonderful setting and opportunity for needed verbal praise and social reinforcement.

This is added confirmation of the child's movement toward a nonencopretic pattern. A technique I have used in conjunction with this is to have the child draw a picture of the desired reward. If he or she is not able to draw the reward, I have the child and parent find a picture that can represent it. These pictures are to be cut up as a puzzle. A pre-agreed upon number of stars or checks will then earn a piece of the puzzle. When the puzzle is complete, the patient has earned the event and is often well on their way. Remind the child and family that the moderate or severe encopresis has become established over a long period of time. Therefore, it will not quickly resolve. Six to eight weeks of increasingly successful management of these categories of behavior (bowel movements in toilet and clean pants) are usually necessary to achieve initial substantial success. These patients should be maintained on mineral oil (or another stool softener) for 2 to 3 months before tapering.

It is also important to predict and expect regressions for all categories of encopretics. This ensures that no one is surprised or overly dismayed by it. Occasionally it may be necessary to go back to the old intensified interventions including oral laxatives, but only for a short period of time. The resumed normal defecation pattern will then usually be quickly reestablished. I then share with the patient and family that it has been my experience that the next nonencopretic period will be longer than the one completed.

The most common causes of treatment failure as noted by Sondheimer are: treatment of the patient with stool softeners without adequately cleaning the bowel; adequate bowel clean-out, but without follow-up maintenance of stool softeners; and poor or inadequate patient education, guidance, and follow-up.

A psychiatric interview is recommended if these interventions fail and physiologic causes have been ruled out. A developmental history with milestones should be reviewed with an emphasis on control struggles and aggressive expression (e.g., the 2-year-old's autonomy struggle, toilet training, temper tantrums, and mealtime and sleep-time behavior). Situational alterations should also be pursued. These might include, but are not limited to, parental disruption, job loss, separation, divorce, family illness, death of a close family member or friend, a family move, school changes, sibling births, and hospitalizations.

There is a strong interface between psychology and medicine in encopresis. A psychologically proactive stance by the pediatric practitioner will often combine all the elements necessary for a bimodal attack of psychology and medicine on this challenging problem.

INDICATIONS FOR REFERRAL

Psychiatric referral should be considered in children who present with a concomitant learning disability or hyperactivity; children with marked fearless, risk-taking, and disobedient behavior; and children with frequent incontinence in school. Children who have fecal incontinence without impaction or adolescent encopresis should also receive psychiatric consultation.

ANNOTATED BIBLIOGRAPHY

American Psychiatric Association: Diagnostic and Statistical Manual of Mental Disorders, III-R. Washington, DC, American Psychiatric Association, 1987. (The authoritative source of definitions.)

Bemporad JR, Kresch RA, Asnes R, Wilson A: Chronic neurotic encopresis as a paradigm of a multifactorial psychiatric disorder. J of Nervous and Mental Dis 166:472–479, 1978. (Useful review of psychological perspectives of encopresis.)

Bornstein PH, Balleweg BJ, McLellarn RW et al: The "bathroom game": A systematic program for the elimination of encopretic behavior. Behav Ther Exp Psychiatry 14(1):67–71, 1983. (Behavioral intervention using intermittent positive rewards for bowel movements in the toilet and for clean pants.)

Levine MD: Encopresis: Its potentiation, evaluation, and alleviation. Pediatr Clin North Am 29(2): 315–330, 1982. (Thorough, excellent review; comprehensive presentation of inpatient and outpatient medical management of all ranges of problems.)

Sondheimer JM: Helping the child with chronic constipation. Contemp Pediatr 12–28, March 1985. (Succinct treatment approach; strong on patient education.)

35
Attention Deficit Hyperactivity Disorder

Michael S. Jellinek

Children of various ages and temperaments have a range of behavior related to motoric activity, attentiveness, self-control, and socialization. At the extremes, children who are motorically hyperactive, inattentive, and impulsive disrupt structured settings such as a classroom and often impair their own ability to develop friendships and self-esteem. In the early part of the century, the term "organic drivenness" was applied to children with neurologic damage after encephalitis or trauma. From the 1940s through the 1960s, the diagnosis of hyperactivity broadened to include children with various difficult behaviors, especially motoric hyperactivity. Over the last 20 years, extensive research efforts to validate many child psychiatric disorders have led to a narrowing of diagnostic criteria and an emphasis on the cognitive component of these children's difficulties. Despite the many years of research and experience with the cluster of symptoms that include inattention, impulsivity, motor hyperactivity, and learning difficulties, the diagnosis remains based on somewhat imprecise clinical judgment, and the treatment is largely remedial rather than curative.

The cause of *attention deficit hyperactivity disorder (ADHD)* remains unknown. The diagnosis, as currently applied, probably includes several distinct disorders with multiple neurologic, genetic, temperamental, environmental, and behavioral factors variously contributing to the etiology of the yet-to-be-defined subgroups. There has been much speculation that sugar or food additives contribute to or even cause ADHD. Although case report data suggest that a small group of children may respond to an elimination diet, formal studies of groups of children with ADHD have shown little or no effect of limiting sugar or food additives. ADHD symptoms are infrequently caused by medical disorders but are occasionally manifested as a part of seizure disorders, postconcussion syndrome, thyrotoxicosis, and hypoglycemia. Rarely, medications (e.g., sympathomimetics), environmental factors such as lead, or an adverse reaction to phenobarbital may be contributory or etiological. Pediatricians should also consider other psychiatric disorders that may be associated with ADHD, especially learning disabilities, conduct disorder, depression, anxiety disorder, and Gilles de la Tourette's syndrome.

With use of the current criteria for ADHD, there is strong suggestive evidence of a genetic pattern for a substantial percentage of children. The pattern of inheritance is currently being elucidated and has not been differentiated from other tentatively defined genetic influences in depression, alcoholism, and conduct disorder. The male-to-female ratio for ADHD is approximately 5 to 10:1, and the estimated prevalence is approximately 3% to 5% with use of the strict diagnostic methodology.

PRESENTATION

Usually an early age of onset heralds a more severe form of the disorder. The preschool child is usually brought to the pediatrician by exhausted parents who complain that their child acts as if "driven by a motor." The parents must provide constant surveillance and cannot risk being only in "earshot"; they must be at arm's length. No toy holds the child's attention. The risk of dangerous falls is always present, and routines such as holding hands near streets is a struggle. Many of these young children are interpersonally aggressive, and this adds to the burden of babysitters or daycare providers. The constant need to supervise and limit readily takes on a negative tone and may initiate or contribute to the child's sense of low self-esteem. A shortened attention span and impulsivity will be manifested as accidental disobedience rather than intentional destructiveness. Some parents will try to adapt to the child's disorder by lowering expectations for activities that require the child to sit still (e.g., at dinner or at religious services) or by providing additional child-proofing in the home. The parents may also have a greater tolerance for the child's need for supervision, structure, and outlets for physical activity. Other parents are less accepting of a young child's ADHD and will interpret the child's behavior as inconsiderate and intentional misbehavior. These parents, because of their beliefs or because they are exhausted, may maintain unreasonable expectations and thus become trapped in cycles of repeated disappointment and punishment.

The school-aged child usually presents in kindergarten or first grade when higher expectations stress their cognitive and behavioral abilities. The child with ADHD will have a shorter attention span than his peers and will require frequent teacher intervention to keep him or her "on task." Despite the teacher's efforts, the child will withdraw from work that requires sustained attention. He or she may daydream, walk around the room, talk out of turn, engage others to join him or her in play, or (possibly in a manner similar to that used by children with conduct disorder) begin to misbehave and disrupt the class. The short attention span, impulsivity, and occasional destructive behavior will also be disturbing at home because it will prevent the family from relaxing during the "prime time" of 5:00 PM to 8:00 PM and will set up daily arguments about homework or chores. School-aged children with ADHD will also often have motor hyperactivity with fidgetiness and an intense need "to get the energy out."

Adolescent-onset ADHD in the absence of obvious neurologic insult is not a primary diagnosis. It usually represents continuing symptoms from childhood, ADHD-like symptoms secondary to a learning disability elicited by academic demands for abstract/organizational thinking, or one symptom of a primary psychiatric diagnosis (e.g., anxiety, agitated depression, mania, and so forth).

DIFFERENTIAL DIAGNOSIS

The current *Diagnostic and Statistical Manual of Mental Disorders*, published by The American Psychiatric Association, lists criteria for ADHD. The most reliable diagnosis of ADHD requires that children have symptoms present in every setting (e.g., home, school, and clinic) and usually with an earlier age of onset (preschool). The younger onset and aggressive interpersonal behavior both indicate a more virulent course and a poorer prognosis.

Attention deficit hyperactivity disorder is a clinical diagnosis based primarily on a history and secondarily on observation and psychological testing. After the rarer neurologic, physiologic, and environmental etiologies are excluded, the most valid diagnoses of ADHD depend on a consistent pattern of short attention span, impulsivity, and motor hyperactivity that is present both at home and at school. It is not unusual for the child to be able to override ADHD symptoms for short periods of time or under highly structured circumstances such as individual tutoring, although the same set of symptoms is present on other days. The age of onset can be as late as 7 years, but earlier onset is common.

Although observation in the office and a neurologic examination may be contributory factors, these procedures are insufficient to confirm or rule out the diagnosis. Many children will have ADHD-like symptoms in a physician's office or even in several settings for a short duration secondary to stress or anxiety. Neurologic "soft" signs are not pathognomonic. The diagnosis depends on meeting criteria. Clinically, the child should demonstrate the hallmarks of the disorder consistently, on a daily basis, in the major settings (home and school) of a child's life. If the child is older than 7 or is symptomatic in school, other diagnoses such as learning disability should be thoroughly considered; if the symptoms are manifest only at home, then anxiety and family discord require thorough evaluation.

The differentiation of learning disabilities and ADHD can present a complex problem. A child with an undiagnosed specific learning disability can, secondary to the frustration of not meeting classroom expectations, begin to manifest ADHD symptoms, especially fidgetiness, short attention span, and "calling out in class" impulsively. An appropriate education plan for such a child will relieve the stress, and the ADHD symptoms will ease or disappear. In addition, studies have shown that up to 80% of children with ADHD have associated learning disabilities; therefore, all children presenting with ADHD symptoms require intelligence and achievement testing. Projective psychological tests can help define the impact of the disorder on the child's defenses and self-esteem. Neuropsychological testing can help confirm the diagnosis by carefully assessing the child's cognitive style; this is also helpful for children with complex learning disabilities. Working with the school to implement an appropriate education plan is essential.

PRINCIPLES OF MANAGEMENT

Attention deficit hyperactivity disorder is a 24-hour-a-day disorder, and its management includes psychological/family issues, an educational plan, and frequently psychopharmacologic intervention. Given the complexity, chronic nature, and changing impact of the child's development, the management of ADHD requires a substantial initial time commitment and follow-up at regular intervals.

Children with ADHD are at serious risk for an ongoing sense of failure, rejection, and damaged self-esteem. The child is difficult to manage in the home and requires special planning for physical activity, increased parental presence for supervision, and daily support for academic work. Often, a conscientious effort must be made to set limits for disruptive behavior. In school, the child is constantly being reminded to pay attention, complete assignments, sit still, and stop disrupting the class. Given the likelihood of associated learning disabilities, the child may also be under major stress trying to keep up with the rest of the class, having to work especially hard to understand assignments, and being identified as "a poor student" or as "not trying" either by the teacher or because of having to leave the room for special help.

Managing any child, especially a preschooler with ADHD, is a challenge. Self-esteem is fragile, energy level is high, and judgment is often poor. Parents should be helped to decide what is reasonable to expect and to limit the number of rules to those needed for health and safety. Younger children need much time for vigorous play in safe settings. Parents often will need relief provided by tolerant baby-sitters.

The pediatrician must look at the child's entire day and carefully assess the parent's and teacher's level of expectations. Using the severity of ADHD, the key trouble points at home as identified by the history, and the insights available from the psychological testing, the pediatrician should help to establish a specific, reasonable set of expectations. The pediatrician should ascertain what the parents' expectations are regarding the time allowed for dinner, homework, music or religious lessons, the orderliness of the child's room, or how long a friend can visit. Children with ADHD will do best with increased parental structure and support that is titrated so as not to be overbearing or inhibit potential autonomy. Usually a period of "mindless" relaxation, such as sports or television, is essential after a school day, with homework organized into manageable 10- to 30-minute subunits. Rules are best divided into "squirrels and elephants," focusing on a few elephants, major rules and goals, and letting the squirrels go. Both parents should agree on the elephants so that manipulation and discord are minimized. A more detailed implementation of these guidelines requires an understanding of any associated learning disabilities, the range of variability in the child's daily performance, the child's developmental level, the parent's personality, and the family background.

Developing the child's educational plan requires careful diagnostic testing that hopefully will be part of the school's evaluation. If the local school system does not seem to have the necessary expertise, or the educational plan does not seem to be effective, then it is often helpful to get a second opinion from an experienced educational consultant or neuropsychologist who can then work with the school to set reasonable expectations for the child's academic program. With changes in teachers, courses, and the child's development, the educational plan should be reviewed on a yearly basis. If stimulant medication is part of the overall plan, it is important to discuss the reasons and minimal risks with the school administration (to assure that the medication will be given) and with the teacher (so that the child is not subtly criticized for needing drugs).

Although the use of stimulants to treat ADHD is considered the first and most successful psychopharmacologic approach, the treatment is not curative or specific. The first step in prescribing a psychotropic drug for ADHD is to clarify the target symptoms that are the goal of the treatment. Psychotropic drugs have several behavioral effects that are helpful for many children, including a decrease in motor hyperactivity, a better control of impulsivity, and an increased attention span. Therefore, for many children, the use of medication will improve daily school performance, limit disruptive behavior, and, if used in the evening, make the child more "livable" during valuable family time. A secondary benefit of medication may be an improvement in self-esteem (secondary to any decrease in criticism). There is no strong evidence that stimulant drugs improve long-term educational achievement or remedy specific learning disabilities.

Stimulants are the first line of pharmacologic treatment. Dextroamphetamine and methylphenidate have a therapeutic effect for 2 to 4 hours (a slow-release preparation of methylphenidate may last longer). For some children, the short length of action is a problem because of mood swings and reemerging misbehavior, and because up to three doses, including one in school midday, may be necessary. Thus, the dose and the decision of whether to use a slow-release form of methylphenidate must be tailored to the child. Pemoline is a longer acting stimulant but may be less effective. It has a delayed therapeutic onset of several weeks. Dosage should be titrated starting at a low dose (dextroamphetamine and methylphenidate 0.3 to 1 mg/kg/day in divided doses; pemoline 0.5 to 2 mg/kg/day as a single dose), with objective tracking of target symptoms on a weekly basis to assess for optimum therapeutic effect. Adverse effects from stimulant medication are usually mild and tolerable (e.g., decreased appetite, sleep disturbances, equivocal effect on growth). Occasionally children do not tolerate stimulants because they suffer a mood disturbance and become tearful and dysphoric, usually in the late afternoon. Reports suggest that the use of stimulants may be associated with the onset of Tourette's syndrome and thus may be contraindicated in families with a history of tics. If discontinued, stimulants such as other psychotropic drugs should be tapered to assess for behavioral change and to prevent side effects.

For some children, stimulants may not be well tolerated and the length of action may be too short. Antidepressants, especially desipramine, have been tested for the treatment of ADHD. These antidepressants seem to have the same behavioral benefits as the stimulants and require only one dose a day because of a 10- to 17-hour half-life, which also permits blood level measurement to assess for toxicity and compliance. This treatment approach, however, is not approved by the FDA and should be undertaken only within a specialized treatment center, by those expert in this area, or under a protocol. Recently, heightened concerns about cardiac toxicity have led to stricter, still-evolving guidelines on EKG monitoring.

Clonidine and multiple drug regimens have been used in the treatment of ADHD. As with antidepressants, the use of clonidine, antipsychotics, or several drug combinations should be limited to those specializing in pediatric psychopharmacology.

Even with the best efforts of interventions in the home, interventions at school, and the use of medications, the child with ADHD will have, and be aware of, his shortcomings (which will also be pointed out by peers or siblings). As the child gets older, certainly when in grade school, the pediatrician should try to develop a relationship with the child and include the child's perspective in assessing the efficacy of the treatment plan. Most children with ADHD will identify what is useful. For example, despite their inclination not to take medication, they will readily affirm the need for stimulants if they are helpful. In addition, it is essential to find areas of special interest (e.g., sports, mechanical ability, hobbies) that the child can gradually develop into real areas of skill that will foster self-esteem or become positive shared experiences with parents or peers.

INDICATIONS FOR REFERRAL

Caring for a child with ADHD requires time and expertise, and some pediatricians may refer the patient to a child psychiatrist, psychologist, or behaviorist for the comprehensive treatment of the child and family. If the pediatrician has the expertise and is able to devote the time necessary for interviewing, reviewing psychological test results, contacting the school, assessing the medication, and providing follow-up, then the care of the child with ADHD can be among the most interesting and gratifying aspects of pediatric practice. Some children with ADHD seem to mature out of the disorder by adolescence, others are less motorically hyperactive but still have the cognitive deficit, and a third group has persistent ADHD in adulthood. Recent follow-up studies have shown that providing comprehensive care does have a real impact on the child with ADHD. Self-esteem can be preserved, an appropriate level of educational achievement is possible, and outcome in adult life after graduating from the special demands of a school setting can be successful. In adult life, patients with persistent ADHD can find a niche that fits their cognitive ability and style.

If the pediatrician is the primary care-giver, referral should be selective to meet special needs, or if an aspect of the treatment plan is not effective. Specific criteria for referral include help in addressing a persistent behavioral problem, family counseling, or the trial of alternative medication.

ANNOTATED BIBLIOGRAPHY

American Psychiatric Association: Diagnostic and Statistical Manual of Mental Disorders, 3rd ed. Washington, DC, American Psychiatric Association, 1980. (Official diagnostic manual that sets criteria for all psychiatric disorders for adults and children; supporting sections give current perspectives on diagnostic methodology.)

Barkley R: Attention Deficit Hyperactivity Disorder: A Handbook for Diagnosis and Treatment. New York, Guilford Press, 1990. (Up-to-date comprehensive overview of ADHD.)

Biederman J, Jellinek M: Psychopharmacology in children. N Engl J Med 310:968–972, 1984. (Well-referenced review of psychiatric medications in children; covers the practical use of stimulants and antidepressants in the treatment of children with ADHD.)

Biederman J, Steingard R: Psychopharmacology of Children and Adolescents: A Primer for the Clinician. Washington, DC, World

Health Organization, 1989. (State-of-the-art brief review of pediatric psychopharmacology.)

Silver L: The relationship between learning disabilities, hyperactivity, distractibility, and behavioral problems. J Am Acad Child Psychiatry 20:385–390, 1981. (Excellent study demonstrating the frequency of learning disabilities in children with ADHD.)

Taylor E: Syndromes of overactivity and attention deficit. In Rutter M, Hersov L (eds): Child and Adolescent Psychiatry, Modern Approaches, 2nd ed, pp 424–441. London, Blackwell Scientific Publications, 1985. (Outstanding review of ADHD emphasizing a sophisticated, critical review of the literature; helpful start for an in-depth review of any aspect of ADHD, with an extensive bibliography.)

Weiss G, Hechtman L: Hyperactive Children Grown Up: Empirical Findings and Theoretical Considerations. New York, Guilford Press, 1986. (Thoughtful review of what is known about the long-term outcome of children with ADHD.)

36

Depression and Suicide

Richard M. Sarles and Mohammad Haerian

Depression during the childhood and adolescent years is not uncommon and represents between 10% and 20% of patients seen in child psychiatric outpatient settings. In "normal" school samples, approximately 1.5% to 4% of children and adolescents meet the diagnostic criteria for depression.

Depression may be defined broadly as a condition in which painful feelings of loss are accompanied by a lowered sense of self-esteem, with feelings of helplessness and hopelessness and a sense that the world has lost its meaning. Depression must be differentiated from sadness, which is a normal human emotion. With sadness, the painful feelings of hopelessness, helplessness, and worthlessness are absent. Depression may also be defined from a biologic perspective as a genetically vulnerable central nervous system that is depleted of biogenic amines (serotonin and norepinephrine).

The *Diagnostic and Statistical Manual,* 3rd edition (DSM-III), published by the American Psychiatric Association, defines depression as a dysphoric or irritable mood or pervasive loss of interest or pleasure accompanied by at least four of the following symptoms: change of appetite, difficulty in sleeping, psychomotor agitation or retardation, loss of interest in usual activities, loss of energy, feelings of self-reproach or guilt, complaints or evidence of diminished ability to concentrate, and recurrent thoughts of death or suicide. Associated features, such as separation anxiety and fears in the prepubertal age group, and restlessness, sulkiness, withdrawal from social activities, reluctance to cooperate with family activities, lack of attention to schoolwork, and lack of attention to personal appearance in the adolescent age group, are also listed.

A sustained feeling of sadness and dysphoria is an essential part of adult depression, but because young children are usually so exuberant and playful, they may not appear depressed for a long period of time. For example, they often can be cheered up by the interviewer, playmates, or joyful events. In young children, therefore, any change in mood or a serious mood may be regarded as a symptom of depression.

The concept of "masked" depression popular in the 1970s listed symptoms such as the following: an increase in psychosomatic complaints that are unsubstantiated by a careful physical examination and laboratory data (e.g., recurrent headaches or recurrent abdominal pain); reversal of affect in which the child or adolescent takes an uncharacteristic, foolish, provocative, or clowning behavior; a sense of feeling rejected by peers, teachers, or family; low frustration tolerance; self-punitive behaviors; aggression; a decrease in school performance and grades; listlessness; and a loss of interest in friends, hobbies, and school. Although many clinicians do not accept the concept of masked depression, children, in addition to having the core symptoms of depression (dysphoric mood and pervasive loss of interest or pleasure), present with a variety of unsubstantiated somatic complaints, agitation, irritability, decline in school performance, and other symptoms listed above. Adolescents may also manifest symptoms that may "mask" the underlying depression, such as delinquency, runaway behavior, substance abuse, and dangerous (abusive) sexual behavior (see also Chap. 44, "Rebelliousness and Out-of-Control Behavior"). Many normal adolescents may also demonstrate periods of feeling "blue" or "confused" as part of their developmental struggle. These periods, which may be considered "normal depression," may be the reaction of the adolescent to the dependence–independence struggle in which they vacillate between feeling that their independence is not being achieved fast enough and feeling that it is approaching too fast. The normal adolescent is also confronted with the struggle for self-identity and self-image in which he or she often cannot meet his or her own (and often his or her parents') goals and expectations professionally, scholastically, and sexually, which leads in many cases to "normal" feelings of depression. As the adolescent moves toward young adulthood and the adult world, he or she may experience anger toward the adult world, which is often directed at the "mess the world is in," inflation, war, famine, and pollution. Depression, anger, and guilt may also result from the values and restrictions their parents place on them. The adolescent, in the consolidation of the developmental concept of death, begins to understand the finiteness of life, which is often reinforced by the deaths of peers in automobile accidents.

The DSM-III-R recognizes several forms of depression, namely, major depression, bipolar disorder (manic depressive illness), and dysthymia. The onset of major depression may be acute, and the illness usually causes a significant change in the emotional and behavioral state of the youngster who often has good premorbid functioning. The average duration for a *major depression* is 32 weeks. Most patients recover fully within 18 months; however, 70% of these patients will have another episode of major depression within 5 years.

In contrast, a *dysthymic disorder* manifests only mild to moderate impairment, generally has an earlier age of onset than major depression, and usually demonstrates a long history of emotional problems and family discord. The average duration of a dysthymic episode is approximately 36 months, and 70% of these patients will have an episode of major depression within 5 years. The chronicity of dysthymia often significantly interferes with social and emotional growth. Thus, children suffering from dysthymia are more prone to develop lasting characterological problems.

Both major depression and dysthymic disorder have a high correlation with other childhood disorders, especially anxiety disorders and conduct disorders. This association is not fully understood. The differential diagnosis, therefore, is often complex and unclear, and it may include overlapping symptoms of attention deficit hyperactivity disorder (ADHD), anxiety disorders, and conduct disorders. Unfortunately, even child psychiatrists are hampered in the differential diagnostic work-up because of these overlapping conditions and by the lack of reliable laboratory tests for children and adolescents. For example, tests such as the EEG Sleep Study, the dexamethasone suppression test (DST), urinary methoxyhydroxyphenylglycol (MHPG), and growth hormone assay, which are often helpful in the diagnosis of adult depression, are unreliable in children and adolescents. However, certain psychological tests, including projective tests, may provide additional diagnostic help, as may the semistructured diagnostic interviews, such as the Beck's Depression Inventory (BDI) and the Depression Inventory Schedule for Children (DISC).

Mania is very rare in prepubertal children. Therefore, in the absence of mania, it is difficult to establish the diagnosis of *manic depressive illness*. The distinction between major depression and depression as a part of bipolar disorder, however, is important, because the latter has a stronger genetic basis and responds favorably to lithium. Some children presenting as ADHD may be suffering from a bipolar disorder. However, the change to the more characteristic bipolar presentation usually manifests only after puberty.

SUICIDE

Suicidal behavior in children and adolescents covers a spectrum of behaviors and may be defined broadly as thoughts and actions that, if carried out, may lead to serious self-injury or death.

The spectrum of behaviors begins with the benign, almost universal, *nonsuicidal thought about death* coinciding with the developmental understanding of death and dying as the child matures. The *wish to be dead* is also probably a normal occurrence in many children and adolescents when, on occasion, feeling so bad, upset, humiliated, or angry they wish to be dead. Suicidal ideation, however, represents a quantum leap from normal thoughts of death to the actual thinking of killing oneself. *Suicidal threats* are usually well beyond the scope of normality and usually indicate serious signs of danger that may lead to overt or covert suicidal gestures and attempts. Lastly, and most tragically, in the spectrum of behaviors is *completed suicides*.

RISK FACTORS

No single factor can dictate the appropriate treatment or predict the outcome for the suicidal patient. How, then, can the busy primary care physician identify the child or adolescent who is at risk for suicidal behavior, and how does the practitioner deal with the patient who expresses suicidal thoughts, actions, and behaviors?

Disturbed family background; parental separation, divorce, or death; and inadequate social support are suicide risk factors. In comparison with the general population, the suicidal youngster has a higher prevalence of family emotional problems (particularly alcoholism and depression) and a higher number of relatives with a history of suicide. The immediate events precipitating a suicide attempt usually include loss of a close friend or confidant and humiliating experiences with loss of self-respect.

If the primary care physician suspects signs of depression, it is important to determine if the patient experiencing suicidal thoughts is contemplating suicide, or if he has previously attempted suicide. A series of empathetic questions can often elicit important information that the patient is often eager to share in his quest for help, because the suicidal patient often feels that no one is willing to listen and no one wants to help or understand.

The physician can begin by commenting that the patient appears "blue," "down in the dumps," or depressed. The patient can be asked if they ever felt so depressed that they wished they were dead. Then the patient can be asked if he or she has ever thought of killing him- or herself. The practitioner should not be fearful of asking this question. If the child is not suicidal, such a question will not put suicidal ideas in his or her mind, and if the patient is actually feeling suicidal, this simple question may save his or her life. If the patient denies such thoughts, it is helpful to ask why the patient has not been depressed or has not thought of killing him- or herself. The answer may indicate coping skills and ego defense mechanisms providing strengths to the patient in times of stress. Should the patient admit to suicidal thoughts, it is important to ask how far the thoughts have been taken; for example, is there a plan or method and a date? It is also critical to learn if the patient has made previous attempts, in what fashion, who knew, and what response was elicited. Verbalizations by the patient such as

"Nothing matters anymore, it's too late," "I won't be a problem much longer," or "I'd be better off dead" should signal the need for mental health intervention. If the patient gives away favorite possessions, stating, "I won't need these anymore," there is considerable cause for alarm, because this may indicate a serious suicidal potential. Each of these questions and statements provides important data for the practitioner to use in determining an appropriate treatment plan and recommendation.

Thirty percent of people who have attempted suicide have made previous attempts, and the risk of a successful suicide increases with each attempt. Fifty percent of adolescents who attempt suicide abuse drugs or alcohol, 50% are "in trouble with the law," and 66% not only abuse substances but also are in legal difficulties. In addition, 30% of suicidal patients demonstrate signs of depression during the 3 months preceding the suicidal behavior.

For those patients contemplating suicide or who have attempted suicide, the method of the attempt gives some indication of the intent and lethality; therefore, the more lethal the method, the greater the risk factor. Wrist cutting, house gas, and nonprescription pills are of relatively low lethality compared to highly lethal carbon monoxide, hanging, and firearms. The patient who has a well-thought-out plan, method, date, place, clothes, and so forth, and who has the means to carry out the attempt (e.g., a gun, a noose, or a long bayonet knife, or a high building or a bridge), is at high risk for lethality. Suicide is rather rare before the age of 10. The incidence increases steadily through puberty and adolescence. Boys outnumber girls in the number of completed suicides, whereas attempted suicide is five times more common in girls. In young children who do not have access to firearms or pills, some accidents may actually be suicide attempts (e.g., running in front of a car, falling off a ledge). The clinician, therefore, must be alert when dealing with these situations.

INDICATIONS FOR REFERRAL AND TREATMENT

In general, treatment of the depressed or suicidal child or adolescent is usually beyond the expertise or interest of most pediatricians. Even those practitioners who have had significant behavioral pediatric training or elective training in child psychiatry and have a particular interest in the psychosocial aspects of pediatrics find that the time demands involved in intensive psychotherapeutic intervention preclude this type of work in a busy pediatric practice.

The pediatrician who strongly suspects a major depression, a dysthymic disorder, or suicidal behavior in a child or adolescent should present his or her honest appraisal of the situation. Appropriate recommendations for mental health consultation and intervention should be made without trying to please or appease the patient or parents; a discussion of the clinical situation should not be avoided. The physician should explain to the patient and the parents that the patient's behavior signals a marked departure from the norm. Nonargumentative firmness on the part of the physician concerning the need for consultation is essential. Although the primary care physician may acknowledge the patient's anger or dismay about needing to see a "shrink" or other mental health professional, the practitioner needs to assert his professional responsibility to render the best medical opinion, even if it is not to the liking of the patient. It may seem paradoxical, but a firm stance is reassuring to the patient because it conveys the idea that someone (the practitioner) is listening to and hearing the patient's trouble and is concerned.

The patient and the parent often question the primary care physician regarding what treatment should be offered to the depressed or suicidal patient. Should the patient be given an antidepressant? Is the preferred treatment hospitalization, family therapy, individual or group therapy, cognitive or behavioral therapy, or a combination of these treatment modalities? Is a special day school for the emotionally disturbed indicated, or is a brief or long-term intensive hospital treatment necessary? What should be the professional background of the consultant, physician, psychologist, or social worker? All of these important questions must be addressed, and the answers vary widely, depending on the nature and severity of the problem, the family support systems, financial considerations, and the availability of mental health resources within the community.

It is beyond the scope of this chapter to discuss treatment modalities. However, the referring physician should be familiar with the mental health resources that exist in his community. This knowledge should include the therapeutic approach that is used, the level of professional competency, and the fee structure. It is highly desirable for the physician to have an ongoing personal relationship and contact with a specific mental health facility or professional. The selection of, and ongoing relationship with a mental health professional are critical to optimal patient care and may represent the most important role that the primary physician can assume in caring for a child or adolescent with emotional difficulties.

ANNOTATED BIBLIOGRAPHY

Curran BE: Suicide. Pediatr Clin North Am 26(4):737–746, 1979. (Directed specifically to the practicing pediatrician; provides a good overview of the problem, with important diagnostic issues and treatment strategies.)

Kashani JH, Husain A, Shekim WO et al: Current perspectives in childhood depression: An overview. Am J Psychiatry 138(2):143–153, 1981. (Excellent overview and summary of the issues of diagnosing childhood depression; discusses the historical background leading up to current thinking.)

Pfeffer CR: Suicide Among Youth. Washington, DC, American Psychiatric Press, 1989. (Collection of ongoing empirical studies on youth suicide covering many issues, including risk factors, epidemiologic studies, role of media, and so forth.)

Poznanski E, Mokros HB, Grossman J, Freeman LN: Diagnostic criteria in childhood depression. Am J Psychiatry 142(10):1168–1173, 1985. (Good overview on the diagnostic aspects of childhood depression.)

Rutter M: Depression in Young People. New York, The Guilford Press, 1986. (Comprehensive collection of papers on the developmental and clinical aspects of depression by a very distinguished group of authors.)

Sarles RM, Friedman SB: The process of consultation and referral. In Gellert E (ed): Psychosocial Aspects of Pediatric Care, pp 145–154. New York, Grune & Stratton, 1978. (Discusses broad indications for consultation and referral and gives specific suggestions to facilitate the selection of a consultant.)

6

DEVELOPMENTAL PEDIATRICS AND SCHOOL HEALTH

37

Detection and Assessment of Developmental Disabilities

Bruce K. Shapiro

Developmental disorders are a group of disorders whose common factor is a dysfunction resulting from a "static" central nervous system (CNS) disorder that manifests in childhood and that has a chronic course with a high likelihood of functional limitations. There is no universally accepted classification of developmental disorders; most are based on the disorder's most obvious functional limitations. Classification is difficult because CNS lesions are likely to be diffuse in children (e.g., from asphyxic, genetic, or metabolic disorders) and multiple disorders may coexist. Diagnoses may also be accompanied by lesser degrees of dysfunction that do not result in additional diagnoses but are important for management. Classification is further limited by CNS maturation. Children may "grow into" disorders. For example, the neurologic substrate for a specific learning disability exists before school, but the diagnosis cannot be established until academics commence. Children may also "outgrow" disorders; however, residual dysfunction is common. Early delays in motor or language areas may not prove handicapping but may be "markers" for other dysfunctions in learning and behavior. Early diagnosis is important in order to group children with similar disorders and thereby further delineate the natural history of the disorder, identify etiologic factors, design treatment programs, and prognosticate. A clinically applicable classification is presented in Table 37-1.

PRESENTATIONS

Efforts to detect developmental disability as early as possible have been an integral part of treatment programs, schools, and legislation (e.g., Public Law 99-457—The Education of the Handicapped Act Amendments of 1986). As part of these efforts, screening of asymptomatic populations during well-child visits has been advocated. It is unclear that this action substantively improves the detection of a developmental disability. However, screening focuses attention on the development of infants and young children, and this may result in children being identified earlier.

The age at which developmental disabilities can be detected is decreasing despite a lack of routine screening. Postulated reasons for this include the better visibility of handicaps, an increased awareness on the part of pediatricians, greater availability of services, preschool experiences, and more stringent parents who are unwilling "not to worry" in the expectation that their child will "outgrow it."

Formal screening tests are limited by applicability to only certain ages or poor test qualities. Most initial screenings are done by the parent. The results of these screenings will be shared if the pediatrician inquires whether there are concerns about the baby or if he or she asks the mother to estimate how old the baby/child is acting (divide this age by the chronologic age to obtain a reliable overall rate of development).

Developmental disabilities usually present as a result of the failure of the child to meet age-related expectations. The earliest presentations are those related to a dysfunction in major organ systems (e.g., coarctation of the aorta in Turner's syndrome), physiologic anomalies (e.g., Down syndrome), or physiologic imbalance (e.g., maple syrup urine disease). Slightly later presentations are failure to establish proper feeding, periodicity, and colic. Poor interaction with care-givers or the environment may indicate vision and

Table 37-1. Classification of Developmental Disorders (Prevalence/1000)

A. Disorders primarily manifesting a motor handicap
   1. Cerebral palsy (2)
B. Disorders primarily manifesting a cognitive handicap
   1. Mental retardation 13
C. Disorders having globally normal cognition but showing specific deficits in processing
   1. Peripheral disorders of processing
      a. Deafness (1)
      b. Blindness (0.4)
   2. Central processing disorders
      a. Motor
         1. Minimal cerebral palsy
         2. Central hypotonia
         3. Apraxia
         4. Clumsy child syndrome
         5. Complex tic disorders
      b. Language
         1. Autism (0.4)
         2. Preschool communication disorders (40)
         3. Articulation disorders (?)
         4. Developmental dysphasias (?)
            a. Expressive
            b. Receptive
            c. Mixed
         5. Specific learning disability
      c. Minor perceptual dysfunction (visual motor dysfunction) (?)
      d. Behavioral
         1. Attention deficit hyperactivity disorders (ADHD; Strauss syndrome) (100)
         2. Oppositional disorders (?)
D. Seizures (10)

hearing deficits. Gross motor failures, such as an inability to sit, predominate after 9 months, with most children referred by 15 months. Although a motor dysfunction is the presenting symptom, these children commonly have additional abnormalities in thought and language. At this age, however, moderate degrees of dysfunction in nonmotor areas are usually not evident to the care-givers. However, language delay becomes the major reason for referral between 21 and 30 months. These children may also show behavioral disorders, which are usually dismissed as "terrible twos." Behavioral and preacademic areas are the major concern with 3- to 5-year-old children, and problems often result when a child is unable to match the performance of his peers in preschool. Underachievement is a major reason for evaluating young school-aged children for developmental disabilities. Behavioral dysfunction may accompany academic underachievement and may be severe enough to mask a learning dysfunction.

DIFFERENTIAL DIAGNOSES

Developmental Disability Syndromes

Cerebral Palsy. Cerebral palsy is the most common movement disorder of childhood. It is a disorder of movement or posture and results from a static lesion to the immature central nervous system. In addition to physiologic and topographical categories, cerebral palsy is also classified by other, associated neurologic defects. In cerebral palsy, the motor disability may not be the greatest handicap.

Mental Retardation. There is a significant subaverage intellectual functioning manifested during the developmental period and associated with deficits in social/adaptive function. Most retarded people are mildly affected. Behavioral dysfunction is usually the major impediment to successful adaptation.

Blindness and Deafness. These categories do not refer to total end-organ failure. Thus, the definitions for these disorders (vision less than 20/200 corrected or visual fields less than 20°, and hearing loss to a level of 100 dB) can be viewed as arbitrary. Although these disorders affect peripheral organs, the etiology may also cause a central dysfunction.

Central Processing Disorders. Central processing disorders preclude function at a level predicted by intelligence (IQ) alone. Thus, a bright child with an IQ of 125 may not learn to read. The central processing disorders form a spectrum of presentation and severity across age: autism to preschool communication disorder to developmental dysphasia to specific learning disability. Some disorders change category with time (e.g., preschool communication disorder to specific learning disability). A more precise definition of the neural mechanism of these dysfunctions awaits a better understanding of how humans learn. Most of these disorders (except the most severe) are compatible with independent life function. Aberrant behavior, however, may be more of a problem than the neurologic dysfunction. Attentional peculiarities (ranging from short attention to perseveration), hyperactivity, impulsivity, and emotional lability may be part of abnormal neurologic development and not secondary reactions to disability.

WORK-UP

If there are concerns about a child's development, an assessment should be performed. An assessment entails the quantification of the child's abilities for the purpose of a diagnosis and, if indicated, a comprehensive management (habilitation) program. A proper assessment will yield clues regarding the etiology of the child's condition, provide a diagnosis, and delineate areas of strength and weakness. An assessment of areas other than those of primary concern is required because neurologic dysfunction in children is diffuse. An incomplete assessment leads to incomplete counseling, incorrect treatment goals, unsuccessful programs, and frustration.

In developmental disorders, the history usually gives the diagnosis. A diagnosis, however, reveals little about the etiology and degree of impairment. Developmental disabilities are functional descriptors and may result from many etiologies. Thus, the history should also review family, prenatal, and perinatal histories, past medical history, and current functioning, and it should assess behavioral disturbances. Processes that result in neurodegeneration must be distinguished from static encephalopathies. Prenatal disorders may masquerade as asphyxic injury. Genetic, metabolic, and structural causes of dysfunction should be considered. Some of these disorders, such as fragile X syndrome, do not have specific symptomatology in early childhood. Toxic effects of lead, alcohol, and other common environmental exposures must also be weighed. Physical examinations should be comprehensive, with particular attention to dysmorphisms, pigmentary abnormalities, and an expanded neurologic examination. Unfortunately, the list of etiologies is long, and there is no work-up that will guarantee that all important etiologies are excluded. Therefore, no "routine" laboratory battery can be employed for developmental disorders. The yield of individual tests is low, although more

severely affected children are more likely to have an etiology determined.

An assessment is usually based on the child's "best" performance on standard tests. An alternative means of obtaining data is through parental recall of the child's developmental milestone attainment (Table 37-2). Historical milestones are not widely used for several reasons: (1) they may not be recorded accurately; (2) practitioners are not taught how to use them; and (3) their variability in the normal population obscures their consistency in delayed children. This technique depends on parental recall but requires less time and obviates the need to secure the child's cooperation. Old records and baby books may supplement poor memory.

Milestones can be grouped into four major categories: gross motor, language, fine motor/problem solving, and personal/social. *Gross motor milestones* are directed toward independent locomotion. Gross motor delay is necessary for the diagnosis of cerebral palsy, but the age of motor mile-

Table 37-2.   Usual Ages of Attainment of Developmental Milestones

1 mo	GM	Head up in prone	9 mo	GM	
	FM			FM	Object constancy
					Bangs cubes together
	LAN	Social smile (6 wks)			Rings bell for fun
2 mo	GM	Chest up in prone		LAN	Gesture games
	FM	Follows across midline			
	LAN	Coos	10 mo	LAN	Dada (discriminately)
3 mo	GM	On elbows in prone	11 mo	FM	Plucks pellet
	FM	Follows in a circle		LAN	First word (other than ma/da)
		Blinks to visual threat	12 mo	GM	Walks independently
	LAN			FM	Places pellet in bottle
		Up on wrists in prone			Voluntary release
4 mo	GM	Rolls prone to supine			Marks with a crayon
		Orients to voice (E)		LAN	Immature jargon
	LAN	Laughs out loud (4½)			Imitates squeezing a doll (E)
5 mo	GM	Rolls supine to prone		P.S.	Drinks from a cup
	FM	Transfers			Assists with dressing
		Pulls down ring	15 mo	GM	Runs
	LAN	Orients to sound (E)		FM	Dumps pellet from bottle
6 mo	GM	Sits (unsupported)		LAN	Directed pointing
	FM	Unilateral reach			4–6 words
	LAN	Babbles	18 mo	FM	Scribbles spontaneously
7 mo	GM	Comes to sit (7.5)			Uses tools
	FM	Attempts pellet			3-cube tower
	LAN			LAN	3 body parts
8 mo	GM	Crawls; pulls to stand			Parallel play
	FM	Attains pellet			Domestic imagery
		Inspects bell			7–20-word vocabulary
		Understands "no"			Mature jargon (16 mo)
	LAN	Dada (indiscriminate)		P.S.	Uses spoon
			21 mo	LAN	2-word phrases
					50-word vocabulary
					Points to pictures (E)
			24 mo	FM	3-cube train
				LAN	2-word sentences

FM = fine motor/problem solving; GM = gross motor; LAN = language; P.S. = personal/social. Gross motor and personal/social milestones are historical. Fine motor/problem solving are elicited. Language milestones are historical save where noted by examiner (E).

Table 37-3. Dissociation: An Aid to Early Diagnosis

DISORDERS	STREAMS OF DEVELOPMENT			
	Gross Motor	Language	Problem Solving	Personal/Social
Cerebral palsy	D	N	N	N to D
Mental retardation	N	D	D	D
Communication disorder	N	D	D	N to D

The table demonstrates the use of rates of development to achieve early diagnoses. N = normal, D = decreased. *Normal* and *decreased* are relative terms because developmental disabilities that occur multiply, and therefore the number of combinations is greater than that shown on the table.

stone attainment is not predictive of later cognition. *Language milestones* relate to the development of symbolic thought. They can be further subdivided into expression (that which is said), reception (that which is understood), speech (the manner in which things are said), and visual language (nonverbal communication—e.g., play). Language is the best predictor of later cognition. *Fine motor/problem solving milestones* interweave visual maturation, hand function, problem solving, and visual motor abilities. These milestones are not easily obtained by a history but do have a good relationship to cognition. They form the basis for most of the infant intelligence scales. *Personal social abilities* are the end result of problem solving, motor and language. These milestones reflect an increasing mastery of the child over his environment and relate to feeding, dressing, and hygiene. These depend on environmental factors but are associated with cognitive thresholds.

Pediatricians should record milestone attainment data at each well-child examination. Usually four or five questions need to be asked about language, motor, and personal social development. If concerns arise from the questions, then fine motor/problem solving skills can be elicited. Ascertaining milestone achievement in the various categories of development permits a rate to be assigned to each category. Rates can be calculated by dividing the expected age of achievement by the actual age of achievement. Viewing developmental rates across time allows the detection of degeneration or acceleration.

Quantification of milestone achievement can yield three types of abnormalities: delay, dissociation, and deviance. *Delay* is the most common reason for referral and indicates a significantly subaverage (usually less than 75%) rate of development. Delay is a symptom and requires further evaluation. The delay can be global or may affect only one stream of development. Infants and toddlers with delays of 25% or more in their development are eligible for early intervention services under Public Law 99-457.

Dissociation is the state that exists when one phase of development is out of synchrony with the others. Table 37-3 demonstrates the use of dissociation to achieve early diagnosis. *Deviance* refers to nonsequential development, as in the case of the child who walks without crawling, and is most commonly seen in processing disorders.

Limitations

Diagnoses are not fixed until the CNS matures. Variability of diagnosis is particularly true of children with normal or near-normal rates (greater than 65%). (A change in diagnosis is possible in children with slower rates but is less likely.) Prognostication in young infants is difficult because conclusions are based on small amounts of observed behavior. Repeated measures over time are indicated if prognosis is the goal of assessment.

Prematurity affects developmental assessment inconsistently. As a result, there can be no single formula to correct for "preemie catch-up." Correcting for most preemies (over 32 weeks' gestation) is not critical after 12 months of age because there will be little effect on clinical decisions. Children with unstable baselines (e.g., those who fail to thrive, who are oxygen dependent, and who are in compensated heart failure) may also demonstrate developmental delays. Although an assessment is important to document their current level of function and to decide if developmental interventions are required, prognostication is poor if the child is not physiologically stable.

Some children will not perform when asked. Shy children are often noncompliant. Studies have shown that excessively shy children may be unable rather than unwilling to perform. Both of these scenarios point to the value of historically derived data. Having the parent participate in the assessment may also be helpful.

Although gifted children generally attain milestones at a faster rate, developmental assessments in the first 2 years are not able to reliably detect gifted children. No harm is done to the gifted child if detection is delayed until giftedness is obvious; however, problems are likely to ensue in the child who is incorrectly identified as "gifted." Thus, an assessment for giftedness is unwarranted in the first few years.

INDICATIONS FOR REFERRAL

Children with a *motor dysfunction* require delineation of the motor deficit by a developmental pediatrician, neurologist, or motor therapist. They also require an evaluation of cognitive processes by a psychologist, with or without a speech pathologist. Audiologic, ophthalmologic, and orthopedic referrals may be required. The child with *language delay* requires an audiologic evaluation to exclude significant hearing loss and psychologic testing to rule out mental retardation. A pediatric speech pathologist may assist in defining the nature of a language disorder and developing a treatment program. Professionals trained in neurobehavioral problems can teach parents techniques for dealing with behavioral disorders. Children with *academic underachievement* require an expanded neurologic examination to assess subtle abnormalities, and an evaluation of their cognitive potential (IQ) and achievement (academic performance) is warranted if a specific learning disability is suspected. Psychiatric intervention may be indicated if secondary behavior disturbances are significantly interfering with the child's function.

TREATMENT AND MANAGEMENT

There is no cure for developmental disorders; therefore, treatment should be viewed as palliative. The broad goals of treatment are to allow the child to function to the maximum level permitted by his impairment and to prevent secondary dysfunctions (social or biologic). These goals, however, must be further refined based on the knowledge of the diagnosis and the constellation of problems with which the patient presents. Short-term objectives must be clearly defined and be consistent with long-term goals.

The pediatrician's role in management/treatment is not limited to prevention, diagnosis, evaluation, and treatment of medical conditions (including pharmacotherapy). Comprehensive management (habilitation) plans transcend traditional health issues, and interaction with educational and social agencies is frequently required. As a result, competing management goals underscore the need to prioritize these plans. The pediatrician is in an ideal position to coordinate services and act as an advocate for the patient because of his or her knowledge of the family and ability to view the "total" child.

Chronic disorders require ongoing monitoring. Treatment programs need to be reviewed to ensure that they are still relevant. Goals may need to be readjusted. Periodic reviews afford the opportunity to assess health status, family function, school performance, and behavior. New information, reflecting therapeutic advances or age-appropriate concerns, may be provided during these visits. Reviews should be undertaken by pediatricians whenever a child is not meeting expectations, or at least semiannually in infants, annually in preschoolers, and biannually in school-aged children.

Early Intervention

The early intervention is predicated on three assumptions: the condition being intervened upon can be modified by the intervention; earlier intervention is more effective than later intervention for the primary disorder; and secondary prob-

lems may be avoided. Early intervention can be categorized as an intervention designed to offset social disadvantage (e.g., Head Start), biological risk (e.g., prematurity), or developmental disability. It is in this latter group that the assumptions about early intervention are the least well proved. While the goal of achievement of normal function is unlikely in children with developmental disability, early intervention seeks to assist parental acceptance of the child and to prevent secondary disorders.

Despite the lack of a firm scientific foundation, Public Law 99-457 (The Education of the Handicapped Act Amendments of 1986) has mandated service to toddlers (3–5 year olds) who demonstrate developmental delays or who are at risk for such delays. The exact criteria for receipt of services is set by the state, but children who show a 25% delay in any of five areas of their development (cognitive, speech/language, motor, self-help, or psychosocial) or have conditions that have a high likelihood of resulting in developmental disorders are included. The provision of early intervention services under this law must include a multidisciplinary assessment and a written Individualized Family Service Plan (IFSP). The IFSP must contain: (1) a statement of the child's present level of development, (2) a statement of the family's strengths and needs related to enhancing the child's development, (3) a statement of expected outcomes for the family and child, (4) a list of the specific early intervention services required to meet the needs of the child and family, (5) the name of the case manager responsible for implementing the plan, and (6) the procedures for transition from early intervention to preschool services. Programs for infants from 0 to 2 years of age are still discretionary. It is anticipated that between 5% and 10% of children will be eligible for early intervention services under this legislation.

ANNOTATED BIBLIOGRAPHY

Accardo PJ, Capute AJ: The Pediatrician and the Developmentally Delayed Child: A Clinical Text Book on Mental Retardation. Baltimore, University Park Press, 1979. (Presents an approach to developmental disabilities and questions for language assessment [see also Clin Pediatr 17:847, 1978].)

Capute AJ, Shapiro BK, Palmer FB et al: Normal gross motor development I: The influence of race, sex and socioeconomic status. Dev Med Child Neurol 27:635–643, 1985. (Contains questions for assessment of motor development and current motor milestones.)

Drillien CM, Drummond MB: Neurodevelopmental Problems in Early Childhood. London, Blackwell, 1977. (Basic text describes a neurodevelopmental examination, specific entities, and therapies.)

Glascoe FP, Martin ED, Humphrey S: A comparative review of developmental screening tests. Pediatrics 86:547–553, 1990. (Description of 19 developmental tests for children 0–3 and/or 3–5 that sample multiple domains.)

Illingworth RS: The Development of the Infant and Young Child, 7th ed. Edinburgh, Churchill Livingstone, 1980. (Comprehensive review of development and assessment focusing on children under 5 years of age.)

Shapiro BK, Palmer FB, Wachtel RC, Capute AJ: Issues in the early identification of specific learning disability. J Dev Behav Pediatr 5:15–20, 1983. (Reviews temporal components of development.)

Thompson G, Rubin IL, Bilenker RM: Comprehensive Management of Cerebral Palsy. New York, Grune & Stratton, 1983. ("Total child" approach to cerebral palsy and its manifestations.)

White K, Casto G: An integrative review of early intervention efficacy studies with at-risk children: Implications for the handicapped. Analysis and Intervention in Developmental Disabilities 5:7–31, 1985. (Results of 162 early intervention efficacy studies with disadvantaged, at-risk, and handicapped populations.)

Wing L (ed): Early Childhood Autism: Clinical Education and Social Aspects, 2nd ed. New York, Pelham Press, 1976. (Best single source on the topic.)

38

School Readiness

Bruce K. Shapiro

Failure to develop school readiness at the appropriate time frequently portends serious academic and behavioral dysfunctions in the primary grades and has been associated with difficulties extending through adolescence into adulthood. Hyperactivity, language processing disorders, visual perceptual disorders, and other central processing disorders exist in preschool children, but school readiness has not been a major pediatric issue. Two reasons given for the traditional lack of involvement are that most children perform adequately in school and that the pediatric role in school problems is not clear. School readiness has become an area of concern because parents are more aware of deviant development: unready children can be identified, and alternatives to traditional school may be implemented earlier.

School readiness indicates that the child has the necessary psychoneurologic processes for academic learning to proceed. Psychologic abilities are developing rapidly during this period. Language abilities expand from limited communication (750 words, 3-word sentences) to nearly mature usage. Visual skills show marked maturation, particularly in visual motor areas. Abstract reasoning appears. Expectations are specific not to the individual but to a group; performance is measured against peers. The determination of school readiness uses psychoneurologic processes to predict educational progress. This approach to school readiness is based on two hypotheses: (1) deviations can be detected and (2) these processes relate to school performance. Further delineation of predictive processes and charting of their natural history in preschool children represent a major research direction.

PRESENTATIONS

Unreadiness for school may be associated with delays in motor or language areas. These delays are usually not handicapping and are modest in degree (associated with developmental rates above 75%). Delays may occur in only one aspect of development (e.g., expressive language).

Gross motor dysfunction is usually associated with abnormalities of tone. Hypotonia is most common and is reflected in clumsiness. Awkward running or reticence in engaging in motor activities may result from minimal spasticity or asymmetric tone. Preschool children who "trip over the cracks in the sidewalk" or experience multiple episodes requiring sutures may have motor dysfunction, hyperactivity, or attentional problems.

Fine motor/visual motor dysfunction may be seen in children who experience difficulty with buttoning, delayed shoe tying (over age 5 years), or poor cutting or pencil grasp. An inability to copy figures or solve puzzles may reflect a motor dysfunction or a lack of the brain's ability to interpret visual information accurately (visual motor dysfunction). In preschool children, reversing letters occasionally is not unusual, although excessive reversals should be investigated.

Language and behavior are the major areas of developmental concern in preschool children. By this time, most mild to moderate motor disorders have resolved, although central hypotonia may persist. Clumsiness is difficult to define, and other motor dysfunctions (e.g., tic disorders) present at a latter age. Visual perceptual delays may coexist with language and behavioral problems but go unnoticed unless the child has had a school experience.

Delayed language abilities are common in preschool children, with an estimated prevalence of 3%. Disorders may affect articulation (clarity of speech), expression (that which is said), or reception (understanding). Most articulatory and expressive disorders resolve, but receptive disorders are usually associated with deficits in expression and articulation. Defining articulatory disorders is best done by speech pathologists. Subtle manifestations of receptive disorders may be reflected by difficulty in following instructions or a poor memory (see Chap. 32, "Speech Disorders").

Although language disturbances are common, disordered behavior is the most common presenting symptom of school unreadiness. Behavioral disturbances may not be fully recognized in the preschooler. Disobedience, increased activity, and temper tantrums characterize this developmental period. However, as the child approaches school age, his aberrant behavior is no longer seen as prolonged terrible twos. Poor play skills, unwillingness to share or take turns, or inability to play by the rules may be seen. Other components of behavior contributing to poor peer interaction may also be present, such as emotional lability, "negativeness," impulsivity, or activity that is excessive for age. Attentional peculiarities such as a short attention span, "tuning out," or perseveration may be present but are more difficult to note in unstructured situations. These behavioral aberrations frequently lead to suboptimal responses to discipline and create major parental stress.

"Late bloomers" cause transitory concern to their parents and physicians. These are children whose development has been delayed sufficiently to raise concerns but who prove not to have handicaps (e.g., 20-month-old walkers or 30-month-old talkers). They achieve a functional level (threshold), and concern may diminish incorrectly because they have "closed the gap." In some children, if abilities are measured carefully, the gap persists. Many "late bloomers" are evidencing abnormal CNS maturation and not simply individual variation. Late bloomers commonly have difficulties in academic areas.

Perhaps the most dramatic presentation of school unreadiness is the child who is expelled from nursery school because he "isn't ready" because of "immaturity." Immaturity is not well defined but is generally applied to the child who has sufficient delay to prevent effective competition with age peers but not enough to be called "delayed." Immaturity is most commonly used to describe behavior but may be applied to other aspects of development.

DIFFERENTIAL DIAGNOSIS OF SCHOOL UNREADINESS

School readiness is not a single entity. It is a concept that is not easily measured because it is the end result of multiple processes that mature at different rates. Although many etiologies are responsible for failure to achieve school readiness, school unreadiness is usually expressed as dysfunctions in processing or intellectual limitation.

A hearing loss should also be considered among the causes of school unreadiness, although this is not common. Preschool children constitute a "high-risk" group for mild intermittent hearing loss because of the large number of children with fluid in the middle ear. Whether an intermittent hearing loss can result in lasting dysfunction in language processing is unclear. The child with a sensorineural hearing loss is less controversial. These children may have a communicatively significant hearing loss that interferes with language processing. Even minimal losses of this type should be monitored because their hearing loss may progress (see also Chap. 78).

Eye problems are usually *not* a primary cause of school unreadiness. Major visual deficits are usually detected in infancy. Although the preschool period is important for detecting preventable/treatable conditions, such conditions are not causes of, but are associated with, school unreadiness. Most of the problems with visually presented material result from a neurologic rather than an ophthalmologic dysfunction (see also Chap. 91).

In the past, mental retardation was a major cause of school unreadiness. Although mentally retarded children

are still delayed in their attainment of school readiness, they are being identified earlier and therefore infrequently present de novo. The intellectual limitation now associated with school unreadiness is usually in the borderline range (IQ equivalent 70–80).

Minimal brain dysfunctions (MBD) or processing disorders are the most common causes of school unreadiness. These disorders represent deficits in CNS function that express themselves in a more limited fashion than do the more global disorders (e.g., cerebral palsy, mental retardation). The classification of these disorders is descriptive. However, symptomatology is not specific, and it is likely that each cerebral dysfunction represents a family of disorders. Classification is further clouded by the coexistence of disorders (e.g., hyperactivity and communication disorder). Further definition of the neural mechanisms of these disorders may lead to a more useful classification (see also Chap. 35).

Social deprivation, or inadequate prior experiences, is commonly invoked as an etiology of school unreadiness; however, this is an unproven cause. In the absence of extremes, it is unclear that experience exerts a major influence on the development of school readiness. The argument (e.g., Head Start) is more compelling in those children who also border on intellectual limitation, have processing disorders, or are from socially unstable situations. However, the type and amount of experiences needed to ensure school readiness remain to be defined.

Intellectual limitation, minimal brain dysfunctions, and hearing loss may each result from many etiologies. Although usually associated with static encephalopathies arising in early life, these conditions may be acquired later (e.g., brain infection or automotive trauma) or result from progressive processes. Central nervous system degeneration, infection, ischemia, metabolic and nutritional disorders, neoplasia, physical agents and toxins, and immunologic processes have all been implicated in the failure to achieve school readiness.

WORK-UP

The basic work-up for the child whose school readiness is questioned is a comprehensive history and physical examination. Modifications of usual techniques may be necessary because of the age of the child and because the history may reflect varying views (e.g., parents and teachers, mother and father) of the child. Further evaluations and tests will depend on the clinical findings.

Although some clinicians attempt to develop a history of the present illness, this may prove difficult if there is no clear onset of the child's problem. Others find that reviewing the child's development from the earliest beginnings to the present is the most useful technique. Regardless of the approach, the clinician should be able to detail the nature of the problem, know when the parents became concerned, establish a course (worsening/improving), and delineate associated problems.

The family history should focus on the academic progress of first- and second-degree relatives. Parents should be queried about their academic attainment, grades repeated, early school performance, and whether they are recreational readers. Early school performance of siblings, uncles, aunts, and cousins should also be reviewed. Late walkers (over 18 months) and late talkers (over 30 months) should be noted, as should "late bloomers." Cerebral palsy, mental retardation, learning disorders, and early childhood deaths should be noted.

Pregnancy, birth, and neonatal histories may be of limited value, although conditions arising during this time have been related to adverse developmental outcomes. Questions should review maternal factors (e.g., age, infertility, chronic diseases), pregnancy factors (e.g., glycosuria, abnormalities of placentation), potentially toxic agents (e.g., infections, alcohol), labor and delivery complications, gestational age, birth weight, and neonatal disorders. Special attention should be paid to early feeding difficulties.

The past medical history is usually unremarkable; however, a pattern of repeated episodes of minor trauma, sutures, or ingestions occasionally emerges. The past history should also identify factors (significant illnesses or hospitalizations) that might be responsible for altering a child's developmental rate (e.g., head trauma or seizures).

A developmental history documents the child's pattern of development. Early delays are noted in the acquisition of motor, language, and self-help skills, as is the presence of deviant (nonsequential) development. Some children who lack school readiness show a pattern of plateaus and spurts. A history of a loss of skills suggests a degenerative disease.

The behavioral history attempts to detect abnormalities in the development of behavior and to assess components of current behavior. Unusual fetal activity, prolonged colic, and difficulty in establishing periodicity may be noted. Excessive or prolonged stranger and separation anxiety is not uncommon. Delays in interactive play and socialization are common. Qualitative aspects of behavior (e.g., lability, hyperactivity, and distractibility) may be difficult to quantitate because these criteria are age dependent and parents show wide variations in their judgments. Parents and teachers may have discordant views of the child that reflect the differences in home versus group behaviors.

A complete review of systems and previous evaluations is indicated to more completely delineate the scope of the problem and identify other disorders that may contribute to the lack of school readiness.

The goals of a comprehensive physical examination of the child who exhibits school unreadiness are to detect possible etiologies for the clinical picture, identify curable conditions, and assess brain function. Growth parameters (including head circumference) may indicate chronic disease, fetal alcohol syndrome, or Soto's syndrome. Mild dysmorphisms (e.g., high palate or posteriorly tipped ears) are more frequent in children with cerebral dysfunction.

An assessment of brain function includes examination of the cranial nerves, motor function, sensation, and other aspects of processing. A cranial nerve examination may reveal strabismus, facial asymmetry, or decreased tongue movements. Vision and hearing assessments are indicated. Motor assessment may show abnormality of tone, focality of findings, or difficulty in modulating movement. The sensory examination in the preschool child is visually limited to the primary modalities. Higher cortical functions such as laterality, stereognosis, extinction, and finger identification are not reliably assessed in preschool children. Processing may be addressed by various pencil and paper tasks, block constructions, and memory tasks.

The Sprigle School Readiness Screening Test (Sprigle and Lanier, 1967) and the Pediatric Examination of Educational Readiness (Meltzer LJ et al, 1981) were developed to identify children who lack school readiness. Both tests show good correlation with selected aspects of kindergarten function. However, the ability of these tests to predict school performance has not been demonstrated. Studies of the Denver Developmental Screening Test also show a relationship with school performance; however, there is disagreement over how well it predicts later school problems. None of these tests permits a diagnosis to be made, nor do they define a specific course of treatment.

INDICATIONS FOR REFERRAL

The major differential diagnoses of school unreadiness are cognitive limitation and MBD. A pediatric psychologist can provide an estimate of the child's cognitive potential and make qualitative statements about processing. Although a large number of instruments may be used, the minimum should include either the Wechsler Preschool and Primary Scale of Intelligence—Revised (WPPSI-R) or the Stanford Binet, a measure of social-adaptive behavior (e.g., Vineland), quantitation of the child's behavior, and a screening of family function. Supplemental tests are frequently used to assess language and visual processing abilities.

Although the differential diagnoses are few, the manifestations are many. Consequently, consults must be brokered carefully to prevent the "gang" approach to management. Audiologic and ophthalmologic referrals may be indicated if office screening tests were failed. Speech pathologists may help if articulation problems are significant, and they may help to further define language disorders detected by psychological testing. Psychiatrists, behavioral pediatricians, psychologists, and social workers may assist with associated behavioral problems. Motor therapists are available to try to diminish the clumsiness and improve the quality of movement.

PRINCIPLES OF MANAGEMENT

Children who fail to successfully make the transition into school are likely to experience lasting difficulty. Unfortunately, there is no method to instill readiness. Treatment is aimed primarily at the prevention of secondary problems while ensuring that the child is in a situation that will allow his potential to be achieved.

Children who lack school readiness commonly exhibit dysfunctions in several areas. A comprehensive treatment program is needed to deal with the varied manifestations of an abnormal CNS. Attempting to treat each manifestation as a separate problem fails to prioritize treatment goals and mandates that even trivial (in terms of long-range function) problems be treated. This may lead to delays in parental acceptance of the developmental dysfunction, because focusing on transitory phenomena may obscure the true nature of the deficit. Unless a comprehensive plan is instituted, parents are frequently overwhelmed by the number of "problems," confused when new problems appear (e.g., reading difficulty), and frustrated by the therapist's inability to cure their child.

Although each program must be individualized, certain general principles of treatment can be delineated: (1) Parents must have a clear understanding of the child's dysfunction. (2) They must be reassured that the child's problems are not primarily the result of inept parenting. (3) Questions of etiology, inheritability, and prognosis need to be answered. (4) Alternate strategies for dealing with the child's behavior and techniques for saying "yes" should be established. (5) The child's strengths must not be lost in his or her dysfunctions.

Children who lack school readiness may be eligible for special educational services. Public Law 99-457 (The Education of the Handicapped Act Amendments of 1986) has mandated service to toddlers (3- to 5-year-olds) who demonstrate developmental delays or who are at risk for such delays. The exact criteria for receipt of services is set by the state, but children are included if they show a 25% delay in any of five areas of their development (cognitive, speech/language, motor, self-help, or psychosocial) or have conditions that have a high likelihood of resulting in developmental disorders. While the most unready children will receive services, the majority of children with school unreadiness are not sufficiently delayed to receive services, and the legislation does not address lesser delays in multiple areas of development. The eligibility criteria and type of service are determined by the local educational agency.

The role of pharmacotherapy in preschool children is controversial. Approximately one half of preschool children who show increased levels of activity show resolution of their hyperactivity in elementary school. Children with associated deficits in language, cognition, or socialization are more likely to show persistence of preschool hyperactivity.

It should also be noted that substantial numbers of hyperactive children are not recognized in the preschool period; their hyperactivity is not clearly manifested until the child is in school. Stimulant medication may assist distractibility, attentional problems, and hyperactivity, although most parents initially prefer to try a behavioral approach. Dextroamphetamine sulfate may be used in children older than 3 years of age and is available as an elixir. Methylphenidate is not approved by the FDA for children younger than 6 years. However, Barkley showed both a decrease in maternal use of commands during a free-play situation on a low dose (0.15 mg/kg b.i.d.) of methylphenidate and significant increases in the length of time of sustained compliance with maternal commands and decreases in off-task behavior on a higher dose (0.5 mg/kg b.i.d.). Major tranquilizers may have adverse effects on learning. If used, medications should be an adjunct to a comprehensive program.

Unless the child's progress is monitored, the program is likely to fail. Parents will need to have questions answered about their child's progress. Aspects of the treatment program will need modification. For example, the diagnosis of a specific learning disability may be made. Special programming in school is likely to be needed. The latest "fad" cures will require discussion.

The management of the preschooler who lacks readiness is not the end of the process; the unready preschooler is likely to need management as a school-aged child with learning disorders. However, properly identifying and managing preschool issues is likely to make the transition into school easier.

ANNOTATED BIBLIOGRAPHY

Barkley RA. The effect of methylphenidate on the interactions of preschool ADHD children with their mothers. J Am Acad Child Adolesc Psychiatry 27:336–341, 1988. (See above text for results of this study.)

Drillien C, Drummond M: Development Screening and the Child with Special Needs. Clin Dev Med 86. Philadelphia, JB Lippincott, 1983. (Population study of over 5000 children; follows a cohort into school. Bibliography is selective, fairly current, and useful in determining the outcome of preschoolers who lack readiness.)

Meltzer LJ, Levine MD, Palfrey JS et al: Evaluation of a multidimensional assessment procedure for preschool children. J Dev Behav Pediatr 3:67–73, 1981. (Outlines development of this test.)

Shapiro BK, Palmer FB, Wachtel RC, Capute AJ: 1981 Issues in the early identification of specific learning disability. J Dev Behav Pediatr 5:15–20, 1984. (Suggests that neurologic substrate for learning disability is detectable before school age and reviews studies suggesting relationships between early development and learning problems; extensive bibliography.)

Sturner RA, Green JA, Funk SG: Preschool Denver Developmental Screening Test as a predictor of later school problems. J Pediatr 107:615–621, 1985. (Bibliography contains articles for and against the use of DDST to detect school problems.)

39

School Refusal

David Van Buskirk

When a physically healthy child fails to attend school, the primary care physician often finds the child unconcerned, the parents greatly frustrated, and the school ready to take action. The pediatrician must determine the origins and nature of the reaction in order to assess such a complicated situation. Despite varied manifestations, issues relating to separation underlie *school phobia, school withdrawal,* and *school refusal*—all of which are now termed *school refusal*—to encompass the wider range of disorders. The peak incidences occur when children leave a familiar situation to begin elementary or junior high schools.

PSYCHOLOGICAL MECHANISMS

Separation anxiety is normal in the infant and toddler. A child cries, clings, refuses to get out of the car, and may develop somatic symptoms such as a stomachache in response to the anxiety over separation. The very young child links survival to the availability of mothering, and the loss of the mother is as terrifying as the prospect of death. The first encounter of the child with the extended and regular separations demanded by nursery school or kindergarten tests how well the child mastered earlier, briefer separations.

The child who is vulnerable to separation anxiety is so overwhelmed by the stress of such separation that he or she activates an intertwined series of defense mechanisms, particularly regression, displacement, and avoidance. Being regressed, he or she functions in the psychic state of a 2-year-old, an age when feelings and thoughts have magical powers. His anger is so intense that he fears it may destroy the mother who sent him away to school. Displacement diverts the strong feelings of upset and rage from his mother to his school. This defensive step amounts to converting the school into the cause of overwhelming feelings, where the school is perceived as a hostile and dangerous place. Thus, the school is the incidental recipient of this displacement of the child's intolerable feelings. (On other occasions, the hostile or dangerous object might be a strange dog or a dark room.) No logic can dislodge such phobic conviction. Once the vulnerable child has created a phobia incorporating all the power derived from his belief that loss of the mother is tantamount to death, a most formidable pattern of avoidance has entered the life of the child, his family, and his school.

The young child who becomes school phobic has a pre-existing temperamental and presumably biological vulnerability antedating symptoms connected to school. Current symptoms may have their roots in life experiences that occurred during the second year of life, which is a crucial time for the mastery of separation and individuation. Severe stresses during that developmental period, such as the birth of a sibling, the departure of a father, a life-threatening illness, or the death of a grandparent, leave an indelible imprint on the psychological development of the toddler. Such interruptions in the flow of preschool life hinder smooth separations and reunions.

The older child who fails to attend school presents a different picture. While progressing through primary school, he or she has outgrown much of his parents' influence on his or her behavior. By puberty, the child's own control over school attendance is far greater. For preteens and high-school students, the preferred diagnostic label is now *school refusal*, to emphasize the conscious motivation of such children not to attend school. Thus, in the younger children, one presupposes a predominantly unconscious mechanism with anxiety and fear; older children demonstrate a *dislike* of school.

There are two dissimilar groups among older school refusers. One group of the older *refusers* is conduct-disordered young teenagers who may already be substance abusers or involved with the juvenile courts. Their school refusal is often referred to as truancy, because there appears to be minimal anxiety or fear related to school avoidance. In the second group, early separation anxiety disorder has persisted, and as they enter adolescence these children become more anxious, constricted, and avoidant.

Immediate Precipitating Stresses

Children who suffer early losses will be more vulnerable to regression when such trauma occurs subsequently. Because separation is so important to the syndrome of school phobia and refusal, it is not surprising that the recent loss of a parent (by disease, death, marital disruption, or geographic distance) is the most common immediate precipitant or stressor. In susceptible children, a phobic reaction may develop subsequent to any illness, even one as minor as an upper respiratory infection. Physical symptoms are usually far out of proportion to the immediate stress.

The school itself may play a central role in the development or the attenuation of the symptom of school refusal. Starting school (phobias are most common in the first months of the school year), transferring to a new school, or changing teachers raises the anxiety of a susceptible child. Occasionally the loss of an important friendship with a schoolmate after a fight or an argument may precipitate the refusal. The capacity of the school to react with support while expecting that the child will soon display age-appropriate behavior may arrest the onset of the phobic avoidance.

PRESENTATION

The initial complaint to the primary care physician is frequently of a somatic nature. The sore throat, stomachache, anorexia, or vomiting that may be symptoms of a separation anxiety disorder may distract the physician temporarily from the underlying situation. A careful history unmasks the crucial timing. For example, the stomachache occurs before breakfast and disappears when the child is back home at the end of the school day, or the headache never occurs on a weekend. It is important for the physician to reconstruct the essential family and life events behind these symptoms. It is useful to inquire about the loss of a parent by death or family disruption, about the arrival of new siblings, about illness in any family member, about a move to a new dwelling, and about a change at school.

DIFFERENTIAL DIAGNOSIS AND WORK-UP

Somatic Illnesses

Because the child who presents as phobic most frequently will have somatic complaints, laboratory tests such as complete blood counts and throat cultures are the first step both to rule out organic illness and to assist the physician in communicating the degree of his own concern to parents whose fears of organic disease are sometimes very concrete. School-initiated behavioral programs begin with the premise that the physical symptoms are emotionally induced and that sending a child to school will not neglect the treatment of the child's physical illness. Nonmedical care-givers responsible for subsequent management need reassurance (often repetitively) that there is no evidence for somatic illness.

Childhood Depression

Failure to attend school may occasionally be observed as a manifestation of a major depressive disorder, even when the more common signs of depression are not apparent. The presence of withdrawal, isolation from peers, sleep disturbances (difficulty falling asleep, awakening in the midst of sleep, as well as difficulty arising), tearfulness, vulnerability to rejection, low energy, and low self-esteem are strongly suggestive of this syndrome in children as well as in adults. In a childhood depressive reaction, persistent sad facial expressions, erratic moods with periods of great activity, and aggressive behavior may also be present.

Disruptive Disorders

Aggressive or disruptive behavior with late-onset school refusal points toward a conduct disorder diagnosis, although attention deficit hyperactivity disorder (ADHD) may be a previous or concurrent disorder. The prognosis for return to school, despite community sanctions through court intervention, is worse for this group than for those with anxiety disorders.

Psychoses

Bizarre behavior accompanied by delusions, hallucinations, thought disorders, and severe difficulty in relationships is the common presenting symptom for psychotic children. The symptom of school refusal may seem minor by comparison with the manifestations of the psychotic process.

Anxiety Disorders

As many as three fourths of school-refusing children may be classified as having anxiety disorders, particularly separation anxiety disorder. They lack the capacity to bear intense anxiety, and follow-up studies reveal that they develop more panic attacks and anxiety disorders in adulthood than do others. Whatever the combination of nature (central nervous system proclivity) and nurture (prior stresses), these children are vulnerable to stresses that involve separation.

Sexual or Physical Abuse

The avoidance of school may stem from persistent trauma at home or from abuse at school. The intimidation of the child by an abusing parent or other adult can become a way of life. Inhibition may spread to any area of the child's existence where incest, alcohol, or domestic violence might be revealed, and the child stays home to keep secrets hidden.

PRINCIPLES OF MANAGEMENT

Recent-onset school phobia is an emergency. Studies of this condition have demonstrated that the younger phobic child with recent onset of school refusal responds to immediate interventions, while any delay in intervening leads to greater resistance. In his or her first telephone contact with the parents, the pediatrician can discuss steps toward identifying possible physical illness, and he or she should support immediate school collaboration to bring about a rapid return of the child to class.

After further evaluation and familiarity with the situation, the pediatrician may suggest tolerance for symptomatic behavior. For example, permission to have pain (or perhaps to vomit) will give the child support in his or her mastery of the fear of separating. The pediatrician's message is that strong feelings as well as physical discomfort can be lived with as part of growing up. Precipitating events (e.g., a recent marital quarrel, a fight at school, or a viral illness) should not be pursued in depth until after steps have begun to correct the avoidant behavior.

Parental Involvement

The parents of a child with a school attendance problem should be involved immediately and urgently in the attempt to return the child to school. When the primary care pediatrician encounters a child who has been out of school, it is important to include both parents in helping to develop a comprehensive plan. For example, the pediatrician might suggest a shift of the responsibility for taking the phobic child to school from mother to father. It is important to support the parents' participation in whatever team approach the school may initiate. The unconscious fostering of avoidance by the anxious parent can be counterbalanced when parents join with other adults who share the objective of returning the child to school at the earliest possible time. Panic and anxiety disorders are significantly more common in the parents of school-phobic children, and consequently such parental disorders influence the course of the illness both interpersonally and genetically.

School Intervention

In many communities, public schools are sensitized to the need for rapid intervention and may rely on the pediatrician only to assess the physical state of the child. Once that assessment demonstrates no organic disease, the school system, through an integrated team including parents, teacher, school psychologist, nurse, and administrator, may develop a series of increasing expectations of attendance using a behavioral protocol. Home tutoring is usually contraindicated because it reinforces avoidance of school. An experienced school system is ready to go to court for legal support if the parents fail in their efforts to get a child back into school.

INDICATIONS FOR REFERRAL

Two weeks is an adequate trial for unassisted school-based intervention in situations where there is no immediate physical illness or emotional trauma. If progress has not occurred during that interval, the pediatrician should consider referral to a mental health specialist.

Other indications for referral relate more to the nature of the child or family than to the failure of an initial concerted effort to correct behavior. The suspicion of either childhood depression or psychosis, as well as the possibility of abuse or other substantial family issues, is reason for referral to a child psychiatrist. Comprehensive psychiatric care progresses from treating the acute phobic symptoms to dynamic therapy with the aim of lessening the impairment of emotional and cognitive development. The pediatrician has a key role in supporting the commitment of the family during the process of transition from crisis to long-term care.

Pharmacotherapy is effective for school phobia. A child psychiatrist might choose an antianxiety agent (e.g., alprazolam 1–3 mg/day) or an antidepressant (e.g., imipramine to therapeutic blood levels). The choice would be determined by the symptoms of the disorder diagnosed, the prospect of compliance, and routine blood chemical screening tests (liver, kidney, and thyroid). Cardiotoxic effects of the tricyclic antidepressants necessitate regular electrocardiograms during initiation and when doses are increased. Full therapeutic benefits may not be seen for 8 weeks.

Psychotherapy, as family or as individual behavioral or dynamic therapy, is usually indicated for phobic or school-refusing children. Working through irrational fears often requires weeks or months of play therapy; therefore, the return of a child to school cannot await a psychotherapeutic resolution. Because the phobic child may turn out to be the expressor of an overwhelming family discord, the focus of care may shift from the child's fear of school to the mother and father's troubled relationship.

The longest follow-up studies of school-refusing children with separation anxiety disorder indicate that as many as one third follow a deteriorating spiral from primary school phobia to high-school refusal to adult behavioral constriction, including agoraphobia and panic disorder. An early working through of the dynamics of separation and loss may prevent such future disability. Only 36% of the older-onset school refusers return to school, and these children also have a poor prognosis for healthy adaptation as adults.

ANNOTATED BIBLIOGRAPHY

Bernstein GA, Garfinkel BD, Borchardt DM, et al: Comparative studies of pharmacotherapy for school refusal. J Am Acad Child Adolesc Psychiatry 29(5):773, 1990. (Findings show alprazolam is more effective than imipramine, but both are superior to placebo.)

Blagg NR, Yule W: The behavioral treatment of school refusal—A comparative study. Behav Res Ther 22(2):119, 1984. (Carefully designed protocol for school refusal with rapid and successful results.)

Coolidge J, Brodier D, Feeney B: A ten-year follow-up study of sixty-six school phobic children. Am J Orthopsychiatry 34:674–684, 1964. (Group was followed through acute and long-term difficulties; study demonstrates the need for a guarded prognosis where phobia or refusal persists.)

Hersov L, Berg I (eds): Out of School. New York, John Wiley & Sons, 1980. (The most comprehensive overview of the subject with excellent chapters on several aspects; see particularly: Waller D, Eisenberg L: School refusal in childhood—A psychiatric–pediatric perspective; Lewis M: Psychotherapeutic treatment in school refusal; Gittleman-Klein R, Klein D: Separation anxiety in school refusal and its treatment with drugs [An overview of the psychopharmacologic management].)

Kolvin I, Berney TP, Bhate SR: Classification and diagnosis of depression in school phobia. Br J Psychiatry 145:347, 1984. (Older children with school phobic symptoms reveal a disproportionate number of symptoms consistent with childhood depression.)

Perugi G, Deltito J, Soriani A, et al: Relationships between panic disorder and separation anxiety with school phobia. Compr Psychiatry

29(2):98, 1988. (School-phobic children go on to panic attacks and phobic avoidance such as agoraphobia more frequently, at a younger age, and with more severe symptoms than do normals.)

Waldron S Jr, Shrier DK, Stone B, et al: School phobia and other childhood neuroses: A systematic study of the children and their families. Am J Psychiatry 132:8, 1975. (Twice as many school-phobic children compared with other neurotic children show excessive separation anxiety, dependency, and depression.)

40

Learning Disabilities

Charles N. Swisher

Learning disability represents a large area of morbidity in the pediatric population, estimated from 3% to 7% of the general population. Its presentation is multifaceted. School failure, behavioral disorders, and clumsiness are common presenting features.

The focus in this chapter is on "cognitive" learning disability as opposed to the learning disabilities resulting from attention deficit hyperactivity disorders (ADHD; see Chap. 35) and the learning disabilities resulting from global developmental delay or retardation. However, it should be clearly understood that there is a considerable overlap between these various etiologies, and the "final common pathway" of a learning disability has several possible precursors in addition to the cognitive problems discussed in this chapter.

PATHOPHYSIOLOGY

From the neurologic perspective, the most concrete data have come from the work of Geschwind and Galaburda (Duffy and Geschwind, 1985). "Disconnection syndromes" in the brain have been demonstrated in adults following stroke, and "disconnections" in the form of heterotopias have been found in the brains of learning-disabled individuals following accidental death. This neuropathologically demonstrated anatomic variability may relate to the behavioral characteristics delineated by the neuropsychologist, including such specific areas of difficulty as attention, memory, reasoning, communication, reading, writing, spelling, calculation, social competence, and emotional maturation. Learning disabilities are not due primarily to visual, hearing, or motor handicaps, mental retardation, emotional disturbance, or environmental disadvantage, although they may occur concurrently. A strong familial pattern has been noted in the expression of learning disability, and, as with infantile autism and ADHD, males are predominantly affected. However, it is obvious that environmental factors

have a considerable influence on the phenotypic expression of various learning disabilities, and parental attitudes and behaviors as well as parental genes influence the success or failure of a child with learning disabilities.

CLINICAL PRESENTATION

Recognition of the child with a cognitive learning disability, in contrast to the child with ADHD, occurs when the parent or educator assesses skills at the preschool or early school level. Approximately one third of children with cognitive learning disabilities have motor problems characterized by clumsiness, left–right confusion, and eye–hand coordination difficulties, so they may be slightly delayed in walking and may develop expected motor skills (such as throwing or catching a ball or riding a bicycle) poorly or late. They are frequently the last chosen in intramural athletics, and their problems with motor performance add to the low self-esteem they develop quickly when confronted with their learning problems in the school setting.

In view of the paucity of data on the intrinsic nature of learning disabilities, various classifications are available. Perhaps the most widely used, if not the most sophisticated from an etiologic standpoint, is the current classification in the *Diagnostic and Statistical Manual of Mental Disorders* (DSM-III):

1. Attention deficit hyperactivity disorder
2. Developmental reading disorder
3. Developmental arithmetic disorder
4. Developmental language disorder
   a. Expressive type
   b. Receptive type
5. Developmental articulation disorder
6. Mixed specific developmental disorder
7. Atypical specific developmental disorder

This classification equates developmental reading disorder with dyslexia and considers there to be a significant reading impairment in children between 8 and 13 years of age if there is a 1- to 2-year discrepancy in reading skill to chronological or mental age. Because the time of acquisition of basic reading skills varies widely, it is preferable to avoid a clear designation of dyslexia or reading disability prior to the age of 7 or 8. Although not a component of learning disability per se, emotional problems such as low self-esteem, depression, and withdrawn and apathetic behavior are frequently present. There may also be aggressive or acting-out behavior as a result of frustration with the education process or parental expectations. Recently, there has been increased interest in a group of children who, although of normal verbal intelligence, have particular difficulty in interpreting social signals, making abstractions, and learning math. This has been termed "nonverbal learning disability" and appears to relate primarily to dysfunction in the right hemisphere.

DIFFERENTIAL DIAGNOSIS

By definition, cognitive learning disabilities exclude specific causes that make the acquisition of reading, arithmetic, language, or articulation skills difficult or impossible, such as vision, hearing, or motor handicaps, as well as psychiatric disturbance, global mental retardation, and environmental disadvantage.

The most controversial differential diagnosis is that of an underlying neurologic disorder. In the 1960s, the term *brain damage* was frequently used interchangeably with learning disability because certain patterns of functioning ("scatter" or variable performance) on psychological subtests were considered similar to the patterns of performance demonstrated in patients who had recovered from acquired traumatic injury to the brain. Subsequent study has more strongly suggested a pattern of developmental delay in the development of certain cognitive skills such as reading and arithmetic, although some inconsistent performance is seen occasionally in both the injured brain and the learning-disabled child. However, there is not a strong correlation between prior brain injury, such as perinatal asphyxia, postnatal meningitis, or head trauma, and cognitive learning disability.

Psychiatric disturbance is another controversial differential diagnosis. All too frequently the child with poor cognitive performance in the classroom is considered to have a motivational or discipline problem suggesting an underlying psychiatric disturbance. Determining the primary condition is often a chicken-or-egg problem because school failure quickly leads to low self-esteem, depression, frustration, and acting-out behavior.

Global mental retardation is distinguished from learning disabilities by a uniform delay in all areas of cognitive development, in contrast to the scattered areas of strength and weakness shown by the learning-disabled child. The mentally retarded child acts more or less like a younger child, whereas the learning-disabled child has striking inconsistencies in performance.

WORK-UP

The evaluation and treatment of learning disabilities is best managed by an interdisciplinary team approach ideally including teachers, psychologists, pediatricians, and pediatric neurologists, as well as speech and language pathologists, psychiatrists, occupational therapists, and social workers. This interdisciplinary activity may be informal or formal depending on the location of one's practice. Informally, one should utilize past evaluations and recognize that medical evaluation and management is only one part of a multifaceted approach to the learning-disabled child. Formally, there exists in many communities the opportunity for comprehensive interdisciplinary evaluation of learning-disabled children through specialized programs based in school districts, hospital outpatient clinics, or private settings. Although the primary care pediatrician cannot expect to master the intricacies of psychological testing, he or she can prove valuable or detrimental in the proper management of the child. As long as the pediatrician explores community resources and selects competent services for referral, together with maintaining an active interest as the child's advocate, the child will benefit; if the pediatrician abdicates this role and fosters a pessimistic approach, the child will remain either incompletely evaluated or improperly managed. Alternatively, the parents may gravitate to practitioners with unproven therapies and expensive, fad-oriented approaches that prey on parents anxious for remediation.

History

A careful family history often reveals learning disabilities and should be carefully explored. The history of development of motor and language milestones is also important because language and motor delays are frequently present. Additionally, one should inquire into current patterns of behavior, peer relations, school strengths and weaknesses, and home activities and hobbies.

Physical Examination

A physical examination may show some mild dysmorphic features, such as abnormal dermatoglyphics. Particular attention is paid to the visual, auditory, and tactile sensory examination, because specific sensory deficits can mask learning disabilities. Subtle motor signs suggestive of delayed maturation (such as clumsiness), choreoathetoid movements of the upper extremities (particularly when the arms are held outstretched or when the patient is asked to run), difficulty with rapid alternating motions and other tests of fine motor coordination, and errors in cortical sensory tests (such as stereognosis and graphaesthesia) are often present. Hearing and vision screening evaluations are, of course, essential components of the examination.

Laboratory Tests

Even though psychological testing is expensive and time-consuming, any child in whom there is a strong suspicion of learning disabilities should be evaluated by a qualified clinical psychologist. The tests selected by the psychologist depend on the age of the patient and the presenting learning difficulties but frequently include the Stanford–Binet or Wechsler intelligence test or the Peabody Picture Vocabulary Test. These tests, however, may be inappropriate for a child with a language deficit; thus, more specialized tests may be administered. A school psychologist is frequently available to perform these tests at no additional cost to the parents.

An aid to referral is a screening evaluation by the pediatrician. Such a screening evaluation may include a test of reading, such as the Gilmore Oral Reading Test (reading and answering questions regarding short, grade-appropriate paragraphs); a test of perceptual-motor skills, such as the Berry–Buitanika Test of Visual Motor Integration (copying figures of increasing complexity such as a circle for 3-year-olds, a triangle for 5-year-olds, a diamond for 8-year-olds); and the Denver Developmental Screening Test for children under the age of 6. Any interpretation of test results should be tentative and should take into account the child's past history of educational progress and environmental stress.

At present, electrophysiologic evaluation of children with learning disabilities has limited diagnostic usefulness. An electroencephalograph (EEG) may be useful to distinguish between children who are inattentive from those with seizures (either abortive focal seizure activity or generalized [petit mal]), and those who are unresponsive because of anxiety, auditory processing problems, or distractibility. A number of EEGs in normal children may be read as "borderline," and unless convincing paroxysmal unresponsiveness or inappropriate behavior is noted, anticonvulsant medication is not indicated. Evoked potential testing, primarily of use in the testing of vision and hearing in very young or retarded children, has research interest but little clinical use at this time. Likewise, the Brain Electrical Activity Mapping (BEAM) has considerable research interest but presently has unproven clinical use.

PRINCIPLES OF MANAGEMENT

Allocation of the pediatrician's time in the office setting is an important initial consideration in the management of the learning-disabled child. Because learning disabilities are complex and controversial and present a chronic pattern of school difficulties interspersed with crisis periods relating to new school settings, parent–teacher controversies, and secondary emotional distress, these issues are difficult to resolve in the usual length of time for general pediatric visits. Depending on the interests and practice patterns of the pediatrician, special time may be set aside for a 1-hour initial session, and subsequent visits may be half an hour or more. Regardless of where the evaluation is performed, the pediatrician should have a good knowledge of the community resources available for the evaluation and subsequent management of the child. By law (PL 94-142), school districts are required to evaluate and provide an adequate program of remediation for all children with prominent learning disabilities. Private programs have a distinct advantage as mediators when controversy exists (as is not infrequently the case) between parental expectation and school assessment of a child's appropriate educational placement.

Considerable controversy exists regarding the "correction" of motor deficits as an aid to enhancing educational progress. Eye movement exercises and vestibular stimulation are two therapies in which efficacy is currently questioned.

Unlike the use of medication in the treatment of many children with ADHD disorders, the role of medication in children with cognitive learning disabilities is much more limited. If attention deficits coexist and do not appear to be secondary to anxiety or problems with language or memory difficulties, medications may be used. Medication may again be indicated if emotional lability or depression is a feature. In the former case, methylphenidate, pemoline, or imipramine may be used. In the latter, imipramine or amitriptyline may be useful (see Chap. 35).

INDICATIONS FOR REFERRAL

As discussed, the evaluation and management of the learning-disabled child is an interdisciplinary process and depends on the local facilities and the nature and degree of the learning disability. Children over 2 years of age with language delays and normal hearing should be referred for a speech and language evaluation. Children with gross and fine motor delays and apparent difficulty with following directions and socialization may benefit from a "zero-to-three" infant stimulation program. After the age of 3, if speech and language or learning problems are present, a preschool program including a psychological assessment and input from special educators, speech and language pathologists, and physical and occupational therapists may be indicated. Subsequent school programs for learning-disabled children include both self-contained classrooms for children with prominent learning disabilities who require a full-time program of remediation and resource room placement for one or several hours each day where the learning-disabled child receives assistance in reading or other cognitive tasks. Ongoing assistance is also usually available in the school from clinical psychologists, social workers, and counselors who periodically evaluate or offer supportive psychotherapy for the child.

PATIENT EDUCATION

After psychological testing has been reviewed, it is important to emphasize the child's areas of strengths to the parents and to encourage successful experiences for the child in those areas in which he does well. For example, a child with poor coordination and good cognitive but poor reading skills may not enjoy competitive team sports. However, this child may enjoy individual sports such as swimming or hiking and activities such as Scouts and museum visiting. The parent frequently assumes the role of the tutor for the learning-disabled child. Although tutoring has some limited value, it often leads to frustration and recrimination on both sides when things do not go well. The parent should be advised to limit, if possible, extra academic work at home, and if special homework projects are required, a tutor (who could be an interested high-school student) could be engaged as a more objective enhancer of the child's progress.

ANNOTATED BIBLIOGRAPHY

Accardo P: A Neurodevelopmental Perspective on Specific Learning Disabilities. Baltimore, University Park Press, 1980. (Excellent critical review of the neurodevelopmental perspective in learning disabilities.)

Brutten M, Richardson SO, Mangel C: Something's Wrong with My Child. New York, Harcourt Brace, 1973. (Excellent guide for the parent and other interested lay people regarding learning disabilities.)

Duffy H, Geschwind N: Dyslexia, A Neuroscientific Approach to Clinical Evaluation. Boston, Little, Brown, 1985. (Presentation of recent research and new diagnostic aids as well as a historical perspective of learning disabilities.)

Frederiks JAM (ed): Handbook of Clinical Neurology, vol 2 (46): Neurobehavioral Disorders. Chaps 4, 5, and 7. New York, Elsevier, 1985. (Comprehensive discussions of clinical presentation and evaluation of aspects of learning disabilities.)

Gabel S, Erickson M: Child Development and Developmental Disabilities. Boston, Little, Brown, 1979. (Comprehensive textbook written from the interdisciplinary standpoint with various specialists contributing to an overview of normal and pathologic development, including learning disabilities.)

Gaddes WH: Learning Disabilities and Brain Function, 2nd ed. New York, Springer, 1985. (Learning disabilities viewed from the neuropsychological perspective with much information on the appropriateness and effectiveness of test results.)

Kinsbourne M, Kaplan P: Children's Learning and Attention Problems. Boston, Little, Brown, 1979. (Sensitive and practical guide to evaluation and management.)

Rapin I: Children with Brain Dysfunction. New York, Raven, 1982. (Well-written perspective on some of the more complex areas of language and cognition from the standpoint of etiology and evaluation; written for the practicing pediatrician.)

Rourke BP: Nonverbal Learning Disabilities: The Syndrome and the Model. New York, Guilford Press, 1989. (Review of current thinking on "social" learning disabilities.)

41

School Failure

Murray M. Kappelman

In addition to providing for the child's physical and emotional health, parents correctly expect that the primary health care-giver will also advocate for the child's educational health with equal expertise and enthusiasm. If one considers the community within which the child and family live and interact, who better should take the objective role as an investigator and source finder in cases of school failure than the child's personal physician? It therefore becomes imperative that the pediatrician become aware of and knowledgeable regarding the potential "failure factors" in children whose grades plummet and whose achievement is inadequate. Much of what follows is based on the framework created by Zuckerman.

LEVEL OF MATURITY

Could the child have entered school at too early an age (see Chap. 38, "School Readiness")? This is a fairly common problem in the early grades. The child whose birthday is in November or December, but who is registered for school with other children born potentially 11 months earlier, may be less prepared for the pace or the social and educational demands of a system geared for children at a more advanced age and level of maturity. Each child develops educational skills at his or her own pace; some move quickly, others more slowly. The ultimate result is usually the same—each reaching a satisfactory range of assimilating and adapting information at some point during the first few years of school. If a youngster has entered school at an early age and has normal but relatively sluggish learning skills or emotional adaptability, the child may find the peer group advancing at a more rapid pace. This child could easily fail despite serious and earnest efforts to succeed. This child wants to be like his or her peer group, to do well in school, and not to be the slowest in the class; however, he or she cannot "put it all together" at quite the same rate as the slightly older peers. The result may be anger, frustration, withdrawal, and, ultimately, failure that may adversely influence the child's later education.

The child's pediatrician must balance the potential impact on the child of "holding him back" one year versus the continuing frustration of the youngster trying to race with a peer crowd faster and more mature. If social and learning maturity is the key factor in the child's early grade failure, then suggesting that the child be retained to repeat the early grade successfully could have several positive features. Having experienced the material before, the child will likely experience success and esteem the second year. In addition, the child's age will be more in keeping with that of the older youngsters in the new cohort in terms of social maturity, peer acceptance, and coordination in games and sports. When appropriate, the immature child could benefit clearly from repeating the year. The key issue for the pediatrician is to be sure that this recommended approach is not viewed as a failure on the part of the teachers, parents, or child but rather as a reassignment to a more appropriate group according to the age and level of learning maturity. A vital rule of communication between parent and the failing child in this situation is optimism. The pediatrician's role after suggesting the potential school response is to protect the child's self-esteem.

NEUROLOGICALLY BASED SENSORY AND MOTOR DISTURBANCES

Hearing Impairment

Many professionals and parents are unaware what an isolating handicap severe hearing impairment can be to the growing child. This is particularly true with congenital deafness or severe hearing loss with associated impaired language development.

The child with congenital deafness and poor speech formation is usually diagnosed long before entry into school. These youngsters are often sent to separate classes or schools within which attention is paid to the child's need for alternative teaching techniques, speech development, and socialization skills enhancement.

The youngster who presents the challenge to the pediatrician is the child who is failing because of diminished hearing acuity due to congenital or acquired reasons that are not serious enough to identify the child during preschool play. Acquired diminished hearing may result from trauma, sequelae to bacterial meningitis, persistent or recurrent otitis media, or foreign material in the outer ear canal. It is the pediatrician's responsibility to diagnose these losses *before* the school failure and not to overlook this possibility after the child receives poor grades (see also Chap. 78, "Hearing Loss").

Visual Impairment

Serious visual impairment or blindness will be diagnosed long before school in most cases; however, more subtle but significant visual abnormalities such as myopia, hyperopia, astigmatism, and significant strabismus can be missed and can form the basis of a child's failure within the school situation. Appropriate office screening at 4 years of age and attention to eye muscle movement and coordination with each physician/child contact will alert the pediatrician to the possibility of reduced visual acuity. Thus, a through assessment of potential visual impairments using a history and an examination and visual screening should be a part of every pediatrician's work-up of the failing child (see also Chap. 90, "Visual Testing").

Motor Impairment

The child with cerebral palsy or hypotonic syndromes is rarely missed before entrance into school. The pediatrician faces the task of working with the parents and the school system to find the educationally and motorically ideal school setting for the child with motor handicaps. So much can be accomplished by these children as they grow into productive adulthood that anything less than a herculean effort by parent, child, pediatrician, and school system to help the child reach maximum potential is unacceptable (see also Chap. 147, "Muscle Weakness," and Chap. 154, "Cerebral Palsy").

COGNITIVE DISORDERS

Mental Retardation

The pediatrician will find the differentiation between the child with mild mental retardation and the child with learning disabilities or emotional/situational problems to be difficult. Generally, the youngster whose development has been sufficiently slow to warrant the label of moderate to severe and profound retardation has come to the attention of the parents and the pediatrician during regular office visits when history, observation, and such tests as the Denver Developmental Screening Test are employed as part of the child's assessment. Moderate to severe brain dysfunction resulting in childhood autism must also be distinguished from mental retardation because of the somewhat different prognosis in some cases and the educational approach in most. Mental retardation is static but deserves the correct educational approach; autism (usually neurologic rather than emotional) can be dynamic, and correct approaches may make a considerable difference in the ultimate educational and social level of performance.

The pediatrician should be alerted to the potential of mild mental retardation when there is a lag or dysfunction in the growing youngster's levels of fine-motor coordination and more complex speech development (use of pronouns, syntax development, association of words and shapes). School failure may be the first sign of slow development at the level of mild mental retardation. The work-up of the failing child should include referral to a clinical psychologist. The pediatrician becomes the child's advocate for maximal mainstreaming with appropriate resources in areas needing special assistance in learning. Vocational training that begins early to create independent citizens may also require encouragement from the pediatrician working closely with the school system.

Minimal Brain Dysfunction

Specific Learning Disabilities. It is estimated that between 5% and 10% of school children suffer from specific learning disabilities sufficiently serious to affect their learning. Specific learning disabilities are covered in Chapter 40; however, in this section, consideration must be given to prevention and diagnosis because they relate so clearly to school failure. The learning-disabled child awakens every morning painfully aware that he or she will be going to class to "fail" often despite an innate sense that better work could be done but is being blocked and detoured outside of the child's control.

Preventing failure from specific learning disabilities is based on early suspicion and diagnosis. Language development plays a key role not only in the expressive language area but also in the area of reading. Dyslexia is more often a result of abnormalities in the auditory-verbal perceptual axis than related to visual-motor difficulties as previously believed. Delayed speech development, early signs of poor coordination, clumsiness beyond the norm, impaired use of writing instruments and toys, and delayed fine-motor development (tying shoes, buttoning buttons) are only a few of the clues that alert the pediatrician to watch this child for school problems. Overt developmental signs pointing to future learning disability can be referred earlier than the preschool years; however, most youngsters can wait until peer group interaction and expectations suggest the diagnosis.

This means early action so that proper educational assistance can be programmed for the learning-disabled child.

Currently, there are two nonstandardized but useful screening tests that measure the neuromaturational development of children at various ages. They have been designed for pediatricians to administer and score. These tests are Levine's Pediatric Early Educational Readiness (PEER: ages 5 to 7) Test and the later Pediatric Early Elementary Examination (PEEX: ages 7 to 9) as well as Shaywitz's Yale Neuromaturational Screening Test. These instruments do not provide valid "numbers". They are designed to make the pediatrician more aware that a specific child may have learning disabilities and that further investigation may be required with the use of standardized instruments. They are screening instruments for the pediatric office and do not replace the psychologist's standardized tests, the educator's instruments, or the speech pathologist's important screening.

The longer the pediatrician waits to make this diagnosis and begin remediation, the more often the child will see "Failure" on his or her report card, and the more educational and emotional hurdles will be created to prevent satisfactory educational and emotional outcome for the child.

Attention Deficit Hyperactivity Disorder. Too many overly active youngsters who are doing poorly in school are labeled as attention deficit hyperactivity disorder (ADHD) children. The challenge to the pediatrician is to analyze carefully each case and, if appropriate, refer to other professionals expert in learning and behavior problems in children. The diagnosis of ADHD is best made after considerable thought and after working with a team of experts. Poor attention span, impulsivity, inability to finish tasks, and easy distractibility are components of this "syndrome" that may be present without overactivity or misdirected activity (then known as ADD—attention deficit disorder). Any one or combination of these behaviors can lead to poor performance in the school setting and eventual failure (see Chap. 35).

Psychoactive drugs (Ritalin, Dexedrine, Cylert) and newer drugs such as desimpramine and clonidine have demonstrated satisfactory results in controlling the activity and attention issues in most children if monitored carefully; however, unless the other elements often associated with this problem (specific perceptual weaknesses, peer and family rejection, emotional overlay, speech problems, medical issues, sense of low self-worth) are addressed simultaneously with the medication, the pediatrician may merely be slowing the child down to better recognize his failures.

ENVIRONMENTAL INTERFERENCE
Poor School Environment

Several issues may play a role in creating a school environment that is conducive to failure in a specific child, and these possibilities should be investigated. Poor instruction looms large as a potential for inadequate information transfer; however, this is too often the first accusation made by the parent without a school visit and first-hand observation. In actuality, poor teaching ranks low on the list of frequent causes of school failure among children in the educational system. The adequate child often learns despite the teacher. A poorly controlled, noisy classroom is another cause. Personality conflicts, real or imagined, between teacher and child can form the basis of diminishing motivation to perform, which can then result in a poor report card. If a child is bullied or shunned, this may create emotional barriers to learning in an environment perceived by the child to be hostile. The pediatrician, by talking to the parent, teacher, and child (alone), may uncover one of these as a possible reason for the school failure.

Education Not in the Dominant Language

This has become a serious problem in our current school system, particularly in the lower grades. The young child is confronted with English as the dominant language of communication after preschool years of another language being the primary or exclusive form of verbal interchange. The parents' English is often poor to nonexistent. Quick answers cannot be given to this problem. The school must start with these youngsters as bilingual, with English clearly the weaker of the two languages. The pediatrician can alert parents of the impending problem and encourage them to teach their children to speak English. If no progress is made in the bilingual equilibrium of the child, the pediatrician needs to alert the school of the child's special language needs. Schools often make accommodations; occasionally, the family is isolated in an English-speaking world.

School Absence

This problem has three basic causalities requiring investigation by the pediatrician. The first reason for persistent significant school absence is chronic illness in the child. At times, these absences are unavoidable (e.g., severe asthmatics), but too frequently the parents keep the chronically ill child away from school too long after an illness and too often when he or she has only minor symptoms. In the former, home teaching can be suggested by the pediatrician; in the latter, the pediatrician needs to educate the parents and lower their level of anxiety. Parents must realize that their child is subject to the serious potential problem of educational deprivation.

The second reason for school absence occurs when the parent, because of personal or social crises, is unable or unwilling to ensure that the child attends school. The depressed parent, the recently separated single parent, and the rural farming parent needing extra hands are examples of parents who inappropriately and willingly encourage or suggest school absence. The pediatrician will need assistance from the social work professional to deal with these parents. Poverty and lack of school clothing is another social reason why children stay away from school, re-creating the cycle of lack of education, poor job potential, and low incomes.

Truancy is the third reason for frequent school absences. This increases with an increase in age and grade. Truancy need not be sociopathic behavior; it may indicate trouble within the school environment. This trouble could be learning disabilities with persistent failure, serious emotional or physical taunting or teasing, sexual harassment or panic, drugs or alcohol, unannounced pregnancy, or merely a serious problem with self-esteem realistically or unrealistically based on intellect, appearance, or sociability. It is essential to regard truancy as a signal and work with the parents and the school to discover the basic reasons behind the willing withdrawal from the learning environment. Returning the young person to the same environment without working on remediating the underlying concerns only leads to further truancy, recidivism, and early school dropout. This is the ultimate school failure.

Family Dysfunction

The child who has family issues on his mind and cannot concentrate on schoolwork will most likely have problems with his school performance. Poor school performance commonly accompanies parental separation or divorce, illness of a close family member, the death of a loved one, physical violence within the household, the involvement of a family member with police with or without incarceration, family incapacity due to drugs or alcohol, and disruption due to a family member moving away (e.g., father in the service). These family issues are examples of common child concerns that crowd out the information to be learned from the child's thought processes. These problems often require only quick medical and educational assessment of the family situation. However, on occasion, a one-on-one interview with the child (sometimes several to build trust) will be necessary to uncover the basic anxiety that is preventing learning and precipitating school failure.

As noted above, the very dysfunctional family often cannot see school as a priority; therefore, the child misses school so often that failure ensues. Another serious issue in this type of family is the poor role modeling toward educational achievement and often the low priority given to educational achievement. This is a "no-win" situation as long as the child remains in such a household.

The pediatrician often makes the diagnosis and may be able to assist in the resolution of some family issues; more often, however, he needs the assistance of other professionals (e.g., social worker, protective services, psychiatrists, lawyers) to deliver the comprehensive family remediation needed to relieve the child's anxiety and permit the youngster's attention to be redirected toward learning in school.

EMOTIONAL DISORDER

Lack of Motivation

Motivation often stems from family enthusiasm over learning and solid home role models. Even with these in place, however, some children appear to lack the motivation to learn. More careful investigation will often reveal that the lack of motivation shields the child from his or her own poor self-concept as a learner, his or her fear of failure in a family with high standards, competition from siblings, underlying undiagnosed learning disabilities, or interest in areas far removed from those taught within the school environment. "He just doesn't care about getting good grades" may be one of the most dangerous statements that can be made about a failing child. Of course he cares; why he is doing poorly in school is the issue that must be discovered by the team of parent, teacher, and pediatrician.

"Bad Crowd" Syndrome

A frequent complaint by parents and teachers is that a young person has begun to do poorly in school because he or she associates with a group of peers who are also doing poorly in school, who are truant, or who are school dropouts. This argument does have a solid basis in the school performance slide of some youngsters; however, the pediatrician must remember that the young person may have selected friends because of his or her perception of their similarity to him- or herself. He or she is living a self-fulfilling prophecy of his or her own learning inadequacy. The reasons for this may need the pediatrician's attention rather than the "bad crowd."

Depression

Poor school performance is a cardinal sign in the depressed youngster and adolescent. It may be one of the first and only signs before the child takes major self-destructive action. The unexpected decline in school grades in the older child clearly points toward an investigation of the young person's state of emotional well-being. Whether the depression is endogenous or acutely situational in origin, the sudden falling school grades must cause the team of parent, teacher, and pediatrician to investigate the young person's status and refer for treatment expediently if depression is the apparent cause of the poor school performance (see also Chap. 36, "Depression and Suicide").

Psychosis/Thought Disorder

Again, one of the early signs of serious emotional illness may be withdrawal from learning within the school environment and school failure. Careful questioning by the teacher and pediatrician should uncover a child with disordered thinking and a dysfunctional mental status who requires intensive therapy, often within residential settings where the young person's educational needs are addressed simultaneously with the emotional rehabilitation. The pediatrician has the responsibility to make the diagnosis and initiate the expedient referral. School failure in this youngster is just an indication of many problems.

It is a large challenge to reverse school failure in the pediatric patient; in many ways it turns the pediatrician into a detective teaming with other professionals and the parents, and often the child, to discover the clues that will lead to the diagnosis or multiple diagnoses regarding the causes behind the poor grades on the child's report card. This investigation can take considerable time, but it gives the pediatrician his or her distinctive role in the care of the "total" child.

ANNOTATED BIBLIOGRAPHY

Feagans L: A current view of learning disabilities. J Pediatr 102(4):487–493, 1983. (Provocative and controversial article by a psychologist.)

Hartzell H, Compton C: Learning disability: 10 year follow-up. Pediatrics 74(6):1058, 1984. (Long-term effect of learning disabilities addressed in a sensible manner.)

Learning Disabilities. Pediatr Clin North Am 31:2, 1984. (Excellent compendium of articles on the subject.)

Levine M et al: The dimension of inattention among children with school problems. Pediatrics 70(3):387, 1982. (Interesting perspective on the issue of attention deficit disorder.)

Levine M et al: The pediatric early elementary examination: Studies of a neurodevelopmental examination for seven- to nine-year-old children. Pediatrics 71(6):894, 1983. (Levine's neurodevelopmental testing instrument for early detection of learning disabilities offers help to the pediatrician.)

Shaywitz S et al: Current status of the neuromaturational examination as an index of learning disability. J Pediatr 104(6):819, 1984. (Another pediatric screening instrument of some value for learning disabilities.)

Zuckerman B, Chase C: Specific learning disability and dyslexia: A language-based model. Adv Pediatr 1984. ("Ground-breaking" article that predicts subsequent findings.)

7

ADOLESCENT MEDICINE

42

Pregnancy Prevention

Arthur B. Elster

The dramatic changes in sexual behavior of American youth since the 1960s have been well documented. More adolescents are having sexual intercourse and at earlier ages. By age 16, 29% of boys and 17% of girls have had sexual intercourse. These figures jump to 65% and 51% by age 18 for boys and girls, respectively. The average age of first sexual intercourse is now around 16. With the downward trend in the age of puberty and the upward trend in the age of marriage, the "culturally based" sexual abstinence and infertility period imposed by society has lengthened. It is difficult (and unusual) for adolescents to pass through the interval from menarche to marriage without engaging in sexual intercourse. The AIDS epidemic has now necessitated that efforts at pregnancy prevention be broadened to include HIV prevention. Although less than 1% of AIDS patients are adolescents, 20% of people with AIDS are between the ages of 20 and 29. Considering the interval between infection with the HIV virus and the acquisition of AIDS, many of these young adult AIDS patients acquired the virus during adolescence.

REPRODUCTIVE PROFILE

A "reproductive profile" of sexually active 15- to 19-year-old girls shows that 51% used contraception at last intercourse, 23% have been pregnant, 10% had an abortion, and 11% gave birth. Because of the high rate of sexual behavior and the low rate of contraceptive usage, the United States has one of the highest adolescent pregnancy rates of all

Western countries. Overall, approximately one million teenagers (representing about one girl in ten aged 15–19) become pregnant each year in the United States. Half of these pregnancies occur within 6 months of the first sexual encounter. With the dual problem of pregnancy and HIV prevention, the primary care physician assumes an expanded and increasingly important role in adolescent health.

ETHICAL ISSUES

Providing pregnancy prevention services to adolescents is made complex by an array of ethical and practical issues that clinicians treating this population must face. Central are issues of legal restraint and confidentiality, parental involvement, reimbursement for services, and communication style.

Legally, physicians can provide unemancipated minors services related to the diagnosis and treatment of sexually transmitted diseases and the diagnosis of pregnancy. Depending on state jurisdiction, physicians may also be permitted to counsel confidentially about birth control devices and prescribe a contraceptive method. Some states explicitly define under what conditions an adolescent may be considered an "emancipated minor" or a "mature minor," thus permitting physicians the opportunity to provide a full range of services without parental involvement. Other states, however, leave these issues ill-defined. Physicians should inquire about the statutes in their state prior to providing reproductive services.

Adolescents' sexual activity is often known by their parents. In these situations it is usually best to have the parents involved in, or at least broadly informed of, the types of issues discussed with their adolescent. Involvement of parents is more important for younger adolescents who need a greater degree of supervision than do older adolescents. A greater degree of independence is appropriate for older adolescents. It is essential that the ground rules be set at the first clinic visit so that both the adolescent and the parents are aware of what information will be shared and what will remain confidential. Many sexually active adolescents, however, are living in situations estranged from parents, are victims of physical or sexual abuse, or already have had a pregnancy. In these situations, the involvement of parents may be impossible, unrealistic, or unwarranted.

Associated with the issue of parental involvement is the question of who provides the financial reimbursement for pregnancy prevention services. Because adolescents usually lack adequate financial resources to pay for clinic visits as well as prescription contraceptives, physicians must decide on one of three options: accept whatever reimbursement is possible either directly from the adolescent or from Medicaid, if eligible, and treat the adolescent confidentially; involve the parents and bill them for the services; or refer the adolescent to a community clinic that can provide confidential services either free or on a sliding fee scale.

The nature of the physician–patient communication style is especially important to adolescents who are evolving from the emotional and physical dependency of childhood to the autonomy of adult life. Helping youth make appropriate decisions about the management of their health is an important task for the physician. Whenever possible, adolescents should be provided the rationale for health care decisions and given the opportunity to choose among options. This "empowerment" may lead to a greater level of emotional commitment to the preventive intervention plan, to greater compliance, and to an improved feeling of self-worth. Empowerment is best fostered when physicians use an authoritative, rather than an authoritarian, style of interaction. The former style recognizes that, within limits of physical safety, adolescents should play an active role in their health care decisions. Because of the varied safe options, sexually active adolescents without major medical contraindications can be provided the opportunity to choose between using a diaphragm or oral contraceptives. Regardless of their choice, they can then provide their written "assent" documenting that they understand the possible side effects of the method and that all of their questions have been answered. An authoritative style, on the other hand, is one in which decisions are made for the adolescent for which she has little or no input. This is the predominant style used with younger children and one with which physicians are usually the most acquainted. Because of familiarity with this latter style and the need to keep patient visits relatively short, physicians need to actively work at making the transition from an authoritarian to an authoritative approach.

ROLE OF THE PHYSICIAN IN PREGNANCY PREVENTION

Primary care physicians can play a major role in helping adolescents prevent pregnancy. The level of involvement physicians have with pregnancy prevention depends on their knowledge and skill managing adolescent patients, their personal comfort dealing with adolescent health issues, and time restraints of their office practice. Physicians should decide whether they view their role as providing essential care or more advanced care for adolescents regarding sexual health issues.

Essential care consists of those health services that all adolescents should receive. This includes a basic sexual history; the provision of health-promotion information regarding sexual development, pregnancy, and sexually transmitted diseases; the identification of sexually active teens who need reproductive health services (e.g., those not using contraception or those who might be pregnant); and coordination with other private or public clinics to ensure that adolescents receive the reproductive health services they need. For adolescents who are sexually active, essential care also includes promoting the use of condoms to prevent not only pregnancy but also HIV infection and other sexually transmitted diseases.

All physicians treating adolescents should be aware of the early symptoms of pregnancy, such as nausea, breast tenderness, fatigue, and increased frequency of urination. When the adolescent reports a missed menstrual period along with symptoms of early pregnancy and has a history of a recent sexual encounter, a urine pregnancy test should be performed. With the identification of purified human chorionic gonadotropin, rapid agglutination tests have been developed that are highly sensitive and able to detect pregnancy within 2 to 3 weeks of conception. These tests are relatively inexpensive, have a low rate of false-positives, and are easy to perform in the office. Urine pregnancy tests produce results in several minutes and, because of the need to provide the anxious adolescent immediate counseling, are more desirable than blood tests. Home pregnancy tests are also quite reliable. During their early pubertal years, however, the menstrual periods of adolescents are easily disrupted. In addition to pregnancy, rapid changes in weight, stress, extreme exercise, and acute illness can also cause irregular menses. Because adolescents frequently experience irregular menstrual periods and perceive pregnancy as an emotional crisis, the use of home pregnancy tests for this population should be discouraged.

In addition to the services described above, advanced care involves obtaining a more in-depth evaluation of sexual health, counseling about specific ways to prevent pregnancy, the provision of contraceptive services, and the provision of gynecologic care. Basic skills for the delivery of advanced services include performing a pelvic examination, interpreting the findings, medically managing adolescents on birth control pills and diaphragms, and diagnosing and treating sexually transmitted disease. There are various effective methods of contraception available for the sexually active adolescent (see Table 42-1). Younger adolescents and those who have a less stable relationship with their partner are usually best served by oral contraceptive agents. Older

Table 42-1. Contraceptive Methods Used by Adolescents*

METHOD	FAILURE RATE[†]	ADVANTAGES	DISADVANTAGES	COMMENT
Rhythm	28% (white) 34% (nonwhite)	Safe No cost	Requires: Regular ovulation Self-discipline Self-monitoring	Not realistic for teens
Withdrawal	18%	Safe No cost	Requires discipline Sperm in pre-ejaculate fluid	Gives teens a false sense of security
Diaphragm	12% (white) 35% (nonwhite)	Use-related: Few side effects Minimal use of doctor	Requires: Medical visit Preplanning Emotional maturity	A good method for older or multiparous teens
Condom	13% (white) 22% (nonwhite)	Use-related: No side effects Low cost Prevents HIV & STD	Requires: Preplanning Support of partner Interrupts sex	Should be promoted for all teens
Spermicide	35% (white) 34% (nonwhite)	Safe Low cost May help prevent STD	Not effective when used alone	Should be used with other method
Pills	9% (white) 18% (nonwhite)	Effective Acceptable to most teens	Expensive Many side effects Requires monitoring	Usually the most agreeable method for teens
Implants	Less than 1%	Lasts for 5 years	Irregular menstrual bleeding Requires minor surgery	Use not studied in teens

*Figures based on studies by Jones EF, Forrest JD: Contraceptive failure in the United States: Revised estimates from the 1982 National Survey of Family Growth. Fam Plann Perspect 21:103–109, 1989; and Trussell J, Hatcher RA, Cates WC et al: Contraceptive failure in the United States: An update. Stud Fam Plann 21:51–54, 1990.

[†]Failure rates are those that would be found in typical users, not rates found when the method is used optimally.

adolescents often have the emotional maturity to effectively use a diaphragm. All adolescents should be counseled to use condoms, regardless of other methods of contraception.

DEVELOPMENTALLY APPROPRIATE SERVICES

Because adolescent biopsychosocial development is a gradual process that occurs over a 7- to 10-year period, physicians are advised to tailor health care services to the unique issues and needs of the age of the adolescent. Although age is not always an accurate measurement of level of development, for practical purposes it is helpful to consider three stages of adolescence—early, middle, and late. The general approach, sexual history, and direction of health promotion are best considered in terms of these three stages.

Early Adolescence (Ages 10–14)

General Approach. Information must be obtained from both the adolescent and the parents. In order to establish an effective provider–patient relationship, however, at least a portion of each visit should be with the adolescent alone. It is important to not only establish the stated expectations for the visit but also uncover any "hidden agenda" of either the parent or the adolescent. Physicians should be aware of subtle cues, such as embarrassment, shyness, or reluctance

discussing sexual issues. If present, these issues should be addressed with parents. Because sexual abuse increases at the time of puberty, physicians should be suspicious when they see a young adolescent with a sexually transmitted disease, venereal warts, recurrent and unexplained abdominal pain, or excessive anxiety about the physical examination.

Sexual History. The sexual history should be incorporated as part of the general health assessment. The following information should be obtained during the clinic visit:

- Knowledge, expectations, and feelings regarding pubertal changes
- Anxiety regarding physiologic and behavioral changes surrounding puberty, such as menarche, wet dreams, masturbation, and sexual fantasies
- Sources and extent of sexual information
- Involvement in sexual behavior (e.g., petting, sexual intercourse)
- History of sexual abuse

Health Promotion. Because adolescents want to know if they are "normal," time should be spent discussing issues related to sexual development. Although not usually expressed directly as a concern by the adolescent, physical changes are on the minds of all adolescents as they go through puberty. Discussion might focus on:

- The normal physical and emotional events that occur during puberty. It is best to include a discussion of timing and the sequence of emergence of secondary sexual characteristics.
- Information to help young adolescent females prepare for menarche. This is usually best done in association with the adolescent's mother. Having the mother relate her own experiences of menarche and menstruation is a good way to begin the discussion.
- A brief mention of the role of both wet dreams and masturbation in adolescent development. These two issues can cause adolescents considerable anxiety and should be addressed proactively.
- Information to parents to help them become better health educators of their children.

Middle Adolescence (Ages 15–17)

General Approach. Most, if not all, of the interview should be done with the adolescent alone. Important to the middle adolescent is having a relationship with an adult they can trust. Confidentiality and use of a communication style that is open and neither condescending nor condemning are ways that physicians can promote trust among their adolescent patients.

Sexual History. Many, but not all, sexually active adolescents engage in other health risk behaviors. The sexual history, therefore, should assess a range of behavioral possibilities:

- Social relationships, including the degree of involvement with friendship groups, the recreational behaviors of these friends, and pressures to participate when friends engage in health risk behaviors (e.g., drugs, drinking, smoking, sexual behavior)
- Attitudes about, knowledge of, and involvement in other health risk behaviors, such as drug, alcohol, and tobacco use
- Sexual behaviors, including involvement with same-sex as well as opposite-sex partners, number of partners, use of contraception, and whether sexual favors are used to purchase drugs

Health Promotion.

- Replace myths about sexual behavior with facts by providing information on normative behavior. Discussing these issues does not increase an adolescent's sexual behavior.
- Encourage adolescents to be sexually responsible. For some this may mean abstinence, while for others it may mean maintaining monogamous relationships and using appropriate contraception in an effective manner.
- Empower adolescents by helping them to understand the motivation behind their behavior. Regardless of the popular appeal of single-focused motivational messages to change behavior, such as "Just Say No" and "Just Do It," adolescent behavior is influenced by a more complex set of factors. Health education could also address the social factors that affect behavior by discussing the intent of some advertising campaigns to link sexuality with use of a product and the inappropriate portrayal of sexism and violence against women contained in some rock music and movies, and by encouraging adolescents to resist negative peer influence.

Late Adolescence (Ages 18–21)

General Approach. Older adolescents are more comfortable with their sexuality, less influenced by peer group behaviors, and more interested in making the transition to responsible "adult" behaviors. Questions about sexuality should be phrased in a gender-neutral, nonthreatening manner, such as, "Although not everybody your age has had sex, many have. I was wondering if you have had sex." Until more information is provided, it is best not to make a judgment regarding whether an adolescent has had sex or, if sexually active, that his or her partner is heterosexual.

Sexual History. The sexual history of the older adolescent should address the following:

- Sexual relationships and measures used to prevent pregnancy or infection with HIV
- Anxieties about their sexual behaviors and about HIV infection
- Involvement in drug, alcohol, and tobacco use
- History of previous pregnancy and outcome

Health Promotion. Health promotion should be directed at transition to an adult health care setting, prevention of HIV and other sexually transmitted diseases, and responsible sexual behavior. Because of its dual protection against pregnancy and sexually transmitted diseases (including HIV infection), condom use should be promoted to all adolescents, even if another method is already being used.

Physicians can help influence the behavior and health of adolescents in their practice, but they must choose whether they want to deliver basic, essential services to adolescents or whether they have the interest, time, and training to provide more in-depth, advanced care.

ANNOTATED BIBLIOGRAPHY

American Academy of Pediatrics, Committee on Adolescence: Contraception and adolescents. Pediatrics 86:134–138, 1990. (Brief background of adolescent sexual behavior and contraception, and recommendations for pediatricians.)

Gans J, Blyth D, Elster A, Gaveras LL: America's Adolescents: How Healthy Are They? AMA Profiles of Adolescent Health. Chicago, American Medical Association, 1990. (Description of current health problems and health-compromising behaviors of adolescents and how these have changed over time.)

Hatcher RA, Stewart F, Trussell J, et al: Contraceptive Technology 1990–1992. New York, Irvington Publisher, 1990. (Still a good "cookbook" for approaches to adolescent sexual health and for use of each contraceptive method.)

Neinstein LS, Katz B: Contraceptive use in the chronically ill adolescent female: Parts I and II. J Adolesc Health Care 7:123–133, 350–360, 1986. (Provides a review of the interaction between contraceptive methods and a variety of chronic diseases of adolescents.)

43

Eating Disorders of Adolescents

Richard M. Sarles and Mohammad Haerian

Eating disorders of adolescents are usually more prevalent in women who are preoccupied with weight and food and who develop abnormal eating patterns. The two most prevalent eating disorders, anorexia nervosa and bulimia, are the primary disorders within this category, and although somewhat related and overlapping, they appear to be distinct and different entities.

ANOREXIA NERVOSA

The term *anorexia nervosa* is actually a misnomer. Anorexia means loss of appetite, yet most of these young women do not experience loss of appetite but a profound disorder of body image and eating patterns. The German word *pubertätmagersucht* better defines this condition as a relentless pursuit of thinness or a seeking or passion for the leanness of puberty.

Case (Clinical) Presentation

Laura M, a 15½-year-old high-school sophomore, was examined by her pediatrician because of a marked weight loss over a 3-month period. Laura insisted that she felt well and that she had no physical complaints.

Laura was a tenth-grade student, a class officer who generally achieved an A to B average. She was an avid tennis player, competed on the school swimming team, and had a part-time job at a fast-food chain. She was described by her parents as a happy teenager who never gave them any trouble and who seemed like the "perfect child." Laura seemed to be liked by her peers and often received phone calls from them each evening. She helped in the house and often prepared meals for the family. Laura's early childhood growth and development were completely normal.

During the summer vacation, Laura felt that her thighs were too large and decided to "cut back" on sweets and junk food. Her routine preschool sports physical examination revealed that her weight had dropped from 118 to 112 lbs and that her menstrual periods had stopped for the prior 2 months, but she appeared in good physical health and still fell easily within normal limits on the growth chart.

In early November, Laura's mother accidentally saw her undressing and was shocked by Laura's marked thinness. Laura could not understand her mother's great concern, insisting instead that she still had fat thighs and a pot belly, and, in fact, she admitted to running 5 to 7 miles each day and doing calisthenics each evening prior to bed. When Laura stood on the bathroom scale, she weighed only 82 lbs. She had lost approximately 36 lbs.

Mr M, her father, was a 41-year-old insurance executive who owned his own agency and had gained professional recognition and marked financial success through real-estate dealings. He was president of his fraternity and captain of the tennis team in college. He maintained his interest in sports as an avid spectator at professional baseball and football games and as an active participant in tennis.

Mrs M was a 39-year-old successful member of a large advertising agency. She had graduated from college cum laude, Phi Beta Kappa, and had won two journalism awards. She entered graduate school to pursue her master's degree and doctorate work in journalism but completed only 1 year before getting married. She became pregnant soon after being married.

Mr and Mrs M were an attractive couple. Mrs M always dressed stylishly, expensively, and impeccably; Mr. M dressed conservatively and neatly. Both admitted that appearances were important to them and achievement was the mark of success. They admitted to being "wed to their work," managing to go out to dinner together or spending time alone only "once in a great while." Family vacations had denied them time to vacation alone as a couple for the past 7 years.

When Laura was examined by her pediatrician, the following physical findings were noted. Laura appeared as a very thin and wasted but well-groomed adolescent with absent normal female body contours. Her axillary and pubic hair patterns were normal, and a thin, silky body hair was present. Her skin was cold, dry, and cracked. Her temperature was 96.2°F; her blood pressure was $^{68}/_{48}$; her pulse was 52. Laboratory studies including hemoglobin; hematocrit; WBC and differential; urinalysis; stool specimen for blood, ova, and parasites; and liver studies were all within normal limits.

Laura represents a typical example of the adolescent girl with anorexia nervosa. A well-behaved girl in a high-achievement family, she developed an overwhelming need for thinness of delusional proportions resulting in profound weight loss.

The American Psychiatric Association's *Diagnostic and Statistical Manual (DSM-III)* Criteria for Anorexia Nervosa include an intense fear of becoming obese with an age of onset prior to age 25, which does not diminish as weight loss progresses; a disturbance of body image; a refusal to maintain body weight over a minimal normal weight for age and height; a weight loss of at least 15% of original body weight; and no known illness that would account for the weight loss. Amenorrhea is usually present, although 25% of these girls cease their menstrual periods prior to the onset of weight loss. Bradycardia; hypotension; hypothermia; dry, cracked, red skin; thinning of scalp hair with an increase in fine body hair; and loss of female body contours are other physical signs. Petechiae and ecchymoses are frequently seen in severely emaciated patients and are probably due to increased capillary permeability rather than thrombocytopenia. The presence of edema is troublesome but rarely life threatening.

Laboratory data usually show no major abnormalities until severe starvation and physical deterioration result. Then, electrolyte abnormalities, hypoglycemia, leukopenia, lymphocytosis, low ESR (erythrocyte sedimentation rate), and low T_3 (triiodothyronine) may occur. Electrocardiograms may reveal cardiac arrhythmias.

Other signs and symptoms include excessive ritualistic exercising that may be in addition to organized school sports and an excessive preoccupation with food, such as preparing the family dinner, working in food establishments, and gourmet cooking. The adolescent often has a marked disturbance of body image and a body concept of delusional proportions, claiming absolute denial of pathologic weight loss or thinness. Anorectic adolescents often see themselves as fat even with a marked weight loss and often misjudge their own waist size as overly large by at least 50%. Curiously, these adolescents can correctly observe other persons' body size and the size of inanimate objects. Anorectic adolescents often have an inaccurate or confused perception of body stimuli in that they often believe that food, once in the stomach, will multiply. The adolescent, for example, may think that four Cheerios for breakfast is ample and filling.

The marked and progressive weight loss despite parental or physician intervention is often so striking that the diagnosis of anorexia nervosa is usually made without difficulty.

BULIMIA

Bulimia is defined as episodic binge eating followed by vomiting (usually self-induced), abdominal pain, use of laxatives, and deep sleep. Like anorexia nervosa, the age of onset is usually prior to age 25, and it is found predominantly in women. However, unlike the anorectic patient whose weight loss is most profound and noticeable, weight loss is not obvious with bulimic patients, and marked overt physical symptomatology is usually absent. The binge-eating bulimic often consumes large amounts of high-calorie, usually sweet, soft, and easily digested food in rapid fashion with little chewing. Eating is usually secretive and inconspicuous and is often unknown to families or

friends. Excessive binging is terminated by intense abdominal pain, social interruption, or sleep. Self-induced vomiting often occurs, which helps relieve the abdominal pain. Bulimia is often associated with substance abuse, particularly barbiturates, amphetamines, and alcohol use. There is a high correlation with depression, and self-deprecating thoughts and a depressed mood often precede and follow the binge period. In contrast to the anorectic, the bulimic has a clear awareness that his or her eating habits are abnormal and has an ingrained fear of not being able to stop and control his or her eating.

On physical examination, the primary care physician is often able to discern side effects of the bulimic behavior, such as parotid enlargement, hypokalemia, rectal bleeding, destruction of dental enamel, and alopecia.

Although anorexia nervosa and bulimia share broad, general characteristics and often coexist, personality features have been described that distinguish the two groups. Anorectic patients tend to be more perfectionistic, compliant, conforming, academically successful, and generally well liked by their teachers, yet they often have difficulty in forming relationships outside of the family, and social isolation is a common occurrence. Anorectic patients are also more introverted, display little overt psychiatric symptomatology, and deny hunger more often than do their bulimic counterparts.

Bulimics, on the other hand, are more extroverted and exhibit more somatic complaints. The bulimics also manifest greater anxiety, depression, and guilt. Of special importance, *kleptomania*, an impulse control disorder, is a common problem among bulimic patients but is seldom, if ever, seen with anorectic patients. In general, bulimic patients also show more characterological and personality problems. A specific personality disorder, *the borderline personality*, is quite common in patients with bulimia. These patients usually manifest symptoms of impulsivity, unpredictability, unstable and intense relationships, intense anger, and physically self-damaging acts (e.g., suicidal gestures and self-mutilation).

ETIOLOGY OF EATING DISORDERS

Although many etiologic factors have been offered to explain the various eating disorders, no single theory is universally applicable or accepted. The concept of biopsychosocial etiology can best be applied to the eating disorders. Biologic factors have been demonstrated in case reports of anorexia nervosa occurring in twins, siblings, and parent–child pairs. Further evidence of biologic factors points to the temporal relationship between the pubertal endocrine changes and clear findings of hypothalamic dysfunction in anorectic patients. Whether any of these hypothalamic alterations is primary and precedes the anorexia, or is secondary to starvation effects, is not completely understood. Further evidence for biologic factors contributing to eating disorders includes the high preponderance of affective disorders in patients with eating disorders and their families. Bulimic patients, in particular, appear to be at significant risk for primary affective disorder, and in one study, more than 40% of bulimic patients had previously sought therapy for depression.

Sociocultural Factors

The eating disorders are most commonly found in the upper socioeconomic classes of industrialized nations. Certain religious and ethnic groups (Jewish, Italian, and Catholic populations) have higher prevalence rates and may be at greater risk of developing the disorder. Social displacement or upward socioeconomic mobility may be essential to the development of anorexia nervosa in minority groups, especially blacks and Hispanics. The minority group anorexic adolescent is usually the child of professional upper-middle-class parents. Among other sociocultural factors is the Western culture's pursuit of and preoccupation with thinness. Unfortunately, young women are bombarded with multimedia messages to remain thin and "perfect." A recent United States National Health survey of 17-year-old girls revealed that 50% would like to be thinner. A survey of friends and relatives of anorectic patients demonstrated envy in 50% of those questioned for the self-control and discipline the anorectic exerts toward food. In addition, the mass media is bombarded with advertisements for diet sodas, diet foods, and diet drugs. One seldom sees an overweight model, actress, or Miss America.

Family Theories

Although family theories suggesting destructive forces within the family were popular a decade ago, the contribution of these theories to the understanding of eating disorders is not clear. These theories generally suggest that the anorectic is often the identified patient in a family that is described as enmeshed, overprotecting, and rigid.

Developmental Theories

Many adolescent and young adult anorectics clearly state that they do not wish to grow up. Most authors have emphasized the anorectic patient's rejection of adult femininity and her intense neediness. Psychodynamic theories share the same point of view, suggesting that the anorectic patient's behavior and starvation can be viewed as a mechanism to deny the assumption of the female sexual role and mature adult role. The loss of the normal hourglass feminine curve, the diminution of apparent breast fullness, and the amenorrhea all contribute to the "negative" feminine image. Additionally, the normal biologic urges of puberty may be defended against by the intense obsessive–compulsive control that the anorectic directs toward dieting and food intake.

Early Personality Characteristics

Some researchers believe that social insecurity, excessive dependency, limited spontaneity, and perfectionism are probably among the early signs that predispose to the development of eating disorders, particularly anorexia nervosa. Patients who binge and purge, on the other hand, are more likely to have a history of childhood maladjustment and increased psychopathology in the family.

Others, such as Garfinkel, believe in a more integrated etiologic model in which biologic, cultural, family, and individual factors contribute to the onset of the eating disorder.

TREATMENT

Eating disorders represent a biopsychosocial disorder and therefore demand both medical and psychiatric treatment.

The first priority of treatment, however, is a complete and thorough medical evaluation that may be accomplished on an outpatient basis or, if weight loss is severe, on an inpatient basis. Medical personnel must inform the patient and the parents that the eating disorder is not of organic etiology but that serious physical consequences can and do occur. In addition, the medical team should emphasize the biopsychosocial nature of this disorder and the importance of cooperative work between the medical and psychiatric personnel. The decision to hospitalize a patient must take into account the patient's physical condition and if there is profound weight loss with physical symptoms, such as marked hypotension or bradycardia. Hospitalization should also be considered if the patient or family refuses to comply with the medical and psychiatric treatment and a significant and serious weight loss continues. Depending on the severity and the nature of the presenting symptoms, a decision can be made regarding the use of family therapy, group therapy, individual therapy, antidepressant medication, behavior modification, or cognitive therapy. Because there is no single precise etiology for the eating disorders, there is no single clear-cut effective therapy.

The type of psychotherapy and the possible use of antidepressant medication should be left to the expertise of a professional involved in the mental health aspects of eating disorders. Although many patients can be successfully treated by the primary care physician, the very nature of this biopsychosocial disorder suggests that a cooperative venture between physical health care specialists and mental health care specialists would lead to an optimal treatment program and a greater potential for a successful outcome.

ANNOTATED BIBLIOGRAPHY

Bruch H: The Golden Cage. Howard University Press, 1978. (By one of the leading authorities in the field of eating disorders; vignettes of almost biographical flavor are balanced by keen clinical insights into the illness of anorexia nervosa; applicable to both the professional and lay public.)

Dickstein LJ: Anorexia nervosa and bulimia: A review of clinical is-sues. Hosp Community Psychiatry 36(10):1086–1092, 1985. (Summary of theoretical and clinical issues concerning eating dis-orders, with an excellent bibliography.)

Garfinkel PE et al: Eating disorders: Implications for the 1990's. Can J Psychiatry 32:624–631, 1987. (Interesting paper proposing a risk factor model, perpetuating factors and their implications for treatment.)

Lucas RL: Toward the understanding of anorexia nervosa as a disease entity. Mayo Clin Proc 56:254–264, 1981. (Provides an interesting historical review of anorexia nervosa and presents the clinical ma-terial from a broad and varied point of view.)

Minuchin S, Baker L, Rossman B et al: A conceptual model of psy-chosomatic illness in children. Arch Gen Psychiatry 32:1031–1038, 1975. (Classic paper in the psychosomatic literature; gives an interesting family dynamic perspective to eating disorders.)

Yates A: Current perspectives on the eating disorders. J Am Acad Child Adolesc Psychiatry 28(6):813–828, 1989. (Excellent overview of literature on current thinking about eating disorders.)

44

Rebelliousness and Out-of-Control Behavior

Joseph J. Jankowski

Rebelliousness may be defined as an externally directed be-havior against parents or their surrogates, including the es-tablishment, society, authority in general, teachers, or a therapist. It can be difficult to evaluate clinically because within a behavioral spectrum it could be considered both normal and abnormal. At points along this spectrum, rebel-lious behavior changes imperceptibly from being acceptable to being of increasing concern. As this occurs, parents, teachers, and other human service providers tend to refer the child initially for a medical examination. As a result, the pediatrician is often the first clinician to examine such children, and he or she is expected to make clinical judg-ments regarding the seriousness of the behavior and the need for intervention. This chapter is intended to help the pediatrician make these clinical decisions.

According to Offer, all forms of adolescent rebellious-ness should be taken seriously. His studies, which have gained wide acceptance, reveal that the majority of adoles-cents get along well with their parents and do not perceive major problems between themselves and their parents. His studies dispute the normal adolescent phase of "intergen-erational conflict." In fact, normal teenagers feel good about their families, are proud of them, and like them. This work has shed a new light on "the natural rebellion of ado-lescents against their parents," which is now felt to be pathological. As a result, rebellious behavior currently is

considered to be clinically significant, even if that behavior is mild in its initial presentation. It begins as a mild problem but can potentially develop into a severe reaction leading to out-of-control behavior.

PRESENTATION

Rebellious behavior usually occurs initially at the develop-mental stage of identity formation, around the age of 13, when the adolescent is struggling to become an individual separate from his or her parents. Rebelliousness often begins insidiously and escalates slowly until it either reaches a resolution with psychological integration or progresses to a more serious problem manifested by out-of-control behavior.

The course of clinically significant rebellious behavior is not predictable. In some, it occurs intermittently and does not become serious; in others, it smolders for several years before either slowly burning out or progressively leading to a more serious problem.

Adolescents separate from their parents and develop their own identities at variable rates. Both intrapsychic and interpersonal factors influence this process. Reality issues such as acute and chronic medical problems, sexual or physical abuse, disfigurement, physical and emotional handi-caps, and the loss of a parent through separation, divorce, illness, or death often play critical roles.

Rebelliousness is less serious when it involves the selec-tion of clothing, music, and grooming styles that are at variance with parental expectations. A progression toward more serious behavior includes experimentation with drugs and alcohol, irritability, unprovoked fighting with the par-ents, or assuming a life-style totally different from that of the parents. If left unchecked, this later behavior might es-calate to lying, cheating, stealing, truancy, and running away. If it becomes out of control, the patient might run away, overdose on drugs, talk about suicide, or become as-saultive. At the extremes, the patient can demonstrate overt homicidal or suicidal behavior and can lose contact with reality. Such patients are unable to care for themselves and are at high risk of being injured, arrested, hospitalized, or incarcerated. Thus, what appears at times to be rebellious behavior might actually represent symptoms of a more se-rious underlying psychiatric disturbance, such as anxiety, panic, depression, mania, or psychosis (see also Chap. 36, "Depression and Suicide").

DIFFERENTIAL DIAGNOSIS

The differential diagnosis of rebellious and out-of-control behavior is as follows:

- *Developmental disorders* are usually first present in the early grades. If reading, arithmetic, and language deficits are still prominent in adolescence, the patient will invari-ably have problems in relating to parents, peers, and teachers. These adolescents are more likely to develop a poor self-esteem and become rebellious because they are frustrated by not being able to function adequately in a learning environment and by not being understood by others.

- *Personality disorders* occur in adolescents suffering from personality deficits that result in an impairment of social relationships with parents, peers, teachers, and others with subsequent oppositional, rebellious, or withdrawn behavior. Stress superimposed on such disorders usually exaggerates the symptoms and can mimic more serious psychiatric illnesses.
- *Oppositional disorder* includes a pattern of disobedience, negativism, and oppositional reactions—for example, temper tantrums, argumentativeness, and stubbornness.
- *Identity disorder* encompasses the impairment of social or academic functioning as a result of difficulty in identity formation such as definition of goals, career, moral values, and friendship choices, sexual orientation, and group loyalties.
- *Attention deficit disorder* includes attentional deficits with or without hyperactivity in acute or residual states. Such children display problems with impulse control as manifested by acting before thinking, quick shifts from one activity to another, difficulty organizing one's work because of competing external stimuli, and difficulty in postponing gratification (see also Chap. 35, ''Attention Deficit Hyperactivity Disorder'').
- *Adjustment disorder* is the result of a poor adaptation to psychosocial stressors. Symptoms often include a depressed mood, anxiety, anger, disregard for rules or societal norms, work inhibition, or withdrawal.
- *Substance abuse disorder* includes patients abusing drugs or alcohol either socially or continuously. They are often secretive, untruthful, and committed to continuing their pattern of abuse with physiologic or psychological dependency. Personality changes and deterioration in school attendance, grades, work, and interpersonal relationships are usually observed.
- *Conduct disorder* is characterized by a repetitive aggressive pattern of violating another's rights, such as the destruction of property, vandalism, rape, assault, and breaking and entering, or by a repetitive nonaggressive pattern of violating societal norms or rules—for example, lying, stealing, persistently running away, truancy, substance abuse, and disregard for rules at home and at school. Rebelliousness is often confused with conduct disorder.
- *Anxiety disorders* are usually noted as the adolescent separates from the parent. Symptoms of anxiety can manifest as fighting with parents, siblings, or peers, school avoidance, phobias, or increased fear during separation experiences such as changing schools, graduation, moving, or parental separation or divorce.
- *Post-traumatic stress disorder* is manifested by symbolic behavioral events that represent the re-experience of psychological trauma that was severe enough initially to evoke significant reactions of distress. This may occur after being sexually abused. Post-traumatic symptoms often include promiscuity, hypersexualized behavior, or perpetrating sexual abuse on others. Those who have been physically abused often express post-traumatic symptoms of overaggressiveness, self-destructiveness, and injurious or violent behavior directed at others.
- *Affective disorder* indicates an abnormal variation of two moods—manic and depressive. During manic phases, the patient is unusually active, demonstrating a physical restlessness, a flight of ideas, grandiosity, a decreased need to sleep, and easy distractibility. Depressive patients report a decreased appetite, insomnia, loss of energy, loss of libido, unusual fatigue, feelings of poor self-esteem, and an inability to concentrate. In a bipolar disorder, manic and depressive phases often alternate.
- *Schizophrenic disorders* present as social isolation, bizarre ideation, blunted affect, peculiar behavior, and impairment in personal hygiene progressing to the point of bizarre, controlling, somatic, grandiose, or persecutory delusions. Auditory or visual hallucinations may also be present. Such patients frequently cannot achieve or maintain prior levels of functioning in school or work and become embattled with parents, peers, and teachers.
- *Other psychotic disorders* include such entities as schizophreniform disorder and brief reactive psychosis, both presenting as schizophrenic-like disorders. Schizophreniform patients have no prior recognizable psychosocial stressors. The illness lasts for more than 2 weeks but less than 6 months. Brief reactive psychosis appears immediately following a stressor. Symptoms last from days to weeks, and there is a general return to premorbid levels of functioning. Included in this category are schizoaffective disorders that combine schizophreniclike and affective symptoms.

WORK-UP AND DIAGNOSTIC EVALUATION

Before an evaluation can proceed, the clinician must develop a trusting relationship and an alliance with the adolescent and an assurance of confidentially. Once these prerequisites are in place, essential components of the work-up include the following:

- *Chief complaint* defines the adolescent's problem by establishing the level of rebelliousness or out-of-control behavior. Information can be obtained by meeting both with the adolescent alone and together with the parent(s) as well as relatives, school personnel, or other human service providers.
- *Past history of patient* includes a past medical, developmental, educational, and psychiatric history obtained from the patient, parents, and records of other human services providers.
- *Past family history* includes the development of a genetic history of medical and psychiatric illnesses to help establish a differential diagnosis. This history should include data on parents, aunts, uncles, cousins, and grandparents and can be provided by the patient and parent.

- *Current family functioning* is determined through interviews with the patient and parents. An assessment is made of the family's capability to allow the patient to separate gradually. Is the family so enmeshed that it cannot allow a member to separate without a severe disruption, or is separation perceived as an abandonment? Are there current problems within the family that might negatively affect separation experiences (e.g., medical or psychiatric illness, death, marital separation, or divorce)?

- *Psychosocial environmental influences* include the type of activities experienced in the peer group and the patient's personal interests (e.g., sports, music, acting, photography). The type of community in which the patient lives and the social factors inherent in such a locale (e.g., poverty, affluence, and expectations) can be important forces in shaping behavior. It is also helpful to know whether adequate supervision is provided in the environment.

- *Medical examination* should include observation for birth defects, physical deformities, and highly visible problems (e.g., acne that has a high psychological impact). It is also important to determine the use of prescription and over-the-counter medications. Screening for venereal disease is mandatory if the examiner suspects sexual abuse or promiscuity.

- *Mental status examination* is used to evaluate the patient's pattern of thinking, including the presence of delusions, hallucinations, and suicidal or homicidal behavior. A determination should also be made regarding whether the adolescent is oriented to time, place, and date. Abnormalities in the patient's mood (e.g., depressed, agitated, hypomanic or manic states) should be described.

PRINCIPLES OF MANAGEMENT

- *Mild rebellion* includes behavior at variance with parental expectations, such as choice of music, hairstyle, dress, and clothing. An increased amount of time is also spent with peers. This behavior is within the range of normal, and parents are cautioned not to overreact or interfere with it. In most cases, the parents can benefit from support to help them tolerate these behaviors and not reject the adolescent or overinterpret the behavior as negative.

- *Moderate rebellion* includes behavior that might have an adverse effect on the adolescent, such as experimentation with alcohol, smoking, staying out late, provocativeness, and fighting with parents. In this stage, it is necessary to set firm limits to help prevent the adolescent's behavior from becoming self-destructive. The parents often require professional help to understand and respond appropriately to their child's behavior. They must be cautioned against fighting with their child as if he were a peer.

- *Severe rebellion* includes behavior that has an adverse effect on the adolescent, such as truancy, substance abuse, stealing, promiscuity, and lying. Parents will need professional help to deal with these symptoms before their child becomes alienated or driven out of the home. Such ado-

lescents can be treated psychiatrically as outpatients if the parents are understanding and stable. The child must, however, be capable of responding to limits and using the anxiety generated in outpatient psychotherapy to progress developmentally without severe regression. If severe regressive behavior occurs, the child may need to be hospitalized psychiatrically. Parental rejection is often a reaction to this phase of adolescent rebellion.

- *Out-of-control behavior* has a self-destructive effect on the adolescent. Examples include suicidal, assaultive, or running away behavior, school dropout, pregnancy, or living on the streets. During this stage, the child will likely require inpatient hospitalization and, afterward, placement in a residential treatment facility. Their needs for intensive psychiatric treatment usually necessitate a special clinical setting where a therapeutic milieu, psychotherapy, and psychopharmacologic agents are available. Treatment hopefully will avoid criminalization and placement in a correctional facility.

INDICATIONS FOR REFERRAL

- *Mild rebellion*—The pediatrician can discuss the adolescent's behavior with the parents and help them to understand and better tolerate these changes. It must be pointed out to parents that with this behavior, their child is slowly separating from them. These children do not usually require a referral. However, the pediatrician must follow them in case the rebellious behavior worsens.

- *Moderate rebellion*—The pediatrician can meet with the child and parent together or separately to discuss the rebellious behavior and attempt to help the parent set appropriate limits. Follow-up meetings with the child and parent on a weekly basis for several months is important. A child psychiatrist should be consulted. Early intervention is important because procrastination often leads to more severe problems.

- *Severe rebellion*—The child and parents should be referred to a child psychiatrist for diagnosis and development of a treatment plan. Severely rebellious adolescents require a complete psychiatric evaluation including assessments of the individual child, child–family interaction, and current family functioning. In most cases, the child will require individual and family psychotherapy that can be provided on an outpatient basis.

- *Out-of-control behavior*—In this extreme clinical condition, the child should be referred immediately to a child psychiatrist or to a child psychiatry emergency service or inpatient psychiatric facility. In this stage, the child will require a comprehensive diagnostic assessment followed by intensive psychiatric treatment including psychotherapy and psychopharmacologic medication. This treatment is best provided within an inpatient child psychiatry setting that has the capacity to contain the child and prevent him or her from running away and harming him- or herself. Children in this stage of rebellion often do not accept psychiatric services of their own volition. They often need to be court-ordered into a treatment facility with the help of a child psychiatrist and attorney.

Children at any stage of rebellion can be referred to a clinical psychologist for cognitive assessments and projective testing.

- *Cognitive assessments*—A battery of psychological tests are used. The results of the Wechsler Intelligence Scale for Children—Revised (WISC-R) allows the clinician to determine a patient's current cognitive and potential intellectual functioning. Learning disabilities can be assessed by the Diagnostic Reading Scales (also referred to as Spache), the Halstead Neuropsychological Test, and the Gates–MacGinitie Reading Test. Achievement tests such as the Gray Oral Reading Test, Wide-Range Achievement Test (WRAT), and Key-Math Diagnostic Arithmetic Test can also be helpful.
- *Projective tests*—Tests such as the Rorschach Test help to either determine the existence of or establish the parameters of psychopathological thinking.

ANNOTATED BIBLIOGRAPHY

Blos P: The function of the ego ideal in adolescence. Psychoanal Study Child 27:93–97, 1972. (Important developmental paper on understanding adolescent behavior including rebelliousness.)

Freud A: Adolescence. Psychoanal Study Child 13:255–278, 1958. (Treatise on general adolescent development with a section on rebellious behavior.)

Freud S: Three essays on the theory of sexuality. Standard Edition 7:132–243, 1905. London, Hogarth, 1953. (Earliest reference to adolescent rebellion.)

Johnson A, Szurek SA: The genesis of antisocial acting out in children and adults. Psychoanal Q 21:323–343, 1952. (Landmark paper concerning etiology of antisocial and rebellious behavior as related to unconscious parental influences.)

Offer D, Astrov E, Howard KI: Adolescence—What is normal? Am J Dis Child 143:731–736, 1989. (Updated version of what constitutes normal behavior/mental health among teenagers.)

Offer D, Offer JB: From Teenage to Young Manhood: A Psychological Study. New York, Basic Books, 1975. (Study of normal adolescent behavior including a section on rebelliousness.)

45

Street Drugs

Michael A. McGuigan

Street drugs are defined as psychoactive chemicals that can be purchased without medical authorization from a non-licensed dispenser for the purpose of sensory alteration. Street drugs, therefore, may be legal as well as illicit drugs or chemicals. Drugs that are commonly used illicitly include cannabis (marijuana, hashish), hallucinogens (LSD, PCP, peyote, mescaline), depressants (barbiturates, benzodiazepines, and other hypnotic–sedative medications), stimulants (amphetamines, cocaine, phenylpropanolamine), opiates (heroin), and inhalants (gasoline, glues, trichlorethane, and other solvents). Legal drugs that are widely used by young people are ethanol and tobacco.

Many studies have established the use, prevalence, and demographics of young drug users. Because the drug-use epidemic may well be a series of overlapping miniepidemics, one can anticipate that both the choice of the drugs and their popularity will vary with geography, time, and the age of the population studied.

Although recent surveys have documented an apparent stabilization or even decrease in drug-use prevalence among children, there is still cause for concern. Ethanol is still widely consumed (more than 50% of high-school students reported using alcohol at least once during the month prior to a 1987 survey), and more than one third of adolescent non–problem drinkers became problem drinkers in adulthood. Thus, not only is drug use a contemporary concern, but the pediatrician has a responsibility for practicing preventative medicine.

The discussion in this chapter has two goals. The first is to provide guidelines to help the practicing pediatrician identify and treat children with drug-related problems. The second is to provide an overview of the syndromes of acute overdose with cannabis products and with cocaine.

PATHOPHYSIOLOGY

The child, adolescent, or teenager begins to use legal drugs (ethanol or tobacco) in an experimental or recreational way. Street drugs may be encountered as early as the late elementary school grades. Peer pressure and a desire to be accepted may be contributing causal factors in the initiation of drug use. One of the strongest influences on a child's decision to use marijuana is that he has a friend who uses it. Other factors that influence children or adolescents to try marijuana include prior unapproved use of ethanol or cigarettes. Parental influence appears to be important for the initiation of ethanol use and the use of illicit drugs other than marijuana. It must be stressed, however, that the use of "legal drugs" (ethanol, tobacco) does not mean that the child will progress to the use of illicit drugs. The converse is also true: a certain number of teenagers will initiate marijuana use without prior use of either ethanol or tobacco.

The pleasure and excitement derived from "recreational" use may reinforce further use of the drug. A progression in drug use and a predisposition to dependence is recognized when the frequency of use increases, when the use of drugs interferes with normal daily activities, or when the drug is used for the purpose of dealing with stress.

As drug dependence becomes established, school, social, and family situations deteriorate. Depression and suicidal thoughts may be manifest. Full dependency on drugs occurs when the adolescent no longer uses drugs for their pleasurable effects but uses them to maintain a feeling of normalcy. By this stage, the victim's social environment has deteriorated and the physical health of the individual may be declining.

CLINICAL PRESENTATION

The adolescent drug user may present to the pediatrician in several ways. The child may come forward spontaneously or upon questioning with an admission of drug use. Indirect clues to the diagnosis of drug use may include a deterioration in family life or functional or behavioral problems in a younger sibling. Social problems consistent with, but by no means diagnostic of, drug use include deteriorating school or athletic performance, truancy, and law breaking. The difficulty in coping that many of these children have may lead to suicidal gestures. Adolescents who have drug problems may also present to the hospital emergency room with trauma or overdose.

Not infrequently, the pediatrician may examine young drug users for drug-use-related "functional" complaints such as fatigue, sore throat, cough, chest or abdominal pain, or headache. In any adolescent or teenager with these complaints, a contributing diagnosis of drug use should be considered.

The complications of chronic drug abuse are more commonly seen in adult populations but may also be found in older teenagers. Some of these problems are hepatitis, streptococcal arthritis, anorexia, weight loss, bacterial endocarditis, osteomyelitis, fever, convulsions, and renal disorders.

DIFFERENTIAL DIAGNOSIS

None of the clinical presentations are pathognomonic for drug use. Because drug-related medical problems have protean manifestations, drug use should be considered in the differential diagnosis of each specific complaint or presenting symptom or sign.

WORK-UP

Once it has been established that an adolescent is using drugs, the pediatrician must identify the drug(s) and assess the extent of use. An inquiry into the adolescent's drug history may include general questions about drug use at school or about social functions. Areas to explore are the settings in which the drugs are used and the amount of disruption in social, academic, athletic, or work-related life that can be attributed to the drugs. It is also important to try to identify the perceived benefits from using drugs. During this assessment phase, it is necessary to establish certain drug-related facts, such as which drugs, how much of each drug, and how often the drugs are used.

If the answers to direct questions appear misleading or the patient is uncooperative, the extent or degree of drug involvement may need to be established indirectly from the history of behavior. The pediatrician may have to seek information from the parents and the school representatives to obtain a history about an uncooperative child. Parents may be able to give a history of cigarette smoking, argumentative behavior, refusal to accept responsibility, irritability, and mood swings. Asking the parents about their child's friends may elicit negative feelings. The parents themselves may be feeling stress at their child's drug use, and this stress may be manifested as insomnia, short temper, or altered sexual performance. Interviews with school representatives may reveal a deteriorating school performance, such as declining grades, truancy, drowsiness in class, poor memory, lack of motivation, or the need for special classes. A review of the patient's past medical history is important and may reveal numerous functional complaints, involvement with a child psychiatrist or psychologist, or that the child has been and still is developmentally immature.

A physical examination is less likely to be revealing. There may be a recent weight loss or other evidence of the complications of drug abuse.

Laboratory identification of the drug(s) in question in blood or urine is likely to be unrewarding. A sophisticated analytical laboratory is required and, even then, the chemical assays are not reliable for some of the substances in question. Furthermore, many of the drugs used are eliminated rapidly from the body so that the analysis may be negative even in the face of regular use. Cannabis is relatively unique in that tetrahydrocannabinol, the active ingredient, is stored in the body for long periods of time, and metabolites may be detected in the urine for 1 to 2 weeks after use.

TREATMENT

Prevention may be the most important aspect of treatment. Although the use of any street drug should not be condoned, there is evidence that the younger the child is at the age of initiation, the greater the risk of progression in use and the subsequent development of serious drug problems. It may be sufficient only to postpone the initial illicit drug exposure until late adolescence to prevent significant drug dependency.

Once street drug use is identified, the pediatrician has the obligation to intervene therapeutically. Even for a cooperative child, clear-cut, detailed, and successful therapeutic approaches have not been established for the management of adolescent drug users, although certain general guidelines can be formulated. The therapeutic approach chosen will depend on the perceived severity of the drug use and the availability of resources.

In the early stages, before dependency and deterioration have occurred, physician-guided parental intervention may be successful. Lacking capable parents, a surrogate (social worker, counselor, teacher, athletic coach, or physician) may be effective. The emphasis at this stage is on educating the child and the parents regarding the adverse, and perhaps unappreciated, aspects of drug use. It is also necessary to help the parents and child build the child's self-image and to teach social and communication skills. These aspects may help the child to resist the pressure to use drugs that comes from his social environment. The clear relationship between drug use and automobile accidents must also be discussed.

Other approaches to the therapy of adolescent drug users include keeping daily records, self-assessment of leisure activity, and routine drug screening. Daily records should include the number, the time, and the activity associated with drug cravings, drug refusals, and drug uses. It is important that the patient learn to identify the triggers or stimuli for his or her drug use. Special emphasis may be put on the methods that the patient used to refuse drug use at any time. The adolescent who uses drugs generally has a problem in using free or leisure time constructively. Time needs to be spent in evaluating how unstructured time is spent, the degree to which drugs are used during these periods, and how and to what extent drug use is acting as a barrier to doing what he wants. Daily urine samples should be collected. The treatment period must be drug-free. Although spontaneous confessions of drug use should be encouraged, the requirement of a daily urine sample for drug analysis will help the adolescent achieve and maintain a drug-free state. Of course, not every sample needs to be analyzed.

More severely affected children may require more aggressive therapy, and the pediatrician should be aware of the local facilities available for treatment purposes. Outpatient or ambulatory care services such as social services, peer counseling groups, psychiatry, or adolescent medicine may be useful. Inpatient drug treatment facilities for adolescents may be unavailable. The adolescent who requires hospitalization for drug use will usually be admitted to a general pediatric ward or to an adolescent medicine or psychiatric unit. The ultimate goals of therapy are to change or dampen the stimuli for drug use, to establish alternate methods for achieving the rewards that drugs provided, and to change the adolescent's peer group.

Because there is no one clearly successful approach to treating adolescent drug abusers, the pediatrician must constantly monitor the effectiveness of whatever treatment program is started. Relapses are common. Treatment must be individualized, and the physician must consider both the child and his family.

INDICATIONS FOR ADMISSION OR REFERRAL

Inpatient therapy or referral to a tertiary care specialty center may be necessary if ambulatory care is unsuccessful or cannot be followed. Adult treatment centers usually do not accept adolescents and young teenagers and would not be appropriate for these patients. Unfortunately, many pediatric medical centers are not equipped for treating such patients.

CANNABIS

Cannabis generally refers to the active substances (primarily Δ-9-tetrahydrocannabinol or THC) that come from the plant *Cannabis sativa*. Marijuana refers to the flowering tops and leaves of the *Cannabis sativa* plant and is 1% to 3% THC. Sensimilla is the seedless unpollenated flowering tops of the female plant and has a higher concentration of THC (3% to 5%). Hashish, the crude resin from the plant, may range in THC content from 2% to 15%. Hash oil is a dark viscous liquid extracted from the flowering tops of the plant; it contains up to 22% THC.

Pathophysiology

The mechanism of action of THC is unknown. The psychotomimetic and physiologic effects are related to the amount of drug absorbed and the experience of the user. The potentially lethal dose of THC is in the range of 30 mg/kg.

Clinical Presentation

Patients who suffer from an acute overdose of THC demonstrate a nonspecific syndrome. Conjunctival hyperemia is common. Tachycardia and mild hypertension or postural hypotension may be noted. Skeletal muscle jerking and a fine tremor may occur, but convulsions are a risk only in individuals who have a preexisting convulsive disorder. Occasionally, a patient will demonstrate a panic reaction or rapid extreme swings in mood. The most common features of acute overdose are euphoria and central nervous system depression, poor coordination, ataxia, slurred speech, lethargy, and stupor. Frank coma and respiratory depression may occur in toddlers who ingest cannabis products or in adolescents who have also ingested other drugs. Significant symptoms and signs usually last for no longer than 6 to 12 hours.

Treatment

Most serious acute overdoses are due to the ingestion of THC; thus, the administration of activated charcoal orally or by nasogastric tube is recommended. Most patients will do well with just quiet observation in a normally lighted room. Panic reactions that do not respond to nonpharmacologic care may be treated with small doses of a short-acting benzodiazepine.

Indications for Admission or Referral

Significantly symptomatic patients may need short-term observation in the hospital. Infants or small children who inadvertently ingest THC should be hospitalized if any symptoms or signs develop within 2 hours. It is unlikely that a patient with an acute overdose of THC will require a transfer to a referral center.

COCAINE

Cocaine is a white, crystalline, water-soluble powder obtained from the leaves of the plant *Erythroxylan coca*; as yet, there is no "synthetic" cocaine. A major concern about illicit cocaine is its purity. Most street samples contain other chemicals, including, but not limited to, sugars, local anesthetics, caffeine, amphetamines, and phenylpropanolamine.

Pathophysiology

Cocaine is absorbed from all routes. Peak blood levels occur 30 to 60 minutes after intranasal application. The half-life of the drug in the plasma is in the range of 20 to 90 minutes. The pertinent pharmacologic effects are on the central nervous system, where cocaine interferes with the neurotransmitters, producing first stimulation and then depression of function. Peripherally, cocaine stimulates the sympathetic nervous system.

Clinical Presentation

The development of symptoms of cocaine intoxication is rapid. Symptoms and signs begin within 5 to 10 minutes. They reach a maximum within 30 minutes, and they may last for another 30 minutes. In a case of extreme overdose, the time between the onset of symptoms and the development of coma may be only a few minutes. Central nervous system abnormalities include excitement, euphoria, confusion, and apprehension. Mydriasis, hyperpyrexia, nausea, and vomiting may occur. Hyperreflexia and convulsions may give way to muscular paralysis, areflexia, and coma. Cardiovascular effects include tachycardia and hypertension. The respiratory rate and depth may be increased. Death has been reported from cardiovascular collapse, convulsions, or respiratory insufficiency.

Differential Diagnosis

The syndrome produced by acute cocaine overdose is similar to that of bacterial or viral meningitis/encephalitis, or poisoning with salicylates, antihistamines, amphetamines, or phenylpropanolamine.

Work-Up

The minimum toxic dose of cocaine has not been established. Even if it were, an accurate application to the impure cocaine bought illicitly would be impossible. Exposure to any amount should be considered as potentially serious. Because cocaine is absorbed from any mucous membrane, the route of administration must be established. The time of administration is also important. The duration of existing symptoms should be established. In a physical examination, the physician should try to document objective signs of cocaine intoxication, especially the vital signs and the degree of central nervous system excitation, in order to be able to appreciate future changes. Routine laboratory evaluations are not helpful in the diagnosis or management of cocaine intoxication.

Treatment

Because cocaine is absorbed rapidly, gastric decontamination procedures such as ipecac-induced emesis or gastric lavage are not warranted. If an ingestion has occurred within 1 hour, the administration of activated charcoal may be beneficial. If the overdose has occurred through the nose, the nasal mucosa should be irrigated to remove unabsorbed drug. Supportive care should include frequent determinations of vital signs, a cardiac monitor, and the establishment of a secure intravenous (IV) line. Significant hypertension should be treated with rapidly acting hypotensive agents such as nitroprusside, phentolamine, or diazoxide. The treatment of cocaine-induced cardiovascular abnormalities has included the administration of propranolol or chlorpromazine. However, the usefulness of either drug has not been demonstrated satisfactorily in the clinical setting. Convulsions should be treated vigorously with IV diazepam or phenytoin. If the convulsions fail to respond to these drugs within 30 minutes, thiopental anesthesia should be considered.

Indications for Admission or Referral

Any patient with a history of exposure to cocaine should be examined by a physician. All symptomatic patients should be admitted to a hospital for observation and care. The rapidity of the clinical course may preclude the transfer of the patient to a distant medical center.

ANNOTATED BIBLIOGRAPHY

AAP Committee on Adolescence: The role of the pediatrician in substance abuse counselling. Pediatrics 72:251–252, 1983. (Good review and approach to the subject.)

AAP Committee on Drugs: Marijuana. Pediatrics 65:652–656, 1980. (Good coverage of the basic concerns regarding marijuana use.)

Anonymous: Adverse effects of cocaine abuse. Med Lett Drugs Ther 26:51–52, 1984. (Brief rundown of adverse effects of cocaine use.)

Farrar HC, Kearns GL: Cocaine: Clinical pharmacology and toxicology. J Pediatr 115:665–675, 1989. (Good review of the pediatric aspects of cocaine.)

Kandel DB et al: Patterns of drug use from adolescence to young children. Vols I to III. Am J Public Health 74:660–681, 1984. (Excellent, though somewhat technical, epidemiologic study covering three aspects: periods of risk for initiation, continued use, and discontinuation; sequences of progression; predictors of progression.)

MacDonald DI: Drugs, drinking and adolescents. Am J Dis Child 138:117–125, 1984. (Insights, advice, and an approach from an experienced individual.)

Robins LN: Editorial: The natural history of adolescent drug use. Am J Public Health 74:656–657, 1984. (Summarizes and comments on DB Kandel's three-part study.)

Schwartz RH: Marijuana: A crude drug with a spectrum of underappreciated toxicity. Pediatrics 73:455–458, 1984. (Discussion of some of the lesser appreciated effects of marijuana.)

Weinberg D, Lande A, Hilton N et al: Intoxication from accidental marijuana ingestion. Pediatrics 71:848–850, 1983. (Case reports and brief discussion of common management problems.)

8

ALLERGY, IMMUNOLOGY, AND DRUG REACTIONS

46

Allergic Rhinitis

Irving W. Bailit

Of the estimated 17 million people in the United States with allergic rhinitis, 10% to 20% are children. Symptoms usually begin in the pediatric age group and often in the preschool period. Early recognition and treatment will provide necessary control measures. Only 5% to 10% of children with allergic rhinitis "outgrow" their sensitivity. Allergic rhinitis may be seasonal, perennial, or both. Genetically predisposed children in the temperate climates may develop seasonal hypersensitivity to trees (April through May), grass (May through July), ragweed (August through October), or molds (spring through fall). Perennial causes include animal dander, feathers, house dust, and indoor molds. The dust mite is probably the most antigenic factor in house dust. Sensitivity may be to a single allergen, but more often multiple allergens are involved. Foods are seldom causes of nasal allergy.

Nasal allergy causes increased hyperresponsiveness to nonallergic stimuli, such as sudden temperature changes, positional changes, smoke, aerosols, odors, and airborne particulate matter. Food allergy, atopic dermatitis, and bronchial asthma are also often present.

PATHOPHYSIOLOGY

Sensitization to inhalant antigens produces specific IgE antibodies that attach to the abundant mast cells found in conjunctival and nasal tissues and to the circulating basophils. On reexposure to the antigen, a series of enzymatic reactions occurs, causing the disintegration of the mast cells and the release of chemical mediators (histamine, kinin, prostaglandin D_2, leukotriene C, and TAME esterase). The effects are increased nasal edema, vasodilation, mucorrhea, and infiltration of eosinophils. Reactions may be both immediate- and late-phase responses occurring 3 to 12 hours after provocation. Added parasympathetic responses increase nasal obstruction and rhinorrhea.

CLINICAL PRESENTATION

Rhinorrhea is clear and bilateral. Because of the congestion, nasal speech and mouth breathing are common, as are manifestations of postnasal drip, such as throat clearing and nocturnal and early morning coughing. Paroxysmal sneezing and nasal itching are characteristic of the allergic nose. Ophthalmic symptoms (redness, itching, tearing) are especially bothersome in seasonal allergic rhinitis.

DIFFERENTIAL DIAGNOSES

Acute and chronic respiratory infections are the most common causes of upper airway symptoms. In the presence of purulent secretions, one should look for foci of infection in the ears, nose, throat, and sinuses. Nasal smears and cultures may indicate infection.

Sinusitis is a complication and a differential diagnosis of chronic allergic rhinitis. Approximately half of allergic children with chronic nasal symptoms have abnormal sinus films. Chronic purulent nasal discharge, fever, and cough are suggestive of sinusitis. A Water's view of the sinuses may be necessary for diagnosis (see Chap. 80, "Sinusitis").

Nasal obstruction from choanal atresia, foreign body, septal deviation, or hypertrophied adenoids must be considered. A lateral x-ray view of the nasopharynx may be necessary to exclude adenoidal hypertrophy.

Eosinophilic nonallergic rhinitis may present with the classical symptoms of allergy and with nasal eosinophilia.

An allergy work-up is completely negative. This condition is seen less frequently in children than in adults. *Vasomotor rhinitis* is a nonallergic rhinitis associated with profuse rhinorrhea and nasal obstruction caused by an autonomic nerve imbalance. It is also only rarely seen in the pediatric population.

Nasal polyps are uncommon in childhood but do occur in 10% to 20% of children with cystic fibrosis. A sweat test should be performed when polyps are identified. The triad of nasal polyps, aspirin hypersensitivity, and asthma appears occasionally in the adolescent.

The overuse of topical nasal decongestants may produce rebound swelling (*rhinitis medicamentosa*). Local vasoconstrictor drops should not be used for more than 3 to 5 days.

WORK-UP

History

A comprehensive history should indicate the relationship of symptoms to season, place, time of day, activity, and exposure to both specific allergens and nonspecific irritants. The onset, duration, and progression of symptoms, the response to previous management, and the complications are important details. The family history and past history of allergy will help confirm the presence of atopy. An environmental history should disclose potential allergens in the home, school, and outdoor environments.

Physical Examination

Although somewhat variable, findings associated with acute seasonal allergic rhinitis are pallor and edema of the nasal turbinates, clear nasal secretions containing eosinophils, conjunctival injection, tearing, and lid swelling. An examination for chronic allergic rhinitis may reveal frequent swiping of the nose (the "allergic salute"), a transverse nasal crease (the "allergic crease"), and facial elongation, gaping mouth, and malocclusion from chronic nasal obstruction ("allergic facies"). Darkening beneath the eyes ("allergic shiners") may result from venous engorgement.

Laboratory Tests

Children with suspected allergy should be skin tested. The prick method of testing to the inhalant antigens is safe, accurate, and noninvasive and is more sensitive and cost-effective than in vitro radioimmunoassays (RAST). With a strong clinical history, follow-up selected intracutaneous testing may be necessary. Food tests are less reliable and should be performed by prick test only. Positive skin test reactions are meaningful only if there is a clinical correlation. There is no age limitation to skin testing for allergies. However, in the preschool child, testing should be limited to those allergens that relate to the history of exposure or symptoms. Prick skin testing should be considered for iden-

tifying the atopic child, for determining the presence of specific allergens for avoidance, and for measuring the intensity of skin reactions prior to immunotherapy.

The presence of eosinophilia and elevated IgE may be helpful but not necessarily diagnostic or necessary as part of a routine work-up. Serum IgE levels over 20 IU/ml at 1 year of age and over 100 IU/ml at 3 years of age suggest atopy. Nasal eosinophilia may help distinguish an allergy from an infection.

TREATMENT AND MANAGEMENT

The control of allergic symptoms should be directed toward the avoidance of exposure and the use of symptomatic medication and immunotherapy when indicated.

The avoidance of indoor allergens such as animals, feathers, and house dust will often be sufficient to alleviate symptoms. Parents should be provided with detailed instructions for environmental control, especially of the child's bedroom. Nonspecific irritants such as aerosol sprays, tobacco smoke, and wood-burning stoves should be avoided. Humidification in the winter and air conditioning in the summer may be helpful. Electronic air cleaners are seldom necessary.

Antihistamines that competitively inhibit the effects of mediator release by binding to the H_1 receptors are the primary sources of symptomatic relief. The effects of these drugs are unpredictable, and trials with representatives of the six classes of antihistamines may be necessary. The addition of an oral nasal decongestant (pseudoephedrine, phenylpropanolamine, or phenylephrine) may be beneficial. Tachyphylaxis and excessive sedation may limit the use of oral antihistaminics. Several newer agents, such as terfenadine (Seldane) 60 mg b.i.d., may also provide relief. They do not cross the blood–brain barrier and do not usually cause sedation.

Allergic conjunctivitis may require flushing with artificial liquid tears or may require topical ophthalmic antihistamine-decongestants to supplement the antihistamines. Ophthalmic cromolyn sodium 4% is an effective prophylactic agent (one drop in each eye four times/day). Ophthalmic corticosteroids are not usually necessary or recommended.

Cromolyn sodium 4% (Nasalcrom) is available in a pump spray and should be used locally in each nostril four to six times a day for the prevention of nasal symptoms. There are no significant side effects, but supplementary antihistamines may be needed for optimum effect.

The topical nasal corticosteroids have proved to be effective when other measures fail. Hypothalamus-pituitary-adrenal axis suppression, mucosal atrophy, or candidiasis rarely occurs. A therapeutic trial should extend at least 2 weeks. The usual dose is two sprays to each nostril twice daily (beclomethasone [Vancenase]; Beconase 400 μg/day; or flunisolide [Nasalide] 200 μg/day). Alternatively, beclomethasone may be administered as one spray in each nostril two to four times a day. The dose should be reduced to the lowest effective amount. Short-term side effects of capillary bleeding and local irritation may occur, but tachyphylaxis has not been reported. Dexamethasone nasal spray (Decadron Turbinaire) may be used short-term only because one third of this drug is absorbed systemically.

Many double-blind placebo-controlled studies have shown that immunotherapy is over 80% effective in children with seasonal allergic rhinitis. Perennial nasal allergy often responds to immunotherapy with house dust mites but is less responsive to animal dander injections. Monthly maintenance injections should continue for 3 to 5 years. Immunotherapy should be reserved for those children who have a proven sensitivity, those who have intense and prolonged symptoms, and those who are unresponsive to other forms of treatment.

Otitis media and serous otitis occur more frequently in the allergic child secondary to eustachian tube obstruction and dysfunction. Hearing, speech, and learning may be affected and should therefore be monitored carefully.

Approximately 3% to 10% of children with allergic rhinitis will develop allergic asthma. In addition, up to 40% of children will have exercise-induced wheezing.

INDICATIONS FOR REFERRAL

A referral to an allergist should be considered for children with symptoms of sufficient intensity and duration, and those who are unresponsive to treatment. Children with chronic or recurrent infections might need to be referred for possible underlying allergic hypersensitivity, especially in the presence of a past or family history of allergy. Although some pediatricians do skin testing, allergy diagnosis must not be based solely on positive skin tests. Follow-up intracutaneous testing (usually best performed by an allergist) is often necessary to uncover suspected allergens.

ANNOTATED BIBLIOGRAPHY

Bailit IW: Pediatric aspects of allergic rhinitis. Allergy Proc 3:468–471, 1982. (Review of the incidence, causes, complications, and treatment of allergic rhinitis in the child.)

Kawabori I, Pierson W, Conquest L et al: Incidence of exercise-induced asthma in childhood. J Allergy Clin Immunol 58:447, 1976. (Study of the high incidence of exercise-induced asthma in childhood allergic rhinitis.)

Naclerio, RM: Allergic rhinitis. N Engl J Med 325: 860–869, 1991. (Excellent review of therapy for allergic rhinitis.)

Rachelefsky G, Goldberg M, Katz R et al: Sinus disease in children with respiratory allergies. J Allergy Clin Immunol 61:310–314, 1978. (Demonstrates the high incidence of sinus disease in the allergic child.)

Siebohm P: Allergic and nonallergic rhinitis. In Middleton E, Reed CE, Ellis EF (eds): Allergy Principles and Practice, pp 868–876. St. Louis, CV Mosby, 1978. (Lucid classification and description of allergic, nonallergic, and vasomotor rhinitis.)

47
Asthma

Allen Lapey

Asthma is the most common chronic lung disorder of children and the most frequent cause of medical hospital admission for children in the United States. Prevalence studies show that 5% to 10% of all children are affected. The incidence peaks from ages 10 to 12 and then gradually subsides during adolescence and young adulthood. Recent epidemiologic data suggest an increasing prevalence, especially in black children and in urban areas. There is convincing evidence of steadily increasing urban mortality as well. Correspondingly, increasing numbers of children are being hospitalized with asthma. Risk factors include a history of atopy, bronchiolitis, parental smoking, recurrent croup, and a home environment conducive to house dust mite proliferation. Over 50% of asthmatic children have their first attack of wheezing before 2 years of age. The common perception that most children grow out of their asthma is unfortunately a misconception. Although over 50% of intermittent childhood wheezers are asymptomatic by the age of 21, most retain their bronchial hyperresponsiveness on methacholine challenge and are apt to become symptomatic with viral, exercise, or antigen provocation in later years. The natural history is discouraging for those children who are persistent wheezers or highly atopic. Less than 5% have any likelihood of a long-term remission.

PATHOPHYSIOLOGY

The fundamental abnormality shared by asthmatic patients of all ages is airway hyperreactivity, resulting in varying degrees of smooth muscle spasm, increased mucous secretion, and inflammation. Normal subjects may demonstrate a similar response following an appropriate infectious or inflammatory insult. Hyperresponsiveness, however, always returns to normal in time. This does not occur with the asthmatic airway; it always demonstrates an abnormal response to a cholinergic, cold air, or immunologic challenge. This clear distinction between normal and asthmatic is the rationale for methacholine challenge, the infrequently used but highly specific test of bronchial hyperreactivity.

The theories of β-adrenergic unresponsiveness and increased cholinergic airway responsiveness have been proposed as alternative explanations for a basic underlying genetic defect common to all asthmatic patients. Neither fits well with known data.

Viral infections, especially respiratory syncytial viruses, parainfluenza viruses, and rhinoviruses, are the most important triggers of asthma in children, especially those under

5 years of age. Bacterial infections, on the other hand, have not been implicated as triggers of acute bronchospasm. It is important to differentiate between the mechanism of airway obstruction induced by viral insults and that from cold air or methacholine challenge. The latter is characterized almost entirely by spasm and hyperirritability of large airway smooth muscle. The former is an inflammatory insult with mucous membrane disruption and a tremendous mucous hypersecretion.

The hyperpnea of exercise is another common trigger of asthma and is most bothersome in adolescents with increased physical activity and those involved in competitive athletics. The bronchospasm is associated with heat loss from the airway surface and is, therefore, more pronounced in cold, dry air.

Airborne antigens, notably ubiquitous perennial indoor agents, begin to play a more important role in school-aged and adolescent children. Animal dander, dust, and house dust mites are frequently implicated, whereas seasonal pollens have yet to be conclusively implicated in pure childhood asthma without rhinitis.

Many nonspecific, poorly defined environmental irritants are also involved. Passive exposure to cigarette smoke, strong fumes or odors, smoke from defective wood stoves, and outdoor air pollution are frequently mentioned. A sudden change in the weather appears to be another factor and may be the explanation, along with viruses, for the epidemic of childhood asthma that peaks every October and November. Emotional factors must also be considered; for example, joy and sorrow can both precipitate bronchospasm.

Characteristically, the asthmatic response to an antigenic challenge is immediate (occurring within 5 to 10 minutes), mediated by IgE, and associated with the release of preformed and membrane-bound mediators that bring about smooth muscle spasm, mucus hypersecretion, and recruitment of neutrophils and eosinophils. This is often followed by a *late asthmatic response,* which is more likely to occur in patients with frequent or chronic asthma. The late response peaks 8 to 10 hours after challenge, long after the subject has recovered from the immediate phase.

In clinical practice, early and late responses most likely coexist and blend into one another. Late responses involve an inflammatory and cellular mechanism. They are more persistent and difficult to treat, and they respond poorly to both theophylline and β-agonist drugs.

Several physiologic and anatomic considerations can help differentiate the small child's asthmatic reaction from that of the adult. First, there is the application of Poiseuille's law: the resistance to airflow through a tube varies inversely with the fourth power of the radius. Small airways are more easily obstructed. Second, collateral ventilation through pores of Kohn and channels of Lambert is poorly developed in early childhood. This may help explain why the child's lung is more susceptible to atelectasis. Third, anatomic studies have shown that there is an increased percentage of mucous glands in the bronchial mucosa of children compared to adults. The increased secretions are another factor predisposing to obstruction.

CLINICAL PRESENTATION

A typical presentation of acute asthma is the rapid onset of wheezing, cough, tachypnea, and retractions in a previously well child 2 days after the first signs of an upper respiratory infection (URI). Other common scenarios include the athlete who runs without stopping up and down the field and who cannot catch his breath 15 minutes into the game, and the allergic child who has recently been exposed to an animal and has both an early and a late response. The child develops itchy eyes and sneezing associated with a constant irritative cough within an hour. The cough responds to a β-adrenergic inhalant. That night, however, 8 to 10 hours later, the patient develops progressive chest tightness and wheezing but has little relief from the inhaler.

Many children with asthma respond with cough or perhaps mucous hypersecretion rather than wheezing. Such patients typically cough at night; they seem better during the day, but they cough again with hard play or excitement. The diagnosis is established when the cough responds to maintenance bronchodilator therapy. Other asthmatic children are apt to be mislabeled as having recurrent pneumonia because every viral URI results in a cough, patchy segmental infiltrates on a chest x-ray, and perhaps a fever. Infiltrates are frequently in the right middle lobe or lingula. In reality, these infiltrates represent atelectasis from retained secretions, characteristically in those lobes that drain the least efficiently. Most of these patients have a history of wheezing, though not necessarily with each illness.

DIFFERENTIAL DIAGNOSIS

Just as not all asthmatic children wheeze, all children who wheeze are not asthmatics. The differential diagnosis between *bronchiolitis* and asthma in the young child is difficult, even when a documented respiratory syncytial viral infection exists. On the other hand, if clinical bronchiolitis recurs, the infant more than likely has asthma. *Cystic fibrosis* is an important cause of wheezing and cough and is often exacerbated by respiratory viral infections. Such patients can be recognized because they generally respond slowly and incompletely to bronchodilators. The diagnosis of cystic fibrosis is confirmed by a positive sweat test.

The wheeze and cough of *foreign body aspiration* begin abruptly. The chest examination generally yields asymmetric findings. Nonradiopaque objects are suspected when supine films or fluoroscopy shows asymmetric emptying due to trapped air on the involved side. Bronchoscopy with a rigid scope is indicated if suspicion exists.

Gastroesophageal reflux has been incriminated as a cause of chronic or recurrent pulmonary disease, but its role in otherwise healthy children remains unsettled. The pediatrician should remember that gastroesophageal reflux is a normal age-related phenomenon. The tests for pathologic reflux are often inconclusive, and the medical management of reflux is generally safe, allowing the physician to "buy time." Surgical intervention, with potentially serious sequelae and no proven pulmonary benefits, should be avoided if possible.

Several anatomic lesions can sometimes be confused with asthma. Although many congenital and acquired airway lesions can cause wheezing, they are not common. *Tracheomalacia* is caused by hypercompliant tracheal cartilage that collapses during expiration and may vibrate during inspiration. Expiratory stridor characteristic of tracheomalacia may be confused with wheezing. Premature airway collapse during expiration or cough causes incomplete clearance of secretions. The patients are chronically noisy breathers, which is accentuated by excitement, but they have no retractions or respiratory distress. They are frequently labeled "happy wheezers" and outgrow their problem. Extrinsic airway compression can be caused by vascular anomalies impinging on the airway, hilar nodes, or mediastinal masses. The wheezing is characteristically fixed. In the case of vascular rings, it is both inspiratory and expiratory. Chest fluoroscopy with barium and possibly a CT scan will confirm the diagnosis.

Finally, mention should be made of "pseudoasthma," a functional problem more common in female adolescents. Inspiratory wheezing is simulated by paradoxical vocal cord motion and is usually more noticeable when the patient is under stress. The obstruction can usually be overcome by asking the patient to *pant* rapidly, at which time the noise will clear. The clue in these patients is the unusually noisy and occasionally stridorous nature of their breathing, and their total unresponsiveness to standard aggressive bronchodilator therapy. Such patients are invariably symptom-free at night or when involved with activity, which is the opposite of asthma. An evaluation should include laryngoscopy to confirm normal glottic structure and function followed by a referral for speech therapy.

WORK-UP

History

The history is the most important aspect of the asthma work-up. Past wheezing episodes are carefully reviewed for age of onset, time of year, associated illnesses or allergic exposures, response to and side effects from therapy, and patient status between attacks. Are there other features to suggest atopy, such as eczema or rhinitis? Is there a past history of bronchiolitis or recurrent croup? Is there asthma or atopy in the family? Do the parents smoke? Is the child in day care? The answers to these questions should give the pediatrician a good sense of the mechanism triggering the child's asthma. Remember, the hallmark of the twitchy airway is cough, characteristically at its worst at night and during hard play or excitement. The frequency and severity of past episodes, as well as the status between attacks, will

guide the decision of whether to use maintenance drugs or medication as needed.

Physical Examination

Between episodes, the child with asthma may appear entirely normal. Airway lability can often be brought out, however, by insisting that the patient expire forcefully, which frequently uncovers end-expiratory wheezing. Chest deformities may develop when asthma becomes chronic. Pectus carinatum, increased anteroposterior diameter of the thorax, elevated shoulders, and slouching habitus are not uncommon. Despite chronic hypoxemia, digital clubbing is rare and should suggest cystic fibrosis.

The allergic child with asthma generally has facial clues: allergic shiners (bluish discoloration beneath the lower eyelids), a transverse nasal crease (secondary to chronic upward rubbing because of an itch), and gaping facies due to nasal obstruction and chronic mouth breathing. The nasal mucosa may be pale and swollen with a clear discharge. Sinusitis is suggested if the nasal mucosa is red with purulent discharge. The presence of nasal polyps in a young child who is wheezing should suggest cystic fibrosis.

An examination of the acutely ill asthmatic reveals a marked prolongation of the expiratory phase and air hunger. A pulsus paradoxus of over 20 mm Hg indicates severe airway obstruction. The pediatrician should remember to check for neck crepitus caused by subcutaneous emphysema and precordial crunch caused by pneumopericardium. Asymmetry of breath sounds between the right and left lung is not unusual in uncomplicated asthma, but unless it resolves promptly with treatment, this should suggest pneumothorax or a foreign body.

Laboratory Tests

The complete blood count may reveal eosinophilia but is otherwise usually normal. Total IgE is helpful in clarifying the allergic component of the patient's disease. Pulmonary function testing to determine the degree of airflow obstruction and its reversibility is the single most important test in evaluating the asthmatic patient. Pulmonary function tests, including at least FVC, FEV_1, and reversibility with inhaled bronchodilator, are repeated annually and more frequently if necessary. (For a further discussion on pulmonary function tests, see Chap. 172.) In complicated or refractory cases, a sweat test to rule out cystic fibrosis and sinus films to rule out sinusitis should be obtained.

TREATMENT AND MANAGEMENT
Acute Asthma

For the therapy of acute bronchospasm, repeated inhalations of nebulized $\beta 2$-adrenergic agents have become the preferred initial therapy. Isoetharine 0.5 ml, albuterol 0.5 ml, or metaproterenol 0.2 to 0.3 ml in 2 ml saline has consistently been shown to be as effective as subcutaneous epinephrine but with considerably less tachycardia, pallor, excitement, and nausea. Aerosol therapy is effective even in severe bronchospasm with little air movement and in patients who have become unresponsive to inhaled β2-agonists on the outside. In uncooperative subjects, many physicians now prefer terbutaline 0.01 mg/kg subcutaneously instead of epinephrine because of fewer side effects and a longer duration of action. Tremor may be a problem, however.

Inhalation treatments are continued every 20 minutes as necessary. Clinical response should be monitored by both repeated physical exam and peak flow measurements. If there has not been a sufficient improvement following the second treatment, intravenous access is established and corticosteroids along with theophylline are initiated. (There is controversy over the additive benefit of theophylline plus β-agonist and corticosteroids in emergency asthma management. Side-effects and the frequent need to monitor blood levels must be weighed against benefits; this has not been consistently demonstrated. For this discussion, theophylline will be included.) Methylprednisolone 1 mg/kg or hydrocortisone 5 mg/kg IV is effective. The patient should then be "bolused" with IV aminophylline, 7 mg/kg over 20 minutes, but it should be remembered that every 1 mg/kg in the loading dose will raise the serum theophylline level by 2 μg/ml. Patients who have received oral theophylline over the past 24 hours should first have a stat theophylline level and the loading dose adjusted to achieve a final serum concentration of 14 μg/ml. Aminophylline can then be continued at a constant infusion rate of 1.1 mg/kg/hr for ages 1 to 6 and at 0.9 mg/kg/hr for ages 7 to 12. Treatment with an aerosol β2-agonist should be continued, because the steroid bolus should begin to restore β-receptor responsiveness after 1 hour. If, after 4 hours of observation, there is no satisfactory improvement, hospitalization for continued IV therapy is indicated. All aspects of the acute management plan described above can be carried out in an office setting, with the possible exception of stat theophylline level determinations.

Once satisfactory acute control is achieved, the patient can be sent home receiving one drug more than he had previously been using at the time of the attack. For example, the physician should prescribe a β-agonist if the patient was on nothing previously, a β-agonist plus maintenance theophylline if the patient was previously on a β-agonist, and both of the above plus prednisone if the patient was previously on a β-agonist and theophylline. Any patient requiring steroids in the past for acute asthma can generally be assumed to need steroids again for subsequent acute attacks. Finally, patients using aerosolized beclomethasone who break through with asthma must be considered steroid dependent, and they should be treated with systemic prednisone until the airway obstruction has subsided and aerosolized medications can again be reintroduced.

Many preschool patients are seen with recurrent episodes of cough, some fever, diffuse wheezing, and, at times, rales. Segmental infiltrates on chest x-rays are common, more likely the result of atelectasis than pneumonia. Although acute bronchospasm is not usually associated, this nonetheless represents asthma. Therapy should involve an aggressive use of bronchodilators with consideration of corticosteroids acutely and anti-inflammatory prophylaxis with nebulized cromolyn chronically. It appears that most of these episodes are triggered by viral illnesses. Despite the radiographic abnormalities, there is little to justify the use of antibiotics.

Chronic Asthma

The goals of long-term asthma management are to prevent hospitalization and emergency room visits, to minimize school absenteeism, to encourage full physical activity and sports participation, to discourage secondary gain from chronic illness, and to do all this with the least amount of medication and minimal side effects. The major components of asthma therapy are patient education, avoidance of environmental triggers, and pharmacotherapy. The major groups of asthma drugs, bronchodilators, and anti-inflammatory agents will be discussed separately.

Asthma Triggers. Provocative stimuli vary from one patient to the next; however, certain principles apply and need constant reinforcement. Cigarette smoke exposure is a known irritant in children with reactive airways and must be avoided. In atopic children, indoor pets (particularly cats) should be avoided, both for the antigens present in dander and saliva and for the increased level of dust mites that they will attract. Dust mites have received increased attention as a possible important risk factor for the development of chronic asthma in children. Global epidemiologic studies suggest that asthma prevalence is increasing more rapidly in those countries where high humidity, wall-to-wall carpeting, and cold-water phosphate detergents encourage dust mite proliferation. Accordingly, carpeting should be discouraged, with appropriate vinyl dust covers (envelopes) provided for mattresses. In midsummer, when humidity favors mite replication, air conditioning and/or dehumidification may be helpful. Mitocidal sprays for carpets and upholstery have also recently been developed, but their clinical efficacy is unproved.

Upper respiratory viruses trigger the vast majority of asthma attacks in preschool-aged children. Day care places the susceptible asthmatic child at considerable risk. Whenever possible, asthmatic children should be placed in small groups in which contagious illness can be monitored.

Finally, asthmatic children should be steered away from sports that demand sustained exertion because of the likelihood of exercise-induced difficulty. Sports such as soccer may not be as preferable as swimming, for example.

Self-Management. Parents and eventually patients are instructed to monitor the cardinal signs of asthma (i.e., repetitive cough, tachypnea, retractions, and wheeze). In algorithmic fashion, they intensify therapy until control is again achieved. Home peak flow meters are invaluable and essential tools for objective assessment. All patients with chronic asthma are asked to document their peak flow twice daily and to establish their "at best" value. Any reading that is >70% of the "at best" value is considered good function; values of 50% to 70% necessitate additional maintenance therapy (e.g., increasing b.i.d. cromolyn to t.i.d. and adding a t.i.d. β-agonist as well). Peak flows <50% generally require intervention with systemic steroids and a call to the physician.

Pharmacotherapy

The pharmacologic approach to asthma has changed dramatically in recent years with the realization that, even in its mildest form, asthma is considered an inflammatory disease. Furthermore, there is growing concern that the steady upward trends in asthma morbidity and mortality reflect patient overreliance on β-agonist inhalers and theophylline. (Indeed, the prescribed therapy may be contributing to the disease.)

Cromolyn. Long-term maintenance therapy with inhaled antiinflammatory medication is now considered first-line therapy for asthma. With the exception of the otherwise healthy child with intermittent asthma triggered *only* by infectious insults or exercise, maintenance cromolyn sodium has become the drug of choice. Much of the interest in cromolyn has grown from the realization that theophylline is not tolerated by many patients, even in subtherapeutic doses. In contrast, cromolyn is essentially free of any side effects, which increases compliance and relieves parents.

Furthermore, it has become increasingly clear that cromolyn is effective in controlling nonspecific airway hyperreactivity. For smaller children, cromolyn is available as a 20% aerosol solution for use with a power-driven nebulizer. By age 6, children can advance to a metered dose inhaler with the help of a spacer; by age 10, the inhaler alone will usually suffice. Many comparative studies have consistently shown that cromolyn is as effective as maintenance theophylline.

As a first-line drug roughly equivalent to theophylline in efficacy, cromolyn is less likely to benefit the poorly controlled asthmatic who is already requiring full doses of β-adrenergic agents and theophylline. Such a patient will more likely require systemic followed by inhaled corticosteroids. Cromolyn is not indicated for acute asthma; its use is strictly prophylactic and as such has been shown to prevent both the early and late bronchial response to inhaled antigen challenge.

Corticosteroids. Reluctance to initiate steroid therapy in the setting of persistent or worsening asthma has eased considerably in recent years with the appreciation of the central role of airway inflammation. Indications for systemic steroid use now include: loss of β-agonist responsiveness; patients with respiratory difficulty despite optimal inhaled steroids; chronic low-grade asthma that persists despite full therapy; and patients who have consistently required steroids with previous episodes. One regimen is prednisone 2 mg/kg/day in two divided doses—up to 40 mg/day for 3 to 5 days until the asthma resolves, then tapering quickly over 3 to 4 more days. The tapering process prevents the psychological withdrawal and muscular aching that patients experience occasionally, even following 7-day courses of therapy. A brief steroid course is remarkably effective in clearing asthma and restoring responsiveness to β-agonist agents, and the risks are minimal. For the occasional severely involved chronic asthmatic, low-dose alternate-day prednisone can free the child to lead a relatively normal life without the major side effects of daily therapy. The patient is generally cleared with a 7-day course of prednisone. He or she then remains on 15 to 20 mg given at or about 8:00 AM every 48 hours. The dose can be slowly withdrawn in increments of 2.5 mg every 1 to 2 weeks, depending on the patient's response.

In adolescents and adults, inhaled beclomethasone, triamcinolone, or flunisolide has become first-line, long-term maintenance therapy for chronic asthma, even in its milder forms. Patients treated as such have consistently better lung function and less need for bronchodilators for symptomatic relief. In beclomethasone doses of up to eight inhalations a day, hypothalamic-pituitary-adrenal suppression is absent or insignificant. This is because the drug is extremely surface-active in small doses; although absorbed, it is rapidly metabolized by the liver. The only notable side effects are oral candidiasis and dysphonia due to deposition of larger aerosol particles in the oropharynx and upper airway. If the drug is prescribed with a spacer device, these problems are markedly reduced.

Reduced growth rate in prepubertal children is another potential adverse effect of concern; this is due presumably to inhibition of insulinlike growth factors. On the other hand, chronic asthma itself suppresses growth and delays the onset of puberty. In such a case, topical antiinflammatory therapy can actually stimulate growth.

At the present time, concerns about growth lead to greater reliance on cromolyn in prepubescent children, with topical steroids reserved for refractory cases. Clearly, more information is needed in this age group.

The effectiveness and relative safety of steroid therapy in the treatment of asthma, whether in alternate-day doses, topical doses, or short-course high doses, must be emphasized. The most tragic outcomes in childhood asthmatics come from a lack of treatment, not from the therapy itself.

β-Agonists. For mild asthma with intermittent wheezing less than half the time, an oral or inhaled β-agonist is the preferred drug. Either albuterol or terbutaline is preferred, given their enhanced β2 selectivity and longer duration of action. Children over the age of 8 years are encouraged to use metered-dose inhalers rather than oral drugs because systemic side effects are fewer and bronchodilation is prompt at one tenth the oral dose. Most children with mild asthma can be effectively controlled on two inhalations every 6 to 8 hours. Optimal airway deposition of the inhaled agent, which at best is no more than 15% of that expelled from the device, is dependent on a proper inhaler technique; this must be demonstrated and patiently reinforced by the physician and his staff. The correct method involves a single slow inhalation from end expiration (FRC) rather than from residual volume, with the mouthpiece held 1 inch from the open mouth. The lips should not touch the inhaler. Inhalation is followed by a 10-second breath hold, and the entire procedure is repeated 3 minutes later. In younger patients or those who find inhaler coordination difficult, various useful spacer devices have been developed. For the pre-school-aged child, many parents much prefer the improved control they can enjoy using a home compressor and nebulizer to administer β-agonist aerosol by mask or mouthpiece. With this equipment, β-agonist inhaler solution such as isoetharine 0.5 ml, albuterol 0.5 ml, or metaproterenol 0.2 to 0.3 ml is diluted in 2 ml of cromolyn or saline and the medication is nebulized for a 5- to 10-minute treatment of quiet breathing. This procedure requires essentially no cooperation from the child other than sitting reasonably still.

β2-adrenergic aerosols are also the preferred drug for preventing exercise-induced asthma. Two inhalations from a metered-dose inhaler immediately before anticipated activity frequently permit the athlete to participate successfully in strenuous physical exercise that he or she would otherwise have to avoid. Inhalers have the potential for abuse, especially when used by adolescents. The danger with the newer selective β2-agonists is not as much the direct toxicity of the drug as it is the failure of the patient to recognize that an inadequate short-lived response to therapy is an immediate indication to seek medical attention, not to continue taking more of the drug. This problem can be avoided with proper education and reinforcement.

Theophylline. The development of sustained-release theophylline preparations with essentially total bioavailability has greatly simplified the management of childhood asthma. There are still many physicians who consider theophylline the preferred bronchodilator for maintenance therapy of moderate (i.e., persistent or frequently intermittent) asthma. However, the drug has a low therapeutic index (i.e., a narrow range between therapeutic and toxic serum concentrations) (see also Chap. 173, "Therapeutic Drug Monitoring in Pediatric Practice"). Furthermore, many patients, not infrequently younger children, experience side effects of hyperactivity, gastrointestinal upset, and insomnia at therapeutic or even subtherapeutic serum levels. Finally, the drug

is at best a bronchodilator probably with little or no anti-inflammatory activity.

It is prudent to begin therapy with one half the recommended dose. The dose can be increased in incremental steps every 3 to 4 days until a satisfactory clinical response is achieved or a peak recommended dose is attained. Children aged 1 to 9, with relatively shorter theophylline half-lives, usually require t.i.d. administration of a sustained-release preparation with a maximal dose of 24 mg/kg/day, up to 600 mg/day. Older children and adolescents can usually be managed with b.i.d. administration at a dose of 18 to 20 mg/kg/day up to 800 mg/day. Theophylline levels should be checked when the conventional dose causes signs of toxicity or it fails to produce a good response. Standard anhydrous theophylline liquid or tablet preparations are rarely indicated in asthma management. There are many reliable sustained-release products now available, including bead-filled capsules that can be opened and sprinkled on food for younger children. Both Slo-BID and Theodur are particularly reliable in their absorption characteristics and can provide continuous therapeutic levels with b.i.d. administration in older children and t.i.d. administration in children ages 1 to 9. Although the therapeutic range of serum levels is stated as 10 to 20 µg/ml, it is preferable to aim for levels in the lower end of the range. Otherwise, a temporary reduction in clearance could result in toxicity. To complicate matters, several common drugs (such as erythromycin), diet, and coexisting conditions can influence clearance. It must be remembered that there is nothing magical about a therapeutic level. Many mildly involved patients have complete control of their asthma with no side effects on low doses and "subtherapeutic" levels. When to stop the drug is usually not completely clear; it is wise to have the patient symptom-free for at least 1 week before maintenance therapy is discontinued.

INDICATIONS FOR REFERRAL

Asthma is often a chronic disease requiring a comprehensive and long-term therapeutic approach. Episodic intervention must be replaced by anticipatory care. For physicians willing to devote the time, long-term asthma management can be one of the most gratifying experiences in pediatrics. In this respect, referrals are generally unnecessary and may actually interfere with physician–patient communication. This is certainly true of mild and moderate asthma. Referral is more likely necessary for management of severe chronic, steroid-dependent asthma, and for diagnostic clarification of suspected allergic factors in asthma.

It should be remembered that there is no evidence that therapy of any sort, even by the most sophisticated subspecialist, influences the natural history of the disease. Nonetheless, proper patient and family education, stressing anticipatory care and self-management, has been effective in improving patient self-esteem and the overall quality of life.

ANNOTATED BIBLIOGRAPHY

Cropp GJA: Special features of asthma in children. Chest 87:555, 1985. (Particularly strong discussion of epidemiology, risk factors, and prognosis.)

Ellis EF: Asthma in childhood. J Allergy Clin Immunol 72:526, 1983. (Lucid, concise discussion by one of the acknowledged leaders in the field.)

Gergen PJ, Weiss KB: Changing patterns of asthma hospitalization among children: 1979 to 1987. JAMA 264:1688–1692, 1990. (Disturbing epidemiologic data.)

Guidelines for the diagnosis and management of asthma. Washington, DC: US Department of Health and Human Services; 1991. US Dept of Health and Human Services publication 91–3042. (The expert panel's long-awaited and comprehensive report on the diagnosis, treatment, and prevention of asthma.)

Reed CE: Aerosol steroids as primary treatment of mild asthma. N Engl J Med 325:425–426, 1991. (Cogent summary of arguments for and against inhaled steroids as first-line asthma therapy.)

Sears MR, Taylor DR, Print CG et al: Regular inhaled beta-agonist treatment in bronchial asthma. Lancet 336:1391–1396, 1990. (Makes a strong case that our therapy may actually be contributing to asthma morbidity.)

Sporik R, Holgate S, Platts-Mills T, Cogswell J: Exposure to house dust mite allergen and the development of asthma in childhood: A prospective study. N Engl J Med 323:502–507, 1990. (10-year follow-up study that links the development of chronic asthma with high levels of dust mite exposure; cause and effect?)

Weiss KB: Changing patterns of asthma mortality: Identifying target populations at high risk. JAMA 264:1683–1687, 1990. (More disturbing epidemiologic data.)

48

Anaphylaxis—Outside the Emergency Room

Irving W. Bailit

Anaphylaxis is the most frightening unanticipated and potentially fatal hypersensitivity reaction. Reaction may occur within minutes of provocation. The rapidity of the reaction is related directly to the intensity. Because of the imminent danger of such reactions, the physician must be knowledgeable of the causes and the means of prevention, and he or she must be prepared to offer emergency treatment.

PATHOPHYSIOLOGY

A massive release of the chemical mediators of anaphylaxis may be the result of specific antigen–antibody (IgE) interaction from prior sensitization or may occur from a number of non-IgE–mediated mechanisms. In either type of reaction there is a basophil and mast cell disintegration and a release of histamine, leukotrienes, prostaglandins, and platelet activating factors. Nonallergic responses may involve immune complexes and the activation of complement (anti-IgA reactions), the direct basophil and mast cell release of mediators (radio-contrast reactions), or arachidonic acid metabolism (aspirin hypersensitivity). The major pathologic findings are edema of the larynx and upper airway (the primary cause of death in children), acute pulmonary hyperinflation, and cardiovascular collapse secondary to hypovolemia and shock. The site of the reaction is dependent more on the host than on the provoking source.

CLINICAL PRESENTATION

Initial symptoms begin with flushing, increased warmth, and generalized pruritus followed by urticaria and angioedema. Reactions may lead to stridor and hoarseness, dyspnea and wheezing, dysphagia, vomiting, cramps and diarrhea, lightheadedness, and loss of consciousness.

WORK-UP
History

The following is a list of the most common causes of anaphylaxis, and the history should explore recent exposure to these offending agents:

- Drugs—Penicillin and its synthetic derivatives are the most common causes of anaphylaxis, followed by aspirin and the nonsteroidal antiinflammatory agents. The cephalosporins may cross-react with penicillin. Other drugs include insulin, ACTH, codeine, morphine, and the non–β-lactam antibiotics (see Chap. 49, "Drug Allergy").
- Biologicals—Antiserum, toxoids, egg-based vaccines, gamma globulin, and chymotrypsin
- Diagnostic agents—Radiocontrast materials
- Foods—Especially milk, eggs, nuts, legumes, fish, shellfish, and berries (see Chap. 50 "Adverse Reactions to Food")
- Hymenoptera venoms—Honeybee, yellow jacket, hornet, wasp, and fire ant (see Chap. 71 "Insect Bites and Infestations")
- Allergy extracts—Diagnostic and therapeutic allergens given by injection
- Physical agents—Cold-induced anaphylaxis, exercise-induced and postprandial exercise-induced anaphylaxis
- Injectables—Dextran and nitrofurantoin. Blood transfusion in sensitized IgA-deficient patients
- Idiopathic—Despite extensive studies, the cause of many anaphylactic reactions is unknown.

Physical Examination

Depending on the severity and duration of an episode, an examination will reveal flushing and regional or generalized urticaria with or without associated angioedema. Edema of the tongue, uvula, or larynx may cause stridor, retraction, or cyanosis. Lower airway obstruction will be manifested by a cough and wheezing. Cardiovascular effects are hypotension, a thready or irregular pulse, and signs of shock.

The presence of these clinical manifestations, combined with the history of a compatible temporal association with a likely etiologic agent, is diagnostic of an anaphylactic reaction. However, it should be remembered that many such episodes are idiopathic in origin. The diagnosis of the cause is based on a history and studies to determine allergic antibody. Laboratory studies are not usually necessary for diagnosis of the acute episode but may be helpful in monitoring the reaction.

TREATMENT

The possibility of an anaphylactic reaction must be anticipated in all patients receiving drugs or diagnostic or therapeutic materials. The atopic patient is more susceptible to anaphylaxis. Early identification and treatment are important. Necessary medications and equipment should be readily available for monitoring and treatment. Necessary office equipment should include tourniquets, needles and syringes, an arm board, intravenous tubing, parenteral fluids, oxygen, an ambu bag, oral airways, and a cricothyrotomy tube or No. 12 needle (see Appendix E.)

The most important drug is epinephrine (Adrenalin) 1:1000 0.1 to 0.5 ml max (0.01 ml/kg) given subcutaneously or intramuscularly. The dose may be repeated at 15- to 20-minute intervals three times. In the presence of cardiovascular collapse, epinephrine is diluted in 10 ml saline, and 1 to 2 ml is given slowly over several minutes intravenously. If the antigen is introduced by injection or venom sting on an extremity, then epinephrine may be given subcutaneously (0.1–0.2 ml) at the site. A tourniquet should be applied proximally to reduce antigen absorption.

In the presence of urticaria and angioedema, epinephrine should be followed with diphenhydramine (Benadryl). This drug may be administered orally or intramuscularly 10 to 25 mg in younger children and 25 to 50 mg in older children. With severe reactions, one should treat intravenously (2 mg/kg) up to 50 mg/dose over several minutes. Benadryl should be continued orally for the next 48 hours (5 mg/kg/day).

In the presence of wheezing unresponsive to epinephrine, isoetharine (Bronkosol) or $\beta2$ agonists such as metaproterenol (Alupent) or albuterol (Ventolin, Proventil) may be given by nebulization. Continued wheezing warrants the use of aminophylline (5–7 mg/kg) in IV solution over 20 minutes, followed, if necessary, with an infusion of 0.6 to 1.0 ml/kg/hr. Theophylline levels should be monitored.

Treatment of hypotension is by rapid infusion of intravenous saline or volume expanders. Dopamine or dobutamine may be infused at 2–20 μg/kg/min to treat shock. Alternatively, vasopressor agents such as metaraminol (Aramine) 0.4 mg/kg given slowly in 500 ml of 5% D/W, or

levarterenol bitartrate (Levophed) 1 mg (1 ml) in 250 ml of 5% D/W at 0.5 ml/min in children or 4 mg (4 ml) in 1000 ml of 5% D/W at a rate of 1 to 2 ml/min in adults, may be necessary to control hypotension. Blood pressure and cardiac rate should be closely checked.

Corticosteroids are not useful as initial treatment of anaphylaxis but may be indicated for secondary or delayed symptoms. Either hydrocortisone (Solu-Cortef) 7 mg/kg followed by 7 mg/kg/24 hr at 4- to 6-hour intervals or methylprednisolone (Solu-Medrol) 2 mg/kg followed by 2 mg/kg/24 hr may be used.

It is important that vital signs be monitored frequently. Oxygen should be available and used when needed. Acute upper airway obstruction may require a cricothyrotomy tube or a No. 12 needle to establish a temporary airway. Initial treatment of anaphylaxis should take place in the office. Unresponsive patients should be transferred to hospital intensive care units for continued care.

PREVENTION

Most anaphylactic reactions are preventable. A complete history should uncover previous history of anaphylaxis, adverse drug reactions, and allergic reactions to foods, venoms, vaccines, and diagnostic agents.

Drugs

Any history of adverse drug reactions must be considered as a possible cause of anaphylaxis. A review of previous medical records or skin testing may rule out drug allergy. Alternative drugs should be used whenever possible. Oral medications are less likely to cause systemic reactions. In serious clinical situations where penicillin is mandatory, testing to both the major and minor antigenic determinants of penicillin is both safe and accurate. Children with negative reactions may be safely treated with penicillin. Positive skin reactors should avoid penicillin and its derivatives or undergo oral desensitization. Unfortunately, testing to most drugs is not possible.

Vaccines

Routine childhood immunizations should be maintained so that heterologous antiserum does not become necessary. Children with known egg hypersensitivity may react to viral vaccines grown on chick embryo. Skin testing with diluted vaccine should precede administration. One should test first by the prick method with a 1:10 dilution of vaccine. If there is no reaction after 15 minutes, one should proceed to intradermal testing with a 1:100 dilution. If there is still no reaction (less than 5 mm), the vaccine may be safely administered. If the reaction is positive, desensitization can be done. It is best performed by trained personnel who are prepared to treat anaphylaxis. For further details, see the current Red Book of the American Academy of Pediatrics.

Foods

Foods should be introduced cautiously to atopic children. Known food reactions should be avoided. Questionable reactions may be proved by prick skin testing or by radioimmunoassay testing (RAST), although delayed reactions may require dietary elimination and challenge for diagnoses. Although most food sensitivity clears with increasing age, certain food allergies, such as to nuts and fish, may persist for a lifetime.

Radiocontrast Material

Previous reactors should avoid reexposure. However, when repeated studies become necessary, one should pretreat with prednisone 50 mg orally every 6 hours for three doses before the study, and diphenhydramine (Benadryl) 50 mg IM 1 hour before the procedure. The use of nonionic contrast media will also reduce anaphylactic reactions.

Hymenoptera

Children with urticarial responses only to venom stings are not believed to be at risk for systemic anaphylaxis, and immunotherapy is not recommended. Children with upper or lower airway obstruction or with cardiovascular symptoms and reaction to venom testing should be immunized to the specific venoms.

IMMUNOTHERAPY

Physicians who administer inhalant antigens and venoms by injection must be prepared to treat systemic reactions. Such reactions may be reduced by observing the size of local reactions as a guideline to antigen tolerance, reducing antigen dose during high pollen seasons and with new extracts, and observing the patient for 30 minutes after injection.

EXERCISE-INDUCED ANAPHYLAXIS

This physical condition is now being recognized with increasing frequency. Incidence is greater when exercise occurs after meals and sometimes after specific foods (e.g., celery, shrimp). Treatment includes limitation of exercise duration, avoidance of foods for 4 hours prior to exercise, and the availability of an epinephrine syringe.

Children with a history of anaphylaxis should wear an identifying bracelet. This may be obtained from the Medic-Alert Foundation in Turlock, California. These children should also have an epinephrine kit available (Epi-pen, Epipen Jr. from Center Laboratory Port Washington, NY, or an AnaKit from Hollister–Steir Laboratory West Haven, CT) for emergency use. The parent and child should be instructed regarding the technique of administration and indications for use.

Annotated Bibliography

Sale SR, Greenberger PA, Patterson R: Idiopathic anaphylactoid reactions. JAMA 246:2336, 1984. (Excellent treatise on idiopathic anaphylaxis—the scope of the problem, work-up, and management.)

Sheffer AL: Anaphylaxis. J Allergy Clin Immunol 75:227–233, 1985. (Current knowledge of immunologic mechanisms of anaphylaxis.)

Yaffe SJ et al: Anaphylaxis. Committee on Drugs, American Academy of Pediatrics. Pediatrics 51:137–140, 1973. (Review of causes and treatment by the Committee on Drugs of the American Academy of Pediatrics.)

49
Drug Allergy
Steven M. Matloff

Adverse drug reactions are an important clinical problem. This chapter focuses on the small subset of adverse drug reactions that can be demonstrated to have an immunologic mechanism, and the term *drug allergy* is used to refer to these reactions. Allergic drug reactions account for the minority (5%–10%) of all adverse reactions to drugs, whereas the majority (~90%) of all drug reactions are not immunologically mediated. Most of these latter reactions are due to either excessive dosage (leading to toxicity), side effects, intolerance, idiosyncrasy, or drug interactions.

An exact incidence of adverse drug reactions is not known, but estimates in hospitalized patients indicate a prevalence of as high as 6% to 15%, and drug-induced reactions may account for as many as 3% of hospital admissions. Thus, these reactions cause significant morbidity and mortality.

Epidemiologic data on drug allergy are difficult to obtain for several reasons. First, it is not always possible to determine if a symptom or sign is caused by the drug or by the disease being treated. Second, many patients are often treated with more than one medication concurrently, and it is difficult to determine which medication is responsible for the reaction. Third, ambulatory patients who have drug reactions are seldom reported, and therefore accurate statistics are difficult to obtain.

Certain factors may be important in determining whether an individual will have a greater chance of developing an allergic drug reaction, although in most instances it is not clear why a drug allergy occurs in a particular patient. Those individuals who have had a history of an allergic reaction to one drug seem to be at increased risk for developing repeated allergic reactions to the same drug and also to other drugs. The drug itself is important because some drugs (e.g., penicillin) appear to be more allergenic than others. Genetic factors may play a role, but this relationship is still not clear. Atopic patients do not appear to have a higher incidence than nonatopic patients. Multiple courses of a drug increase the chances of developing an allergic reaction to that drug. Certain disease states may increase the risk of reactions to certain drugs.

PATHOPHYSIOLOGY

Allergic drug reactions are characterized by an immunologic response to a drug or drug metabolite. This, in turn, produces a reaction that is manifested by the appearance of various signs or symptoms that do not resemble the known pharmacologic effects of the drug. Most immunologic reactions can be categorized according to the well-known Gell's and Coombs' classification. *Type 1* reactions, manifested as anaphylaxis, are those mediated by an IgE antibody directed against specific drug-related antigens. IgE is bound to the surface of mast cells and basophils, and when the drug antigens attach to specific antidrug IgE, vasoactive mediators (e.g., histamine, leukotrienes) are released from these cells, leading to anaphylaxis that can vary in severity from trivial to fatal. The manifestation and treatment of anaphylaxis are discussed in Chapter 48. These reactions occur within minutes to several hours of initiation of drug treatment, but reactions may also appear days after the drug is started. There is usually a history of prior exposure to the drug, but often this history cannot be elicited. The most common medication to cause severe and fatal anaphylaxis is penicillin.

Anaphylactoid reactions have symptoms similar to those of IgE-mediated anaphylactic reactions. In these cases, the drug is capable of directly or indirectly causing non–IgE-dependent vasoactive mediator release. The spectrum of symptoms is the same as that seen with true anaphylaxis. Examples of diagnostic agents and medications that may cause these types of reactions include radiographic contrast material, codeine and other narcotic analgesics, aspirin, and the nonsteroidal anti-inflammatory drugs.

Type 2 immunologic reactions are those mediated by the production of cytotoxic antibody (IgG, IgM), which binds to cell membranes, causing complement activation or inducing mononuclear cell activation. Penicillin-induced hemolytic anemia is an example of this type of reaction.

Type 3 reactions are caused by an immune complex formation (drug antigen–antibody complexes) that subsequently activates the complement cascade, leading to the generation of anaphylotoxins C3a and C5a, with subsequent mediator release and inflammation. Serum sickness is the classical clinical presentation and can be caused by several medications, but it occurs most commonly with penicillin and other antibiotics. Manifestations include lymphadenopathy, fever, urticaria, exanthem, arthralgia or arthritis, and general malaise.

Type 4 reactions are classical delayed hypersensitivity reactions and include T-cell–mediated immunity. Delayed skin reactions and contact dermatitis from topical medication exposure are examples of this type of drug-induced immunologic reaction.

WORK-UP

The diagnosis of a drug allergy is clinical in most instances because there are usually no immediate diagnostic tests that can help confirm the diagnosis. The history and physical examination are the most important tools in diagnosing a drug allergy. A clear history of the symptoms and their temporal relationship to drug administration, prior drug use, and prior history of drug reaction are all important. Symptoms or signs of drug allergy may be present while an individual is taking a drug. The drug dosage, the duration of therapy, the disease being treated, and concomitant medication use should be determined. Other underlying medical disorders (e.g., hepatic or renal dysfunction) should be known.

The patient will often have a history of drug allergy. It is best to avoid the drug, unless it is considered essential for treatment and no acceptable alternatives are available, or if the alternative medications themselves have caused unacceptable adverse reactions.

If no acceptable alternative therapy is available that is well tolerated and equally effective, the patient should then be referred for further evaluation and diagnostic testing (if available) or desensitization or test dosing (if appropriate). The following discussion reviews selected aspects of the most common allergic drug reactions. (For an exhaustive review, see any of the four references listed in the bibliography.)

PENICILLIN

Although penicillin and other β-lactam antibiotics may cause various adverse reactions, their propensity to cause immediate anaphylactic reactions is a major concern. Anaphylactic reactions may occur when the drug is administered for the first time, implying that the patient was sensitized by an occult source (foods, or by intrauterine exposure). Patients will often give vague histories of penicillin allergy but are unable to recall the details. These patients should often be assumed to be allergic, and penicillins should be avoided, as they should be in those patients with more convincing histories.

If a patient with a positive history requires penicillin, penicillin skin testing should be performed with both the major and minor metabolites of penicillin. The three reagents currently in use for skin testing include benzylpenicilloyl polylysine, penicillin G, and a minor determinant mixture (MDM) containing benzylpenicilloate and benzylpenicilloyl-n-propylamine (MDM is not commercially available at this time).

A positive skin test to any reagent, but especially the minor determinant, indicates that the patient is at high risk (50%–70%) for developing an anaphylactic reaction if penicillin is administered. Patients with positive skin tests can be desensitized by administering small amounts of penicillin and cautiously increasing the dose until full therapeutic doses are achieved. This procedure involves considerable risk and should be performed only in an ICU setting with an open IV line in place, resuscitation equipment available, and personnel in attendance. It must be made clear in the medical record that no acceptable alternative therapy is available to the patient; it is best if this is stated by an Infectious Disease Consultant. Most patients can be successfully desensitized, but it must be emphasized that the desensitization applies only to the present course of antibiotic therapy, and the patient would need to be reevaluated at a later time if it became necessary to readminister penicillin. There are few clinical situations in which penicillin would be the only acceptable alternative medication, and these situations occur generally in hospitalized patients with serious life-threatening systemic infections.

If the skin tests are negative, patients are at low risk of developing immediate (i.e., within the first 72 hours of penicillin administration) IgE-mediated reactions. However, false-negative results occur rarely, and for this reason patients with negative test reactions should also be given penicillin cautiously, starting with small test doses and gradually increasing to full therapeutic doses. Skin test results cannot predict the likelihood of developing delayed adverse reactions, which may occur more than 72 hours after the initiation of penicillin treatment. This should be made clear to patients before beginning a course of treatment.

An urticarial reaction will often occur while a patient is taking both penicillin and another drug, and in this situation, penicillin testing may be useful to help determine if penicillin is the likely offending agent. However, penicillin skin testing should not be done if alternative non–β-lactam antibiotics can be used in a patient. Penicillin testing should be considered only if alternative therapy has failed or is not well tolerated.

Caution should be exercised in administering cephalosporins and semisynthetic penicillins to patients with documented penicillin allergy. These antibiotics should be avoided in such patients if an alternative therapy is available, but they could be cautiously administered if necessary by using similar test dosing or desensitization schedules. The exact incidence of cross-reactivity between cephalosporins and penicillin is not known but is believed to range between 10% and 15%.

Serum sickness can be a manifestation of drug allergy and is caused by a variety of antibiotics, including penicillin, cephalosporins, and sulfonamides. There appears to be a greater incidence of serum sickness reactions with the use of cefaclor than there is with amoxicillin (see also Chap. 51, "Urticaria, Angioedema, and Serum Sickness").

AMPICILLIN

Ampicillin can cross-react with penicillin and cause anaphylactic reactions. A major cause of concern is its frequent cause of delayed skin rashes (usually maculopapular), which may occur after several days of therapy. These are usually not IgE mediated and may not reappear on subsequent administration. They occur more frequently in patients with infectious mononucleosis or hyperuricemia, or if taken concomitantly with allopurinol. Alternative therapy would be recommended. Skin testing can help in assessing the risk of developing immediate IgE-mediated reactions.

ASPIRIN AND NONSTEROIDAL ANTI-INFLAMMATORY DRUGS

These medications can cause severe life-threatening anaphylactoid reactions, bronchospasm, and generalized urticaria. There is a significant degree of cross-reactivity between aspirin and the nonsteroidal anti-inflammatory drugs (NSAIDs). It is therefore advisable for an individual who is sensitive to aspirin to avoid NSAIDs unless the drugs are considered absolutely necessary because of their anti-inflammatory effects and because no acceptable alternative agents are available.

If there is doubt about the clinical diagnosis of aspirin hypersensitivity, and it is essential to use this medication, the patient can be tested by cautious oral challenge, beginning with small doses (1 mg or less) and gradually increasing the dose every 30 minutes. It must be emphasized that this is a high-risk procedure and should be performed only by individuals skilled in its administration, and it should be done in a hospital ICU setting. Informed consent is necessary, and unequivocal indications for performing the challenge must be clearly recorded in the medical record.

SULFONAMIDES

These antibiotics commonly cause immunologic reactions, manifested primarily by generalized skin eruptions ranging from minor urticaria to life-threatening exfoliative dermatitis or Stevens-Johnson syndrome. Other manifestations, such as serum sickness, blood dyscrasias, and anaphylaxis, are also observed.

The treatment involves withdrawal of the medication and strict avoidance of sulfa-containing medications in the future. Test dosing can be performed, but it involves considerable risk and should be done only if there are no acceptable alternative medications. Cross-reactivity may occur with the thiazide diuretics, some oral hypoglycemic agents, and acetazolamide, and they should be avoided in sulfa-allergic patients.

LOCAL ANESTHETICS

Patients with a history of an adverse reaction to a local anesthetic will often be referred by dentists or other health care providers. In most instances, the reactions that have occurred have been nonimmunologic. Many of these reactions are due to vasovagal reactions, hyperventilation, central nervous system stimulation or depression, cardiovascular side effects, or side effects from other components of local anesthetics such as epinephrine. IgE-mediated hypersensitivity occurs rarely, and it is almost always possible to find an alternative local anesthetic that the patient will be able to tolerate by performing appropriate subcutaneous challenges. It is important to perform challenges with this group of drugs, if appropriate, so that they will not unnecessarily be avoided because of a history of a nonallergic adverse reaction. When true immediate (IgE-mediated) hypersensitivity can be demonstrated, other agents may at times need to be substituted, such as a local injection of Benadryl or general anesthesia.

IMMUNIZING AGENTS

Various adverse reactions to both passive and active immunizing agents have been reported. These can be either immunologic or nonimmunologic, and fortunately they are seen rarely. One major concern is the use of egg protein–containing vaccines in the patient with known or suspected egg allergy manifested by anaphylactic symptoms after eating eggs. These vaccines include MMR, measles, mumps, influenza, and yellow fever. (Rubella vaccine alone does not contain egg protein.) Patients who can eat eggs without allergic symptoms can be immunized with these vaccines without prior testing. Those with definite adverse reactions to egg ingestion or suspected reactions should be evaluated on an individual basis, weighing the risks of vaccination and the risks of not being immunized against the benefits of immunization.

Skin testing can be performed with measles vaccine. There is a desensitization protocol to administer measles vaccine to children with a history of egg allergy and a history of positive skin tests to measles vaccine. (See the Red Book of the American Academy of Pediatrics.)

Some vaccines such as MMR and OPV contain trace amounts of neomycin. A history of anaphylaxis to neomycin would contraindicate the use of these vaccines. DPT may rarely induce urticarial or anaphylactic reactions.

Immune globulin is rarely associated with adverse reactions of the anaphylactoid type. Patients with IgA deficiency are at increased risk for adverse reactions with immune globulin.

RADIOGRAPHIC CONTRAST MATERIAL

Radiographic contrast material (RCM) may cause anaphylactoid reactions in a small percentage of patients. Patients with a prior history of anaphylactoid reaction to RCM should avoid future use if possible because they are at increased risk of developing repeat reactions. If a diagnostic study is considered absolutely necessary, and no acceptable alternative diagnostic procedure can be performed, patients can be treated with diphenhydramine, corticosteroids, and (if not contraindicated) ephedrine before RCM administration. It is recommended that a low-osmolality RCM be used because of its lower incidence of adverse reactions. This will significantly reduce but not eliminate their risk of anaphylactoid reactions. If emergency RCM administration is necessary in patients with prior reactions to RCM, pretreatment is also recommended, but its effectiveness is still uncertain. Informed consent and documentation of the absolute need for the procedure must be clearly recorded in the chart.

PREVENTION

The best treatment of drug allergy is prevention. Patients should be questioned carefully before drugs with a propensity to cause allergic reactions are prescribed. It is important to establish a definite need for a drug before it is prescribed so that unnecessary drug administration can be avoided. On the other hand, it is important not to unnecessarily withhold appropriate drug therapy if indicated for fear of a possible drug reaction.

Immediate treatment of acute reactions is best managed by withdrawal of the suspected drug and symptomatic control with antihistamines. Epinephrine should be used if the reaction is life-threatening. (The reader is referred to Chap. 48 for elaboration of the treatment of anaphylaxis.) Corticosteroids should be considered for the more serious drug allergies to ameliorate late-phase reactions.

Patients should be made aware of their history of drug allergy and advised of the importance of future avoidance. Medical records should have drug allergies prominently displayed. Patients should be encouraged to obtain a Medic-Alert bracelet to identify drug allergy in the event of emergency treatment.

INDICATIONS FOR REFERRAL

Referral to an allergist should be considered for the following situations: limited or no therapeutic alternatives; desensitization; clarification of whether the reaction was drug-induced, or, if multiple medications were taken simultaneously, to help determine the offending one; severe parental anxiety; and any severe or life-threatening drug reactions. Unstable patients, and those who have had major anaphylaxis reactions, should be hospitalized. Those whose symptoms appear to be progressing should be referred immediately to an Emergency Department.

ANNOTATED BIBLIOGRAPHY

DeSwarte RD: Drug allergy. In Patterson R (ed): Allergic Diseases: Diagnosis and Management, 3rd ed, pp 505–661. Philadelphia, JB Lippincott, 1985. (State-of-the art review; well referenced.)

Goldstein RA, Patterson R (eds): Supplement symposium proceedings on drug allergy: Prevention, diagnosis, treatment. J Allerg Clin Immunol 74(4), 1984. (Excellent coverage of various clinically relevant topics.)

VanArsdel PP Jr: Adverse drug reactions. In Middleton E Jr, Reed CE, Ellis EF (eds): Allergy: Principles and Practice, 3rd ed. St. Louis, CV Mosby, 1988. (Excellent overall review of drug reactions.)

VanArsdel PP Jr: Drug hypersensitivity. In Bierman CW, Pearlman DS (eds): Allergic Diseases From Infancy to Adulthood, 2nd ed, pp 684–709. Philadelphia, WB Saunders, 1988. (Another excellent review.)

50

Adverse Reactions to Foods

Steven M. Matloff

The primary care physician is often consulted by patients or their parents because of a symptom or group of signs and symptoms believed to be caused by food ingestion. The physician's task is to determine if the symptoms are related to food, or if there is another cause of the symptom complex. If the adverse reaction is found to be food related, the physician must then also determine if the etiology is immunologic or nonimmunologic. The term *food allergy* is reserved for those reactions that have an immunologic mechanism. *Food intolerance* is the term applied to nonimmunologic mechanisms.

An accurate prevalence of food allergy is not known, but food allergies are estimated to be present in 1%–3% of the pediatric population. In general, this problem seems to be more common in children, but the onset of allergic and nonallergic reactions can occur at any age. Many children will outgrow their food allergy, although this is often dependent on the type of food involved. For example, it is not uncommon to see a child outgrow a food allergy to milk or eggs. However, a food allergy to peanuts, tree nuts, or fish is more likely to remain for life.

PATHOPHYSIOLOGY

The most common immunologic reaction that leads to classical food allergy is the Type I immediate hypersensitivity reaction, mediated by food allergen–specific IgE. An IgE antibody directed toward a specific food allergen is probably produced as a result of a poorly defined genetic or acquired susceptibility. There may be an alteration in the normal gastrointestinal immunologic or nonimmunologic processing of food antigens in these individuals. It is not clear what predisposes an individual to develop an allergic response to food. The food-specific IgE will not, by itself, cause direct symptoms but will strongly adhere to specific receptors on the membrane surface of mast cells and basophils. When the patient is reexposed to the same or a similar cross-reactive food allergen, these allergens will bind to cell-bound IgE, initiating a cascade of biochemical events that results in the local or systemic release of histamine and other vasoactive mediators. These chemical mediators, in turn, exert their effects on the blood vessels, respiratory tract, myocardium, and gastrointestinal tract, accounting for the range of symptoms of anaphylaxis.

Nonallergic reactions may produce symptoms by the direct, non–IgE-mediated release of mast cell mediators, or they may produce symptoms by other mechanisms that are not mast cell–dependent. A detailed discussion of these nonallergic mechanisms is beyond the scope of this discussion.

CLINICAL PRESENTATION

The symptoms may be localized to one site or one organ system or may include the full constellation of anaphylactic symptoms. The latter includes cutaneous symptoms (angioedema, urticaria, pruritus), respiratory symptoms (laryngeal edema, oropharyngeal pruritus, or swelling, wheezing, chest tightness, or cough), gastrointestinal symptoms (nausea, vomiting, crampy abdominal pain, diarrhea), and vascular symptoms (lightheadedness, hypotension).

Anaphylactic food reactions are the easiest to recognize because the symptoms and signs are generally well-defined and often striking, and the presence of allergen-specific IgE can almost always be confirmed. The most common foods that produce this type of allergic reaction include (but are not limited to) peanuts, nuts, shellfish, eggs, milk, seeds, and fruits. The clinician will typically see the patient either during the acute episode, when clinical symptoms are manifest, or after their resolution, when the signs and symptoms have abated. It is important to establish the temporal relationship between the time of food ingestion and the onset of symptoms, because the shorter this time interval is, the more likely that the food can be confirmed to be the trigger of the adverse reaction (allergic or nonallergic).

DIFFERENTIAL DIAGNOSIS

Adverse reactions to foods can be produced by many medical conditions (see display entitled "Differential Diagnosis of Adverse Food Reactions"). Various gastrointestinal disorders such as reflux esophagitis, gastric or duodenal ulcer, celiac sprue, lactose intolerance, cholelithiasis, and achalasia will present with food-induced symptoms. Many infectious diseases produce prominent gastrointestinal symptoms, such as infection with *Salmonella, Shigella, Vibrio parahaemolyticus, Giardia,* and *Trichinella,* and hepatitis and botulism. Various food toxins, both endogenous and exogenous, may be implicated. Examples are scombroid poisoning, mushroom poisoning, and paralytic shellfish poisoning. Many foods contain endogenous pharmacologi-

Differential Diagnosis of Adverse Food Reactions

1. Food allergy
   a. IgE mediated
   b. Other immunologic mechanisms
2. Pseudoallergic conditions
   a. Foods containing vasoactive mediators
   b. Foods causing direct histamine release
3. Additive reactions
4. Gastrointestinal disorders
5. Infectious diseases
6. Metabolic conditions
7. Toxins
8. Psychogenic conditions
9. Postprandial exercise-induced anaphylaxis

cally active ingredients, such as histamine, dopamine, and serotonin, that may produce symptoms indistinguishable from classical IgE-mediated symptoms.

WORK-UP

The history is the most important diagnostic aid in the work-up of food-induced reactions. Meticulous attention should be given to the presenting signs and symptoms, their severity, their temporal relationship to the intake of concomitant foods, beverages, or drugs, and the state of the food (e.g., processed, cooked, fresh, or uncooked). The relationship between exercise and eating, the presence of atopic disease, and the potential contamination of the food by toxins, additives, or antibiotics are important historical features. A thorough analysis, if possible, of a food or meal may be necessary to elucidate the source of a food reaction. It should be determined if the child has had consistent or similar reactions to the same food. This will identify the patient who is having either an allergic or a nonallergic reaction. A patient may be having adverse reactions to various apparently unrelated foods, but in fact the reaction may be to a preservative or additive that is contained in, and common to, different foods. The physician can often make a diagnosis by examining the list of offending foods and attempting to link them, knowing that they may contain the same preservative.

Patients with immediate IgE-mediated reactions to foods will often describe an immediate awareness of something being seriously wrong after a bite or slight taste of the food. Extremely sensitive patients may develop symptoms by merely inhaling the odors from the food, such as fish or peanut butter.

Physical Examination

During an acute allergic episode, the following may be observed: urticaria, angioedema, oropharyngeal or laryngeal edema, hyperactive bowel sounds, abdominal distention, bronchospasm, rhinoconjunctivitis, hypotension, and symptoms of generalized systemic anaphylaxis with shock. The physical examination is usually normal when the patient presents for a diagnostic evaluation.

Laboratory Tests

Immediate hypersensitivity skin testing detects the presence of a food allergen–specific IgE antibody. Skin test results should not solely be relied upon to make a diagnosis of food allergy. A negative skin test will usually exclude a severe IgE-mediated food allergy, but coupled with a strikingly positive history, the latter should be assumed to be diagnostically reliable. The skin test has very good negative predictive value but will often yield false-positive results. If correlated with the history, the skin test will generally provide sufficient information to recommend a trial of elimination from the diet, with anticipated improvement. If the patient is able to unequivocally tolerate a food that gives a positive skin test reaction, the skin test result should be disregarded.

The patient with a history of anaphylaxis to a specific food should not be skin tested unless the specific cause of the reaction is unclear (e.g., when the patient ate several foods at the same time, each being a potential offending agent) and other, safer methods of diagnosis (i.e., radioallergosorbent test, or RAST) have failed to reveal a likely cause.

The RAST, which detects allergen-specific IgE in the patient's serum, should be performed as the initial diagnostic procedure in a patient with a history of severe anaphylaxis, or in individuals who are unable to be skin tested because of severe eczema or dermatographism. These tests are more expensive than skin tests, and the results take longer to obtain. They are also only as good as the quality of the allergen used in the assay, and because they measure allergen-specific IgE in the serum, patients with significant amounts of cell-bound IgE, but small amounts of circulating IgE, may be missed.

ORAL CHALLENGE

If the history and results of skin or RAST tests are still equivocal, oral challenges with the food or additive in question may be necessary. The challenge is usually performed in either an open (physician and patient aware of the food), single-blind (patient not aware), or double-blind (patient and physician not aware) fashion. The latter approach is the most objective because patient and physician biases are eliminated. Oral challenges should never be performed if the history reveals anaphylaxis. Freeze-dried food inserted into opaque dye-free capsules is generally used for the testing.

It is beyond the scope of this chapter to describe these methods in detail. In office practice, the physician seldom needs to proceed to an oral challenge. However, in many cases, particularly where psychogenic factors are felt to be causative, this is a useful method to refute or confirm the diagnosis of an adverse food reaction.

ELIMINATION DIETS

Various types of elimination diets, ranging from the elimination of a single food to instituting an elemental diet, may be used both as a diagnostic and as a therapeutic trial. The patient needs to be reliable and compliant in order for an accurate assessment to be made. Foods can be added back gradually and removed a second time if the symptoms reappear. This approach can be time-consuming but is often worth the temporary inconvenience.

CONTROVERSIAL TECHNIQUES

Cytotoxic testing and provocative subcutaneous and sublingual testing are unproven diagnostic techniques, and they should not be performed.

TREATMENT AND MANAGEMENT

When a particular food has been confirmed to be the cause of an adverse food reaction, avoidance is obviously the primary treatment. It is important for the patient to be aware of potentially cross-reacting foods (see display entitled "Partial List of Cross-Reacting Food Groups"). If a suspected food cannot be confirmed as causing the adverse reaction, it is best to eliminate that food for a limited time. The food should be permanently eliminated if the symptoms do not improve or return when the food is reintroduced.

Particular vigilance must be enforced when the child is eating away from home (e.g., at restaurants, friends' or relatives' homes, school parties). In these settings, patients may not be aware of all the ingredients used in cooking (e.g., walnuts contained in a coffee cake), and severe anaphylactic reactions will most commonly occur in individuals already known to be allergic to a particular food. The patient should be clearly warned that when in doubt, he or she should avoid the food in question. Health education must emphasize that future reactions could be lethal. This warning is generally well-accepted by patients who have had a severe anaphylactic reaction, and these patients usually become appropriately cautious. Again, it is important to emphasize that elimination of the specific food(s) is central to effective treatment.

In the case of adverse reactions to additives and preservatives, it is important to become aware of those foods that contain them. This information will often not be on the label of a food or indicated on menus in restaurants. Therefore, awareness is necessary to avoid these reactions. Consultation with a nutritionist is helpful in learning which foods to avoid.

It is important for the physician not to induce a state of unnecessary caution and elimination, unless specifically indicated, particularly in the adolescent and young adult who

Partial List of Cross-Reacting Food Groups

1. Dairy Products	5. Nightshade Family
Milk	Pepper
Butter	Eggplant
Cheeses	Tomato
Yogurt	Potato
Ice cream	6. Parsley Family
2. Legumes	Caraway
Peanut	Carrot
Pea	Celery
Soybean	Dill
Lentil	7. Walnut Family
Licorice	Walnut
Bean	Pecan
3. Cashew Family	Hickory nut
Cashew	Butternut
Mango	
Pistachio	
4. Plum Family	
Plum	
Prune	
Almond	
Apricot	
Cherry	
Peach	
Nectarine	

Patients should be given a list of all foods that are in the same food group, because they can all potentially cross-react, producing allergic symptoms of greater or lesser severity. The degree of cross-reactivity in a particular patient is variable. (Adapted from Adverse Reactions to Foods, AAAI and NIAID Report, US Department of Health and Human Services, NIH Publication No. 84-2442, July 1984, pp 21–25.)

might be at risk for, or is presently suffering from, an eating disorder. Some of these patients may rationalize their eating disorders because of confirmed or unconfirmed food allergies, and they begin to feel, without foundation, that they are allergic to virtually all foods. To avoid exacerbation of an underlying eating disorder, psychiatric referral is necessary in these atypical cases.

All patients with documented food-induced anaphylaxis should be given an H_1 antihistamine and self-injectable epinephrine to use in the event of accidental ingestions and subsequent reactions. (The treatment of acute anaphylaxis is reviewed in Chap. 48.) Gastric lavage is rarely necessary because most patients will spontaneously vomit the residual gastric food contents. An osmotic cathartic, such as magnesium citrate, may sometimes be used. Observation for 24 hours or longer for delayed symptoms may be necessary, depending on gastrointestinal transit time and the severity of the symptoms.

The young child with a food allergy should be reevaluated every year by the allergist, because a food allergy presenting at a young age is more likely to spontaneously remit with time than is a food allergy that has its onset in late childhood or adulthood. However, a food allergy in some individuals may remain for life.

A Medic-Alert bracelet should be worn by the patient so that the recognition and treatment of a reaction will be immediate.

Some patients may have food allergies that are linked to exercise. These individuals should not exercise for 4 to 6 hours after eating.

Immunotherapy with the use of food extracts has not been demonstrated to be effective. Preventative pharmacologic treatment may need to be tried in rare refractory cases, but this cannot be recommended as a standard treatment, and it is usually ineffective.

Reassurance and psychological support for the patient and family are important aspects of the overall treatment plan.

INDICATIONS FOR REFERRAL

The patient with confusing symptoms, an unclear association of symptoms with food, and a lack of response to treatment should be referred to an allergist for an appropriate work-up. An allergist should be consulted in all cases where the diagnosis of a food allergy is seriously entertained but not easily confirmed, or when a patient has had a severe anaphylactic reaction to a food. If an allergy evaluation fails to reveal an immunologic etiology, other nonimmunologic causes of adverse food reactions need to be considered, particularly if the symptoms recur.

A multidisciplinary team approach with consultation by a gastroenterologist, infectious disease specialist, food technologist, nutritionist, and psychiatrist may occasionally be necessary.

With the continuous introduction of new food additives, flavorings, colorings, and sweeteners, the clinician should be aware of their possible role in the production of food-related symptoms. An understanding of the heterogeneity of adverse food reactions will help the clinician focus the work-up in an appropriate direction without performing numerous expensive and unnecessary tests.

ANNOTATED BIBLIOGRAPHY

Adverse Reactions to Foods, AAAI and NIAID Report, NIH publication No. 84-2442, July 1984. (Excellent, state-of-the-art reference source reviewing all aspects of adverse food reactions, including pathophysiology, diagnosis, and treatment; excellent appendix of diseases transmitted by foods that is well referenced and indexed.)

Bock SA: Prospective appraisal of complaints of adverse reactions to foods in children during the first 3 years of life. Pediatrics 79:683–688, 1987. (Two important findings: [1] most reactions are non–IgE-mediated, and [2] most reactions occur during the first year of life and with rechallenge; by the third year, they don't usually recur.)

Metcalfe DD, Sampson HA, Simon RA: Food Allergy: Adverse Reactions to Foods and Food Additives. Oxford, Blackwell Scientific Publications 1991. (Thorough and current general reference.)

Symposium Proceedings on Adverse Reactions to Foods and Food Additives. J Allergy Clin Immunol 78(1), July 1986. (Excellent overview of the subject.)

51

Urticaria, Angioedema, and Serum Sickness

Raoul L. Wolf

Urticaria and angioedema are common occurrences in pediatrics; as many as one quarter of the general population will experience an episode. The two conditions are examples of an acute allergic reaction, initiated by several allergenic substances. The response manifests itself by an accumulation of fluid in the epidermal or dermoepidermal regions.

By contrast, serum sickness is an unusual problem, predominantly occurring in response to drug administration. It is important to recognize the condition when it occurs and to remove the offending agent when possible.

PATHOPHYSIOLOGY

The development of *urticaria* and *angioedema* is similar in both conditions. The response is mediated by IgE and depends on prior sensitization. These molecules of IgE are fixed to mast cells. With cross-linking by a specific antigen, they initiate the release of potent vasodilator substances, such as histamine and leukotrienes (previously known as slow-reacting substances). The result of this is local edema and swelling; in urticaria, these lie within the epidermis, and in angioedema, they occur at the dermoepidermal junction and in the subcutaneous tissue. The resultant stimulation of nerve endings gives rise to pruritus.

Serum sickness arises because of a completely different mechanism. It is an IgG-mediated reaction that occurs mostly with injected antigens (such as penicillin) or occasionally with ingested substances. Antigens and antibodies normally form complexes in the presence of excess antibody, giving rise to an insoluble lattice that is removed by the action of phagocytic cells. When antigen is present in excess, or when there is deficient or delayed antibody production, the complexes remain soluble. This phenomenon is an example of a circulating immune complex disease. The complexes deposit in blood vessels and tissues, primarily skin, joint tissues, and lung. This activates the serum complement cascade, releasing substances that are chemotactic for polymorphonuclear cells. With the resultant release of enzymes and prostaglandins, an inflammatory response occurs. This gives rise to the characteristic fever, rash, and joint pain. This type of reaction was a common result of injections of vaccines prepared in horse serum (hence the name), but now the penicillin group is probably the most common cause.

CLINICAL PRESENTATION

The patient with urticaria usually has an abrupt onset of symptoms, often within 10 to 15 minutes of exposure to antigen. Pruritus is the first sign and may be intense. This is followed by the appearance of macular or elevated multiform lesions, ranging from 2 mm to several centimeters in size, with wide surrounding erythema. Even apparently uninvolved areas of skin may be pruritic. Fever is not a usual accompaniment to the condition and, if present, should raise suspicion about an underlying disease process.

Chronic urticaria is present when the condition has persisted for longer than 6 weeks. This problem is more common in adults than in children. The cause is usually difficult to determine, and the condition is often refractory to therapy.

Angioedema may have a more gradual onset and is often associated with drug reactions. Pruritus is not as prominent; rather, a burning or painful sensation is noted. Swelling often begins about the lips or hands and is diffuse. The swelling may spread to involve the tongue and, in extreme cases, may cause laryngeal edema and acute respiratory distress. The time from exposure to emergence of the lesions can vary, and it is often more difficult for the patient to pinpoint the offending agent than it is in urticaria. The patient, however, will sometimes note lip and tongue swelling that occurs almost immediately upon tasting a food that causes an allergic reaction. Angioedema on an allergic basis is usually associated with urticarial reactions at the same or at distant sites, making identification easier.

The clinical pattern of serum sickness is distinct from that of urticaria and angioedema. Fever is the initial event, and the temperature may be high ($103°-105°F$), often spiking in nature, returning to the baseline or below between spikes. A headache is usual. A rash accompanies the fever. This is usually red, diffuse, and punctate but is often urticarial. The lesions may involve the palms and soles. Lymphadenopathy is seen and may involve any nodes, including the supraclavicular and epitrochlear nodes. Arthritis involves large joints, especially knees and hips. This feature may be prominent, causing significant pain and discomfort. Encephalitis and peripheral neuropathy are rare manifestations. Renal involvement presenting with hematuria occurs rarely and is seldom a major feature.

DIFFERENTIAL DIAGNOSIS

The lesions of urticaria are characteristic and easy to distinguish. The difficulty is in determining the cause. Examples of the more common causes are listed in the display. The distribution and pattern of the lesions may be helpful. Lesions that start around the lips and tongue may indicate sensitivity to a food. The usual foods involved are nuts, peanuts (not themselves nuts), dairy products, fish, and shellfish. In considering the possible foods that might be causative, one

---

Common Causes of Urticaria and Angioedema

Foods
  Peanuts
  Nuts
  Dairy products
  Shellfish
  Berries
Drugs
  Penicillins
  Sulfa drugs
  Iodides
Insect stings
Physical stress
  Heat
  Cold
Infestations

---

should keep in mind that cross-reactivity occurs within families of foods; for example, peanuts belong in the legume family (see Chap. 50, "Adverse Reactions to Foods"). Insect stings are a relatively common cause of urticaria and angioedema, but the patient is often aware that this is the cause of the problem. *Physical urticaria,* such as cholinergic or solar, often forms a characteristic pattern with fine punctate wheals in clusters. There is usually a history of exposure to heat or cold or a history of strenuous activity.

The swelling seen in angioedema is less typical of an atopic reaction than it is in urticaria. Other causes of diffuse swelling, such as hypoproteinemia, must be excluded. The intermittent nature of angioedema is a clue, as is the uneven distribution of the lesions. The area of greatest involvement may provide an indication of cause (e.g., the lips and tongue suggest a food source).

Many diseases, especially those with an immunologic basis, such as rheumatoid arthritis, can present with urticaria. Because this is a relatively uncommon subgroup, it is difficult to decide when to investigate for these disorders. The presence of fever, especially with high spikes and a return to the baseline, should indicate the possibility of an autoimmune disorder. Chronic or recurrent episodes of urticaria should suggest infectious hepatitis, infectious mononucleosis, or a parasitic infestation. The latter is usually accompanied by eosinophilia. Repeated ingestion of or exposure to a drug should be looked for when the lesions are recurrent.

Recurrent angioedema, especially on cold exposure, raises suspicion of *hereditary angioedema.* In this autosomal-dominant condition, there is a deficiency of an inhibitor (C_1 esterase inhibitor) of activation of the complement pathway. As a result, there is spontaneous complement activation with formation of active vasodilator substances. This condition can be life-threatening because of laryngeal edema. The measurement of serum complement and C_1 esterase levels will confirm the diagnosis.

Serum sickness is less typical in appearance than are urticaria and angioedema, making definitive diagnosis difficult. Systemic inflammatory diseases such as juvenile rheumatoid arthritis (JRA) may also present with joint swelling and fever. This onset is generally slower, and a migratory pattern of joint involvement is noted. There are often nodules associated with rheumatoid diseases. The ultimate differential usually is made only by long-term observation; signs and symptoms persist in JRA. Systemic lupus erythematosus (SLE) presents with fever and arthritis, but multiple organ systems are involved. Renal involvement is frequent, whereas it is rare in serum sickness. The rapid onset and history of drug or infectious exposure indicate serum sickness. The absence of positive rheumatoid serologic tests does not exclude JRA, because these tests are often negative in this form of the disease. On the other hand, negative serology does exclude SLE. In distinguishing the various causes of serum sickness, drug reactions are the most common, especially reactions to penicillin and phenytoin (Dilantin). Vaccines and various sera are also common causes (see also Chap. 49, "Drug Allergy").

WORK-UP

History

A careful history is the key to diagnosing urticaria and angioedema. Most identifiable causes can be traced to within 30 minutes of onset of the lesions. For example, the patient may describe a shrimp dinner that ended abruptly when his or her lips and tongue became swollen and urticarial lesions appeared. Other examples include exposure to a drug or contact agent, such as a cat, with rapid emergence of the lesions. A history that is helpful in determining a diagnosis could be a reaction to iodides in soap or contrast media. This is predictive of a severe reaction with the use of injected radiocontrast media and must be sought in all patients who will undergo these procedures (see Chap. 49, "Drug Allergy"). In a case where the history is not so helpful, and a reaction to a food is suspected, the patient may be asked to keep a food diary, recording everything eaten and annotating the log with the times and dates of allergic reactions. Theoretically, this is a helpful procedure; in practice, it often fails because patients do not keep the record or attempt to fill it in from memory a week later. Thus, this technique is useful only if the patient is diligent.

A history of drug reactions should be sought. Other atopic diseases such as allergic rhinitis, eczema, contact reactions, and asthma should be elicited. Although not diagnostic, such a history increases the possibility that a suspicious reaction is urticarial.

In evaluating serum sickness, the onset of symptoms 10 days to 2 weeks after drug exposure or an infectious episode is suggestive of the condition. There is often a history of previous episodes with spontaneous resolution or in response to therapy. Family history or a history of atopic disease does not correlate with serum sickness.

Physical Examination

The clinical appearance of urticaria has already been noted. Some aspects of the physical presentation may be helpful. The distribution of the lesions may indicate the source. Lesions beginning around the mouth or tongue imply that an ingested agent, such as nuts or berries, may be responsible. The location on the skin, such as in the underwear area, suggests a reaction to a laundry detergent. Hand, mouth, and tongue involvement, especially an exposure to cold or physical stress, should raise suspicion of hereditary angioedema. Pruritus is the most helpful sign associated with urticaria.

Physical causes for urticaria can be excluded by hot or cold contact tests or by applying pressure. Signs of systemic disease, such as splenomegaly, lymphadenopathy, and hepatomegaly, are unusual in urticaria and should be taken as indicators of an underlying disorder such as rheumatoid disease. These features are not uncommon in serum sickness. They do not, however, indicate a need for extensive investigation.

Laboratory Tests

Laboratory investigations are generally of limited value in these conditions, and tests should be reserved for specific indications. Allergy skin testing is unlikely to be helpful, other than to confirm the lack of a suspected IgE-mediated response to a food. A positive skin test has less than a 50% sensitivity (true positive), but a negative reaction has more than a 90% specificity (true negative). It will not be of any value in detecting food or other allergens unsuspected from a careful history. The skin test assay is a sensitive measurement of specific IgE bound to mast cells in the skin. In urticaria, however, the reaction may not correlate well with actual causes for the condition. Specific IgE can also be measured from serum by means of a radioallergosorbent (RAST) test. This test is sensitive. It, too, may not be helpful in delineating the cause, and it is a more expensive assay than skin testing. A complete blood count (CBC) with differential may reveal a high eosinophil count, suggesting a parasitic infestation or underlying atopic state. Where a suspicion of systemic disease is entertained, an erythrocyte sedimentation rate (ESR) is a good screening test. More specific assays, such as rheumatoid factor and antinuclear antibody, should be done if there is an elevated ESR with a prolonged course for the disease.

Low serum complement levels, namely total hemolytic complement, C4 level, and C3 (BIC) levels, indicate hereditary angioedema. All will be reduced during an acute attack, but between episodes only C4 will be low. Definitive diagnosis is made on the basis of a low C_1 esterase inhibitor.

The investigation of serum sickness should include CBC and ESR. The CBC may show eosinophilia, neutropenia, or thrombocytopenia in response to the etiologic agent. A positive Coombs' test and anemia should arouse suspicion of SLE. A urinalysis is essential to differentiate from conditions that more frequently involve the kidney, such as SLE, although mild proteinuria is seen in serum sickness. Other investigations should be conducted to either confirm or disprove clinical suspicion, such as rheumatoid serology if rheumatoid disease seems likely. Serum complement values may be transiently low in serum sickness, but it is not usually necessary to perform this test.

TREATMENT AND MANAGEMENT

The initial therapy for urticaria and angioedema consists of removing the patient from the cause, if possible, and preventing a progression of the condition. If an insect stinger is present, it should be removed with a scalpel blade, not tweezers or fingers, to avoid breaking it off and thereby injecting more venom.

Where there is a significant swelling or a threat that swelling may spread, epinephrine 0.01 ml/kg of a 1/1000 dilution to a maximum of 0.3 ml is given subcutaneously. This can be followed by diphenhydramine (Benadryl) 12.5 mg–25 mg tid (maximum dose of 300 mg/day) for 3 to 5 days (see also chapter 48, "Anaphylaxis—Outside the Emergency Room"). In cases where pruritus is a major symptom, this is better controlled by hydroxyzine (Atarax, Vistaril) at 0.5–2 mg/kg/24 hours. This should also be continued for 3 to 5 days or longer if resolution of the lesions is delayed.

Chronic urticaria is much more difficult to treat and is often refractory to antihistaminics. Some authors have indicated that histamine H_2 receptors are present in skin blood vessels. (H_1 receptors are found on smooth muscle, and H_2 receptors are part of the regulation of gastric acid secretion and are found on mast cells.) Cimetidine, an H_2 blocker, has been used in conjunction with an H_1 blocker with some success in refractory cases of urticaria. Astemizole (Hismanal), a long-acting, selective histamine H_1-receptor antagonist, may also be effective.

Steroid therapy does not have a place in acute urticaria, although it may be helpful in refractory cases. In angioedema, the presence of laryngeal edema or severe swelling of the face and lips is an indication for using prednisone 1–2 mg/kg/day or dexamethasone (Decadron) 0.1 mg/kg/day in a short course of 4 to 5 days. The drug can be discontinued without tapering if such a short course is used.

Serum sickness is usually self-limited and requires supportive therapy. Salicylates at 80 mg/kg/day are effective in controlling joint symptoms and fever and may be used for about 1 week beyond the resolution of symptoms. Diphenhydramine is useful to treat an urticarial component. In the presence of severe symptoms, neurologic involvement, or significant renal involvement, prednisone 2 mg/kg/day should be used. Following the resolution of symptoms, the prednisone dose can be tapered over 2 to 3 weeks.

INDICATIONS FOR REFERRAL OR ADMISSION

Most patients with urticaria will recover spontaneously and will not have another episode. In recurrent or refractory episodes, a consultation and an extensive work-up and history may be beneficial.

Admission is indicated in the patient with angioedema or serum sickness accompanied by a low or unstable blood pressure. Severe reactions, even with a stable circulatory system, are an indication for admission and observation for 24 hours. The patient who does not respond or who has further episodes will benefit from a work-up for an underlying disease. At times, this may be accomplished best in a hospital.

ANNOTATED BIBLIOGRAPHY

Bock SA: The natural history of food sensitivity. J Allergy Clin Immunol 69:173–177, 1982. (Important review of the natural history of food sensitivity.)

Casale TB, Samson HA, Hanifin J et al: Guide to physical urticarias. J Allergy Clin Immunol 82:758–763, 1988. (Excellent review of less common urticarias.)

Fauci AS: Serum sickness. In Parker CW (ed): Clinical Immunology, pp 486–490. Philadelphia, WB Saunders, 1980. (Overall review.)

Goldstein RA, Patterson RJ (eds): Drug allergy: Prevention, diagnosis, treatment. Symposium. J Allergy Clin Immunol (Oct suppl) 74:549–644, 1984. (Wide coverage of the topic.)

Kaplan AP: Urticaria and angioedema. In Middleton E Jr, Reed CE, Ellis EF (eds): Allergy, Principles and Practice. Philadelphia, WB Saunders, 1988. (Broad-based discussion of the problem.)

Metcalfe DD: Food hypersensitivity. J Allergy Clin Immunol 73:749–766, 1984. (Sober look at a topic fraught with myth and misunderstanding.)

Sheffer AL: Anaphylaxis. J Allergy Clin Immunol 75:227–236, 1985. (Recommended as a postgraduate review.)

52

Acquired Immunodeficiency Syndrome (AIDS) in Children

Anthony B. Minnefor, James M. Oleske, and Edward C. Connor

Given the origins of the AIDS epidemic in the United States, it seemed unlikely that infants and children would be affected. Once it became apparent that the causative agent could be transmitted by blood products and that women could become infected through intravenous drug abuse (IVDA) and through sexual contact with infected men, the potential for pediatric involvement increased. Indeed, by late 1982, the Centers for Disease Control (CDC) had received reports of sporadic cases involving infants and children with clinical and laboratory findings compatible with AIDS. Over the next 10 years, the human immunodeficiency virus (HIV) had infected an estimated 10,000 to 20,000 children in the United States alone.

Vertical spread from infected mother to infant has emerged as the main mode of transmission. The vertical transmission rate is approximately 30%. Pediatricians may also encounter infected hemophiliacs and other recipients of blood products, as well as those whose route of acquisition is sexual (including sexual abuse). Clinical and laboratory features may vary markedly over what is generally considered the pediatric age group. The CDC's classification system for patients with HIV disease who are less than 13 years of age is as follows: (1) P-0, indeterminate infection, (2) P-1, asymptomatic infection with or without laboratory evidence of immunosuppression, and (3) P-2, symptomatic infection.

PATHOPHYSIOLOGY

The causative agent for AIDS (HIV, a human retrovirus) is tropic for T lymphocytes, specifically the subpopulation termed *helper cells* (T-helper/inducer, CD4). Infection can occur by cell-associated or cell-free virus that attaches to the CD4 antigen that defines T-helper lymphocytes. The virus is typically cytolytic or, under certain circumstances, may integrate as a provirus. Consequently, HIV infection is considered to be chronic and lifelong.

Because of the quantitative depletion of CD4 cells, along with functional defects, these lymphocytes are no longer capable of effectively modulating B-lymphocyte antibody production directed by triggering antigens. Similarly, suppressor T-lymphocytes (cytotoxic, CD8) are also no longer regulated in a normal fashion. Thus, the immunologic dysfunction may be profound. Normal humoral immune and specific cytotoxic responses are not possible. Autoantibodies and circulating immune complexes result in tissue injury. This broad defect results in the development of the opportunistic infections (OI) and malignancies that characterize AIDS.

Unfortunately, HIV is neurotropic as well. The evidence includes detection of HIV genome by in-situ hybridization, intrathecal synthesis of anti-HIV antibodies, the presence of HIV antigen in cerebrospinal fluid, and virus isolation from brain tissue.

CLINICAL PRESENTATION

Acquisition of HIV occurs both prenatally and at the time of delivery, with no differences noted between women delivering by caesarean section and those delivering vaginally. Transmission rates have been reported to be higher in premature infants and those with mothers having low anti-gp

Table 52-1. Clinical Manifestations of Pediatric HIV Infection

Failure to thrive	Chronic interstitial pneumonitis
Hepatosplenomegaly	Severe or recurrent infections
Lymphadenopathy	Recurrent febrile episodes
Recurrent diarrhea	Encephalopathy
Chronic parotid swelling	Skin rashes (eczema-like)
Nephropathy/nephritis	Cardiomyopathy
Hepatitis	Dysmorphic syndrome
Malignancies	

120 antibody (an important antigenic determinant on the virus).

There is a growing appreciation of the diversity of presentations. Onset may be abrupt or slowly progressive. Patients presenting in the first year of life (about one third) generally have severe illness and high early mortality. The other patients with perinatal HIV infection and later onset have more indolent courses and a prolonged survival after diagnosis. Dysfunction of one organ system may dominate the clinical picture, or there may be a combination of problems. The triad of failure to thrive (or wasting syndrome), chronic interstitial pneumonitis, and hepatosplenomegaly is a common presentation. The most frequently encountered clinical manifestations are listed in Table 52-1. Table 5-2 contrasts HIV infection in adults and children.

Invasive bacterial infections may be severe and recurrent and, when present, are considered an AIDS-defining infection in pediatric patients. *Streptococcus pneumoniae*, *Haemophilus influenzae*, *Salmonella* spp., and *Staphylococcus aureus* are the most common pathogens. The fevers may be protracted and of high grade without apparent explanation, in part presumably because of reactivation of latent agents such as cytomegalovirus (CMV), Epstein–Barr virus (EBV), *Mycobacterium avium-intracellulare* (MAI), or HIV itself. The immunologic defect is such that multiple

Table 52-2. Differences Between Pediatric and Adult HIV Infection

1. Kaposi's sarcoma and B-cell lymphoma are rare in children.
2. Hepatitis B infection is less frequent in children than in adults.
3. Hypergammaglobulinemia is more pronounced in children.
4. Peripheral lymphopenia is uncommon in children.
5. Lymphocytic interstitial pneumonia (LIP) is much more common in children.
6. CD4 counts have age-specific normal values.
7. Serious bacterial sepsis is a major problem in children.
8. Dysmorphic features may be found in some children (embryopathy).
9. Acute mononucleosis-like presentations are rare in children.
10. Progressive neurologic disease secondary to primary HIV CNS infection may be more pronounced in children.
11. Opportunistic infections and tumors of the CNS are less common in children.

pathogens may be present simultaneously at the same or different body sites. Dermatologic lesions occasionally reflect systemic illnesses (e.g., disseminated candidiasis or cryptococcosis) and may be atypical in appearance and/or progression (e.g., herpes simplex virus [HSV] or varicella-zoster [VZ]). Related conditions include condylomata, molluscum contagiosum, and fungal skin/nail infections.

The lung is the most common site of clinically recognizable infection, with *Pneumocystis carinii* pneumonia (PCP) the most frequent indicator of disease and OI. Even with treatment, mortality is high for this condition, and PCP prevention is central in a management scheme. Lymphocytic interstitial pneumonia (LIP) is the next most important pulmonary condition and represents one part of the spectrum of lymphoid hyperplasia seen with HIV infection. The genomes of both EBV and HIV have been identified in sections of lung from children with LIP, but the exact etiology is uncertain. Less common pulmonary opportunists include CMV, MAI, HSV, and *Candida*.

The gastrointestinal tract is the next most common site for an OI, with *Candida* esophagitis the most frequent infection. Thrush, while not a classic OI, is nearly universal in AIDS. The more severe the thrush, the greater the likelihood of esophagitis, although one may be present without the other. Cryptosporidiosis is responsible for most of the chronic diarrhea seen in AIDS patients when a specific organism is identified. Gastrointestinal and hepatobiliary disease may also appear as periodic abdominal pain and distention. Enterocolitis may be caused by OI with MAI or CMV, colonic polyps, biliary obstruction, and rarely Kaposi's sarcoma (KS) or other tumors/malignancies.

The central nervous system (CNS) involvement in pediatric HIV is a primary, persistent, and progressive retroviral infection of the brain. It may precede other manifestations of the disease. In older patients, an acute HIV meningoencephalitis with or without seizures may be part of an acute mononucleosis-like illness associated with recent acquisition of HIV infection. In infants and children, a progressive loss of developmental milestones or an arrest in development is perhaps the most common early sign. There may be secondary microcephaly. In older children, it may be possible to discern an AIDS dementia comparable to that in the adult. Other features are truncal ataxia with pyramidal tract signs, paraparesis, incontinence, and peripheral neuropathy.

Because intrauterine infection is an accepted mode of transmission of HIV, investigators have sought and apparently identified an HIV embryopathy. The following abnormalities were noted in the initial 20 patients reported: growth failure (75%), microcephaly (70%), and craniofacial abnormalities: ocular hypertelorism (50%), prominent boxlike forehead (75%), flat nasal bridge (70%), mild upward or downward obliquity of the eyes (65%), long palpebral fissures with blue sclerae (60%), short nose with flattened columella and well-formed, triangular philtrum

(65%), and patulous lips (60%). The children ranged in age from 5 months to 7½ years at the time of evaluation. Expression of the embryopathy appears variable. It is uncertain how early in life the stigmata can be discerned. They appear to be distinguishable from the fetal alcohol syndrome and ethnic variability.

DIFFERENTIAL DIAGNOSIS

Given the possibility of the protean manifestations noted earlier, the differential diagnosis is widely varied depending on the organ system(s) affected. In general, the two most important diagnostic considerations are congenital immunodeficiency state and congenital infections. The former usually has distinct genetic patterns and diagnostic clinical and/or laboratory features. The clinical and laboratory abnormalities associated with congenital infections are usually limited to that particular infection. It is generally possible to exclude a secondary immunodeficiency seen with severe malnutrition, immunosuppressive chemotherapy, and malignancy.

WORK-UP

History

The key element is to establish whether a patient can be considered at risk for HIV infection. A personal or parental history of "high risk" (i.e., sexual exposures, blood/blood products transfusion, IVDA, and signs and symptoms consistent with HIV infection) should be sought. It must be emphasized that HIV-positive mothers need not be ill to transmit the infection to their offspring.

Despite careful histories, the first indication that a pregnancy has been complicated by HIV may be the development of illness in the infant. Children seem to have a shorter incubation period than adults following transfusions, ranging from 1 month to 2 years or longer (median, ≥ 8 months). Adolescents generally follow a more adult pattern, with incubation periods of 5 years or longer, regardless of the route of transmission. The history should emphasize those features of HIV infection outlined in Table 52-1.

Physical Examination

Examination may be entirely normal. When present, physical findings (although almost never diagnostic), coupled with a positive history for HIV "exposure," will often trigger an expedited AIDS work-up. Untreated patients almost always have thrush. Lymphadenopathy is nontender, and nodes are usually large (greater than 1 cm) and present at two or more noncontiguous sites. Growth and development are generally impaired. Children with PCP are often febrile, with tachypnea and retractions, and have diminished breath sounds, wheezes, and rhonchi on auscultation. Patients with

LIP are less hypoxic than are those with PCP and have digital clubbing, parotid enlargement, and generalized lymphadenopathy. Hepatosplenomegaly is common.

The neurodevelopmental status should be assessed. The skin manifestations of invasive infections or KS may be present. The latter are papulonodular, red-purple lesions, but on occasion they can closely resemble pigmented, cystic acne. They may involve any area of the skin (as well as the gastrointestinal tract or other viscera). Skin lesions (e.g., HSV) may be atypical in appearance.

Laboratory Tests

Screening for HIV antibodies with use of the ELISA technique, with positive tests confirmed by Western Blot analysis, remains the most common initial study. Paradoxically, antibody positivity to HIV denotes *infection* with the virus and *not* protection, as is the case with most other antigen–antibody systems. Because these are IgG antibodies, they will not distinguish between actual perinatal infection and maternal transfer of antibody until 15 months of age, when maternal antibody is gone.

Viral culture for HIV, if available, has a sensitivity of over 90% in patients 4 months of age or older. Polymerase chain reaction (PCR), IgM and IgA ELISA assays, antigen capture assay, and in-vitro antibody production assays are being evaluated in children. In any of these other assays, a negative test does not exclude HIV infection. Determination of the CD4 count and CD4/CD8 ratio is the next most important test. These differ from values in adults, are age-specific, and are essential in the timing of PCP prophylaxis and antiretroviral therapy. Other baseline studies include urinalysis, complete blood count (CBC) with differential, platelet count, erythrocyte sedimentation rate (ESR), and quantitative immunoglobulins. Most patients have hypergammaglobulinemia secondary to polyclonal B-cell stimulation, although the antibody is functionally inadequate. Anemia is common, as are leukopenia and immune-mediated thrombocytopenia. Chest x-ray may detect unsuspected pathology. All febrile patients should have blood and other appropriate cultures performed.

A gallium scan can be useful in determining "hot spots" in the lung that are likely to yield a diagnosis if biopsy is contemplated. Comprehensive stains and cultures for the full range of potential pathogens are mandatory on all surgical specimens.

TREATMENT AND MANAGEMENT

Early identification of HIV-infected and at-risk infants permits early PCP prophylaxis and antiretroviral therapy. PCP prophylaxis with trimethoprim-sulfamethoxazole (TMP-SMX) is given at a dose of 150 mg/TMP/m²/day in two divided doses, three times a week. This regimen should be given to children 1 to 11 months of age with CD4 counts

below 1500 cells/mm³, those 12 to 23 months old with CD4 counts under 750, and those 24 months to 5 years of age with CD4 counts below 500. Only at 6 years of age and older is the adult criterion of CD4 counts of 200 or lower used to initiate prophylaxis. All children, irrespective of age, should be treated if the CD4 percent is less than 20.

Zidovudine (AZT) in a dose of 180 mg/m² every 6 hours is safe and results in clinical, immunologic, and virologic improvement when given to children with advanced HIV disease. All children with symptoms (Class P-2) and those who meet criteria for PCP prophylaxis should also receive AZT. For children 6 years of age or older, the adult guideline of CD4 counts of less than 500 is used to begin treatment. Two other antiretroviral drugs have been studied in children—ddI and ddC—with promising preliminary results.

It has recently been shown that the use of intravenous immune globulin (IVIG) is safe and significantly increases the time free from serious bacterial infections for those children with CD4 counts of 200 or more. It can be given in a dose of 400 mg/kg over several hours and can be repeated every 28 days. Serodiagnostic studies should be obtained before an IVIG program is begun, because antibodies in the preparation will render most subsequent results uninterpretable.

The immunization schedule for HIV-infected children should be modified. Inactivated polio vaccine (IPV) is given to eliminate the potential of paralytic polio from the live virus in oral polio vaccine (OPV). Children over 3 months of age should receive annual immunization with influenza vaccine, and those older than 2 years should receive pneumococcal vaccine. DTP and *H. influenzae* type b vaccine can be given in accordance with standard schedules. Despite often inadequate antibody responses, MMR is routinely recommended for children. Fortunately, no serious side effects have been reported. Despite immunization, postexposure prophylaxis should be given for measles (immune serum globulin), except for those children receiving monthly IVIG. The latter group also need not receive MMR. Susceptible children exposed to varicella should be given varicella-zoster immune globulin (VZIG).

Details concerning the management of OIs are for the most part beyond the scope of this chapter. Routine infections should be managed aggressively. For bacterial infections requiring hospitalization, either cefuroxime or cefotaxime (150 mg/kg/day, given IV in three divided doses every 8 hours) has been efficacious empiric treatment. Short courses of prednisone (2 mg/kg/day) are administered for patients with LIP and pO₂ of less than 65 mm Hg. Trimethoprim-sulfamethoxazole (TMP-SMX), calculated as 20 mg/kg/day of the TMP component, is given IV in four divided doses every 6 hours for known or suspected PCP. An alternative for patients who fail to respond in 72 to 96 hours, or those with allergic reactions to TMP-SMX, is pentamidine. It is given in a 4 mg/kg/day single dose by the IV route.

For a variety of reasons, nutritional intake in these patients may be inadequate. Many children require nasogastric feeding, but if chronic diarrhea is present, parenteral hyperalimentation is accomplished by placement of central lines (e.g., Broviac catheters) if necessary.

Pain management is an important but often neglected component of overall care. Pain can come in various ways. All care-givers should be sensitive to this issue, and every effort should be made to control pain medically and psychologically.

INDICATIONS FOR REFERRAL AND/OR ADMISSION

The primary care physician has an important role to play in the evolving team approach to management of HIV-infected infants and children. Treatment protocols have become increasingly standardized, and centers providing services to patients and their families continue to proliferate. Accordingly, even the very symptomatic patient can remain under the care of his or her primary physician. The physician can, in most circumstances, coordinate treatment in consultation with other specialists or a center, and with social services. This includes attempting to assure that his or her patient has access to new treatments and investigational drugs as they become available. Severe opportunistic infections are common causes for admission, but the increasing availability of outpatient service systems has obviated the need for lengthy hospital stays, particularly with "permanent" central IV access. Physicians are advised to follow recommendations put forth by various scientific or regulatory bodies affecting HIV children.

ANNOTATED BIBLIOGRAPHY

Bernstein L, Krieger B, Novick B et al: Bacterial infection in the acquired immunodeficiency syndrome of children. Pediatr Infect Dis 4:472, 1985. (Reviews the type, frequency, and basis of bacterial infections in pediatric HIV infection.)

Centers for Disease Control: Classification system for human immunodeficiency virus (HIV) infection in children under 13 years of age. MMWR 36:225, 1987. (Well-referenced scheme to assist in categorizing patients in pediatric age groups.)

Centers for Disease Control: Guidelines for prophylaxis against Pneumocystis carinii pneumonia for children infected with human immunodeficiency virus. MMWR 40:1, 1991. (Excellent summary of the subject with data on age-specific CD4 counts.)

Goedert J, Mendez H, Drummond J et al: Mother-to-infant transmission of human immunodeficiency virus Type 1: Association with prematurity or low anti-gp 120. Lancet 1:13519, 1989. (May help explain why only a minority of infants exposed to HIV in utero actually become affected.)

Gwinn M, Pappaioanou M, George J et al: Prevalence of HIV infection in childbearing women in the United States: Surveillance using newborn blood samples. JAMA 265:1704, 1991. (Provides information regarding scope and regional variability in prevalence of HIV in this population.)

Krivine A, Yakudima A, LeMay M et al: A comparative study of virus isolation, polymerase chain reaction and antigen detection in children of mothers infected with human immunodeficiency virus. J Pediatr 116:372, 1990. (Describes newer assays and approaches to early diagnosis in perinatally acquired infection.)

Marion R, Wiznia A, Hutcheon G, Rubinstein A: Human T-cell lymphotropic virus Type III (HTLV-III) embryopathy. Am J Dis Child 140:638, 1986. (Initial publication dealing with the dysmorphic syndrome. Includes illustrations.)

McKinney R, Maha M, Connor E et al: A multicenter trial of oral zidovudine in children with advanced human immunodeficiency virus disease. N Engl J Med 324:1018, 1991. (Pivotal study showing AZT benefits children as it does adults.)

National Institute of Child Health and Human Development Intravenous Immune Globulin Study Group: Intravenous immune globulin for the prevention of bacterial infections in children with symptomatic human immunodeficiency virus infection. N Engl J Med 325:73, 1991. (Corroborates earlier clinical impression that IVIG reduces frequency and severity of bacterial infections.)

Oxtoby M: Perinatally acquired human immunodeficiency virus infection. Pediatr Infect Dis J 9:609, 1990. (Reviews the natural history of the condition.)

9

CARDIOVASCULAR PROBLEMS

53

Cholesterol and Prevention of Coronary Artery Disease

Charlene Gaebler-Uhing
and L. Gerard Niederman

Parents are increasingly aware that risk factors for cardiovascular disease, particularly coronary artery disease (CAD), may be present in their children. Pediatricians are frequently asked to provide guidance and recommendations for healthy diets and exercise, and they may be asked to perform and interpret blood cholesterol tests.

There is no consensus regarding the efficacy of universal cholesterol screening in children. Pediatricians are challenged to critically appraise the conflicting literature published in both the pediatric and lay presses. There is, however, unanimity that the incidence of cardiovascular disease would decline with dietary improvements; reduction in smoking; early and sustained management of hypertension, diabetes, and obesity; and a decrease in sedentary lifestyles.

PATHOPHYSIOLOGY

The results of the Framingham Heart Study and other clinical, epidemiologic, and biochemical studies have given support to the cholesterol hypothesis. Levels of total cholesterol (TC), and more specifically low-density lipoprotein cholesterol (LDL-C), are directly and continuously related to the risk of CAD. Increasing evidence also supports the corollary that reducing TC and LDL-C will decrease the incidence of CAD.

Cholesterol Lipoproteins

Lipid and lipoprotein levels are primarily determined by genetic and nutritional factors, although they may be secondarily altered by disease states and medications. The low-density lipoproteins (LDLs) serve as the major protein carrier of cholesterol in fasting patients. Specific cell surface receptors bind LDL-C. With altered receptor function or increased endogenous production of LDL-C, the excess plasma cholesterol enters scavenger cells through a low-affinity mechanism that is LDL-receptor independent and nonregulated. These cells accumulate excessive amounts of intracellular cholesterol, become foam cells, and are incorporated into atherogenic plaques. High-density lipoproteins (HDLs) carry 25% to 30% of the plasma cholesterol, and facilitate the entry of cholesterol into cells by acting as a substrate and a cofactor for two of the enzymes involved in the metabolism of cholesterol at the cell surface. Increased high-density lipoprotein cholesterol (HDL-C) protects against CAD. The very-low-density lipoproteins (VLDLs) function as a triglyceride carrier protein. Excess VLDLs are catabolized into LDLs. In obesity, VLDL-C is increased, indirectly elevating LDL-C. A number of apolipoproteins participate in the metabolism of lipoproteins and have been related to the pathophysiology of dyslipoproteinemias.

Dyslipoproteinemia

The understanding of genetically determined abnormalities of lipid metabolism is rapidly evolving. Familial hypercholesterolemia, the best understood dyslipoproteinemia, is an autosomal dominant disease resulting from defective LDL-C receptors. Homozygous familial hypercholesterolemia is extremely rare. These patients have plasma cholesterol levels ranging from 400 to over 1000 mg/dL and, characteristically, develop cutaneous planar xanthomas during the first 6 years of life and atherosclerosis involving the aortic valves

205

and aortic root. Eighty percent experience symptomatic CAD prior to 20 years of age.

Heterozygote familial hypercholesterolemia has an incidence of 0.2% to 0.5%. Total cholesterol levels in these patients are one and one-half to three times normal. These patients have thickening of the Achilles tendon in their teens and develop xanthomas in their late 30s. Ischemic heart disease develops in 80% of males before age 50 and in 50% of females by age 60.

SCREENING/CASE FINDING

The issues addressing pediatric cholesterol screening (population-based sampling) and case-finding (office-based sampling) have been discussed and debated for over a decade with no resulting consensus. Uncertainty exists in several important areas: (1) the accuracy of identifying children at increased risk for later cardiovascular disease; (2) the magnitude of the effect of intervention; and (3) the cost and public policy implications of a childhood program similar to the current adult-targeted National Cholesterol Education Program.

Childhood cholesterol levels, although correlated (in the aggregate) with adult levels, have marginal individual predictive value. A child in the upper quintile has, at best, only a 50% risk of having a similarly elevated cholesterol level as an adult. If the cutoff point at initial childhood screening were lowered, a greater fraction of future hypercholesterolemic adults would be identified but there would also be a significant increase in the number of children receiving dietary intervention unnecessarily (false positives). Using family history to select children for cholesterol testing would not increase the discrimination.

Opponents of universal screening in childhood also argue that although the risk of cardiovascular disease increases directly with TC or LDL-C, only a small fraction of the total future premature cardiovascular events would occur in children in the highest decile. Although the relative risk might be lower in children in the lower four quintiles, these children will experience the majority of premature events, and in fact will experience the bulk of all future cardiovascular events.

The lead time of 3 to 5 decades between intervention and resultant morbidity and mortality most likely will prohibit empiric evaluation of cholesterol-lowering interventions begun in children. Theoretically, dietary counseling would result in significant (10% to 15%) reductions in TC levels, although school-based studies have shown more modest (4% to 7%) decreases. Whether such reductions can be sustained over decades, or if sustained, what the impact will be on future CAD, is unknown. Equally uncertain is whether present or future interventions capable of lowering blood cholesterol during adulthood or modifying CAD will be more or less effective than years of management begun in childhood.

Despite the contention of proponents of universal screening that the opportunity to prevent the next generation's CAD will be lost if we do not intervene now with more intensive management on the highest risk group, only universal risk reduction measures are indicated. In the absence of more information, the practitioner would be prudent to advise a low-cholesterol, low-saturated fat diet (i.e., American Heart Association's Step One Diet) for all children older than age 2 and to counsel families regarding other risk factors of cardiovascular disease. Selective measurement of cholesterol levels is indicated when a family history of dyslipoproteinemia exists and may be indicated when other risk factors for CAD are present.

WORK-UP

History and Physical Examination

The evaluation should separate primary and secondary hypercholesterolemia and identify additional risk factors for CAD. Diabetes mellitus, hypothyroidism, chronic renal failure, nephrotic syndrome, biliary atresia, and cholestatic liver disease may elevate cholesterol levels. Medications that raise cholesterol include anabolic steroids, oral contraceptives, cyclosporine, anticonvulsants, and 13-*cis*-retinoic acid.

Family history of premature cardiovascular events in first- and second-degree relatives should be obtained. Dietary history, exercise patterns, and active and passive smoking habits also need to be assessed. It is essential to inquire about and update all risk factor data at each visit because of the dynamic nature of these risk factors in the patient and his or her family.

The physical examination should focus on identifying additional risk factors. Accurate heights and weights will assess obesity; accurate blood pressure measurements will identify hypertension. Planar cutaneous xanthomas, often at sites of injury, and thickening of the Achilles tendon may occur in children and adolescents with familial hypercholesterolemia.

Laboratory Tests

Clinical decisions are usually based either on TC or LDL-C values. Laboratory accuracy and precision as well as individual biologic variation will affect the classification and, ultimately, the management of children. Duplicate or triplicate measurements performed in a laboratory with standardized quality control is recommended to reduce misclassification when treatment is considered.

Children considered for dietary management on the basis of an elevated TC should have a fasting lipoprotein profile consisting of TC, HDL-C, and triglycerides. The LDL-C can then be estimated by the following formula:

$$\text{LDL-C} = \text{TC} - \text{HDL-C} - (\text{Triglycerides} \div 5)$$

Table 53-1. Lipid Reference Values (mg/dL)*
for Children Ages 3 to 19

LIPID	PERCENTILE			
	50	75	90	95
Cholesterol	155	175	190	200
LDL-C	95	110	125	135
HDL-C	52	60	68	73
Triglycerides	60	80	100	115

*Values are extracted and rounded from sex- and age-specific charts in the Lipid Research Clinic Population Studies Data Book, Vol 1, The Prevalent Study. US Department of Health and Human Services Report No. NIH-80-1527. Bethesda, MD, National Institutes of Health, July 1980.

From 5% to 15% of children with an elevated TC value will also have an elevated HDL-C, resulting in an LDL-C concentration that would suggest no intervention. Reference values for TC, LDL-C, HDL-C, and triglycerides are listed in Table 53-1.

Recent literature suggests evaluating thyroid function since some children with elevated TC, although appearing euthyroid, will be chronically hypothyroid. Other studies should be performed based on clinical suspicion of conditions causing secondary hypercholesterolemia.

TREATMENT

Dietary Management and Risk Reduction

All children and their families should receive counseling and education regarding risk reduction. Nutritional advice should ensure a diet adequate for a child's growth and activity levels. The American Heart Association's Step One Diet is appropriate for children older than 2 years old. Its salient goals include achieving ideal body weight; limiting total fat intake to 30% of total calories and total saturated fat intake to no more than 10% of total calories; limiting daily cholesterol intake to no more than 100 mg/1000 kcal; and providing 10% to 20% of calories as protein and 50% to 60% as carbohydrates. Pediatricians should also advocate an active life-style rich in strenuous activities and avoidance of smoking.

If cholesterol or lipid profiles are obtained, treatment is most often based on TC or LDL-C percentiles. This approach categorizes patients as *low risk*—usually considered for values less than the 75th percentile; *moderate risk*—values between the 75th percentile and the 90th or 95th percentile; and *high risk*—values greater than the 90th or 95th percentile.

Patients at low or moderate risk should be counseled as described previously, with children in the moderate-risk category having repeated testing of cholesterol levels. These families should have access to nutritional education, such as brochures and workshops, to help implement appropriate dietary changes. High-risk patients should receive more in-

tensive management. Dietary intervention is more successful if dietary changes are made for the entire family rather than for an individual within the family. Screening the family may identify others at increased risk.

To maximize dietary intervention, families should be referred to a registered dietitian for nutritional counseling. The focus of the nutritional education should be on teaching families how to recognize foods high in fat, how to substitute low-fat foods, how to read labels and screen for hidden fats while purchasing foods, and how to use low-fat cooking techniques. This education is crucial in making the conversion from a family with good intentions to one that actually makes the dietary changes. Goals for the TC and LDL-C levels should be set, and reevaluation should be done periodically. Throughout the first year of dietary intervention, the patient's growth and weight should be monitored closely. Usually a minimum of two measurements should be obtained the first year of treatment and annually thereafter to ensure adequate growth.

Lipid-Lowering Medications

Anticholesterol medications have limited use in children and primarily are used for the management of genetic dyslipoproteinemias. The resin-binding agents, cholestyramine and colestipol, in conjunction with diet management, are necessary in most children with heterozygous familial hypercholesterolemia. The starting dose varies between 4 and 20 g/d and is adjusted by the child's decrease in LDL-C. Constipation, the major side effect of resin binding agents, rarely limits therapy. Supplementation with vitamins, iron, and folic acid is recommended. Growth, liver enzymes, folic acid, fat-soluble vitamins levels, and a complete blood cell count should be checked annually. There is limited pediatric experience with other drugs such as nicotinic acid and lovastatin.

INDICATIONS FOR REFERRAL

Children with markedly elevated lipids (TC > 300 mg/L, LDL-C > 200 mg/L, or triglycerides > 250 mg/L) should be referred to an appropriate specialist for evaluation and specialized management. Success with dietary management often will be increased when nutritional counseling is performed by a registered dietitian.

ANNOTATED BIBLIOGRAPHY

American Heart Association: Dietary Treatment of Hypercholesterolemia: A Manual for Patients. Dallas, American Heart Association, 1988. (Excellent and practical guide for low-cholesterol, low-fat meal planning.)

Berwick DM, Cretin S, Keeler E: Cholesterol, Children and Heart Disease. New York, Oxford University Press, 1980. (An extensive, objective analysis of alternative public policy decisions regarding screening and treatment of children based on cholesterol values.)

Griffin TC, Christoffel KK, Binns HJ, McGuire PA, and the Pediatric Practice Research Group: Family history evaluation as a predictive screen for childhood hypercholesterolemia. Pediatrics 84:365, 1989. (Admirable pediatric practice-based study of utility of family history for identification of children with elevated TC and LDL-C.)

Jacobson MS, Lillienfeld DE: The pediatrician's role in atherosclerosis prevention. J Pediatr 112:836, 1988. (A review article on the use and issues of cholesterol screening, dietary intervention, and pharmacologic intervention in the hypercholesterolemic pediatric patient.)

Kwiterovich PO: Biochemical, clinical, epidemiologic, genetic, and pathologic data in the pediatric age group relevant to the cholesterol hypothesis. Pediatrics 78:349, 1986. (A commentary that reviews and summarizes the supporting data for the cholesterol hypothesis in pediatric patients.)

Kwiterovich PO: Diagnosis and management of familial dyslipoproteinemia in children and adolescents. Pediatr Clin North Am 37:1489, 1990. (Comprehensive review of genetic and metabolic basis as well as clinical diagnosis and management of dyslipoproteinemias.)

Lauer RM, Lee J, Clarke WR: Factors affecting the relationship between childhood and adult cholesterol levels: The Muscatine study. Pediatrics 82:309, 1988. (Population-based cholesterol tracking study.)

Lipid Research Clinics Population Studies Data Book, Vol I, The Prevalent Study. US Department of Health and Human Services Report No. NIH-80-1527. Bethesda, MD, National Institutes of Health, July 1980. (Reference lipid values by age, sex, and race.)

Newman TB, Browner WS, Hulley SB: The case against childhood cholesterol screening. JAMA 264:3039, 1990. (Three necessary screening principles—differentiation of "diseased" from borderline or nondiseased, improvement of prognosis with early intervention, and absence of harm to the nondiseased—are critically discussed, with the conclusion that universal screening is not justified.)

Report of the Expert Panel on Blood Cholesterol Levels in Children and Adolescents, National Cholesterol Education Program. Pediatrics (suppl) 89:525–584, 1992. (Detailed and current guidelines for both a population and individualized approach on this topic.)

Wynder EL, Berenson GS, Strong WB et al: Coronary artery disease prevention: Cholesterol, a pediatric perspective. Prev Med 18:323, 1989. (Comprehensive monograph that argues for universal childhood cholesterol screening.)

54

Cardiac Disease in the Newborn

Victor C. Baum

Congenital heart disease is relatively common, affecting approximately 0.8% of all newborns. This figure excludes lesions diagnosed in later life (e.g., mitral valve prolapse, nonstenotic bicuspid aortic valve) and patent ductus arteriosus in premature infants. Congenital heart disease can present in the infant as congestive heart failure, cyanosis, dysrhythmia, airway obstruction, or as an asymptomatic murmur. An evaluation of infants is particularly difficult for various reasons. Up to 60% of newborns will have a murmur on the first day of life, about 1% of infants will have a dysrhythmia noted on a 10-second electrocardiographic rhythm strip, and up to 13% of infants will have ectopic beats. Most of these murmurs and dysrhythmias are asymptomatic and resolve spontaneously. Signs of congenital heart disease may be mimicked by various noncardiac disease processes. The degree of findings (e.g., loudness of murmurs) may bear no relation to the severity (present or future) of the underlying cardiac defect, and murmurs themselves may be due to normal transitional physiologic processes. Almost all electrocardiographic variables have age-related normal values that change rapidly in the first few weeks of life. A stable physiologic state may change drastically with spontaneous closure of a patent ductus arteriosus if certain congenital defects are present. The normally rapid neonatal heart rate makes auscultation difficult for the inexperienced, and finally some clinicians are intimidated by the complex anatomy and physiology of the neonatal cardiovascular system and the complex congenital cardiac lesions.

This chapter is not intended to cover all of the possible congenital cardiac diseases; rather, it is an overview of lesions presenting in the neonatal period and those problems that can masquerade as cardiac disease in the newborn.

PATHOPHYSIOLOGY AND DIFFERENTIAL DIAGNOSIS

Since heart disease in the newborn involves several distinct entities, the pathophysiologies must be considered separately.

Structural Abnormalities

A direct etiologic agent or disease can only be ascribed in about 10% of cases of congenital heart disease. These are due to chromosomal (e.g., Down syndrome, Turner syndrome, trisomy 13, trisomy 18) and single gene (e.g., Holt-Oram and Ellis-van Creveld syndromes) abnormalities, in utero infection (e.g., rubella), and maternal teratogens (e.g., ethanol, lithium). Rare families have been described in which a ventricular septal defect (VSD), atrial septal defect (ASD), patent ductus arteriosus (PDA), or primary pulmonary hypertension are transmitted as autosomal dominant characteristics. Cardiac abnormalities may also be included as components of a recognizable and named dysmorphic syndrome. In most of the congenital cardiac malformations, the etiology is attributed to multifactorial inheritance. The fetal pulmonary arteries normally see only a small fraction of the cardiac output because of shunting by way of the foramen ovale and the ductus arteriosus. When these close, the branch pulmonary arteries must remodel to accommodate the increased blood flow. Until this process is completed after the first few months of life, a murmur may be generated by a turbulent flow across these vessels (peripheral pulmonic stenosis).

Cyanosis

Visible cyanosis is present when greater than 3 to 5 g/dL of desaturated hemoglobin is present. Cyanosis, given a constant hemoglobin oxygen saturation, is more readily apparent with polycythemia and less readily apparent with anemia or the presence of fetal hemoglobin, which shifts the oxygen-hemoglobin saturation curve. A newborn may not be visibly cyanotic until the arterial PO_2 falls below 35 mm Hg. Cyanosis in the infant with congenital heart disease is almost always caused by right-to-left shunting of blood so that systemic venous blood returning to the heart bypasses the lungs before returning to the systemic circulation. This shunting may be at the atrial (ASD or patent foramen ovale), ventricular, or great vessel (PDA) level. The shunting is accompanied usually by decreased pulmonary blood flow. However, some specific lesions, such as the transposition of the great arteries (TGA), total anomalous pulmonary venous return (TAPVR), and truncus arteriosus may have normal or increased pulmonary blood flow because of their specific physiology. Uncommonly, a congenital heart defect may result in pulmonary edema that may itself contribute to cyanosis in an otherwise acyanotic lesion. Cyanosis may also be caused by increased pulmonary arterial pressure, for example, from pulmonary disease or polycythemia, resulting in right-to-left shunting through a normally patent ductus arteriosus or foramen ovale. When pulmonary arterial hypertension results in cyanosis from right-to-left shunting in an otherwise normal heart it is known as *persistent fetal circulation (PFC)*, or more accurately as *persistent pulmonary hypertension*. Pulmonary disease is always in the differential diagnosis and usually results in respiratory distress, an abnormal chest roentgenogram, and hypercapnea. Increased venous pressure may result in decreased local blood flow with venous suffusion and cyanosis. (See Chap. 194 for a detailed discussion of noncardiac causes of cyanosis.)

Heart Failure

Congestive heart failure in the older neonate is most often caused by lesions producing a large left-to-right shunt through a VSD or PDA. However, in the newborn, shunting through these defects is severely restricted by the normally elevated pulmonary vascular resistance, and these lesions do not produce signs of heart disease until shunting is increased coincident with the fall in pulmonary vascular resistance, typically at 1 to 2 months of age. Heart failure on the first day of life is commonly due to metabolic abnormalities

(e.g., anemia, polycythemia, neonatal thyrotoxicosis, hypothyroidism, hypocalcemia, hypomagnesemia, and hypoglycemia) or in utero dysrhythmias (usually paroxysmal supraventricular tachycardia [PSVT] or complete heart block). Structural defects that result in heart failure on the first day of life are those of severe left-sided outflow obstruction (critical aortic stenosis, hypoplastic left heart) and large arteriovenous malformations (cerebral or hepatic). Various disease processes may result in a cardiomyopathy with resultant heart failure in the neonatal period. A peripartum asphyxial insult may result in myocardial damage with resultant heart failure, predominantly of the right ventricle with transient tricuspid insufficiency. Myocarditis can affect persons at any age, including newborns. Endocardial fibroelastosis is a disease of unknown etiology characterized by a marked thickening of the endocardium. Although uncommon, it may produce heart failure from birth. If the left coronary artery arises anomalously from the pulmonary artery rather than from the aorta, it will result in inadequate myocardial perfusion and myocardial ischemia as the pulmonary arterial pressure falls at 1 to 2 months of age. Hypertrophic cardiomyopathy (idiopathic hypertrophic subaortic stenosis) is typically a disease of the ventricular septum and left ventricle in older children and adults. Occasionally, however, it may be present in the newborn. Pompe's disease, one of the glycogen storage diseases (À-1, 4-glucosidase deficiency) is the only glycogen storage disease that has a major cardiac as well as voluntary muscle involvement. Finally, infants of mothers with poorly controlled diabetes may have massive cardiomegaly and decreased myocardial function at the time of birth.

Dysrhythmias

Dysrhythmias may not have a known etiology. Paroxysmal supraventricular tachycardia is most common during the first month of life. The involved bypass tract is manifest as the Wolff-Parkinson-White syndrome only about one half of the time. Congenital heart block may be associated with maternal connective tissue disease with anti-R_o/SSA antibodies, most commonly systemic lupus erythematosus.

CLINICAL PRESENTATION

The signs of heart failure in infants are somewhat different than in older children and adults. Tachypnea is a common early sign. Other common signs are tachycardia, diaphoresis (especially with feeding), hepatomegaly, poor feeding and easy tiring with feeding, and failure to thrive. When heart failure is advanced, pulmonary crackles and a gallop may be noted and the infant will be oliguric. Unlike adult patients, peripheral edema is rare and the distinction between right-sided and left-sided heart failure is not clear. Since the liver is normally easily palpable in the infant about 2 cm below the right costal margin at the midclavicular line, palpation of liver size tends to be a good indicator of the degree of heart failure.

Cyanosis may not be present until low arterial PO_2 values are reached. A differentiation should be made between central cyanosis and peripheral cyanosis or acrocyanosis. Central cyanosis may be normal until 2 to 3 hours of life, but persistence beyond that time should raise concerns that the infant may have cyanotic congenital heart disease. Infants with cyanotic lesions are often tachypneic and hyperpneic but without respiratory distress. Their arterial PCO_2 is typically normal or even low.

Although not all of the congenital cardiac lesions can be discussed, salient points for the most common lesions are presented below.

Acyanotic Lesions

Ventricular Septal Defect. Although the most frequent congenital cardiac defect seen in childhood, an isolated VSD is usually asymptomatic in the nursery and may cause only a trivial or even no murmur. Similarly, the chest roentgenogram will be normal in the newborn. Only as pulmonary vascular resistance falls in the first 1 to 2 months does increasing shunting through the defect and increasing pulmonary blood flow result in a murmur and, if the shunt is great enough, signs of increasing congestive heart failure. These are often first noted on a routine well-baby examination.

Atrial Septal Defect. Simple, uncomplicated (secundum) ASDs are not symptomatic in the newborn period and do not generate a murmur. They are not detected on a routine physical examination, electrocardiogram, or chest roentgenogram in the neonatal period.

Patent Ductus Arteriosus. In the term newborn, PDAs are usually asymptomatic because of the normally elevated pulmonary vascular resistance, similar to VSDs. At 1 to 2 months of age a murmur, which was previously very soft or absent, becomes the typical PDA murmur in the left infraclavicular fossa. If there is major shunting through the PDA, congestive heart failure develops. In the newborn the murmur, if present, tends to be softer, systolic only, and heard lower down along the left sternal border than in older infants and children. It may be impossible to differentiate the murmur of a PDA in the newborn from that of a VSD at this age. Because much of the pulmonary arterial musculature develops at the end of gestation, pulmonary vascular resistance in the premature infant falls more rapidly than in term infants. This explains the development of congestive heart failure in premature infants with a PDA as they recover from respiratory distress syndrome in the first 1 or 2 weeks of life. It must always be remembered that a PDA in a premature infant does not exclude the presence of other congenital cardiac defects that may be masked by the PDA and that may even be "ductal dependent" (i.e., pulmonary or aortic blood flow depends on patency of the PDA).

Coarctation of the Aorta. Infants with coarctation typically present at 7 to 14 days of age, coincident with obstruction to descending aortic blood flow with closure of the ductus arteriosus. The hallmark of coarctation is the disparity of arterial pulses and blood pressure between the arms and the legs, although the left subclavian artery, supplying the left arm, may be variably involved by the narrowed area. Occasionally, the difference in pulses may not be apparent by palpation, and blood pressures must always be obtained in both arms and one leg to exclude the presence of a coarctation.

Aortic Stenosis. Only the most severe degrees of stenosis ("critical aortic stenosis") result in problems in the neonatal period. It is a rapidly life-threatening defect when it becomes manifest so early in life. These infants have poor cardiac output with poor peripheral pulses throughout. There may be a systolic ejection click. A murmur will not be generated if cardiac output is low.

Peripheral Pulmonic Stenosis. This asymptomatic condition has a murmur similar to a soft neonatal VSD or PDA murmur but is heard particularly well at the periphery of the lungs.

Endocardial Cushion Defect. This lesion, or more precisely, group of lesions (primum ASD ± basal VSD ± cleft mitral valve ± cleft tricuspid valve) has a variable presentation depending on its specific components. If a major atrioventricular valve insufficiency is present, the infant may present with early heart failure. Endocardial cushion defects are common in infants with Down syndrome and are present in approximately 25% of these children (approximately one half of those infants with Down syndrome who have congenital defects).

Arteriovenous Malformations. Although not strictly cardiac defects, large arteriovenous malformations present with severe congestive heart failure in the first few days of life. Infants with these lesions have a markedly hyperdynamic precordium and bounding pulses with a wide pulse pressure. A bruit is often, but not always, heard over the affected organ (typically the brain or liver).

Hypoplastic Left Heart. Hypoplastic left heart is due to atresia of the mitral or aortic valve and results in heart failure in the first few days of life. These infants have poor pulses throughout, poor peripheral perfusion, metabolic acidosis, and early death.

Anomalous Origin of the Left Coronary Artery. The left coronary artery may originate from the main pulmonary artery. The low oxygen content in this blood supplying the myocardium is surprisingly well tolerated. However, inadequate myocardial perfusion occurs at the time of the normal fall in pulmonary arterial resistance at 1 to 2 months of age. The increased exercise and energy expenditure associated with feeding may cause angina in these young infants, which may manifest itself as crying, pallor, and diaphoresis.

Vascular Rings, Pulmonary Arterial Sling. Vascular rings and pulmonary arterial sling defects cause difficulty by encircling the trachea alone or in combination with the ductus arteriosus or ligamentum arteriosum. These infants may have evidence of upper airway obstruction with inspiratory stridor in the nursery, or they may develop it in the first few months. This obstruction may be mild with episodic acute exacerbations.

Pompe's Disease. Infants with Pompe's disease present with hypotonia and cardiomyopathy usually at a few months of age.

Infant of a Diabetic Mother. Infants of mothers with poorly controlled diabetes may have a murmur and cardiomegaly. It is uncommon for the newborns to be symptomatic from cardiac involvement, and the cardiomegaly resolves spontaneously over several weeks.

Myocarditis. Myocarditis presents as profound, rapidly progressive heart failure. The newborn has poor peripheral pulses, a quiet precordium, and cardiomegaly. There may be a murmur of mitral insufficiency.

Transient Myocardial Ischemia. Occasionally, infants who have undergone a peripartum anoxic insult will develop ischemic injury to the myocardium. Unlike older patients with ischemic insults, these infants have predominantly right ventricular involvement and present with cardiomegaly and tricuspid insufficiency. As in other cases of myocardial injury, the blood levels of the MB fraction of creatine phosphokinase are elevated.

Hypertrophic Cardiomyopathy. Uncommonly, hypertrophic cardiomyopathy may present with heart failure in the newborn.

Cyanotic Lesions

Transposition of the Great Arteries. Typically these large predominantly male infants present with cyanosis from the time of delivery without the normal resolution over the first few hours. They are surprisingly without distress despite their profound cyanosis. Their physical examination, electrocardiogram, and chest roentgenogram can be close to normal. If there are associated lesions that allow for increased shunting between the pulmonary and systemic circulation, they may be less cyanotic.

Tetralogy of Fallot. The age at presentation of tetralogy of Fallot depends on the severity of the pulmonary stenosis. Most often, pulmonary stenosis is not well developed at birth and these infants do not become cyanotic until several months of age, or they may present only with the murmur of a VSD. If pulmonary stenosis is severe, they will present with cyanosis from birth. Hypercyanotic "Tet spells" are distinctly unusual in the first few months of life.

Total Anomalous Pulmonary Venous Return. If associated with obstruction to pulmonary venous return, typically with TAPVR below the diaphragm, infants present in the first week of life with cyanosis and tachypnea. The chest roentgenogram looks much like that of pulmonary edema, but the cardiac silhouette is normal or small. The arterial PO_2 of these infants can increase significantly in response to increases in the inspired oxygen concentration.

Persistent Fetal Circulation. These infants have already had another insult such as peripartum asphyxia or aspiration. A cardiac examination is essentially normal, although there may be a differential cyanosis of the upper and lower body with a large right-to-left ductal shunt. This differential cyanosis may not be discernible, particularly if there is also a significant atrial right-to-left shunt.

Tricuspid or Pulmonary Atresia. These infants present with cyanosis. There may be adequate pulmonary blood flow by way of the PDA to allow them to remain stable, but these newborns can deteriorate rapidly on ductal closure at 7 to 10 days of age.

Ebstein's Anomaly. This defect of tricuspid valve formation presents with signs related to tricuspid insufficiency and right-to-left atrial shunting. The newborns have cyanosis, massive cardiomegaly, and possibly atrial dysrhythmias related to atrial distention. The dysrhythmias and often the cyanosis resolve with the fall in pulmonary vascular resistance and decreasing tricuspid insufficiency. Ebstein's anomaly is often associated with the Wolff-Parkinson-White syndrome.

Dysrhythmias

Protracted in utero tachycardia or bradycardia can result in nonimmune hydrops fetalis. The specific cardiac rhythm can be determined by fetal echocardiography. Perhaps the most common "dysrhythmias" detected in the nursery are sinus arrhythmia and sinus bradycardia. Sinus arrhythmia is a normal finding that is more pronounced in children than in adults. There is sinus slowing during inspiration. Sinus slowing can be so pronounced that junctional or even ventricular escape beats are noted on the electrocardiogram. Although newborns are typically considered as having relatively high resting heart rates, healthy term newborns can have sleeping heart rates descend into the 70s. Sinus bradycardia can also accompany yawning, defecation, or apnea. If the heart rate responds appropriately to stimulation of the infant, and is not associated with apnea, the bradycardia is of no concern. As mentioned earlier, over 10% of newborns will have atrial or ventricular premature beats. Some of these will be noted on routine auscultation of the chest or palpation of the pulses. Almost all ectopy will resolve spontaneously by 1 month of age.

The most common pathologic dysrhythmia in the newborn is PSVT. The heart rate in infants with PSVT is higher than that in older children and adults and is usually over 210 beats per minute. In addition to hydrops fetalis, heart failure

Diagnostic Clues in Neonatal Heart Disease

Cyanosis (severe), pulmonary blood flow normal or increased ± narrow mediastinum:
    TGA

Mild cyanosis, increased pulmonary blood flow:
    TAPVR, truncus arteriosus, TGA with large VSD, double-outlet right ventricle, common ventricle

Cyanosis, pulmonary venous congestion, small heart:
    TAPVR

Cyanosis, decreased pulmonary blood flow:
    Massive cardiomegaly: Ebstein's anomaly, pulmonary atresia with tricuspid insufficiency
    Left ventricular hypertrophy: pulmonary atresia
    Superior QRS axis [0–(−90)]: tricuspid atresia
    QRS axis 30–90, no murmur: pulmonary atresia with intact ventricular septum
    Right ventricular hypertrophy, QRS axis 30–90, murmur: pulmonary stenosis
    Right ventricular hypertrophy, QRS axis >90, systolic murmur: VSD with pulmonary stenosis (tetralogy of Fallot)
    Right ventricular hypertrophy, QRS axis >90, continuous or no murmur: pulmonary atresia with VSD

Cyanosis, normal cardiac examination, upper to lower body Po_2 difference:
    PFC

Cyanosis, abnormal abdominal situs:
    Heterotaxy, usually asplenia

Heart failure, first week:
    Metabolic
    In utero dysrhythmia
    Tricuspid insufficiency murmur, elevated CPK-MB: transient myocardial ischemia
    Bounding pulses, hyperactive precordium ± bruit: arteriovenous malformation
    Upper to lower pulse disparity: coarctation
    Decreased pulses, left ventricular hypertrophy ± ejection click: critical aortic stenosis
    Decreased pulses, right ventricular hypertrophy, active precordium: hypoplastic left heart

Heart failure, 2–4 weeks:
    Acyanotic, murmur: VSD, PDA, endocardial cushion defect
    Acyanotic, no murmur:
        Left ventricular hypertrophy: endocardial fibroelastosis
        Low-voltage QRS: myocarditis
        Q-wave or T-wave inversion leads 1, aVL, and V5–V6: anomalous origin of left coronary artery
        Left ventricular hypertrophy, short PR interval, hypotonia: Pompe's disease
    Desaturated or cyanotic:
        No murmur or soft murmur: TAPVR
        VSD murmur, right ventricular hypertrophy: double-outlet right ventricle, TGA with VSD
        Biventricular hypertrophy: truncus arteriosus

and tachycardia may occur at any time. Since these infants cannot complain of tachycardia, they often do not come to medical attention until they have developed congestive heart failure. Although it may be difficult to differentiate the rhythm at this time from an appropriate sinus tachycardia, the heart rate in PSVT tends to be higher, and there is little if any beat-to-beat and second-to-second variability in the heart rate.

Exact diagnosis of the structural cardiac malformations depends on rigorous physical, roentgenographic, electrocardiographic, and echocardiographic examinations, as well as cardiac catheterization in difficult cases. However, a simplified approach using the presence of a murmur, cyanosis, or heart failure, the age at presentation, the pulmonary blood flow on chest roentgenogram, and the electrocardiogram is offered in the chart on Diagnostic Clues in Neonatal Heart Disease. These are guidelines; significant individual variation may exist.

WORK-UP

In evaluating these patients, one must steer a careful course between early and appropriate referral to a pediatric cardiologist and needless transfer of infants who have stable or no heart disease. Primary physicians must always keep in mind that electrocardiographic, radiologic, and physical examination findings in this age group may be nonspecific and even completely normal in the presence of significant structural heart disease. A specific diagnosis using the basics of the history, physical examination, electrocardiogram, and chest roentgenogram is often possible. This allows appropriate therapeutic measures to be begun at an earlier stage, after consultation with a pediatric cardiologist.

History

The history may provide clues to various lesions even in newborns. Specific points include maternal drug usage (licit and illicit), connective tissue disease, rashes or other infectious diseases during pregnancy, diabetes, thyroid disease, and a family history of heart disease. The presence of in utero tachycardia or bradycardia should be investigated, and the chart should be reviewed for evidence of peripartum asphyxia (e.g., low Apgar score). The age at onset of heart disease provides an important clue to the specific lesion.

Physical Examination

A complete physical examination is crucial. Is there gross evidence of a dysmorphic syndrome? Are the vital signs normal for age? The blood pressure must be taken in both arms and in a leg. This is easily done manually or with available automated machines. If cyanosis is present, is it acrocyanosis or central cyanosis? If it is central cyanosis, is it generalized or does it affect primarily just the upper or the lower body? Is the skin warm and well perfused, or is it cold and mottled, suggesting heart failure? Are there cutaneous hemangiomas that might be accompanied by internal arteriovenous malformations? Are the peripheral pulses symmetrical in the arms and the legs? Are the pulses weak and thready, or are they bounding, suggesting an aortic runoff lesion? Although an examination of the jugular veins is often not productive in infants because of their short fat necks, the scalp veins may become distended in severe congestive heart failure. Are the lungs clear, or is there evidence of pulmonary disease or pulmonary edema? Is the precordial activity increased? Are there bruits heard over the skull or liver?

Despite the normally rapid heart rate in newborns, cardiac auscultation is made easier by the routinely loud cardiac sounds transmitted by the thin chest wall. The first heart sound is normally narrowly split, and this should be differentiated from a systolic ejection click. The second sound is normally more narrowly split, and the pulmonic component is louder than in older children because of the elevated pulmonary vascular resistance and pulmonary arterial pressure in newborns. Murmurs should be listened for and characterized as in older patients. If the infant is connected to a ventilator, disconnecting the ventilator tubing from the endotracheal tube for a few seconds will markedly increase the quality of the auscultatory examination at no risk to the infant. The abdomen should be examined for hepatosplenomegaly. The liver is normally palpable approximately 2 cm below the right costal margin in the midclavicular line. It is best palpated by gentle pressure of the fingers on the abdomen and moving the hand cephalad and caudad. The fingers will fall off the edge of the liver, which will be felt better than by direct, deep palpation.

Laboratory Tests

Chest Roentgenogram. A single frontal view of the chest will suffice. Very little useful information regarding heart disease is obtained from the lateral chest roentgenogram in young infants. The film should be examined for cardiac size and position, evidence of abdominal situs (manifested by stomach and liver position), a narrow mediastinum, pulmonary blood flow, and the side of the aortic arch (right-sided arches are associated with tetralogy and double-outlet right ventricle). In addition, the pulmonary vascular pattern can be examined to see if it looks like the cascading pattern of normal pulmonary arteries or the more horizontal pattern of bronchial collateral vessels. Films taken in exhalation and the normally large neonatal thymus may both give the appearance of cardiomegaly. The pulmonary blood flow in an expiratory film will also appear to be increased.

Electrocardiogram. All patients with congenital heart disease should have an electrocardiogram. It must be remembered that all electrocardiographic variables have age-, and sometimes rate-related normal values. Some of the more important values are listed in Table 54-1. The change in R wave predominance with age reflects the gradual resolution of the normal fetal right ventricular predominance. The T wave is normally upright in lead V_1 until the fourth day and then again after about 10 years of age. Persistence or resumption of its upright position is a sign of right ventricular hypertrophy. The Qt_c interval (<0.4 second) is the same in

Table 54-1.   Selected Age-Related Normal ECG Values

	1 DAY	1–30 DAYS	1–3 MONTHS
QRS axis	110–170	70–120	30–110
PR interval (sec)	0.11	0.11	rate 91–110: 0.14 rate 111–130: 0.13 rate 131–150: 0.12 rate >150: 0.11
QRS duration (sec)	0.08	0.08	0.09
R V_{4R} (mm)	5–13	4–8	2–9
R V_1 (mm)	6–19	5–17	6–17
R V_5 (mm)	5–15	4–22	12–25
R V_6 (mm)	2–10	3–15	7–19

infants as in older children. The electrocardiogram of the premature infant shows a shorter PR interval (0.10 seconds) and QRS duration (0.05 seconds) with lower QRS amplitude and a more rapid shift to left ventricular predominance. The P-wave axis should be the same as in older patients. An upright or rightward P-wave axis may be seen with the heterotaxy syndromes.

Arterial Blood Gas Analysis. Arterial blood gas analysis is critical, particularly to confirm a clinical diagnosis of cyanosis and to monitor response to therapy. Severe heart failure will result in metabolic acidosis. Cyanosis and a normal arterial PO_2 suggest methemoglobinemia or an abnormal hemoglobin. If congenital heart disease is suspected, samples should be obtained from preductal (right radial or right temporal arteries) and postductal (umbilical artery) sites to assess right-to-left ductal shunting. The arterial PO_2 is normally 45 mm Hg by 1 hour of age and 60 mm Hg by 1 day of age. If the sample is obtained with the infant crying, the PO_2 may be much lower than a resting sample even in normal infants. Oxygen saturation by pulse oximetry is easily done and may substitute for PO_2 measurements.

Echocardiography. Echocardiography, often combined with Doppler evaluation of blood flow, has made major contributions to the early, noninvasive diagnosis of even the most complex congenital cardiac defects. Unfortunately, all of these tests, with the exception of the echocardiogram, may be normal. If there are any questions, a pediatric cardiologist should be consulted.

MANAGEMENT

The specific surgical approach to structural heart disease depends on the specific lesion, as well as the current practices of the cardiac surgeon. However, some general approaches to medical management can be made.

Ductal-Dependent Lesions. Any time there is a concern that a congenital cardiac lesion is present that requires ductal patency for supply of either systemic or pulmonary blood flow, ductal patency should be maintained pharmacologically with prostaglandin E₁ (PGE₁, Prostin VR) until a definitive diagnosis and surgical palliation or correction is undertaken. This procedure can be life saving. Even if a later examination (echocardiography, catheterization) shows that a ductal-dependent lesion is not present, PGE₁ can be discontinued with little if any detriment. Ductal-dependent cyanotic lesions include TGA, pulmonary atresia or severe pulmonary stenosis, and tricuspid atresia. The acyanotic lesions include coarctation of the aorta, hypoplastic left heart, and critical aortic stenosis. The beginning dose of PGE₁ is 0.1 μg/kg/min. After a therapeutic response is achieved (as determined by increased PO_2 or increased peripheral pulses), the dose can be decreased to 0.05 μg/kg/min, and in some infants the disorder may even be controlled with lower doses. The most common complications of PGE₁ are apnea, fever, and cutaneous flushing.

Heart Failure. The general approach to the newborn with heart failure is the same as for any patient. Efforts should be directed at optimizing the four determinants of cardiac output: rhythm, inotropy, preload, and afterload. In the nursery, specific additional measures include using supplemental oxygen and an infant seat, ensuring a neutral thermal environment, correcting acidosis, hypoglycemia, or infections if present, and normalizing hematocrit. Critically ill newborns will occasionally require intubation, mechanical ventilation, and rarely even sedation and paralysis to control severe heart failure with metabolic acidosis. Other measures applicable to all young children include a salt-limited diet, diuretics, and digoxin. Fluid restriction should not be used if it results in a diminished intake of calories. Caloric supplementation, either by use of 24 cal/oz formula or by supplementing regular formula with medium-chain triglycerides will provide much needed extra calories. Several commercially available infant formulas have a lower salt content than others. The most widely used diuretic is furosemide (Lasix) at a dose of 1 mg/kg two to three times per day intravenously or orally, although some infants will require more, particularly if this drug is given orally. Potassium depletion is a concern as in older patients. The schedule for digitalization depends on the age of the infant and the mode of administration. One half the total digitalizing dose is given followed by one fourth in 8 hours, and one fourth 8 hours after that. It may also be given in three equal doses 8 hours apart. After the total digitalizing dose has been given, the maintenance dose is begun. The normal maintenance dose is one fourth the digitalizing dose, if both are administered by the same route (orally or parenterally). If the infant was digitalized intravenously and the maintenance dose is given orally, the daily maintenance dose is one third the total digitalizing dose. The daily dose is usually given in two divided doses, every 12 hours (Table 54-

Table 54-2. Digoxin Doses (mg/kg)

AGE	DIGITALIZING PARENTERAL	DIGITALIZING ORAL
Premature	0.02	0.03
Term−2 weeks	0.03	0.05
2 weeks−6 months	0.05	0.06

2). Digoxin levels are usually not useful in newborns. The usual therapeutic levels are higher than in adults.

Infants who have lesions that could result in congestive heart failure in the first few months (e.g., VSD, PDA) should be seen at least monthly for the first 3 months. Infants with significant heart failure due to surgically correctable lesions should have surgical correction relatively early, rather than undergoing protracted medical therapy, if appropriate surgical care is available.

Indomethacin (Indocin), useful for ductal closure in the preterm infant, is not useful in term and post-term infants.

Congenital Heart Block. If congenital heart block is diagnosed prenatally, a pediatric cardiologist or a pediatric surgeon should be notified in case emergent transvenous pacemaker placement is required. If the heart rate is more than 60 beats per minute, no therapy is usually required. An isoproterenol (Isuprel) infusion may be used as a temporizing measure, but results are usually minimal.

Paroxysmal Supraventricular Tachycardia. The therapy for PSVT is the same as for older children, using vagal maneuvers, digoxin, β-adrenergic antagonists, and, in critically ill children, electrical cardioversion. Verapamil, although very effective, is contraindicated in newborns because of the high incidence of profound hypotension. The diving seal reflex (application of ice water to the face) tends to be more effective in newborns than in older children. The dose of digoxin is the same as for treating heart failure. The dose of intravenous propranolol is 0.1 mg/kg. Conversion by overdrive pacing, either transvenous or transesophageal, should be reserved for use in specialized centers. Once the rhythm is successfully terminated, these infants are usually maintained on digoxin for 6 to 12 months. It is then discontinued if the infant has no further episodes.

Persistent Fetal Circulation. PFC is treated by hyperventilation to produce a significant respiratory alkalosis. Occasionally these infants also require treatment with tolazoline (Priscoline), a vasodilator. The dose is 1 mg/kg intravenously into a vein draining to the superior vena cava (arm or scalp) followed by an infusion of 1 to 2 mg/kg/h. In most infants the disorder is controlled successfully with hyperventilation alone.

PATIENT EDUCATION

Parents of infants who are at risk of developing heart failure should be given a list of the signs of congestive heart failure with instructions to contact the physician should any of these signs develop. Parents should also be reassured that if heart failure develops, it will be over a period of days to weeks and not as an acute emergency. It might also be worthwhile to explain that the term *heart failure* is not as ominous as it may sound. The families of all infants with congenital heart disease should receive appropriate counseling regarding the risk of recurrence in future pregnancies.

ANNOTATED BIBLIOGRAPHY

Braudo M, Rowe RD. Auscultation of the heart—early neonatal period. Am J Dis Child. 1961;101:67-78. (Describes the common occurrence of murmurs in normal newborns.)

Davignon A, Rautaharju P, Boisselle E, et al. ECG standards for children: Percentile charts. Pediatr Cardiol. 1979-1980;1:133-152. (Lists age-related normal values for a wide range of ECG variables.)

Lees MH. Cyanosis of the newborn infant. Recognition and clinical evaluation. J Pediatr. 1970;77:484-498. (Discusses the pathophysiology of cyanosis, particularly in the neonate.)

Southall DP, Johnson AM, Shinebourne EA, et al. Frequency and outcome of disorders of cardiac rhythm and conduction in a population of newborn infants. Pediatrics. 1981;68:58-66. (Discusses the incidence, distribution, and prognosis of abnormal rhythms noted in the nursery.)

Long WA, ed. Fetal and Neonatal Cardiology. Philadelphia, Pa: WB Saunders, 1990. (An extensive text exclusively covering cardiology of the neonate.)

55

Heart Murmurs

Herbert E. Cohn

The incidence of congenital heart disease is 6 to 8:1000 live births or less than 1 in 100 children. Cardiac murmurs are noted in 50% to 70% of children who are active, healthy, and asymptomatic. Most of the latter have insignificant or *functional* cardiac murmurs that represent vibrations of normal structures within the heart. It is essential to differentiate these from the significant cardiac murmurs that reflect underlying congenital heart lesions and that warrant referral to a pediatric cardiologist for further evaluation. One should be able to do this by means of a history, cardiovascular examination, and basic laboratory information consisting of an electrocardiogram, chest roentgenogram, and hemoglobin determination.

PATHOPHYSIOLOGY AND CLINICAL PRESENTATION

The *vibratory murmur* is produced at the aortic valve as blood ejected in systole passes over the free margins of the open aortic valve leaflets. An open aortic valve is not cir-

cular but triangular. It is the valve leaflets that form the sides of the triangle that vibrate in systole. The pulmonary systolic ejection murmur takes its name from its chest wall location at the upper left sternal edge over the pulmonic valve. Some phonocardiographic studies have suggested that this murmur's origin is actually in the left ventricular outflow tract and that its mechanism is similar to that of the vibratory murmur. In both cases, the cardiac murmurs reflect vibrations of normal structures. There are no pressure or volume overloads. No compensatory mechanisms operate, thus no additional physical or laboratory findings should be present.

The murmurs of *valvular aortic* and *pulmonic stenosis* stem from significant turbulence as blood is ejected from a ventricle in systole across thickened, stenotic valve leaflets. When sufficient vibration occurs, it causes the anterior chest wall to vibrate; this palpable sensation is called a *thrill*. The area of greatest turbulence is distal to the stenotic valve, and dilatation of the arterial wall occurs there. As the thickened valve domes or pops open in systole causing a jet of ejected blood to strike the dilated, tensed arterial wall distal to the valve, a high-frequency sound called an *ejection click* is produced.

Atrial septal defects produce systolic ejection murmurs at the pulmonic valve. Blood flows from left to right through the defect at the atrial level and produces a right ventricular volume overload. As right ventricular volume increases there is a relative stenosis at the pulmonic valve. Thus, more blood is presented to the pulmonic valve orifice than can readily pass, which accentuates the physiologically occurring vibrations at the pulmonic valve. Since right ventricular volume is increased on an absolute basis, right ventricular ejection time and pulmonic valve closure are delayed and there is wide splitting of the pulmonic component of the second heart sound. If the degree of left-to-right shunting is significantly large (a pulmonary to systemic flow ratio above 2:1), a relative tricuspid stenosis also occurs and an early diastolic flow murmur is audible at the tricuspid area (lower left sternal edge). This diastolic murmur is referred to as a *flow rumble*.

The murmur of a *ventricular septal defect* reflects the turbulence of blood flow through the defect itself, commonly located in the membranous ventricular septum. The vibrations are harsh and pansystolic (i.e., they have almost the same pitch and intensity throughout systole as opposed to peaking in intensity in midsystole as do ejection murmurs). Blood flow produces a right ventricular pressure and volume overload, increased pulmonary arterial pressure and flow, and a left ventricular volume overload as it flows from left to right through the defect. If the blood flow is sufficiently large (a pulmonary to systemic flow ratio above 2:1), a relative mitral stenosis occurs and a mid-diastolic murmur or flow rumble is audible at the apex.

The murmur of *hypertrophic subaortic stenosis* is associated with a diamond-shaped systolic ejection murmur heard along the lower left sternal edge. The hypertrophied

Differential Diagnosis of Systolic Ejection Murmurs in Childhood

Vibratory, musical murmur (innocent, functional)
Basal pulmonic ejection murmur
Valvar aortic stenosis
Valvar pulmonic stenosis
Atrial septal defect
Ventricular septal defect
Hypertrophic subaortic stenosis

---

muscular portion of the ventricular septum obstructs the left ventricular outflow tract in systole. Events such as the Valsalva maneuver that transiently decrease left ventricular filling intensify the obstruction and accentuate the murmur. A bifid pulse wave is palpable at the radial pulse and reflects the pattern of left ventricular emptying during systole. (See the display, "Differential Diagnosis of Systolic Ejection Murmurs in Childhood.")

WORK-UP

History

The detection of a cardiac murmur frequently leads the pediatrician to conduct a more thorough evaluation of the cardiovascular system. A careful history and cardiovascular system review, including a review of the prenatal and perinatal history, should be obtained including inquiry into the child's level of activity and endurance, which often reflect cardiovascular performance. A history of recurrent pneumonitis or lower respiratory infections may be found, especially in patients with left-to-right shunt lesions. The rate of linear growth and weight gain can be reduced in the presence of increased caloric expenditure associated with increased cardiovascular workload or congestive heart failure. Linear growth is not usually affected, but slower than normal weight gain is common. Cardiovascular signs and symptoms such as syncope or chest pain may indicate significant left or right ventricular outflow tract obstruction. Cyanosis associated with exposure to cold or prolonged bathing, chest pain that is "sticking" in quality and brought on by deep inspiration, and palpitations associated with anxiety may appear to reflect cardiac disorders but are rarely of cardiac origin in childhood.

Previous cardiologic evaluations, previous hospitalizations, or studies such as electrocardiograms and chest roentgenograms may provide baseline data for comparison with current findings. A review of the family history is important. A parent or sibling with known congenital heart disease increases the probability of a patient having a congenital heart lesion.

Physical Examination

Clinical findings that reflect structural cardiac lesions are often present but may be subtle. Neither the intensity nor the quality of sound of most cardiac murmurs provides reliable criteria by which the significance of the murmur can be determined. Furthermore, lesions such as mitral valve prolapse or bicuspid aortic valve may not produce a cardiac murmur. A child with a significant congenital heart lesion requiring surgery may be asymptomatic. Therefore, an approach that includes a search for other physical findings such as abnormal precordial impulses or chest deformities, an assessment of the second heart sound components in terms of intensity and movement with respirations, and the presence of ejection clicks or diastolic flow murmurs is necessary to yield an accurate assessment of the child's cardiovascular status.

An inspection of the child's chest for an asymmetric precordial bulge may reflect underlying ventricular hypertrophy. A palpable ventricular impulse reinforces the high index of suspicion for ventricular hypertrophy. Abnormalities of the second heart sound, both in terms of intensity and movement with respiration, are valuable means of assessing right ventricular hemodynamics. A widened split of the second heart sound generally indicates a right ventricular volume overload. An increased intensity of the second heart sound indicates an elevated pulmonary arterial pressure. When the pulmonary arterial pressure is sufficiently elevated, an increased intensity often results in a palpable second heart sound along the upper left sternal edge. The presence of an ejection click generally reflects a dilated aorta or pulmonary artery in the vicinity of the click. This is commonly found with obstructive valvular lesions such as aortic or pulmonic stenosis. Clicks are found in other conditions and cause dilatation of a great vessel, such as truncus arteriosus when the aortic root is dilated.

The assessment of a cardiac murmur should include at least six characteristics: (1) timing; (2) quality; (3) intensity; (4) duration; (5) location; and (6) radiation of sound. *Timing* may be described as systolic, diastolic, or continuous, the latter referring to a murmur being present in systole and continuing beyond the second heart sound into diastole, even if it is not present throughout all of diastole. *Quality* refers to the characteristics of the sound, such as "harsh," "soft," "vibratory," or "musical." The *intensity* of systolic murmurs is graded on a scale of 1 to 6, whereas the intensity of diastolic murmurs is graded on a scale of 1 to 4. The *duration* refers to the amount of systole or diastole in which the murmur is heard, such as holosystolic or midsystolic. The *location* refers to the area where the murmur is loudest. The *radiation* of sound is usually in the direction of flow. Murmurs of pulmonic stenosis, for example, are heard in the pulmonary area and over both lung fields posteriorly, and murmurs of mitral insufficiency are heard in the left axilla.

The most common *innocent* or functional murmur is a *vibratory systolic ejection murmur*. It is of low to medium pitch with a musical quality and is best heard along the lower left sternal edge, at the third to fourth left interspace, and toward the apex. It is short, midsystolic, and ends well before the second heart sound. It is heard best when the patient is in the supine position, diminishes in the upright position, and is intensified by fever or excitement. There are no precordial impulses or deformities, normal first and second heart sounds are present, and no clicks or extra sounds are noted.

The *basal or pulmonary systolic ejection murmur* is higher in pitch and less uniform in quality than the vibratory murmur. This functional murmur is best heard when the patient is in the supine position and is intensified by fever or excitement. These systolic murmurs are usually less than grade 3/6 in intensity and are usually not transmitted to the back. They are associated with a normal second heart sound whose two components widen in inspiration and narrow with expiration. As noted, there are no associated cardiovascular findings on physical examination. The electrocardiogram and chest films are normal.

The continuous murmur known as a *venous hum* is also considered a functional murmur. It extends through systole into diastole. It is best heard at the upper left or right sternal edge with the patient in the upright position and can be obliterated by placement of a thumb over the external jugular vein just above the clavicle or by having the patient turn his or her head laterally. This murmur disappears with the patient in the supine position, and there are no other associated physical findings.

Diastolic flow murmurs are noted with large left-to-right shunt lesions associated with a pulmonary to systemic flow ratio of greater than 2:1. Similar phenomena occur if there is a left-to-right ventricular volume overload associated with mitral or tricuspid valve regurgitation and relative stenosis at either valve.

The murmurs reflecting atrial septal defects and mild valvular pulmonic stenosis may closely resemble the pulmonary systolic ejection murmur. The associated findings, however, differentiate these lesions. Atrial septal defects have wide splitting of the second heart sound components that do not narrow to a single sound on expiration. The tapping impulse of the right ventricular volume overload is felt over the left precordium along the left sternal edge. A slight left precordial bulge may be evident. The electrocardiogram shows a minor right ventricular conduction delay or incomplete right bundle branch block pattern and evidence for a right ventricular hypertrophy. Chest roentgenograms show increased pulmonary vascular markings and a fullness to the pulmonary arterial segment. The heart size is generally normal but may be slightly increased. Valvular pulmonic stenosis is associated with an ejection click along the left sternal edge from the fourth left intercostal space to the pulmonic area. The click precedes the systolic ejection murmur, which is harsh, diamond-shaped, and is best heard along the upper left sternal edge at the second to third left interspace. A palpable impulse reflects right ventricular hypertrophy. A thrill reflects turbulence at the pulmonic valve but does not convey reliable information about severity. The electrocardiogram shows evidence of right ventricular hypertrophy. The chest posteroanterior and lateral roentgenograms may show decreased or normal pulmonary vascular markings, and the overall heart size is generally normal.

The ventricular septal defect, uncomplicated by pulmonary arterial hypertension, may have a harsh pansystolic murmur beginning with the first heart sound and lasting throughout the aortic component of the second heart sound. This murmur is often associated with a thrill and is best heard at the lower left sternal edge, radiating to the xiphoid region. The pulmonary component of the second heart sound is neither accentuated nor obscured and is best heard at the lower left sternal edge. If the magnitude of left-to-right shunting is sufficiently large, a diastolic flow rumble may be audible at the apex. There is no ejection click unless the ventricular septal defect is closing by aneurysm formation in the ventricular septum. Electrocardiographic findings may show left ventricular hypertrophy or combined ventricular hypertrophy. The chest posteroanterior and lateral films show increased pulmonary vascular markings and ventricular enlargement.

Laboratory Tests

The electrocardiogram provides several different kinds of information. The heart rate and rhythm can be determined by inspection. The intervals of the P, QRS, and T waves and characteristics of the electrical conduction system can be measured. The presence and severity of ventricular hypertrophy can be interpreted by voltage criteria and pattern recognition. The type of physiologic adaptations, such as pressure or volume overload made by each ventricle, can be distinguished. The electrical axis in a three-dimensional plane can be determined, and is valuable in understanding both the conduction system and the adaptations of ventricular hypertrophy.

The chest roentgenogram provides information on cardiac size and silhouette, the pulmonary vasculature, and the location and configuration of the aortic arch. The boot-shaped upturned apex of right ventricular enlargement and the figure-eight or snowman configuration of supracardiac total anomalous pulmonary venous return are two examples.

The hemoglobin determination provides information on anemia or polycythemia and is a sensitive indicator for chronic hypoxemia.

These laboratory studies are readily available in the primary care setting and provide independent sources of information that may support information derived from the history and physical examination. For example, the presence of a right ventricular impulse, evidence for right ventricular hypertrophy on the electrocardiogram, and an upturned apex on the cardiac silhouette all support the impression of a real abnormality in cardiovascular function and help to distinguish the patient with a structural congenital heart lesion from a patient with an insignificant cardiac murmur.

Noninvasive Studies

The various forms of echocardiography provide much detailed physiologic data on cardiovascular anatomy and function that can be obtained noninvasively. The M-mode echocardiogram gives information on chamber dimensions and wall thicknesses, as well as the pericardial space and the presence of an effusion. The information is printed on paper, and assessment of ventricular function can be made.

The two-dimensional echocardiogram provides a videotape picture of intracardiac anatomy (e.g. the septal and valvular structures, chamber walls, and chamber dimensions.) Septal defects, thickened valve leaflets, or membranous structures can be visualized directly.

Doppler echocardiography can detect specific sites of turbulence within the heart or circulation. It can measure the velocity of blood flow at an obstructive site. From these data, one can estimate the pressure difference across the obstructive site that produced the increased flow velocity. This technique provides a graphic picture, on screen or on paper, of the turbulence associated with increased blood flow.

Doppler color flow imaging combines the use of Doppler echocardiography with two-dimensional echocardiography by displaying the flow data in color, in real time, on the two-dimensional echocardiographic image, all being recorded on videotape. Hence, one can visualize blood flow patterns of interest and can localize a source of turbulence to specific anatomic structures, such as stenotic valves or septal defects.

Echocardiographic studies are not generally available in the primary care setting and are costly. The application of these techniques is best reserved for the pediatric cardiologist when the patient's clinical findings require these studies.

INDICATIONS FOR REFERRAL

The primary care provider can generally differentiate patients with insignificant murmurs from those with structural congenital heart lesions. Children identified as having structural congenital or acquired heart disease should be referred to a pediatric cardiologist for further evaluation and therapy as necessary. Children with borderline findings in which a more definitive evaluation is necessary to distinguish whether they have a significant congenital heart problem should also be referred. Children with known congenital heart disease whose disease severity and course need to be monitored with respect to medical management, the timing of surgery, or changes in the patient's clinical course also warrant referral to a pediatric cardiologist.

PATIENT EDUCATION

If the cardiovascular evaluation detects structural congenital heart disease, the child should receive appropriate bacterial endocarditis prophylaxis. If the child is found to have a cardiac murmur that is insignificant and no real structural congenital heart lesion is noted, it is important to emphasize that the child does not have any cardiac disease. The emphasis should be on health and fitness rather than on an insignificant finding that may mistakenly carry undertones of morbidity and negative psychosocial values.

ANNOTATED BIBLIOGRAPHY

Adams FH, Emmanouilides GC, Riemenschneider TA, eds. Moss' Heart Disease in Infants, Children and Adolescents. 4th ed. Baltimore, Md: Williams & Wilkins, 1989. (Exhaustive, multiauthored reference for pediatric cardiologists.)

Caceres CA, Perry LW, eds. The Innocent Murmur, A Problem in Clinical Practice. Boston, Mass: Little, Brown & Co, 1967. (Interesting book that relates diverse views on the characteristics and causes of an innocent murmur.)

Gooch AS, Maranhao V, Goldberg H. Clues to Diagnosis in Congenital Heart Disease. Philadelphia, Pa: FA Davis, 1969. (150 diagnostic puzzles based on clinical findings in patients with congenital heart disease.)

Fyler DC. Nadas's Pediatric Cardiology. 3rd ed. Philadelphia, Pa: Hanley and Belfus, 1992. (Concise, thorough discussion of cyanotic and acyanotic congenital heart disease and a useful reference.)

Perloff JK. The Clinical Recognition of Congenital Heart Disease. 3rd ed. Philadelphia, Pa: WB Saunders, 1987. (Emphasis on physical examination findings and relationship to physical measurements, such as carotid pulse tracings, phonocardiography, and cardiac catheterization data.)

Stein PD. A Physical and Physiological Basis for the Interpretation of Cardiac Auscultation: Evaluations Based Primarily on the Second Sound and Ejection Murmurs. Mount Kisco, NY: Futura Publishing Company, 1981. (Detailed discussion on turbulence and cardiac murmurs that reflect it.)

56

Hypertension

Jerold C. Woodhead

Diagnosis and management of hypertension require an understanding of the changes in normal blood pressure associated with growth from infancy to adolescence. Early detection of hypertension and its effective, long-term management can greatly reduce its associated morbidity and mortality. This goal can be achieved by including regular blood pressure measurement in routine preventive health care for *all* children 3 years of age and older. In addition, selective screening of infants and young children with known risk for hypertension, and recognition of symptomatic hypertension at any age, will allow detection of those who need close monitoring or treatment. However, a single modestly elevated blood pressure reading does not justify the diagnosis of hypertension. Care must be taken to assign this diagnosis only to patients for whom blood pressure elevation has been documented by repeat measurements. Although the medical consequences of hypertension can be serious, the social and psychological morbidity of a diagnosis of hypertension in a normotensive person is great. Too often, a person mislabeled "hypertensive" in childhood or adolescence finds insurance impossible to obtain or job opportunities closed as an adult.

PATHOPHYSIOLOGY

Control of Blood Pressure

Modulation of blood pressure involves the interaction of renal and nonrenal mechanisms. The principal renal factors active in blood pressure control include the renin–angiotensin system, the renal–blood volume–pressure control mechanism, the renal response to hormones such as aldosterone, antidiuretic hormone, and others, and the renal response to the sympathetic nervous system. These combine with cardiac, central nervous system, and vascular mechanisms to control blood pressure. Renal mechanisms, overall, have the major effect. A detailed discussion of the central, integrative role of the renal–blood volume–pressure control mechanism in the maintenance of long-term blood pressure control is beyond the scope of this chapter.

Normal Blood Pressure

Blood pressure increases with growth and differs among boys and girls at all ages; but, unlike adult blood pressure, it does *not* differ by race. Prospective cohort studies in the United States and Great Britain provided the data used by the Second Task Force on Blood Pressure Control in Children to develop standards for blood pressure from infancy to adolescence (Fig. 56-1). The Task Force also provided definitions of the different blood pressure levels (Table 56-1), an age-based classification of hypertension (Table 56-2), and recommendations for detection, evaluation, and management of hypertension. The blood pressure nomograms in Figure 56-1 represent an extremely practical tool for clinical use. They provide age-specific blood pressure norms and the weight and stature parameters for which the norms are valid, and they can serve as a permanent record when used to plot blood pressure measurements.

Blood pressure also varies with body habitus, being higher for tall or heavy persons than for their shorter or leaner peers. The nomograms in Figure 56-1 are valid only for persons whose height and weight fall between the 10th and 90th percentiles for age and sex. When a child's body size falls outside this range, blood pressure should be compared with the norms for older or younger children as appropriate. Obesity, however, merits a special note: Obese persons have higher blood pressure and a higher incidence of hypertension than do those who are lean.

Hypertension

Elevated blood pressure in childhood is a risk factor for development of true hypertension. Hypertension in adults predisposes to premature cardiovascular disease and complicates many other diseases, especially hyperlipidemia and diabetes mellitus. The relationship between childhood hypertension and adult hypertensive cardiovascular disease has not been proven, although most investigators assume that adult primary (essential) hypertension begins in childhood. Because no risk data exist on which to base a rigorous definition of hypertension (or, for that matter, normal blood pressure), the definitions in Table 56-2 were developed from clinical experience. According to these definitions, persons having blood pressure between the 90th and 95th percentiles have *high normal* blood pressure. Blood pressure readings are not labeled *hypertensive* until they equal or surpass the 95th percentile on three repeated measurements. *Significant hypertension* reflects blood pressure that does not reach the 99th percentile, and *severe hypertension* has blood pressure readings at or above the 99th percentile for age and sex. The risk of adverse outcomes increases as the blood pressure progressively deviates above the normal range. Hypertension, thus, has a statistical definition, validated by clinical observations that associate adverse outcomes with the level of blood pressure.

In addition to severity, hypertension is classified by cause into two etiologic groups: *primary* and *secondary*. Primary hypertension, also known as *essential* hypertension, has no identifiable cause. Secondary hypertension, as the name implies, results from an underlying anatomical abnormality or disease process. Secondary hypertension has its greatest incidence in infancy and childhood, while primary hypertension becomes increasingly common in older children and adolescents. Hypertension may be symptomatic or asymptomatic, whether primary or secondary. Symptoms occur more commonly when blood pressure exceeds the 99th percentile.

CLINICAL PRESENTATION

Hypertension may be sustained, transient, or labile. It typically presents with elevation of both systolic and diastolic pressures, although occasionally, an adolescent will be identified with elevation of systolic blood pressure only. In addition, hypertension may present as an acute, symptomatic blood pressure elevation that requires prompt identification and management. Sustained hypertension causes the most problems for the patient and the physician, although the transient hypertension associated with an acute illness or disease process may require medical management. Labile hypertension is often hard to identify and has uncertain consequences for children and adolescents. Isolated systolic hypertension probably does not have the same significance for children and adolescents that it does for adults and does not usually require treatment with antihypertensive medications.

(Text continues on p. 222)

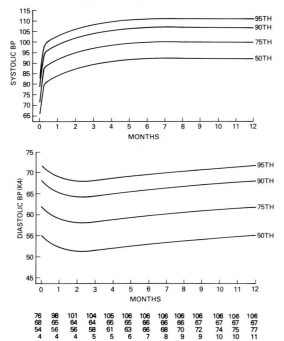

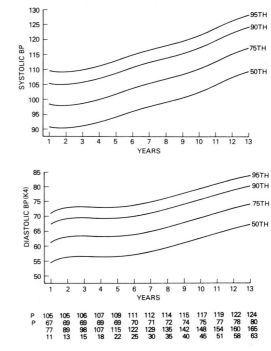

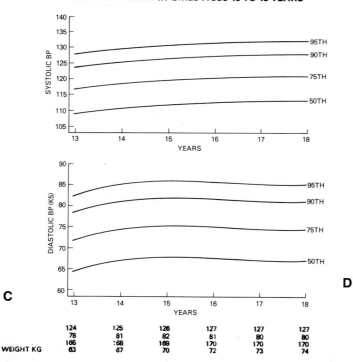

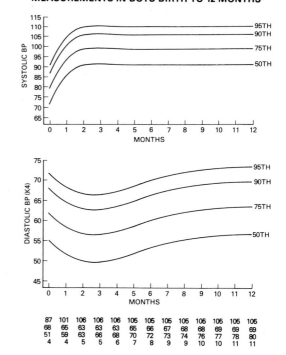

A

76	98	101	104	105	106	106	106	106	106	106	106	106
68	65	64	64	65	65	66	66	66	67	67	67	67
54	56	56	58	61	63	66	68	70	72	74	75	77
4	4	4	5	5	6	7	8	9	9	10	10	11

B

P	105	105	106	107	109	111	112	114	115	117	119	122	124
P	67	69	69	69	69	70	71	72	74	75	77	78	80
	77	89	98	107	115	122	129	135	142	148	154	160	165
	11	13	15	18	22	25	30	35	40	45	51	58	63

C

124	125	126	127	127	127
78	81	82	81	80	80
166	168	169	170	170	170
WEIGHT KG	63	67	70	72	73	74

D

87	101	106	106	106	105	105	105	105	105	105	105	105
68	65	63	63	63	65	66	67	68	68	69	69	69
51	59	63	66	68	70	72	73	74	76	77	78	80
4	4	5	5	6	7	8	9	9	10	10	11	11

Figure 56-1.

**AGE-SPECIFIC PERCENTILES OF BLOOD PRESSURE
MEASUREMENTS IN BOYS AGES 1 YEAR TO 13 YEARS**

**AGE-SPECIFIC PERCENTILES OF BLOOD PRESSURE
MEASUREMENTS IN BOYS AGES 13 TO 18 YEARS**

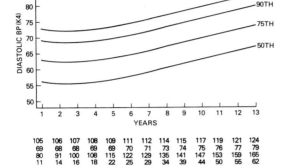

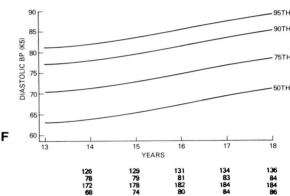

105	106	107	108	109	111	112	114	115	117	119	121	124
69	68	68	69	69	70	71	73	74	75	76	77	79
80	91	100	108	115	122	129	135	141	147	153	159	165
11	14	16	18	22	25	29	34	39	44	50	55	62

126	129	131	134	136
78	79	81	83	84
172	178	182	184	184
68	74	80	84	86

Figure 56-1. (**A**) Age-specific percentiles of blood pressure (BP) measurements in boys—birth to 12 months of age; Korotkoff phase IV (K4) used for diastolic BP. (**B**) Age-specific percentiles of BP measurements in girls—birth to 12 months of age; Korotkoff phase IV (K4) used for diastolic BP. (**C**) Age-specific percentiles of BP measurements in boys—1 to 13 years of age; Korotkoff phase IV (K4) used for diastolic BP. (**D**) Age-specific percentiles of BP measurements in girls—1 to 13 years of age; Korotkoff phase IV (K4) used for diastolic BP. (**E**) Age-specific percentiles of BP measurements in boys—13 to 18 years of age; Korotkoff phase V (K5) used for diastolic BP. (**F**) Age-specific percentiles of BP measurements in girls—13 to 18 years of age; Korotkoff phase V (K5) used for diastolic BP. (From Task Force on Blood Pressure Control in Children: Report of the Second Task Force on Blood Pressure Control in Children, 1987. Pediatrics 79:1-25, 1987

Table 56-1. Definitions

BLOOD PRESSURE LEVEL	AVERAGE SYSTOLIC AND/OR DIASTOLIC BLOOD PRESSURE FOR AGE AND SEX
Normal	<90th percentile
High normal	≥90th but <95th percentile
Hypertension	≥95th percentile
Significant	≥95th but <99th percentile
Severe	≥99th percentile

Adapted from Task Force on Blood Pressure Control in Children: Report of the Second Task Force on Blood Pressure Control in Children—1987. Pediatrics 79:1–25, 1987.

Table 56-2. Classification of Hypertension

AGE GROUP	SIGNIFICANT HYPERTENSION		SEVERE HYPERTENSION	
	Systolic	Diastolic	Systolic	Diastolic
Newborn	96		106	
8–30 days	104		110	
<2 y	112	74	118	82
2–5 y	116	76	124	84
6–9 y	122	78	130	86
10–12 y	126	82	134	90
13–15 y	136	86	144	92
16–18 y	142	92	150	98

Adapted from Task Force on Blood Pressure Control in Children: Report of the Second Task Force on Blood Pressure Control in Children—1987. Pediatrics 79:1–25, 1987.

Table 56-3. Most Common Causes of Sustained
Hypertension From Infancy Through Adolescence

AGE GROUP	CAUSE OF HYPERTENSION
Newborn	Renal artery thrombosis or stenosis Congenital renal malformations Coarctation of the aorta Bronchopulmonary dysplasia Intracranial hemorrhage
Infancy–6 y	Renal parenchymal diseases Coarctation of the aorta Renal artery stenosis Neuroblastoma
6–10 y	Renal artery stenosis Renal parenchymal diseases Primary hypertension
Adolescence	Primary hypertension Renal parenchymal diseases

Adapted from Task Force on Blood Pressure Control in Children: Report
of the Second Task Force on Blood Pressure Control in Children—1987.
Pediatrics 79:1–25, 1987.

Sustained Hypertension. Table 56-3 lists the most common causes of sustained hypertension at different ages. Most hypertension in infants and children younger than 3 years of age will be identified in symptomatic patients or because a diagnosis prompts blood pressure measurement. Symptomatic and/or secondary forms of hypertension predominate into late childhood, but by adolescence, most hypertension is asymptomatic and primary, detected by routine screening. Secondary hypertension at all ages usually declares itself by its severity or the associated physical findings or laboratory test results. The elevated blood pressure of obesity, if measured correctly, represents true hypertension caused by the obese state, not artifact; a successful weight reduction program often results in normalization of blood pressure.

Transient Hypertension. An acute, short-lived elevation of blood pressure accompanies many illnesses and usually does not persist after resolution of the illness. Renal diseases, hypervolemia, hypovolemia, neurologic disorders, lead poisoning, drug therapy or overdose, and seizures are some of the conditions associated with transient hypertension. Use of oral contraceptives by adolescent girls and of anabolic steroids by adolescent boys are especially important causes of transient hypertension. Discontinuance of the medication or treatment of the underlying disorder generally results in normalization of blood pressure. Occasionally, medical management of hypertension may be necessary during the acute phase of the underlying process.

Labile Hypertension. Adolescents, particularly, may react to stressful situations with blood pressure elevation into the hypertensive range but remain normotensive when not stressed. Whether this predicts development of sustained, primary hypertension later in life is not known. The stress that triggers the blood pressure elevation may be physical or emotional. Tendency to labile hypertension may be identified by comparison of blood pressure measurements in stressful environments, such as the physician's office, and those in a less stressful place, such as the home. In addition, physical or psychoemotional stressors may be used during blood pressure measurement. *Physical stressors* include such activities as squeezing a hand grip device for 3 to 5 minutes or placing one hand in ice water; *psychoemotional stressors* include recalling number sequences or performing serial subtractions of 3 or 7 from 100. Persons with labile hypertension will have a marked increase of blood pressure during such stressful situations.

Isolated Systolic Hypertension. Isolated systolic hypertension predicts development of cardiovascular disease in adults, but no data exist about the predictive significance for children and adolescents of systolic blood pressure readings above the 95th percentile *without* corresponding elevation of diastolic blood pressure. Such patients usually do not need medical treatment, although careful monitoring is warranted, and counseling, as discussed later, seems reasonable.

Hypertensive Emergency. The abrupt onset of severe hypertension in a previously asymptomatic or minimally symptomatic person may cause encephalopathy, cardiac failure, loss of vision, or acute renal failure. Such a hypertensive emergency occurs most commonly in a poorly controlled chronic hypertensive patient but may also result, for example, from head trauma, drug reactions, acute glomerulonephritis, pregnancy, and pheochromocytoma. Diastolic blood pressure in adolescents typically exceeds 140 mm Hg; levels may be lower in younger patients. Rapid identification of the hypertensive state and reduction of pressure by approximately 30% (e.g., to a diastolic blood pressure of about 100 mm Hg in an adolescent) will minimize morbidity and allow time for evaluation.

WORK-UP

Measurement of Blood Pressure

Careful attention to details will ensure reliable measurement of blood pressure. Unfortunately, some of these details are not always controllable, especially when an ill, agitated infant or young child or an anxious adolescent must have blood pressure measured. Controllable factors include proper technique, a quiet, nonthreatening setting, the instrument, the cuff, and the choice of the proper Korotkoff sound for systolic and diastolic pressure. Many blood pressure measurements at health fairs and by most automatic blood pressure machines (e.g., those in drug stores and shopping malls) are made with "one size fits all" cuffs *not* appropriate for children (and frequently inappropriate for adults, as well). Any elevation of blood pressure so detected must be confirmed, and families should be cautioned to avoid labeling children and adolescents hypertensive on the basis of such "screening" activities.

Technique. By convention, blood pressure measurements are made on the right arm, although, at times, measurements on the left arm and/or the legs may be appropriate. Infants may have blood pressure measured while sitting in a parent's lap with the arm held at the level of the heart or while supine with the arm held at a slight angle to the table. Routine blood pressure measurements in children and adolescents should be made with the patient sitting and the arm held at the level of the heart. Occasionally, measuring blood pressure with the patient standing or supine will be necessary. Attempts to reduce anxiety and to avoid discomfort will enhance the likelihood of obtaining valid measurements.

Instrument. The mercury-filled sphygmomanometer is the standard for comparison of all other noninvasive blood pressure measurement methodologies. The aneroid sphygmomanometer has comparable accuracy and precision plus the advantage of portability but requires regular calibration. Doppler and oscillometric devices are greatly useful for infants and small children but provide accurate measurements only of systolic blood pressure (with the exception of the Dynamap oscillometric device, which can determine diastolic pressure accurately).

Cuff Size. The label on the cuff (e.g., "infant," "child," "adult") bears little relationship to its use at a specific age. The size of the inflatable bladder in the cuff determines the cuff's suitability for a person. The bladder length should allow it to completely encircle the arm, preferably without overlapping, or, at a minimum, to enclose 75% of the arm's circumference. The bladder width should cover 75% of the arm from the axilla to the antecubital fossa, leaving enough room for the bell of the stethoscope over the brachial artery and avoiding obstruction of the axilla.

Korotkoff Sounds. The Korotkoff sounds represent turbulent blood flow and vibration of the wall of the artery during the process of blood pressure measurement. The first Korotkoff sound (K1) corresponds to systolic pressure. Diastolic pressure is defined by the fourth (K4, low pitched, muffled sound) and/or fifth (K5, disappearance) Korotkoff sounds. The lack of precision in the definition of diastolic pressure results from variability in occurrence of the sounds: K4 may be extremely hard to hear or may occur simultaneously with K5, and in young children K5 may not occur at all. The nomograms in Figure 56-1 use K4 as the marker for diastolic pressure in infants and children up to age 13; for adolescents, K5 represents diastolic pressure.

Identification of Hypertension

Blood pressure above the 90th percentile for age and sex demands repeat measurement. In general, three blood pressure measurements above the 95th percentile support the diagnosis of hypertension. Timing of the repeat measurements will be dictated by the blood pressure; the higher the blood pressure, the more rapid will be the response of the physician. *Never ignore elevated blood pressure, even though most blood pressure elevations do not persist on repeat measurement.* Approximately 20% of children with an initial blood pressure greater than the 95th percentile will have a second measurement greater than the 95th percentile, while 50% of children with two blood pressure measurements greater than the 95th percentile will have persistently high blood pressure on the third and fourth measurements. Blood pressure persistently above the threshold values in Table 56-2 should trigger an evaluation leading to management that may or may not include antihypertensive agents. Severe hypertension (≥99th percentile) has a strong association with an underlying disease process, most commonly of renal, cardiac, or endocrine origin, especially in infancy, and demands prompt attention and intervention.

Evaluation of Hypertension

The evaluation of elevated blood pressure involves multiple steps dictated by the severity of the hypertension. A careful history is the first step in almost all cases, except for hypertensive emergencies. As the second step, a thorough physical examination will provide clues to the diagnosis of secondary hypertension or document the absence of physical abnormalities in primary hypertension. Sustained blood pressure elevation, whether primary or secondary, will damage "target" organs. Third, a diagnostic evaluation, including basic screening laboratory tests, imaging studies, and other diagnostic procedures, will corroborate and expand the findings of the first two steps. More detailed evaluation will require consultation.

History. The evaluation for persistent hypertension includes a careful review of the patient's current and past medical history (Table 56-4). Special attention should be given to evidence of cardiac, renal, or genetic disorders and to possible sequelae of prematurity. All patients should be queried about medication or drug use, especially adolescents who may be using oral contraceptives, anabolic steroids, or illicit drugs.

Because blood pressure demonstrates family aggregation and because many disorders that produce hypertension have familial or hereditary distribution, the family history of both first- and second-degree relatives provides essential information (see Table 56-4). In addition, family members should all have blood pressure measured, since the index case often identifies a previously unknown family predilection to hypertension.

Physical Examination. A thorough general physical examination should include blood pressure measurements in all extremities and should focus on the organ systems "targeted" by elevated blood pressure (eyes, heart, kidneys, nervous system) (Table 56-5). In addition, a careful search

Table 56-4. Conditions Associated With High Risk of Hypertension

Family History (First- and second-degree relatives)
Hypertension
Premature cardiovascular disease
Hereditary renal disease
Lipid abnormalities
Preeclampsia or toxemia of pregnancy
Obesity

Personal History
Neonatal
  Birth asphyxia
  Complications of labor and delivery
  Physical abnormalities
  Prematurity and its sequelae
    Bronchopulmonary dysplasia
    Indwelling umbilical catheter
    Intracranial hemorrhage

General
  Abdominal pain
  Drugs
    Medications (e.g.,
        corticosteroids,
        pseudoephedrine,
        oral contraceptives)
    Anabolic steroids
    Other illicit drugs (e.g., amphetamine, LSD)
  Dysuria
  Edema
  Enuresis
  Nocturia
  Toxic exposures
    Lead
    Mercury
    Licorice
  Urinary frequency or infection

for the physical findings of the diseases or disorders that produce hypertension will provide valuable diagnostic clues and baseline information (Table 56-6).

Laboratory and Imaging Studies. Choice and timing of laboratory and imaging studies will depend, in part, on the history and physical examination. If no clinical clues direct this part of the evaluation, the initial studies should search for abnormalities of renal and cardiac function (Table 56-7). Further studies (Table 56-8) will be determined by the results of the initial screening evaluation unless already suggested by the degree of hypertension or the patient's diagnosis. Consultation is recommended at any stage of the evaluation but is especially valuable if the initial screening does not provide diagnostic clues or if the blood pressure is severe and/or symptomatic.

MANAGEMENT

Nonpharmacologic Management

Some hypertensive patients require antihypertensive medications, but *all* hypertensive patients will benefit from non-

pharmacologic intervention including dietary modification, an age-appropriate exercise prescription, stress reduction, and counseling about risk factors such as smoking, weight loss, and lipid levels. Nonpharmacologic intervention is also appropriate for those identified with *high normal blood pressure*, since this group may eventually develop higher blood pressure. Many of the following recommendations are not practical for infants and small children, although parental education about these issues may have great importance for the child's future, as well as for the parents.

Dietary. Recommendations should emphasize modification of family cooking and eating habits to enhance compliance and to avoid singling out the hypertensive person within the family. Familial aggregation of blood pressure and obesity increases the likelihood that the parents or siblings of the index case will also benefit from the dietary modifications (and other recommendations).

Weight reduction by obese patients and maintenance of ideal body weight by nonobese patients have a central role in management of hypertension. Normalization of blood pressure for many obese persons accompanies weight loss. Any weight-loss program for growing children or adolescents must include age-appropriate dietary modifications, plus increased aerobic (dynamic) exercise.

Another dietary change worth considering is a no-added-salt diet (or at least reduction of excessive salt intake), even though the precise role of salt in the etiology of hypertension is unclear. Reduction in blood pressure may result from dietary salt reduction alone or in conjunction with medications. Dietary counseling should also include information about the cardiac risk associated with high-fat diets, especially if there is a familial predisposition to hy-

Table 56-5. General Physical Findings Suggestive of Hypertension

FINDING	SUGGESTIVE OF:

Adolescent
  Female
  Male
	Primary hypertension
	Oral contraceptive use
	Anabolic steroid use

Altered mental status	Drugs, encephalopathy, toxins
Cushingoid features	Excess glucocorticoids
Failure to thrive in infancy	Cardiac, renal, endocrine disorders
Genetic syndromes	Neurofibromatosis, Riley-Day syndrome, Turner syndrome
Newborn	Cardiac, renal, endocrine disorders
Obesity	Obesity-caused hypertension
Pubertal delay	Cardiac, renal, endocrine, genetic disorders
Trauma (especially head trauma)	Intracranial bleeding or increased pressure
Vomiting/dehydration	Brain tumor, congenital adrenal hyperplasia, renal disease

Table 56-6. Specific Physical Findings Suggestive of Hypertension

FINDING	SUGGESTIVE OF:
Abdominal	
Bruit	Renal artery stenosis
Mass	Hydroureteronephrosis, tumor
Burns	Fluid balance problems
Cardiac/chest	
Murmur	Aortic coarctation
Pulses	
Absent	Aortic coarctation
Bounding/prominent	Hypertension
Rales	Congestive heart failure
Venous hum	Aortic coarctation with collateral circulation
Snapping second heart sound	Hypertension ("target organ")
Eyes	
Papilledema	Increased intracranial pressure
Retinal vessel hemorrhage, nicking, tortuosity	Hypertension "target organ"
Visual field cuts	Increased intracranial pressure, tumor
Genitourinary	
Absent abdominal muscles	"Prune belly" syndrome (obstructive uropathy)
Ambiguous genitalia (newborn)	Congenital adrenal hyperplasia
Distended bladder	Bladder outlet obstruction
Dribbling or weak urinary stream	Posterior urethral valves
Infection (sepsis, urinary tract infection)	Vesicoureteral reflux
Head	
Bruit	Arteriovenous malformation
Shape	Genetic syndrome, prematurity
Neurologic	
Ataxia	Brain tumor, increased intracranial pressure
Cranial nerve paralysis	Brain tumor, hypertension, increased intracranial pressure,
Peripheral neuropathy	Guillain-Barré syndrome
Nuchal rigidity (meningeal irritation)	Meningitis
Seizure	Brain tumor, head trauma, lead poisoning
Pulmonary	
Hyperinflation/wheezing	Bronchopulmonary dysplasia
Rales	Congestive heart failure
Skin	
Café-au-lait macules	Neurofibromatosis
Ecchymoses/petechiae	Henoch-Schönlein purpura, hemolytic uremic syndrome
Striae	Excess glucocorticoids

Table 56-7. Basic Diagnostic Evaluation of Hypertension

Laboratory Tests	Imaging Studies
Complete blood cell count	Chest roentgenogram
Serum	Echocardiogram
Creatinine	**Other Studies**
Electrolytes	Electrocardiogram
Urea Nitrogen	
Uric acid	
Urinalysis with specific gravity	
Urine culture	

Table 56-8. Further Diagnostic Studies

Renal imaging studies	Hormone studies
Ultrasound	Catecholamines
Radionuclide scan	Plasma
Intravenous pyelogram	Urine
Renal arteriography	Serum
Digital subtraction angiography	Aldosterone
Voiding cystourethrography	Peripheral vein renin
	Renal vein renin
24-Hour urine collection	Other hormone assays (serum and urine)
Creatinine clearance	
Protein	
Computed tomography	
Abdomen	
Adrenal glands	
Kidneys/ureters/bladder	

perlipidemia. The diet recommended by the National Cholesterol Education Program is a good starting point, since it reduces total fat, saturated fat, and cholesterol and recommends moderation of salt intake (see Chap. 53, "Cholesterol and Prevention of Coronary Artery Disease"). Interestingly, vegetarian diets may protect against hypertension. The benefits of increased dietary potassium and calcium have not been evaluated in children and adolescents.

Exercise. Regular aerobic exercise has a salutary effect on health in general, as well as on elevated blood pressure at all levels. Coaches, parents, educators, and physicians often mistakenly assume that hypertension precludes participation in physical activity. However, it is *not* necessary to restrict participation in physical education or competitive sports for most hypertensive children or adolescents. All but the most severely hypertensive persons may participate in supervised aerobic exercise. Although preparticipation exercise stress testing has been recommended by some authorities for hypertensive adolescents who wish to participate in competitive sports, there are no available guidelines. The dilemma of isometric exercise remains. Theoretically, such activity causes increased diastolic blood pressure, but no long-term studies exist to provide guidance about the benefits or risks to hypertensive persons of isometric exercise such as weight lifting and wrestling (see also Chap. 17, "Sports Medicine and Physical Fitness").

Stress Reduction and Lifestyle Changes. Identification of specific stressors in the life of a hypertensive person can occasionally assist in their modification. Use of stress reduction techniques such as biofeedback and self-hypnosis has proven effective for many patients with hypertension, as well as those with other psychosomatic illnesses.

Pharmacologic Management

Regardless of age, patients with secondary hypertension usually require antihypertensive medications, and adolescents with primary hypertension may also require medications. Oral antihypertensive therapy should be started when diastolic blood pressure exceeds the 95th percentile, when symptoms or signs related to hypertension develop or when "target organ" damage is identified. Although the long-term risks of antihypertensive therapy for infants, children, and adolescents are unknown, the short-term benefits have been extensively documented; hypertensive morbidity and mortality are markedly reduced by effective therapy. The goal of antihypertensive therapy should be to reduce diastolic blood pressure below the 90th percentile using the lowest possible dose of medication and a regimen that minimizes medication side effects and enhances compliance.

Infants. Most hypertensive infants will require initiation of management by a nephrologist or cardiologist. Primary care physicians will often participate in management after blood pressure has been controlled. A thorough understanding of the specific antihypertensive drugs prescribed will be necessary in such cases.

Children and Adolescents. After infancy, hypertensive patients are likely to have hypertension managed by a primary care physician, although consultation with a specialist will be necessary for complicated or refractory cases and for hypertensive emergencies. To ensure optimal control of hypertension, the management scheme must emphasize compliance with all its facets, especially medications. The simplest possible medication regimen has the greatest chance of success because it promotes compliance.

Medications. Advances in the medical management of hypertension in adults have greatly expanded the pharmacopeia of antihypertensive medications. Unfortunately, few have been rigorously evaluated in patients younger than age 21, but clinical experience is available to guide their judicious use in treating pediatric hypertension (Table 56-9). Many of the newer antihypertensive medications may be used alone, often in a single daily dose. In general, single-drug therapy (monotherapy) begins with an angiotensin converting enzyme inhibitor, a β-adrenergic blocker, *or* a calcium channel antagonist. A diuretic may be added if control of blood pressure has not been achieved in 2 weeks. Failure to respond to maximal doses of the combined drugs should lead to replacement of the diuretic with a direct vasodilator. Initial therapy with an angiotensin converting enzyme inhibitor *plus* a calcium channel antagonist provides excellent blood pressure control, usually without the need for a diuretic. Poor response to such medical management will prompt referral to a specialist familiar with complicated hypertension in childhood. Details of therapy for specific variants such as low-renin or high-renin hypertension and for hypertension associated with specific diseases or disorders are beyond the scope of this discussion. In general, control of secondary hypertension requires attention to any correctable features of the disease or disorder as well as to antihypertensive medication.

Treatment of Hypertensive Emergencies

Primary care physicians must be able to manage hypertensive emergencies. The choice of treatment depends on the urgency of the situation, the availability of medications and knowledge of their use, and availability of monitoring equipment. Reduction of diastolic pressure by approximately 30% should be the goal of therapy.

Two medications that may be used in the outpatient setting while arranging transfer to an intensive-care unit are nifedipine and diazoxide. Other medications act more slowly or require complex administration and monitoring. *Nifedipine,* administered orally or sublingually in a dose of 2.5 to 20 mg (0.3 mg/kg/dose), generally provides prompt blood pressure reduction within 5 to 15 minutes and may be

Table 56-9. Antihypertensive Medications

| MEDICATION | ORAL DOSE (mg/kg/dose) | | FRE-QUENCY (doses/day) |
	Initial*	Maximum	
α-Adrenergic Blocking Agent			
Prazosin (Minipress)	0.05	0.2	2
α- and β-Adrenergic Blocking Agent			
Labetolol (Trandate)	1.0–1.5	5.0–6.0	2
β-Adrenergic Blocking Agents			
Atenolol (Tenormin)	0.5	1.0	2
Metaprolol (Lopressor)	1.0	3.0	2
Propranolol (Inderal)	1.0	3.0	3
Angiotensin Converting Enzyme Inhibitors			
Captopril (Capoten)	0.1	2.0	3
Enalapril (Vasotec)	0.2	1.0	1
Lisinopril (Zestril)	0.2	1.0	1
Calcium Channel Antagonists†			
Diltiazem (Cardizem)	1.0	1.75	2
Nifedipine (Procardia)	0.1	0.3	3
Verapamil (Calan)	1.5	3.5	2
Diuretics			
Bumetanide (Bumex)	0.01	0.4	1
Furosemide (Lasix)	0.5	7.0	2
Hydrochlorothiazide (Hydrodiuril)	0.5	2.0	2
Metolazone (Zanex)	0.2	0.4	1
Spironolactone (Aldactone)	1.0	3.0	1
Triamterene (Dyazide)	1.0	3.0	2
Vasodilator			
Hydralazine (Apresoline)	1.0	2.5	3
Minoxidil (Loniten)	0.1	3.0	2

*Begin with the recommended initial dose and increase as necessary and tolerated to the maximum dose.
†Calcium channel antagonists are also available in sustained-release forms.

repeated. Duration of action is 2 to 3 hours for sublingual nifedipine and 4 to 8 hours when the drug is administered orally. Administration of less than 10 mg of nifedipine requires withdrawal of the drug from the capsule with a fine-gauge needle and a syringe. *Diazoxide,* 300–500 mg/kg/dose given as an infusion over 30 minutes, likewise provides prompt blood pressure reduction with a duration of action of 4 to 12 hours. Repeated doses may result in hyperglycemia.

INDICATIONS FOR REFERRAL OR HOSPITALIZATION

Hypertensive emergencies require prompt hospitalization and aggressive treatment. Patients with symptomatic hypertension may require hospitalization and will benefit from the expertise of a pediatric cardiologist or nephrologist. Asymptomatic patients may have their evaluation and therapy initiated without consultation, although most newborns, infants, and young children will eventually require management by a specialist because of the high incidence of secondary hypertension in this group. Patients with primary hypertension that do not respond to the stepped management scheme outlined previously will also need referral.

ANNOTATED BIBLIOGRAPHY

Barkin RM, Rosen P. Emergency Pediatrics. 3rd ed. St. Louis, Mo: C.V. Mosby, 1990:124–132. (Discussion of the management of hypertensive emergencies.)

Dillon MJ. Clinical aspects of hypertension. In: Holliday MA, Barratt TM, Vernier RL, eds. Pediatric Nephrology. 2nd ed. Baltimore, Md: Williams & Wilkins, 1987:743-757. (Review of the presentation, causes, evaluation, and management of hypertension. Emphasis on secondary hypertension.)

Guyton AC. The kidney in blood pressure control and hypertension. In: Holliday MA, Barratt TM, Vernier RL. eds. Pediatric Nephrology. 2nd ed. Baltimore, Md: Williams & Wilkins, 1987:729-737. (Review of the multifactorial causes of hypertension with emphasis on the kidney. Extensive and lucid discussion of the renal–blood volume–pressure control mechanism.)

Hanna JD, Chan JCM, Gill JR Jr. Hypertension and the kidney. J Pediatr. 1991;118:327-340. (Review of the causes of hypertension and its medical management. Discussion of single antihypertensive therapy.)

National Cholesterol Education Program. Highlights of the Report of the Expert Panel on Blood Cholesterol Levels in Children and Adolescents. Bethesda, Md: National Heart, Lung and Blood Institute, 1991. (Review of the childhood origins of adult atherosclerosis and recommendations for dietary and life-style modifications for children and adolescents.)

Task Force on Blood Pressure Control in Children. Report of the Second Task Force on Blood Pressure Control in Children—1987. Pediatrics. 1987;79:1-25. (Age-specific blood pressure nomograms, recommendations for detection, evaluation, and management of hypertension. References for the studies on which the nomograms are based.)

57

Chest Pain

Herbert E. Cohn

Chest pain in children is a common complaint in primary care settings and creates anxiety in patients, their parents, and pediatricians. Although a physician evaluating a child with chest pain may think first of angina pectoris or myocardial infarction, these are unlikely since chest pain in childhood infrequently stems from heart disease. In assessing chest pain, one must be careful not to increase the child's anxiety level. This can best be done by a careful history with an emphasis on letting the patient express the symptoms in his or her own words. The physical examination may yield a full explanation but is usually normal.

PATHOPHYSIOLOGY, CLINICAL PRESENTATION, AND DIFFERENTIAL DIAGNOSIS

Musculoskeletal causes of chest pain can occur through muscle strain, as in an overuse injury producing chest wall pain. Direct trauma to the chest (e.g., from diving, swimming, gymnastics, or soccer) has often been forgotten by the patient when the bruising becomes symptomatic.

Costochondritis may arise through exercise, coughing, or sneezing and causes a tenderness or inflammation over the junction between the anterior ribs and the sternum. It is associated with sharp, anterior chest pain at the costochondral junctions. In *Tietze's syndrome* there is a local swelling of a particular costochondral junction. Rib fracture is often associated with severe chest pain and follows chest trauma or a period of severe or protracted coughing. *Slipping rib syndrome* is believed to be a sprain disorder produced by trauma to the costal cartilages of the eighth, ninth, or tenth ribs. The patient describes a slipping movement of the ribs and can sense a clicking and popping when bending or flexing the trunk. One can reproduce the pain by performing a "hooking" maneuver in which the affected rib margin is grasped and then pulled anteriorly.

Pleural causes of chest pain usually manifest as a pain worsened by deep inspiration and coughing and include such entities as the "precordial catch" syndrome, pleurisy, and pneumothorax. *Precordial catch syndrome* refers to a pattern of left anterior chest pain in young, healthy persons. The pain is sharp, severe, sudden in onset, and localized to the left precordium near the apex. It occurs at rest, especially with bending, and is worsened by attempting to take a deep breath, as if something "catches" or sticks. The pain most likely arises from the parietal pleura, although there is no apparent correlation with previous illnesses, physical abnormalities, or evidence of a cardiac origin. In *pleurisy* there is inflammation of the parietal pleura innervated by intercostal nerves carrying pain fibers. The pain is made more intense by deep and rapid breathing that causes greater excursions of the lung against the inflamed parietal pleura. In *pleural effusion* the pain usually arises from pressure on the diaphragm. Pain is felt posteriorly in the shoulder when the central part of the diaphragm is involved and in the side or back when the anterior part of the diaphragm is involved. Marked inflammation of the lung parenchyma does not produce chest pain unless the parietal pleura is involved. The pain of pneumonitis is the pain of pleurisy.

Inflammation of the bronchi may manifest in several different forms. Tracheobronchitis may be associated with a burning pain on coughing. "Asthmatic bronchitis" may be associated with a sensation of pain or tightness in the chest during inspiration.

Intercostal nerve pain is most commonly seen in a child with *herpes zoster infection* and follows a specific dermatome distribution. It may be sensed as an ache over a portion of the chest wall. Its distribution can be mapped by touch or pinprick. In herpes zoster the pain may precede the appearance of skin lesions by several days.

Cardiovascular causes of chest pain, although the least common, are among the most serious. Structural congenital heart lesions that can cause chest pain include the left ventricular outflow tract obstructive lesions such as *valvular* and *subvalvular aortic stenosis,* and cardiomyopathies including *idiopathic hypertrophic subaortic stenosis.* To a lesser extent, pulmonic stenosis can also be associated with chest pain. These lesions are not generally associated with chest pain at mild or even moderate degrees of severity, and one is not likely to find symptomatic left ventricular outflow tract obstruction if cardiac signs have not been noted previously on physical examination. Children with worsening aortic or pulmonic stenosis may begin to complain of chest pain on a cardiogenic basis and need surgical relief of their severe obstructive lesions. The pain is caused by myocardial oxygen deprivation leading to myocardial insufficiency and ischemia. Coronary arterial anomalies, such as an *anomalous left coronary artery* arising from the pulmonary artery, are rare. Although they may be difficult to diagnose, the usual signs and symptoms are those of myocardial ischemia and congestive heart failure. Thus, the patient is often acutely and severely ill and needs urgent care. Pallor, irritability, chest pain, and signs of acute congestive heart failure, together with the characteristic electrocardiographic pattern (deep Q waves in lead I and aVL) usually assist in making the diagnosis in an infant younger than 1 year old.

Mitral valve prolapse is often associated with chest pain in the adult population but is much less frequently associated with chest pain before adolescence. The pain occurs with or without exertion. Its etiology is not clear; it may result from papillary muscle dysfunction or through noncoronary causes such as autonomic dysfunction and instability.

Pericarditis and *myocarditis* can occur in any child. In pericarditis the chest pain is due to a large effusion causing great tension on the pericardial sac. It is associated with a dull ache over the heart, especially the mid to left precordium. Acute pericarditis is also associated with severe, sharp midsternal pain and can be referred to the left intraclavicular or subscapular areas of the chest. These children often appear sick and uncomfortable and have other findings of cardiovascular involvement.

Supraventricular tachycardia, at rates above 200 beats per minute, may cause chest pain and hypotension through inadequate myocardial oxygen delivery, leading to myocardial insufficiency and ischemia. At rates of 140 to 200 beats per minute, supraventricular tachycardia is unlikely to cause chest pain. Extrasystoles do not usually cause chest pain unless they are occurring successively or in runs of ventricular tachycardia. Palpitations may be felt by the child if the cardiac rhythm is irregular.

Esophageal reflux of gastric contents may be associated with a retrosternal burning sensation referred to in lay terms as *heartburn*. This sensation is usually in the xiphoid region of the upper abdomen. In adults, this area is a frequent source of confusion in differentiating between gastrointestinal and cardiogenic causes of pain. In childhood, this area is an infrequent source of pain.

Psychogenic causes of chest pain are common in childhood. The pain can mimic angina pectoris in its characterization, and the distribution may be similar to that described by an adult in the child's family.

Miscellaneous causes of chest pain include sickle cell crises with anginal pain secondary to vascular occlusion, tumors involving the lung and chest wall such as Hodgkin's disease, or bony infiltration of ribs and sternum by sarcomas or leukemic involvement. Inflammatory myopathies such as trichinosis can also produce intercostal myalgia.

Idiopathic causes of chest pain make up a large percentage of pediatric complaints of chest pain (45% in one prospective study). This group includes the complaints of chest pain not associated with exercise or syncope and present in a child with an otherwise normal history, physical examination, and laboratory studies such as an electrocardiogram, a chest roentgenogram, and a hemogram. In most cases, symptoms appear to be self-limited and tend to diminish or resolve within 1 year.

Differential Diagnosis of Chest Pain in Childhood

1. Musculoskeletal causes
   a. Muscle strain
   b. Direct trauma
   c. Costochondritis
   d. Rib fracture
   e. Slipping rib syndrome
2. Pleural causes
   a. Precordial catch syndrome
   b. Pleurisy
   c. Pleural effusion
3. Pulmonary parenchymal causes
   a. Referred pain from pneumonitis
   b. Tracheobronchitis
   c. "Asthmatic bronchitis"
4. Intercostal nerve causes
   a. Herpes zoster infection
   b. Radiculitis
5. Cardiac causes
   a. Left ventricular outflow tract obstructive lesions
      1. Aortic stenosis, valvular and subvalvular
      2. Hypertrophic cardiomyopathy
   b. Right ventricular outflow tract obstructive lesions
      1. Pulmonic stenosis, valvular and subvalvular
   c. Coronary artery anomalies
      1. Anomalous left coronary artery arising from the pulmonary artery
   d. Mitral valve prolapse
   e. Pericarditis
   f. Myocarditis and other inflammatory disorders
   g. Kawasaki disease, including coronary arteritis
   h. Dysrhythmias
      1. Supraventricular tachycardia
      2. Extrasystoles, ventricular and artrioventricular junctional in origin
6. Esophageal causes
   a. Esophageal reflux
   b. Esophagitis
7. Psychogenic causes
8. Miscellaneous causes
   a. Sickle cell crisis
   b. Thoracic tumors, including lung parenchyma and chest wall
   c. Inflammatory myopathies
9. Idiopathic

WORK-UP

History

A careful history is necessary in differentiating the causes of chest pain in childhood. One should have a description of the chest pain: what it feels like and its precipitating factors, as well as its location and duration. Is it exercise-induced and associated with other symptoms such as lightheadedness? Has the chest pain been associated with syncope? Chest pain associated with exercise or syncope is likely to reflect an underlying structural cardiac lesion, such as a left ventricular outflow tract obstruction. Has there been prior drug use? Has there been recent illness, a heart attack, or death in a relative or friend? Is there an underlying source of anxiety in the child's daily life? Family, friends, and school-related stresses should be asked about. It is especially important to observe and listen as much as to ask. Anxiety may be reflected in a worried expression, a quiet child, a tachycardia, hyperventilation, or a lack of congruence between the child's appearance and behavior. An active child, who is talkative and eager to play, is probably well. Have you noted differences from prior interactions during the visit (child–parent, child–physician, and parent–physician)? Who is most stressed? Is the atmosphere tense and emotional or relaxed and more rational? Have you considered your own feelings and openness to any diagnosis? Have you prejudged that there is nothing wrong?

Physical Examination

Clinical findings that reflect the etiology of chest pain are not usually evident. The child's appearance is important and can be assessed as the physician measures the pulse, respiratory rate, and blood pressure. The respiratory rate and effort may reflect the degree of illness and discomfort. A dyspneic child has driven, hard respirations and is likely to have an underlying respiratory or cardiovascular problem. The clinical picture of hyperventilation, sweaty palms, and a dry mouth is likely to reflect anxiety (which could also be caused by the patient's concern about his or her chest pain). Asthma, with its prolonged expiratory phase and greater use of the accessory muscles in breathing, is usually easily diagnosed. An inspection of the patient's chest may yield signs of recent trauma. A prominent or tender costochondral junction may reflect costochondritis. Chest wall asymmetry due to an underlying cardiac lesion is easily missed unless the physician looks at the supine patient from the feet toward the head.

Palpation of the midsternal area may elicit tenderness over the costochondral junctions. Palpation over the supraclavicular areas may elicit crepitus from subcutaneous air secondary to a pneumomediastinum. Palpation of the precordia for abnormal cardiac heaves, impulses, or thrills may provide evidence of a structural congenital heart lesion. An examination of the breast tissue and other soft tissue of the chest for tenderness, particularly in the adolescent, may provide an explanation for the chest pain. Anteroposterior or lateral compression of the chest wall may reproduce the pain of recent rib cage trauma.

Percussion of the chest provides information on the lung parenchyma. Dullness to percussion is often associated with underlying consolidation, atelectasis, or pleural effusion. Tympany may reflect hyperaeration, most commonly from asthma. Resonance to percussion suggests a normal quality of the underlying lung parenchyma.

Auscultation provides evidence of bilateral air exchange. Wheezing reflects bronchospasm. Decreased breath sounds may reflect pneumonitis, atelectasis, or pneumothorax.

The cardiovascular examination should be directed toward evidence of an inflammatory disorder such as pericarditis or myocarditis, a dysrhythmia, and findings of a structural congenital heart lesion. Tachycardia, muffled heart sounds, or the presence of a pericardial friction rib are useful clues for pericarditis. The quality of the heart sounds and the presence of a gallop rhythm might also reflect a myocarditis. The rhythm should be described as regular or irregular, and if the latter, its pattern should be noted. Children with supraventricular tachycardia may experience chest pain during a period of rapid heart rate. Patients with ventricular or supraventricular extrasystoles are generally asymptomatic but may describe palpitations. Insignificant cardiac murmurs are common in childhood. Few congenital heart lesions are likely to produce chest pain, and it is more likely that a child with chest pain from any cause could have a cardiac murmur of the insignificant type that is wholly unrelated to the chest pain. On the other hand, the presence of an ejection click, a prominent cardiac impulse, or hepatomegaly related to congestive heart failure would be important clues to an underlying structural congenital heart lesion. Any of the left or right ventricular outflow tract obstructive lesions are likely to be associated with significant cardiac murmurs as well as ejection clicks, ventricular impulses, alterations of the second heart sound, and other positive cardiac findings.

Laboratory Tests

An electrocardiogram should not be considered a routine study as part of an evaluation of chest pain but is valuable if clinical clues suggest its usefulness. It can document the cardiac rate and rhythm, the electrical conduction pattern, and the presence of chamber hypertrophy. It may also provide clues in the presence of an anomalous coronary artery from the pulmonary artery or other coronary abnormalities such as seen in Kawasaki disease. ST-segment and T-wave changes suggest pericarditis or myocarditis. However, early in the illness the electrocardiogram may be entirely normal in any of these conditions; subtle changes may be appreciated only when several studies are obtained sequentially as the illness evolves.

The chest roentgenogram is also valuable in the assessment of chest pain, but it should be considered only if the history and physical findings warrant it. The chest film may corroborate the physical findings of a pulmonary process such as pneumonitis, effusion, or pneumomediastinum. A chest film might also show evidence of chest trauma such as rib fracture, displacement, or bony callus formation.

Noninvasive Studies

Additional noninvasive cardiovascular studies may be useful, particularly in the child whose chest pain is associated with exercise or syncope. Two-dimensional echocardiography is valuable in assessing ventricular function and anatomic abnormalities such as aortic or pulmonic stenosis, other intracardiac abnormalities, and coronary artery anomalies. It is also valuable in documenting the presence and magnitude of a pericardial effusion. A treadmill electrocardiogram (stress test) is valuable in assessing cardiac dysrhythmias such as supraventricular tachycardia. The acute stress of the study may provoke and hence document the dysrhythmia. This type of study may also demonstrate the degree to which the child can perform before evoking chest pain and may provide some degree of reassurance to the child and parents regarding strenuous activity in the face of a recent complaint of chest pain.

MANAGEMENT AND INDICATIONS FOR REFERRAL

Any child in acute distress complaining of chest pain should be evaluated in the emergency department where cardiovascular support can be provided if the patient develops circulatory collapse. The child with recurring chest pain associated with exercise, syncope, lightheadedness, palpitations, easy fatigue, or a history of known congenital heart disease should be referred to a pediatric cardiologist for further evaluation. Children with findings suggestive of an acute inflammatory process such as pericarditis or myocarditis should also be referred. Patients in whom esophagitis is secondary to reflux, caustic ingestion, or a foreign body ingestion leading to retrosternal chest pain, as well as patients with chest wall trauma, pleural effusion, or pneumothorax may be managed by the pediatrician in conjunction with a pediatric surgeon for further evaluation and treatment of the underlying condition. Children whose chest pain is on a musculoskeletal basis secondary to trauma, but not associated with a bony fracture, can generally be managed with rest, analgesics, and simple supportive measures. Those children whose chest pain is on a psychogenic basis can be

helped as they are listened to and allowed to believe that their symptomatology is being taken seriously. Gentle questioning as to what the child sees as the cause of the chest pain often leads to acceptance of the physician's reassurance that the child's pain is not on a cardiogenic basis and that he or she is not in imminent danger (see also Chap. 26, "The Constant Complainer").

Despite the descriptions of each of these entities, nearly one half of childhood complaints of chest pain are called "idiopathic" since no specific explanation can be given. A course of watchful observation usually shows that the child remains free of impairment of cardiovascular function or performance.

ANNOTATED BIBLIOGRAPHY

Coleman WL. Recurrent chest pain in children. Pediatr Clin North Am. 1984;31:1007. (Extensive discussion of the causes and pathophysiology of recurrent chest pain in childhood.)

Driscoll DJ, Glicklich LB, Gallen WJ. Chest pain in children: A prospective study. Pediatrics. 1976;57:648. (This prospective study concludes that chest pain in children rarely signals serious disease that is not apparent from a thorough history and physical examination.)

Fyfe DA, Moodie DS. Chest pain in pediatric patients presenting to a cardiac clinic. Clin Pediatr. 1984;23:321. (This study shows that in pediatric patients, chest pain is infrequently due to underlying cardiac disease.)

Miller AJ, Texidor TA. Precordial catch, a neglected syndrome of precordial pain. JAMA. 1955;159:1364. (Thorough description of this common source of chest pain in young, healthy persons.)

Selbst SA. Evaluation of chest pain in children. Pediatr Rev. 1986;8:56. (Clearly written review of the subject with a rational approach to the management of children with chest pain.)

DERMATOLOGIC PROBLEMS

Amy Paller, Section Editor

58

Topical Preparations and Applications: General Principles

Amy Paller

Dermatologic problems seen by pediatricians are often responsive to topical agents, but the pediatrician must be aware of the most appropriate agent to select. The absorption of topical preparations is increased greatly by occlusion, whether from plastic wraps or natural occlusion of skinfolds (axillae, inguinal), and the strength of the agent must be tailored accordingly. Agents that are well tolerated on intact skin, such as corticosteroid creams and topical tars, are often irritating to acutely inflamed or denuded skin, and only bland emollients and compresses may be tolerated. The pediatrician should be aware that topical agents may aggravate an underlying condition by irritation or by causing allergic contact dermatitis. The allergic contact dermatitis is often not caused by the active ingredient itself but by the vehicle, stabilizers, preservatives, or perfumes present in the medication. Among the most common allergens found in medications are ethylenediamine, lanolin, parabens, thimerosal (merthiolate), diphenhydramine (Benadryl), "caines," and neomycin (see Chap. 62). If a dermatologic condition appears to be aggravated by an agent that contains one or more of these common sensitizers, the preparation should be changed to one without the allergen.

When choosing a topical preparation, the vehicle and ingredients should be chosen to suit the individual patient. Ointments or emollient creams are most appropriate for patients with dry skin. The less occlusive creams or lotions are preferable if the skin is not very dry or in summer when

excessive occlusion may cause blockage of normal sweating and miliaria (prickly heat). Acute weeping dermatitis is dried and relieved by cool compresses.

In general, preparations of lower concentrations should be used first if appropriate. Although it would be ideal to have the pharmacist compound ingredients to individualize each preparation, the cost is usually prohibitive and the most appropriate available agent is preferable. Generic agents are often just as effective as the more expensive brand names.

One of the most common patient complaints is itching, and various topical agents, in addition to systemic antihistamines, may be helpful. Environmental factors that may cause or exacerbate the pruritus should be identified. Excessive bathing, especially with bubble baths, is often a cause of dryness and irritation and may be easily eliminated. Other frequently implicated irritants include wool (in clothing, blankets, and rugs), cold, sweat, dryness, and retained laundry products. Home remedies may aggravate the condition. The pruritus of dry skin may be relieved by the use of mild soaps (such as Dove), bland emollient creams and lotions, and topical preparations with antipruritics. Topical antihistamines (especially Benadryl) and "caine" anesthetics should be avoided, since they often cause contact sensitization, but menthol 0.125% to 0.25% may be added to ointments or lotions and pramoxine 1% is a nonsensitizing topical anesthetic. Topical corticosteroids are helpful for patients with moderate to severe pruritus.

AVAILABLE TOPICAL AGENTS

Topical therapeutic agents may be applied as liquids (wet dressings, lotions) or solids (powders, creams, ointments).

Wet dressings cool and dry oozing and vesicular eruptions, debride crusts, and help relieve itching. Medications applied to the moist skin after compresses are more effectively absorbed. Plain tap water, saline solution (parents may add 1 teaspoon of salt to 1 pint of lukewarm water), or Burow's solution (one Domeboro tablet in 1 pint of water makes a 1:40 solution) are the most frequently used compressing solutions. Potassium permanganate or silver nitrate 0.5% are other antiseptic drying solutions, but they stain. Wet dressings are best applied with strips of clean sheets or handkerchiefs to promote evaporation. The total time of compressing should be 20 minutes, with dressings applied three to four times daily. The cloth should be soaked in the lukewarm solution (cool solutions cause heat loss), wrung out, and applied. After 5 minutes, before the dressing is dry, the cloth should be wetted again and reapplied. After the compresses, the skin should be gently patted dry. The child should be distracted during the sessions to increase compliance. *Baths* are useful for widespread skin eruptions. Baking soda, oatmeal, or Aveeno colloidal oatmeal may be added to bathwater to ease pruritus. Bath oils, such as Alpha-Keri, Lubath, or Domol, are lubricating but should not be used in young children and must be used with care in older children because they cause the bathtub to become slippery. Tar baths (Zetar, Polytar bath, Balnetar) are useful adjunctive agents for psoriasis.

Lotions are mixtures of powder in liquids and are best used to provide cooling by evaporation for acute dermatitis. Shake lotions, such as calamine, are effective in drying as well as cooling and soothing and are often discontinued when the acute dermatitis has subsided after a few days. *Emulsion lotions* are lotions with oil that are less occlusive and more drying than creams or ointments. Corticosteroids and antifungal agents are available in these forms.

Creams and ointments are the most commonly used bases for topical medications. Creams are mixtures of oil droplets in water, and ointments are water in oil or pure preparations of oils (i.e., petrolatum). The oil component is usually lanolin or petrolatum. When the emollient agent is applied to the skin, the water evaporates, leaving the protective or occlusive film of oil. Various bland ointments and creams, such as Aquaphor, Eucerin, and Nivea, may be used as lubricants or as bases for adding corticosteroids, antibiotics, keratolytics, and other active ingredients. *Gels* are combinations of propylene glycol, hydrocarbon polymers and water, acetone, or alcohol that are best used for hairy areas. Benzoyl peroxide, corticosteroids, tars, and keratolytics are available in a gel form. *Oils,* such as mineral oil, may be useful as mild keratolytics (removing psoriatic scalp scale) or to clean surfaces (removing zinc oxide paste in the diaper area of patients with irritant dermatitis) but are too occlusive to be recommended as emollients.

Powders are finely divided solids that are absorptive and reduce friction. Cornstarch is useful for diaper dermatitis, but talcum powder should be avoided for infants because of the risk of inhalation. Powders, such as Zeasorb, are effective agents for hyperhidrosis. *Pastes* are combinations of powders and oils that are drying (powder) and protective (oil). Pastes are thick, sticky, and difficult to apply and re-

move but are useful for irritant diaper dermatitis (zinc oxide paste, Lassar's paste—25% zinc oxide, 25% talc, 50% petrolatum, or a combination of Burow's solution, Aquaphor, and zinc oxide paste in a ratio of 1:2:3). Forty percent salicylic acid *plaster* is incorporated into an occlusive backing for treating warts, calluses, and corns.

Mild *shampoos,* such as Castille soap, DHS, Ionil, Sebulex, and Neutrogena, may be preferable for patients with atopic dermatitis and scalp dryness. Tar shampoos are useful for psoriasis and seborrhea. Superfatted *soaps* with lanolin, oils, cold cream, or Aquaphor added are less drying, as are glycerine soaps (e.g., Neutrogena). Nonsoap bar cleansers, such as Lowila, and Cetaphil cleanser are alternatives. Sulfur or salicylic acid is added to acne soaps to remove oil and peel skin. These soaps alone will not control acne and may cause irritant dermatitis.

ACTIVE INGREDIENTS IN TOPICAL AGENTS

Of all the available topical preparations, *corticosteroids* are most important for their anti-inflammatory, antipruritic, and vasoconstrictive properties. Pediatricians should not avoid corticosteroids if they are indicated but must be careful in choosing their strength, especially in infants, and to stop their use as soon as the condition is adequately treated. Local side effects include atrophy, telangiectasias, folliculitis, striae, hypertrichosis, acneiform eruptions, hypopigmentation, and secondary infections. Topical corticosteroids may mask the erythema of bacterial, fungal, yeast, or mite infections or infestations while encouraging the proliferation of organisms.

Very mild corticosteroids, such as hydrocortisone, should be used on the face and intertriginous areas (Table 58-1). Fluorinated corticosteroids on the face produce atrophy and acneiform eruptions. Mild corticosteroids are usually also effective on the body for dermatitis in infants, but moderate strength or even strong corticosteroid preparations may be required for limited periods of time in older children for more severe eruptions. The vehicle chosen should be appropriate for the underlying condition (e.g., ointment for dry skin and cream for exudative dermatitis). Occlusion may be indicated for recalcitrant plaques in chronic conditions. The corticosteroid (usually in ointment form) should be applied and topped with occlusive plastic film (such as Saran wrap). Gauze wrap, socks, gloves, or stockinettes may be used to maintain occlusion.

Tars and anthralin preparations are useful in older children and adolescents, especially for psoriasis, but should only be prescribed by a dermatologist. Tars may darken skin and stain light-colored hair yellow. Potential side effects include irritation, folliculitis, and photosensitivity.

Many cutaneous infections require systemic antibiotics. *Topical antibiotics* should be used alone for minor infections, but otherwise as adjunctive agents to systemic medications. Topical antibiotics that contain neomycin (e.g.,

Table 58-1. Examples of Topical Corticosteroid Preparations

POTENCY (%)	GENERIC NAME
Lowest Potency	
1.0	Hydrocortisone
2.5	Hydrocortisone
Low Potency	
0.05	Alclometasone dipropionate (Aclovate)
0.2	Hydrocortisone 17-valerate (Westcort)
0.1	Hydrocortisone butyrate (Locoid)
0.1	Clocortolone (Cloderm)
0.01	Fluocinolone acetonide (Synalar)
0.05	Desonide (Tridesilon)
Moderate Potency	
0.025	Fluocinolone acetonide (Synalar)
0.1	Betamethasone valerate (Valisone)
0.1	Triamcinolone acetonide (Kenalog)
0.1	Mometasone furoate (Elocon)
Potent	
0.05	Fluocinonide (Lidex)
0.25	Desoximetasone (Topicort)
0.1	Amcinonide (Cyclocort)
0.1	Halcinonide (Halog)
0.05	Diflorasone diacetate (Maxiflor)
0.05	Betamethasone diproprionate (Diprosone)

Neosporin) may cause contact allergies. Topical erythromycin, clindamycin, meclocycline, and tetracycline in alcohol, cream, and gel vehicles are frequently effective for patients with mild inflammatory acne.

Topical antifungal and *antiyeast agents* are effective, but systemic agents such as griseofulvin or ketoconazole should be used if lesions are widespread or if the scalp or nails are involved. Imidazole (miconazole, clotrimazole, econazole) creams, lotions, or solutions are used to treat dermatophyte, candidal, and *Pityrosporum* infections. Nystatin is available as a cream, ointment, or powder for cutaneous candidal infections, but the imidazoles are of equal or greater efficacy. Less expensive agents, such as selenium sulfide lotion, are equally effective for *Pityrosporum* (tinea versicolor) infections (see Chap. 66, "Superficial Dermatophyte and Yeast Infections"). *Topical acyclovir* is helpful for treating herpetic infections but is most useful for primary infections and is expensive. Immunocompromised children should be treated with systemic acyclovir; topical acyclovir has minimal additional value. *Antiparasitic agents* may be used topically for lice and scabies. Elimite (5% permethrin) is a new scabicide that is at least as effective as other scabicides (lindane, crotamiton) and is believed to be safe for use in infants and lactating mothers. Pyrethrin (RID) or lindane shampoos are used for head or pubic lice infestations (see Chap. 71, "Insect Bites and Infestations").

Sunscreens protect the skin from ultraviolet light and are important for use in children, especially those with fair skin, to help prevent the later development of cutaneous aging changes, precanceroses, and skin cancers. The most widely used chemical sunscreens contain *p*-aminobenzoic acid (PABA) or PABA esters and are most effective against ultraviolet B light (290 to 320 nm). Presun is a PABA-containing sunscreen. Water Babies is a hypoallergic (PABA-free) sunscreen. Benzophenones block ultraviolet A light (320 to 390 nm) and include Solbar and Uval. Some sunscreens contain both PABA or PABA esters and benzophenones. Physical sunscreens, such as zinc oxide paste, RVPaque, and A-Fil, protect the skin from all wavelengths of ultraviolet light. Sunscreens that offer high sun protection factors (SPF 15 and higher) are most effective.

Masking preparation such as Covermark (Lydia O'Leary) and Dermablend cover disfiguring lesions. They are especially useful for teenagers with port wine stains, areas of hypopigmentation or hyperpigmentation, and scars.

59
Atopic Dermatitis

Amy Paller

Atopic dermatitis is a chronic, severely pruritic disorder characterized by dry skin, eczematous patches, lichenification, and a predisposition to staphylococcal pyodermas. The term *atopic* refers to the fact that affected children frequently have elevated IgE levels and a family or personal history of other atopic disorders, especially allergic rhinitis or asthma. The disorder usually begins in infancy but occasionally occurs later in childhood or even in adulthood. Atopic dermatitis affects 1% to 3% of the pediatric population. The diagnosis is made by the characteristic distribution and clinical features of the rash.

PATHOPHYSIOLOGY

Despite considerable strides in studying atopic dermatitis, the primary cause remains unknown. Abnormalities of the adrenergic/cholinergic axis, IgE levels, and cell-mediated immunity have been noted. Basophil and mast cell histamine and perhaps other chemical mediators, such as prostaglandins and leukotrienes, are thought to participate. The decreased levels of cyclic adenosine monophosphate have been related to increased levels of leukocyte phosphodiesterase. The elevation of IgE may be due to deficient T-lymphocyte suppression of IgE-producing B cells. Whether the T-cell anomalies are primary or secondary to increased histamine and decreased cyclic adenosine monophosphate levels is unclear.

CLINICAL PRESENTATION

Atopic dermatitis begins between 2 and 6 months of age in 60% of affected children. Lesions are typically intensely pruritic, dry, scaling, erythematous patches, often characterized by edema and linear excoriations. The lesions are poorly defined; their borders fade gradually into the surrounding normal skin sites. In some children, especially black children, the rash may be papular. Rarely, the dermatitis takes the form of an exfoliative erythroderma. In infants, the rash is frequently exudative, even without a secondary infection. In older children and adolescents, well-circumscribed patches of eczema (*nummular eczema*) may develop and evidence of chronic changes, such as areas of thickened skin with exaggerated skin markings (lichenification) and hyperpigmentation, may be seen (Fig. 59-1). If the atopic dermatitis becomes secondarily infected with bacteria, yellow exudate and crust overlie the rash.

As the child gets older, the areas of predilection change. In infancy, the eruption may be widespread or limited to areas with maximal irritation, such as the perioral area and cheeks. By the second half of the first year of life, the crawling infant is most severely affected on the extensor surfaces of the arms, wrists, and legs. By childhood and adolescence, the rash localizes to the flexural areas at the antecubital and popliteal folds, the wrist, and around the neck. Not uncommonly, the hands and feet become involved during childhood with extreme dryness, erythema, and hyperkeratosis with fissure formation. *Dyshidrotic eczema* may occasionally develop with tiny vesicles and pustules on the palms, soles, and interdigital areas, probably due to exposure to sweat and other irritants.

The rash of atopic dermatitis is aggravated by several factors. The process of rubbing or scratching leads to more rash and more pruritus. Patients with the disorder have extremely dry skin, due at least in part to increased transepidermal water loss. The dermatitis often becomes aggravated by the low humidity in winter. The skin is easily irritated so that exposure to wool, saliva, and sweat can markedly exacerbate the dermatitis. Some patients have an exacerbation

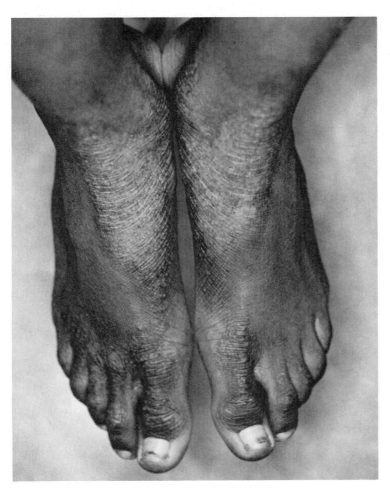

Figure 59-1. Lichenification on the dorsal aspect of the feet of a teenager with atopic dermatitis.

of the eczema in the summer as a result of the irritant reaction to sweat and sweat retention. Other flare factors include infections and superimposed allergic contact dermatitis.

OTHER FEATURES OF ATOPIC DERMATITIS

Besides the generalized dryness, dermatitis, and excoriations, patients with atopic dermatitis display various other clinical features that are not pathognomonic to the disorder. On the face, an extra line may be found under the eyelid (Dennie's pleat, Morgan's fold), presumably due to lower eyelid edema or chronic dermatitis. The eyelids may also appear hyperpigmented (allergic shiners). In addition, affected children show midfacial pallor, probably because of increased vascular permeability and edema (see also Chap. 46, "Allergic Rhinitis"). *Pityriasis alba* presents as slightly scaly, hypopigmented circular patches that are most commonly found on the face, trunk, and upper arms due to mild inflammation. *Follicular hyperkeratosis* with mild to moderate inflammation (*keratosis pilaris*) is common and usually found on the upper anterior thighs, the upper extensor arms, and the cheeks in younger children. The palmar creases of affected persons are accentuated because of dryness and thickening of the skin. *Ichthyosis vulgaris* with fine white scaling, which is most prominent on the lower legs, and *palmoplantar keratoderma* have been associated with atopic dermatitis. Children with atopic dermatitis also demonstrate the phenomenon of "white dermographism." When the skin of a dermographic person without atopic dermatitis is stroked firmly, the "triple response of Lewis" occurs, characterized by a red line, a flare, and then a wheal. Children with atopic dermatitis have a paradoxical response with the initial red line replaced by a white line without any wheal within approximately 10 seconds. This phenomenon helps in making the diagnosis of atopic dermatitis but may also be observed in nonatopic persons. Finally, there appears to be an increased risk of the development of asymptomatic bilateral, central anterior subcapsular cataracts (<5% and usually in adults) even without corticosteroid use and keratoconus (elongation of the corneal surface, <1%).

Atopic dermatitis clears by school age in 50% of the patients who develop the disorder in early infancy. In an additional 25% of children, the dermatitis may resolve by puberty, but 25% of patients continue to have difficulty into adulthood.

The most common complication of atopic dermatitis is secondary bacterial infection of affected areas of skin, especially at excoriated sites. The usual organism is *Staphylococcus aureus,* followed by *group A β-hemolytic streptococci.* Studies have shown that 93% of lesions of atopic dermatitis harbor *S. aureus* and that 76% of samples of uninvolved skin also yield the organism by culture. Although children may show complicating bullous impetigo (coagulase-positive *Staphylococcus*), the typical lesions of impetigo are erythematous with superficial yellow crusts and sometimes small superficial pustules. Patients with a secondary infection will often not respond to appropriate therapy for the underlying eczema unless the infection is cleared with systemic antibiotics.

Eczema herpeticum (*Kaposi's varicelliform eruption*) is a severe complication of atopic dermatitis, characterized by the abrupt development and rapid spread of the vesicles of herpes simplex. The lesions are usually multiple groups of intact or umbilicated vesicles and pustules overlying erythematous bases. The diagnosis may be confirmed by the finding of multinucleated giant epithelial cells (and occasionally intranuclear viral inclusion bodies) on a Tzanck test. This rapid test is performed by lifting the roof of the vesiculopustule, by scraping the base, and by applying the material to a slide that is stained with Giemsa. Viral cultures of lesional material and antibody testing will further verify a herpes infection. The high risk of *eczema vaccinatum* that was once associated with having a smallpox vaccination or being exposed to a vaccination recipient has been virtually eliminated since the vaccination is no longer given.

Children with atopic dermatitis have an increased risk of the development and spread of molluscum contagiosum, dermatophyte infections (tinea), and warts. This propensity appears related to T-lymphocyte abnormalities, the abnormal cutaneous barrier, and the tendency toward easy spread because of pruritus and scratching.

DIFFERENTIAL DIAGNOSIS

The diagnosis of atopic dermatitis is facilitated by the intense pruritus and characteristic pattern and appearance of lesions. Other types of cutaneous inflammation in children may resemble that of atopic dermatitis. *Seborrheic dermatitis* is a common eruption of infants that often develops within the first month of life. It tends to be nonpruritic with greasy, yellow scales that are typically found on the scalp (*cradle cap*) and in intertriginous areas. Seborrheic dermatitis usually clears by the second year of life. *Irritant contact dermatitis,* although it is frequently one of the manifestations of atopic dermatitis, may be noted in normal infants and children after exposure to saliva (cheeks), to urine and feces (groin area), or to harsh soaps, detergents, and sheets (cheeks, extensor surfaces). Irritant dermatitis without associated atopic dermatitis is less dry and less pruritic. *Allergic contact dermatitis* is rare in young children and often involves well-circumscribed erythematous vesicles and papules that follow the distribution of the contactant. The dry, scaly, fissured eruption of *juvenile plantar dermatosis* may resemble eczema on the feet of children with atopic dermatitis. The eruption occurs symmetrically at pressure sites on the plantar surface of the feet and does not involve other sites.

Psoriasis commonly develops during childhood but may be distinguished from atopic dermatitis by the minimal pruritus and well-circumscribed brightly erythematous lesions topped with the thick white scale of psoriasis. Areas of predilection include the scalp, elbows, knees, and intertriginous areas. The nails may be pitted and dystrophic. The perioral and acral vesicular lesions of infants with *acrodermatitis enteropathica* may be distinguished by the associated failure to thrive, alopecia, diarrhea, irritability, and lethargy. Patients frequently have secondary candidal and bacterial infections and respond rapidly to zinc administration. Many infants and children with *scabies* develop eczema from rubbing and scratching. The clues for making a diagnosis of scabies are the clinical characteristics and distribution of the lesions and the associated linear burrows. The mite, eggs, or feces may be found in skin scrapings with mineral oil.

The most common cutaneous manifestation of *histiocytosis X* in infants (Letterer-Siwe disease) is a scaly, erythematous eruption on the scalp and intertriginous areas. The rash may be differentiated from atopic (and seborrheic) dermatitis by the hemorrhagic character, vesicles, and ulcerations as well as the simultaneous occurrence of gingival and visceral abnormalities. The *Wiskott-Aldrich syndrome* is an X-linked recessive disorder characterized by severe eczema, thrombocytopenic purpura, an increased susceptibility to recurrent pyogenic infections, and abnormalities of both humoral and cell-mediated immunity. The eczema closely resembles that of atopic dermatitis but also has petechiae and purpuric areas. Interestingly, the atopic dermatitis—like eruption resolves in patients treated successfully by bone marrow transplantation with T-lymphocyte engraftment. The severe eczematous rash of the *hyperimmunoglobulin E syndrome* tends to be more intertriginous and is associated with cutaneous abscesses.

WORK-UP

The history of a child with atopic dermatitis will often include a family (70%) or personal history of allergic rhinitis, asthma, atopic dermatitis, or hives. Questions regarding the time of onset (after the first 2 months), the degree of pruritus, and the sensitivity to irritants and seasonal variations may help to establish the diagnosis. Determining the bathing habits and past experiences with trials and topical corticosteroid preparations and antibiotics will help in management. Attention should be paid to the distribution and character of lesions on physical examination as well as to the coexistence of secondary infection or other abnormalities that may suggest a systemic abnormality (see Differential Diagnosis). No routine laboratory tests are necessary. Suspected bacterial, herpetic, or fungal infections should be cultured. Tests to eliminate the possibility of other disorders, such as Wiskott-Aldrich syndrome and the hyperimmunoglobulin E syndrome, may be considered.

TREATMENT

Physicians should discuss the exacerbating factors and therapeutic measures with parents and children. Families must understand that the disorder is chronic and that quick cures do not exist. They should be reassured, however, that therapy can result in dramatic improvement and prevent the disfiguring lichenification. Teenagers should avoid choosing occupations that involve frequent hand washing or exposure to irritating chemicals. Personal or family counseling is advisable for persons in emotionally stressful home situations.

General Measures

Many patients with atopic dermatitis benefit from a daily bath or shower, which adds water to the outer layer of skin, followed immediately by the application of lubricants. In winter the skin tends to be particularly dry because of the decreased ambient humidity, and heavy emollient creams, such as Eucerin or Nivea, or petroleum jelly (Vaseline) may be required. Harsh soaps should be substituted with mild or superfatted soaps. The bath water should be lukewarm, because hot water increases skin dryness. Bubble baths are best avoided because they irritate the skin. Older children may benefit by the addition of bath oils. Humidifiers are also helpful during dry winter months; however, they must be cleaned regularly to avoid the dissemination of molds.

The treatment of a patient with atopic dermatitis should be tailored to the individual child. Although most patients are more troubled by the dryness and pruritus in winter, some children have more difficulty in summer and find that the irritation of sweat is a major problem. These patients may experience more pruritus with thick lubricants and benefit from lubricating lotions, such as Shepard's lotion, which are less occlusive. Such patients are also helped by the use of air conditioners in the summer. Similarly, most patients improve with the regimen of daily baths followed immediately by lubrication. Other children, especially with many excoriated sites, cannot tolerate water at all and benefit from avoidance of water and the use of Cetaphil lotion as a cleansing and lubricating agent.

Corticosteroids

Anti-inflammatory topical corticosteroid preparations are usually necessary to clear the inflammatory lesions. The strength and base of topical preparation depend on the location and severity of the rash and also on the age and tolerance of the patient. Fluorinated corticosteroids should never be used for more than a few days on the face or intertriginous areas because of the risk of skin atrophy. Younger children and patients with milder eruptions may clear with the weak, nonfluorinated agents only, whereas patients who are older or who have more severe pruritus and inflammation may require a moderate or high-strength corticosteroid (see section on Topical Preparations and Applications in Chap. 58). Most children with dry skin prefer ointment bases or emollient bases, especially during the winter, whereas some prefer to use cream bases covered with lubricating agents. Corticosteroid gels and lotions are usually too drying for patients with atopic dermatitis. Systemic corticosteroids are rarely indicated and should be used only for short periods of time by patients with a severe, generalized, intractable disease. Exacerbations resulting from discontinuation of systemic corticosteroid therapy are a further disadvantage of this therapeutic approach.

Other Topical Agents

Other topical agents that have been helpful for children with atopic dermatitis include ultraviolet light, mild tar preparations, and keratolytics, such as urea or salicylic acid, for lichenified plaques.

Weeping dermatitis is often caused by a secondary infection and requires compresses to dry and cool the areas and to remove crusts and debris. Burow's solution or cool saline compresses should be applied two to three times daily for 20 to 30 minutes using a large handkerchief or torn bed sheets to allow for evaporative loss. Topical corticosteroid or lubrication may be applied after the compresses. If *bacterial infection* is suspected and involves more than a small area, the patient should be treated with systemic antistaphylococcal antibiotics, such as erythromycin or dicloxacillin. The treatment of *herpetic infections* depends on the extent of involvement. Compresses and topical antibiotics (e.g., Polysporin) should be used in all patients. If patients have rapidly spreading vesicles, fever, or evidence of visceral involvement, such as elevated transaminases levels, systemic acyclovir should be administered. The use of topical acyclovir five times daily will also decrease the spread and duration of lesions, but it is not needed along with systemic acyclovir. Secondary bacterial infection of herpes simplex lesions should be treated with systemic antistaphylococcal antibiotics.

Antipruritics

Antihistamine preparations, such as hydroxyzine and diphenhydramine, may be valuable, especially for their sedative effects. Many children cannot tolerate antihistamines during the day because of sedation but find these agents invaluable at night when scratching is most intense. It is also advisable to keep one's nails short.

Diet Therapy

Dietary therapy is helpful in a small percentage of patients and is best reserved for patients with severe eczema who do not respond to more traditional measures, because compliance with dietary manipulation is difficult. The foods most commonly implicated are milk and eggs. By 3 or 4 years of age, many children no longer require food restriction and the avoided foods may be added gradually. Skin testing and hyposensitization are of minimal value.

Other Therapy

Subcutaneous gamma-interferon has recently been shown to be effective for patients with severe atopic dermatitis. Experimental therapies, such as topical phosphodiesterase inhibitors, oral evening primrose oil, and papaverine, require more study before they can be recommended.

INDICATIONS FOR REFERRAL AND ADMISSION

Patients who are difficult to manage or who require more than moderate-strength topical corticosteroid preparations should be referred to a dermatologist for management. Patients with severe atopic dermatitis who cannot be managed effectively as outpatients may respond to the intensive topical or systemic management of brief hospitalization. Patients with eczema herpeticum or severe secondary bacterial infections may also require observation and treatment in the hospital.

ANNOTATED BIBLIOGRAPHY

Buckley RH, Matthews KP: Common "allergic" skin diseases. JAMA 248:2611, 1982. (Includes a good review of the clinical features of atopic dermatitis.)

Dahl MV: Atopic dermatitis: The concept of flare factors. South Med J 70:453, 1977. (Reviews the flare factors that patients should be counseled to avoid.)

Hanifin JM: Atopic dermatitis. J Am Acad Dermatol 6:1, 1982. (Excellent review of the histopathologic, immunologic, and pharmacologic features of atopic dermatitis.)

60

Seborrheic Dermatitis

Amy Paller

Seborrheic dermatitis is a common disorder characterized by scaling and erythema in a "seborrheic" distribution, involving areas with the highest concentration of sebaceous glands and sebum production, such as the face, scalp, upper chest, and retroauricular and intertriginous areas. The disorder occurs in infancy and adolescence.

PATHOPHYSIOLOGY

Despite the localization of lesions of seborrheic dermatitis, there is no clear relation between sebum and dermatitis, and the cause of seborrheic dermatitis remains unknown. Some authors have postulated that sebum or a breakdown product irritates the skin. Recent evidence suggests an association between the inflammatory reaction and *Pityrosporum orbi-*

culare, a lipophilic yeast that is a normal inhabitant of the skin. The yeast is found in increased numbers, and therapy with topical ketoconazole decreases both the yeast and the inflammation. However, other investigators consider that the yeast is a secondary invader without any etiologic role.

CLINICAL PRESENTATION

In infancy, the dermatitis usually begins between the second and tenth week of life. "Cradle cap" and diaper dermatitis with erythema and greasy yellow or dry white scaling of the scalp and inguinal region, respectively, are the most common manifestations. Some infants have more widespread involvement with lesions across the entire face and scalp and intertriginous and presternal areas. Secondary bacterial or candidal infections are common. Pruritus is minimal, and the child is otherwise well. Most infantile cases either clear spontaneously after weeks to months or respond quickly to topical medication. Seborrheic dermatitis is rarely seen in prepubertal children older than 18 months of age.

In addition to infancy, the disorder may begin in adolescence during or after the onset of puberty. The scalp is the most common site, and seborrheic dermatitis is found in the form of fine white scaling or dandruff. In addition, the nasolabial folds, eyebrows, forehead, external ears, and retroauricular areas are frequently inflamed and scaly. Intertriginous sites and the presternal area may become involved. The dermatitis is bilaterally symmetric. Blepharitis and conjunctivitis are occasional complications. Although often asymptomatic, the rash is pruritic for some persons. Lichenification is unusual, and oozing and crusting, especially of intertriginous sites and the ear canals, suggest secondary bacterial infection.

Leiner's disease is a severe, exfoliative form of seborrheic-like dermatitis associated with diarrhea, failure to thrive, and gram-negative bacterial and candidal infections. Most affected infants are breast fed. Within the first weeks of life, scales and erythema resembling seborrheic dermatitis develop on the scalp, face, and intertriginous areas, followed by a generalized extension of the rash. This disorder has been shown to be a heterogeneous group of immunodeficiency disorders, including severe combined immunodeficiency, hyperimmunoglobulinemia E, and C_3 deficiency in addition to C_5 dysfunction.

DIFFERENTIAL DIAGNOSIS

The differential diagnosis of seborrheic dermatitis and dandruff in infants and teenagers includes tinea capitis and tinea corporis, atopic dermatitis, pediculosis, contact irritant and allergic dermatitis, psoriasis, drug eruptions, and histiocytosis X. In teenagers, tinea versicolor, lupus erythematosus, other photosensitivity disorders, pityriasis rosea, Darier's disease, and pemphigus foliaceus should be considered. *Tinea capitis* may manifest as fine white scaling of the scalp

without erythema or alopecia. *Atopic dermatitis* may mimic scalp seborrhea, but the flexural lichenification and positive family history of atopy help to confirm the diagnosis. *Pediculosis* may be differentiated by the nits and excoriations. *Contact dermatitis* shows sharp borders, conforming to the distribution of the offending agent. Plaques of *psoriasis* tend to be well demarcated in contrast to the erythema and scaling of seborrheic dermatitis; the clinical course, predilection for sites of trauma, and skin biopsy are helpful in the differential diagnosis. The lesions of *pityriasis rosea* tend to follow skin lines and are not typically found in sites of seborrheic dermatitis. Plaques and patches of *lupus erythematosus* have telangiectasia, and the superficial crusting of *pemphigus* can be differentiated from infected seborrheic dermatitis by skin biopsy and immunofluorescence microscopy. *Darier's disease* is an autosomal dominant condition characterized in adolescence by greasy, scaly papules in a seborrheic distribution but with oral and nail changes as well. The hypopigmented and hyperpigmented circular macules of *tinea versicolor* may be confused with seborrheic dermatitis, but microscopic examination of skin scrapings reveals the spores and hyphae of *Pityrosporum orbiculare.*

The most important disorder to distinguish from seborrheic dermatitis in infants is the Letterer-Siwe form of *histiocytosis X.* The cutaneous eruption usually begins as scaling and erythema on the scalp, retroauricular, axillary, and diaper areas. The concomitant petechiae and purpuric papules, pustules, and ulcerations should lead one to suspect the diagnosis. Not infrequently, the palms and soles are affected, in contrast to the typical sparing of palms and soles in seborrheic dermatitis. Other manifestations of histiocytosis X include gingival ulcerations, fever, hepatosplenomegaly, adenopathy, lytic lesions of bone, pulmonary infiltration, and hematologic suppression. Histopathologic examination of cutaneous lesions shows a proliferation of well-differentiated histiocytes with other inflammatory cells, especially neutrophils and eosinophils. The greatest mortality occurs in infants with widespread visceral involvement and thrombocytopenia.

TREATMENT

The therapy for seborrheic dermatitis depends on the site and extent of involvement. The disorder is self-limited in infants but chronic and recurrent when it begins in adolescence. If moderate or symptomatic inflammation and scaling are present in infancy, the scalp is best treated with a mild antiseborrheic shampoo, such as those with ketoconazole, selenium sulfide, or zinc pyrithione. The shampoo should be used three to four times a week and left on the scalp for 5 minutes before rinsing. If the crusts of "cradle cap" are thick, warm mineral oil or baby oil applied for 10 minutes prior to shampoo may be helpful. Skin lesions are best treated with hydrocortisone 1% cream or ketoconazole cream twice daily. For teenagers, the same general measures are employed, but more vigorous therapy may be necessary, such as tar shampoos or the use of preparations for cutaneous lesions with stronger nonfluorinated topical corticosteroids. Secondary infection with bacterial or candidal organisms should be treated with compresses and antistaphylococcal antibiotics or antifungal agents, respectively.

INDICATIONS FOR REFERRAL AND ADMISSION

Infants or adolescents who do not respond readily to antiseborrheic shampoos, topical ketoconazole, and nonfluorinated topical corticosteroids should be referred for dermatologic consultation. Hospitalization is indicated only in patients with severe seborrheic dermatitis with secondary infections, Leiner's disease, or disorders that may resemble seborrheic dermatitis but do not respond to routine therapeutic measures, such as histiocytosis X.

ANNOTATED BIBLIOGRAPHY

Ford GP, Farr RM, Ive FA et al: The response of seborrheic dermatitis to ketoconazole. Br J Dermatol 111:603–607, 1984. (Reports good response to ketoconazole therapy, suggesting that yeast contributes to the disorder.)

Gianotti F, Caputo R: Histiocytic syndromes: A review. J Am Acad Dermatol 13:383–404, 1985. (Review of histiocytic syndromes and their evaluation.)

Glover M, Atherton D, Levinsky R: Syndrome of erythroderma, failure to thrive and diarrhea in infancy: A manifestation of immunodeficiency. Pediatrics 81:66–72, 1988. (Lists immunodeficiency disorders that are associated with Leiner's disease.)

Lipton JM: The pathogenesis, diagnosis, and treatment of histiocytosis syndromes. Pediatr Dermatol 1:112–20, 1983. (Current review of the manifestations, therapy, and prognosis of histiocytosis X.)

Marks R, Pearse AD, Walker AP: The effects of a shampoo containing zinc pyrithione on the control of dandruff. Br J Dermatol 112:415–422, 1985. (Significant results with zinc pyrithione on clearance of seborrhea, correlated with significant reduction in the number of *Pityrosporum orbiculare* organisms.)

Ruiz-Maldonado R, Lopez-Martinez R, Perez Chavarria EL et al: *Pityrosporum ovale* in infantile seborrheic dermatitis. Pediatr Dermatol 6:16–20, 1989. (Further investigation of the role of this yeast in seborrheic dermatitis.)

61

Diaper Rash

Amy Paller

One of the most common problems of infants is diaper dermatitis. Irritant contact dermatitis is the usual underlying cause, but the dermatitis is frequently superinfected with candidal organisms.

PATHOPHYSIOLOGY

Several factors encourage the development of diaper rash. Infants with an atopic or seborrheic diathesis tend to be more susceptible. The diaper area is occluded, especially by plastic pants or plastic-covered diapers, and moisture is trapped with resultant alteration of the stratum corneum layer, maceration, and cutaneous erosion. Irritation is produced by friction in the inguinal area and further promoted by the wetness of the area. The moist, warm environment encourages the overgrowth of *Candida albicans* and bacteria. In the past, urinary ammonia was thought to be a prime factor in causing irritant diaper dermatitis. Although ammonia does produce more inflammation on wet skin with altered barrier properties than saline solution, it is now known that the concentration of ammonia and the *p*H of the urine are the same in infants with and without diaper dermatitis.

CLINICAL PRESENTATION AND DIFFERENTIAL DIAGNOSIS

The history and physical examination provide the clue to the underlying cause of a diaper rash. It is often necessary to culture the inguinal area, since secondary candidal or bacterial infections of irritant dermatitis are common.

Primary irritant contact dermatitis appears on convex surfaces with sparing of the folds. It is usually not seen until after 3 months of age and relates to trapped moisture and to friction at sites of contact with the diaper. Ammonia and its irritant products from bacterial enzyme catabolism may contribute to the irritation. Tightly applied diapers, especially with occlusive edges, and rubber or plastic pants that overlie diapers increase the risk of irritant contact dermatitis. The erythema has a shiny appearance and tends to wax and wane. Pustules, nodules, and erosions are frequently found, and erythematous papules may be present, especially at the periphery of the rash. Infants with frequent diarrheal stool may have intense perianal and even medial buttock inflammation. If the inguinal area folds are affected by a rash as well as by convex surfaces, *intertrigo* due to the heat, maceration, and sweat retention of folds must be considered. Intertrigo appears in the folds as erythema with maceration and erosions. The hot humid diaper environment may also cause prickly heat with tiny vesicles (*miliaria crystallina*) or erythematous papules and pustules (*miliaria rubra*) due to sweat retention, often in association with intertrigo. *Allergic contact dermatitis* is unusual in infants but has been reported following the use of contact sensitizers, such as neomycin (in Neosporin) and parabens (preservatives in creams). The diaper rash of allergic contact dermatitis from a topical medication often manifests itself as an exacerbation of the previous rash under treatment despite adequate therapy, and involves sharply demarcated areas exposed to the sensitizing agent. Allergic contact dermatitis begins as tiny superficial vesicles that rupture and appear eczematous within a few days after the onset of the eruption (see Chap. 62, ''Contact Dermatitis'').

Candidal infections are the most characteristic of the diaper rashes. The infection may be the primary cause of dermatitis or secondary to other inflammatory processes, especially irritant dermatitis or seborrheic dermatitis. The rash is intensely red, has sharp borders with satellite pustules and papules beyond the borders, and involves the inguinal folds. The infant may have concomitant oral thrush or *Candida* in the gastrointestinal tract or have been exposed to maternal vaginal candidiasis. Perianal erythema with papules and pustules suggests candidal infection with seeding from the gastrointestinal tract. Many infants with candidal infections have a recent history of antibiotic use, often for recurrent otitis media. Occasionally, scattered plaques or patches of scaly erythema are seen elsewhere in conjunction with a candidal diaper rash. This ''id'' reaction is a hypersensitivity response to the candidal antigens and no organisms can be cultured from the plaques (see Chap. 66, ''Superficial Dermatophylic and Yeast Infections'').

Seborrheic dermatitis commonly occurs in the diaper area of infants, beginning at 3 or 4 weeks of age. The rash (usually nonpruritic) starts in the folds and extends to convex surfaces with a poor demarcation from surrounding skin. The scale is yellow and greasy, and other sites, such as the scalp (cradle cap), face, retroauricular areas, axillae, neck folds, and umbilicus may be affected. In infancy, secondary yeast infections are common. Seborrheic dermatitis usually clears by 6 months of age and almost always by 18 months. *Histiocytosis X* often involves the diaper area and resembles seborrheic dermatitis. The concurrent erosions and purpuric areas help to distinguish the conditions. Infants may have gingival erosions, hepatosplenomegaly, lymphadenopathy, pulmonary interstitial infiltrates, and hematologic abnormalities as well. The lesions of histiocytosis X do not respond readily to mild topical corticosteroids, in contrast to the rash of seborrheic dermatitis. A skin biopsy is diagnostic. The severe seborrheic dermatitis of *Leiner's disease* is much more extensive than only in the diaper area and is associated with diarrhea, failure to thrive, and gram-negative bacterial and candidal infection. Affected infants may demonstrate a variety of immunologic abnormalities (see Chap. 60, ''Seborrheic Dermatitis'').

Atopic dermatitis may first become manifest in the diaper area due to the increased susceptibility to irritation, although the diaper area is often spared in atopic dermatitis because the infant cannot scratch there. The eruption begins after 2 months of age and is characterized by marked pruritus and secondary bacterial infections with oozing and crusting. Frequently, other sites are affected by the dry, pruritic rash, especially the face and extensor surfaces. *Psoriasis* occasionally begins in infancy, usually in the diaper area since it is the site of greatest trauma (Koebner phenomenon). The typical well-demarcated scaly plaques of psoriasis may not be scaly in the diaper area because of maceration and moisture. Other sites of involvement, including the scalp and nails, as well as characteristic skin biopsy changes may be found, but often the diagnosis only becomes apparent by a recurrence of the rash beyond infancy (see Chap. 59, ''Atopic Dermatitis.'')

Large vesicles or bullae in the diaper area may be due to infection with *Staphylococcus aureus* (bullous impetigo). The bullae tend to be flaccid and rupture easily, leaving a denuded red base. *Staphylococcal scalded skin syndrome* is most commonly found in infants and is due to a blood-borne toxin produced by the organisms in a localized infected site. Exfoliation typically begins around orifices, including the perineal and perianal areas. The rash begins as tender patches of erythema. Superficial vesicles and pustules develop and rapidly rupture to form yellow crusts overlying the erythema. Infants with widespread blistering may develop fluid and electrolyte imbalances as well as sepsis (see Chap. 65, ''Bacterial Skin Infections'').

Granuloma gluteale infantum is characterized by large, firm, dusky red nodules in the perineal area, buttocks, and inner thighs. The condition tends to resolve spontaneously after several months. Although the cause of this disorder is not known, in many affected infants topical fluorinated corticosteroids had been used for long periods of time before the appearance of lesions.

Acrodermatitis enteropathica is a rare autosomal recessive disorder because of abnormal absorption and metabolism of zinc. Affected infants have erythema and crusting at acral and periorificial sites, as well as hair loss, diarrhea, and failure to thrive. Secondary candidal infections are common. Infants with zinc deficiency due to inadequate zinc intake (hyperalimentation without trace minerals, hypozincemia in breast milk) exhibit identical manifestations. The response to zinc supplementation is rapid. Finally, infants with *scabies* frequently have papules, burrows, and secondary dermatitis in the inguinal area. Usually other sites are affected, especially the trunk and axillae, and the mites, eggs, or feces are found in mineral oil scrapings of affected areas.

TREATMENT

The treatment of diaper dermatitis is most successful if the cause of the rash is determined. Since friction and occlusion are detrimental in all forms of dermatitis, the diaper area should be kept dry and occlusive pants should be eliminated. Some double-blind studies have found that superabsorbent disposable diapers decrease the incidence of rashes. The diaper area should be dried gently and exposed to air to dry completely following urination. Washing of the diaper area with each urination is excessive and may be irritating. Cleansing after bowel movements is necessary, but only mild soaps should be used. Commercial wipes should not be used if they prove irritating.

Ointments such as zinc oxide paste or A & D ointment may be helpful to reduce friction and prevent the skin from contact with irritants. Petrolatum may be too occlusive and may encourage the trapping of moisture. Cornstarch may be useful for decreasing friction and does not encourage the growth of *Candida* as was once thought. Talcum powder should be used carefully because it has been associated with aspiration pneumonitis in infants. Baking soda should be avoided because its use in diaper rash has led to metabolic alkalosis.

Irritant and allergic contact dermatitis are best treated with avoidance of the offending agent and twice-daily application of a mild nonfluorinated topical corticosteroid cream, such as 1% hydrocortisone. The diaper dermatitis of seborrheic dermatitis and psoriasis also responds to topical preparations of hydrocortisone and other nonfluorinated corticosteroids. Fluorinated corticosteroid preparations should not be used in the groin area because of the high risk of local side effects, especially skin atrophy.

Candidal infections are best treated by keeping the area dry and by application of a topical antifungal preparation, such as clotrimazole, for 3 weeks. If thrush is present or the gastrointestinal tract is suspected of being the source of candidal organisms, oral suspensions of nystatin 200,000 units four times daily for 7 days is helpful. Possible sources of candida should be identified and eliminated (e.g., treatment of maternal mastitis or vaginal infection). The id reactions are best treated by anticandidal therapy to the diaper region and other involved intertriginous sites and 1% hydrocortisone cream to the plaques. Preparations of topical corticosteroids and antifungals, such as Mycolog and Lotrisone creams, should be avoided because they contain fluorinated corticosteroids.

INDICATIONS FOR REFERRAL AND ADMISSION

Infants with diaper dermatitis that is not responsive to general measures and selected anti-inflammatory or anticandidal therapy should be referred to a dermatologist for further evaluation and management. Patients with severe generalized dermatitis, staphylococcal scaled skin syndrome, or histiocytosis X may require hospital admission.

ANNOTATED BIBLIOGRAPHY

Gonzalez J, Hogg RJ: Metabolic alkalosis secondary to baking soda treatment of a diaper rash. Pediatrics 67:820–822, 1981. (Reminder of the potential development of metabolic alkalosis from the use of baking soda.)

Leyden JJ: Cornstarch, *Candida albicans,* and diaper rash. Pediatr Dermatol 1:322–325, 1984. (Cornstarch did not encourage the growth of *Candida albicans.*)

Leyden JJ, Katz S, Stewart R et al: Urinary ammonia and ammonia-producing microorganisms in infants with and without diaper dermatitis. Arch Dermatol 113:1678–1680, 1977. (No difference was found in the amount of ammonia in the diaper area of infants with and without dermatitis.)

Mofenson HC, Greensher J, DiTomasso A et al: Baby powder—a hazard! Pediatrics 68:265–266, 1981. (Good review of the problem of baby powder inhalation.)

Stein H: Incidence of diaper rash when using cloth and disposable diapers. J Pediatr 101:721–723, 1982. (Less diaper rash found with use of disposable rather than cloth diapers.)

62
Contact Dermatitis

Amy Paller

Dermatitis caused by exogenous agents may be irritant (nonimmunologic) or allergic (delayed hypersensitivity). In infants, most contact dermatitis is irritant. In older children and adolescents, it is more likely to be due to a contact allergy.

Irritant contact dermatitis in infants usually involves the diaper area and is due to contact with urine or feces (see Chap. 61). Saliva or fruit juices are the most common irritating agents on the face or neck. In older children and adolescents, irritant dermatitis is less common because of thicker, less irritable skin but may occur after exposure to irritating solvents, deodorants, or medications (e.g., acne preparations). Other agents that may produce primary irritant dermatitis include harsh soaps, detergents, bubble baths, bleaches, fiberglass, acids, and alkalis. Children with atopic dermatitis are most susceptible to irritant dermatitis. The development of irritant dermatitis depends on the concentration, duration, frequency, and site of exposure to the contactant, as well as local factors, such as occlusion and sweating.

Allergic contact dermatitis, in contrast to irritant dermatitis, only requires a brief exposure to a small amount of the causative agent. It is much less common in children than in adults. The incidence clearly increases as the child gets older, but documented contact allergic dermatitis has been described in young infants.

PATHOPHYSIOLOGY OF ALLERGIC CONTACT DERMATITIS

Allergic contact dermatitis is a cell-mediated (type IV) hypersensitivity response. A sensitization period of exposure of the allergen to skin takes at least a week. For many cutaneous allergens, this sensitization phase requires antigen processing by the epidermal Langerhans cells and complexing to a haptenic carrier before proliferation of specific T lymphocytes occurs. On second exposure to the antigen, the elicitation phase occurs with activation of the T lymphocytes, release of inflammatory mediators and subsequent erythema, edema with occasional blister formation, and cellular infiltration. Typically, the dermatitis may be seen within 24 hours after subsequent exposure to the allergen and persists for approximately 2 weeks.

CLINICAL PRESENTATION

Allergic contact dermatitis may be acute, subacute, or chronic, and the appearance of lesions depends on the phase. Acute dermatitis is characterized by intense erythema, papules, vesicles, and oozing. In subacute dermatitis, the lesions are scaling and crusting with less vesiculation, and in chronic dermatitis, the reaction may include mild erythema, scaling, fissures, pigmentary alteration, and lichenification. The reaction is usually limited to the site of contact with the allergen, and the distribution provides a clue to the cause of the dermatitis. For example, reactions to nickel appear on the ear lobes, fingers, midabdomen (at belt buckle), and neck. Reactions to leather tanning agents or to the rubber of shoes are seen on the dorsa of the feet, and reactions to cosmetics, nail polish, or topical medications occur on the face and eyelids.

Common Allergens

The most common cause of contact allergy in children is *Rhus plant dermatitis* (poison ivy, poison oak, poison sumac) (Fig. 62-1). The poison ivy plant has three notched leaflets. Poison sumac is a shrub or tree with 7 to 13 leaflets arranged in pairs along a central stem and is found east of the Mississippi in wooded areas. Poison oak is an upright shrub found on the West coast. The eruption follows contact

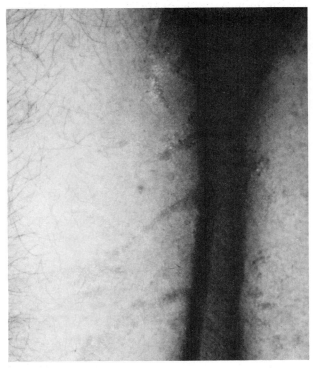

Figure 62-1. Linear pattern of contact dermatitis due to poison ivy.

with damaged leaves, roots, or stems, which contain the plant oleoresin and its active compound pentadecylcatechol. The oleoresin is spread on the skin by scratching, and vesicles and erythema often have a linear distribution. The face, hands, and feet are usually affected, although boys will commonly have lesions over the genital and perigenital area. Commonly, the dermatitis becomes secondarily infected with streptococcal or staphylococcal organisms.

Besides allergy to the *Rhus* group of plants, the frequency of allergy to specific agents is determined by patch testing. In the United States, the most common contact allergens in children are nickel, rubber chemicals, formaldehyde, ethylenediamine, balsam of Peru, benzocaine, mercuric bichloride, paraphenylenediamine (PPD), potassium dichromate, *p*-aminobenzoic acid (PABA) preservatives, and neomycin. The major sources of these agents are jewelry, shoes, cosmetics, and topical medications.

The incidence of contact sensitivity to *nickel* is 2.5% in children aged 5 to 13. Sources of nickel allergy include jewelry, eyeglass frames, metal fasteners, and belt buckles. The patient is often not aware that metal (such as in earrings) contains nickel. The presence of nickel may be ascertained by painting the metal with 10% dimethylglyoxine, which causes a pink color. Although stainless steel is an alloy of nickel and chrome, the two metals are tightly bound and stainless steel does not cause contact allergy. If nickel cannot be eliminated, sensitivity may be diminished by coating the nickel with several layers of clear nail polish.

Shoe dermatitis is usually caused by contact with *rubber chemicals*, including accelerators (mercaptobenzothiazole and thiurams) and antioxidants. The reaction most commonly involves the dorsa of the feet with sparing of the interdigital webs and plantar surface. *Adhesive agents* and *potassium dichromate*, a chemical used to tan leather, may also be responsible for shoe dermatitis. Sweating exacerbates the dermatitis by increasing percutaneous absorption of the allergen or causing superimposed irritant dermatitis. The rubber compounds may also be found in bandages and adhesive tape. In susceptible children, nonrubber acrylate bandages, Dermicel or Micropore tape, and Steri-strips may be used.

Cosmetic dermatitis often affects the eyelids, even when the agents are applied to the hands or scalp, by transfer of the allergen to an area of greater permeability. Allergy to the organic dye *PPD* usually develops in teenage girls after exposure to hair dyes, with erythema, edema, and vesiculation of the posterior neck, ears, face, and scalp. Occasionally, PPD may be used to dye textiles, stockings, and shoes with resultant contact allergy. *Formaldehydes* are used as preservatives in shampoos, cosmetics, and glues. Topical medications may contain contact allergens, and disorders may appear to be aggravated because of the development of a superimposed contact allergic dermatitis. *Balsam of Peru* is occasionally found in topical medications. It cross reacts with fragrances in cosmetics and can cause hand or facial dermatitis in children. *Parabens* are antimicrobial preservatives found in cosmetics and topical medications. Although the use of *mercury compounds* has decreased, they are strong sensitizers and are still used as disinfectants in topical preparations, such as Merthiolate. *Benzocaine* is a topical anesthetic that is used for relief of sunburn and pruritus. *Neomycin* is a topical antibiotic, most commonly found in Neosporin. Topical preparations that contain *diphenhydramine,* such as Caladryl, may cause contact reactions when the topical agent is applied or with later use of the oral antihistamine.

Clothing dermatitis is usually irritant, but allergic contact dermatitis occasionally occurs. *Formaldehyde* and *formaldehyde-releasing substances* in permanent press fabrics (polyester-cotton) may cause clothing dermatitis, especially in areas with a tight fit, such as the axillae and the inner thighs. *Rubber compounds* may cause waistband dermatitis from the elastic waistband of underwear following washing with bleach.

DIFFERENTIAL DIAGNOSIS

Conditions that may resemble allergic contact dermatitis include irritant dermatitis, dyshidrotic eczema, bacterial or candidal infections, juvenile plantar dermatosis, and phytophotodermatitis. The distribution, history of exposure, and later results of patch testing aid in confirming the diagnosis. Bacterial and candidal infections may be ruled out by culture of lesions. Juvenile plantar dermatosis is usually found in school-aged, prepubertal children and is characterized by symmetric erythema, scaling, and fissuring of the weight-bearing areas of the feet with sparing of the insteps and interdigital spaces. Most affected children are athletic, have hyperhidrosis, and wear occlusive socks and shoes. Allergic dermatitis due to shoes, atopic dermatitis, and tinea pedis must be considered in the differential diagnosis. The treatment of juvenile plantar dermatosis includes topical corticosteroid ointments, antibacterial ointment to fissures, and agents, such as aluminum chloride, to decrease hyperhidrosis. *Phytophotodermatitis* is a toxic reaction due to exposure to certain plants and sunlight. The furocoumarins that cause phytophotodermatitis are released on crushing the plant and are found in limes, lemons, figs, celery, and parsnip plants. Lesions are typically well-circumscribed patches or linear streaks of hyperpigmentation, occasionally following erythema, in a sun-exposed site.

WORK-UP

The history of exposure to the allergen is critical in suspecting the diagnosis. The distribution and appearance of lesions by physical examination further confirms the diagnosis of contact allergy and suggests the contactant. Patch testing by the dermatologist provides corroborative evidence that a suspected allergen is responsible. Patch testing should be deferred until the acute reaction has cleared to prevent exacerbation from absorption of the test material. Aluminum-backed strips with disks containing the individual allergens are applied to the back for 48 hours and read 30 minutes after removal. Reactions are graded on the basis of erythema and edema. For patients with nickel allergy, applying dimethylglyoxine to a suspected metal will determine nickel content.

TREATMENT

Management of contact allergy, whether irritant or allergic, involves treatment of the dermatitis and elimination of the offending agent. Topical corticosteroid creams of moderate potency (unless the lesions are on the face or intertriginous sites) should be applied two to three times daily until the rash has cleared. If extensive areas are involved, such as in widespread *Rhus* dermatitis, prednisone 1 mg/kg/d for 10 to 14 days is the most effective treatment. Weeping lesions should be compressed with saline solutions or Burow's solution 1:20 to 1:40 (one Domeboro tablet to 1 pint of lukewarm water is a 1:40 solution). Shake lotions, such as Calamine, are also helpful to dry lesions and decrease oozing. Systemic antihistamines may decrease pruritus. Secondary bacterial infection should be treated with systemic antistaphylococcal antibiotics.

To minimize exposure to the *Rhus* group of plants, affected children should be taught to recognize the plant and to remove clothes and wash rapidly and thoroughly after exposure to remove the oleoresin from fingers and other body parts. The fluid within vesicles does not contain allergen. Nickel should be avoided or coated with nail polish. Hypoallergenic shoes are available for patients with allergic contact dermatitis to shoe components. These include vinyl and canvas tennis shoes without rubber, moccasins, wooden clogs, and polyvinyl shoes. Special shoes may be ordered from the Musebeck Shoe Company, Foot-So-Port Shoe Division, Forest and Westover, Oconomowoc, WI, 53066. Rubber-free insoles or agents used to diminish sweating of the feet, such as tea baths or aluminum chloride solutions, may also help.

INDICATIONS FOR REFERRAL

Any patient suspected of having allergic contact dermatitis that requires patch testing or patients with widespread or recalcitrant dermatitis should be referred to a dermatologist.

ANNOTATED BIBLIOGRAPHY

Coffman K, Boyce T, Hansen RC: Phytophotodermatitis simulating child abuse. Am J Dis Child 139:239–240, 1985. (Two cases of phytophotodermatitis in children.)

Fisher AA: Contact Dermatitis, 3rd ed. Philadelphia, Lea & Febiger, 1986. (Extremely complete text of contact allergens, their manifestations, and cross-reactivity.)

Heskel NS: Contact dermatitis in children. Dermatol Clin 2:579–584, 1984. (Review of allergic contact dermatitis in children, citing the overdiagnosis of the condition.)

Mackie RM: Juvenile plantar dermatosis. Semin Dermatol 1:67–71, 1982. (Review of juvenile plantar dermatosis.)

Weston WL, Weston JA: Allergic contact dermatitis. Am J Dis Child 138:932–936, 1984. (Review of contact dermatitis, suggesting that allergic contact dermatitis is more common than suspected.)

63

Papulosquamous Eruptions

Amy Paller

Papulosquamous eruptions include various childhood dermatologic problems that are all characterized by small, elevated lesions with scaling. Among the more common papulosquamous disorders of children are psoriasis, pityriasis rosea, Mucha-Habermann disease, lichen nitidus, and lichen striatus.

PSORIASIS

Psoriasis is one of the most common dermatologic abnormalities (affecting 1% to 3% of the population), and 37% of patients first develop the disorder during childhood, especially during the second decade of life. The diagnosis, nevertheless, is often missed by pediatricians. The disorder is chronic with periods of spontaneous remissions and recurrences. Although there is a familial predisposition, the inheritance pattern of psoriasis appears to be multifactorial.

The underlying cause of psoriasis is unknown. Both epidermal alterations with accelerated epidermal proliferation and dermal vascular abnormalities are believed to be contributory. Research has focused on the role of leukotrienes in causing the inflammation. It is clear that environmental factors may improve or exacerbate psoriasis. Cutaneous trauma may induce lesions after a lag time of 1 to 3 weeks, a phenomenon called the *isomorphic response* or *Koebner phenomenon*. The sudden appearance of small widespread psoriatic plaques (acute guttate psoriasis) can follow streptococcal infections, especially in adolescent patients (Fig. 63-1). Although sunlight in moderate amounts may help to clear psoriatic lesions, sunburn is another environmental response that is associated with the Koebner phenomenon. Certain drugs may also aggravate the condition, such as systemic corticosteroids (especially on withdrawal), lithium, and some of the nonsteroidal anti-inflammatory agents.

Psoriasis may manifest in various cutaneous alterations, some of which are found only in children. The most common variant is typical plaque-type psoriasis (psoriasis vulgaris) with well-circumscribed erythematous papules and plaques with loosely adherent shiny white scale concentrated at the center of lesions. The plaques of children are usually less scaly and thinner than those of adults. When the scale is removed, pinpoint sites of bleeding are uncovered (Auspitz sign). The lesions are symmetric and are found at sites of trauma, especially the elbows, knees, and buttocks, the umbilical, intergluteal, and presacral areas, and the palms and soles. The scalp is another common site and may be the only site of initial involvement. Lesions frequently encircle the hairline and are found on the retroauricular area and external ears. Well-demarcated, thick adherent crusts are found occasionally on the scalp (tinea amiantacea). Seborrhea and fungal infections of the scalp must be differentiated from the well-defined plaques and thick scaling as well as by potassium hydroxide examination and cultures. In contrast to its rarity in adults, the face is commonly involved in children. Many patients with psoriasis have dystrophic nails with discoloration, thickening, distal fractures, ridging, and pitting (Fig. 63-2). In patients with nail alterations but no cutaneous psoriatic plaques, fungal or bacterial infections, trauma to the nail, lichen planus, alopecia areata, atopic dermatitis, and 20-nail dystrophy of childhood must be considered.

Psoriasis in the diaper area of infants (napkin psoriasis) usually appears eczematous and is often mistaken for seborrheic dermatitis, irritant dermatitis, or candidal infection. Just as psoriasis vulgaris is seen at the sites of trauma in children and adolescents, psoriasis in infants is most commonly manifest in the diaper area, a site of considerable trauma. Napkin psoriasis is more recalcitrant to mild topical corticosteroids than contact dermatitis and seborrheic dermatitis. The rash usually affects the inguinal and intergluteal folds. Psoriatic plaques are also often found on the scalp and trunk. They must be differentiated from seborrheic dermatitis and the id reaction of candidal diaper dermatitis. All lesions in the diaper area should be cultured for *Candida albicans* because yeast is a common cause of secondary infection in infants with psoriasis.

The acute *guttate* (teardrop) form of psoriasis is the first sign of psoriasis in 15% of patients, although it occurs more frequently in patients with known psoriasis. Teenagers and young adults are commonly affected. The lesions are round to oval erythematous scaling papules that range in size from 2 to 10 mm. The papules are widespread and symmetric. Lesions may be present on the face and are more common on the trunk and proximal extremities, but the palms and soles are usually spared. Two thirds of patients report pharyngitis 2 to 3 weeks before the eruption develops, and streptococcal organisms are often found by pharyngeal cultures. Guttate psoriasis should be differentiated from psoriasiform drug reactions, pityriasis rosea, and secondary syphilis.

Pustular psoriasis is an unusual form in childhood and may be generalized or localized. Although pustular psoriasis in adults usually follows years of plaque-type psoriasis,

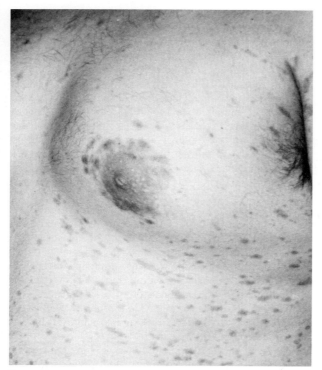

Figure 63-1. Acute guttate psoriasis in a teenager following streptococcal pharyngitis.

pustular psoriasis in children is often the initial manifestation of psoriasis. Some children have a history of psoriasiform seborrheic dermatitis. Episodes of generalized pustular psoriasis are frequently accompanied by malaise, fever, and leukocytosis. Sheets of 1- to 2-mm pustules appear suddenly and overlie erythema and scaling. Cultures of the pustules yield no organisms. The localized form of pustular

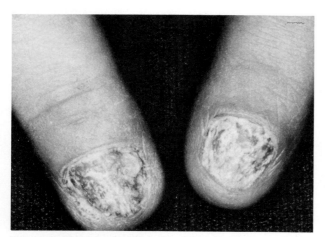

Figure 63-2. Psoriatic nails of a child with a single psoriatic plaque in the periungual area.

psoriasis involves the palms and soles, often in association with more typical plaques elsewhere on the body. Staphylococcal pustulosis, dyshidrotic eczema, contact dermatitis, infantile acropustulosis, and fungal infections should be considered.

Exfoliative erythroderma is a rare form of psoriasis that is characterized by generalized desquamation and erythema. Children who are most affected have a past history of psoriasis. Drug reactions, severe seborrheic or atopic dermatitis, contact dermatitis, and pityriasis rubra pilaris must be considered.

Psoriatic arthritis in children is unusual but has been recognized with increasing frequency. It is defined as an inflammatory arthritis beginning before the age of 16 years associated with psoriasis, either preceding the onset of psoriasis or occurring within the subsequent 15 years, usually with the absence of rheumatoid factor in the serum. The peak age at onset is 9 to 12 years, and the arthritis is more prevalent in girls. Nearly one half of the patients have a positive family history of psoriasis. Cutaneous psoriasis may be absent or mild, and patients are frequently given the erroneous diagnosis of juvenile rheumatoid arthritis (see Chap. 133, "Juvenile Rheumatoid Arthritis"). Joint disease is usually asymmetric and monoarticular or oligoarticular, although polyarticular arthritis often develops later. Sausage digits, tendon sheath involvement, and distal interphalangeal joint changes are typical. Some patients have sacroiliitis or spondylitis (especially with HLA-B27). Iridocyclitis is the most common extra-articular feature (9%), but other systemic manifestations, such as fever, hepatosplenomegaly, lymphadenopathy, and cardiopulmonary alterations, are rare. The long-term prognosis is good, with minimal permanent joint destruction for most patients. Most children who have psoriatic arthritis respond to aspirin and nonsteroidal anti-inflammatory agents in addition to physical and occupational therapy.

A histopathologic examination of lesional skin supports the clinical diagnosis of psoriasis, although many biopsy specimens, especially of treated lesions, may not show classic features. The typical microscopic features of psoriatic plaques include a thickened stratum corneum with layers of retained keratinocyte nuclei (parakeratosis), hyperplastic epidermis, dilated capillaries, and intracorneal and subcorneal collections of polymorphonuclear leukocytes (Munro abscesses).

Psoriasis tends to be a chronic disorder, and onset in childhood often suggests a more complicated, recalcitrant course in adulthood. Many patients tend to have a mild form of the disease, however, and spontaneous remissions occur for variable periods of time in almost one half of patients.

Management

One of the most important aspects of management is the education of parents and patients that psoriasis is a chronic disorder with remissions and recurrences. Injury to the skin should be avoided (Koebner phenomenon) by protective guards when participating in contact sports and by choosing occupations that minimize cutaneous injury. Tight elastic undergarments, clothing, and shoes should also be avoided. Patients must be careful to avoid excessive exposure to the sun so that sunburn does not occur.

Since psoriasis is a chronic disease, therapy should be conservative, especially in children. Topical therapy is usually successful, especially corticosteroids, tars, and anthralin. Fluorinated corticosteroids are usually required (except on the face and intertriginous areas) and should be applied up to three times daily. Arthralin or coal-tar preparations are also useful as adjunctive agents but may cause irritation, folliculitis, and staining of the skin and clothes. These preparations are available as ointments, pastes, body oils, bath oils, and gels. Topical vitamin D has been shown to be useful for adults with psoriasis; trials in children are in progress. Thick plaques may require keratolytic agents, such as 3% sulfur or 6% salicylic acid preparations, or intralesional injections of triamcinolone. Scalp psoriasis is best treated with shampoos containing tars and keratolytics used at least every other day. Thick plaques may be softened with mineral oil covered by a warm towel or phenol and saline solutions. Corticosteroids in solutions or ointments may also be useful for scalp psoriasis.

More complicated therapy for psoriasis is rarely needed for children. Patients with lesions that are recalcitrant to topical medications may improve with a combination of tar and ultraviolet B light (Goeckerman regimen). Psoralens and ultraviolet A light may be used in older children and adolescents. Methotrexate, cyclosporin, and systemic retinoids may be valuable for children with resistant generalized pustular psoriasis or erythroderma. Systemic corticosteroids are almost never indicated, except in rare cases of erythroderma for acute therapy. Any patient who does not respond to regimens of topical corticosteroids should be managed by a dermatologist. Hospitalization may be required for Goeckerman regimens and initiation of systemic medications.

PITYRIASIS RUBRA PILARIS

Pityriasis rubra pilaris is a rare skin disorder in children characterized by salmon-colored scaly plaques surrounding islands of normal skin, pointed follicular papules, and palmoplantar keratoderma. Some juvenile cases are hereditary with an autosomal dominant mode of inheritance. Three forms are described in children and account for 45% of cases. Juvenile forms often relapse but may remit completely after 3 years. Pityriasis rubra pilaris is most commonly mistaken for psoriasis, and there is an intrafamilial (or even personal) occurrence of both disorders. The clinical and histologic appearance of lesions are very similar. Occasionally other disorders, including seborrheic dermati-

tis, lichen planus, vitamin A deficiency, follicular eczema, atypical keratosis pilaris, and drug eruptions, must be considered in the differential diagnosis.

Pityriasis rubra pilaris is often recalcitrant to topical corticosteroids and keratolytic agents, including topical vitamin A derivatives. Oral vitamin A in doses of 50,000 to 150,000 units daily may be effective in children with pityriasis rubra pilaris, but its use is limited by potential side effects. Success has also been reported with systemic retinoids (13-*cis*-retinoic acid and etretinate) and methotrexate, but these agents can only be administered intermittently and cautiously in children.

PITYRIASIS ROSEA

Pityriasis rosea is a common papulosquamous eruption that occurs frequently in children and adolescents. Although a virus is suspected to be causative, no agent has yet been isolated and the risk of contagion is minimal. The eruption often begins with a 1- to 5-cm scaly erythematous patch (*herald lesion*) that is often mistaken for tinea. A few days to a few weeks later, generalized lesions typically develop, especially on the neck, upper arms and legs, and trunk. The lesions are oval with a collarette of scale at the periphery and follow a typical distribution along skin lines to produce a "Christmas tree" pattern on the back. Lesions are occasionally papular (especially in black children), vesicular, hemorrhagic, or urticarial. The rash may be limited to the extremities and intertriginous areas (inverse pityriasis rosea) or may be localized. Palms and soles are rarely affected, but facial involvement is more common in children. Most patients are asymptomatic or complain of mild pruritus. Pruritus is occasionally intensive and patients have mild constitutional symptoms, such as malaise, pharyngitis, fever, or headache. The eruption is self-limited and tends to clear after 6 to 8 weeks, although transient pigmentary changes may remain.

When pityriasis rubra is atypical in distribution, especially with lesions on the palms and soles, the diagnosis of secondary syphilis must be considered. Other disorders that may resemble pityriasis include drug eruptions, parapsoriasis, seborrheic dermatitis, widespread tinea infections, psoriasis, lichen planus, and scabies with eczematization. Therapy is symptomatic, because the disorder is self-limited and includes antihistamines, emollients, and mild topical corticosteroids.

MUCHA-HABERMANN DISEASE

Mucha-Habermann disease (*acute parapsoriasis, pityriasis lichenoides et varioliformis acuta*) is a self-limited disorder that occurs frequently in children and especially in adolescents. The disorder is characterized by crops of papules and vesicles with central necrosis and crusts. The papulovesicles are usually on the trunk and extremities. Lesions may heal with scars or pigmentary alterations. Each episode lasts for weeks to months, with resolution and recurrences for a few years.

   Mucha-Habermann disease must be differentiated from chickenpox, pityriasis rosea, scabies, and impetigo. A histopathologic examination of skin shows a heavy infiltrate of lymphocytes and histiocytes, erythrocyte extravasation into the dermis, and epidermal edema with necrosis and vesicle formation. Pruritus may be decreased by lubricants, mild topical corticosteroids, antihistamines, and lubricants. Tetracycline or erythromycin administered for 3 to 6 months and ultraviolet B light have been helpful in many cases.

   Pityriasis lichenoides chronica may evolve from the acute form or de novo and usually lasts for 6 months to years. The firm, hyperpigmented papules are more scaly than those of the acute form and resolve without scar formation. Pityriasis rosea, psoriasis, and secondary syphilis should be considered. Many patients improve during the summer and with exposure to ultraviolet B light.

LICHEN PLANUS

Lichen planus is a pruritic dermatosis that occurs occasionally in children. The typical lesion is a small flat violaceous papule covered with a shiny white scale. Fine white lines (Wickham's striae) cross the surface of the papules. Several variants with atrophic, hypertrophic, vesiculobullous, annular, and ulcerated lesions have been reported. Lesions are most commonly found on the flexural surfaces of the extremities, anterior lower legs, dorsa of the hands, and genitalia. Mucous membranes, especially the buccal mucosae, are covered by lacy patterns of white papules in most patients and may be the only site of involvement. Up to 10% of patients have nail dystrophy with thinning of the nail plate, longitudinal ridging, and distal splitting. Pterygium formation with fusion of the proximal nail fold with the nail bed is the most typical nail change.

   The histopathologic changes of lesional skin are fairly specific. They include hyperkeratosis, focal increase of the granular layer, degeneration of the basal cell layer, a "saw-toothed" appearance of the epidermis, and a linear band of lymphocytes and histiocytes in the upper dermis and lower epidermis. Direct immunofluorescence of skin sections shows ovoid globular deposits of immunoglobulins and complement and a linear band of fibrinogen at the dermal-epidermal junction that suggests an immunologic etiology. Several drugs have caused lichenoid reactions, but none are commonly used in childhood.

   Lichen planus tends to resolve spontaneously after months to years. Systemic antihistamines, lubrication, and topical corticosteroids may help to diminish the intense pruritus experienced by most patients. Severely affected children may require a short course of systemic corticosteroids. Griseofulvin has occasionally been reported to be helpful.

LICHEN NITIDUS

Lichen nitidus is a benign, asymptomatic dermatosis that is seen usually in children. The papules of lichen nitidus are tiny, sharply demarcated, and skin colored. The papules are usually hypopigmented in black children. Papules may have a central depression and are often linear in distribution. The forearms, trunk, genitalia, and abdomen are the most common sites of involvement. The histopathology of lichen nitidus is distinct, with compressed epidermis encircling discrete dermal nests of lymphocytes, histiocytes, and giant cells. In children, the differential diagnosis includes flat warts, keratosis pilaris, and the lichen spinulosus pattern of papular eczema. No known therapy is effective, but the disorder clears spontaneously within a few years.

LICHEN STRIATUS

Lichen striatus is a rare dermatosis that is seen usually in school-aged children. A unilateral linear band of violaceous papules develops suddenly, especially on an extremity, and may extend for a few months. The eruption is often asymptomatic, but may be pruritic, and regresses spontaneously after 6 months to 1 year. The histopathologic changes are not specific, and biopsy is only helpful to eliminate the possibility of other disorders that may resemble lichen striatus, such as inflammatory linear epidermal nevus, flat warts, linear lichen planus, tinea, and psoriasis. Treatment is not necessary, but topical corticosteroids may decrease the inflammation and encourage clearance of the lesions.

ANNOTATED BIBLIOGRAPHY

Cohen PR, Prystowsky JH: Pityriasis rubra pilaris: A review of diagnosis and treatment. J Am Acad Dermatol 20:801–807, 1988. (Review of pityriasis rubra pilaris.)

Fox BJ, Odom RB: Papulosquamous diseases: A review. J Am Acad Dermatol 12:597–624, 1985. (Well-written review of the various papulosquamous disorders.)

Gelmetti C, Rigoni C, Alessi E et al: Pityriasis lichenoides in children: A long-term follow-up of eighty-nine cases. J Am Acad Dermatol 23:473–178, 1990. (Good discussion of pityriasis lichenoides.)

Periman HH, Lubowe II: Pityriasis rosea in children. J Pediatr 40:109–129, 1952. (Study of pityriasis rosea in a large population.)

Shore A, Ansell BM: Juvenile psoriatic arthritis—an analysis of 60 cases. J Pediatr 100:529–535, 1982. (Review of psoriatic arthritis in children with the suggestion that it is more common than we think.)

Watson W, Farber EM: Psoriasis in children. Pediatr Clin North Am 18:875–895, 1971. (Complete review of psoriasis in children.)

Zelickson BD, Muller SA: Generalized pustular psoriasis in childhood. J Am Acad Dermatol 24:186–194, 1991. (Review of childhood pustular psoriasis.)

64

Vesicular, Bullous, and Pustular Eruptions

Amy Paller

The cutaneous disorders with vesicles, bullae, and pustules that occur in infancy and childhood may be benign and self-limited, as transient neonatal pustular melanosis, or chronic and potentially severe, as epidermolysis bullosa. By definition, a *vesicle* is an elevated lesion filled with clear fluid that measures less than 1 cm in diameter, whereas a *bulla* is larger than 1 cm in diameter. A *pustule* is a vesicle or bulla that is filled with purulent material.

TRANSIENT NEONATAL BLISTERING DISORDERS

The most common transient cutaneous abnormality in the newborn is *erythema toxicum neonatorum,* a disorder of unknown cause characterized by erythematous macules and papules, vesicles, and pustules. The lesions usually appear at 2 to 3 days of age and clear spontaneously at the end of the first week of life. The face, trunk, and extremities are usually affected, and the palms and soles are almost always spared. The diagnosis may be confirmed by performing a smear of a vesicle or pustule that will show eosinophils without polymorphonuclear leukocytes, multinucleated giant cells, or bacteria by Wright, Giemsa, or Gram stains. A histopathologic examination of a skin biopsy specimen shows that the pustule filled with eosinophils is follicular and beneath the horny layer of skin. *Transient neonatal pustular melanosis* is noted usually at birth or within the first 24 hours of life in 5% of all black infants but in less than 1% of white infants. The neck, chin, palms, soles, and groin area are most commonly affected. The typical lesions are pustules and vesicles with a collarette of scale that resolve as hyperpigmented macules. The vesicles and papules clear spontaneously by 3 days of age, and the hyperpigmented macules clear by 3 months. Scrapings from the vesicles or pustules show neutrophils without multinucleated giant cells or bacteria. A histopathologic examination of a skin biopsy specimen demonstrates that the neutrophils are in and beneath the horny layer of skin.

Miliaria rubra and miliaria crystallina result from obstruction of the immature eccrine sweat ducts and occur in newborns during the first few weeks of life. *Miliaria crystallina* is an asymptomatic eruption characterized by tiny clear vesicles, especially in intertriginous areas, that rupture easily. The duct obstruction in miliaria crystallina is superficial, and the vesicle forms beneath the horny layer. There is minimal inflammation, and special stains show no organ-

isms. *Miliaria rubra* is a pruritic eruption that is often found on areas of skin covered by clothing and is characterized by erythematous papulovesicles and rarely pustules. The sweat duct obstruction is deeper, and histopathologic examination of a skin biopsy specimen shows inflammation surrounding the epidermal eccrine ducts. Special stains for organisms are negative. Miliaria also occurs in older children at areas with excessive sweating that are occluded by clothing. Miliaria may be prevented by regulation of environmental temperature. In newborns, avoidance of overheating and application of lukewarm compresses facilitate the clearing of lesions and decrease discomfort. Older children benefit from the application of cool compresses, calamine lotion, and preparations of ¼% menthol in lotion.

Eosinophilic folliculitis is a pustular disorder that occasionally occurs in infants and newborns. The scalp is the most commonly affected site, especially near the vertex. Lesions may be pruritic, and smears show many eosinophils. Biopsy of a lesion shows infiltration of tissue by eosinophils, especially at hair follicles. Patients often respond to systemic antibiotics and topical erythromycin. Topical corticosteroid preparations may decrease the associated pruritus.

Acropustulosis of infancy is a rare disorder, most commonly seen in black male infants. The disorder usually begins by 10 months of age but may be manifest at birth. The dorsal and plantar aspects of the hands and feet develop pruritic erythematous papules that evolve rapidly into vesicles and pustules. Smears of vesiculopustular contents show neutrophils and occasionally eosinophils but no organisms by special stains. Histopathologic examination of skin biopsy specimens shows that the pustules are located beneath the horny layer. The lesions tend to remit and recur every few weeks for 2 to 3 years, and the associated pruritus may be severe. Topical corticosteroids are often not effective. Oral antihistamines and dapsone may help, but hematologic tests must be monitored if dapsone is used.

Several infectious processes may develop in the newborn period that are associated with vesicles, bullae, and pustules and must be distinguished from the more benign transient disorders. These are reviewed in detail elsewhere in this text (ee Chap. 196). *Impetigo neonatorum* is staphylococcal bullous impetigo in the neonatal period and is characterized by vesicles, bullae, or pustules on an erythematous base (see also Chaps. 65 and 196). The lesions erode, leaving a moist base with crusting. The intertriginous areas are most commonly affected. Smears of the lesions show polymorphonuclear leukocytes, and cultures grow *Staphylococcus aureus*. Impetigo neonatorum must be treated with systemic antistaphylococcal antibiotics. The vesicles and pustules of *congenital cutaneous candidiasis* must also be considered (see also Chap. 66). The lesions are generalized without accentuation of the diaper and oral areas and are present at birth or appear within a day after birth. The palms and soles are usually involved. The yeast may be found on potassium hydroxide examination of smears from the lesions and in culture. Congenital cutaneous candidiasis should be treated by the application of topical anticandidal creams and oral nystatin for 10 days. *Herpes simplex* infection in the newborn is the most devastating of the vesiculopustular eruptions and must be considered (see also Chaps. 68 and 196). Lesions may be single, but some grouped vesiculopustules should be noted. Tzanck smears of lesional contents show multinucleated epidermal cells and occasionally intracytoplasmic inclusion bodies. Viral cultures are confirmatory. Administration of intravenous acyclovir should be initiated if the diagnosis of herpes simplex is suspected. *Congenital varicella* infections may also manifest as vesiculopustules in the neonatal period and demonstrate multinucleated giant epidermal cells, but cultures yield the varicella-zoster virus (see also Chaps. 196 and 204). Finally, vesiculobullous hemorrhagic lesions, especially on the palms and soles, are rare but diagnostic of *congenital syphilis* in the newborn or young infant (see also Chaps. 196 and 200).

MASTOCYTOSIS

The group of disorders characterized by mast cell infiltration of skin is called *mastocytosis.* In children, *urticaria pigmentosa* is the most common form. Urticaria pigmentosa is characterized by solitary or multiple red-brown macules, papules, and nodules that become urticarial or frankly bullous after the lesions are stroked firmly (Darier's sign). The lesions are usually 1 to 3 cm in diameter and are located most commonly on the trunk. The lesions may resemble bruises, and affected children are occasionally mistakenly considered to be victims of child abuse. The reaction is believed to relate to the release of mast cell contents, especially histamine. A histopathologic examination of skin biopsy specimens shows large numbers of mast cells in the dermis and subcutaneous tissues. The mast cell granules stain well with toluidine blue or Giemsa stains.

Most patients develop the lesions of urticaria pigmentosa by school age, and the lesions usually clear spontaneously by puberty. With advancing age there is less of a tendency for blistering of lesions to occur. Systemic involvement, including flushing, gastrointestinal symptoms, headaches, tachycardia, hypotension, and coagulation abnormalities, is rare in children who develop the disorder before they reach 10 years of age. Ten to 30% of older children have systemic symptoms, although these are usually mild. Ninety-five percent of children with systemic mastocytosis have cutaneous lesions. In the systemic form, mast cells may infiltrate almost any organ, although the bone, gastrointestinal tract, liver, and spleen are most frequently affected. Patients may have bone pain with lytic lesions, gastrointestinal ulcers, hepatosplenomegaly, anemia, and eosinophilia.

Most patients with urticaria pigmentosa are asymptomatic and require no therapy. Patients with pruritus, urticaria, flushing, or more severe symptoms are best managed by antihistamine administration and the avoidance of exacerbating factors. Affected infants and children should avoid hot baths and vigorous exercise. Medications that may stimulate mast cell histamine release include salicylates (except in low doses), codeine, morphine, procaine, polymyxin B, and atropine. Cheeses and alcoholic beverages (including cough syrups with alcohol) may also exacerbate the disorder. H_1-blocking antihistamines and combinations of H_1 and H_2 blockers (e.g., cimetidine) may help in preventing or ameliorating systemic symptoms. Topical corticosteroids have been shown to decrease pruritus and clear lesions in adults with urticaria pigmentosa. Oral disodium cromoglycate, a drug that blocks histamine release, has been used successfully in patients with gastrointestinal reactions. Psoralens and ultraviolet A (PUVA) light therapy decreases the number of mast cells in cutaneous lesions but is not recommended for children. The administration of aspirin in low doses has been suggested, but trials must be attempted with great caution because aspirin also stimulates mast cell release of histamine.

In the newborn and young infant, collections of mast cells usually manifest as *mastocytomas,* nodules that increase in size for months and disappear spontaneously within the first few years of life. The lesions are usually solitary, slightly elevated red-brown nodules that are most frequently located on the trunk or arms. Not uncommonly, the nodules have a pebbly, thickened appearance, and the Darier's sign is positive. Mastocytomas must be distinguished from juvenile xanthogranulomas and, if on the head or neck, from nevus sebaceus. Systemic symptoms are rarely associated. Some cases have been reported to have progressed to generalized urticaria pigmentosa.

ERYTHEMA MULTIFORME AND TOXIC EPIDERMAL NECROLYSIS

Erythema multiforme minor, erythema multiforme major, and toxic epidermal necrolysis are now considered to be related hypersensitivity reactions that are immunologically mediated. *Toxic epidermal necrolysis* is unusual in children, almost always occurs after 10 years of age, and is usually a complication of drug use. The most common etiologic agents in children are sulfonamides, penicillins, barbiturates, phenytoin, and salicylates. Toxic epidermal necrolysis is a rapidly progressive, potentially life-threatening disorder characterized by the development of large flaccid bullae that rupture to reveal denuded tissue. Occasionally, patients initially have the rash and mucosal changes of erythema multiforme, with a rapid evolution into the bullae of toxic epidermal necrolysis. The mucosal surfaces are also usually covered by blisters and crusting. The cleavage of toxic epidermal necrolysis is at the dermoepidermal junction (in contrast to the intraepidermal level of blistering in the *staphylococcal scalded skin syndrome,* which was formerly considered to be a form of toxic epidermal necrolysis). This level of cleavage can be easily suspected clinically in black patients by the loss of pigmented skin, consistent with a loss of the entire melanin-containing epidermis.

Erythema multiforme is more common than toxic epidermal necrolysis, and 20% of cases of erythema multiforme occur in children and adolescents. The lesions of erythema multiforme begin as erythematous macules that enlarge and develop circumferential pallor. The central portion develops epidermal necrosis and turns a dusky purple, leading to the characteristic "target" lesions or "iris" lesions, with concentric zones of color surrounding zones of pallor. Occasionally, central vesicles or bullae develop. The lesions are symmetrically distributed and begin acrally over the extensor surfaces of the extremities and the dorsa of the hands. The palms, soles, and later the flexural areas, trunk, and ears often become involved. The skin lesions evolve during a 3- to 5-day period. Mild involvement of mucous membranes, especially the lips and oral mucosa, may be seen with the minor form of erythema multiforme. The cutaneous lesions heal in 2 to 4 weeks with desquamation, crusting, and transient pigmentary alterations but without scar formation. Symptoms of an upper respiratory tract infection are described in the week preceding the skin eruption in one third of children.

Erythema multiforme major (*Stevens-Johnson syndrome*) is characterized by more severe mucosal lesions and considerable morbidity. Inflammatory lesions develop suddenly after a prodromal period of up to 2 weeks that includes malaise, fever, sore throat, cough, chest pain, headache, vomiting, diarrhea, myalgias, and arthralgias. The mucosal vesicles and crusts are most commonly found on the lips, oral mucosa, and bulbar conjunctivae. The ocular involvement may be severe and may progress from purulent conjunctivitis to corneal ulceration, anterior uveitis, panophthalmitis, synechiae, and blindness. The nasopharynx, esophagus, respiratory mucosa, and genitourinary tract may also be involved, resulting in refusal to eat, trouble with breathing, and urinary retention due to pain on urination. Pneumonitis and renal disease with hematuria and tubular necrosis have also been reported. High fever and weakness are commonly associated.

The skin lesions of erythema multiforme major are variable in appearance and include the typical "target" lesions of erythema multiforme minor, confluent areas of erythema, and the large bullae with desquamation of toxic epidermal necrolysis. A histopathologic examination of skin from lesions of erythema multiforme major or minor shows epidermal necrosis and perivascular infiltrates of mononuclear inflammatory cells in the upper dermis but no vasculitis. The lesions of erythema multiforme major continue to erupt for 10 days to 1 month and heal after 4 to 6 weeks.

Erythema multiforme may be associated with infections or drugs. The drugs that cause erythema multiforme reactions in children include sulfonamides (including thiazides), barbiturates, phenytoin, and penicillins. The two infectious diseases that have clearly been associated with erythema multiforme are *herpes simplex* and *Mycoplasma pneumoniae* infection. The erythema multiforme usually follows the infectious processes by about 10 days. As a drug reaction, erythema multiforme also occurs 10 days after initiation of a drug for the first time, but may appear within hours after beginning a drug that has been previously administered.

The management of erythema multiforme and toxic epidermal necrolysis in children is controversial. The most critical therapy is the removal of an offending drug, if one is discovered. In general, erythema multiforme minor is self-limited and should be treated conservatively with cool compresses and oral antihistamines. Topical corticosteroids are usually not helpful, even for associated pruritus. Children with erythema multiforme major and toxic epidermal necrolysis should be hospitalized because of the extensive associated tissue necrosis and debilitation. Lukewarm compresses or whirlpool baths are helpful and should be followed by the application of antibacterial ointments to promote re-epithelialization and prevent secondary bacterial infection. If secondary infection occurs, antistaphylococcal antibiotics should be administered, but otherwise any unnecessary systemic drugs should be withheld. An ophthalmologist should be consulted to manage ocular involvement. The use of systemic corticosteroids for severe erythema multiforme major and toxic epidermal necrolysis in children is controversial, and no good prospective studies have been described. Since the disorders can lead to extensive fluid and electrolyte imbalances and secondary bacterial infections with a mortality of up to 50%, some dermatologists recommend high-dose corticosteroid therapy, especially if the corticosteroids can be started early in the course and infection as a cause of the erythema multiforme is eliminated or adequately treated. The corticosteroids should be tapered during the following weeks as healing occurs. Most investigators have suggested that corticosteroids have no beneficial effect and only lead to complications, especially infection.

CHRONIC BULLOUS DISEASE OF CHILDHOOD

Immunologically mediated blistering disorders in children are rare, although pemphigus, bullous and cicatricial pemphigoid, dermatitis herpetiformis, and epidermolysis bullosa acquisita have all been described in children. The most common blistering disorder in childhood is *chronic bullous disease of childhood*. This disorder usually occurs before the age of 6 and is characterized by blisters with variable pruritus in the perioral area, lower trunk, upper thighs, and perineum. The blisters are often hemorrhagic and may be large or small and clustered in annular or sausage-shaped patterns. A histopathologic examination of skin sections shows a subepidermal blister with a variable amount of mixed inflammatory cell infiltration. By immunofluorescence microscopy, linear deposits of IgA are seen at the basement membrane zone.

In contrast to other blistering disorders, chronic bullous

disease of childhood is self-limited and clears spontaneously after months to a few years. The preferred management is administration of sulfapyridine or dapsone with or without supplemental prednisone. These drugs should be tapered to a maintenance dose as soon as possible and discontinued when the patient tolerates withdrawal without a recurrence of blisters.

EPIDERMOLYSIS BULLOSA

Epidermolysis bullosa is a group of inherited disorders in which blistering occurs at sites of mechanical trauma. Subgroups are distinguished by the clinical manifestations, the mode of inheritance, and the level of blistering. The pathophysiology of most forms of epidermolysis bullosa is poorly understood. The most common forms are the autosomal dominant *simplex* and *Weber-Cockayne* forms. In both of these disorders the blistering occurs within the epidermis and no scarring results. Blisters in patients with the Weber-Cockayne form are localized to the hands and feet, whereas blisters of the simplex form are usually more generalized. Blisters tend to occur readily after trauma and are increased with hyperhidrosis during the summer. Patients with the simplex form of epidermolysis bullosa may have blisters at birth or in early infancy, whereas patients with the Weber-Cockayne form often do not develop blisters until later childhood or adolescence.

Junctional epidermolysis bullosa is a group of autosomal recessive disorders with cleavage through the lamina lucida region of the dermoepidermal junction. The most common and most severe type is *epidermolysis bullosa letalis*. Newborns almost always have blisters at birth, especially of the extremities, as well as intraoral blisters and a loss of nails. The lesions resolve with atrophy, but without scarring or milia formation. These infants are at a great risk of fluid loss and sepsis. Subsequent blisters may develop spontaneously or after minimal trauma. Not uncommonly, the gastrointestinal, upper respiratory, and genitourinary tracts develop blisters that may resolve with tissue stenosis.

The diagnosis of junctional epidermolysis bullosa may be made by demonstration with electron microscopy or immunofluorescence mapping of blister formation through the lamina lucida zone of the cutaneous basement membrane. Most affected infants die of the complications of extensive blistering. The few reported infants with the letalis form who have survived into later childhood have growth retardation, anemia, and extensive granulation tissue, especially in the perioral area.

The scarring or dystrophic forms of epidermolysis bullosa may be autosomal dominant or autosomal recessive. The *dominant dystrophic types of epidermolysis bullosa* may manifest at birth or in early childhood. Lesions resolve with scar formation and milia. The mucous membranes and nails are rarely affected. The *recessive dystrophic form of epidermolysis bullosa* is severe and mutilating. The blisters are almost always present at birth as large tense, deep blisters that heal slowly, leaving scars and milia. Repeated blistering and scar formation lead to syndactyly (mitten deformity) of the hands and feet by early childhood. Dysphagia due to esophageal involvement is common, and blisters of the pharynx, larynx, and trachea have resulted in hoarseness and upper airway obstruction. Eating may be impaired because of intraoral involvement. Squamous cell carcinomas of the scarred skin or mucosae may develop and are the most common cause of death in patients who survive early childhood.

Patients with forms of epidermolysis bullosa except the mildest of the epidermal forms should be managed by a dermatologist, as well as by other specialists in the care of patients with epidermolysis bullosa, including pedodontists, pediatric and plastic surgeons, and dietitians. Therapy is primarily supportive and includes wound dressings, the prevention of secondary infection, the management of complications, and the assurance of optimal nutrition. Compresses should be applied to open wounds two to four times a day, followed by the application of topical antibiotics, such as bacitracin—polymyxin B, mupirocin, or silver sulfadiazine. Artificial skin barriers, such as Vigilon or Opsite dressings, may be helpful for some patients. Staphylococcal colonization of skin may be diminished by adding chlorhexidine to the bath water. In all patients, trauma must be avoided by using nontraumatic nipples, shoes that fit well, and padding over extensor surfaces and other sites of trauma.

Systemic antibiotics are crucial in patients with secondary infections. Brief courses of topical corticosteroid preparations may decrease inflammation. For patients with the recessive form of dystrophic epidermolysis bullosa, phenytoin, a drug that decreases collagenase production by fibroblasts, may be useful, although multicenter trials of phenytoin for these patients suggest that phenytoin does not decrease blistering for most patients. Surgical repair of the syndactyly should be performed in early childhood and repeated as necessary to restore hand function. Finally, referral of families to the Dystrophic Epidermolysis Bullosa Research Association of America (DEBRA), 2936 Avenue W, Brooklyn, NY 11229, is invaluable.

ANNOTATED BIBLIOGRAPHY

Cooper TW, Bauer EA: Epidermolysis bullosa: A review. Pediatr Dermatol 1:181–188, 1984. (Practical, comprehensive review of the subgroups of epidermolysis bullosa and their management.)

Huff JC, Weston WL, Tonnesen MG: Erythema multiforme: A critical review of characteristics, diagnostic criteria, and causes. J Am Acad Dermatol 8:763–775, 1983. (Good review of erythema multiforme.)

Lucky AW, Esterly NB, Heskel N et al: Eosinophilic pustular folliculitis in infancy. Pediatr Dermatol 1:202–206, 1984. (Discussion of this benign entity in infants.)

Rasmussen JE: Erythema multiforme in children: Response to treatment with systemic corticosteroids. Br J Dermatol 95:181–186,

1976. (Retrospective study of the effect of systemic corticosteroids in the Stevens-Johnson syndrome.)

Schachner L, Press S: Vesicular, bullous and pustular disorders in infancy and childhood. Pediatr Clin North Am 30:609–629, 1983. (Comprehensive review of the various vesicular, bullous, and pustular disorders in children.)

Surbrugg SK, Weston WL: The course of chronic bullous disease of childhood. Pediatr Dermatol 2:213–215, 1985. (Review of chronic bullous disease of childhood.)

65

Bacterial Skin Infections

Amy Paller

The normal skin of infants and children provides an effective barrier against bacterial invasion. When the skin is damaged, pathogenic bacteria can easily invade and proliferate. Spontaneous blistering, as in epidermolysis bullosa, or localized alteration of host defenses due to trauma, as in insect bite reactions and scalp trauma due to traction, are often associated with secondary bacterial infections. The most common organisms are staphylococci and streptococci. Children with underlying inflammatory dermatoses, especially seborrheic dermatitis and atopic dermatitis, are also prone to secondary infections. Maceration and abnormally moist skin permit both gram-positive and gram-negative bacterial infections. Children with alterations in physiologic defenses risk recurrent bacterial infections. Children with alterations in lymphatic drainage, as in chronic familial lymphedema, have chronic infections of the feet and lower legs. Patients with immunologic disorders, especially agammaglobulinemias, chronic granulomatous disease, and deficiencies of the alternate complement pathway or terminal sequence, have severe bacterial infections of viscera and skin. Children who are immunocompromised by a neoplastic disease or immunosuppressive drugs have an increased susceptibility to bacterial infections from both common and unusual organisms. Finally, infants are more subject to bacterial infections because of an immature immunologic system. The higher frequency of the staphylococcal scalded skin syndrome in infants is believed to be due to inadequate renal clearance and metabolism of the staphylococcal toxin.

GRAM-POSITIVE BACTERIAL INFECTIONS

Most bacterial skin infections of infants and children are due to *Staphylococcus aureus* and group A *Streptococcus pyogenes* infections. *Impetigo* is the most common manifestation and accounts for 10% of all skin problems in pediatric clinics. Impetigo may be bullous, caused by phage group II staphylococcus, or vesiculopustular, caused by streptococ-

cus or staphylococcus. The bullae of bullous impetigo are tense and filled with purulent material. They rupture, leaving a moist, erythematous base (Fig. 65-1). The superficial vesiculopustules of impetigo rupture easily to form thick yellow crusts and are found most commonly on the lower extremities during the summer. Either form of impetigo may be associated with fever and lymphadenopathy.

Staphylococcal organisms produce the exotoxin exfoliatin, which is responsible for the bullae of bullous impetigo. Staphylococcal organisms also cause furuncles and carbuncles, invade the hair follicles to produce folliculitis, and disrupt the epidermis in the staphylococcal scalded skin syndrome. In newborns, staphylococcus is also responsible for omphalitis, dacrocystitis, mammary abscesses, and paronychia, probably because these are sites of trauma. Streptococcus is responsible for the generalized rash of scarlet fever and local infections, including erysipelas and ecthyma.

Folliculitis in children usually affects the superficial portion of the hair follicle and is characterized by a tiny pustule and erythema centered in a hair follicle. Folliculitis usually occurs on the face, scalp, extremities, and buttocks. Lesions frequently appear in crops and are nontender but may be pruritic. Most folliculitis is due to *Staphylococcus aureus*, but streptococcus may occasionally be responsible. *Gram-negative folliculitis* caused by klebsiella, proteus, or enterobacter may occur on the periorificial region of the face of teenagers who use broad-spectrum systemic antibiotics for acne. *Hot tub dermatitis* caused by pseudomonas may be follicular and has been reported in children who are exposed to infected hot tubs or pools. Superficial folliculitis may also be noninfectious from the occlusion of follicles by oils (as in hair pomades), tars, and occlusive dressings.

Folliculitis barbae is a deep folliculitis caused by staphylococcal infection of the beard area that occasionally affects adolescent boys. Pruritic follicular papules and pustules with erythema may progress to form crusts and boggy edema (sycosis barbae). Scratching and shaving spread the infection. Warm compresses, topical or systemic antibiotics, and the use of an electric razor or avoidance of shaving are helpful. *Pseudofolliculitis barbae* is an inflammatory process of the hair follicle due to curly hair (especially in black patients) with repenetration of the skin by hair. Pathogenic bacteria are not responsible. Pseudofolliculitis barbae may respond to changing the manner of shaving, use of chemical depilatories, shaving less closely, or keratolytic agents such as topical vitamin A acid (tretinoin [Retin-A]).

Acne keloidalis (folliculitis keloidalis nuchae) is a chronic perifollicular infection that is common in black adolescents and young adults. Collections of pruritic, firm, skin-colored or hyperpigmented papules are found at the nape of the neck. Many patients harbor pathogenic staphylococcus organisms, but it is not clear that there is any relation between the organisms and the folliculitis. Patients respond to systemic antibiotics, as in the treatment of acne, and to intralesional or strong topical corticosteroids to diminish keloid formation.

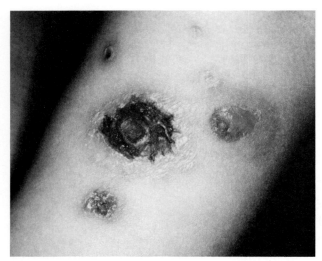

Figure 65-1. The bullae of staphylococcal impetigo rupture leaving a moist, denuded base.

Furuncles are painful, circumscribed, perifollicular, staphylococcal abscesses that extend from folliculitis. They occur most commonly in older children on hairy areas subject to trauma—especially on the thighs, buttocks, perineum, face, scalp, nape of the neck, and axillae. They may reach a diameter of 5 cm, become fluctuant, and eventually rupture to release a purulent, sanguineous discharge. *Carbuncles* are deeper staphylococcal abscesses formed by interconnecting furuncles that drain from many sites at the skin surface. The lesions are larger than furuncles and are often associated with extreme tenderness, fever, chills, and malaise. Patients with chronic granulomatous disease have recurrent staphylococcal abscesses that often require repeated incision and drainage procedures as well as systemic antibiotics. Children with the hyperimmunoglobulin E syndrome (and Job's syndrome) also have recurrent abscesses but are not able to mount a normal inflammatory response so that the abscesses are only mildly tender and inflamed.

Paronychia, or inflammation around the nails, is often due to *Staphylococcus aureus.* Streptococcus or pseudomonas is occasionally causative. Pseudomonal paronychia is characterized by a green discoloration of the nails. Patients who have paronychia and nail dystrophy and whose hands are frequently in contact with water may have candidal paronychia.

The *staphylococcal scalded skin syndrome* is an exfoliative condition most common in infants because of the diminished ability to excrete the responsible toxin produced by phage group II *Staphylococcus aureus.* Three phases occur: erythematous, exfoliative, and desquamative. Many parents report cutaneous tenderness and restlessness before erythroderma is seen. Cutaneous erythema and tenderness initially develop periorificially and spread rapidly to involve the trunk and limbs. One to 2 days later exfoliation devel-

ops, with yellow crusts around the mouth, eyes, umbilicus, perineum, and perianal area. Two to 3 days later, the skin begins to shed spontaneously or with light stroking (Nikolsky's sign). The palms and soles shed last. Affected children are uncomfortable and experience malaise but are often without fever or other complaints.

The diagnosis of staphylococcal scalded skin syndrome is made by the typical clinical course and appearance of affected infants and the superficial blistering at the granular level of the epidermis, in contrast to the dermoepidermal separation of toxic epidermal necrosis. *Staphylococcus* is usually recovered from the nasopharynx and occasionally the conjunctivae and impetiginous areas of skin but rarely from the blood or erythematous areas of skin. Many cases are aborted at the erythematous or exfoliative stage by the prompt institution of systemic antistaphylococcal antibiotics. Although the mortality is low, infants may have considerable loss of fluid and electrolytes. Systemic corticosteroids are contraindicated.

The *toxic shock syndrome* is another disorder with cutaneous manifestations due to a staphylococcal toxin that may be seen by the pediatrician, especially in adolescent girls who use tampons. Patients have fever, hypotension, or postural dizziness, and there is evidence of multiple visceral involvement, especially diarrhea, vomiting, myalgia, and renal failure. The mucocutaneous abnormalities include a diffuse *scarlatiniform* (rough texture with red-brown fine papules) or macular erythematous eruption and subsequent desquamation, edema of the hands and feet, and conjunctival hyperemia. The conditions that are most commonly mistakenly diagnosed are scarlet fever and Kawasaki disease.

Scarlet fever is a diffuse erythematous eruption due to a toxin produced by β-hemolytic streptococci, usually in association with streptococcal pharyngitis. Other features are lymphadenopathy, nausea and vomiting, headache, abdominal discomfort, and occasionally splenomegaly. The disease occurs most commonly in children and begins with fever and pharyngitis. One to 2 days later the rash appears, first on the neck and then on the trunk and extremities. The eruption is characterized by dusky red, blanching tiny papules that have a rough texture. Papules are usually absent from the face, palms, and soles, but the face characteristically shows flushing with circumoral pallor. On the body, the rash is intensified in skin folds and at sites of pressure. In the antecubital and axillary fossae, linear petechiae are seen with accentuation of the erythema (Pastia's lines). The exanthem usually lasts 4 to 5 days and then begins to desquamate, first on the face and last on the palms and soles. *Staphylococcus aureus* and viral infections may also be associated with scarlatiniform rashes.

Ecthyma, a condition that is usually streptococcal in origin, is characterized by superficial vesicles that rapidly become ulcers with necrotic central crusts. The ulcer spreads centrifugally if it is left untreated. The lesions heal slowly and usually leave scars. The lower extremities are usually affected, and associated lymphadenopathy is common. Insect bites and varicella lesions may be precursors of ecthyma.

Cellulitis is an acute inflammation of the dermis and subcutaneous tissues characterized by tenderness, warmth, and erythema with a poorly defined border. Usually *Staphylococcus aureus* or group A hemolytic streptococcus is the causative agent. Periorbital cellulitis is often due to *Staphylococcus aureus* or *Streptococcus pneumoniae.* Buccal (facial) cellulitis in infants has often a violaceous hue and may be due to *Hemophilus influenzae.* Violaceous cellulitis has also been described with pneumococcal infections. Tender regional adenopathy is commonly associated with cellulitis, and patients may have malaise, fever, and chills. Cellulitis with superficial blisters is usually caused by streptococcus. *Blistering distal dactylitis* is an uncommon form of cellulitis in children caused by *Streptococcus pyogenes* with purulent blisters and a rim of erythema localized to the volar fat pad of the distal phalanx of the finger. The differential diagnosis includes blisters from friction and burns, herpetic whitlows, staphylococcal bullous impetigo, and epidermolysis bullosa. *Erysipelas* is a distinctive type of cellulitis caused by streptococcus with a sharply demarcated, elevated advancing edge. Affected sites in young children and infants include the face, abdomen, legs, and intertriginous areas.

Erythrasma is a superficial infection due to the gram-positive bacterium *Corynebacterium minutissimum* characterized by well-circumscribed, dusky-red, scaly patches in axillae, groin, and interdigital spaces. Fifteen percent of cases occur in prepubertal children, and the disorder is more common in adolescents. Erythrasma may coexist with candidal infections. The treatment of choice is erythromycin 50 mg/kg/d ÷ g/d for 10 days. *Trichomycosis axillaris* is a benign infection of the axillary and pubic hairs due to *Corynebacterium tenuis.* Only postpubertal adolescents are affected. Concretions that are usually white or yellow are found on the hair shaft, and patients may complain of hyperhidrosis with an unpleasant odor or red-stained perspiration. Management includes shaving the affected hairs and the use of antibacterial soaps and deodorants.

THERAPY FOR STAPHYLOCOCCAL AND STREPTOCOCCAL INFECTIONS

Most cutaneous infections require treatment with systemic antibiotics. Although topical antibiotic ointments may be used as adjunctive agents, they are only appropriate as single agents for very localized impetigo. Mupirocin, however, has been shown to be as effective as oral antibiotics for the treatment of impetigo. Usually oral antibiotics suffice for impetigo, folliculitis, and paronychia (except in young infants), but parenteral antistaphylococcal antibiotics must be administered in newborns with any bacterial infection and for more serious infections, such as buccal and periorbital cellulitis, staphylococcal scalded skin syndrome, and toxic shock syndrome. Furuncles and carbuncles often respond to incision and drainage procedures in addition to

systemic antibiotics. In the acute phase of impetigo, saline or Burow's solution compresses help to decrease oozing and debride the crusts. Emollient lotions are useful during the desquamation phase of infections, such as the staphylococcal scalded skin syndrome and scarlet fever.

GRAM-NEGATIVE BACTERIAL INFECTIONS

The major gram-negative bacteria that cause infections with cutaneous manifestations are *Neisseria meningitidis, Neisseria gonorrhoeae,* and the gram-negative rods that cause gram-negative folliculitis and hot tub dermatitis. *Gram-negative folliculitis* is an infection with gram-negative rods, especially enterobacter, klebsiella, escherichia, serratia, and proteus, that usually occurs as a complication of acne vulgaris. Affected persons have taken oral antibiotics for prolonged periods. Most patients have superficial pustules without comedones on the cheeks, chin, and philtrum. Deep nodulocystic lesions are occasionally seen. Patients respond within weeks to ampicillin or trimethoprim-sulfamethoxazole treatment, which eliminates the causative bacteria. Isotretinoin (Accutane) has also been effective.

Hot tub dermatitis is a rash due to *Pseudomonas* that appears within 2 days after exposure to infected hot tubs, whirlpool baths, and swimming pools. The eruption may be follicular, maculopapular, vesicular, pustular, or polymorphous and is distributed primarily on the lateral aspects of the trunk, the proximal extremities, and the buttocks and in the axillae. Patients often have malaise, pruritus, discomfort of the eyes and throat, axillary adenopathy, and occasionally fever, external otitis, mastitis, nausea, vomiting, and abdominal cramps. The disorder is self-limited and lasts 7 to 10 days. Other cutaneous lesions caused by pseudomonas include otitis externa, toe web infections, cellulitis of the foot, and ecthyma gangrenosum. *Ecthyma gangrenosum* causes ulceration with a necrotic black eschar and surrounding erythema. The lesion is frequently located in the anogenital or axillary region and may be associated with pseudomonal septicemia. Debridement and systemic antibiotics are required.

Skin lesions develop in approximately two thirds of patients with meningococcemia or meningococcal meningitis. The cutaneous lesions may be macular and erythematous, morbilliform, urticarial, purpuric, or petechial. The petechiae are pinpoint lesions that may have a raised vesicular or pustular center. Lesions are most common on the trunk and extremities but may also occur on the palms, soles, and mucosae. More fulminant meningococcal infections are often associated with extensive purpuric lesions and with large, well-circumscribed ecchymotic patches covering large areas of the body. Necrotic bullae may develop within the ecchymotic patches with resultant sloughing. Other features of acute meningococcemia include fever, irritability, myalgia, arthralgia, and hypotension. The cutaneous and visceral lesions are due to vasculitis of capillaries and venules.

Cutaneous lesions occur in more than 90% of patients with chronic meningococcemia, although this disorder is uncommon in children. Crops of erythematous macules and papules often appear with fever and develop purpuric, ulcerated centers. Myalgia and arthralgia are commonly present. The differential diagnosis of the cutaneous lesions includes Henoch-Schönlein purpura, Rocky Mountain spotted fever, gonococcemia, purpura fulminans, erythema multiforme, and typhoid fever. Intravenous penicillin (alternatively, chloramphenicol) is the preferred antibiotic, and patients with shock must be supported with fluids to increase circulating blood volume and vasopressor agents.

The skin lesions of gonococcemia resemble those of meningococcemia. They are small erythematous, hemorrhagic papules or vesiculopustules or petechiae found primarily overlying the joints of the distal extremities. Lesions are also associated with fever, arthralgia, and myalgia and resolve spontaneously within a week. *N. gonorrhoeae* may be found by a smear or culture of early cutaneous lesions. The preferred treatment is parenteral penicillin (alternatively, ceftriaxone or tetracycline).

ANNOTATED BIBLIOGRAPHY

Bach MC: Dermatologic signs in toxic shock syndrome—clues to diagnosis. J Am Acad Dermatol 8:343–347, 1983. (Review of the skin changes in the toxic shock syndrome.)

Blankenship ML: Gram-negative folliculitis: Follow-up observations in 20 patients. Arch Dermatol 120:1301–1303, 1984. (Discussion of the complication of gram-negative folliculitis in patients with acne.)

Chandrasekarm PH, Rolston KVI, Kannangara DW et al: Hot-tub associated dermatitis due to *Pseudomonas aeruginosa:* Case report and review of the literature. Arch Dermatol 120:1337–1340, 1984. (Review of the skin and systemic changes of hot tub dermatitis.)

McCray MK, Esterly NB: Blistering distal dactylitis. J Am Acad Dermatol 5:592–594, 1981. (Discussion of this streptococcal infection of children.)

Tunnessen WW: Practical aspects of bacterial skin infections in children. Pediatr Dermatol 2:255–265, 1985. (Review of cutaneous bacterial infections and their management.)

66

Superficial Dermatophyte and Yeast Infections

Amy Paller

Superficial fungal and yeast infections are limited to the epidermis, hair, nails, and mucous membranes. The three common causes of these infections are dermatophytes (especially *Trichophyton tonsurans*), *Pityrosporum orbiculare* (tinea versicolor), and *Candida albicans.*

DERMATOPHYTOSES

The dermatophytoses can be subdivided, based on the location of the fungal infection, into *tinea capitis* (scalp), *tinea corporis* (face and body), *tinea cruris* (groin), *tinea pedis* (feet), and *tinea unguium* (nails). Of these, tinea capitis and corporis are commonly seen in prepubertal children. Tinea cruris, tinea pedis, and tinea unguium almost always occur beyond the onset of puberty or in immunocompromised children.

Tinea Capitis

Tinea capitis is the most common dermatophytosis of childhood and usually affects prepubertal children from 2 to 10 years of age. Fewer than 5% of cases of tinea capitis occur in adults. More than 90% of cases are due to *Trichophyton tonsurans,* passed from human to human (anthropophilic), whereas the remaining less than 10% are mostly due to the zoophilic *Microsporum canis. T. tonsurans* affects black children much more commonly than white children.

Pathophysiology. Fungal hyphae are transmitted from fallen hairs, scale, and shared fomites, such as combs, towels, and hats. The hyphae spread and penetrate the hair follicles from the site of initial infection. *T. tonsurans* spores are formed within the hair shaft (endothrix infection), whereas *M. canis* spores form on the surface of the hair shaft (ectothrix infection). Endothrix infections cause significant weakening of the hair shaft with fracture of the hair near the scalp, resulting in the "black dots" on the scalp. The hair bulb is usually preserved.

Clinical Presentation. The manifestations of tinea capitis due to *T. tonsurans* differ considerably from those of *M. canis* infections. Children with *M. canis* infections have well-demarcated areas of alopecia that fluoresce on Wood's lamp examination. *T. tonsurans* is more variable and often subtle in its appearance. It does not fluoresce. Approximately 20% of children with noninflammatory tinea capitis have the seborrheic type of *T. tonsurans* tinea capitis with fine white scaling and associated pruritus. Alopecia may only occur after years of scaling and infection and is then slowly progressive (Fig. 66-1). The scaling may be localized or generalized and is commonly mistaken for seborrheic dermatitis or atopic dermatitis. The black dots that are characteristic of *T. tonsurans* tinea capitis are seen in 40% of patients and are the best material for diagnosis. The black dots may be hidden under scale or may be almost imperceptible so that alopecia areata is mistakenly diagnosed. *Kerions* are boggy, erythematous, tender nodules with perifollicular pustules that develop on the scalp in 5% to 30% of patients as a hypersensitivity reaction to the fungus. They may be associated with lymphadenopathy, a generalized papular rash ("id" reaction), fever, and leukocytosis. They are often incorrectly thought to be bacterial cellulitis or folliculitis and are treated with antibacterial antibiotics. Cultures may grow *Staphylococcus aureus,* but only antifungal

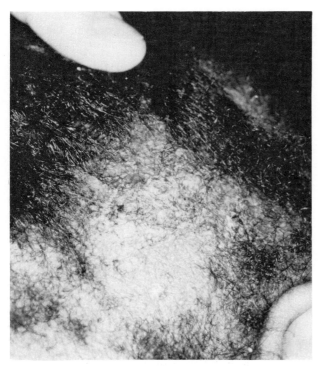

Figure 66-1. Alopecia and scaling of tinea capitis due to *Trichophyton tonsurans*.

agents eliminate the kerions. Many patients with tinea capitis have concurrent tinea corporis.

Differential Diagnosis. The scaling and pruritus of *T. tonsurans* infections may be confused with seborrheic dermatitis, atopic dermatitis, or even with psoriasis. In alopecia areata, the scalp is usually totally normal with a well-demarcated area of alopecia and no scaling, inflammation, or black dots. The black dots may be mistaken for the broken hair shafts of trichotillomania, but perifollicular hemorrhage is not present in tinea capitis. The kerions must be distinguished from bacterial folliculitis and cellulitis, and the appearance of a healing kerion may resemble morphea or the alopecia of discoid lupus erythematosus.

Work-Up. Wood's lamp has been used for years for making a diagnosis of tinea capitis, based on the fluorescence of hairs infected with *Microsporum*. With the marked preponderance of infections due to the nonfluorescent *T. tonsurans,* Wood's lamp examination is of minimal value. The diagnosis depends on the results of a potassium hydroxide (KOH) examination of infected hairs and fungal cultures. The most reliable source of infected hairs is the black dot, which may be found with a magnifying glass and extracted by forceps or gentle scraping with a scalpel or sterile toothbrush. Other hairs that are long enough to be pulled are rarely infected but may have spores and hyphae at the base. KOH preparations are made by placing the specimens on a glass slide, adding a drop or two of 10% to 20% KOH,

heating gently, and examining them under the microscope. The KOH dissolves the cellular material and enables hyphae and spores to be seen. The hyphae and spores are aligned within the hair shaft in parallel orientation in *T. tonsurans* endothrix infections. The fungi surround the hair shafts in *M. canis* infections.

Despite the result of KOH examination, a fungal culture should be performed. Specimens should be inoculated onto Sabouraud's agar with cycloheximide and chloramphenicol (Mycosel). Fungal growth is usually seen within 2 weeks. Dermatophyte test medium (DTM) contains a phenol red indicator that changes from yellow to red and allows a rapid diagnosis but has a high rate of false-positive reactions from saprophytic fungi or bacteria.

When a diagnosis of tinea capitis is made, the entire body should be examined for evidence of tinea corporis. In addition, all family members should be examined for tinea, because untreated family members provide a continuing source of reinfection following adequate therapy.

Treatment. Tinea capitis infections must be treated with systemic griseofulvin. Ketoconazole appears to be equally effective but may cause liver abnormalities. Topical antifungal agents are not curative and have no additive value. The microsize form of griseofulvin is available in a suspension of 125 mg/5 mL. The medication should be administered with fatty meals or milk at a single or twice-daily dose of 15 mg/kg/d for 6 to 8 weeks. Patients should be followed at 3- to 4-week intervals to evaluate progress.

Children with tinea capitis may transmit the disorder until all spores are cleared. Spores may be cultured for 8 weeks after the initiation of griseofulvin alone. The use of sporicidal shampoos decreases the time that the child must be kept home from school or wear protective head covering. Sporicidal shampoos with selenium sulfide 2.5% (Selsun) clear spores after approximately 2 weeks. These shampoos should be left in contact with the scalp for 5 to 10 minutes after lathering and used two to three times weekly. Oiling of the hair after shampooing prolongs the carriage of infectious spores.

The use of systemic or intralesional corticosteroids for children with kerions is controversial. Most dermatologists find that the incidence of scarring is negligible and hair regrowth is excellent after kerion resolution with griseofulvin alone. Secondary infection should be treated with oral antistaphylococcal antibiotics in four divided doses and Burow's compresses to the site to decrease oozing and crust formation.

Tinea Corporis

Tinea corporis is a superficial tinea infection of non-hair-bearing areas that is now usually caused by *T. tonsurans*, often in association with tinea capitis. Tinea corporis is characterized by one or more well-circumscribed scaly patches with a papular, vesicular, or pustular border ("ringworm") and central clearing. Lesions must be differentiated from the papulosquamous plaques of pityriasis rosea, nummular eczema, psoriasis, seborrheic dermatitis, contact dermatitis, tinea versicolor, and granuloma annulare. Any lesion suspected of being fungal should be scraped at the border and examined with KOH and culture. Limited tinea corporis is treated effectively with topical antifungal agents, such as clotrimazole, miconazole, and econazole, for 3 to 4 weeks or until 2 weeks after the clinical manifestations have cleared. For more extensive lesions, a course of griseofulvin should be administered.

Tinea Cruris

Tinea cruris (jock itch) is common in adolescent boys and affects the groin, intertriginous folds, and upper thighs. It is often pruritic, especially during hot, humid weather or physical exercise or when wearing tight clothing. *Epidermophyton floccosum* and occasionally *Trichophyton rubrum* or *T. mentagrophytes* are the responsible dermatophytes. Tinea pedis is commonly associated. The rash of tinea cruris is usually bilaterally symmetric, well circumscribed, erythematous, and scaly with a raised border. Tinea cruris must be differentiated from seborrheic dermatitis, intertrigo, irritant or allergic contact dermatitis, psoriasis, and erythrasma. The diagnosis is confirmed by KOH examination and culture of scales from the periphery. The fungal infection responds rapidly to topical antifungal agents, applied two to three times daily for 4 weeks. Adjunctive measures include the use of absorbent powders and wearing of loose-fitting clothing.

Tinea Pedis

Tinea pedis or athlete's foot is the most common tinea infection of adolescents and adults but is rarely found in prepubertal children. *T. rubrum* and occasionally *E. floccosum* and *T. mentagrophytes* are the usual causative dermatophytes. Tinea pedis may manifest as a chronic scaling disorder with or without an increased horny layer, intertriginous inflammation, or vesiculopustules. The interdigital area is almost always involved with peeling and maceration of surrounding skin. The dorsum of the foot usually remains clear in contrast to the eruptions of contact and atopic dermatitis. Occasionally, erythema, scaling, and vesicles occur as an "id" reaction on the palms and sides of the fingers and less commonly on the trunk and extremities. Atopic dermatitis, dyshidrotic eczema, juvenile plantar dermatosis, and contact dermatitis must be distinguished by KOH examination and fungal culture. Tinea pedis may be treated with topical antimycotic agents. The warm, moist environment of the feet, however, predisposes patients to recurrent infections. Absorbent powders, such as Zeasorb or powders with undecylenic acid (Desenex) or tolnaftate (Tinactin), are helpful in decreasing moisture. Acute vesicular lesions should be dried and cooled with compresses (e.g., Burow's solution) three times daily for 3 to 5 days. Severe tinea pedis infections may require systemic griseofulvin. "Id" reactions are best treated with compresses and topical corticosteroids.

Tinea Unguium

Tinea unguium is a chronic infection of the nails caused by *T. rubrum, T. mentagrophytes,* or *E. floccosum.* Tinea unguium is rarely seen in prepubertal children unless they are immunocompromised. The infection usually begins distally as a white or yellow patch of the nail. The nail becomes thickened and with subungual debris and is friable. The most commonly confused entity is onychomycosis due to *Candida albicans,* which is usually associated with paronychia. Fungal infections in children must also be distinguished from nail dystrophy associated with atopic dermatitis, psoriasis, trauma, lichen planus, twenty nail dystrophy of childhood, and ectodermal dysplasias, such as pachyonychia congenita and the nail-patella syndrome. Scrapings for KOH and culture should be taken from underside of the nail. Tinea unguium is difficult to eradicate and has a high recurrence rate. Topical agents are rarely curative but help to control spread of the infection. Griseofulvin must be administered for 6 to 9 months for infections of the fingernails and 12 to 18 months for toenail infections. Patients taking griseofulvin for longer than 2 to 3 months should be monitored every 3 months for the rare development of hematologic and hepatic abnormalities.

Tinea Versicolor

Tinea versicolor (pityriasis versicolor) is a common infection caused by *Pityrosporon orbiculare,* a lipophilic yeast that is a normal inhabitant of the epidermis. The infection is most prevalent in adolescents but may also occur in prepubertal children. Lesions appear during warm, humid weather because of overgrowth of the yeast and are characterized by multiple, coalescent, round, scaly erythematous macules (Fig. 66-2). The macules usually occur on the anterior and posterior trunk and on the proximal arms. The lesions become more pronounced because of pigmentary changes that result from postinflammatory hyperpigmentation or hypopigmentation due to the production by yeast of azelaic acid, an inhibitor of tyrosinase, an important enzyme for melanin synthesis. The eruption is occasionally pruritic but is otherwise benign.

The differential diagnosis of tinea versicolor includes postinflammatory hypopigmentation or hyperpigmentation, pityriasis alba, vitiligo, pityriasis rosea, and secondary syphilis. The diagnosis of tinea versicolor can usually be made clinically because of the characteristic appearance of the eruption. A KOH examination should be performed to confirm the diagnosis. Fungal hyphae and spores overlie epidermal cells in a typical, tightly clustered "spaghetti and

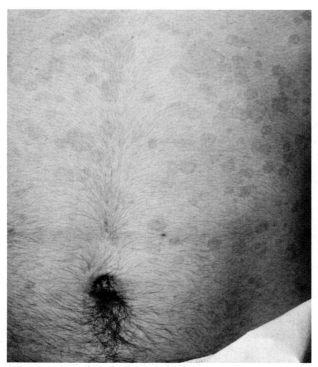

Figure 66-2. Round, scaling erythematous macules of tinea versicolor.

meatballs'' pattern. Fungal cultures should not be performed because the yeast is difficult to grow. Lesions fluoresce by Wood's lamp examination.

Tinea versicolor responds well to many topical agents. Selenium sulfide lotion 2.5% (Selsun lotion) is the most commonly used preparation. A thin layer may be applied to all affected areas, left on for 30 minutes and washed. The lotion should be applied daily for 1 week, weekly for the next month, and then monthly for 3 months. Since the infection is due to overgrowth of normal inhabitants of the skin, the lotion should also be applied once monthly during warm months (April through October in northern climates). Alternate therapies include twice daily application for 4 weeks of 25% sodium thiosulfate with 1% salicylic acid (Tinver lotion) or topical antifungal agents, such miconazole, econazole, and clotrimazole, and the monthly administration of a single oral dose of 400 mg of ketoconazole for adolescents.

CANDIDAL INFECTIONS

Candidiasis (moniliasis) is an infection of the skin, mucous membranes, and occasionally the viscera caused by *Candida albicans*. Although not normally found on the skin, candidal organisms may be normal inhabitants of the mucosal surfaces. Candidal infections are more common in newborns; children with endocrinologic disorders (especially diabetes mellitus), trisomy 21, immunologic deficiencies, acrodermatitis enteropathica, leukemia, or lymphoma; and children who are administered corticosteroids or other immunosuppressive agents and long-term systemic antibiotics. Candidal mucocutaneous infections may manifest in various forms.

Oral candidiasis or thrush is especially common in infancy and is noted at the end of the first week of life in 5% of infants, presumably acquired from an infected maternal vaginal area. The lesions are white, curdlike adherent plaques that overlie inflammation of the tongue, buccal and gingival mucosae, and hard and soft palates. They may be confused with a milk coating, but unlike milk the lesions are more adherent, when rubbed away often produce punctate bleeding, and are frequently surrounded by erythema. KOH preparations demonstrate egg-shaped budding yeast and hyphae or pseudohyphae (nonseptate). Nystatin oral suspension, 200,000 units, used four times daily for 1 to 2 weeks is effective therapy. One milliliter should be swabbed on each side of the mouth with each dose. In rare instances of treatment failure, 1% gentian violet solution may be applied directly onto the lesions once a day for up to 3 days. Because gentian violet may cause ulcerations, it should be used with caution.

Cutaneous candidiasis usually affects warm, moist intertriginous areas. In the newborn, cutaneous candidiasis usually takes the form of diaper dermatitis, especially after the first week of life, with fiery erythema, scaling, and satellite papulovesicles in the diaper area (see Chap. 61). Occasionally, a congenital form occurs in which the lesions appear within a few days of birth, presumably from intrauterine exposure to candidal organisms. The lesions of congenital candidiasis are scattered diffusely over the trunk, extremities, scalp, palms, and soles without aggregation in the diaper area. The oral mucosa is usually not involved. The lesions begin as erythematous macules that become papular, then pustular. Constitutional symptoms or signs of visceral involvement are rare, and the papulopustules tend to clear spontaneously with residual desquamation after approximately 1 week.

Erythema toxicum, staphylococcal pustulosis, transient neonatal pustulosis, neonatal herpes simplex, congenital syphilis, and Letterer-Siwe disease are included in the differential diagnosis and may be distinguished by smears and cultures of pustules and scales, as well as by lack of other clinical features. Although the eruption clears spontaneously, oral nystatin and topical anticandidal agents (nystatin, miconazole, clotrimazole) should be applied to decrease the number of cutaneous and gastrointestinal organisms.

Candidal vulvovaginitis is not an uncommon infection of adolescent girls who take contraceptives or systemic antibiotics or have diabetes mellitus. The labia are pruritic and brightly erythematous with white patches on the mucosae. There is often a thick white vaginal discharge. The infection may spread to the perineal and perianal areas and upper thighs. Miconazole cream inserted into the vagina nightly or vaginal tablets inserted twice daily are effective therapies.

Perleche or angular cheilitis is an irritant dermatitis of the corners of the mouth due to saliva. The dermatitis most commonly affects teenagers with braces and is best treated with petroleum jelly and hydrocortisone ointment. Secondary infection by *Candida* occasionally occurs and should be assessed by KOH examination and culture.

Candidal paronychia develops most commonly in patients who immerse their hands frequently in warm water. It may also occur in newborns and infants in association with thrush and thumb sucking. The paronychial area is red and swollen but is often painless. The nail is thickened and discolored. Secondary bacterial infection due to *Staphylococcus aureus* or pseudomonas may occur. *Erosio interdigitalis blastomycetica* is also encouraged by moisture and is frequently associated with candidal paronychia. The eruption affects the interdigital space and is pruritic, erythematous, macerated, and fissured. Treatment includes the avoidance of moisture and the application of topical antibiotics and anticandidal preparations.

Chronic mucocutaneous candidiasis is a rare disorder due to a dysfunction of the immunologic response to candidal organisms. The disorder is often seen in children with AIDS and is occasionally associated with other immunologic deficiencies or with endocrinopathies, especially hypoparathyroidism and Addison's disease. Widespread candidal infections of the skin, mucous membranes, and nails begin in infancy or childhood. In addition to oral thrush and vaginitis, cutaneous lesions develop that are red and markedly scaly with serpiginous borders, especially on the extremities. The nail folds are chronically red and swollen with dystrophy of the nails. Associated visceral candidiasis is uncommon. In the past, anticandidal agents were either ineffective or dangerous. Ketoconazole clears the infections effectively and rarely causes side effects. Oral clotrimazole may also be efficacious.

INDICATIONS FOR REFERRAL

KOH examinations and cultures should be performed on all patients with suspected fungal and yeast infections. Unless a pediatrician feels competent in performing these examinations, both diagnosis and treatment should be managed by a dermatologist.

ANNOTATED BIBLIOGRAPHY

Chapel TA, Gagliardi C, Nichols W: Congenital cutaneous candidiasis. J Am Acad Dermatol 6:926–928, 1982. (Report of a case of congenital candidiasis and review of the clinical features.)

DeVillez RL, Lewis CW: Candidiasis seminar. Cutis 19:69–83, 1977. (Review of the various clinical manifestations of candidal infections.)

Krowchuk DP, Lucky AW, Primmer SI et al: Current status of the identification and management of tinea capitis. Pediatrics 72:625–631, 1983. (Well-written review of the evaluation and management of tinea capitis.)

Solomon LM, Rippon JW, Lucky AW et al: Tinea capitis: Current concepts. Pediatr Dermatol 2:224–237, 1985. (Discussion by several dermatologists of how each treats tinea capitis.)

Wyre HW, Johnson WT: Neonatal pityriasis versicolor. Arch Dermatol 117:752–753, 1981. (Case of tinea versicolor in a 2-week-old infant.)

67
Warts and Molluscum Contagiosum
Amy Paller

Warts and molluscum contagiosum are among the most common skin lesions in children. Both are caused by DNA viruses that remain restricted to the epidermis and are transmitted by skin to skin contact. Both may be autoinoculated from one area of skin to another.

WARTS

Warts affect up to 10% of school-aged children, with a peak incidence during adolescence. The virus that causes warts is a papillomavirus and has an incubation period of 1 to 6 months. The wart viruses have now been classified into almost 50 subgroups based on DNA homology, each one associated with a particular clinical type of wart.

Clinical Types

There are four common clinical types of warts: verruca vulgaris, verruca plantaris, verruca plana, and condyloma acuminatum. Verrucae vulgaris, or common warts, are found usually on the hands of children and adolescents, although they may be found anywhere on the body, especially at sites of local trauma and autoinoculation. *Verrucae vulgaris* are most commonly round with finger-like projections initially (papillomatous) and become markedly rough and hyperkeratotic (verrucous) with time. Within the warts are multiple, tiny black dots that represent thrombosed capillaries. *Filiform verrucae vulgaris* are long, thin, filamentous warts that are found usually on the face, neck, nasolabial region, and eyelids. *Periungual* and *subungual verrucae vulgaris* occur around and under the nails, especially on the hands. Because of the location of periungual and subungual warts at sites of trauma, these warts grow easily and become irritated. They may become secondarily infected and are difficult to eradicate.

Verrucae plantaris or *plantar warts* occur on the weight-bearing areas of the heels, soles, and metatarsal heads. Because of the location of weight-bearing areas, they extend deeply into the epidermis and develop a smooth horny surface, rather than becoming raised and verrucous. They may become extremely uncomfortable as they enlarge. Plantar warts may be single, but more commonly are mother–daughter warts (primary central warts with satellite warts) or mosaic warts (thick plaques of coalescent small warts, usually found on the heels and soles). Plantar warts must be differentiated from calluses, corns, and scars. Calluses and corns are localized areas of hyperkeratosis that form at points of pressure, especially at the metatarsophalangeal joints. The distinction may be made by paring the lesions. Calluses and corns have a central hard core but no thrombosed capillaries, which appear as tiny black dots. In addition, calluses and corns tend to be most tender to direct pressure, in contrast to maximal tenderness with lateral pressure to warts. Scars result from thickening of the dermis and are thus not hyperkeratotic and easily pared. They have neither a central core nor thrombosed capillaries. *Talon noir* or *black heel* must also be distinguished from plantar warts. This condition is most common in teenaged athletic boys and is caused by capillary rupture. Clusters of brown or black pinpoint hemorrhages are found on the heel or lateral aspects of the feet. The hemorrhages are localized to the horny layer, and when the skin is pared the hemorrhages disappear.

Verrucae plana or *flat warts* are flat, smooth, slightly elevated warts that range in size from 2 to 5 mm (Fig. 67-1). They are most commonly found on the face, arms, and

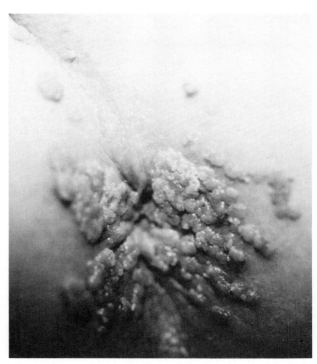

Figure 67-2. Perianal condyloma acuminatum in a 2-year-old boy who was sexually abused.

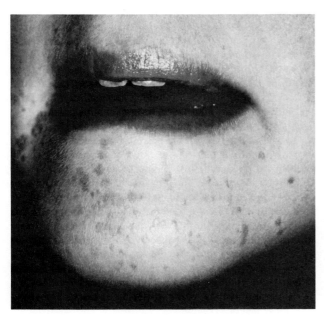

Figure 67-1. Flat warts on the chin of a teenager.

legs. Flat warts are usually multiple, and hundreds may be present. Flat warts often coalesce to form small plaques or spread in a linear array by autoinoculation.

Condylomata acuminata, or genital warts, are moist, cauliflower-like warts that are found on the mucous membranes and mucocutaneous junctions of the anogenital and inguinal areas (Fig. 67-2). Less commonly, these warts are seen in the mouth, at the urethral meatus, and on the conjunctivae. Genital warts become white and macerated rather than scaly because of their location in moist occluded areas. In patients younger than 20 years of age, condylomata acuminata are usually found on sexually active adolescents but they may also be noted on younger children. Although infants may develop the warts after an incubation period of 1 to 20 months from contact with maternal genital warts during delivery, any child with condylomata acuminata must be suspected for child abuse and medical and social investigations for abuse must be performed. *Laryngeal papillomatosis* in infants is contracted during passage of the infant through a maternal genital area that is infected with papillomavirus. The laryngeal papillomas occur on the vocal cords and laryngeal mucosa and may extend into the trachea and bronchi, leading to hoarseness and airway obstruction. Condylomata acuminata must be distinguished from condylomata lata of secondary syphilis. Condylomata lata are more broad-based, flattened, and smooth than condylomata acuminata.

Treatment

Warts in children have a high rate of spontaneous involution. Twenty-five percent of warts disappear within 6 months, and 65% of warts clear without therapy by 2 years. Warts that are painful, subject to trauma, enlarging, or cosmetically objectionable should be treated.

No single therapy is effective for warts. Regardless of the form of management selected, warts have up to a 10% recurrence risk. Plantar, periungual, and subungual warts are the most recalcitrant to therapy. Treatment must be adjusted to the maturity and tolerance of the child. Therapies such as liquid nitrogen and electrodesiccation are painful, whereas treatment modalities such as cantharidin, salicylic acid, and podophyllin are painless on application.

The most commonly used agents for treating warts are *keratolytic preparations* with salicylic and lactic acids. These preparations (such as Duofilm, which is a combination of 16.7% salicylic acid and 16.7% lactic acid in flexible collodion) are best applied nightly, or twice daily for thick warts, after soaking the affected area to increase permeability. High concentrations of salicylic and lactic acids are most useful for verrucae vulgaris and plantar warts and are often used alone or in conjunction with cryotherapy. Preparations with lower concentrations of acids (5%) are useful for flat warts. The acids should be applied with a toothpick or wooden applicator directly to the wart with avoidance of surrounding normal skin. If irritation develops, the medication should be stopped for a few days and subsequently applied less frequently. Results are usually noticeable within 3 to 4 weeks. *Forty percent salicylic acid plasters* and plasters that deliver salicylic acid transdermally are useful for plantar warts. The plasters should be cut to the size of the wart and left on as instructed. Between applications of the plaster, the foot should be soaked in water and pared or rubbed with a pumice stone to remove the excessive horny layer. *Tretinoin (Retin-A)* may be effective for flat warts, probably because it is irritating and causes peeling. The cream or gel may be applied twice daily in increasing concentrations until mild irritation develops.

All other therapy must be applied at the physician's office, preferably by a dermatologist. *Cryotherapy with liquid nitrogen* (−197°C) is highly effective for all forms of warts, although it is painful. Liquid nitrogen is applied to the lesion until the wart and the area surrounding the wart are white. The freezing induces intraepidermal blistering within a week, which removes the wart but leaves the junctional zone of skin intact. Pigmentary changes may result, especially in dark-skinned children, but scarring does not occur.

Cantharidin is a potent blistering agent that is extracted from beetles and is available as a 0.7% solution in acetone and flexible collodion (Cantharone). Cantharidin in solution with acids and podophyllum resin is particularly effective for plantar warts and periungual warts but may induce a ring of satellite warts at the periphery of the primary lesion.

Cantharidin is applied with a toothpick or wooden applicator and is allowed to dry. An intraepidermal blister is formed that eliminates the wart and causes no scarring.

Bleomycin injected directly into warts is a highly effective therapy but should be used only for warts that are resistant to more conventional means of treatment. The lesions become necrotic and clear within a few weeks. Scarring rarely occurs. Bleomycin is especially useful for plantar and periungual warts.

Podophyllum resin is a antimitotic cytotoxin that is useful for condylomata acuminata on mucosal surfaces. A 20% solution in tincture of benzoin is applied to lesions and washed after 4 to 6 hours. Podophyllum is toxic to the kidneys and nervous system and should not be used in large amounts, especially in children. Podophyllum is contraindicated in pregnant women. The therapy may be repeated weekly to monthly, but alternate methods of treatment, such as cryotherapy, electrodesiccation and curettage, or the application of trichloroacetic acid, should be used for condylomas if the lesions do not respond readily. In addition, recurrent or recalcitrant condylomata acuminata should prompt investigation for condylomas of the rectal mucosae by proctoscopy.

The excision of warts is not recommended, but other methods of removing wart tissue, including *electrodesiccation* and *curettage* and *laser,* are highly effective. Electrodesiccation and curettage are especially useful for large single warts and require preceding injection with lidocaine (Xylocaine). Laser therapy has been highly effective for plantar warts and recalcitrant condylomata acuminata.

MOLLUSCUM CONTAGIOSUM

The lesions of molluscum contagiosum are caused by a poxvirus that replicates in the cytoplasm of epidermal cells. The lesions are seen most commonly in children between the ages of 3 and 16, although it has been reported as early as the first week of life. The incubation period is 2 weeks to 6 months. The virus may be contracted in swimming pools as well as by direct skin-to-skin transmission.

Clinical Presentation

Molluscum contagiosum is characterized by discrete, smooth, pearly, or flesh-colored papules on a mildly erythematous base (Fig. 67-3). The center is often umbilicated, especially in larger lesions, and contains a milky white material with virus and epidermal cells. The papules are usually found on the trunk, in axillary, antecubital, and crural areas, and on the face. The lesions begin as tiny papules and enlarge up to 3 cm in diameter. Papules may be seen in a linear array due to autoinoculation. Hundreds of papules may be found on patients with atopic dermatitis and in immunologically compromised children. Molluscum contagiosum is found occasionally on mucosal surfaces, including the oral mucosae and conjunctivae.

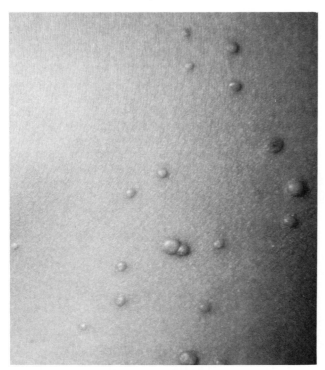

Figure 67-3. Dome-shaped papules of molluscum contagiosum, some with central umbilication.

Patients may complain of pruritus, and excoriations may be seen, especially in children with atopic dermatitis. Dermatitis often surrounds the lesions. The disorder may occur near the eyelids and on the conjunctival mucosa, leading to conjunctivitis and superficial keratitis. In addition, lesions may become secondarily infected with staphylococcal or streptococcal organisms.

The differential diagnosis of molluscum contagiosum includes chickenpox, intradermal nevi, juvenile xanthogranuloma, warts, and milia. Secondarily infected lesions may be confused with primary pyoderma. Characteristic eosinophilic intracytoplasmic inclusion bodies (molluscum bodies) are found on histopathologic specimens of lesions or smears of the central white material.

Treatment

The treatment of molluscum contagiosum depends on the age of the patient and the size and distribution of lesions. Although the lesions are self-limited and last from 2 weeks to more than 1 year, they spread readily, are a source of secondary bacterial infection, and are cosmetically objectionable. As a result, removal should be considered.

Most therapeutic regimens for molluscum contagiosum require destruction of the lesions. Cantharidin is useful for younger children because its application does not cause pain. In contrast to the response of keratotic warts to can-

tharidin, molluscum contagiosum lesions blister easily, often within hours after application, and must be washed as soon as blistering begins. Cantharidin should never be used in intertriginous areas or on the face, because the extent of blistering may be poorly controlled. As with warts, cryotherapy is helpful and light freezing at intervals of 2 to 3 weeks will eradicate lesions effectively. Individual lesions may be removed by piercing the center of each papule with a needle to remove the viral material or by curettage. Cryotherapy and removal of individual lesions by physical means are both acceptable for facial lesions.

Indications for Referral

Children with warts and molluscum contagiosum may be referred to a dermatologist if the primary care physician is uncomfortable with the therapy or if the treatment has been unsuccessful. A gastroenterologist may be consulted to perform proctoscopy in children with condylomata acuminata in the perianal area. Patients with warts and molluscum contagiosum should be followed for a period of months for the development of more lesions or recurrent lesions, in view of the viral incubation periods.

ANNOTATED BIBLIOGRAPHY

Cohen BA, Honig P, Androphy E: Anogenital warts in children: Clinical and virologic evaluation for sexual abuse. Arch Dermatol 126:1575–1580, 1990. (Seventy-three percent of the children with anogenital warts in this study were not abused.)

DeJong AR, Weiss JC, Brent RL: Condyloma acuminatum in children. Am J Dis Child 136:704–706, 1982. (Review of 34 cases of condylomas in prepubertal children with emphasis placed on the need to consider child abuse.)

Jarratt M: Viral infections of the skin. Pediatr Clin North Am 25:348–355, 1976. (Review of the clinical features and treatment of warts and molluscum contagiosum.)

Lutzner MA: The human papillomaviruses. Arch Dermatol 119:631–635, 1983. (Discussion of the different subgroups of papillomaviruses.)

Sanders BB, Stretcher GS: Warts: Diagnosis and treatment. JAMA 235:2859–2861, 1976. (Well-written review of the clinical features of warts and their therapy.)

68

Viral Exanthems

Amy Paller

Viral exanthems are generalized or localized cutaneous eruptions that are commonly confused with drug reactions. The rashes may take the form of macules, papules, vesicles, petechiae and purpura, and urticaria. An enanthem and other evidence of viral infection may be associated.

PATHOPHYSIOLOGY

Viral exanthems are often generalized and result from hematogenous dissemination of virus to the skin and cutaneous blood vessels. Alternatively, the rash may represent a hypersensitivity reaction to the virus. Viruses may also reach the skin by nerve fibers, leading to the cutaneous localization of herpes simplex or herpes zoster infections. The reason for the specific distribution of certain viral exanthems, such as the peripheral distribution of coxsackievirus A16 in the hand-foot-and-mouth disease or the central localization of echovirus infections, is unknown.

CLINICAL MANIFESTATIONS

Erythematous macular exanthems without papules are unusual and are most commonly related to echovirus infections. Occasionally, the rash of infectious mononucleosis noted in association with ampicillin administration is generalized, macular, and confluent. More commonly, the rash is maculopapular. *Maculopapular eruptions* are the most common form of viral exanthem. The rash may be discrete maculopapules (*rubelliform*) or confluent maculopapules (*morbilliform*). The most common cause of maculopapular exanthems is enterovirus, especially echovirus 9. The eruption is usually rubelliform. It starts on the head and upper trunk and spreads peripherally. Fever and aseptic meningitis may be associated. Adenoviruses are a common cause of upper respiratory tract infections in children. Two to 8% of infections are associated with maculopapular rashes that are usually rubelliform. Rhinovirus, influenza viruses, respiratory syncytial virus, and parainfluenza viruses also cause rubelliform eruptions that clear within 2 to 3 days.

Papular eruptions associated with viral infections may manifest as *papular acrodermatitis of childhood,* a self-limited disorder of children characterized by the sudden appearance of nonpruritic flat-topped, flesh-colored to erythematous papules on the extensor extremities, face, and buttocks. Papular acrodermatitis of childhood was originally described with hepatosplenomegaly, lymphadenopathy, and anicteric hepatitis due to hepatitis B (*Gianotti-Crosti syndrome*). It has also been associated with several other viruses, including Epstein-Barr virus, parainfluenza virus, coxsackievirus A16, and hepatitis A. The eruption is often preceded by upper respiratory tract symptoms, including fever, cough, and rhinitis. The lesions clear spontaneously after about 2 weeks to 2 months. Children with the eruption of papular acrodermatitis should be questioned about a recent history of an upper respiratory tract infection and should be evaluated for hepatosplenomegaly and lymphadenopathy. Liver enzyme levels and serologic studies for hepatitis A and B virus, Epstein-Barr virus, coxsackieviruses, and parainfluenza viruses should be performed as deemed appropriate. No treatment is necessary.

The most common *vesicular exanthem* is chickenpox (see Chap. 204). Generalized vesiculopustular exanthems

that heal without crusting have been described with enterovirus infections. Localized vesicles are typical of hand-foot-and-mouth disease and herpes simplex and zoster infections. *Petechiae* and *purpura* may be due to direct damage or immunologic damage by the virus. Alternatively, petechiae may be the manifestation of thrombocytopenia, most common with rubella infections. Petechiae and purpura may be seen with echovirus 9 infections. Bacterial infections, particularly meningococcemia, and rickettsial infections must be considered in the differential diagnosis. *Urticarial eruptions* have been described with infectious mononucleosis, enterovirus infections, mumps, and hepatitis B virus infection.

SPECIFIC VIRAL INFECTIONS WITH DISTINCT MORPHOLOGIES

Measles (rubeola) is a disorder of considerable morbidity and mortality that is due to a paramyxovirus. The incubation period is 10 to 14 days. The prodromal phase, the period of greatest contagion, begins with malaise, headache, cough, coryza, photophobia, conjunctivitis, and a fever that rises during a 4-day period. The classic enanthem (Koplik spots) appears 2 days after the onset of other symptoms and is often gone by the time that the exanthem develops. Koplik spots are tiny white papules, resembling grains of salt, overlying bright red buccal and lower labial mucosae. The vivid red-purple maculopapular rash is discrete at first but quickly becomes confluent. It begins on the scalp, forehead, and neck and spreads toward the feet over a 3-day period. The rash begins to clear after 4 days, first on the face, and resolves with fine branny desquamation and hyperpigmentation. Generalized lymphadenopathy, especially of the cervical nodes, pharyngitis, otitis media, pneumonia, laryngotracheitis, vomiting, and diarrhea may be seen in association. Subacute sclerosing panencephalitis and encephalitis are rare complications. *Atypical measles* occurs in patients who have been immunized against measles, especially with inactivated virus, and are subsequently exposed to measles. The inactivated virus has not been used since 1967, except in immunocompromised patients. The disorder begins with marked fever for 2 to 3 days, headaches, and myalgia. The exanthem starts peripherally and either does not progress or advances in a cephalad direction, in contrast to the course of typical measles. In addition to erythematous maculopapules, vesicles and petechiae may be noted. Koplik spots do not occur, but edema of the extremities and a typical nodular pneumonia are common. The illness lasts for 1 to 3 weeks.

Rubella (German measles) is now uncommon because of vaccination. The virus is spread by respiratory droplets with an incubation period of 14 to 21 days. The exanthem is usually the first sign of the illness and lasts between 1 and 5 days. It is characterized by generalized, discrete pink maculopapules that first appear on the face and then spread to the trunk and extremities as the facial rash fades. An enanthem (Forchheimer's sign) is characterized by petechiae on the soft palate and may be seen in up to 20% of patients early in the course. In younger children, slight fever and lymphadenopathy, especially of the suboccipital and post-auricular nodes, are associated features. Adolescents and adults often have a prodromal period with fever, headache, coryza, sore throat, mild conjunctivitis, and malaise. Arthritis, particularly of the small joints of the hands and feet, is occasionally a complication of older children and adults. Purpura and encephalitis are also rarely reported.

The most severe complication of rubella is *congenital rubella* by transplacental infection of the fetus during pregnancy. Affected infants are small for gestational age and may have a typical triad of deafness, congenital cataracts, and congenital heart disease. Other features include hyperbilirubinemia, hepatosplenomegaly, thrombocytopenic purpura, pneumonia, bone defects, and meningoencephalitis. "Blueberry muffin" lesions are multiple purple palpable macules or nodules that are noted at birth or within the first 24 hours. Blueberry muffin lesions are located usually on the head, neck, extremities, and trunk and range in size from 2 to 8 mm. On histopathologic examination, the lesions show aggregates of nonnucleated and nucleated erythrocytes in the dermis, due to dermal erythropoiesis. Dermal erythropoiesis and blueberry muffin lesions may also be seen in newborns with toxoplasmosis, cytomegalovirus infection, leukemia, and Rh incompatibilities. In rubella, the lesions clear after approximately 1 month. (For a more extensive discussion on these and other congenital infections, see Chap. 196.)

Roseola infantum (exanthem subitum) is the most common exanthem of children younger than 3 years of age. The infection has recently been attributed to herpesvirus type 6. The disorder is characterized by high fevers with rapid defervescence when the rash appears on the third or fourth day. The exanthem consists of small pale pink discrete macules or maculopapules that last only 1 to 2 days. The child is otherwise well, but periorbital edema is common. Leukopenia with relative lymphocytosis is common at the time of the rash. Febrile seizures may be associated.

Erythema infectiosum (fifth disease) is caused by parvovirus B19, and is characterized by three stages. The first stage develops suddenly as an erythematous blush of the malar area (slapped cheek appearance). The next day the second stage develops, which is a maculopapular rash on the extensor surfaces of the extremities and occasionally on the trunk and buttocks. After about 6 days as this rash fades, the third stage develops and the characteristic lacy pattern of macular erythema is seen. The lacy pattern persists for a few days to a week but frequently reappears after sun exposure, friction, or temperature change. Constitutional symptoms are mild, and no enanthem is associated.

Hand-foot-and-mouth disease is a distinctive disorder caused by coxsackievirus A16 and occasionally coxsackievirus A5 or A10. The illness is characterized by a fever and a vesicular eruption that follows a 3- to 6-day incubation period, occasionally associated with malaise, low-grade fever, sore throat, and abdominal discomfort. The enanthem begins first with small red macules that rapidly progress to vesicles and then ulcers on an erythematous base. The oral lesions may be seen on the buccal mucosae, tongue, gingivae, soft and hard palates, uvula, and tonsillar pillars. Up to two thirds of affected children have characteristic vesicular lesions on the hands and feet, especially on the dorsal surfaces. The lesions begin as maculopapules and progress to superficial elliptical vesicles surrounded by a red border. Occasionally, high fever, diarrhea, arthralgias, and adenopathy are associated.

Infectious mononucleosis is a common infection in adolescents but is rare in younger children. It is caused by the Epstein-Barr virus. The illness begins with headache, fever, and malaise followed by pharyngitis. Lymphadenopathy is generalized, although most notable of the cervical nodes. Over one half of patients have splenomegaly, and hepatomegaly is not uncommon. A maculopapular (or occasionally macular) confluent eruption develops in 10% to 15% of patients after approximately 5 days. The trunk and upper arms are most frequently involved, and the eruption tends to persist for a few days. Other cutaneous manifestations of infectious mononucleosis include urticaria, eyelid edema, and the development of a generalized maculopapular rash in almost 90% of patients after ampillicin, and occasionally penicillin, administration. Twenty-five percent of patients develop an enanthem 1 to 2 weeks after the onset of the disorder characterized by discrete petechiae at the junction of the hard and soft palates.

Herpes simplex cutaneous and mucosal infections may be "primary" in patients without previous exposure or circulating antibodies or "recurrent" when the infection develops again in the area of the primary infection. Primary infections occur most commonly in children between 1 and 5 years of age by close contact with infected adults and other children. Primary infections tend to be more painful, extensive, and of longer duration than recurrent infections. The incubation period is 3 to 10 days. Most children and adolescents have primary herpetic gingivostomatitis or recurrent herpes labialis, and the infection is usually due to type 1 herpes simplex. Primary gingivostomatitis begins with fever, sore throat, and irritability followed by the development of painful grouped vesicles overlying erythema on the gingivae, buccal mucosae, tongue, palate, and lips. The vesicles ulcerate and form white plaques overlying marked mucosal erythema. Cervical lymphadenopathy is associated. The fever disappears after approximately 4 days, but the oral lesions of primary herpes persist for up to 2 weeks. Primary herpetic gingivostomatitis must be differentiated from aphthous stomatitis, hand-foot-and-mouth disease, erythema multiforme, Vincent's infection, and Behçet's disease (see Chap. 82).

The recurrent infection is due to reactivation of quiescent viruses from regional spinal ganglia and usually manifests as a "cold sore" or "fever blister" with localized grouped vesicles on the lower lip. A few hours to a few days before the eruption appears patients complain of a burning sensation or itching at the site. Erythema and swelling develop first, followed by vesicles that rapidly become pustular and crusted after 2 to 3 days. Trauma to the lips, sun exposure, menstruation, and stress often precipitate recurrent lesions. Systemic toxicity is not usually associated, and the lesions resolve after 7 to 10 days. Erythema multiforme may be associated with recurrent herpes labialis as a hypersensitivity reaction that follows the herpetic eruption by 7 to 10 days. Painful erosions in the mouth and on the lips and the classic target lesions of the extremities and trunk are the manifestations of erythema multiforme (see Chap. 64).

Herpetic vulvovaginitis and *herpes progenitalis* are rare in children but are occasionally found in sexually active adolescents. Usually herpes simplex virus type 2 is responsible. The primary forms are characterized by burning pain, edema, grouped vesiculopustules, and ulcerations, usually on the vaginal mucosa, labia, or perineum in girls and on the penile shaft or perineum in boys. Fever, malaise, and regional lymphadenopathy are usually associated. The lesions form crusts within 7 days and clear in 2 to 4 weeks. Recurrent genital infections in boys are usually on the prepuce, glans, or sulcus, and in girls on the labia, vulva, clitoris, or cervix. The lesions tend to be more localized than in the primary forms, and constitutional symptoms or lymphadenopathy are mild. Recurrent lesions usually heal after about 8 days (see Chap. 119).

Primary cutaneous inoculation herpes may appear anywhere on the body but is most common on the finger (*herpetic whitlow*). The virus is inoculated into traumatized skin of the finger and develops into a painful vesiculopustule or bulla with surrounding erythema. The pain subsides after approximately 1 week, but lesions commonly take up to 3 weeks to resolve.

Eczema herpeticum or Kaposi's varicelliform eruption is a widespread eruption of cutaneous herpes lesions in patients with underlying atopic dermatitis, Darier's disease, or bullous ichthyosiform erythroderma. Clusters of vesicles develop on areas of abnormal skin and spread during a period of about a week (Fig. 68-1). The coalescence of grouped vesicles into sheets of pustules overlying erythema is not uncommon. The lesions often become secondarily infected with bacteria. Lymphadenopathy and fever are usually associated, especially in primary herpetic infections. The lesions heal spontaneously in 2 to 3 weeks. Visceral dissemination is unusual, but occasionally patients demonstrate evidence of hepatic involvement or meningoencephalitis.

Neonatal herpes infections occur in 1 in 3000 to 1 in 15,000 deliveries. The disease is usually caused by type 2 herpes simplex virus, acquired at or immediately before de-

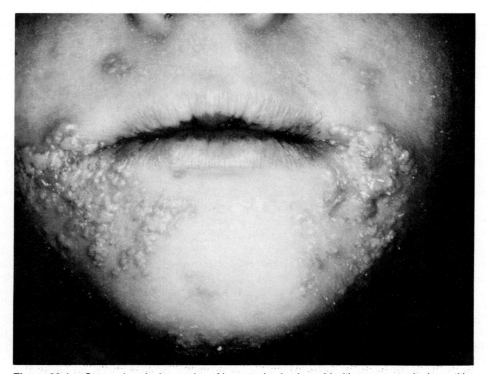

Figure 68-1.   Grouped vesiculopustules of herpes simplex in a girl with severe atopic dermatitis and eczema herpeticum.

livery. Infections may be disseminated, involving the viscera with or without involvement of the central nervous system, or may be localized, involving the central nervous system, skin, eyes, or mouth. Skin vesicles are seen in 70% to 80% of affected newborns and are often the initial manifestation and the clue to the correct diagnosis. Other features include microcephaly, seizures, respiratory distress with pneumonitis, hepatitis with jaundice, conjunctivitis, and petechiae and ecchymoses (see Chap. 196).

DIAGNOSIS OF HERPES SIMPLEX

Rapid diagnosis of herpes simplex can be made by a Tzanck smear or by testing of scrapings with antibody. For a Tzanck smear, the base of the vesicle is scraped and applied to a slide, which is stained with hematoxylin and eosin, methylene blue, Wright's stain, or Giemsa stain. Multinucleated giant cells and occasionally intranuclear inclusion bodies may be seen. The Tzanck smear is usually not positive once the lesions have become crusted and cannot differentiate herpes simplex from varicella and herpes zoster. Viral isolation by a culture of scrapings from the base of vesicles is the definitive diagnostic method and distinguishes herpes simplex from herpes zoster. A rising serum antibody titer between acute and convalescent sera is necessary to distinguish between primary and recurrent infections.

THERAPY FOR HERPES SIMPLEX INFECTIONS

Mucocutaneous herpetic infections are best treated topically by compresses (e.g., Burow's solution 1:20 to 1:40) three times daily to decrease drainage and relieve discomfort, followed by the application of topical antibiotics, such as Polysporin ointment. If secondary bacterial infection develops, oral antistaphylococcal antibiotics, such as erythromycin or dicloxacillin, must be administered. Oral and topical administration of acyclovir decreases the duration and shedding of infections. Oral acyclovir for preventing recurrent genital herpes may be indicated in particularly severe cases. Topical acyclovir must be applied five to six times daily. Oral acyclovir is now available for children at a concentration of 200 mg/tsp. The use of acyclovir for primary infections does not prevent recurrences. Oral anesthetics, such as liquid diphenhydramine (Benadryl) or 2% viscous lidocaine (Xylocaine), decrease the discomfort of oral lesions.

Intravenous acyclovir and vidarabine decrease the morbidity and dissemination of virus in immunocompromised patients. Intravenous acyclovir is currently the preferred drug for immunocompromised patients, including patients receiving immunosuppressants or chemotherapy, patients with eczema herpeticum with evidence of cutaneous or visceral dissemination, and newborns with herpes infections.

Despite the fact that intravenous acyclovir and vidarabine decrease the morbidity and mortality of herpes simplex infections in the newborn, prevention remains the best management. Infants are at greatest risk of developing neonatal herpes if maternal infection is primary, i.e., lack of transfer of maternal antibodies. If an infant is delivered vaginally from a high-risk mother, fetal scalp monitoring should be avoided to prevent direct inoculation at the site of the monitor. If any suspicion exists that an infant may have been exposed to herpes from an infected mother, serial viral cultures should be obtained from the eyes, mouth, and any skin vesicles. Caregivers should wear gloves and gowns, and the newborn must be kept from contact with other newborns.

Chickenpox (varicella) is a highly contagious disease of children caused by the herpes varicella-zoster virus. After an incubation period of 10 to 14 days, low-grade fever, malaise, and the characteristic exanthem appear. The exanthem consists of nongrouped erythematous macules that become papular, then vesicular, and, within 24 hours, ulcerated and crusted. Typically, lesions of various sizes and stages are found in the same vicinity and continue to appear during a 3- to 5-day period. Lesions begin on the trunk, scalp, and face and are pruritic. Involvement of the distal extremities is minimal. Secondarily infected or deeply excoriated lesions may become scars. Ulcers may be present on mucous membranes, especially on the pharynx, palate, and tonsillar pillars. In adults and immunocompromised persons, chickenpox is usually more severe with hemorrhagic or bullous lesions and disseminated infection, including viral pneumonitis. Oral acyclovir has recently been approved for the treatment of chickenpox. It has limited clinical benefit and is probably unnecessary in most uncomplicated cases (see Chap. 204).

Herpes zoster (shingles) is the recurrent form of varicella due to reactivation of virus in the dorsal root ganglia through peripheral nerves to the skin. Herpes zoster in children is uncommon and is usually associated with less morbidity than in adults. The risk of developing herpes zoster is greater in children with acute lymphocytic leukemia and children who had chickenpox during the first year of life. Grouped dermatomal erythematous papules rapidly become vesicles and then pustules. New vesicles continue to appear for approximately 7 days and then become crusted. The thoracic and lumbar dermatomes are usually involved. Scattered lesions may be seen outside the dermatomal borders. In contrast to adults, children with herpes zoster rarely have a prodrome of discomfort or erythema at the dermatomal site. The eruption clears after 2 to 3 weeks. Lymphadenopathy is common, but children rarely develop fever, headache, or postherpetic neuralgia. The lesions of herpes zoster have varicella-zoster virus, so that chickenpox may be transmitted to a susceptible person. There is no evidence that herpes zoster itself is transmissible. Immunosuppressed persons may develop dissemination of herpes zoster with widespread lesions, pneumonitis, hepatitis, meningoencephalitis, and purpura fulminans.

The treatment of varicella and herpes zoster is similar to

that of herpes simplex. Shake lotions, such as calamine, or compresses may be useful in drying the lesions of varicella and decreasing pruritus. The dermatomal vesicles of herpes zoster should be managed with compresses and topical antibiotics. Topical corticosteroid creams are useful in diminishing pruritus and inflammation after lesions have crusted. The risk of developing varicella zoster in immunocompromised patients who are exposed to the varicella-zoster virus may be decreased by the administration of zoster-immune globulin. Patients who develop disseminated varicella zoster should be given intravenous acyclovir. A varicella vaccine is being tested.

ANNOTATED BIBLIOGRAPHY

Cherry JD: Viral exanthems. Curr Probl Pediatr 13:5–44, 1983. (Review of viral exanthems, including skin manifestations.)

Gianotti F: Papular acrodermatitis of childhood and other papulovesicular acrolocated syndromes. Br J Dermatol 100:49–59, 1979. (Discussion of the association of papular acrodermatitis and hepatitis B infections.)

Jarratt M: Herpes simplex infection. Arch Dermatol 119:99–103, 1983. (Review of the clinical and epidemiologic features of herpes infections.)

69

Vascular Nevi

Amy Paller

Vascular disorders occur in 20% to 40% of newborns. These lesions are benign tumors caused by faulty communication of angioblastic tissue with surrounding vessels. Telangiectasias are ectatic vessels, and hemangiomas and lymphangiomas are a collection of proliferating endothelium-lined vessels. Although usually confined to the skin, vascular nevi are occasionally associated with systemic complications or as a feature of various syndromes.

STRAWBERRY AND CAVERNOUS HEMANGIOMAS

Hemangiomas vary from small harmless patches to large mutilating and occasionally life-threatening lesions. They are proliferations of immature blood vessels, thought to result from abnormalities at about the 30th day of development. The proliferation of hemangiomas may be due to an angiogenesis factor. In addition, mast cells are believed to participate in hemangioma growth because they are found in large numbers in biopsy specimens of proliferating but not involuting lesions.

The most common form of hemangioma is the *superfi-*

cial (*"strawberry"*) *hemangioma* that is characterized as a raised, red, firm, well-circumscribed, partially compressible lesion. The face, scalp, and thorax are the usual sites. Most superficial hemangiomas are not present at birth but appear within the first 1 or 2 months after birth. The initial lesion may appear as fine telangiectasias surrounded by pallor or as an erythematous patch that resembles nevus flammeus. The surface often develops a lobulated texture as the lesion expands and becomes more elevated during the first 3 months of life. Superficial hemangiomas may be confused with *pyogenic granulomas,* which are common vascular lesions that are bright red, firm, raised, slightly pedunculated papules. Pyogenic granulomas are often associated with focal trauma or infection and are believed to present a reactive process of vascular proliferation. The lesions grow rapidly and bleed easily but often clear spontaneously. They usually respond well to electrodesiccation, cryotherapy, and surgical removal. *Deep hemangiomas* are dermal and subcutaneous collections of large, mature blood vessels lined by thick fibrous walls. The depth of the vascular lesion imparts a blue color. Lesions are commonly present at birth and are characteristically red-blue soft, poorly demarcated compressible lesions. A combination of superficial and deep elements often occurs—the *mixed hemangioma.*

Hemangiomas grow rapidly during the first 6 months of life but usually do not more than double in size. Complications may occur during this period of rapid growth. Larger lesions, especially those that are subject to trauma, may ulcerate. Ulcerated lesions do not tend to bleed significantly but may become secondarily infected and result in scarring. Good local care of ulcerated hemangiomas, including topical antibiotics such as polysporin ointment or Silvadene cream to prevent secondary infection, should be initiated. A more serious complication that may occur during the period of rapid expansion is the development of thrombocytopenia, microangiopathic anemia, and disseminated intravascular coagulation, believed to be due to platelet trapping within the growing hemangioma (*Kasabach-Merritt syndrome*). Most involved hemangiomas are large and are located on the extremities. Findings that suggest the Kasabach-Merritt syndrome are a rapidly enlarging hemangioma, pallor, ecchymoses and petechiae (especially near the hemangioma), and a bleeding tendency from mucosae and wounds. The hemangioma becomes tense with overlying shiny, discolored skin. An evaluation for the Kasabach-Merritt syndrome should include a complete blood cell count with blood smear and platelet count, prothrombin and partial prothrombin times, and levels of fibrinogen and fibrin split products. *Disseminated eruptive hemangiomas* develop in crops of up to hundreds of hemangiomas during the first 3 months of life. Visceral hemangiomas, especially of the liver, gastrointestinal tract, spleen, lungs, eyes, and central nervous system, may be associated. Changes on physical examination, especially hepatomegaly, an abdominal bruit or cardiac murmur, and rales, are suggestive of visceral involvement. Further diagnostic evaluation should include a complete blood cell count to check for anemia and thrombocytopenia and a urinalysis and stool examination for blood. If cardiac failure is suspected, a chest roentgenogram, electrocardiogram, and echocardiogram should be obtained. Ophthalmologic examination should be performed if lesions involve the eyes, and computed tomography should be done if central nervous system lesions are suspected. Abdominal roentgenography, ultrasound scanning, liver-spleen scanning, and hepatic angiography may help to locate intra-abdominal hemangiomas if they seem likely on the basis of an examination.

Most hemangiomas do not enlarge after 12 months of life and subsequently begin to involute spontaneously. In the process of involution, superficial hemangiomas become pale centrally with gray regions within the lesion. Clinical regression is complete in 60% of children by the time that they begin school and in more than 90% of children by 9 years of age. Deep and mixed hemangiomas follow a similar course, although deep hemangiomas do not tend to grow as dramatically as superficial hemangiomas.

In general, no treatment is indicated for hemangiomas. The long-term cosmetic result of a spontaneous involution is usually superior to that of treatment with cryotherapy, sclerosing agents, surgery, or radiation, which often leads to scarring or atrophy. Parents, however, need considerable reassurance, and serial photographs with careful measurements and illustrations of the spontaneous resolution of similar lesions are helpful. Hemangiomas occasionally require intervention because their location or size compromise vital structures, including the eyes, airway, and ear canal. Superficial hemangiomas that are near the orbit and eyelids may cause amblyopia and strabismus. Deeper lesions may cause proptosis, glaucoma, and optic nerve compression (Fig. 69-1). Hemangiomas that obstruct the airway, especially laryngeal hemangiomas, may be associated with cutaneous hemangiomas. The lesions usually cause stridor and other evidence of airway obstruction when they begin to grow toward the end of the first month of life and always by 3 months of age. When therapy is needed, prednisone is usually the most effective agent, in a dose of 2 to 3 mg/kg/d for 1 month followed by every-other-day doses and gradual withdrawal as tolerated. Involution usually begins by the second or third week. Infants must be observed carefully for the development of complications of corticosteroid use, especially growth retardation, infections, and cataract formation. Intralesional injections of triamcinolone acetonide may also result in involution and must be administered by an experienced clinician, often using general anesthesia for maximal control. The flashlamp-pumped pulsed dye laser has recently been shown to eradicate superficial hemangiomas without scarring.

The treatment of the Kasabach-Merritt syndrome must be individualized. Infants with moderate thrombocytopenia may not show signs of active bleeding and may be observed

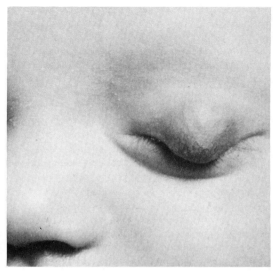

Figure 69-1. Eyelid hemangiomas that obstruct vision or compress the globe require intervention.

and not vigorously treated. A precipitously dropping platelet count with evidence of bleeding requires intervention. A 2-week trial of prednisone may be attempted if the situation is not emergent. Other treatment modes that have been employed include compressive bandages, surgical debulking of the hemangioma, embolization, irradiation, heparin, aspirin and dipyridamole, and the administration of platelets, fresh frozen plasma, and cryoprecipitates. Children with disseminated eruptive hemangiomas without visceral hemangiomas and without signs of cardiac failure do not require therapy. Cardiac failure should be treated with digitalis and diuretics. Corticosteroid therapy should be employed if visceral lesions are present and problematic.

Several syndromes include "hemangiomas", although the lesions are more consistent with vascular malformations. The *blue rubber bleb nevus syndrome* is an autosomal dominant vascular disorder characterized by multiple distinctive vascular lesions of the skin and gastrointestinal tract that are persistent and progressively increase in number. The typical "hemangiomas" of the blue rubber bleb nevus syndrome are elevated, blue or purplish-red papulomodules, or thin-walled sacs that contain blood and are easily compressed. Most patients have gastrointestinal tract vascular lesions, especially of the small intestine, resulting in chronic gastrointestinal bleeding and secondary iron deficiency anemia.

Maffucci's syndrome is the association of multiple vascular lesions and enchondromas. The "hemangiomas" often persist. The enchondromas usually affect the small bones of the hands and feet and the long bones and become apparent in early childhood. Lesions are firm, fixed, easily palpable 1- to 2-cm nodules. The enchondromas increase in size throughout childhood and occasionally progress after puberty, causing considerable deformity. From 23% to 30% of patients with Maffucci's syndrome develop an associated malignancy, especially chondrosarcomas.

The *Bannayan syndrome* is an autosomal dominant disorder characterized by hemangiomas and vascular malformations, lipomas, and lymphangiomas in association with macrocephaly, mental retardation, diminished linear growth, and intracranial tumors. *Gorham's syndrome* is a sporadic disorder characterized by multiple cavernous hemangiomas and massive underlying osteolysis with complete or partial replacement of bone by fibrous tissue. *Riley-Smith syndrome* is an autosomal dominant disorder with multiple hemangiomas, macrocephaly, and pseudopapillomas.

Telangiectatic Lesions

The *salmon patch,* the most common vascular lesion of infancy, is a transient telangiectatic nevus. It occurs in 40% of infants as a flat pink macule on the neck ("stork bite"), glabella, or upper eyelids ("angel kisses"). No treatment is needed. Ninety-five percent of salmon patches on the glabella and eyelids disappear within the first years of life, and 50% of the nuchal lesions clear spontaneously.

Nevus araneus (spider nevus) is a small telangiectatic lesion with a central arteriole from which blood vessels radiate. Spider nevi are common in school-aged children and often disappear during puberty. Typically, spider angiomas appear on the exposed areas of the face and upper half of the body. Destruction of the central vessel results in the disappearance of the radiating peripheral vessels, so that desiccation of the central punctum with curettage usually eliminates the lesion.

Cutis marmorata is a normal physiologic response of transient vascular mottling with chilling that occurs during the first weeks of life in newborns and for longer periods of time in premature infants and patients with Down's syndrome, the Cornelia de Lange syndrome, homocystinuria, and neonatal lupus erythematosus. *Cutis marmorata telangiectatica congenita* is a congenital vascular disorder with prominent venules and capillaries, resulting in a deep red mottling of skin. The telangiectasias often fade with time and may no longer be visible by adulthood. At least 50% of affected patients have associated abnormalities. Most common are limb asymmetry due to hypotrophy or, less commonly, hypertrophy of an involved extremity, macrocephaly, and mental and psychomotor retardation. In contrast to cutis marmorata, the telangiectasias of cutis marmorata telangiectatica congenita are wider, deeper red, and persistent despite changes in environmental temperature.

Hereditary hemorrhagic telangiectasia (*Rendu-Osler-Weber syndrome*) is an autosomal dominant disorder characterized by the progressive development of mucocutaneous and visceral telangiectasias associated with recurrent episodes of hemorrhage. The skin lesions usually appear after puberty, most commonly on the face, ears, hands, palms, fingers, nailbeds, and forearms. The mucosae of the lips, tongue, buccal mucosa, and nasal septum are virtually always involved. Epistaxis is the most common presenting manifestation, usually during childhood, and is a feature in up to 90% of patients. Forty-four percent of patients have gastrointestinal bleeding, especially of the upper gastrointestinal tract and usually as adults. Twenty percent of patients have pulmonary arteriovenous fistulas.

Ataxia-telangiectasia is an autosomal recessive syndrome of progressive oculocutaneous telangiectasias, cerebellar ataxia beginning in early infancy, a tendency toward sinopulmonary infections and selective immunodeficiencies, and chromosomal instability after radiation damage. The initial manifestation is usually cerebellar ataxia, which first becomes apparent when the child begins to walk. Neurologic deterioration is progressive. The characteristic mucocutaneous telangiectasias are usually noted between 3 and 6 years of age, although they have been described at birth. The bulbar conjunctivae are initially affected, and the telangiectasias may appear subsequently on the ears, eyelids, malar prominences, neck, antecubital and popliteal fossae, dorsa of the hands, and palate. Progeric changes have been noted in almost 90% of patients, with early loss of subcutaneous fat and premature graying of the hair. Sinopulmonary infections occur in most patients, and the most common causes of death are from bronchiectasis and respiratory failure. Patients have a 10% risk of developing neoplasms, especially lymphoreticular and epithelial tumors.

A deficient or absent level of IgA is found in 70% of patients, and many have circulating anti-IgA antibodies. Other immunologic defects include low to absent levels of IgE, defective cell-mediated immunity, and an absent or abnormally developed thymus. Almost all patients with ataxia-telangiectasia have elevated levels of α-fetoprotein and carcinoembryonic antigen.

The *port wine stain* (*nevus flammeus*) is a vascular lesion of mature capillaries that is present at birth and grows in proportion to the growth of the child. The lesions are flat and red-purple to blue. They tend to darken in color with advancing age and may develop angiomatous papules. Nevus flammeus does not involute. The vascular lesions may be camouflaged with makeup or treated with laser therapy for cosmetic purposes even in the first month of life.

The *Klippel-Trenaunay-Weber syndrome* combines the triad of nevus flammeus, associated hypertrophy or, less commonly, hypotrophy of the soft tissue and bone, and venous varicosities. The vascular lesion is unilateral in 85% of patients and usually involves a lower extremity. The bone and soft tissue hypertrophy is probably related to augmented arterial flow associated with the vascular nevus and with venous stasis. Varicose veins develop as collateral channels for obstructed deep veins during the first years of life, when the child spends more time in an upright position. The deep veins may be absent, hypoplastic, or occluded by fibrovascular bands. A few patients with features of Klippel-

Trenaunay-Weber syndrome have associated arteriovenous shunts. The most common complications of this syndrome are compensatory scoliosis due to hemihypertrophy of a lower extremity and cutaneous ulcerations, edema, stasis changes, and thrombophlebitis due to the venous varicosities. Children with significant varicosities should use elastic support stockings. Varicotomy and vein stripping are not usually indicated in view of the frequently inadequate deep venous supply. These procedures may lead to ankle edema and a rapid recurrence of the varicosity.

The *Sturge-Weber syndrome* (encephalotrigeminal angiomatosis) is a congenital vascular disorder characterized by vascular malformation of the leptomeninges over the cerebral cortex (usually the posterior parietal and occipital lobes) in association with an ipsilateral nevus flammeus in the distribution of the first trigeminal nerve. Seizures occur in up to 89% of patients, with the majority starting during the first year of life. Typically, the seizures are focal motor seizures or begin with a focus and then generalize. Hemiparesis or hemiplegia contralateral to the nevus is noted in 26% of patients, especially with extension of cerebral atrophy into the major motor portion of the parietal lobe. Intracranial calcifications may be visible by computed tomography within the first few months of life and by roentgenograms after 2 years of age. Ocular abnormalities, especially glaucoma, develop more frequently in patients with involvement of both the second and first trigeminal branches. Telangiectatic hypertrophy of oral mucosae is also common.

Coat's disease includes telangiectasias of the face, conjunctivae, nail beds, and breast with retinal telangiectasias and a massive exudation with retinal detachment. *Cobb syndrome* is characterized by nevus flammeus or angiokeratomas in a dermatomal distribution, associated with angiomas of the corresponding segment of spinal cord. *Von Hippel-Lindau syndrome* is an autosomal dominant condition with cerebellar hemangioblastomas, cyst formation, and occasionally port wine stains.

ANGIOKERATOMAS

Angiokeratomas are asymptomatic, firm, dark red scaly papules that range from 1 to 10 mm. Histopathologic examination of lesions shows a thickening of the epidermis overlying vascular ectasia. Solitary or multiple angiokeratomas may occur in childhood after trauma and are usually located on the lower extremities. Disorders involving angiokeratomas are uncommon and include *Fabry's disease, angiokeratoma circumscriptum, angiokeratoma of Mibelli,* and *angiokeratoma of Fordyce.*

LYMPHANGIOMAS

Tumors of the lymphatic vessels may be classified into four types: lymphangioma simplex, lymphangioma circumscriptum, cavernous lymphangioma, and cystic hygroma. Ninety percent are present at birth or appear during infancy. *Lymphangioma simplex* is a solitary, well-demarcated, skin-colored tumor with a smooth surface that is usually located on the head, neck, or proximal extremities. It is often amenable to surgical removal. *Lymphangioma circumscriptum* is the most common form of lymphangioma. The lesions have the appearance of clustered thick-walled vessels and are usually found on the proximal extremities, neck, trunk, and oral mucosae. Vascular lesions are frequently associated, so that lesions may be deep red. Surgical removal often results in recurrence. *Cavernous lymphangiomas* are large, cystic dilations of the deep dermis and subcutaneous tissue that are poorly defined and involve large areas of the extremities, trunk, and face. Surgery must be extensive and often leads to recurrences. *Cystic hygromas* are large, often unilocular lymphangiomas that are commonly located on the neck, axillae, or inguinal regions. Recurrences after surgical removal are uncommon, and cystic hygromas occasionally undergo spontaneous resolution (see Chap. 84).

ANNOTATED BIBLIOGRAPHY

Esterly NB: Kasabach-Merritt syndrome in infants. J Am Acad Dermatol 8:504–513, 1983. (Review of Kasabach-Merritt syndrome and its treatment.)

Esterly NB, Margileth AM, Kahn G et al: The management of disseminated eruptive hemangiomata in infants. Pediatr Dermatol 1:312–317, 1984. (Discussion of the diagnosis and management of disseminated hemangiomatosis.)

Jacobs AH: Vascular nevi. Pediatr Clin North Am 30:465–482, 1983. (Review of the common vascular nevi.)

Wisnicki JL: Hemangiomas and vascular malformations. Ann Plast Surg 12:41–59, 1984. (Review of the classification, natural history, and treatment of various vascular lesions.)

70

Epidermal Tumors

Amy Paller

Epidermal tumors include benign lesions of the epidermis, malignant lesions of the epidermis, adnexal tumors (i.e., tumors of eccrine gland, apocrine gland, sebaceous gland, or hair follicle origin), and tumors derived from melanocytes.

MELANOCYTIC LESIONS

Pigmented nevi ("moles") are the most common tumors of childhood. *Congenital melanocytic nevi* are present in only 1% of all newborns. Most persons acquire nevi throughout infancy and childhood with a peak average of 20 to 40 nevi per person in later adolescence and young adulthood. Nevi begin to involute later in adulthood. Nevi occur most commonly on sun-exposed areas above the waist and have smooth borders with sharp demarcation from the surrounding skin and usually with homogeneous pigmentation. Pigmented nevi may be classified into three major subgroups: junctional, compound, and intradermal.

Junctional nevi are believed to represent the initial stage of compound nevi and are usually found in children. They are light brown to black macules that are usually devoid of hair but do not retain normal skin lines. Junctional nevi begin as tiny macules and grow to reach a maximum diameter of 4 to 6 mm. Histopathologically, junctional nevi show single melanocytic cells or a nest of nevus cells "dropping off" of the epidermis in an orderly arrangement. *Compound nevi* are usually seen in older children and adolescents, although they are occasionally present at birth. They are more elevated than junctional nevi, have a warty or smooth surface, and often contain dark coarse hairs. Compound nevi show nevus cells at the dermoepidermal border as well as in the dermis. *Intradermal nevi* are seen most frequently in adults but may develop in childhood. These nevi are dome shaped with coarse central hairs and a broad or pedunculated base. Clinical differentiation from compound nevi may be difficult. Histopathologically, intradermal nevi show nests of nevus cells in the dermis only. In adulthood with increasing age, intradermal nevi tend to involute and are replaced by fatty or fibrous tissue.

Most pigmented nevi are benign and are of cosmetic concern only. However, congenital pigmented nevi, especially giant congenital nevi, and dysplastic nevi are precursors for malignant melanomas and surgical removal should be performed. Most congenital nevi are small or medium-sized nevi. Fewer than 1 in 20,000 newborns have giant congenital pigmented nevi with a diameter of greater than 10 to 20 cm. Giant congenital melanocytic nevi are most commonly found on the buttocks, scalp, and paravertebral areas in the distribution of a garment, especially a bathing suit. They are usually deeply pigmented and often have scattered satellite lesions. The nevus is usually covered with hair (Fig. 70-1). The histopathologic appearance of congenital melanocytic nevi differs from that of acquired melanocytic nevi. Congenital nevi have nevus cells that extend deep into the lower dermis and often deep into the subcutaneous tissues with an extension between collagen bundles in single rows. In addition, nevus cells are found within hair follicles, blood vessel walls, the perineurium, eccrine ducts and glands, and sebaceous glands.

Infants with giant congenital nevi have a lifetime risk of at least 6.3% of developing melanomas by transformation. Because 70% of these giant nevi transform during the prepubertal years, their removal as early as possible is encouraged. Because of the depth of congenital nevi, complete excisional removal to the fascia should be performed.

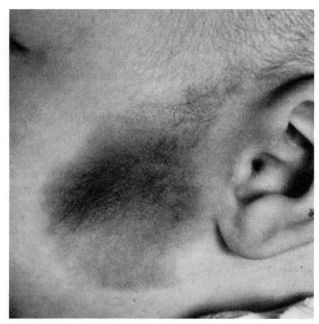

Figure 70-1. Congenital hairy nevus.

Dermabrasion or treatment with phenol often leads to a better cosmetic result but does not usually remove the nevus entirely. Although decreasing the number of nevus cells may lower the risk of transformation into melanoma, melanomas have developed in dermabraded congenital nevi. Giant nevi must be removed using general anesthesia, so that many surgeons prefer to wait until the infant is 3 to 6 months of age to decrease the risks of general anesthesia. Atypical areas within the giant nevus during the first 6 months of life should be excised with local anesthesia and examined for possible melanoma. Most giant nevi must be removed with serial grafting of normal skin. Tissue expansion of contiguous areas with the nevus is being employed as a potential source of skin flaps or grafted tissue. Cutaneous lesions that overlie the head and spinal cord may be associated with leptomeningeal melanocytosis that may lead to hydrocephalus, seizures, and melanoma. Computed axial tomography may demonstrate leptomeningeal involvement, but the complete removal of nevus cells from this site is impossible.

The risk of transformation of small and medium-sized nevi into melanoma is controversial. Anecdotal reports suggest that melanomas arise in these congenital nevi, but good prospective studies to determine the actual risk and the need for removal have yet to be done. Although there does appear to be an increased risk of transformation into melanoma, the time course of this transformation suggests that it occurs after puberty. The recommendations from dermatologists for management range from observation only to removal of all lesions during infancy. Many dermatologists favor removal of all lesions by local anesthesia at or after puberty with annual observation of lesions or removal of selected lesions based on the location and the desires of the patient (e.g., a lesion over a joint is difficult to remove without contracture formation and is easily visible to the patient, but a lesion on the buttocks or scalp is difficult to observe and removal leads to minimal cosmetic defect). Signs of transformation to melanoma include the development of irregular borders, variegate pigmentation, and irregular alteration of topography.

Dysplastic nevi are acquired nevi that are markers of patients who are predisposed to developing malignant melanomas. It has been estimated that approximately 2% of persons in the United States have at least one dysplastic nevus. In addition, 5% to 10% of patients who develop a melanoma have a family history of melanoma. Dysplastic nevi have been found by histopathologic examination in 20% to 35% of all melanomas. The familial types have an autosomal dominant mode of inheritance.

The characteristic clinical features of dysplastic nevi usually appear at puberty, although patients often note large numbers of nevi that develop at 5 to 8 years of age. At puberty and subsequently into adulthood, the number of nevi increases further, so that the patient commonly has 25 to 75 nevi (especially in the familial forms) with atypical features, including irregular borders, variegate pigmentation with mixtures of pink, tan, and brown, and indistinct margins. Dysplastic nevi are usually larger than normal nevi and range in size from 6 to 15 mm. In contrast to the distribution of normal nevi, dysplastic nevi are most commonly found on the trunk and are also located on feet, scalp, and buttocks. The dysplastic nevi may be macular or may have an irregular rough appearance. Features to suggest that a melanoma has developed are black areas within a lesion and a change in topography developing at the edge of a dysplastic nevus. Any lesion that is suspected of being a melanoma must be removed by excision. Histopathologically, dysplastic nevi show atypical melanocytic hyperplasia with dermal mesenchymal changes and usually nevus cells in the dermis. Patients with suspected dysplastic nevus syndrome should have two or three of the most atypical lesions removed by excisional biopsy to confirm the diagnosis. Subsequently, patients should be followed carefully with serial photographs at least every 6 months, such as at a pigmented lesion clinic. Lesions should be assessed histologically if clinical changes occur. Patients should avoid exposure to sunlight and should not use oral contraceptives. All family members should also be examined for the possibility of dysplastic nevi.

OTHER MELANOCYTIC LESIONS

Café-au-lait spots are well-circumscribed, homogeneously light-brown macules that are present at birth or may appear during the first 5 years of life. Ten to 19% of all persons have one café-au-lait spot, although the presence of more than two café-au-lait spots is unusual (less than 0.75%). Café-au-lait spots are associated with *Albright's syndrome* (polyostotic fibrous dysplasia) and *neurofibromatosis*. The café-au-lait spot of Albright's syndrome is usually solitary, large, and segmental. The café-au-lait spots of neurofibromatosis are usually multiple (greater than five), are scattered, and may be associated with generalized or axillary freckling. Although the café-au-lait spots of Albright's syndrome have been distinguished from those of neurofibromatosis by the irregular borders of those in Albright's syndrome, such distinctions are often misleading. *Nevus spilus* is a café-au-lait spot with darker macules or papules of pigmentation overlying the light-brown patch. Histopathologically, the raised papules usually show nevus cells while the macular areas demonstrate melanocyte proliferation.

Spindle cell nevus (Spitz nevus, benign juvenile melanoma) is a firm, smooth, dome-shaped red-brown lesion that is usually solitary and occurs most frequently in prepubertal children. The lesions are occasionally darker brown and may be confused clinically with malignant melanomas. Spindle cell nevi must also be distinguished clinically from intradermal nevi, pyogenic granulomas, and juvenile xanthogranulomas. Histologically, the spindle cell nevus is a variant of the compound nevus. Although the lesion is benign, confusion with the histopathologic appearance of melanoma may result from the disordered appearance of nevus cells and the large number of mitotic figures. The presence of spindle and epithelioid cells, sparsity of melanin, dilated dermal blood vessels, and increased maturation of the deeper nevus cells help to differentiate the conditions. Spindle cell nevi may persist into adulthood or become intradermal nevi.

The *halo nevus* (Sutton's nevus) usually occurs late in childhood or during adolescence. A halo of depigmentation appears around a pigmented nevus, probably due to immunologic destruction of melanocytic cells. Halo nevi appear most commonly on the trunk. In most cases, the central pigmented lesion disappears. Rarely, the depigmentation is associated with melanoma.

Mongolian spots are flat, blue-gray, often poorly circumscribed lesions that are usually found on the buttocks, lumbosacral area, and shoulders of infants, especially in black, Asian, and hispanic infants. The lesions are often large and may be single or multiple. A histopathologic examination of mongolian spots shows spindle-shaped melanocytes and melanin deep in the dermis, and the spots are believed to represent melanocytes that have failed to migrate to the epidermis. The blue color results from the depth of the pigmentation and the reflection of blue light (Tyndall effect). Mongolian spots usually disappear within the first 5 years of life, and fewer than 5% of patients have spots that persist into adulthood. Other variants of dermal melanocytosis are the nevus of Ota, nevus of Ito, and blue nevus. The *nevus of Ota* is usually found in black or Asian female patients and is characterized by patchy blue discoloration of the periorbital area, forehead, and upper cheek. The nevus of Ota is usually unilateral. Approximately 50% of patients have the nevus at birth, while most other patients develop the lesion at puberty or pregnancy. The *nevus of Ito* shares the clinical characteristics of the nevus of Ota but involves the shoulder, upper arms, scapula, and supraclavicular regions. In contrast to the disappearance of mongolian spots, nevus of Ota and nevus of Ito persist and often darken with increasing age. Cosmetic cover-ups are the only indicated treatment. *Blue nevi* are uncommon in children and usually appear during the second or third decades of life, especially in Asians. They are small, round, well-circumscribed nevi that are blue because of the depth of spindle-shaped melanocytes and melanin. Blue nevi are also believed to result from the arrested migration of melanocytes bound for the dermoepidermal junction. A malignant transformation from blue nevi is rare.

Becker's nevus usually appears at the end of the first decade of life in boys but has even been reported at birth and may develop in female patients. Brown macular pigmentation develops on the chest, back, or upper arm and spreads irregularly until a size of 10 to 15 cm in diameter is reached. Within the next few years, coarse hairs develop in the area of pigmentation. The hyperpigmentation and hypertrichosis are persistent.

Lentigines are small, tan to black oval macules that usually appear in childhood (lentigo simplex). In adults, lentigines are usually sun-induced (solar lentigines, "liver spots"). A histopathologic examination of lentigines shows epidermal melanocytic proliferation. In children, lentigines usually fade or disappear with advancing age. Lentigines are important for their association with syndromes. In the *Peutz-Jeghers syndrome,* characteristic lentigines appear during early childhood on the lips and oral mucosa, on the nose and periorbital region, on the palms and soles, and on the dorsa of the fingers and toes. Associated with the lentigines are polyps, especially of the small intestine. The polyps have a low malignant potential but may lead to colicky abdominal pain, melena, and intussusception. The Peutz-Jeghers syndrome has an autosomal dominant mode of inheritance. The *multiple lentigines syndrome,* or *LEOPARD syndrome,* is another autosomal dominant disorder with variable expressivity characterized by generalized *l*entigines that are usually present at birth or in early infancy, *e*chocardiographic abnormalities, *o*cular hypertelorism, *p*ulmonic stenosis, *a*bnormalities of the genitalia, *r*etardation of growth, and *d*eafness.

EPIDERMAL NEVI

Epidermal nevi usually appear at birth or in early childhood. They may occur anywhere but are most common on the head and extremities and are in a patterned distribution. Lesions tend to be 2 to 3 cm or larger; they are usually pigmented to various degrees; and they often appear warty. Epidermal nevi may continue to extend until late adolescence. They do not regress spontaneously and usually become more verrucous in adulthood. Various subgroups of epidermal nevi have been described based on the appearance, distribution, and mixture of epidermal and appendageal components. *Nevus unius lateris* is a linear or curved lesion limited to one side of the body that follows the long axis of the trunk or extremity. The *inflammatory linear verrucous epidermal nevus* is an erythematous, often pruritic linear epidermal nevus that almost always affects a lower extremity and shows eczematous changes histopathologically. These nevi must be differentiated from lichen striatus, a benign inflammatory condition that resolves spontaneously after months (see Chap. 63). If a large area of the body is covered with the epidermal nevus, the lesion is a systematized epidermal nevus. *Ichthyosis hystrix* is a form of systematized epidermal nevus that is widespread and usually bilateral with whorls of hyperkeratosis. Epidermal nevi are difficult to remove and often recur, even after full-thickness excision. Malignant transformation of epidermal nevi, usually into basal cell carcinoma, is rare and attempts to remove the lesions are unnecessary except for cosmetic purposes.

The *epidermal nevus syndrome* is a sporadic condition characterized by the association of acquired deformities of the skeletal system, central nervous system, cardiovascular system, and skin. Cutaneous anomalies include epidermal nevi, café-au-lait spots, hypopigmented macules, melanocytic nevi, and hemangiomas. The epidermal nevi may take the form of localized acanthosis nigricans, nevus unius lateris, ichthyosis hystrix, and, when on the face or neck, linear nevus sebaceus. The most common systemic complications are kyphoscoliosis, mental retardation, seizures, and hemihypertrophy. Patients with the epidermal nevus syndrome must be followed carefully for the development of these systemic abnormalities with careful physical examinations, electroencephalograms, and radiographic studies, as determined by history and examination.

ADNEXAL TUMORS

Adnexal tumors in children are often present at birth or develop in early childhood. Other than the nevus sebaceus, adnexal tumors are usually benign and require removal for cosmetic purposes only. The *nevus sebaceus* (of Jadassohn) is a well-circumscribed, yellow-orange hairless plaque that is usually solitary and located on the scalp, face, or neck. At puberty, the lesion becomes raised and warty. A histopathologic examination of nevus sebaceus shows overgrowth of sebaceous glands and rudimentary hair follicles. Tumors, especially basal cell carcinomas, develop in 10% to 15% of lesions in young adulthood. As a result, it is advisable that all nevus sebaceus be excised by teenage years. *Trichoepitheliomas* are benign, firm, dome-shaped, skin-colored tumors that are most common on the face. They appear occasionally in childhood but more commonly develop in adults and can be confused with basal cell carcinoma. Multiple trichoepitheliomas may be inherited in an autosomal dominant manner as epithelioma adenoides cysticum (Brooke's syndrome). *Trichofolliculomas* are solitary skin-colored papules that are also usually on the face but may be distinguished clinically by a central pore with a woolly tuft of hair. *Syringomas* are benign tumors of the eccrine glands that usually appear during adolescence as skin-colored to yellow tiny papules, usually on the lower eyelids, neck, or upper chest. Syringomas are seen with increased frequency in children with Down syndrome. *Pilomatrixomas* (calcifying epithelioma of Malherbe) are benign tumors of hair that usually develop during childhood as hard, skin-colored, or blue nodules on the face, neck, or upper extremities. Pilomatrixomas are usually solitary but may be multiple, especially in children with myotonic dystrophy.

BASAL CELL CARCINOMA

Basal cell carcinomas are rarely seen in children, except in association with nevus sebaceus, xeroderma pigmentosum, and the basal cell nevus syndrome. The *basal cell nevus syndrome* (Gorlin's syndrome) is an autosomal dominant disorder characterized by multiple basal cell carcinomas that develop in childhood in association with musculoskeletal, neurologic, and endocrinologic abnormalities. The basal cell tumors usually appear between puberty and 35 years of age but may develop as early as the second year of life. The face, neck, and chest are most commonly affected, and the basal cell carcinomas appear as skin-colored to brown dome-shaped papules that erupt in crops. Associated tumors include medulloblastomas in infancy and ovarian fibromas.

ANNOTATED BIBLIOGRAPHY

Greene MH, Clark WH, Tucker MA et al: Acquired precursors of cutaneous malignant melanoma: The familial dysplastic nevus syndrome. N Engl J Med 312:91–97, 1985. (Review of the clinical characteristics of dysplastic nevi, including numerous color illustrations.)

Hurwitz S: Epidermal nevi and tumors of epidermal origin. Pediatr Clin North Am 30:483–494, 1983. (Review of the various epidermal tumors.)

Jacobs AH, Hurwitz S, Prose NS et al: The management of congenital nevocytic nevi. Pediatr Dermatol 2:143–156, 1984. (Discussion by several pediatric dermatologists of the management of congenital nevi.)

Rhodes AR: Pigmented birthmarks and precursor melanocytic lesions of cutaneous melanoma identifiable in childhood. Pediatr Clin North Am 30:435–463, 1983. (Review of congenital nevi and their differential diagnosis.)

Solomon LM, Esterly NB: Epidermal and other congenital organoid nevi. Curr Probl Pediatr 6:2–56, 1975. (Excellent review of epidermal nevi and other tumors derived from adnexal structures.)

71
Insect Bites and Infestations

Amy Paller

Bites and infestations are especially common in children and may manifest as papules, nodules, blisters, urticaria, and hemorrhagic lesions. The correct diagnosis is frequently missed. Recognition of these lesions is based on the distribution and grouping of lesions, and history, including exposure to pets and other affected persons, environmental conditions, childhood habits, seasonal incidence of the lesions, and a recent history of travel. Bites and infestations of dermatologic significance are caused by arthropods, particularly eight-legged arachnids (e.g., mites, ticks, and spiders), six-legged insects (e.g., fleas, mosquitoes, bedbugs, lice, and caterpillars), and helminths.

ARACHNIDS

Mites attack children by burrowing under the skin or by attaching themselves to the skin and causing dermatitis. Mites that most frequently cause dermatologic problems include itch mites (*Sarcoptes scabiei*) and harvest mites (chiggers). The *scabies* mite burrows into the horny layer of skin, especially in areas of skin with a thin horny layer and few hair follicles. The eruption is usually intensely pruritic and manifests as various primary lesions, including burrows, papules, nodules, and vesicles, mixed with secondary excoriations, dermatitis, crusting, and secondary infection (Fig. 71-1). The burrows are the home of the female parasite and the papules represent skin invaded by the scabies larvae. The nodules, vesicles, and pruritus are thought to be hypersensitivity reactions to the mite and do not develop until 3 to 6 weeks after infestation begins. Although adolescents and older children usually have lesions in the interdigital spaces, in flexural regions, at the wrists, at the waistline, on the buttocks, and around the areolae, infants and young children tend to have more widespread involvement, including lesions on the face, neck, scalp, palms, and soles. The red-brown nodules are especially common in children, particularly on covered parts of the body such as the axillae, groin area, and buttocks. The nodules and their associated pruritus may persist for months, despite adequate antiscabetic therapy. The burrows are found on approximately 10% of adult and adolescent patients, but even less frequently on the skin of young children and infants, because of the elimination of visible burrows by vigorous hygiene and secondary eczematization.

Infants and children frequently develop secondary eczema because of vigorous scratching as well as excessive bathing and application of irritating topical preparations.

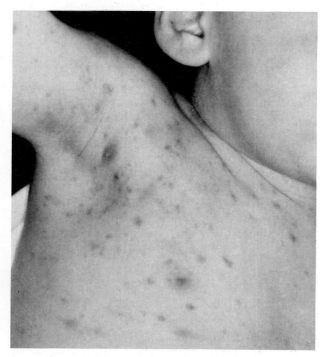

Figure 71-1. Papules, vesicles, and nodules of scabies in an infant.

Atopic children are especially predisposed to develop eczematization and secondary bacterial infections. The administration of topical corticosteroids to unrecognized lesions may diminish the pruritus and erythema but will encourage the proliferation and transmissibility of the organism. This phenomenon has been called *scabies incognito.*

Norwegian scabies (crusted scabies) is a form of scabies characterized by lesions covered with thick crusts and scales that are teeming with mites. The buttocks, scalp, palms, soles, elbows, and knees are most extensively involved. Norwegian scabies tends to be less pruritic than classic scabies and occurs with greatest frequency in children with mental or physical handicaps and immunocompromised children (particularly with Down syndrome). *Canine scabies* is a form of scabies carried by domestic animals, especially the dog. The mite does not reproduce on human skin but may cause a transient eruption in children on the forearms, thighs, chest, and abdomen. The mite is difficult to identify by skin scrapings, and the diagnosis is often made by a history alone. The infestation clears spontaneously after 4 to 6 weeks.

The differential diagnosis of scabies most frequently includes atopic, contact allergic, and contact irritant dermatitis. Papular urticaria, histiocytosis X, seborrheic dermatitis, and dermatitis herpetiformis may also be considered.

The diagnosis of scabies is often based on the history and the distribution and morphology of lesions. A scraping to identify mites, feces, or eggs, however, should always be taken. Fresh papules or burrows are the best sites to scrape after placing a drop of mineral oil on the suspected site. Potassium hydroxide should never be used on scrapings for scabies, since it dissolves the mites, eggs, and feces. Occasionally, a skin biopsy is performed to eliminate the possibility of other diagnoses. A burrow and mite may be found by a histopathologic examination, but this is rare except in Norwegian scabies. Once the diagnosis of scabies is made, all family members must be examined and treated to avoid reinfection.

Scabies may be treated with a variety of preparations, including 5% permethrin (Elimite), 1% gamma benzene hexachloride (lindane, Kwell), crotamiton (Eurax), or 6% precipitated sulfur. Five percent permethrin or lindane is applied from the neck down, unless lesions are present on the head, and is washed off thoroughly 6 to 8 hours later. The skin should not be soaked before applying the medication so that percutaneous absorption is minimal. A second application may be advisable 1 week later to destroy hatched larvae, but no further applications are necessary unless reinfection occurs. Family members who are in close contact with the patient should also be treated. The mite survives up to 48 hours off the body, so that clothing, bedding, and towels that have been used in the 48 hours before treatment should be laundered with hot water. Twenty-four hours after therapy the patient is no longer capable of transmitting scabies. Evidence of hypersensitivity (e.g., pruritus, nodules, and vesicles) may persist for months. Topical tar preparations, antipruritic lotions such as ¼% menthol in Shepard's lotion, and nonfluorinated topical corticosteroids may ameliorate the pruritus. Currently, 5% permethrin is the drug of choice for patients younger than 1 year of age or in pregnant or lactating mothers. Systemic antistaphylococcal antibiotics should be administered to patients with secondary bacterial infections.

Harvest mite (chiggers) infestations are usually found in the southern United States and are characterized by intense itching and discrete, bright-red tiny papules with hemorrhagic puncta. Purpuric lesions, bullae, urticaria, excoriations, and erythema may be noted. The lesions are most commonly located on the legs and at the waistline, although they may be widespread in children. Mosquito repellants are effective against chiggers. For relief of the pruritus, compresses, topical corticosteroids, antihistamines, and clear nail polish applied directly to the bites have been used.

Ticks may cause local inflammation or systemic symptoms or may transmit serious systemic disease. The bite is painless, but within days reactions occur from the introduction of tick saliva. Pruritus and local urticarial reactions are the most common sequelae. A foreign body reaction with nodules may develop if mouth parts are left in the skin. Rarely, patchy hair loss in the area of the tick bite may occur. Serious systemic reactions may result from tick bites, but they subside quickly once the tick is found and removed. These reactions include generalized urticaria, tick bite fever, and tick paralysis. *Tick bite fever* is characterized by fever, headache, nausea, and abdominal cramping. *Tick paralysis* is an ascending paralysis that resembles the Guillain-Barré syndrome. Respiratory failure and death may ensue. Ticks may be removed by various methods but should never be plucked off since body fragments may be left behind. Accepted techniques include covering the area with nail polish, mineral oil, or petrolatum; cryotherapy with liquid nitrogen; heating the area with an extinguished match; and application of a few drops of chloroform or ether.

Ticks may transmit a number of systemic diseases with dermatologic manifestations, particularly *Rocky Mountain spotted fever* and *Lyme disease*. Rocky Mountain spotted fever is an acute exanthematous illness caused by *Rickettsia rickettsii* that is most prevalent in the southeastern United States. The rash begins on the extremities (including the palms and soles) after 3 to 4 days and spreads to the trunk and abdomen as erythematous maculopapules that become hemorrhagic. Other features include fever, headache, conjunctivitis, nausea, and myalgias. Complications include cardiovascular collapse, gangrene, hepatosplenomegaly, disseminated intravascular coagulation, and visceral hemorrhage. Early diagnosis of Rocky Mountain spotted fever is crucial and may be obtained by demonstration of the pathogen by direct immunofluorescence microscopy of skin biopsy sections. Antibodies to *Proteus* OX-19 or OX-2 appear in the second or third week of the illness. The differential diagnosis includes viral exanthems, meningococcemia, and typhoid fever. Tetracycline and chloramphenicol are the preferred antibiotics and should be administered as early as possible.

Lyme disease is caused by a spirochete (*Borrelia burgdorferi*) that is transmitted by ticks. The disorder usually begins in the summer or early autumn with the multiple expanding, erythematous annular lesions of *erythema chronicum migrans*. Constitutional symptoms, nausea, vomiting, myalgias, arthralgias, eye pain, conjunctivitis, and lymphadenopathy may accompany the cutaneous annular lesions. Weeks to months later the erythema chronicum migrans disappear but patients may have neurologic and cardiac abnormalities and migratory polyarthritis or chronic arthritis. Serologic testing with indirect immunofluorescence or the enzyme-linked immunoabsorbent assay usually confirms the diagnosis. (Laboratory testing may not be reliable.) The preferred treatment is tetracycline in teenagers and penicillin or amoxicillin in younger children (see Chap. 206, "Lyme Disease").

Although the black widow spider is a significant cause of morbidity, only the *brown recluse spider* causes notable dermatologic features. The brown recluse spider is distinguished by a dark violin-shaped band on its thorax. The spider's venom contains hemolytic, necrotizing, and spreading factors. Local burning or pruritus occurs after the bite, followed within hours by a painful hemorrhagic blister. Finally, the central portion becomes ulcerated and gangrenous and may not heal for months. Systemic reactions are common in children and include malaise, chills, nausea, vomiting, myalgias, a generalized erythematous or purpuric maculopapular eruption, thrombocytopenia, hemolysis, hemoglobinuria, shock, and coma. Management includes systemic corticosteroids, antihistamines, antibiotics for secondary bacterial infections, and surgical removal of the necrotic area.

INSECTS

Lice are small, wingless insects that proliferate readily through the production of eggs (nits) and depend on a blood meal for survival. When the lice feed, they release a toxin into the skin that produces tiny purpuric macules and later pruritic papules and wheals as a hypersensitivity reaction. Three forms of lice cause infestations (pediculosis): the head louse, body louse, and pubic or crab louse.

Children are most susceptible to *pediculosis capitis*, caused by the head louse. Infestation results from direct contact with an infested person or contact with hats or combs. The nits are attached to the hair shaft and resemble dandruff but cannot be easily removed. Scalp pruritus and eczematization with secondary infection is common. The diagnosis may be confirmed by viewing the nits attached to the hair under the microscope. A single application to the scalp of 1% Permethrin (NIX), gamma benzene hexachloride (Kwell), or pyrethrins (Rid) shampoo for 10 minutes is the preferred treatment. Malathion 0.5% applied for 12 hours and 10% crotamiton used for 24 hours are also effective. Soaking of the hair with vinegar may help the removal of nits with a fine-toothed comb. Combs, brushes, bedclothes, and headgear should be washed with hot water or soaked for an hour in alcohol. Contacts should be examined for lice and treated if affected.

Pediculosis corporis is caused by the body louse, which lives in the seams of clothing or bedding. The primary lesions are tiny red macules, papules, or wheals with a hemorrhagic central punctum but are usually obscured by secondary eczematization associated with intense pruritus. Body areas under belts, collars, and underwear are usually affected, with sparing of sites not covered with clothing. The diagnosis should be confirmed by finding the nits in the seams of clothing. Laundering of all clothing and bedding with hot water or dry cleaning and good hygiene are appropriate and usually adequate therapy. Contacts must also be examined carefully.

Pediculosis pubis is caused by the crab louse, which infests the skin and hair of the genital area, thighs, lower abdomen, and axillae. The crab louse may also infest the eyelashes (*pediculosis palpebrarum*), especially in prepubertal children. The louse is transmitted by sexual contact in the adolescent and by close contact with infested adults in the prepubertal child. Rarely, the crab louse is transmitted by clothing and bedding. Pruritus is often the initial symptom, followed by secondary eczematization or infection. With severe infestations, blue macules (maculae caeruleae) are occasionally noted on the thighs and lower abdomen.

The diagnosis of crab louse infestation is made by demonstrating the nits on affected hairs. For pubic lice, the area should be washed with gamma benzene hexachloride shampoo for 10 minutes and the nits removed, as in pediculosis capitis. Clothes and bedding should be washed. Pediculosis of the eyelashes should not be treated with pediculocides. The application of petrolatum three times daily for a week with removal of nits is the preferred therapy. Contacts should be sought and treated as well.

Mosquitoes are the most common cause of insect bites in children. The bites occur in warm weather on the exposed areas of skin. Erythematous papules and urticaria result, but regional adenopathy and fever are not associated unless secondary infection occurs. Occasionally, chronic papules and nodules develop that may resemble lymphoma by a histologic examination of skin biopsy specimens. The prevention of bites with insect repellents is the best management. If one is bitten, calamine lotion, oral antihistamines, and topical corticosteroids may be of limited value.

Flea bites are a frequent problem of children with cats and dogs. Since fleas may live as long as 2 years and survive for months without a blood meal, children without pets may develop flea bites after moving into a home that is infested with fleas because of pets in the home previously. Fleas live in upholstery, carpeting, and debris in corners and floor cracks. Flea bites are usually located on exposed areas or on body sites where clothing is snug. The lesions are irregularly grouped urticarial papules with a central hemorrhagic punctum. This *papular urticaria* is usually due to flea bites but has also been described following bites by mosquitoes, bedbugs, and other insects. The lesions may occasionally be vesicular, pustular, or bullous. Generalized flea bites may resemble chickenpox. Therapy includes the elimination of the fleas by treating animals and by the spraying of carpets, upholstery, floors, and corners with gamma benzene hexachloride dust or malathion. Calamine lotion, topical corticosteroids, and oral antihistamines may also be helpful.

Bedbugs cause pruritic lesions that are first noted in the morning. These insects live in the seams of mattresses and bed frames but may also be found on the floor and wallpaper near the bed. Grouped urticarial papules with a central punctum develop on exposed sites. Bedbugs can survive for up to a year without a meal. Extermination is the preferred therapy. *Fire ant bites* affect children in the southeastern United States. Painful wheals develop on exposed areas (especially the feet), followed by vesicles and pustules with a central punctum. Lesions are self-limited but often leave scarring. Systemic urticarial reactions may require systemic antihistamines and epinephrine. *Caterpillar dermatitis* is due to contact with hairs and spines. The reactions may range from a localized dermatitis with discrete pruritic maculopapules to painful wheals with vesicular or necrotic centers. Occasionally, marked local swelling, fever, nausea, headache, muscle cramps, seizures, and shock may occur. The hairs travel through air or by way of clothing to cause widespread dermatitis. The hairs can be seen by microscopic examination of skin scrapings, facilitating the diagnosis. Tape may be applied to the lesions to remove the offending hairs. Antihistamines, analgesics, ice packs, and systemic corticosteroids may be beneficial.

HELMINTHS

Swimmer's itch and *seabather's eruption* are due to immune responses to schistosomal cercariae. Seabather's eruption is usually acquired on the coast of Florida or in the Caribbean and manifests as pruritic urticarial papules on sites beneath the swimsuit. Children with seabather's eruption may have systemic reactions, with fever, malaise, nausea, vomiting, and headaches. Swimmer's itch develops after exposure to cercariae in fresh water, especially on the shores of Wisconsin and Michigan. The urticarial papules are usually located on exposed sites. Both reactions subside spontaneously after 1 to 2 weeks, often with transient residual hyperpigmentation. Therapy consists of antipruritic lotions and antihistamines.

Cutaneous larva migrans (*creeping eruption*) is a distinctive cutaneous eruption that results from the migration of larval hookworms (*Ancylostoma braziliense*) through the skin. The infestation is usually acquired from the sands of the Atlantic Ocean and Gulf of Mexico. The eruption begins with pruritus at the site of penetration, usually the buttocks, feet, lower legs, or hands. The lesions are slightly elevated

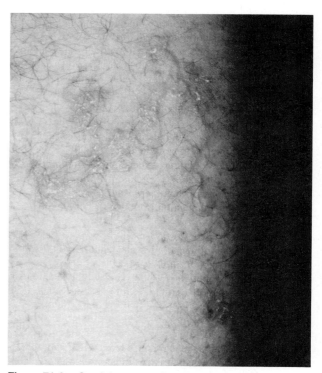

Figure 71-2. Serpiginous eruption of cutaneous larva migrans.

pink or flesh-colored serpentine tracts that progress slowly (Fig. 71-2). Vesicles or bullae may appear along the tract. The eruption may not begin for weeks to months after larval penetration. Systemic eosinophilia may be present. The rash is self-limited and usually clears after 1 to 4 weeks but may last as long as 6 months. Treatment consists of oral thiabendazole (25 mg/kg administered twice daily for 2 to 4 days) or topical 10% thiabendazole suspension applied four times daily for 7 days. Topical corticosteroids may alleviate the pruritus.

ANNOTATED BIBLIOGRAPHY

Honig PJ: Bites and parasites. Pediatr Clin North Am 30:563–581, 1983. (Comprehensive summary of bites and infestations in children.)

Hurwitz S: Erythema chronicum migrans and Lyme disease. Pediatr Dermatol 2:266–274, 1985. (Review of Lyme disease and its cutaneous manifestations.)

Orkin M, Maibach HI: This scabies pandemic. N Engl J Med 298:496–498, 1978. (Review of the diagnosis and management of scabies infections.)

Rasmussen JE: Pediculosis and the pediatrician. Pediatr Dermatol 2:74–79, 1984. (Current review of lice infestations and their therapy.)

Riley HD Jr: Rickettsial diseases and Rocky Mountain spotted fever. Curr Probl Pediatr 11:4–46 (part 1);3–37 (part 2), 1981. (Excellent review for the pediatrician of Rocky Mountain spotted fever.)

Stechenberg BW: Lyme disease: The latest Great Imitator. Pediatr Infect Dis J 7:402–409, 1988. (Good overview on Lyme disease from the pediatric perspective.)

72

Acne

Amy Paller

Acne is one of the most common problems of teenagers. Although it is not a serious medical problem, the psychological effects of inflammation and disfiguring scars may be significant. The typical lesions of acne vulgaris are blackheads, whiteheads, and localized areas of inflammation.

PATHOPHYSIOLOGY

Many factors appear to influence the occurrence and severity of acne. These include (1) increased sebum production by sebaceous glands during and after puberty, (2) bacteria, (3) partial obstruction of the pilosebaceous canal, (4) hormonal influences, and (5) genetics.

The pilosebaceous follicles contain multilobulated sebaceous glands that discharge their contents (i.e., sebum) at the skin surface. Under the influence of androgenic hormones,

sebum production by sebaceous glands increases at the time of puberty. At this time the skin becomes oily and the early lesions of acne begin. The role of sebum in the pathogenesis of acne, however, is poorly understood. In the pilosebaceous canal, the triglycerides of sebum are cleaved into free fatty acids by lipase from the anaerobic bacterium *Propionibacterium acnes,* an organism that also increases dramatically at the time of puberty. These free fatty acids, as well as prostaglandins and other bacterial products, are irritating and chemotactic. Sebum, however, is not the only participant in the formation of acne lesions, since its production continues without change in content or quantity throughout adulthood, despite the disappearance of acne lesions.

Partial obstruction of the follicle also contributes to the formation of lesions. The precursor lesion of acne, the *comedo,* forms in the lower portion of the hair follicle. Rather than the normal disintegration and shedding of horny cells to the surface of the hair follicle, the cells of patients with acne adhere to each other to form the plug of the comedo. The mixture of sebum, horny cells, and *P. acnes* bacteria distends the hair follicle and attracts inflammatory cells. Although the hair follicle is distended, there is not enough pressure to rupture; thus leakage of inflammatory materials, including free fatty acids, results.

Androgens, especially free testosterone and its tissue product dihydrotestosterone (DHT) and the androgenic adrenal steroid dihydroepiandrosterone sulfate (DHEAS) increase the size of sebaceous glands and the production and lipid content of sebum. Finally, genetic factors are involved in determining the occurrence and extent of acne. Identical twins are usually concordant for the expression of acne, and offspring tend to follow the pattern of their parents.

CLINICAL PRESENTATION

Patients with *acne vulgaris* (common acne) may have several types of lesions, any of which may predominate. These include open and closed comedones, inflammatory papules and pustules, and nodulocystic lesions. In early adolescence, acne is usually comedonal and confined to the face. By the mid teens, inflammatory acne with papules and pustules is the most common form, and the chest and back become more involved.

The microcomedo, the initial lesion of acne, represents the hair follicle distended by the accumulated horny cell material, lipids, and bacteria. The closed comedo, or whitehead, is a skin-colored slightly palpable lesion (1 to 3 mm) without a readily visible central pore. Closed comedones have been called "the time bombs of acne" because they often enlarge to form the inflammatory papules or pustules. Alternatively, they may remain quiescent for months or evolve into open comedones. Open comedones, or blackheads, have a wide pore opening filled with black material. This material is melanin and oxidized lipids, not dirt. These open comedones tend to be more stable than the closed comedones and rarely become inflamed.

The papules and pustules of inflammatory acne develop in distended, partially obstructed follicles following the increased permeability of the follicular wall and the influx of inflammatory cells. Although papules and pustules may be superficial and resolve quickly, deeper lesions that form in the lower portion of the hair canal often take weeks to heal. *Nodulocystic lesions* are warm and tender abscesses. They occur most commonly along the line of the jaw, earlobes, and neck and result from the fusion of adjacent deep pustules. Acne cysts require 2 to 3 months to heal by granulation tissue formation and scarring.

Acne scars are the outcome of inflammatory acne. The closed and open comedones may resolve as accentuated pores, but they do not leave scars unless secondary inflammation occurs. The scars may vary in shape and extent. Ice pick scars are small, deep pits that result from inflammatory papules and pustules. Nodulocystic lesions may leave larger disfiguring scars. The most common reason for scarring of superficial lesions is self-inflicted trauma from scratching, squeezing lesions, and extracting them with fingernails (Fig. 72-1). This self-induced trauma tends to leave small, irregular, and often linear scars. Keloids may develop, especially in black teenagers, on the anterior chest, back, and neck and occasionally on the face. Rarely, calcification of scars occurs as small blue nodules that may eventually resolve by extrusion of the calcific material.

In dark-skinned persons, inflammatory lesions often resolve with hyperpigmentation. This postinflammatory hyperpigmentation tends to clear spontaneously after months to years but may be exacerbated by the continued development of inflammatory lesions and sun exposure.

SPECIAL CLINICAL FORMS OF ACNE

Acne conglobata is a form of severe nodulocystic acne that occurs in 3% of white male adolescents. Multiple nodules fuse, forming large, irregular tender purple nodules that discharge purulent material from the resultant sinus tracts. Nontender large multipored open comedones cluster among these draining nodules and sinuses. The back is the typical site of acne conglobata, but the face, upper arms, thigh, and buttocks are also frequently involved. Pustules and cysts may form as well. Acne conglobata often remains active into the third decade of life and leaves severe scarring.

Acne fulminans is a rare form of acne associated with fever, polyarthritis, leukocytosis, and anemia. Large necrotic nodules that drain a gelatinous material are found on the back and upper chest and resolve as deep ulcerations.

Acne neonatorum manifests as tiny yellow papules on the forehead, cheeks, and nose of newborns due to sebaceous gland hyperactivity under the influence of maternal hormones. Papules and pustules are occasionally present. The acne resolves spontaneously when the maternal hormones disappear after 1 or 2 months.

Infantile acne develops after the first 3 months of life and usually resolves spontaneously by 18 months of age. Most commonly, boys with a strong family history of severe acne are affected. Typical lesions are comedones and papules on the cheeks, and occasionally pustules are present. Excessive use of oils and lotions applied to the infant's skin must be considered if there is a predominance of comedones. The pathogenesis of infantile acne is unknown, but a transient increase in gonadal production of testosterone has been postulated. An underlying endocrinologic abnormality should be considered if numerous pustules are present. Therapy is usually not required, and only mild keratolytic agents should be used if the acne is extensive.

Cosmetic acne is caused by oily moisturizers, foundations, and hair preparations. The lesions that result are closed comedones that may become inflammatory papulopustules. Most moisturizers are comedogenic, but cocoa butter is a common cause of comedogenic acne. Makeups that have an oily base and moisturizers will usually cause acne on the cheeks, whereas hair preparations tend to stimulate the formation of acne lesions on the forehead (pomade acne). This form of acne can be puzzling, because patients often use a variety of oily preparations during a period of time and lesions are slow to develop. Cosmetic acne may take 6 to 8 months to resolve following the discontinuation of the inciting agent.

Occlusion-induced acne (mechanical acne) is the exacerbation of mild acne by mechanical factors that rub and occlude. Acne on the chin may be aggravated by resting the

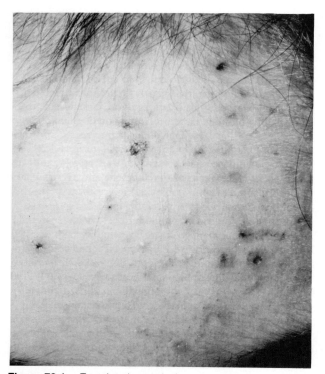

Figure 72-1. Excoriated acne lesions that became scars in a teenaged girl with otherwise mild comedonal acne.

chin on the hand while studying or by chin straps. Forehead lesions may become inflamed by sweatbands, hats, or excessive combing of the hair. Neck lesions may be aggravated by shirt collars or turtle-neck sweaters. Clusters of lesions in a particular pattern may suggest this type of acne.

Occupational acne is prevalent in teenagers who work at fast-food restaurants or as car mechanics. Comedonal acne tends to develop from working over frying oils or contact with greases from car lubricants or other petroleum products. *Chloracne* has rarely developed in children following exposure to chlorinated hydrocarbons at toxic waste dumps near industries.

Drug-induced acne most commonly occurs from the use of oral or fluorinated topical corticosteroids. Within a few weeks after therapy begins, crops of papulopustules without comedones appear. Androgens, gonadotropins, and adrenocorticotropins may produce lesions more typical of the mixed pattern of acne vulgaris. Other drugs that induce or aggravate acne are lithium, phenobarbital, phenytoin, trimethadione, isoniazid, rifampin, iodides, and bromides. Drug-induced acne tends to appear suddenly; it may be characterized by large numbers of lesions and involves unusual areas, such as the upper arms and lower back.

Gram-negative folliculitis develops in patients who have taken oral broad-spectrum antibiotics for long periods of time. As a result of changes in bacterial flora, pustules and cysts appear that do not respond to increased doses of antibiotics. Gram-negative organisms are most common, especially klebsiella, enterobacter, and proteus.

DIFFERENTIAL DIAGNOSIS

The lesions of acne are easily recognizable; the underlying factors that exacerbate the acne may be more difficult to determine. Occasionally, patients with tuberous sclerosis and adenoma sebaceum may be mistakenly thought to have acne. Patients with unusual or severe forms of acne may have endocrinologic abnormalities; other signs include hirsutism, precocious puberty, irregularities in menses, and features of Cushing's disease (see also Chap. 88, "Precocious Puberty").

WORK-UP

Patients with acne should be questioned about the duration and typical severity of their acne and the effect and duration of medications that have been tried in the past, including over-the-counter medications. Possible use of other oral and topical medications must be elicited, especially oral contraceptives and topical fluorinated corticosteroids. Knowledge of the use of moisturizers, makeup, and hair pomades is important for the pediatrician. Finally, the history of other medical abnormalities and menses of adolescent girls should be ascertained. A physical examination may be limited to the face, neck, chest, and back, unless the history suggests an underlying problem that requires a more extensive examination. The predominant lesional types will direct management. Routine laboratory testing is unnecessary. Other evidence of androgenic effects should prompt the evaluation of adrenal and gonadal function.

TREATMENT

Several misconceptions about acne must be dispelled. First, dietary factors including chocolate and carbohydrates are probably insignificant. If a patient believes, however, that a particular food aggravates the acne, it is best to eliminate that food. Second, although topical therapeutic agents cause dryness, they are more effective than harsh soaps, scrubs, and frequent washing. The use of scrubs should be discouraged to lower the risk of irritation by prescribed topical agents and prevent the risk of transformation of comedones into inflammatory lesions. Finally, moisturizers and oil-based makeups exacerbate acne by plugging the follicles and encouraging comedo formation. Patients should be advised to use water-based makeup or none at all. Noncomedogenic lotions, such as Nutraderm lotion, may be used for excessive dryness without causing increased comedonal acne.

Treatment regimens should be directed toward (1) altering the pattern of keratinization, (2) decreasing sebum production, (3) decreasing the population of *P. acnes,* and (4) producing an anti-inflammatory effect. *Benzoyl peroxide* preparations are the most commonly used acne medications. Benzoyl peroxide is an oxidizing agent with bacteriostatic properties. As a primary irritant, it also increases blood flow to the lesional skin and accelerates healing. In addition, benzoyl peroxide is keratolytic and decreases the adherence of follicular horny cells. As a result, benzoyl peroxide is useful for both comedonal and inflammatory acne. Benzoyl peroxide causes contact allergy in 2.5% of patients, resulting in pruritus, erythema, and periorbital edema. The most common reaction is an irritant reaction, which often causes postinflammatory hyperpigmentation in black patients. Improvement in acne may be seen within 1 to 3 weeks.

Retinoic acid, a metabolite of vitamin A, is an exfoliant and irritant that also increases blood flow to the skin. It is best used as a comedolytic agent; it increases the turnover of pilosebaceous epithelial cells and prevents the adherence of horny layer cells. Not uncommonly, pustules may develop as comedones are expelled 3 to 4 weeks after the onset of therapy; this is not an indication to stop the agent. Secondary hyperpigmentation may result in black and Asian patients. Patients using retinoic acid may be more susceptible to sunburn and should be advised to use sunscreens during sun exposure. Good results are seen in up to 70% of patients within 3 months.

Other keratolytic agents, such as 5% to 10% salicylic acid or 3% to 6% sulfur preparations, may be helpful for patients who cannot tolerate benzoyl peroxide or retinoic acid. The effect of sunlight is mostly keratolytic, although lesions may be obscured by the resultant erythema and pigmentation. The routine use of ultraviolet light to treat acne is not indicated in view of the potential carcinogenic effect.

Topical and systemic antibiotics are helpful for inflammatory acne as antibacterial and anti-inflammatory agents. Topical antibiotics should be used for patients with mild to moderate inflammatory acne and for patients who cannot tolerate systemic antibiotics. Topical preparations of clindamycin, erythromycin, and tetracycline are available. The only significant side effect of topical preparations is dryness, especially from those with alcohol bases. The risk of pseudomembranous colitis from topical clindamycin is remote. Topical tetracycline produces a yellow fluorescence under black light.

Systemic antibiotics should be introduced for moderate to severe inflammatory acne. Tetracycline, doxycycline, erythromycin, and minocycline accumulate in the pilosebaceous canal, decrease the population of *P. acnes,* and inhibit neutrophil chemotaxis. Side effects are usually gastrointestinal intolerance and vaginal candidiasis. Unusual side effects of minocycline include dizziness and hyperpigmentation, and photosensitivity is not uncommon with doxycycline. Tetracycline, doxycycline, and minocycline should not be prescribed for pregnant adolescents. Systemic antibiotics must be given for 2 to 3 months before effectiveness is determined. The dosage should be tapered after this time.

Isotretinoin (Accutane) use should be restricted to patients with recalcitrant cystic acne. Accutane causes involution of sebaceous glands, lowers the colonization by *P. acnes,* and limits keratinization of the follicle. Patients are generally treated for 4 to 5 months at doses of 0.5 to 2 mg/kg/d. Facial cysts tend to respond first, often within the first month; truncal lesions usually require 3 to 4 months of medication. The effect of isotretinoin continues, often indefinitely, after discontinuation of the drug. The major side effects are dose related and include dry skin and lips, epistaxis, conjunctivitis, and, occasionally, musculoskeletal complaints, rashes, increased photosensitivity, peeling of the palms and soles, and headache. Triglyceride levels become elevated in 25% of patients; they may be diminished by a low-fat diet and avoidance of alcohol or a lower dosage of medication; and they return to normal following cessation of isotretinoin. Laboratory parameters should be checked monthly while taking the drug. Accutane is absolutely contraindicated in pregnancy because of its teratogenicity. Fertile female patients should be tested for pregnancy and use an effective form of contraception while taking isotretinoin and for at least 1 month following its discontinuation.

Doses of more than 50 μg of ethinyl estradiol or its equivalent suppress sebum production and diminish acne after 2 to 3 months. Therefore, the administration of oral contraceptives with higher amounts of estrogen (e.g., Enovid-E, Ovulen) may be considered for patients who require birth control or adolescent girls with severe, recalcitrant acne. Antiandrogens, such as spironolactone and cyproterone ace-

tate, have controlled acne in women with elevated androgen levels. Dapsone is an anti-inflammatory agent that has proved useful for severe cystic acne or acne conglobata but is too toxic to use before other treatment modalities. Finally, oral zinc sulfate may be a useful adjunctive agent for inflammatory acne.

Several physical modalities are helpful in the management of acne and its sequelae. Severely inflamed papular and cystic lesions respond within 48 hours to intralesional injection of triamcinolone acetonide. Atrophy rarely results if the amount injected is less than 0.5 mg/cm^2. The superficial scarring of acne may be treated with chemical peels, such as trichloroacetic acid. Deeper scars may be eliminated by dermabrasion, in which the epidermis and upper dermis are removed to the level of the scar. Side effects include erythema, milia, pigmentary alterations, and hypertrophic scarring. Finally, bovine collagen may be injected into deep, ice pick scars to raise them to skin level.

INDICATIONS FOR REFERRAL

In most patients acne of mild severity will respond to topical agents. Patients who require long-term systemic antibiotics, isotretinoin, or other systemic agents or physical modalities of treatment are best referred to a dermatologist.

ANNOTATED BIBLIOGRAPHY

Esterly NB, Furey NL: Acne: Current concepts. Pediatrics 62:1044–1055, 1978. (Review with good descriptions of clinical lesions.)

Matsuoka LY: Acne. J Pediatr 103:849–854, 1983. (Includes treatment modalities.)

Stern RS, Rosa F, Baum C: Isotretinoin and pregnancy. J Am Acad Dermatol 10:851–854, 1984. (Good review of the congenital anomalies associated with isotretinoin use during the first trimester of pregnancy.)

Tunnessen WW Jr: Acne: An approach to therapy for the pediatrician. Curr Probl Pediatr 14(5):6–36, 1984. (Well written, general review.)

73

Disorders of Hair and Nails

Amy Paller

The assessment of a child with abnormalities of the hair and nails requires a detailed history and a careful clinical examination, often including a microscopic examination of hair and fungal cultures of hair and nails (see the display, Assessment of the Child With Hair Loss). The hair texture, style, length, and the distribution of hair loss should be noted. The pattern and extent of nail changes should also be

Assessment of the Child With Hair Loss

HISTORY

Duration of hair loss, pattern, breakage vs. "by the roots"
Past health, use of medications, topical preparations, and diet
Use of hair care products and hair treatments
Other abnormalities of skin, nails, teeth, and sweating
Family history of hair problems and ectodermal abnormalities

EXAMINATION

Pattern of hair loss
Underlying scalp abnormalities
Hair texture, breakage, lengths, and hair tips
"Pull test"
Hirsutism elsewhere, acne, and virilization
Other ectodermal defects by examination

MICROSCOPIC EXAMINATION OF HAIR

Potassium hydroxide examination (and culture) if tinea capitis is
suspected
Mount to examine for hair shaft defects

SCALP BIOPSY

For scarring alopecia and some nonscarring alopecia (may help
to diagnose trichotillomania, alopecia areata)

OTHER LABORATORY TESTS

Sweat quantitation and dental radiographs for ectodermal
dysplasia
Thyroid hormones and complete blood cell count for telogen
effluvium
Thyroid hormones and antibodies if indicated with alopecia
areata

determined. Any child with hair and nail abnormalities
should also be questioned and examined carefully for other
defects, especially ectodermal defects.

HAIR DEFECTS

To understand hair disorders, it is important to review the
three phases of the human hair growth cycle. *Anagen* is the
period of hair growth that lasts 2 to 6 years and includes
90% of hairs. *Catagen* is a transition state that lasts a few
days. *Telogen* is a resting phase that lasts about 3 months
and includes 10% of hairs. The resting hair is shed as the
new anagen hair emerges. The normal scalp has about
100,000 hairs and hair grows at a rate of 1 cm each month.
The hair growth cycle is not synchronized, and it is normal
to lose 50 to 100 hairs a day, especially with shampooing.
Before hair loss becomes clinically evident, 25% to 50% of
hair must be lost.

There are two forms of physiologic hair loss: shedding
of the newborn and temporal recession at puberty. In utero,
silky hair called *lanugo* hair develops over the entire fetus.
Lanugo hair is shed in utero and replaced during the sixth
to eighth month of gestation by vellus hair, except on the
scalp, eyebrows, and eyelashes, where lanugo hair is replaced by terminal hair. This hair is shed during the first
year of life and is replaced by thicker, darker hair. The other
physiologic form of hair loss is due to the increase in androgen levels in both boys and girls at puberty that results in
replacement of vellus hairs with terminal hairs, particularly
from the frontal scalp to the vertex.

Most hair loss in children is acquired, as a result of fungal infections, trauma, or alopecia areata. Fungal infections
are usually characterized by focal or diffuse hair loss with
underlying scalp scaling and erythema (see Chap. 66). If
the diagnosis of tinea capitis is considered, potassium hydroxide (KOH) examination and fungal cultures should always be performed. Excessive traction on the hair from
tight ponytails or braiding (especially "corn-rowing") often
results in hair loss at the sites of maximal traction, such as
at the margins of the hairline, at the part line, or scattered
throughout the scalp. The hair usually regrows if the traction is eliminated, unless chronic traction produces fibrosis
and permanent injury. Similarly, hair may be lost by friction
(usually rubbing the occipital scalp on the bed sheets in infants) that results in hair breakage or by avulsion of clumps
of hair by playmates. Chemical or physical trauma to the
hair from hair dyes, straighteners, permanent wave treatments, and ironing the hair may cause hair breakage or contact dermatitis of the scalp, resulting in hair loss that may
take years to resolve. Occasionally, children compulsively
pull out hairs of the scalp, eyelashes, or eyebrows, a condition termed *trichotillomania*. The patches of hair loss are
irregular, with short hairs of various lengths. On the scalp
the occipital hair is usually spared. The disorder may be
confused with alopecia areata, and a scalp biopsy may be
required to differentiate the conditions. The histopathologic
features of trichotillomania include evidence of follicular
trauma, such as hemorrhage, increased numbers of catagen
hairs, soft keratin material within the follicles, and minimal
inflammation. Many cases resolve spontaneously, but it is
important to make the proper diagnosis and to explain to the
parents that the disorder is due to a habit. Children who
are severely affected should be referred for a psychiatric
evaluation.

Alopecia areata is a common disorder characterized by
the sudden onset of well-circumscribed patches of nonscarring alopecia (Fig. 73-1). Ten to 20% of affected persons
have a positive family history of alopecia areata. The cause
of alopecia areata is unknown, but it is suspected to be an
autoimmune disorder because of the high incidence of associated autoantibodies, especially antibodies against thy-
roglobulin, parietal cells, and the adrenal gland, and of associated autoimmune disorders.

The typical pattern of alopecia areata is the sudden de-

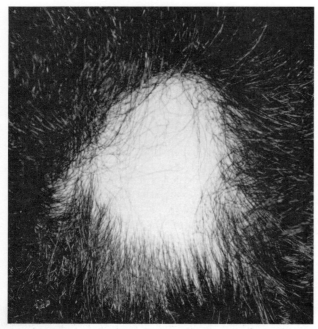

Figure 73-1. Well-demarcated patch of alopecia areata with normal underlying scalp.

velopment of one or more round patches of alopecia with an underlying scalp that is normal. At the margin of the patches, short hairs with an attenuated bulb ("exclamation mark" hairs) may be found. Disease activity can be assessed by the "pull test" in which hair at the periphery is grasped and pulled. Hair comes out easily if the disorder is active at that area. The patches of alopecia usually occur on the scalp but can appear in any hair-bearing area. *Alopecia areata totalis* is alopecia of the entire scalp and *alopecia areata universalis* is the complete loss of all body hair as well. The ophiasis pattern of alopecia areata is alopecia that extends from the occipital area around the sides of the scalp to the front in a band. Rarely, diffuse thinning of the scalp hair occurs and may be confused with telogen effluvium. Nail pitting may develop in 10% to 20% of patients with alopecia areata, but the dystrophy is rarely severe.

The diagnosis of alopecia areata is usually based on the clinical appearance. The disorder may be confused occasionally with the black dot form of tinea capitis or with trichotillomania. A KOH examination, fungal culture, and scalp biopsy aid in distinguishing these disorders. A histopathologic examination of the scalp biopsy of alopecia areata shows small atrophic hair follicles, sometimes with inflammatory cell infiltrates surrounding the hair bulbs. Children with alopecia areata should be examined for the concurrent possibility of Hashimoto's thyroiditis, vitiligo, and collagen vascular disease.

The course of alopecia areata is unpredictable. Most patients show hair regrowth within 1 to 2 years after the onset, especially with the limited forms of alopecia. Children with

alopecia areata need encouragement and, at times, psychologic counseling. The suggestion of a wig may immediately improve the appearance and prevent children from being teased while the disorder resolves or persists. There are no clearly effective forms of therapy, but efficacy may be difficult to assess in view of the high rate of spontaneous resolution. For younger children, moderate- to high-potency topical corticosteroids, topical anthralin preparations, and topical minoxidil are the available treatments. Therapy for at least 6 months is often necessary. In older children, intralesional triamcinolone is most effective if the disease is limited to a few patches. Systemic corticosteroids should not be used. Other possible treatment modalities for older children include the induction of contact allergic dermatitis, such as with dicypterone, psoralens and ultraviolet A light (PUVA) and inosiplex (an immunostimulant).

Anagen effluvium and telogen effluvium are conditions of diffuse hair loss that affect anagen hairs and telogen hairs, respectively. Cancer chemotherapy is the most common reason for loss of anagen hairs in children, with loss of 80% to 90% of the hair occurring 7 to 14 days after use of the drugs. Telogen effluvium occurs 2 to 4 months after injury. The causes in children for later telogen effluvium include high fever, severe infection, illness or psychological stress, surgery, hypothyroidism or hyperthyroidism, pernicious anemia, and nutritional deficiency. In addition, several medications may cause telogen effluvium, such as anticonvulsants, anticoagulants (as in rat poison), retinoids, and hormones. The numbers of telogen hairs increase from 10% to between 30% and 50% in children with telogen effluvium. The hair loss of both anagen and telogen effluvium resolves after the underlying cause is eliminated.

Several congenital disorders are associated with hair loss. The hair may be totally absent (alopecia) or sparse (hypotrichosis). Many of these disorders are due to hair shaft abnormalities, and the diagnosis may be made by an examination of the hair under the microscope. Hair anomalies associated with hair shaft fragility include monilethrix, trichorrhexis nodosa, trichorrhexis invaginata, pili torti, and trichothiodystrophy. Hair shaft abnormalities without associated hair fragility include pili annulati, pseudopili annulati, woolly hair, and the uncombable hair syndrome.

Monilethrix or beaded hair is usually an autosomal dominant condition. The hair is sparse and breaks easily, so that the scalp is covered by short hairs. The scalp tends to have a rough appearance, especially at the occiput, due to follicular hyperkeratosis. Microscopic examination of hair shafts shows uniform beading along the shaft with fractures in internodal areas. Patients may improve spontaneously at puberty. There is no effective treatment.

Trichorrhexis nodosa or trichoclasis is characterized clinically by white nodules on the hair shafts. The condition is usually acquired as a result of trauma, and responds to the elimination of vigorous grooming habits. Patients may have friable, brittle hair that shows the nodules of trichorrhexis nodosa. By microscopy, the hair shafts of trichorrhexis nodosa show brushlike fractures. Trichorrhexis nodosa is seen in patients with arginosuccinic aciduria.

Trichorrhexis invaginata (bamboo hair) is a hair defect characterized by jointlike deformities of the hair shaft. The hair is short, dry, dull, and sparse. The defect tends to be present by infancy and usually persists. This type of hair defect is associated with Netherton's syndrome, an autosomal recessive disorder with nonbullous ichthyosiform erythroderma or ichthyosis linearis circumflex, nail dystrophy, and atopy with eczema, urticaria, angioneurotic edema, asthma, and rhinitis.

Pili torti or twisted hairs is a hair condition characterized by hair shafts that are twisted 180 degrees on their own axes at irregular intervals. The defect is usually present by early infancy, and the hairs are typically fragile. As an isolated defect, pili torti is inherited as an autosomal dominant disorder. Pili torti has also been described in association with Menkes' syndrome.

Trichothiodystrophy (also called low sulfur hair syndrome) is an autosomal recessive neuroectodermal defect with sparse and brittle scalp hair, eyebrows, and eyelashes. Amino acid analysis of hairs shows a low concentration of the sulfur-containing amino acid cystine. The fingernails and toenails of patients are often brittle and dystrophic, with spoon-shaped deformities (koilonychia). Trichothiodystrophy may be part of BIDS syndrome (*b*rittle hair, *i*ntellectual impairment, *d*ecreased fertility, and *s*hort stature).

Pili annulati or ringed hair is an autosomal dominant defect of hair noted shortly after birth. The hair shaft is not fragile, and bands of hair appear to be highlighted. By microscopy, the hair has alternating light and dark bands, due to air-filled cavities within the cortex and medulla of the hair shaft. There is no effective therapy. *Pseudopili annulati* is a variant in which light bands are seen at irregular intervals along the hair shaft, especially in blond persons, due to twisting of the hair shaft and variations in cross-sectional diameter.

Woolly hair is a defect involving the entire scalp with fine, dry, curly hair. This hereditary defect must be differentiated from the woolly hair nevus, which is a localized patch of curly hair and is not a hereditary disorder. The *uncombable hair syndrome* (pili trianguli canaliculi, spun glass hair syndrome) appears soon after birth as thick bundles of hair that grow in all directions and cannot be arranged by combing. The hair is light in color, dry, and has a characteristic sheen, but it grows normally and is not fragile. The main differential diagnosis of the uncombable hair syndrome is woolly hair.

Generalized hair loss may also be due to metabolic abnormalities. *Multiple carboxylase deficiency* is a group of autosomal recessive disorders involving the enzymes that metabolize branched-chain amino acids, including propionyl CoA carboxylase, β-methyl crotonyl CoA carboxylase, and pyruvate carboxylase. All of these enzymes require biotin as a cofactor. Patients with the infantile form exhibit cutaneous manifestations, including sparse hair, periorifi-

cial dermatitis, and severe mucocutaneous candidiasis. Other features include progressive ataxia, seizures, psychomotor retardation, keratoconjunctivitis, and lactic acidosis. Urine testing for organic acids reveals elevated levels of substrate metabolites. Serum biotin levels are decreased or normal, and patients may have hypoglycemia and hyperammonuria. The administration of biotin in doses of 10 to 40 mg daily corrects the immunologic abnormalities and promotes normal hair growth. Alopecia may also be a feature of acrodermatitis enteropathica and arginosuccinic aciduria.

All of the disorders discussed are nonscarring types of alopecia. Scarring alopecia is unusual in children and may be due to developmental defects (such as aplasia cutis congenita), physical injury, infection, lichen planus, lupus erythematosus, scleroderma, sarcoidosis, and neoplasm. *Aplasia cutis congenita* is a rare congenital defect characterized by the absence of circumscribed areas of skin and appendages. The lesion(s) of aplasia cutis are present at birth, usually as a solitary, well-circumscribed hairless area at the midline of the scalp by the vertex or near the sagittal suture. Less commonly, the lesions are located elsewhere on the scalp, and rarely on the face, trunk, or limbs. Lesions on the trunk or limbs are commonly multiple, extensive, and symmetric. The skin usually appears ulcerated with crusting but may be bullous, membranous, or healed at the time of birth. As the aplasia heals, it is replaced by a smooth, atrophic, gray parchment-like scar. Although aplasia cutis is usually an isolated abnormality, 20% of patients have a defect of the underlying cranial bone and 13% have limb malformations.

Aplasia cutis congenita is most easily confused with trauma, usually due to a fetal monitor or to forceps injury. Occasionally, other traumatic injuries due to chemical or thermal burns or scarring from needles or amniocentesis must be distinguished. The well-circumscribed hairless lesion of aplasia cutis can also resemble the congenital hairless sebaceus nevus of Jadassohn. A histopathologic examination of skin biopsy sections allows the diagnosis to be made. The healed, scarred lesions of aplasia cutis must also be contrasted to those of discoid lupus erythematosus, morphea, and the more widespread congenital erosive and vesicular dermatosis.

NAIL DISORDERS

The nails grow continuously throughout life and are not normally shed. The rate of nail growth varies from 0.5 to 1.2 mm per week, with the growth rate of toenails almost one half that of fingernails. Dystrophic nails may result from congenital disorders, such as the nail-patella syndrome and pachyonychia congenita, or may be due to acquired disorders, such as eczema (Chap. 59), infections (Chap. 66), psoriasis (Chap. 64), lichen planus (Chap. 63), alopecia areata, or twenty nail dystrophy. Only the disorders that are not discussed elsewhere in this text are considered here.

The *nail-patella syndrome* (osteo-onychodysplasia, nail-patella-elbow syndrome) is an autosomal dominant defect that is characterized by the absence or hypoplasia of the patella and nails, subluxation of the radial heads, and renal dysplasia with chronic glomerulonephritis. Less common findings are thickened scapulae, iliac horns, and hyperextensible joints. Triangular lunulae are the most characteristic nail abnormality, although softening, spoon nails, discoloration, and narrowing of nails are common as well. The renal abnormalities include proteinuria, hematuria, and decreased renal clearance; these changes are generally asymptomatic, and the prognosis is usually good.

Pachyonychia congenita or the Jadassohn-Lewandowsky syndrome usually follows an autosomal dominant inheritance pattern. The nails show marked subungual hyperkeratosis with thickening of the distal part of the nail so that the nail is lifted off the nailbed. These changes are progressive and often begin as yellowing of the nail or recurrent nail loss at birth or during the first year of life but have been reported to begin as late as the teenage years. All of the nails tend to be involved. Paronychial inflammation may precede or accompany the nail changes. Associated abnormalities include hyperhidrosis and thickening of the palm and soles, follicular keratoses that resemble keratosis pilaris, blisters of the hands and feet, hypotrichosis and multiple cysts (steatocystoma multiplex). Later in childhood, lesions may appear on the trunk, axillae, neck, scalp, and face. Leukokeratosis of the tongue or buccal mucosa is common, and dental and eye anomalies have occasionally been reported in patients with pachyonychia congenita. The nail thickening is persistent, and management may be difficult. Most patients keep the nails short and file the nails down to a more normal thickness for ease of fine manipulation with the fingers and for cosmetic reasons.

Twenty nail dystrophy is an idiopathic nail disorder of childhood that is characterized by whitening and ridging of all 20 nails. The condition is self-limited and resolves within a few years. Therapy is not usually helpful. Other diagnoses, such as psoriasis, lichen planus, and alopecia areata, should be considered. Nail biopsy is traumatic for a child and without other evidence of these mucocutaneous disorders, the diagnosis of twenty nail dystrophy should be made.

DISORDERS OF BOTH HAIR AND NAILS: ECTODERMAL DYSPLASIAS

Ectodermal dysplasia is a term for a number of syndromes that show alterations of ectodermal structures and function, including the skin, hair, nails, teeth, and eccrine glands. Ectodermal dysplasias must be congenital and affect at least two tissues of ectodermal origin. The most common forms of ectodermal dysplasia are *hypohidrotic ectodermal dysplasia* and *hidrotic ectodermal dysplasia*. Hypohidrotic (an-hidrotic) ectodermal dysplasia is the most easily recognizable of the ectodermal dysplasias. The majority of persons who have this complete syndrome are male, with an inheritance pattern consistent with an X-linked recessive mode. Children with hypohidrotic ectodermal dysplasia have a characteristic combination of defective dentition, hypotrichosis, and a typical facies that is so easily recognizable that these affected children more closely resemble one another than they do their own siblings. The most serious feature in affected infants is the inability to sweat adequately because of deficient numbers of eccrine glands. As a result, infants have recurrent high fevers and cutaneous erythema, especially in hot weather following exercise. Febrile convulsions may be associated with the high fevers. The hair is sparse, fine, lighter in color than that of other family members, and often unruly. Complete alopecia is unusual. The nails are usually normal, but the teeth are typically decreased in number and anomalous, with conical or peg-shaped teeth, discolored incisors, and malocclusion. The facial features include frontal bossing, prominent supraorbital ridges, wrinkling and hyperpigmentation of periorbital skin, a depressed nasal bridge (saddle nose deformity), a small nose with hypoplastic alae nasi, underdeveloped maxilla, pointed chin, protuberant lips, and ears that are low lying, anteriorly placed, and pointed. Ectodermal glands other than eccrine glands are also hypoplastic, leading to atrophic rhinitis, dry mouth, pharyngitis, dysphagia, otitis media, recurrent respiratory tract infections, chronic laryngitis, and defective lacrimal gland function. Children with hypohidrotic ectodermal dysplasia have an increased frequency of atopic dermatitis.

The classic form of hidrotic ectodermal dysplasia (Clouston's syndrome) is an autosomal dominant disorder. The major clinical features are dystrophic nails, hypotrichosis, and palmoplantar keratoderma. Sweating is quantitatively normal, and dental abnormalities are rare.

ANNOTATED BIBLIOGRAPHY

Goldsmith LA: An approach to the diagnosis of genetic hair disorders. Prog Dermatol 18:1–7, 1984. (Differential diagnostic approach to hair disorders.)

Mitchell AJ, Krull EA: Alopecia areata: Pathogenesis and treatment. J Am Acad Dermatol 11:763–775, 1984. (Current review of alopecia areata and its management.)

Norton LA: Nail disorders. J Am Acad Dermatol 2:451–467, 1980. (Review of nail disorders.)

Reed WB, Lopez DA, Landing B: Clinical spectrum of anhidrotic ectodermal dysplasia. Arch Dermatol 102:134–143, 1970. (Good discussion of the problems of hypohidrotic ectodermal dysplasia.)

Solomon LM, Keuer EJ: The ectodermal dysplasias. Arch Dermatol 116:1295–1299, 1980. (Review of the various forms of ectodermal dysplasia.)

Stroud JD: Hair loss in children. Pediatr Clin North Am 30:641–657, 1983 (Current review of causes of alopecia in children.)

11

EAR, NOSE, AND THROAT PROBLEMS

74

Diseases of the External Ear

Howard G. Smith

Otitis externa refers to an inflammatory disease of the external structures of the ear including the auricle or pinna and its surrounding skin and both the cartilaginous and the osseous portions of the external auditory canal. The inflammatory process may be produced by primary tissue infections due to bacteria, fungi, yeasts, viruses, or parasites. Inflammation with or without secondary infection may also be produced by various types of trauma or epithelial hypersensitivity reactions. These conditions may produce exquisite pain and tenderness.

PATHOPHYSIOLOGY

Infections of the auricle and periauricular tissues are usually caused by streptococci or staphylococci and are initiated by traumatic epithelial breakdown that permits the entry of the microorganism. This trauma may be produced by penetration of foreign objects or by pressure from prosthetic devices such as hearing aid molds. The resultant infection may be a generalized cellulitis or infection of an obstructed sebaceous gland in the pinna. In either case, the infection may proceed to abscess formation.

Both the auricle and the external ear canal may be injured or invaded by insects. Enzymes, toxins, or microorganisms released by the insect injure the skin directly and may permit other microorganisms to enter and produce secondary infections.

Four factors contribute to the development of external canal infections:

1. The loss of the protective, hydrophobic, acidic cerumen and lipid epithelial coatings following exposure of canal linings to moisture during periods of high environmental temperature and relative humidity, or during periods of skin immersion in water
2. Local penetrating trauma by fingernails or other implements such as cotton-tipped applicators
3. Contamination of the ear canal by pathogenic gram-negative bacteria
4. The immunologic competence of the host

In the cartilaginous outer portion of the external canal, streptococci and staphylococci may invade channels surrounding the hair follicles and produce folliculitis or furunculosis. In more medial portions of the canal, infection is produced by gram-negative organisms such as *Pseudomonas* and *Proteus* species, *Mycoplasma,* fungi such as *Aspergillus* or *Candida* species, or viruses such as herpesviruses. Rarely, the external ear may be invaded by mycobacterial organisms. The infections produced by each class of microorganism have certain unique clinical characteristics.

Habitual scratching of the skin with a fingernail, hairpin, or toy will cause pruritus and a characteristic neurodermatitis of the auricular and external canal skin. This sequence of events may signal the presence of psychological problems that are themselves in need of treatment.

Reactions to chemical or physical agents may occur on the skin of the auricle or the external canal. Chemicals such as cerumenolytic agents (e.g., Cerumenex drops), detergents, or organic solvents will produce an irritant dermatitis after repeated or prolonged exposure. Allergic contact dermatitis may occur after exposure to hair sprays and tinting compounds, pigments used in clothing or linen dyes, metallic compounds containing nickel and chromium, and certain plastic or rubber compounds contained in stereo earphones or hearing aid ear molds. Some agents require light as a catalyst to initiate the reaction. Radiation therapy of the head and neck may also produce a persistent form of otitis externa.

CLINICAL PRESENTATION

Diseases of the external ear become apparent to the patient with the onset of otic pain, a sensation of fullness in the ear, and a hearing loss. Other clinical characteristics such as local tissue changes, exudates, and systemic symptoms and signs may develop depending on the site of disease, the etiologic agent, and host resistance factors.

Ear pain or otalgia may begin gradually or suddenly and progress rapidly to a level poorly tolerated by all but the most stoic child. The sensation of *fullness* in the affected ear occurs early in the disease process as a result of stimulation by the inflammatory process of pressure sense receptors. This perception may continue well after the disease process has clinically resolved.

Hearing loss associated with external ear disease may be conductive or sensorineural. Edematous tissues or canal debris may produce a mild to moderate conductive hearing loss. Viruses such as the varicella-zoster herpesvirus may attack the cochlea, producing sensorineural hearing losses varying in severity from mild to profound. Hearing loss may be perceived as a sense of ear blockage.

Local tissue changes include erythema, edema, and tissue sensitivity. Abscess formation in the external canal is accompanied by fluctuance and spontaneous purulent drainage. Tissue inflammation in the osseous external canal is often accompanied by exudate formation and sometimes by epithelial breakdown and granulation formation.

Systemic symptomatology such as fever, chills, and myalgias is uncommon except in cases of extensive disease, often involving multiple sites. Fatigue is common in both patients and parents because of the sleep deprivation caused by otalgia.

WORK-UP

History

Important historical information to elicit from parent and child includes the following:

- Site of initial pain, discomfort, fullness, and direction of subsequent spread
- Presence of contributory acute or chronic disease such as upper respiratory tract infection, diabetes mellitus, or immunodeficiencies
- Exposure to potential vectors such as contaminated swimming/bathing water or insects
- History of recent ear trauma, including penetrating, blunt, or thermal trauma
- History of cotton-tipped applicator use or habitual insertion of foreign bodies, including fingers
- Occurrence of bleeding or purulent exudate
- Status of hearing in the affected ear
- History of previous episodes of similar disease
- History of middle ear disease, particularly that associated with tympanic membrane perforation
- History of dermatologic disease, particularly eczema, psoriasis, or contact dermatitis from shampoos or metallic products such as earrings

Physical Examination

The clinician should assume that the ear is exquisitely tender. The auricle and periauricular soft tissues should be inspected and palpated in a search for signs of inflammation. The infra-auricular cervical lymph nodes should be examined for evidence of lymphadenitis.

Viewing the canal with the electric otoscope may require use of a smaller than normal speculum because of tissue edema. Epidermal and exudative debris that obstruct the canal must be removed, usually by suction under direct vision using an operating otoscope head. Clinicians without access to otic microsuctions may substitute 18- or 20-gauge plastic intravenous catheters. Gentle irrigation with isotonic saline or topical antibiotic solution may be used to cleanse the canal. The canal epithelium should be examined for evidence of vesiculation, bulla formation, or granular epithelial degeneration, with the latter indicating possible severe underlying disease in the temporal bone.

The tympanic membrane should be observed and manipulated using the pneumatic otoscope. Inflammation of the epithelium covering the tympanic membrane layer may obscure ossicular landmarks and reduce the translucency of the eardrum, but it is possible to determine the presence or absence of middle ear disease.

Both static and active facial symmetry should be noted to assess the function of the seventh cranial nerve. This is critical when the disease presentation suggests deep temporal bone involvement.

Laboratory Tests

The laboratory evaluation includes study of inflammatory exudates obtained from sites of disease and the evaluation of a patient's systemic response to the disease. Although most cases of otitis externa are initially managed empirically, a thorough microbiologic evaluation is imperative for patients with disease resistant to initial management. Cultures should be obtained using microswabs specifically designed for use within the ear canal. Exudates or tissue obtained should be cultured and examined microscopically after staining to demonstrate bacterial and fungal organisms.

Routine hemograms or blood cultures are unnecessary for most patients. Those with advancing external ear disease and with evident systemic toxicity should have white blood cell counts, differentials, and blood cultures.

Audiometry is recommended for those patients who have persistent hearing loss after the resolution of disease. Testing should be delayed for at least 1 month after all signs of acute disease have disappeared. All patients with herpes infections of the external ear should undergo auditory testing during convalescence, since these viruses may attack the cochlea.

MANAGEMENT

Auricular Disease

Primary cellulitis of the auricle should be treated aggressively with systemic antibiotics. It is critical to prevent the spread of infection from the epithelial layers to the auricular cartilage to avoid dissolution of the cartilage and irreversible loss of the auricular structure.

Antibiotics useful for treatment include dicloxicillin, erythromycin, cephalosporins, clindamycin, and trimethoprim-sulfamethoxazole. The presence of perichondritis and chondritis, either primary or secondary, signals the need for adequate gram-negative antibacterial coverage. Application of moist local heat and elevation of the head are adjunctive measures. Fluctuant regions of cellulitic auricles should be promptly incised and drained. Cultures and stains should be obtained. Any necrotic tissue, including cartilage fragments, should be removed. A drain is placed and slowly removed as the perichondrium reattaches to the underlying cartilage. Viral infections should be treated symptomatically to avoid secondary bacterial infection by the use of topical antibiotic ointments such as bacitracin.

Disease of the auricle is often initiated by trauma, and an innocent but firm bump on the ear may produce a hematoma beneath the perichrondrium. If undrained, the hematoma may become organized by fibrous tissue, producing a characteristic "cauliflower" ear deformity. Partially drained hematomas may become infected, leading to abscess formation and ultimate deterioration of the underlying auricular cartilage.

Hematomas of the auricle should be promptly drained. Needle aspiration followed by application of an auricular pressure dressing may be sufficient. Prophylactic treatment with a broad-spectrum antistaphylococcal antibiotic should be given. Reaccumulation of blood or serum indicates the necessity for incision and placement of a drain, usually with the patient under general anesthesia.

BACTERIAL OTITIS EXTERNA

The best treatment is prevention. Children and adolescents with a history of recurrent otitis externa should regularly use an acidifying-antiseptic solution such as 5% boric acid in ethanol after swimming or during hot, humid weather. Excess water in the ear canal should be shaken out or evaporated by adding a few drops of isopropyl alcohol. An antibiotic-corticosteroid topical solution (e.g., Cortisporin otic suspension) may also be used as prophylactic treatment.

Prompt treatment is necessary once infection begins. During the otologic examination, all canal debris must be removed. If edema of the canal skin prevents ready passage of antibiotic drops, a small wick composed of either gauze or absorbent sponge should be inserted into the external canal to carry a topical antibiotic-corticosteroid solution into the ear canal.

The antibiotic-corticosteroid topical solution may contain polymyxin, neomycin, and hydrocortisone. Patients who develop a cutaneous hypersensitivity to neomycin should use commercial preparations without this antibiotic (VoSol or Garamycin otic solution). The patient or parent should insert 4 drops four times a day. If a wick is inserted, the patient places the drops on the wick for the first 2 days. Thereafter, the wick is removed and the ear drops continued for an additional 8 days. The child should be seen after treatment is concluded.

External otitis is painful, and the child should be treated with analgesics, using narcotic compounds sparingly. The ear must be kept dry, and swimming is not permitted. During showers and shampoos, the affected ear is protected using cotton coated with petrolatum jelly. Earplugs that protrude into the canal and irritate the skin should be avoided.

More severe disease requires careful monitoring, and additional suctioning may be required. It may be necessary to reinsert a wick. If the disease spreads to adjacent soft tissue and presents clinically as periauricular cellulitis, a broad-spectrum antibiotic such as a cephalosporin or amoxicillin-clavulanate should be added to the regimen.

Mycotic Otitis Externa

Fungal microorganisms are suspected as the primary etiologic agents or as secondary invaders if the external canal is filled with exudate or a membrane covered by black or white filamentous material. Opportunistic fungi such as *Aspergillus niger* may grow in an ear canal during bacterial infections or after prolonged use of antibiotic-corticosteroid drops. Pathogenic fungal organisms such as *Trichophyton, Microsporum,* and *Candida* species may cause a primary infection.

If there is colonization or superficial infection with minimal epithelial breakdown, 5% boric acid in ethanol may be instilled into the cleansed ear canal as an antiseptic and drying agent. Otherwise, antimycotic agents such as clotrimazole (Lotrimin) and miconazole (Monistat-Derm Lotion) in solution may be instilled alone or in conjunction with topical antibiotic-corticosteroid solutions, if either an accompanying bacterial infection is suspected or the use of a topical corticosteroid is desirable. Patients responding to treatment should be followed at 1- to 2-week intervals, with removal of external canal debris as necessary.

Eczematoid Otitis Externa

Chronic inflammatory changes of the external canal skin are usually accompanied by chronic pruritus. This disease entity occurs most often in older adolescents but may trouble younger patients as well. Hypersensitivity to ingredients in shampoos or cosmetics should be suspected.

If there is infection, treatment should begin with an antibiotic-corticosteroid solution. After infection has resolved, an anti-inflammatory solution of 0.1% betamethasone valerate in ethanol (Valisone Lotion) may be used up to three times a day. After 7 to 10 days of intense treatment, the use of this fluorinated corticosteroid should be tapered to a dose that controls the pruritus.

Bullous or Vesicular Otitis Externa and Myringitis

Bullous or vesicular otitis externa is characterized by the sudden onset of excruciating otalgia relieved as serous fluid escapes from the ear canal. Bullous myringitis often accompanies or follows upper respiratory tract infections. Examination of the ear shows multiple hemorrhagic bullae on the medial external canal wall and on the posterior aspect of the tympanic membrane.

The external walls of bullae should be punctured with either an otic suction or with a spinal needle to relieve severe pain. Extended treatment includes the instillation of an antibiotic-corticosteroid topical suspension three times a day, administration of a broad-spectrum systemic antibiotic (e.g., an erythromycin-sulfa combination [Pediazole]), and the use of adequate analgesics including narcotics for older children and adolescents. The antibiotic should have activity against most gram-positive organisms, *Hemophilus influenzae,* and *Mycoplasma.*

Careful follow-up is necessary since bleb formation continues during the first week after disease onset, and periodic cleansing of the external canal is necessary. As the disease regresses, it is important to reexamine the patient to confirm resolution of tympanic membrane and middle ear disease.

Malignant Otitis Externa

Malignant otitis externa is recognized with increasing frequency in children and adolescents with diabetes mellitus or immunosuppression due to chronic illness or chemotherapy. Beginning as a granular, diffuse otitis externa caused by *Pseudomonas aeruginosa,* the infection rapidly spreads to the underlying temporal bone and the vital structures contained within it. Facial nerve function is often impaired early in the course of the infection. The osteitis and secondary osteomyelitis readily spreads to involve the skull base, and sepsis damages the ninth through twelfth cranial nerves, the sigmoid sinus, and the jugular vein. Preterminal events include progressive cranial neuropathies, jugular vein and sigmoid sinus thrombosis, meningitis, and brain abscess.

Susceptible children with external canal disease should be referred to an otolaryngologist for immediate clinical and radiologic evaluation. Disease unresponsive to parenteral antibiotics alone requires surgical debridement of severely infected or necrotic soft tissue and bone.

INDICATIONS FOR REFERRAL

Children should be referred to an otologist or otolaryngologist if difficulty is encountered in completely cleansing and visualizing the external canal or if the clinician has difficulty inserting a wick to carry topical medication along the length of an infected canal. Referral is also recommended if a child fails to satisfactorily respond to therapy or has marked progression of disease. Children with diabetes mellitus or immunologic depression due to chronic disease or treatment with chemotherapeutic agents should be immediately referred to an otolaryngologist for treatment of otitis externa.

ANNOTATED BIBLIOGRAPHY

Hawke M, Wong J, Krajden S: Clinical and microbiological features of otitis externa. J Otolaryngol 13:289–95, 1984. (Describes the results of a prospective study of both acute and chronic forms of otitis externa along with patient demography, predisposing factors, clinical features, and microbiology.)

Mugliston T, O'Donoghue G: Otomycosis: A continuing problem. J Laryngol Otol 99:327–33, 1985. (Retrospective clinical review of fungal otitis externa in more than 1000 patients of varying ages.)

Nir D, Nir T, Danino J et al: Malignant otitis externa in an infant. J Laryngol Otol 104:488–90, 1990. (Review of a case of a 3-month old with granulocytopenia and malignant otitis externa and comparison with 10 previous cases.)

Rubin J, Yu VL, Stool SE: Malignant otitis media in children. J Pediatr 113:965–70, 1988. (Recent review of the causes, clinical presentations, and management of malignant otitis externa in children.)

Senturia BH, Marcus MD, Lucente FE: Diseases of the External Ear: An Otologic Dermatologic Manual. New York, Grune & Stratton, 1980. (Classic treatise discussing the theoretical and practical aspects of external canal disease.)

75
Acute Otitis Media

Michael Macknin

Acute otitis media, also called suppurative or purulent otitis media, is characterized by the rapid onset of signs and symptoms of inflammation of the middle ear. Middle ear disease is the most common reason for office visits to pediatricians, accounting for one third of all visits. By the age of 3, 83% of children will have experienced one or more episodes of otitis media, and 46% of children will have had three or more episodes.

PATHOPHYSIOLOGY

Eustachian tube dysfunction is the major predisposing factor of acute otitis media. The normal eustachian tube protects, drains, and ventilates the middle ear. Children have shorter, more horizontal, and "floppier" eustachian tubes than adults. Viral infections, particularly respiratory syncytial virus, influenza virus (types A or B), and adenovirus, confer an increased risk of developing otitis media by presumably impairing eustachian tube function. Despite the documented increased risk of developing acute otitis media with an antecedent viral illness, most studies have only isolated viruses from acute otitis media in less than 10% of cases. Bacteria are the major organisms isolated in acute otitis media, and *Streptococcus pneumoniae* is the most common causative organism at any age. *Nontypable hemophilus influenza* is an important pathogen throughout childhood and in adults. *Moraxella catarrhalis* is the third most common isolate in acute middle ear effusions. Other organisms such as *group A β-hemolytic streptococcus* are isolated in less than 5% of cases. *Mycoplasma pneumoniae* is an infrequent cause of acute otitis media and bullous myringitis. Bullous myringitis is generally caused by the same organisms that cause acute otitis media. Neonates, particularly infants with a complicated neonatal course in a neonatal intensive care unit, can have acute middle ear infection with a wide variety of organisms including gram negative enteric rods and *group B β-hemolytic streptococcus* in addition to the more usual organisms.

Risk factors for the development of recurrent otitis media include male sex, American Indians and Eskimos, white race more than black race, enrollment in day care, family history of otitis, siblings at home, low socioeconomic class, possibly bottle *vs* breast-feeding, bottle propping, atopic history in patient or siblings, previous positive history of otitis, winter season, cleft palate, exposure to cigarette smoke and Down syndrome. The precise role of allergies in acute otitis media is poorly defined.

CLINICAL PRESENTATION

The most consistently present abnormalities in acute otitis media are a full or bulging tympanic membrane, absent or obscured bony landmarks due to opacification of the tympanic membrane, and decreased or absent mobility of the tympanic membrane by pneumatic otoscopy due to middle ear effusion. Erythema of the ear drum is an inconsistent finding. By definition, one or more of the following symptoms are present: otalgia (ear pulling in the young infant), fever, or the recent onset of irritability.

DIFFERENTIAL DIAGNOSIS

The classic case of acute otitis media seldom poses a problem in differential diagnosis. Ear pain, however, is not a universal finding in acute otitis media, and there are many causes of ear pain other than acute otitis media. Ear pain may be caused by a furuncle on the external ear or by otitis externa. These conditions usually present with visible inflammation of the external ear or external auditory canal

with pain on manipulation of the pinna or tragus. Temporomandibular joint dysfunction can be detected by palpating the tender joint with a finger in the external auditory canal during opening and closing of the mouth. Cervical lymphadenopathy, pharyngitis, trauma, negative middle ear pressure, tooth infections, foreign bodies, parotitis, sinusitis, tumors, infected sinus tracts or cysts, and mastoiditis can cause ear pain, but can generally be diagnosed by a careful history and physical examination.

EVALUATION

History

Patients often complain of *otalgia* (ear pulling in the young infant). Ear pain, however, is absent in approximately 20% of patients with acute otitis media. Fever is also an inconsistent finding, present in approximately 50% of patients with acute otitis media. Fevers over 104°F occur in less than 5% of cases of isolated acute otitis media. Young children with acute otitis media are often irritable. Hearing loss is generally present in most cases of acute otitis media, but is most commonly noted on history in cases of bilateral disease. Dizziness, unsteady gait, and tinnitus are less frequent complaints. Loose stools and vomiting may occur as a systemic response to acute otitis media. A history of middle ear disease and other infections including sinusitis and pneumonia should be obtained. Risk factors previously outlined under pathophysiology should be discussed.

Physical Examination

The key to the diagnosis of acute otitis media is the physical examination. The tympanic membrane is abnormally full or bulging. Pneumatic otoscopy shows decreased or absent mobility due to middle ear effusion. It is difficult to overemphasize the importance of properly performed pneumatic otoscopy in the evaluation of middle ear disease in children. The bony landmarks are obscured or absent due to opacification of the tympanic membrane. Erythema of the tympanic membrane is an inconsistent finding, as it may also be caused by vascular engorgement due to fever or by crying.

Critical to performing a proper physical examination are: (1) proper equipment including a hermetically sealed otoscopy with a pneumatic attachment. Most otoscopes manufactured prior to 1983 do not maintain a seal adequate for pneumatic otoscopy. The seal can be checked by first squeezing the insufflator bulb, covering the speculum tip with your finger, releasing the pressure on the bulb and checking to see if the bulb remains deflated. A well-charged battery with a bright white, not dull yellow, light source is also essential; and (2) The patient must be still; this can be achieved preferably through gentle persuasion. Some helpful hints are: In a young child demonstrate that looking at ears is not painful by first checking the child's doll, an older sibling, or parent. You may distract a young infant by gentle talking or soft whistling. Give the older child a sense of control by asking, "Which ear should I look at first?" Never ask, "May I look at your ears now?" If the child says "no" you lose credibility and trust when you insist on looking. Emphasize the positive, never say, "This won't hurt." When doing pneumatic otoscopy, let the patient know that, "I will be blowing in your ears and this is going to tickle. Try not to laugh too much, because when you laugh you wiggle and it's hard for me to see your ears." If gentle persuasion fails, the child must be restrained. A young child can sit upright facing to the side on a parent's thigh. The child's legs can be restrained between the parent's thighs. The parent can hold the child's head against the parent's chest with one hand on the child's temple. The parent's other hand can be wrapped around the child's trunk to restrain both arms. If this does not work, the child can have head, arms, and legs restrained (at or above knees and not just at ankles to avoid wiggling) while lying on the examination table.

The external auditory canal must be cleared of cerumen prior to the examination of the tympanic membrane. If the drum is not perforated, this can be accomplished by irrigation with lukewarm water (not too hot or cold to avoid performing calorics) using a water pick or a butterfly with the needle cut off attached to a syringe. Hydrogen peroxide or docusate sodium (Colace) may be instilled in the ear prior to irrigation to facilitate the removal of cerumen. Flushing the ear with water often causes erythema of the tympanic membrane, and cerumen may also still obscure some of the drum surface. This makes pneumatic otoscopy particularly important for an accurate assessment of the tympanic membrane, because the normal appearance of the drum is obscured. Cerumen can also be removed by using a curette. This technique can be safely used only under direct visualization.

Many mistakes are made in performing pneumatic otoscopy. The most common one is not obtaining an adequate seal. It is important to use an ear speculum that is large enough to obtain an airtight seal with the external auditory canal. The seal should be made with the cartilaginous outer one third of the external auditory canal. The bony inner two thirds of the external canal is exquisitely sensitive to pain and should not be touched by the speculum. Soft-tip specula, although not essential to performing a pneumatic otoscopy, have been specifically designed to achieve a comfortable airtight seal with the external auditory canal. All portions of the drum should be checked for mobility. A bulging drum is already maximally stretched toward the examiner and thus will not move when negative pressure (the collapsed bulb is released) is applied in the external auditory canal. Conversely, a retracted drum will not move when positive pressure (a full bulb is squeezed) is applied. Whether a bulging drum will show decreased or no mobility on positive pressure, and whether a retracted drum will show decreased or no mobility on positive pressure, depends on the forces exerted on the drum. Occasionally, particularly with a thinned drum, a hypermobile area may be detected. The large speculum needed to obtain an adequate seal often makes it difficult to completely visualize the entire tympanic membrane simultaneously. Therefore, it will often be necessary to re-position the otoscope to observe multiple segments of the drum to determine the complete appearance of the tympanic membrane.

Laboratory Tests

Laboratory tests are seldom needed in uncomplicated acute otitis media. Indications for performing tympanocentesis for culture and sensitivity of the middle ear effusion in unusual cases of acute otitis media include (1) systemically toxic patients, (2) patients with a suppurative complication of otitis media such as mastoiditis, (3) immune-compromised hosts such as patients on chemotherapy with neutropenia, (4) patients with severe pain unresponsive to oral and topical analgesics, (5) newborns with otitis who do not appear entirely well or who have not had uncomplicated neonatal courses or in whom an excellent follow-up is not ensured, and (6) patients already on "appropriate" antimicrobial therapy or patients who have just completed recent courses of antimicrobial therapy. Gram stain of middle ear effusion obtained at tympanocentesis can be helpful in guiding initial therapy.

Recurrent acute otitis media alone is seldom a presentation of immune deficiency. However, recurrent otitis media in association with other recurrent infections may be indicative of abnormal body defenses. Sinusitis and pneumonia associated with recurrent acute otitis media are among the most common infections associated with detectable immune deficiencies. An initial laboratory evaluation for patients with multiple well-documented episodes of acute otitis media and sinusitis or pneumonia should include a complete blood cell count with differential, sweat test, and quantitative IgG, IgA, IgM, IgE, and quantitative IgG subclasses. A biopsy of nasal mucosa for ciliary abnormalities might also be considered.

TREATMENT

The preferred treatment for acute otitis media is antibiotic therapy. The major pathogens beyond the neonatal period are *Streptococcus pneumoniae,* nontypeable *Hemophilus influenzae,* and *Moraxella catarrhalis.* The choice of antimicrobial agents should be influenced by the geographic prevalence of β-lactamase–producing *H. influenzae* and *Moraxella catarrhalis* causing otitis media. Up to 30% of nontypeable *H. influenzae* and 75% of *M. catarrhalis* produce β-lactamase. Many practitioners, however, find that amoxicillin, 40 mg/kg/d divided three times a day, is still an effective first-line drug and is still generally considered to be the initial drug of choice. Ampicillin need not be used because it offers no advantage over amoxicillin. The drugs have an identical spectrum of activity and comparable cost, but ampicillin causes more diarrhea and must be given four instead of three times a day and on an empty stomach.

Trimethoprim-sulfamethoxazole (Bactrim, Septra), 1 ml/kg/d, has the advantages of a twice-daily schedule and low cost. It is not active against *group A β-hemolytic Streptococcus,* and there are increasing numbers of resistant *Streptococcus pneumoniae* organisms in some areas. It also has the disadvantage of the allergic reactions caused by sulfa drugs.

Erythromycin and sulfisoxazole (combined as Pediazole), 50 mg/kg/d and 150 mg/kg/d, respectively, in divided doses four times a day is another good choice for treating acute otitis media. This combination has a good spectrum of activity. It is more expensive than amoxicillin or trimethoprim-sulfamethoxazole.

Cefaclor (Ceclor), 40 mg/kg/d in three daily doses (although it can be given twice daily), has excellent in vitro activity against major middle ear pathogens. Despite adequate clinical response, there is a poor in vivo bacteriologic response of *H. influenzae* in the middle ear. However, recent data suggest that Ceclor may be less effective in treating AOM than other antibiotics. Ceclor's high cost is also a negative factor in prescribing this drug.

Amoxicillin and clavulanate (combined as Augmentin), 40 mg/kg/d of amoxicillin in three divided doses, has a broad spectrum of activity. Although it has theoretical advantages over amoxicillin in eradicating β-lactamase–producing organisms, a clear clinical superiority has yet to be demonstrated. Augmentin causes a high incidence of diarrhea and is expensive.

Cefixime (Suprax), 8 mg/kg/d, has the advantages of a daily or twice-daily schedule and being highly sensitive against β-lactamase–producing organisms. It has the disadvantages of being expensive, having slightly decreased activity against *streptococcus pneumoniae,* and causing a higher incidence of diarrhea than most other drugs.

Cefuroxime (Ceftin), 125 mg twice daily in children younger than age 2, 250 mg twice daily in children aged 2 to 12, and 250 to 500 mg twice daily in children older than age 12, also has a convenient dosage schedule and broad spectrum of activity. It tastes bitter, has no liquid form, and is expensive.

Cefprozil (Cefzil), 30 mg/kg/d has the advantage of a twice-daily schedule, resistance to β-lactamases, and a less than 10% incidence of diarrhea. Its cost is similar to other cephalosporins.

Analgesics are often important in the initial therapy of acute otitis media until antibiotic therapy can eradicate the infection and decrease pain. Acetaminophen in a dose of 10 to 15 mg/kg every 4 hours is usually effective. Aspirin in doses of 10 mg/kg every 4 hours may be used instead of acetaminophen as long as the patient does not have chickenpox or influenza (i.e., illnesses in which aspirin use is associated with Reye syndrome). Codeine, 0.5 to 1.0 mg/kg, every 4 to 6 hours not to exceed 3 mg/kg/d, may sometimes need to be given with acetaminophen or aspirin for a few doses. Topical Auralgan, or Americaine, which should be used only in the absence of perforation, may also help relieve the ear pain of acute otitis media.

When acute otitis media is effectively treated, symptomatic relief can be expected within 2 to 3 days. Standard treatment continues for 7 to 10 days. If a patient does not respond within several days but is not systemically toxic, antibiotics can generally be safely and effectively switched without performing tympanocentesis for culture and sensitivity. Changing to any of the discussed antibiotics is usually effective. If there is not an acceptable response to a second drug, tympanocentesis to obtain cultures and sensitivities should be performed.

Middle ear effusion commonly persists even after acute otitis media has been effectively treated. Effusion is present in 70% of cases at 2 weeks, 40% at 4 weeks, 20% at 2 months, and 10% at 3 months. Because of the common persistence of middle ear effusion in the first 2 months after an acute infection, follow-up ear checks to ensure complete resolution of middle ear effusion can be scheduled for 2 months after an episode of acute otitis media. Waiting for follow-up for 2 months is appropriate only if the patient can be relied on to return sooner if symptoms return and to keep a 2-month follow-up appointment even if asymptomatic (see Chap. 76, Otitis Media With Effusion). Patients who have recurrent ear infections should probably have their first follow-up visit scheduled near the end of therapy to ensure an adequate initial response to treatment.

Recurrent episodes of acute otitis media are common. In about 25% of the cases, infections occurring within 30 days of the original infection are caused by the same organism that caused the initial infection. Therefore, it is reasonable to empirically use a different antibiotic for a recurrence within 1 month. After 30 days, the infection is usually with another organism, and the infection can probably be treated as an event separate from the initial infection.

Antihistamines and decongestants probably do not help prevent acute otitis media or promote the resolution of acute otitis media. The *H. influenzae* type B vaccine is not helpful in preventing acute otitis media because most *H. influenzae* organisms causing otitis are nontypeable. The pneumococcal vaccine helps prevent some type-specific pneumococcal otitis media. The pneumococcal vaccine, however, does not dramatically decrease the total number of episodes of acute otitis media, and the vaccine is not recommended for routine prophylaxis against ear infections. Myringotomy relieves pain in acute otitis media; however, it has not been proven to promote the resolution of the infection. Gammaglobulin may prove effective in preventing recurrent ear infections in young children, but it should be used only in carefully controlled clinical trials until its safety and possible efficacy are clearly defined.

Antibiotic prophylaxis is effective in preventing acute otitis media. Children with multiple episodes of acute otitis media whose middle ear effusions clear between episodes are ideal candidates for antimicrobial prophylaxis. Criteria for consideration of antimicrobial prophylaxis are three episodes of acute otitis media within 6 months or 2 episodes before 6 months of age. Effective antimicrobial choices include sulfisoxazole, 75 mg/kg/d in divided doses twice daily and once-daily doses of amoxicillin, 20 mg/kg at bedtime, or trimethoprim-sulfamethoxazole, 4 mg/kg/d and 20 mg/kg/d, respectively. (Trimethoprim-sulfamethoxazole has not been formally approved for prophylaxis against otitis media.) Prophylaxis may be for up to 6 months, and the duration is often based on the child's history of seasonal variation of symptoms. Usually winter, when respiratory infections are most prevalent, is the most common period for using antimicrobial prophylaxis. Because middle ear effusion can persist without symptoms of acute otitis media, children on chemoprophylaxis should be examined approximately every 2 months.

INDICATIONS FOR REFERRAL

Complications and sequelae of otitis media often necessitate referral to an otolaryngologist, and less commonly, admission to the hospital. Hearing loss, particularly bilateral loss greater than or equal to 20 dB for more than 3 months, is an indication for otologic referral for possible myringotomy and tube placement and/or adenoidectomy. Recurrent episodes of otitis media unresponsive to medical management is also an indication for referral, as are the less frequent complications of chronic tympanic membrane perforation, chronic suppurative otitis media, retraction pocket, cholesteatoma, adhesive otitis media, ossicular discontinuity, ossicular fixation, mastoiditis, petrositis, labyrinthitis, facial paralysis, and cholesterol granuloma.

Intracranial suppurative complications of otitis media and mastoiditis include meningitis, extradural abscess, subdural empyema, focal otitic encephalitis, brain abscess, lateral sinus thrombosis, and possibly otitic hydrocephalus. These are immediate indications for admission.

PATIENT EDUCATION

Patients should be taught to seek medical care for ear pain. The use of home remedies such as "sweet oil" should be discouraged. Bottle propping may predispose children to recurrent episodes of otitis media and should be avoided. Patients and families should know that acute otitis media means an infection on the inside of the eardrum and that swimming without diving will probably not precipitate or exacerbate acute otitis media if the eardrum is intact. A common misbelief that may need to be dispelled is that going outside in the cold without ear muffs causes acute otitis media. The importance of follow-up examinations to document clearing and to rule out persistent middle ear effusion and hearing loss should be stressed. Parents should know that there will probably be some degree of hearing loss until the ear infection is resolved. Persons who speak to the child, therefore, should face the child and perhaps gently touch the child's shoulder to be sure that the child knows someone is speaking. Until the middle ear effusion is resolved, the child should have preferential seating at the front of the classroom. Parents should also be encouraged to stop smoking because of data suggesting that exposure to smoke predisposes the child to otitis media and prolongs the presence of a middle ear effusion after episodes of acute otitis media.

ANNOTATED BIBLIOGRAPHY

See the references at the end of Chapter 76.

76
Otitis Media with Effusion
Michael Macknin

Relatively asymptomatic middle ear effusion has many synonyms, such as "secretory," "nonsuppurative," or "serous" otitis media, but the most acceptable term is *otitis media with effusion* (OME). The mobility of the tympanic membrane by pneumatic otoscopy is decreased. The appearance of the tympanic membrane, however, may vary from bulging and opaque with no visible landmarks to retracted and translucent with visible landmarks and a clear air–fluid level. Most commonly on otoscopy the tympanic membrane is opaque, making assessment of the type of effusion (i.e., serous, mucoid, or purulent) impossible. The most important distinction between OME and acute otitis media is that signs and symptoms of acute infection such as otalgia or fever are lacking in patients with OME. Because of the imprecision over the definition of terms used to describe otitis media, the terminology used to describe otitis media must be defined clearly and used correctly.

Otitis media with effusion is the most common cause of hearing loss in childhood. The fluctuating hearing losses associated with OME have been linked by some investigators to language and speech delays and poor school performance. Developing an organized approach to the management of OME is essential to the office practice of pediatrics.

PATHOPHYSIOLOGY

Otitis media with effusion most commonly results from eustachian tube dysfunction. Eustachian tube dysfunction can result from various causes, including antecedent viral illnesses, anatomic abnormalities such as cleft palate, barotrauma, and possibly allergies. It may then lead to the development of relatively asymptomatic middle ear effusion without the initial acute inflammatory response seen in acute otitis media.

One series of pathologic events leading to the development of OME begins with eustachian tube dysfunction. This changes middle ear mucosa from ciliated respiratory epithelium with goblet cells and seromucinous glands to a predominantly secretory mucosa with numerous additional mucous glands. Mucus production subsequently arises from goblet cells, and transudation occurs from middle ear blood vessels. The effusion may become increasingly viscous and gluelike as the middle ear mucosa absorbs the effusion's watery component. Resolution can begin with mucous plugging of the glandular tubules with degeneration and the transformation of the secretory epithelium back to the nonsecretory respiratory epithelium.

Another series of pathologic events leading to the development of OME begins with eustachian tube dysfunction, which then develops into acute otitis media. It is the natural history of acute otitis media that middle ear effusion will be present for 2 weeks in 70%, 1 month in 40%, 2 months in 20%, and 3 months in 10%.

Otitis media with effusion had previously been thought of as a collection of sterile and relatively asymptomatic middle ear fluid. Research has shown, however, that approximately one third of all these effusions in children contain pathogenic bacteria such as nontypeable *Hemophilus influenzae, Moraxella catarrhalis,* and *Streptococcus pneumoniae.* The precise role of these organisms in the pathogenesis of OME is poorly understood.

CLINICAL PRESENTATION

By definition, OME is relatively asymptomatic. The most common symptoms are hearing loss, minor ear discomfort or fullness in the ear, tinnitus, the sensation of water rushing or popping in the ear, and, occasionally, impaired balance or dizziness. It is commonly revealed that days or weeks earlier there was a brief episode of ear pain or fever resolving spontaneously. Otitis media with effusion is often discovered during a routine physical examination with no contributory antecedent history.

DIFFERENTIAL DIAGNOSIS

The differential diagnosis for hearing loss in children is extensive and discussed in Chapter 78. The diagnosis of OME, however, is best made by pneumatic otoscopy, and if OME is present, the differential diagnosis of hearing loss is vastly narrowed. In older adolescents and adults, unilateral OME may indicate possible nasopharyngeal carcinoma. Recurrent or persistent middle ear effusion must alert the practitioner to possible anatomic abnormalities.

WORK-UP

History

The history should include the occurrence of previous middle ear disease as well as the presence of risk factors for recurrent otitis media (see Chap. 75).

Physical Examination

The principles of pneumatic otoscopy as outlined under acute otitis media apply to OME (see Chap. 75). The only consistent finding on physical examination in OME is impaired mobility of the tympanic membrane by pneumatic otoscopy. It is impossible to accurately diagnose OME by otoscopy without performing pneumatic otoscopy. The appearance of the eardrum may vary from bulging and opaque to space retracted and translucent.

A careful examination of the head and neck should be done to rule out anatomic abnormalities associated with the development of OME. Cleft palates are easy to detect. A submucosal cleft should be looked for. The normal soft palate forms an arc at its junction with the hard palate. With a submucosal cleft palate, this junction is V-shaped and can be examined easily by palpation. In the uncooperative patient, the examiner can safely palpate by using a stack of tongue blades to prevent the patient from biting down.

Laboratory Tests

Laboratory tests are not always necessary in the diagnosis and treatment of OME. However, confirmatory objective tests for the diagnosis of middle ear effusion and hearing acuity are often helpful in the management of OME (see Chap. 77 for a more detailed discussion).

Tympanometry assesses the change in tympanic membrane compliance as air pressure is varied in the ear canal. The results are plotted on a chart called a tympanogram, which graphically displays compliance as a function of air pressure. This valuable tool can be used to observe the status of a patient's middle ear. The correlation of the tympanogram with the clinical condition of the middle ear, however, has been validated by findings at myringotomy for only a few of the many tympanometers. Thus, the practitioner would be well advised to ask the manufacturer if the clinical validity of the machine has been tested as a prerequisite to purchasing it.

Audiograms can be performed on children of all ages by qualified personnel. A child is never too young to have a hearing test. The specific methods employed at each age group are discussed in Chap. 77. The pediatrician should be able to interpret a conventional audiogram. The audiogram reports hearing threshold for the left and right ear and for air and bone conduction in decibels at different frequencies. Decibels are a log scale, with 0 dB representing normal adult hearing threshold levels. Many children have better than normal adult hearing threshold levels and therefore may have a negative hearing threshold levels, such as -5 dB. Twenty decibels is about as loud as a whisper. Forty decibels is about the normal loudness of speaking. Ninety decibels can become painful. The hearing threshold in decibels on the ordinate is reported at various frequencies given on the abscissa. The normal speaking frequencies of the human voice range from 250 Hz to 4000 Hz.

The symbols for air and bone conduction and left and right ear are always reported on the audiogram. Bone conduction reflects sensorineural hearing. Air conduction reflects conductive hearing, and it is typically adversely affected by OME.

An air–bone gap (i.e., bone conduction better than air conduction) in the same ear at the same frequency of 15 dB or more represents a significant conductive abnormality. Normally, air and bone conduction are similar. A hearing threshold level of 20 dB or more represents a significant hearing loss in a child. (The exact level of decibel loss representing a "significant" hearing loss is controversial.)

If air and bone conduction hearing threshold levels are similarly decreased, there is no air–bone gap and the hearing loss is sensorineural. If bone conduction is normal and air conduction is impaired, there is an air–bone gap and conductive hearing is abnormal. A conductive hearing loss is typical of OME. Combined sensorineural (with impaired bone conduction) and conductive (with an air–bone gap) hearing losses may be present occasionally with OME. The sensorineural component is believed to be due to increased tension and stiffness of the round window membrane. When the OME is resolved, the hearing generally returns to normal. Rarely, permanent sensorineural hearing loss may result from chronic otitis media.

Additional methods of assessing hearing such as electrocochleography and auditory brain stem response are beyond the scope of this review. The auditory brain stem response is preferred over electrocochleography by most clinicians because a surgical procedure performed with the patient under general anesthesia for placing the active electrode is not required for auditory brain stem response as it is for electrocochleography. Candidates with OME for auditory brain stem response testing as outlined by Fria in Bluestone and Stool's text are as follows: (1) infants with recurrent acute otitis media or persistent OME, or both, and (2) children with significant mental retardation, emotional disturbances, or both.

Acoustic reflectometry is a newer method of detecting middle ear effusion and is based on the principle of partial cancellation of incident sound by sound reflected back from the tympanic membrane. It is easy to perform, but its exact reliability and role in clinical medicine have not yet been completely determined.

TREATMENT

The treatment of OME is controversial and can be subdivided into medical and surgical methods.

I suggest that all patients with newly diagnosed OME be given a 14-day course of a systemic antibiotic appropriate for acute otitis media (see Chap. 75). This recommendation is based on the frequently documented presence of pathogenic bacteria in OME. It should be noted, however, that the efficacy of antibiotic treatment of OME is not as well

documented as for acute otitis media and therefore, this recommendation may be subject to controversy.

The patient should be scheduled for a follow-up visit in 2 months or sooner if symptomatic. Meanwhile, the patient should be given preferential seating in school and every effort should be made to have the child face persons when they are speaking.

If the effusion is resolved at the 2-month follow-up visit, the patient should be seen again only for routine well-child visits or if symptoms occur. If the effusion persists, another 14-day course of a different antibiotic may be given and the child scheduled for follow-up in 1 month (i.e., 3 months after initial presentation). The efficacy of treating 2- to 5-year-old children with a minimum 6-week history of middle ear effusion with a 1-month course of trimethoprim-sulfamethoxazole (8 mg/kg and 40 mg/kg, respectively, in two divided doses) has also been demonstrated.

Antibiotics in conjunction with corticosteroids provide another medical option before considering surgical intervention after at least 3 months of OME. Trimethoprim-sulfamethoxazole, or another oral antimicrobial used for acute otitis media, for 2 to 4 weeks can be given in conjunction with a 1-week course of 1 mg/kg/d of prednisone with or without a 1-week taper of the corticosteroids. This regimen probably promotes the acute resolution of OME. Further research must be done to fully evaluate long-term beneficial effects and optimal dosage schedules of antibiotics plus corticosteroids in the treatment of OME. A course of prophylactic antibodies, as outlined in Chap. 75, after a course of antibiotics plus corticosteroids for OME may improve the long-term resolution of OME. Caution must be exercised to avoid adrenal suppression with higher doses or longer duration of the suggested corticosteroid treatment.

Many other medical therapies of OME have been tried. None of the therapies discussed below are of any proven long-term benefit. Antihistamines and decongestants probably do not help the resolution of OME. Nasal corticosteroids and systemic corticosteroids without antibiotics have been shown in some studies to be helpful in promoting the resolution of middle ear effusion. However, the use of nasal and systemic corticosteroids without antibiotics to treat middle ear effusion should be done only in carefully controlled clinical trials until their safety and possible efficacy are established. Controlled middle ear inflation by forcing air up the eustachian tube has no proven long-term efficacy. The role of mucolytic agents is also unsettled. In summary, antibiotics and antibiotics with oral corticosteroids are probably helpful in clearing some OME, but no medical therapy for OME is of proven long-term benefit in most cases of OME. Time is often the best healer.

INDICATIONS FOR REFERRAL

If effusion persists 3 months after initial presentation, an audiogram should be obtained. The precise criteria for referral to an otolaryngologist for possible myringotomy and tube placement and/or adenoidectomy are controversial. I would suggest a bilateral air–bone gap of greater than or equal to 20 dB as criteria for referral to an otolaryngologist. Other important factors that should be considered include the child's language development, seasonal pattern, an associated permanent conductive or sensorineural hearing loss, and the number of previous infections. A child with language delay may be in greatest need of a rapid return of normal hearing acuity, which usually results from myringotomy and tube placement. A child who is most prone to ear infections in the winter and is usually clear during the warm months should preferentially have a myringotomy and tube placement for persistent effusion in October rather than in March. Severe pain, ossicular fixation, mastoiditis, labyrinthitis and vertigo, facial paralysis, cholesterol granuloma, cholesteatoma, chronic tympanic membrane perforation, adhesive otitis media, ossicular discontinuity, and retraction pockets are also indications for referral to an otolaryngologist. The immediate efficacy of myringotomy and tube placement in improving hearing is documented, although the long-term balance of the risks and benefits of myringotomy and tube placement has not yet been clearly defined. Children with persistent middle ear effusion for several months without significant hearing loss, language delay, or the other aforementioned complications can be safely followed by their primary care provider. Repeat examinations and hearing screening tests should be performed at least every 1 to 2 months to monitor for the need for referral.

A tonsillectomy and an adenoidectomy are other surgical interventions used to treat OME. A tonsillectomy probably has no role in the treatment of middle ear disease. Adenoidectomy probably does afford some benefit to selected patients with recurrent middle ear problems. Unfortunately, it is difficult to prospectively identify the minority of patients with recurrent middle ear disease who would benefit from adenoidectomy.

PATIENT EDUCATION

Families with children who have OME should know that there is often a hearing loss associated with this condition. The importance of follow-up examinations to document clearing and to rule out persistent middle ear effusion and hearing loss should be stressed. Families should be reassured that with time, most cases of OME will resolve without any long-term adverse effects on hearing.

ANNOTATED BIBLIOGRAPHY

Bluestone CD: Modern management of otitis media. Pediatr Clin North Am 36:1371–1387, 1989. (Excellent review of management of otitis media.)

Bluestone CD, Stool SE (eds): The Ear and Related Structures: Pediatric Otolaryngology, pp 75–602. Philadelphia, WB Saunders, 1990. (Detailed summary of all aspects of ear disease in the standard pediatric otolaryngology text.)

Cantekin EI, Mandel EM, Bluestone CD et al: Lack of efficacy of a decongestant-antihistamine combination for otitis media with effusion ("secretory" otitis media) in children. N Engl J Med 308:297–301, 1983. (Classic paper proving the lack of efficacy of a decongestant and antihistamine combination in treating otitis media with effusion.)

Lim DJ, Bluestone CD, Klein JO, Nelson JD (eds): Recent Advances in Otitis Media with Effusion. Philadelphia, BC Decker, 1988. (Collection of papers providing an excellent overview of the direction of otitis media research and current knowledge, including Healy's 1984 paper on 1 month of antibiotic treatment for persistent otitis media with effusion.)

Macknin ML: Steroid treatment for otitis media with effusion. Clin Pediatr. 30:178–182, 1991. (Summary of studies on this controversial topic.)

Mandel EM, Rockette HE, Paradise JL, et al: Comparative efficacy of erythromycin-sulfisoxazole, cefaclor, amoxicillin, or placebo for otitis media with effusion in children. Pediatr Infect Dis J 10:899–906, 1991. (Double-blind randomized trial showing amoxicillin group most likely to be effusion-free at 2 weeks, with no other groups better than placebo at 2 and 4 weeks, including amoxicillin group at 4 weeks. This well-done study points out some of the limitations of antibiotic treatment for OME, while also referencing and briefly discussing some successful trials of antibiotics for OME.)

Paradise JL, Bluestone CD, Rogers KD et al: Efficacy of adenoidectomy for recurrent otitis media in children previously treated with tympanostomy-tube placement. JAMA 263:2066–2073, 1990. (Excellent prospective study with previous studies well-referenced.)

Teele DW, Klein JO, Chase C et al: Otitis media in infancy and intellectual ability, school achievement, speech, and language at age 7 years. J Infect Dis 162:685–694, 1990. (Excellent prospective study of a large number of children followed from birth.)

Teele DW, Klein JO, Rosner B et al: Epidemiology of otitis media during the first seven years of life in children in greater Boston: A prospective, cohort study. J Infect Dis 160:83–94, 1989. (Outstanding prospective study of a large group of children enrolled shortly after birth followed until 7 years of age.)

77
Testing Hearing and Middle Ear Function

Marilyn Warren Neault and Howard G. Smith

The human ear and its supporting neural structures represent an ultrasensitive, ultra-high-fidelity sound processing system. The ear can detect both a whisper and a sound 1 million times more intense, such as the roar of a jet engine. A logarithmic unit called the *decibel* (dB) is used to quantify given sound levels. The human ear detects sounds in the frequency range from 20 to 20,000 cycles per second (referred to as *Hertz* [Hz]) but has a different sensitivity to various sound frequencies. The ear is most sensitive to sounds in the range between 1000 to 4000 Hz, within the speech frequency range.

Hearing acuity is tested by exposing the subject to a variety of calibrated sounds and measuring either behavioral or physiologic responses produced by the subject. Tones of specific frequency, called pure tones, are presented in octave intervals from 125 to 8000 Hz. Complex sounds containing energy across a range of frequencies, such as speech, music, or filtered broad-band noises, also may serve as test signals to probe threshold acuity.

The level of hearing or, conversely, that of hearing loss, is a threshold level measured in decibels, referred to as *dB HL* or *decibels relative to normal hearing threshold.* A normal hearing ear demonstrates a threshold for hearing at or very near 0 dB. An ear with a profound hearing loss has a threshold exceeding 90 dB. Purely conductive hearing losses, associated with outer and/or middle ear dysfunction with normal cochlear function, cannot exceed 65 to 70 dB. Sensorineural or mixed (sensorineural and conductive) hearing losses may demonstrate threshold levels of any degree.

The severity of a hearing loss is most commonly determined by averaging the thresholds at 500, 1000, and 2000 Hz for each ear separately and by using these values to enter one of many hearing impairment scales. A typical scale is as follows:

HEARING IMPAIRMENT	HEARING THRESHOLD (dB)	FIDELITY (Discrimination)
None	−10 to 15	Excellent
Slight	16 to 25	Excellent
Mild	26 to 40	Very good
Moderate	41 to 55	Good
Moderately severe	56 to 70	Fair
Severe	71 to 90	Fair to poor
Profound	Above 90	Poor to none

Because the decibel scale is logarithmic, even a "slight" (16 to 25 dB) hearing loss represents a substantial decrease in perceived volume of speech. Hearing loss in the slight or mild range in early childhood can affect speech and language development significantly.

The fidelity or lack of sound distortion decreases with increasing hearing thresholds. Children with sensorineural hearing losses have difficulty understanding and differentiating words that they hear. This situation limits the communication benefit of even the most powerful hearing aids for children with severe to profound hearing losses.

Pure tones and speech stimuli are used to test the neuronal connections from the cochlea to the brain stem and beyond. Other testing routines can determine the integrity of the middle ear sound conduction system.

TESTING TECHNIQUES

Behavioral Audiometry

Behavioral audiometry requires that the child be willing and able to give reliable and reproducible responses to sounds generated by calibrated equipment and presented within a sound-isolated room. To decide whether a child is making a definite behavioral response to sound requires the professional skill of an audiologist experienced in the testing of children, particularly in the case of infants and toddlers. Depending on the age of the child, sounds are presented through loudspeakers or through earphones and a bone conduction phone. For younger children, testing is performed with the parent and often with a second audiologist in the test room to facilitate observation.

The usual audiometric battery includes determination for each ear of (1) a hearing threshold for sounds transmitted through the air of the ear canal and middle ear space called the *air conduction threshold;* (2) a hearing threshold for sounds transmitted directly to the temporal bone bypassing the air conduction system using a vibrator resting on the mastoid process called the *bone conduction threshold;* (3) the *speech reception threshold,* or the lowest sound intensity at which a child can correctly identify selected words in 50% of trials; and (4) the *speech discrimination score,* a measure of hearing fidelity determined by the percentage of a standardized list of monosyllabic words correctly identified if presented at a sound intensity 25 to 40 dB above the speech reception threshold. For infants and toddlers, the goal of behavioral audiometry is to determine the child's *minimal response levels,* or weakest stimulus intensities at which behavioral responses are seen, and to decide whether the child's responses to sound are within the normal range.

The air conduction and bone conduction thresholds are determined and plotted on a standard graphic form called an audiogram, shown in Figure 77-1. The hearing levels are plotted on the vertical axis using an inverse linear scale, and the test frequencies are plotted on the horizontal axis using a logarithmic scale. All audiograms have legends that indicate the symbols used for plotting the data. The audiogram shows the hearing of a child with a moderately severe bilateral mixed hearing loss. The bone conduction threshold is 30 dB. This component of the hearing loss is likely due to cochlear malfunction, although middle ear pathology may also raise the bone conduction threshold a few decibels, adding to the apparent sensorineural hearing loss. The air conduction thresholds are in the 60- to 70-dB range, indicating an overall hearing loss in the moderately severe range, with a 30- to 40-dB potentially treatable conductive hearing loss as a component of the total hearing loss. The speech reception threshold usually approximates the average of the pure tone air conduction thresholds at 500, 1000, and 2000 Hz, which is a useful internal check on the test results.

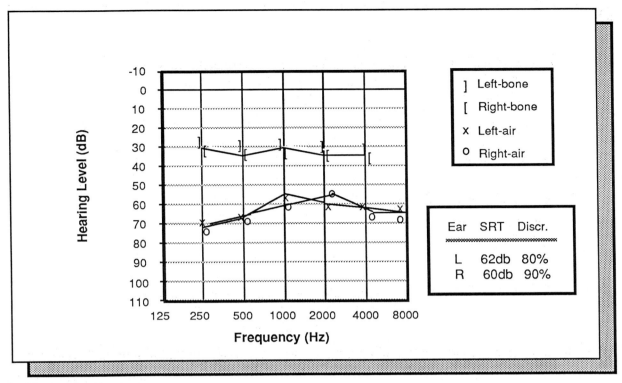

Figure 77-1.   Mixed hearing loss.

If one ear has significantly better hearing than the other when measured by air conduction, it is often necessary to mask the hearing of the better ear to prevent it from interfering with accurate testing of the poorer hearing ear. Masking is accomplished by presenting either white noise (sound including a broad range of frequencies), or narrow band noise at a sufficiently intense level to the better hearing ear. When a conductive hearing loss is present, masking is almost always necessary during bone conduction audiometry, to determine the cochlear sensitivity of separate ears.

The speech discrimination scores indicate the fidelity of the hearing in each ear. Scores normally diminish along with general auditory acuity in the case of sensorineural hearing loss, while scores remain high in the case of conductive hearing loss provided the words are presented at a sufficient intensity. Unusually low or asymmetric scores, particularly in a child with a unilateral or an asymmetric sensorineural hearing loss, may indicate a neural lesion and the need for further evaluation.

Electrophysiologic Audiometry

There are several techniques for measuring the electrophysiologic response of the auditory system to sound. The auditory evoked response measure in most frequent clinical use today is called *auditory brain stem response* (ABR) or *brain stem evoked response* (BSER). This technique measures the initiation of sound-induced electrical signals in the cochlea and their propagation along the auditory nerve into the brain stem during the first 15 to 20 ms after the sound stimulus. The stimuli used are clicks or tone bursts of varying intensities and frequencies delivered to the cochlea through either air or bone conduction with the patient in a shielded sound booth. The resultant electric signals are recorded through noninvasive surface electrodes. The test is performed with infants and young children under sedation with a hypnotic agent such as chloral hydrate, or in an unsedated sleep for infants younger than 6 months. A general anesthetic agent may be used but usually is unnecessary.

With this system it is possible to determine selectively the sound intensity response thresholds for air or bone conduction in each ear. The ABR or BSER evaluation, while accepted as a routine method of hearing assessment in infants and difficult-to-test patients, does require careful interpretation in conjunction with behavioral audiometric data system.

Another technique providing similar information to ABR data is *electrocochleography*. This technique is not widely used for clinical purposes today because ABR is easier and safer to accomplish. Another physiologic technique, the development of which is rapidly approaching clinical usefulness, is the recording of *otoacoustic emis-*

sions (OAEs). These emissions represent acoustic energy generated by outer hair cell activity in the cochlea and are recordable by placing a probe in the ear canal. Although spontaneous OAEs are recordable from many normal hearing ears and absent in cochlear hearing loss, evoked OAEs (elicited by clicks, tones, or pairs of tones) promise greater use for predicting hearing levels, at least in mild and moderate loss ranges. The recording of OAEs bears promise as a neonatal screening tool because of the simplicity of the test, which does not require scalp electrodes.

Immittance Audiometry

Middle ear infections and effusions, as well as ossicular malformations, produce *acoustic impedance*, which may be measured. Sudden intense sound should produce contraction of the stapedius and tensor tympani muscles to protect the cochlea by attenuation of ossicular mobility.

Instruments and procedures have been developed to evaluate middle ear dynamic function. The instrument used for these tests is called an *electroacoustic immittance* (impedance/admittance) *bridge*, and current models can test a number of different middle ear functions. Immittance audiometry requires little cooperation from the child other than the acceptance, with restraint if necessary, of an appropriately sized test probe in the external ear canal.

Tympanometry is a technique that quantifies the change in tympanic membrane mobility or compliance (admittance) as air pressure in the external ear canal is varied. The tympanic membrane is most compliant and able to absorb sound energy when the pressures on either side of it are equal. The test is carried out by placing a three channel probe from the immittance bridge into the ear to be tested. The probe contains (1) acoustic input tubing connected to a tone oscillator that provides a standard sound source, usually 220 or 226 Hz, (2) acoustic output tubing connected to a microphone and amplifier to measure the percentage of input sound energy that is reflected back by the tympanic membrane, and (3) a pneumatic tube connected to an air pump that can control the air pressure within the external ear canal. As the test proceeds, the air pressure within the ear canal is varied from +200 decaPascals (daPa) to −400 daPa (a range of air pressures less than that generated during pneumatic otoscopy). As the air pressure is varied, the sound reflected by the eardrum is measured. A graph called a tympanogram is produced.

Several types of common tympanograms are shown in Figure 77-2. In the *type A tympanogram,* the point of peak tympanic membrane admittance (compliance) is at the point where the air pressure in the ear canal varies from atmospheric pressure or 0 daPa by less than 100 daPa. If the absolute admittance of the tympanic membrane is not within a defined normal range, ossicular pathology may exist. A low admittance peak at atmospheric pressure may indicate that the attached ossicles are partially or completely fixed.

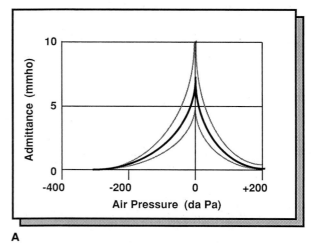

A

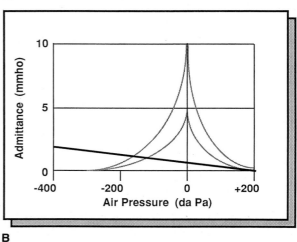

B

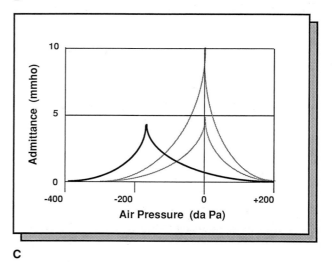

C

Figure 77-2. (**A**) Type A tympanogram, (**B**) Type B tympanogram, (**C**) Type C tympanogram.

High admittance may suggest the presence of ossicular discontinuity or a recently healed tympanic membrane perforation. In a *type B tympanogram,* the tympanic membrane admittance is uniformly low and varies little with change in air pressure within the ear canal. This condition may exist in the presence of an effusion within the middle ear space. The third general type of tympanogram is the *type C,* in which the point of peak admittance occurs when the air pressure within the ear canal is reduced and falls in the -100- to -400-daPa range. This curve indicates that the air pressure within the middle ear space is similarly reduced. Negative peak pressures with normal admittance values are quite variable (even with sniffing) and may or may not be associated with the presence of some degree of middle ear effusion.

The shape of the tympanogram in the region of the peak serves as a good predictor of the presence or absence of middle ear effusion. Middle ear effusion produces either a flat curve or one with an abnormally broad peak. The immittance audiometer can also estimate the physical volume of the external auditory canal from the tip of the probe to the tympanic membrane. If the volume is unusually low, the probe tip may be resting against a cerumen plug or misdirected toward the canal wall. If the volume is abnormally high with a flat curve, there may be a perforation in the tympanic membrane secondary to a middle ear infection or trauma. The patency of tympanostomy tubes also may be determined in this way. It is useful to record a child's canal volume measures prior to myringotomy with tubes; a volume two to three times larger with a pressure equalization tube in place confirms the patency of the tube. When the tympanic membrane is intact, the immittance bridge may be used to demonstrate the *acoustic reflex,* or the contraction of the stapedius and tensor tympani muscles of the middle ear in response to sudden sounds of 70 to 100 dB HL. The absence of this reflex may indicate a significant hearing loss or middle ear dysfunction.

Acoustic Reflectometry

An alternative or adjunct to immittance measures is the use of *acoustic reflectometry,* or sonar impedance analysis, to detect middle ear effusion. Acoustic reflectometry is performed with a hand-held device called an *acoustic otoscope,* the tip of which is inserted into the ear canal. The device emits a multifrequency sound and measures the sum of incident and reflected sound in the ear canal. This sum reaches its lowest value at a frequency for which the quarter wave length equals the distance from the microphone to the tympanic membrane, at which point the incident and reflected sounds are out of phase. The depth of this nadir is related to the presence or absence of middle ear effusion. Reflectivity values from 0 to 9 can be read on the instrument. Low values of 0 to 3 generally are considered normal, 4 to 5, borderline, and 6 to 9, supportive of middle ear

effusion. When this quick reading is supplemented by a printout of reflectivity as a function of frequency, diagnostic accuracy improves, particularly in the case of acute otitis media, which may generate a double-peaked tracing.

From a practical standpoint, acoustic reflectometry bears certain advantages over tympanometry in screening for middle ear effusion. Reflectometry is less aversive to the child because an air-tight seal is not required in the ear canal, as it is for tympanometry. Reflectometry can be performed more readily on a crying child than tympanometry. However, reflectometry is not, at its present stage of development, helpful in assessing the patency of presssure equalization tubes nor the presence of tympanic membrane perforation.

TESTING CHILDREN OF DIFFERENT AGES

Infants and Toddlers

Newborns at high risk for hearing loss (see criteria under Referral to Audiology) are screened by either behavioral or objective audiometric techniques. The behavioral methods require the presentation of a calibrated intense sound through a speaker placed near the child's head. Tone bursts in the 2000- to 4000-Hz frequency range are presented at a 70- to 90-dB level. A trained observer watches for characteristic eye and body movements or arousal responses that indicate that the child has heard the sound. This process has been automated by the use of a device called a *crib-o-gram,* which electronically detects the infant's motor responses to randomly presented sound stimuli. Such behavioral testing yields information only about the child's better hearing ear, if there is an asymmetry, and may rule out deafness but not milder hearing losses.

With increasing availability of auditory evoked response instrumentation, newborns at high risk of hearing loss are now commonly screened either before hospital discharge or within 3 months following discharge. When accomplished prior to discharge, such screening is performed for each ear using clicks at 30 to 40 dB followed by presentation of a higher-intensity stimulus, such as 60 dB, if no response is measured. If the child fails the screen at one or both sound levels, additional ABR threshold testing is recommended. Follow-up behavioral audiometry at age 1 year is advisable for those at-risk children who pass an ABR screening test.

The techniques useful for testing older infants and toddlers depend on the child's chronologic age and cognitive developmental stage. Behavioral audiometry may be accomplished at any age, and the results not only indicate that the child is capable of hearing a sound of a certain frequency and intensity but also that the child is able to process the acoustic information and generate predictable behavior as a result. Behavioral test results may sometimes be difficult to interpret because of random body movements or a child's short attention span. Objective audiometric tests such as evoked response audiometry and immittance audiometry provide reliable physiologic evidence that the auditory pathways are operative. These tests do not indicate whether a child has normal cerebral processing of the auditory information. For this reason, behavioral audiometry is preferred, but objective test procedures are invaluable for certain difficult-to-test persons such as children with mental retardation, emotional or psychiatric disorders, neuromuscular disorders, and newborns younger than 5 or 6 months of age.

The child's behavioral response to sound is age dependent. Children younger than the age of 2½ to 3 years usually are tested by listening to sounds from calibrated loudspeakers, a process known as *sound field audiometry*. In general, younger infants require pure tone or speech sounds of higher intensity to respond, and their responses are more rudimentary. During the first 4 months of life, noise or tones at the 50- to 70-dB level and speech at the 40-dB level should produce the *auropalpebral response,* which consists of such responses as eye widening, eye blink or eye roving in the awake infant, or lid tightening in the sleeping infant. The presentation of sound and determination of response from such behaviors is called *behavioral observation audiometry*. The interpretation of hearing as being "normal" on the basis of behavioral observation audiometry must be taken with caution. Because the likelihood of ruling out a mild degree of hearing loss by behavioral observation audiometry in an infant younger than 5 or 6 months of age is extremely slim, ABR measures are the test of choice for children functioning in this age range.

From 5 to 9 months the noise or tones at the 30- to 50-dB level and speech at the 10- to 20-dB level elicit a more sophisticated localizing response. Because children functioning above the age of 4 months make auditory localization (head turn) responses, they may be conditioned to reproduce the localization response reliably by showing them a visually interesting "reward" just after they turn in the direction of the sound. This technique is called *visual reinforcement audiometry*.

Children of any age may undergo immittance audiometric testing as a screen for the existence of middle ear disease. Some investigators believe that tympanometry is unreliable in infants younger than 6 months of age because of the increased compliance of the cartilaginous external canal. In this age group, the tympanogram may appear normal even when middle ear effusion is present. However, a flat tympanogram in an infant younger than 6 months of age does indicate poor tympanic membrane compliance, assuming patency of the ear canal.

Young Children

Children aged 3 years and older, and some 2-year olds, accept headphones and bone conduction oscillators. This permits the reliable determination of air conduction and bone conduction thresholds for pure tones and speech in each ear rather than for the better ear only. Children aged 2½ to 5 years are often tested using a technique called *play audiometry*. The child is taught to perform a play task such as placing a peg in a pegboard whenever a tone is heard. In this way, a complete audiogram may be generated. Children in this age group will be able to recognize a closed set of words including body parts and common toys so that their speech reception, speech recognition, and discrimination may be tested. Some older children may be able to repeat the words, while others may indicate that they understand the word by pointing to an appropriate object in the sound room or to a picture of the object. Children in this age group should undergo routine immittance or reflectometry testing because of the high incidence of middle ear disease.

Children aged 3 years and older can often be given a hearing screening test in the pediatric office, using an air conduction audiometer, which must receive electroacoustic calibration checks (available from the audiometer vendor or an audiology center) four times a year. The child is seated so that the audiometer controls are not visible. The child is instructed to perform a play task (such as throwing a block in a box) or raise a hand on hearing a tone. Pure tones of 1000, 2000, and 4000 Hz are presented at 20 dB HL. The frequency 500 Hz may also be screened at 20 dB HL if the room is extremely quiet. Failure to hear any one frequency at 20 dB HL requires further investigation. Pure tone audiometric screening may be a useful adjunct to immittance screening, which has proven its usefulness in the pediatric practice for detecting occult middle ear disease and monitoring the resolution of otitis media. Pure tone screening at intensities higher than 20 dB (e.g., 25 or 30 dB) is counterproductive in that half of all slight to mild hearing losses associated with otitis media may be missed.

Older Children and Adolescents

As a minimum, it is recommended that all children who are not at high risk children be routinely screened by audiometry twice: once before starting school and again between 12 and 18 years of age. Children older than the age of 5 or 6 years usually will respond to a standard audiometric test battery, including the determination of air and bone conduction thresholds, speech reception thresholds, and speech discrimination scores for each ear. Older children should also undergo immittance testing. Many children in this age group undergo routine auditory and tympanometric screening in local school screening programs. Children who fail the screening tests require a prompt otoscopic evaluation and an audiometric evaluation, including tympanometry.

Special test routines have been developed to evaluate children who are believed to have a functional hearing loss and children who have *central auditory processing* problems. Children with the latter problem may have difficulty attending to and understanding speech presented in noisy settings, have difficulty synthesizing a sequence of words into linguistic meaning, or have a problem with localizing sounds. Below age 7 years, central auditory processing skills are so closely allied with receptive language development that the assessment of these skills is best accomplished in conjunction with a speech and language pathologist, after hearing loss has been ruled out.

REFERRALS TO AUDIOLOGY

Parental suspicion of hearing loss in an infant is usually correct. Any parental mention of uneasiness regarding an infant or toddler's responsiveness to sound warrants prompt audiologic evaluation, after ruling out cerumen impaction and acute infection. Only two thirds of children with severe sensorineural hearing loss have obvious etiologic risk factors. The remainder tend to be the visually alert children who "don't miss a thing" and are not diagnosed as hearing impaired in the first few months of life.

Regardless of parental impression of hearing, infants having risk factors for permanent hearing loss should receive audiologic evaluation in the first few months of life. Risk factors include family history of permanent hearing impairment in childhood; TORCH infections or syphilis; craniofacial anomalies including minor pinna anomalies; birth weight less than 1500 g, perinatal asphyxia, persistent fetal circulation, treatment with extracorporeal membraneous oxygenation, hyperbilirubinemia exceeding indication for exchange transfusion, treatment with ototoxic medications as a newborn (e.g., aminoglycosides), and bacterial meningitis at any age. In cases of persistent otitis media, a determination of hearing levels may assist in determining candidacy for myringotomy with pressure equalization tube placement.

In a toddler, delayed language development also raises the need to rule out hearing loss. The child who is not babbling or imitating vocal sounds at 12 months, not using single words at 18 months, or not using creative phrases at 24 to 30 months should be referred for audiologic assessment. The advantages of early identification of hearing loss for the child's language, behavioral, and cognitive development are convincing enough to warrant prompt referral when any question is raised.

ANNOTATED BIBLIOGRAPHY

American Speech-Language-Hearing Association: Guidelines for screening for hearing impairments and middle ear disorders. Asha 32 (suppl 2):17–24, 1990. (Reviews the usefulness of various tympanometric measures in the detection of middle ear disease.)

Combs JT: Single vs. double acoustic reflectometry tracings. Pediatr Infect Dis J 8:616–620, 1989. (Presents tympanometric and acoustic reflectivity data for 1005 ears and demonstrates importance of using the acoustic otoscope with a hard-copy printout.)

Joint Committee on Infant Hearing: 1990 position statement. Asha 33 (Suppl 5):3–6, 1991. (Updated risk criteria for detection of hearing loss in infants, with recommendations for identification and management of hearing-impaired infants.)

Keith RW (ed): Audiology for the Physician. Baltimore, Williams & Wilkins, 1980. (Excellent review of current audiologic theory and practice with additional chapters on related otologic subject matter.)

Martin GK, Whitehead ML, Lonsbury-Martin BL: Potential of evoked otoacoustic emissions for infant hearing screening. Semin Hearing 11(2):186–203, 1990. (Reviews types of otoacoustic emissions and discusses their potential for newborn hearing screening.)

Matkin ND: Early recognition and referral of hearing-impaired children. Pediatr Rev 6:151–156, 1984. (Role of the pediatrician in identification of hearing impairment.)

Northern JL, Downs MP: Hearing in Children, 3rd ed. Baltimore, Williams & Wilkins, 1984. (Covers all aspects of diagnostic and rehabilitative pediatric audiology.)

78

Hearing Loss

Howard G. Smith

Current estimates indicate that as many as 15% of school-aged children have significant conductive hearing losses. The incidence of profound sensorineural hearing loss is approximately 1 per 1000 children. Hearing loss is a common childhood problem, and it is a challenge for clinicians to make the diagnosis in a timely fashion. An older child or adolescent who experiences a hearing loss has already acquired sufficient linguistic information to permit serviceable communication using an amplification device and deductive reasoning. In contrast, infants or toddlers with undiagnosed hearing losses are faced with the difficult if not impossible tasks of deciphering and learning spoken language and the cultural rules on which it is based without the ability to hear words clearly.

The identification of hearing loss in children requires that the clinician have a high index of suspicion and be sensitive to the concerns of parents, who are usually the first to become aware of the hearing loss. Parents of children with confirmed hearing losses often bitterly complain that their doctor unnecessarily delayed the diagnosis with comments such as: "Sara is only going through a stage. She will outgrow it."

PATHOPHYSIOLOGY

Hearing losses are characterized by *site of dysfunction* in the auditory mechanism, whether the etiology is genetic and hereditary or environmental and acquired, the age at onset of the hearing loss, the severity of the loss, and the stability of the loss. This latter aspect is discussed in detail in Chapter 77.

Conductive hearing losses occur as a result of interference with sound transmission through the external ear canal, tympanic membrane, or the ossicular chain. Sensorineural hearing losses are caused by malfunctions of cochlear transduction or signal transmission. Mixed hearing losses are the sum total of individual conductive and sensorineural losses.

Conductive Hearing Loss

Acquired conductive losses are the most common types of hearing loss in childhood. Mild to moderate fluctuating hearing losses are caused by cerumen impaction and otitis media. More significant conductive losses are produced by tympanic membrane and ossicular chain fixation, disruption, or destruction by cholesteatoma or by trauma.

Hereditary conductive losses may be congenital or delayed. Congenital deformities of the auricle alone may be inherited as a autosomal dominant or a sex-linked trait. Congenital aural atresia, the partial or complete agenesis of the external auditory canal, the middle ear space, and the ossicles due to malformations of the first and second branchial arch components, occurs in 1 in 10,000 to 20,000 live births. The atresia may be unilateral or bilateral and may be inherited as an isolated finding or as one of many parts of a syndromic constellation. Aural atresia is often associated with the autosomal dominantly inherited dysostoses of both the craniofacial (Crouzon's) syndrome and the mandibulofacial (Treacher Collins-Franceschetti) syndrome. Nonhereditary congenital aural atresia may also occur after fetal exposure to teratogenic pharmaceuticals such as thalidomide or as part of the congenital rubella syndrome. Children who have orofacial syndromes with associated cleft palate often have severe eustachian tube dysfunction, which itself produces secondary acquired conductive hearing losses. Another form of hereditary progressive conductive hearing loss that may first present during adolescence is otosclerosis, which is fixation of the stapes caused by repetitive resorption and redeposition of bone in the otic capsule. Otosclerosis apparently follows an autosomal dominant hereditary pattern.

Sensorineural Hearing Losses

Acquired sensorineural losses may occur either during embryogenesis or at any time after birth. The etiologic agents implicated include microorganisms, toxic chemicals, pharmaceuticals, and metabolic products. These agents cause profound deterioration of labyrinthine structures including the peripheral auditory and vestibular sensory receptors, vascular structures, and supporting membranes. Maternal infection with microorganisms such as the rubella virus, the cytomegalovirus, the protozoan Toxoplasma gondii,

and the spirochete Treponema pallidum may produce mid- to high-frequency hearing losses, dysequilibrium, or rotatory vertigo. Hearing loss due to congenital syphilis may occur suddenly during childhood or may slowly develop during adulthood. Childhood viral infections such as measles, mumps, acute respiratory tract infections, and infectious mononucleosis have been strongly associated with unilateral and bilateral sudden hearing losses in pre-school- and school-aged children. Bacterial meningitis, particularly with Hemophilus influenza type b, has been associated with significant hearing impairment in about 10% of affected children. The recent release of a conjugate protein vaccine for immunizing infants against this microorganism and the addition of corticosteroids to standard therapy for bacterial meningitis should reduce these numbers. Hearing loss is not associated with viral meningitis.

Ototoxic drugs administered either to the embryo or to the newborn may produce labyrinthine damage. The antimalarial drugs quinine and chloroquine, as well as the aminoglycoside antibiotics gentamicin, kanamycin, tobramycin, and amikacin, have profound ototoxic effects. Loop diuretics, such as ethacrynic acid and furosemide, also produce hearing loss, an effect exacerbated by the concomitant use of aminoglycosides. Careful monitoring of drug blood levels, as well as cochlear and vestibular function, will prevent irreversible damage when these agents are used.

Acquired sensorineural hearing losses have also been associated with congenital hypothyroidism, erythroblastosis fetalis, prematurity, hypoxia, prolonged or difficult labor, maternal diabetes mellitus, and toxemia of pregnancy.

Acoustic or head trauma may cause immediate or delayed sensorineural hearing losses. Repeated intense noise, including that emanating from miniature stereo headphones, a sudden explosion, or head trauma with or without a temporal bone fracture produces a characteristic high-frequency hearing loss, often partially or completely reversible, which may later present as a permanent loss. An important, potentially treatable cause of sudden acquired sensorineural hearing loss is perilymph leakage through disrupted membranes at the oval or round windows. A high-frequency hearing loss, with or without accompanying positional vertigo, usually follows vigorous physical activity, marked altitude or barometric pressure changes, or physical trauma to the ear or head. Prompt exploratory surgery and sealing of leaks with soft tissue will often prevent progressive hearing loss and may restore serviceable hearing.

Hereditary sensorineural hearing losses represent 20% to 50% of all cases of severe to profound sensorineural hearing losses. The estimated incidence of hereditary hearing loss is at least 1 in 4000 live births. The hearing loss, often severe to profound, may occur as an isolated finding or may occur in conjunction with other clinical features as shown in Table 78-1. Abnormalities of ocular structures, the renal system, the nervous system, and general metabolism may accompany hereditary sensorineural hearing losses.

Table 78-1.   Types of Hereditary and Genetic Sensorineural Hearing Losses (SNHL)

NAME	INHERITANCE	ONSET	ASSOCIATED FEATURES
SNHL Occuring Alone			
Michel's deafness	AD	C	Complete aplasia of cochlea
Mondini's deafness	AD	C	Partial aplasia of cochlea; associated cerebrospinal fluid leak
Familial progressive deafness	AD	D	Partial aplasia of cochlea at basal turn
Scheibe's deafness	AR	C	Normal bony labyrinth; abnormality of cochlear membranes
X-linked deafness	SL	C	Severe to profound hearing losses
X-linked deafness	SL	D	Moderate to severe hearing losses
SNHL and Metabolic Abnormalities			
Waardenberg's syndrome	AD	C or D	Partial albinism; abnormalities of tyrosine metabolism
Schafer's syndrome	AD	C	Prolinemia; mental retardation
Tietze's syndrome	AD	C or D	Albinism; abnormalities of tyrosine metabolism
Nelson's syndrome	AD	V	Homocystinemia; mental retardation
Albinism	AD, AR, or SL	C	Albinism, strabismus, nystagmus
Hypophosphatasia	AR	V	Decreased bone mineralization
Hyperphosphatasia	AR	V	Dwarfism; other skeletal abnormalities
Hurler's syndrome	AR	D	Lipochondrodystrophy, dwarfism; mental retardation; hepatosplenomegaly
Morquio's disease	AR	V	Osteochondrodystrophy
Onychodystrophy	AR or AD	C	Abnormal nail growth
Tay-Sachs disease	AR	V	Mental retardation; ganglioside lipidosis
Pendred's syndrome	AR	C	Goiter
Wilson's disease	AR	V	Hepatic and ocular lens degeneration
SNHL and Nephropathies			
Alport's syndrome	AD	D	Glomerulonephritis; 1% of hereditary deafness
Muckle-Wells syndrome	AD	D	Nephritis; amyloidosis
Herrmann's syndrome	AD	D	Nephritis; epilepsy; diabetes mellitus; mental retardation
Renal tubular acidosis	AR	D	Metabolic acidosis; failure to thrive
SNHL and Ocular Disease			
Usher's syndrome	AR, SL, or AD	C	Retinitis pigmentosa; 10% of hereditary deafness
Alstrom's syndrome	AR	D	Retinitis pigmentosa; diabetes mellitus; obesity
Cockayne's syndrome	AR	D	Retinitis pigmentosa; dwarfism; mental retardation
Leber's disease	AR	V	Optic atrophy
Norrie's disease	AR or SL	D	Retinal pseudoglioma
Refsum's syndrome	AR	D	Retinitis pigmentosa; ichthyosis; poly-neuritis; ataxia
Biotinidase deficiency	?	D	Retinopathy; dermatoses; neuromuscular abnormalities
SNHL and Nervous System Disease			
Huntington's chorea	AD	D	Progressive chorea
Von Recklinghausen's disease	AD	D	Neural schwannomas

(continued)

Table 78-1. Types of Hereditary and Genetic Sensorineural Hearing Losses (SNHL) *(continued)*

NAME	INHERITANCE	ONSET	ASSOCIATED FEATURES
Friedreich's ataxia	AR	V	Cerebellar ataxia
Richards-Rundle disease	AR	D	Ataxia; mental retardation; muscular dystrophy; absent sexual development
SNHL and Heart Disease			
Jervell-Lange-Nielsen syndrome	AR	C	Prolonged QT interval, heart block
Lewis' syndrome	AR	V	Pulmonic stenosis
SNHL and Skeletal Disease			
Klippel-Feil syndrome	AR	D	Cervical fusion; spina bifida; scoliosis
Paget's disease	AR	D	Deformities of skull and long bones
Chromosomal Abnormalities			
Trisomy 13–15 (D)		C	External and middle ear abnormalities; eye abnormalities
Trisomy 18 (E)		C	External ear abnormalities; micrognathia; digit abnormalities
CHARGE association	?	C	Coloboma; cardiac abnormalities; mental retardation; choanal atresia; genital abnormalities

Mode of inheritance: AD, autosomal dominant; AR, autosomal recessive; SL, sex-linked.
Onset time of SNHL: C, congenital; D, delayed; V, variable.

CLINICAL PRESENTATION

Clinicians have traditionally depended on both their own and parental observations to suggest the existence of a childhood hearing loss. The lack of age-appropriate responses to sound such as eye blink, eye widening, startle response, and head turning in infants and toddlers should prompt referral to an audiologist for formal testing, but the apparent presence of these responses should not delay otherwise indicated testing. Any infant with one or more of the following factors, known to be associated with a higher than normal risk of a hearing loss, should be referred as soon as possible for comprehensive auditory testing if it has not already been done.

1. Birthweight of less than 1500 g
2. Apgar score of 5 or less at 5 minutes
3. Delayed growth and development
4. More than 24 hours in a neonatal intensive care unit, with or without artificial ventilatory assistance
5. Hyperbilirubinemia (>20 mg/dL) requiring prolonged phototherapy or exchange transfusion
6. Seizures or other neurologic abnormalities
7. Known physical abnormalities of the skull or the ear, nose, or throat at birth
8. History of maternal or neonatal infection or sepsis
9. History of head injury at birth or otherwise
10. Family history of hereditary hearing loss

Children of any age with a history of meningitis, encephalitis, severe head injury, or repeated episodes of otitis media should be evaluated for a possible hearing loss.

Hearing losses in preschool children are often heralded by obvious communication difficulties; excessive sound volume on the television, radio, or cassette player; and speech delay or poor speech intelligibility. Children with frequent middle ear problems, even in the absence of other evidence of hearing loss, should also be highly suspect.

School-aged children are often unaware of gradual or even sudden hearing losses. Signs of such losses include failed school screening tests, deterioration of a child's note-taking performance, development of unusual communication problems, and a change in telephone or portable stereo sound system usage patterns. Such a loss should also be suspected if a child complains of noises in the head (tinnitus) or a distortion of hearing.

DIFFERENTIAL DIAGNOSIS

Currently available behavioral testing methods and increasingly sophisticated evoked potential audiometry and impedance audiometry permit an accurate determination of the severity and site of a presumptive hearing impairment at *any age*. These techniques are described in Chapter 77.

WORK-UP

History

The historical review for a child with a suspected hearing loss begins with a review of the prenatal and perinatal periods including maternal exposure to infectious disease; use of prescription, over-the-counter, and recreational drugs; the nature of the gestational period, the labor, and the delivery of the infant including any birth trauma or hypoxia; and the neonatal period including the occurrence of jaundice, sepsis, cardiopulmonary disease, renal disease, and treatment regimens used. Other important information includes the history of the child's middle ear infections, the parent's assessment of the child's responses to sounds and listening skills, the development of communication skills, a history of head injury or acoustic trauma, and a family history of hearing loss or other otologic problems. The parents or older children themselves should be asked about ear pain, changes in hearing level and quality, and signs of balance problems such as clumsiness, stomach upset, or lightheadedness.

Physical Examination

The otologic examination begins with a careful appraisal of the position and anatomy of auricular appendages, the surface anatomy of the temporal bone, the size and shape of the external canal, and the appearance of the tympanic membrane and ossicular landmarks. The mobility of the tympanic membrane and the presence or absence of middle ear air or fluid are determined with the pneumatic otoscope. (For review of technique, see under Physical Examination, Chap. 75.) An intranasal examination should be performed, and, within the oral cavity, the number, position, color, and shape of the teeth should be noted. The structure and function of the hard and soft palate are assessed, looking for evidence of complete, partial, or submucosal clefting and abnormal soft palatal motion. The cervical structures should be evaluated by inspection and palpation for evidence of sinus tracts or embryonic cysts. The thyroid should be palpated to check for enlargement or nodules.

A complete general physical examination should be carried out with particular attention to the eyes, skin, skeletal system, and the nervous system.

Laboratory Tests

An age-appropriate audiometric evaluation should be carried out according to the principles outlined in Chapter 77 if screening tests or clinical presentation suggest the possibility of a hearing loss. To help determine the etiology of a congenital sensorineural hearing loss, infants and toddlers should have serum tested with a TORCH screen to assay their IgM antibody levels to toxoplasma, rubella, cytomegalovirus, and herpesvirus. In an older child, a routine serologic test for syphilis, the fluorescent treponemal antibody-absorption test (FTA-ABS), and a screening heterophil test are drawn. A child with a newly diagnosed hearing loss should have radiographic imaging of the temporal bones by a fine-cut computed tomographic technique.

Serum chemistry tests including determination of random blood glucose, blood urea nitrogen, creatinine, calcium, phosphate, thyroxine, thyroid stimulating hormone, total cholesterol, and triglyceride levels may be performed to discover if a hearing-impaired child has an associated metabolic disorder. Serum biotinidase activity should be assayed, especially in a child with dermatologic disorders and visual problems. An electrocardiogram should be performed. If renal disease is suspected, other tests should include a complete urinalysis, creatinine clearance determination, and abdominal or renal ultrasonography. There is an increased incidence of renal disorders in children with first and second branchial arch syndromes.

MANAGEMENT AND SPECIALIZED CARE

It is not within the scope of this discussion to provide a detailed discussion of the long-term management of hearing loss since services must be individually tailored to the nature and severity of the loss. Middle ear disease, which commonly produces reversible forms of mild to moderate conductive hearing loss, should be actively treated with medical management supplemented by surgical approaches as the longevity or the severity of the disease increases. The approach to this type of otologic disease is discussed in Chapters 75 and 76.

Unilateral hearing losses must be carefully evaluated using auditory brain stem evoked responses and computed tomographic scanning or gadolinium-enhanced magnetic resonance imaging to rule out retrocochlear lesions such as cerebellopontine angle or internal auditory canal lesions. Careful monitoring, preferred classroom seating, and the use of appropriate amplification devices are necessary to minimize the academic impact of the hearing loss.

More severe or irreversible bilateral hearing losses, which are usually sensorineural, present a difficult management challenge and call for a highly organized, multidisciplinary team approach. This team has three goals: (1) to initially assess and periodically monitor the medical and psychological status of the child and his or her family; (2) to provide sufficient background information about deafness and the necessary emotional support for a family to accept the reality of a child's hearing loss and proceed to realistically deal with it; and (3) to help the parents choose suitable educational programs for themselves and their child.

A typical team includes a pediatric otologist, an audiologist experienced with amplification management, a pediatrician with expertise in developmental pediatrics and genetics, a pediatric ophthalmologist, an educational psychologist experienced in evaluating the cognitive skills of deaf children, a speech-language pathologist, a (literally) deaf professional skillful in evaluating gestural language competence, a teacher of the hearing impaired, and a clinical psychologist. Each child undergoes an otologic examination, complete audiologic testing and fitting with appropriate hearing aids, a developmental pediatric evaluation with elective consultation to a pediatric neurologist, an ophthalmic evaluation, a cognitive and psychological evaluation, and a two-part communication evaluation to assess the child's communication skills using verbal and nonverbal language techniques. Monitoring evaluations by selected clinicians are scheduled for every 6 months. When family history or clinical presentation indicates the possibility of a genetic etiology, a complete family pedigree is constructed.

Supportive and therapeutic counseling sessions for family members help them cope with expected initial reactions of grief and denial as well as frequently associated situational crises such as marital strife. Such sessions also permit professionals the opportunity to better understand the psychodynamics operating within the child's family. If a genetic etiology is established, genetic counseling will help family members understand the implications for other family members.

Through reading and discussions with clinicians, other parents, and deaf professionals, family members learn to accept that hearing impairment alone will not prevent their child from leading a happy, rewarding life. The family learns that comfortable communication with severely to profoundly hearing-limited family members may at times only be achieved by the use of sign language. Family members are encouraged to learn about the causes of hearing problems, the measurement of hearing, the effect of hearing loss on child growth and development, historical perspectives about education for hearing-limited children and local educational alternatives, and the legal rights of the hearing impaired child. Parents are strongly urged to enroll themselves and their child in programs with expertise in educating hearing impaired children and that provide a wide variety of ancillary services.

Children with profound sensorineural hearing losses may be eligible for a cochlear implant, which restores a sense of sound rather than hearing with variable degrees of success. Preliminary results of implants in children show that the best results are achieved in post–linguistically deafened children who receive the implant within 4 years of their hearing deterioration. Placing an implant in congenitally deaf children 2 years of age or older remains experimental but may show promise.

Clinicians must be aware of the considerable influence that their factual statements and opinions have not only on the families of hearing impaired children but also on professionals and others within the community. The child's linguistic, intellectual, and emotional development must be carefully monitored to detect and solve problems. When necessary, advocacy on behalf of the child will be essential to ensure the availability and funding of services essential for hearing-limited children to learn strategies that will enable them to reach their full potential in life.

ANNOTATED BIBLIOGRAPHY

Brookhouser PE, Worthington DW, Kelly WJ: Severe versus profound sensorineural hearing loss in children. Laryngoscope 100:349–56, 1990. (Review of 200 children with substantial sensorineural hearing losses highlighting the strategies for selecting appropriate candidates for cochlear implantation.)

Catlin FI: Prevention of hearing impairment from infection and ototoxic drugs. Arch Otolaryngol 11:377–384, 1985. (Review of literature related to the varied causes and the prevention of acquired forms of sensorineural hearing loss.)

Das VK: Etiology of bilateral sensorineural hearing loss in children. Scand Audiol Suppl 30:43–52, 1988. (Review of 1455 cases of sensorineural hearing loss focusing on the causes.)

Davis LE, Johnsson LG: Viral infections of the inner ear: Clinical virologic and pathologic studies in humans and animals. Am J Otolaryngol 4:347–362, 1983. (Review about viral-induced acquired forms of sensorineural hearing loss.)

Freeman RD, Carbin CF, Boese RJ: Can't Your Child Hear: A Guide for Those Who Care About Deaf Children. Baltimore, University Park Press, 1981. (Summarizes the current body of opinion and fact about the causes and consequences of deafness for parents of hearing impaired children and for professionals beginning to learn about deafness.)

Konigsmark BW, Gorlin RJ: Genetic and Metabolic Deafness. Philadelphia, WB Saunders, 1976. (Encyclopedic review of syndromic constellations that include hearing loss.)

Label MH, Frej BJ, Syrogiannopoulos GA et al.: Dexamethasone therapy for bacterial meningitis: Results of two double-blind placebo-controlled trials. N Engl J Med 319:964–971, 1988. (Study showing 14-fold reduction in severe to profound sensorineural hearing losses in children with meningitis treated with corticosteroids.)

79

Epistaxis

Ellen M. Friedman

Nosebleeds, or epistaxis, are relatively common occurrences in the pediatric population. These episodes are usually infrequent, mild, and self-limiting. Nevertheless, epistaxis may be quite frightening and, at times, even life threatening. The highly vascular nasal septum and nasopharynx lend themselves to bleeding. The fragile nasal mucosa lacks surrounding tissue to aid in compression, which may result in persistent and recurrent bleeding.

PATHOPHYSIOLOGY AND CLINICAL PRESENTATION

Epistaxis should be divided into *anterior* and *posterior* nosebleeds. Ninety percent of epistaxis in children is anterior in origin. This is fortunate because anterior nosebleeds are generally less severe and more easily controlled.

Anterior nosebleeds originate in Little's area or Hesselbach's triangle. This highly vascular area is a rich congregation of terminal blood vessels of the anterior ethmoidal artery. The hallmark of anterior epistaxis is for blood to exit almost exclusively from the anterior nares.

Posterior epistaxis is usually more brisk and severe. Vigorous bleeding may occur, usually from a branch of the sphenopalatine artery. Most of the bleeding is in the nasopharynx and mouth. Blood may also exit from the nares.

DIFFERENTIAL DIAGNOSIS

The most common etiology for epistaxis in childhood is trauma and inflammation. The nose is an accessible target for external trauma and the nasal mucosa is highly susceptible to the effects of nose-picking and sneezing. Inflammation from rhinitis can lead to erosion of the tiny blood vessels, and the drying effect of inspiration can further inhibit mucosal healing.

Coagulation defects such as von Willeband's disease are responsible for only approximately 5% of recurrent epistaxis. Other etiologies for epistaxis in childhood are far less common. Juvenile angiofibroma is a benign tumor that occurs in adolescent males and commonly presents as recurrent unilateral nosebleeds. These tumors may originate in the anterior wall of the sphenoidal sinus and may be visualized on intranasal examination. Other nasal and sinus neoplasms, which are even less common in the pediatric population, may also be associated with epistaxis.

Intranasal foreign bodies commonly present as unilateral, foul-smelling, purulent nasal drainage. Epistaxis may occur if the foreign body has developed surrounding friable granulation tissue.

Familial hereditary telangiectasia (Osler-Weber-Rendu syndrome) is a disease with several areas of confluence of dilated arterioles, venules, and capillaries. The nasal and oral mucosa are most frequently involved, although the entire gastrointestinal tract may have lesions.

Systemic disease may also have associated episodes of epistaxis. Leukemias, anemias, hepatic failure, and hypertension may result in nosebleeds.

WORK-UP

It is estimated that 10% of the population experience a significant nosebleed. It is helpful to bear in mind that most cases of pediatric epistaxis are readily controllable at home or by the primary health care provider. Since most cases are due to local trauma or inflammation, an extensive evaluation should be reserved for those cases that are recurrent or particularly severe.

Early assessment of the severity of the blood loss is necessary. A brief family history concerning easy bruisability and coagulopathy should be elicited. Vital signs should be obtained. In general, it is best to control the nasal hemorrhage prior to initiating an extensive search for the underlying etiology.

If, due to the severity of blood loss or the recurrent nature of the problem, a cause other than local trauma is suspected, other tests should be performed. Specialized tests, such as computed tomographic scanning, will be helpful if an intranasal tumor is suspected. If a primary coagulopathy is suspected, screening blood tests should include hematocrit, hemoglobin, prothrombin time, partial thromboplastin time, platelet count, and bleeding time. Further testing for a bleeding defect (e.g., von Willebrand's disease) may be necessary.

TREATMENT

Many pediatric patients with epistaxis can be treated at home. Although many persons apply pressure to the dorsum of the nose, actually the application of pressure to the anterior nasal septum will more effectively result in clot formation. Vasoconstriction through topical drops (e.g., Neo-Synephrine) should be suggested. An ice pack placed around the neck or an ice cube under the lips may also aid with vasoconstriction. The treatment of a patient with severe or recurrent epistaxis will require a visit to a clinic or hospital emergency department. The hemorrhage may be controlled by (1) local cauterizing agents, (2) packing of the nose/nasopharynx, (3) arterial ligation, and (4) treating the underlying blood dyscrasia.

To select the appropriate management, it is essential to determine if the bleeding is anterior or posterior. A nasal examination with good illumination and point suction is necessary to locate the bleeding vessels. In this manner, blood and secretions can be removed to completely visualize the nasal mucosa and septum.

Frequently, topical vasoconstriction, in conjunction with local pressure in Little's area, will control mild bleeding. If dilated blood vessels are easily visualized, silver nitrate cauterization may be necessary. The application of the silver nitrate stick to the dry, dilated vessels will result in the destruction and coagulation of the vessel. Although this procedure causes a stinging sensation, most children can tolerate this procedure if they are told that stinging will occur. Electrocoagulation should be limited in the pediatric population because of the possibility of significant injury to the mucosa or septum (e.g., septal perforation).

If cauterization and pressure do not control the epistaxis, anterior nasal packing is indicated. Various materials may be used. Dissolvable topical agents, such as Gelfoam, topical thrombin, or microfibrillar collagen, may be applied to abraded or oozing areas (the choice of agent is based on the ease of application). This type of packing is most successful when placed on a relatively dry field and direct pressure is immediately applied. If a prolonged compression packing is indicated, 1-inch petrolatum gauze strips may be positioned. It is preferable to use antibiotic-impregnated strips of gauze to avoid associated infection from a blocked sinus ostia. Inflatable balloon-type packs have been used in adults but are of limited use in pediatrics. Compression packs should remain in position for approximately 3 days. Patients are usually placed on oral antibiotics while compression packs are in position to avoid sinusitis.

It is helpful to instruct the patient and family about local measures that may decrease the likelihood of further episodes of epistaxis. A bedside humidifier, the local application of petrolatum to the nares for lubrication, and the reduction of nasal trauma will enhance the healing of the nasal mucosa. If bacterial rhinitis is associated with the local irritation, oral antibiotics for 5 to 7 days may be indicated.

INDICATIONS FOR REFERRAL

Posterior epistaxis is more difficult to control. Cauterization and anterior nasal packing will not be useful. Compression packs positioned in the posterior nasopharynx and anterior nasal cavity are necessary. Considerable skill is required to place a posterior pack and, in a pediatric patient, sedation or general anesthesia may be indicated. Initially, one should use a topical vasoconstrictor in the anterior nasal chamber. A soft catheter should be passed through the nostril into the mouth. A specially designed pack should be used. The antibiotic-impregnated posterior nasal pack should be tied to the catheter with the first string. The second string from the packing will be secured to the outside of the cheek at the end of the procedure and used for the eventual removal of the pack perorally. When withdrawing the catheter from the nose, the pack should be tightly positioned into the nasopharynx. While tensing the string attached to the posterior pack is being done, an anterior nasal packing of petrolatum gauze should be placed. In this manner the posterior pack will be secured and appropriate pressure will be delivered to the nasopharynx. The anterior string exiting from the nose should be tied to a dental roll anterior to the columella. Patients with posterior packs require hospitalization and antibiotic therapy.

Although posterior packs in children have not been known to cause significant carbon dioxide retention, reports of respiratory depression associated with these packs in adults have caused concern. Frequent monitoring of vital signs should be performed. Daily determination of hematocrit and hemoglobin values is indicated to ensure hematologic stability. If bleeding continues following the position of a posterior pack, surgical intervention may be necessary. Ligation of the internal maxillary artery may be achieved by the transantral approach.

In cases of severe recurrent epistaxis, as associated with hereditary hemorrhagic telangiectasia, other surgical procedures may be indicated. Septal dermoplasty may relieve the recurrent epistaxis, although gastrointestinal bleeding and bleeding from the mouth may continue to be a significant problem in this disease.

If an intranasal foreign body is identified, it may be removed in the office setting by an otolaryngologist. Patient cooperation is important so that removal will proceed smoothly and will not result in further impaction of the object or aspiration of the foreign body. General anesthesia is occasionally indicated. A referral to a pediatric otolaryngologist should also be made if an intranasal tumor is suspected. In certain settings a hematologic evaluation, as well as subsequent management, may best be handled by a pediatric hematologist.

ANNOTATED BIBLIOGRAPHY

Bluestone CD, Smith HC: Intranasal freezing for severe epistaxis. Arch Otolaryngol 85:445, 1967. (Excellent description of the technique of inserting nasal packing.)

Montgomery WW: Surgery of the Upper Respiratory System. Philadelphia, Lea & Febiger, 1973. (Excellent discussion concerning the anatomic and surgical considerations in epistaxis.)

80

Sinusitis

Ellen R. Wald

Acute (<30 days' duration) infections of the paranasal sinuses occur in children and adults usually as a complication of viral upper respiratory tract infections or allergic inflammation. *Subacute* or *chronic* (at least 30 days' duration) sinusitis results when the symptoms of acute sinusitis are not recognized as such or when they are inadequately treated. Although there are few data on which to base an estimate of the frequency of these disorders, acute sinusitis probably complicates viral upper respiratory tract infections in 5% to 10% of children.

ANATOMY AND PATHOPHYSIOLOGY

The anatomic relationships of the sinus cavities are shown in Figure 80-1. Three shelflike structures, the superior, middle, and inferior turbinates, protrude from the lateral nasal wall. Beneath each turbinate is a corresponding meatus. The ostia of the maxillary, frontal, and anterior ethmoidal sinuses drain into the middle meatus. The ostia of the sphenoidal sinuses and the posterior ethmoidal air cells drain into the superior meatus. Only the lacrimal duct empties into the inferior meatus.

The maxillary sinus develops as a lateral outpouching of the nasal cavity. As the child grows the maxillary sinus enlarges in width and height and eventually assumes a quadrilateral shape. The position of the maxillary ostium in relation to the body of the sinus is notable. The location of this outflow tract, high on the medial wall of the maxillary sinus, impedes gravitational drainage of secretions; ciliary

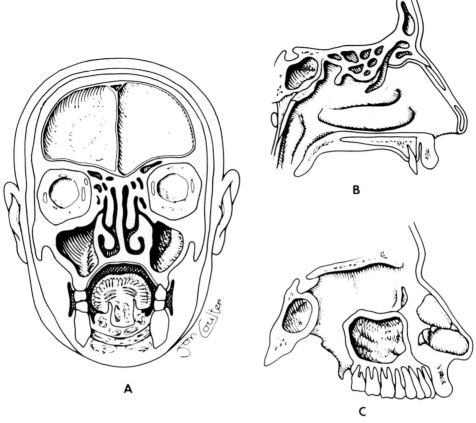

Figure 80-1. Coronal (**A**) and sagittal sections (**B** and **C**) of the nose and paranasal sinuses.

activity is required to move secretions from the body of the maxillary sinus through the ostia to the nose. Secretions are carried from there into the nasopharynx to be either expectorated or swallowed.

The ethmoidal sinuses, as seen on the coronal and sagittal sections (Fig. 80-1*A, B*) are not single large cavities but are divided into 3 to 15 air cells. These air cells, separated from each other by thin bony septa, drain by individual ostia into the middle meatus. The lateral wall of the ethmoidal sinus, the lamina papyracea, is a paper-thin plate of bone that may permit the direct extension of infection from the ethmoidal sinus to the orbit through natural dehiscences in the bone.

The frontal sinus, seen on a sagittal section Figure 80-1*B*), develops either from an anterior ethmoidal cell or from a separate evagination of the anterosuperior portion of the middle meatus. In either case, its drainage is similar to that of the anterior ethmoidal sinuses. The sphenoidal sinuses, which are immediately anterior to the pituitary fossa, are adjacent to the posterior ethmoidal air cells and drain into the superior meatus.

The maxillary sinus is the principal site of disease in most cases of sinus infection in children. The anatomy of the draining ostia probably accounts for its frequent involvement. In most of these patients, the ethmoidal air cells are also involved. The drainage of the ethmoidal, frontal, and sphenoidal sinuses is aided by gravity; on the other hand, the narrow ostia of the ethmoidal sinuses are easily obstructed by mucosal swelling, thus predisposing them to infection. After the age of 10 years, the frontal sinus assumes greater clinical importance because it becomes a more common site of sinus infection and may serve as a focus for rare but serious intracranial complications. Isolated infection of the sphenoidal sinuses is uncommon; however, these sinuses may be involved in cases of pansinusitis.

The predominant bacterial species causing acute sinusitis include *Streptococcus pneumoniae, Moraxella catarrhalis,* and *Hemophilus influenzae.* Both *H. influenzae* and *M. catarrhalis* may be β-lactamase producing and consequently ampicillin resistant. *Staphylococcus aureus* has not been isolated from a child with acute sinusitis; anaerobic flora are also uncommon in acute infection. Several viruses including adenovirus and parainfluenza have been recovered.

The microbiology of chronic sinusitis has been studied

less thoroughly than that of acute sinusitis. Anaerobic bacteria appear to be the predominant pathogens in most studies. The predominant anaerobic organisms are *Bacteroides* species, anaerobic gram-positive cocci, and *Veillonella* and *Fusobacterium* species. The common aerobic organisms isolated include *Streptococcus viridans* and *H. influenzae*. *S. aureus* has occasionally been isolated.

CLINICAL PRESENTATION

Commonly recognized symptoms of sinusitis in adults and adolescents are facial pain, headache, and fever. However, children with acute sinusitis frequently have complaints that are less specific. During the course of apparent viral upper respiratory tract infections, there are two common clinical developments that should alert the clinician to the possibility of bacterial infection of the paranasal sinuses. The first, less common presentation is a "cold" that seems more severe than usual: the fever is high (>39.0°C), the nasal discharge is purulent and copious and there may be associated periorbital swelling and facial pain. The periorbital swelling is gradual in onset and is most obvious in the early morning shortly after awakening. The swelling may decrease and actually disappear during the day, only to reappear once again the following day. A less common complaint is headache (a feeling of fullness or a dull ache either behind or above the eyes), most often reported in children older than 5 years of age. Occasionally there may be dental pain, either from infection originating in the teeth or referred from the sinus infection.

The second, more common clinical situation in which sinusitis should be suspected occurs when the signs and symptoms of a "cold" are protracted. Nasal discharge or daytime cough or both that continue for more than 10 but less than 30 days and are not improving are the principal complaints. Most uncomplicated viral upper respiratory tract infections last 5 to 7 days; although patients may not be asymptomatic by the tenth day, they have usually improved. The persistence of respiratory symptoms beyond the 10-day mark, without appreciable improvement, suggests a complication of the upper respiratory tract infection. The nasal discharge may be of any quality (thin or thick; clear, mucoid, or purulent) and the cough (which may be dry or wet) must be present in the daytime, although it is often worse at night. A cough occurring only at night is a common residual symptom of an upper respiratory tract infection. When it is the only residual symptom, it is nonspecific and does not suggest a sinus infection. On the other hand, the persistence of a daytime cough is frequently the symptom that prompts medical attention. The patient may not appear very ill, and if fever is present it will usually be low grade. Fetid breath is often reported by parents of preschoolers. Facial pain is not usually a prominent complaint; however, intermittent painless morning periorbital swelling may have been noted. In this case it is not the severity of the clinical symptoms but their persistence that calls for attention.

Subacute or chronic sinusitis should be suspected when there are protracted respiratory symptoms—nasal discharge, nasal congestion, or cough that has lasted for more than 30 days. Although the nasal discharge is most often purulent, it may be thin and clear. Once again, the cough should be present during the daytime, although it is usually reported to be worse at night. The patient may complain additionally of facial pain, headache, or malaise. However, unless these less specific complaints are accompanied by respiratory symptoms, they should not be attributed to sinus infection. Fever is less prominent and is found less frequently than in acute sinusitis.

DIFFERENTIAL DIAGNOSIS

The major differential considerations are uncomplicated upper respiratory tract infection or allergic inflammation. The former is discriminated from sinusitis by the severity or duration of symptoms. Allergic inflammation, which may give rise to nasal discharge or cough or both (and may be complicated by a secondary bacterial infection), may be suspected on the basis of family or personal history of atopy. A physical examination may demonstrate the stigmata of allergic inflammation with Dennie's lines, an allergic nasal crease, and pale edematous nasal mucosa. In uncomplicated allergic rhinitis or in bronchospasm (manifested as cough) triggered by upper respiratory tract infection, the sinus roentgenograms will be normal.

WORK-UP

History

The important elements that should be included in the history are the duration and severity of respiratory complaints, the quality of nasal discharge, and the determination of frequency and timing of cough. In addition, an inquiry should be made regarding the presence or absence of malodorous breath (despite good oral hygiene), morning headaches that subside during the daytime if the patient is erect, puffiness about the eyes, dental discomfort, and an allergic history (e.g., asthma, seasonal rhinitis, conjunctivitis, or eczema).

Physical Examination

The important elements of the physical examination include an assessment of the nasal mucosa, nasal septum, tonsillar and pharyngeal areas, and cervical lymph nodes and an inspection of the face for localized swelling. Intranasal instillation of a topical decongestant may shrink the nasal mucosa and permit visualization of purulent material coming from the middle meatus. This is a most helpful clinical observation.

Transillumination may be useful in diagnosing inflammation of the maxillary or frontal sinuses. The patient and examiner must be in a darkened room. The light source, shielded from the observer, is placed over the midpoint of the inferior orbital rim. The transmission of light through the hard plate is then assessed with the patient's mouth open. In judging light transmission, light passing through the alveolar ridges should be excluded. Transillumination of the frontal sinus is accomplished by placing a high-intensity light source inferior to the medial border of the supraorbital ridge and evaluating the symmetry of the blush bilaterally. Transillumination is useful in adolescents and adults if light transmission is either normal or absent. "Reduced" transmission or "dull" transillumination are assessments that correlate poorly with results of sinus aspiration. The increased thickness of both the soft tissue and bony vault in children younger than 10 years of age limits the clinical value of transillumination in the younger age group.

Laboratory Tests

Imaging Techniques. Plain roentgenography has been used traditionally to determine the presence of sinus disease. Standard radiographic projections include an anteroposterior, a lateral, and an occipitomental view. The anteroposterior view is optimal for evaluation of the ethmoidal sinuses, and the lateral view is best for evaluation of the frontal and sphenoidal sinuses. The occipitomental view, taken after tilting the chin upward 45° to the horizontal, allows an evaluation of the maxillary sinuses. Although much has been written about the frequency of abnormal sinus roentgenograms in "normal" children, these studies have been flawed either by inattention to the presence of symptoms and signs of respiratory tract inflammation or by failure to classify abnormal roentgenographic findings into major (significant) and minor (insignificant) categories. One report shows, however, that significantly abnormal maxillary sinus roentgenograms are infrequent in children beyond their first birthday who are without recent symptoms and signs of respiratory tract inflammation.

The roentgenographic findings most diagnostic of bacterial sinusitis are the presence of an air–fluid level in, or complete opacification of, the sinus cavities. An air–fluid level, however, is an uncommon roentgenographic finding in children younger than 5 years of age with acute sinusitis. In the absence of an air–fluid level or complete opacification of the sinuses, measuring the degree of mucosal swelling may be useful. If the width of the sinus mucous membrane is 5 mm or greater in adults or 4 mm or greater in children, it is likely that the sinus will contain pus or will yield a positive bacterial culture. When clinical signs and symptoms suggesting acute sinusitis are accompanied by abnormal maxillary sinus roentgenograms, bacteria will be present in a sinus aspirate 75% of the time. A normal roentgenogram suggests, but does not prove, that a sinus is free of disease.

Computed tomography (CT) of the paranasal sinuses provides a more detailed evaluation than plain roentgenograms. However, CT scans are more expensive and generally less available than plain roentgenograms and are only necessary in patients with recurrent, persistent, or unusually severe illness.

Sinus Aspiration. Although by no means a routine procedure, aspiration of the maxillary sinus (the most accessible of the sinuses) can be accomplished easily in an outpatient setting with minimal discomfort to the patient. The puncture is best performed by the transnasal route with the needle directed beneath the inferior turbinate through the lateral nasal wall. This route for aspiration is preferred to avoid injury to the natural ostium and permanent dentition. In adults, an anterior approach to the maxillary sinus is a Caldwell-Luc antrotomy. If the patient is unusually apprehensive or too young to cooperate, a short-acting narcotic agent can be used for sedation. This procedure is indicated when the infection fails to respond to the usual medical therapy or when the patient presents with intracranial or intraorbital complications of sinus infection.

Surface Cultures. It would be desirable to culture the nose, throat, or nasopharynx in patients with acute sinusitis if the predominant flora isolated from these surface cultures were predictive of the bacterial species recovered from the sinus secretions. Unfortunately, the results of surface cultures have no predictive value; therefore, these cultures cannot be recommended as a guide to the bacteriology of and therapy for acute or chronic sinusitis.

TREATMENT

Antimicrobials

Medical therapy with an antimicrobial agent is recommended in patients diagnosed to have acute maxillary sinusitis. The relative frequency of the various bacterial agents suggest that amoxicillin (40 mg/kg/d, orally, in three divided doses) is an appropriate agent. Amoxicillin is usually prescribed to a maximum dose of 500 or 750 mg three times a day. The prevalence of β-lactamase–positive, ampicillin-resistant *H. influenzae* and *M. catarrhalis* may vary geographically. In areas where ampicillin-resistant organisms are prevalent or when the patient is allergic to penicillin or when there has been an apparent antibiotic failure, several alternative regimens are available. The combination agent sulfamethoxazole-trimethoprim (40 and 8 mg/kg/d, respectively, orally, divided into two doses) has been shown to be efficacious in acute maxillary sinusitis in adults. It is important to remember, however, that this agent may be ineffective in patients with group A streptococcal infections. Cefaclor (40 mg/kg/d, orally, in three divided doses to a maximum dose of 500 mg three times daily) and preferably cefuroxime axetil (125 or 250 mg twice daily) for children who can swallow tablets are additional alternatives. The combination of erythromycin-sulfisoxazole (50 and 150 mg/kg/d, respectively, orally, in four divided doses) is also suitable. Augmentin, a combination of amoxicillin and potassium clavulanate, is another potential therapeutic agent for use in patients with β-lactamase–producing bacterial species in their maxillary sinus secretions. Potassium clavulanate irreversibly binds the β-lactamase, if present, and thus restores amoxicillin to its original spectrum of activity. Augmentin is prescribed in the same dose as amoxicillin. Cefixime (8 mg/kg/d) should be reserved for situations such as clinical failures with amoxicillin, and in which *S. pneumoniae* is an unlikely causative agent.

Clinical improvement is prompt in almost all patients treated with an appropriate antimicrobial agent. Patients febrile at the initial encounter will become afebrile, and there is a remarkable reduction of nasal discharge and cough within 48 hours. If the patient does not improve or worsens in 48 hours, a clinical reevaluation is appropriate. If the diagnosis is unchanged, a sinus aspiration may be considered for precise bacteriologic information. Alternatively, an antimicrobial agent should be prescribed that is effective for β-lactamase–producing bacterial species.

The antimicrobial regimens recommended to treat acute sinusitis are similar (in type and duration) to those used to treat acute otitis media. The usual duration of antimicrobial therapy is 10 to 14 days. When the patient is improved but not completely recovered by 10 or 14 days, it seems reasonable to extend the duration of the antimicrobial agent for another week.

When treating patients with chronic sinusitis, the duration of antimicrobial therapy should be 3 to 4 weeks. Most anaerobes isolated from patients with chronic sinusitis are penicillin sensitive. All *S. viridans* and most *H. influenzae* will be susceptible to amoxicillin. However, there is the potential for the anaerobes or *H. influenzae* to be β-lactamase producing and thus amoxicillin resistant. The list of appropriate antimicrobial agents for chronic sinusitis is the same as for acute sinusitis, unless the patient has already failed to respond to a particular regimen. Amoxicillin or Augmentin at 40 mg/kg/d, orally, in three divided doses is a reasonable initial choice; if the patient does not improve, an alternative antimicrobial should be selected or surgery should be considered.

Decongestants or Antihistamines

The effectiveness of antihistamines or decongestants or combination antihistamine-decongestants applied topically (by inhalation) or administered by mouth in patients with acute or chronic sinus infection has not been adequately studied.

Irrigation and Drainage

Irrigation and drainage of the infected sinus may result in dramatic relief from pain for patients with acute sinusitis. In addition, by relieving pressure in the sinus, oxygenation and blood flow improve, thus restoring compromised defense mechanisms. Drainage procedures are reserved usually for those who fail medical therapy with antimicrobials or who have a suppurative intraorbital or intracranial complication. If an episode of acute or chronic sinusitis cannot be effectively treated by medical therapy alone or medical therapy and simple sinus puncture, more radical surgery may become necessary.

INDICATIONS FOR REFERRAL AND ADMISSION

Complications of sinus disease may cause both substantial morbidity and occasional mortality. Major complications result either from the contiguous spread or from the hematogenous dissemination of infection and result in intraorbital or intracranial suppuration, either of which requires hospital admission and consultation with neurosurgeons, ophthalmologists, and infectious disease experts.

In office practice the only complication that will commonly be found is preseptal cellulitis or, more properly, inflammatory edema. This is not an actual infection of the orbit but rather soft tissue swelling of the periorbital area caused by impedance of the local venous drainage. As such, it is a warning of a potentially serious infection within the sinus. Inflammatory edema about the eye is always associated with an ipsilateral ethmoidal sinusitis. There is usually an ipsilateral maxillary sinusitis and also often a contralateral sinus infection. Frequently, there is a history of intermittent periorbital swelling, which is worse in the morning and improves during the day. The swelling is soft, nontender, and without induration, but there may be prominent erythema. An examination of the globe shows no displacement and full extraocular movements. This latter finding assures the examiner that there is no orbital involvement. The management of these children must be individualized. Those children who have minimal eye swelling and minimal constitutional signs can be managed cautiously as outpatients. If a child has a high fever, or the periorbital swelling has resulted in more than 50% closure of the eye, hospital admission and parenteral antimicrobials are a reasonable treatment decision (see also Chap. 95).

The youngster who presents with an involvement of the frontal sinus must be observed carefully when treatment is undertaken with oral antimicrobials on an ambulatory basis. Infection of this sinus cavity may lead to intracranial, intraorbital, or osseous complications.

ANNOTATED BIBLIOGRAPHY

Brook I: Bacteriologic features of chronic sinusitis in children. JAMA 246:967–970, 1981. (One of the few studies in children on this subject.)

Kovatch AL, Wald ER, Ledesma-Medina J: Maxillary sinus radiographs in children with nonrespiratory complaints. Pediatrics 73:306–308, 1984. (Study showing that children older than 1 year of age without recent respiratory symptoms or current signs of respiratory inflammation infrequently have abnormal maxillary sinus radiographs.)

Rachelefsky G, Katz RM, Siegel SC: Diseases of paranasal sinuses in children. Curr Probl Pediatr 12:1–57, 1982. (Comprehensive review of many aspects of paranasal sinus inflammation.)

Wald ER, Chiponis D, Ledesma-Medina J: Comparative effectiveness of amoxicillin and amoxicillin-clavulanate potassium in acute paranasal sinus infections in children: A double-blind, placebo-controlled trial. Pediatrics 77:795–800, 1986. (Study showing that children with acute sinusitis treated with antimicrobials recover earlier and more often than children on placebo.)

Wald ER, Milmoe GJ, Bowen A et al: Acute maxillary sinusitis in children. N Engl J Med 304:749–754, 1981. (Describes the bacteriology of acute sinusitis in children as learned from maxillary sinus aspirates.)

Wald ER, Pang D, Milmoe GJ et al: Sinusitis and its complications in the pediatric patient. Pediatr Clin North Am 28:777–796, 1981. (Detailed discussion of the serious intraorbital, intracranial, and osseous complications of sinus infection.)

Wald ER, Byers C, Guerra N et al: Subacute sinusitis in children. J Pediatr 115:28–32, 1989. (Reviews bacteriology of sinusitis in patients with respiratory symptoms for 30–120 days.)

81

Sore Throat

L. Gerard Niederman and John F. Marcinak

A sore throat is among the most common complaints seen by the pediatric practitioner, yet its optimal management is both controversial and evolving. Most of the debate focuses around the *group A β-hemolytic streptococcus* (GABHS). The demonstration since the mid 1940s that penicillin treatment of GABHS pharyngitis prevents rheumatic fever has been the basis for widespread diagnostic use of the throat culture for confirming GABHS tonsillitis and guiding treatment. There has, however, been an accelerated decline in the incidence of rheumatic fever in the past 30 years, although focal outbreaks of rheumatic fever have recently occurred in the United States. New data also suggest that early antibiotic treatment shortens the symptomatic course of streptococcal pharyngitis. These considerations, as well as the increasing availability of rapid, although less reliable, diagnostic tests for GABHS, have provoked a reevaluation of the "culture and treat, depending on culture results" approach. The practitioner's task of providing a prompt, accurate diagnosis and treatment for GABHS pharyngitis, while avoiding unnecessary laboratory tests and unnecessary antibiotics for most children who have sore throats

from viral or other non-GABHS agents, is both complex and challenging.

PATHOPHYSIOLOGY AND CLINICAL PRESENTATION

Pharyngitis occurs more often in the colder months, similar to the seasonal pattern of other upper respiratory tract infections. It peaks between 5 and 8 years of age; person-to-person spread of infection in schools is an important source of transmission. Tonsillar tissue increases in size during the years when acute nasopharyngeal infections are most common, reaching maximum size between 8 and 12 years of age and then involuting during adolescence. The temporal association between tonsillitis and tonsillar hypertrophy had been primarily responsible for the widespread practice of performing tonsillectomies on school-aged children.

Bacterial Pharyngitis

Group A β-hemolytic streptococcus is responsible for 15% to 40% of cases of pharyngitis in school-aged children and teenagers. Its onset is usually acute and is characterized by a sore throat (often with dysphagia), fever (often above 101°F), pharyngeal and tonsillar erythema, and tonsillar exudate. Anterior cervical lymph nodes, particularly the jugular-digastric nodes just beneath the angle of the mandible, are tender and enlarged. Erythema of the soft palate is common, and an enanthem of "doughnut" lesions on the soft palate suggests GABHS. If present, the erythematous "sandpaper" rash of scarlet fever and Pastia's lines (petechiae in the flexor skin creases of joints) greatly enhance the likelihood of streptococcal disease. A history of streptococcal exposure also supports this diagnosis. Headache, abdominal pain, and vomiting are common with GABHS, whereas upper respiratory tract symptoms such as cough, rhinorrhea, and conjunctivitis reduce the probability of streptococcal disease. If left untreated, streptococcal pharyngitis usually resolves in 5 to 7 days, although suppurative complications such as otitis media, lymphadenitis, and peritonsillar abscess may occur. GABHS infection in children younger than 3 years old is uncommon and usually presents as common cold symptoms, pharyngitis, or both. Young children may also have associated otitis media or impetigo.

Acute rheumatic fever continues to be a rare complication of untreated GABHS infections, although recent (i.e., mid-1980s) reports indicate that it may be on the rise. An attack rate of 3% was found in untreated military recruits during the 1940s. In the 1950s an attack rate of 0.4% was documented in untreated children. Even with many undiagnosed and untreated streptococcal infections, the annual incidence of acute rheumatic fever in the past decade was between 0.5 and 2.0 cases per 100,000 population, making it a disease that many primary care practitioners will never encounter.

Groups C and G *β-hemolytic streptococci* have also been isolated from children with symptomatic pharyngitis and have, on rare occasions, been implicated in the development of acute glomerulonephritis. Their epidemiologic and clinical importance as an endemic cause of pharyngitis is unclear.

Other causes of bacterial tonsillopharyngitis are uncommon. Tonsillar or pharyngeal diphtheria, caused by *Corynebacterium diphtheriae,* is rare in an adequately immunized child. It is characterized by a gray adherent membranous exudate that bleeds when removed. A careful immunization history and a high index of suspicion are needed to consider this diagnosis. *Gonococcal pharyngitis,* seen in sexually active adolescents and sexually abused children, may present as acute inflammatory, exudative tonsillopharyngitis or as a chronic sore throat. *Tularemia* can cause an exudative tonsillopharyngitis. It is most often associated with ingestion of improperly cooked rabbit meat or contact with an infected animal.

Viral Pharyngitis

A sore throat is a common complaint with viral upper respiratory tract infections, and often there are no clinical features distinguishing the specific etiologic viral agent (see Chap. 163, "The Common Cold"). The associated symptoms of cough and rhinorrhea suggest a viral etiology, particularly in the child who is verbal enough to complain of a sore throat.

Adenoviruses are a frequent cause of exudative pharyngitis, especially in the child younger than 3 years old. Fever, nasal discharge, congestion, and cough are common; laryngotracheobronchitis and pneumonia may occur. The duration of symptoms averages 5 to 7 days. Epidemic adenovirus pharyngitis is usually a winter/spring disease. Pharyngoconjunctival fever, also due to adenovirus, is characterized by a high fever that is sustained for 3 to 4 days, bulbar and palpebral conjunctivitis, and tonsillitis often with exudate. It is usually epidemic during the summer and is frequently transmitted in swimming pools.

Herpangina, due to coxsackieviruses and echoviruses, is an acute illness, often with temperature to 102°F or higher. There may be headache, malaise, as well as sore throat and dysphagia. The typical oral lesions are small vesicles or ulcers on the anterior tonsillar pillars and soft palate, although they may be on the tonsils, pharynx, or posterior buccal mucosa. *Hand-foot-and-mouth syndrome* (due to coxsackie-virus A16) is characterized by oral ulcerative lesions often on the tongue and buccal mucosa, although not infrequently on the palate and anterior pillars of the tonsils. The vesicular and papulovesicular lesions on the dorsa and intraphalangeal areas of the hands and feet, and on the buttocks or diaper area in about one third of children, allow a clinical diagnosis of this syndrome. Both herpangina and hand-foot-and-mouth syndrome occur in the summer and early fall.

Infectious mononucleosis caused by Epstein-Barr virus may present as pharyngitis, with or without exudative tonsillitis. Fever is common, although children rarely appear toxic. Cervical or more general lymphadenopathy, palatal petechiae, splenomegaly, and edema of the eyelids support the clinical diagnosis of mononucleosis. Signs of upper respiratory tract infection, including rhinitis and cough, are more common in children younger than 4 years old. A macular erythematous rash may be present, and if ampicillin is inadvertently administered, the rash may occur more frequently and be more prominent. Other common viral causes of pharyngitis include herpes simplex, parainfluenza, respiratory syncytial and influenza viruses.

Other Agents

Mycoplasma pneumoniae can cause pharyngitis that is clinically indistinguishable from streptococcal disease. It is uncommon in children younger than 5 years of age, but it may account for up to 10% of pharyngitis seen in adolescents. There is little evidence for *Chlamydia trachomatis* as a cause of pharyngitis in children. *Candida* may also cause pharyngitis accompanied by a sore throat.

DIFFERENTIAL DIAGNOSIS

A sore throat may be the presenting symptom of a peritonsillar or retropharyngeal abscess. Anaerobic bacteria, most commonly the *Bacteroides* species, *Peptostreptococcus* and *Fusobacterium,* and aerobic organisms such as group A *streptococcus, Staphylococcus aureus, Hemophilus influenzae,* and viridans streptococci are the most frequent organisms isolated from these abscesses. Mixed aerobic/anaerobic infections are common. *Peritonsillar abscesses* are more common in older children and adolescents and usually follow an episode of tonsillitis. Sore throat, fever, dysphagia, odynophagia, and trismus are frequent complaints. The oropharynx may be difficult to examine in the child with trismus. The tonsil on the affected side is usually displaced medially. There may be edema and erythema of the soft palate contiguous with the tonsil, and fluctuance may be palpable. The tonsillar mucosa may not be significantly inflamed or have exudate. Tender, anterior cervical adenopathy is present.

Retropharyngeal abscesses occur more commonly in young children. Fever, refusal to swallow, drooling, and the development of stridor are due to the abscess and its surrounding edema and cellulitis. An examination may reveal swelling of the posterior pharynx. Meningismus is common because of irritation and spasm of paravertebral muscles. Children with *epiglottis* may complain of a sore throat, but the rapid onset of extreme toxicity and inspiratory stridor makes confusion with uncomplicated tonsillopharyngitis unlikely (see Chap. 166, "Inflammatory Illnesses of the Pediatric Airway").

Trauma from penetrating injuries, thermal injury, chemical injury from a caustic ingestion, foreign body, irritation from dryness and coughing, and, uncommonly, thyroiditis may also present as a sore throat. The PFAPA syndrome has been recently described and includes *periodic fever, aphthous stomatitis, and/or pharyngitis* (with or without cervical *adenitis*). This syndrome usually occurs in young children. Finally, *Kawasaki disease* with rash, mucositis, fever, and toxicity may be confused with scarlet fever.

WORK-UP

History

The physician can suspect GABHS pharyngitis if the history includes streptococcal exposure at home or at school, previous rheumatic fever, and the occurrence of a community outbreak of rheumatic fever. A history of inadequate immunizations or a community outbreak of diphtheria may suggest that diagnosis. Contact with, or ingestion of, rabbits or squirrels should suggest tularemia. Orogenital sexual contact or sexual abuse raises the possibility of gonococcal pharyngitis. Symptoms of cough or rhinorrhea suggest viral pharyngitis. A history of significant dysphagia or odynophagia, drooling, or an inability to open one's mouth should alert the physician to the possibility of a peritonsillar or retropharyngeal abscess or of epiglottis. A history of repeated episodes of fever with pharyngitis may suggest the PFAPA syndrome.

Physical Examination

The physical signs of the common bacterial and viral etiologies of sore throats have been discussed previously. Signs that strongly suggest GABHS are a scarlatiniform rash, Pastia's lines, and a soft palate enanthem. Findings of tonsillar and pharyngeal erythema, tonsillar exudates, and anterior cervical adenitis are frequently present with GABHS tonsillitis but may be seen with mononucleosis, adenovirus, mycoplasma, and other non-GABHS causes of pharyngitis. Ulcerative or vesicular oral lesions, conjunctivitis, or rhinitis suggest viral pharyngitis.

Trismus and displacement of the tonsil and adjacent soft palate, sometimes with palpable fluctuance, are characteristic of a peritonsillar abscess. Airway stridor, stiffness of the neck, and a visible posterior pharyngeal mass point to a retropharyngeal abscess. Stridor, drooling, and fever in a toxic-appearing young child suggest epiglottis.

Laboratory Tests

The diagnosis of streptococcal pharyngitis is confirmed by throat culture. Although considered the "gold standard," it is known to have up to 10% false negatives (usually the result of improper collection or transportation of the specimen) and also up to 50% false positives (carriers of streptococci who are not truly infected). The occurrence of false-positive throat cultures will depend on the prevalence of streptococcal carriers, which has been shown to vary greatly among school-aged children, and also on the selection of children to be cultured. Despite these shortcomings, for children with clinical findings suspicious of GABHS or for children at increased risk for rheumatic fever, the throat culture is the most accurate test to confirm GABHS.

Office kits for the detection of GABHS antigen from throat swabs are commercially available and offer the advantage of a rapid diagnosis and appropriate treatment while the child is still in the office. Most studies have shown high (>95%) specificity but variable sensitivity (60% to 93%). Until improvements provide a test with reliable sensitivity of at least 95%, they may be clinically useful when positive, but cultures should be performed when rapid antigen tests are negative.

Serology (e.g., antistreptolysin O and antideoxyribonuclease B) is rarely useful in the acute management of sore throats but may be useful for documenting recent GABHS infection when rheumatic fever is considered or when the differentiation of streptococcal carriage from infection is necessary.

Diphtheria can be confirmed with isolation of *C. diphtheriae* from the pharyngeal membrane. Fluorescent antibody techniques are available but may be inaccurate in inexperienced laboratories. Tularemia can be confirmed by culture or serologic testing. Pharyngeal gonorrhea is also confirmed by culture for *Neisseria gonorrhoeae*. Viral cultures are usually not useful in the management of uncomplicated pharyngitis, and, except for respiratory syncytial virus, rapid antigen detection for viral agents is currently available only in research laboratories.

A positive heterophil agglutination test when properly performed is highly diagnostic of mononucleosis. Unfortunately, the heterophil test may be negative in children younger than 4 years of age and also negative early in the course of mononucleosis. The mono spot test, a commonly performed test for heterophil antibodies, may remain positive for several months, potentially causing confusion when evaluating acute or recurrent pharyngitis. More specific serologic tests to confirm Epstein-Barr virus infection can be performed if clinically indicated.

The complete blood cell count is helpful; children with a lymphocytosis greater than 50% to 60% or atypical lymphocytosis of more than 10% should be suspected of having mononucleosis. It is also uncommon for children with GABHS pharyngitis to have a white blood cell count less than 12,500 cells/mm^3.

If a retropharyngeal abscess is suspected, a lateral roentgenogram of the neck will often reveal a posterior pharyngeal mass, sometimes with gas formation.

TREATMENT

Optimal management of children with sore throats involves the prompt and accurate differentiation of streptococcal pharyngitis from "viral" nonstreptococcal pharyngitis. It also involves recognizing other uncommon, yet important, bacterial causes of sore throats such as diphtheria and gonorrhea, as well as recognizing the child with symptoms and signs suggesting a peritonsillar abscess, retropharyngeal abscess, or epiglottis.

The two decisions most often faced by the practitioner managing a child with a sore throat are whether to obtain a culture (or rapid antigen test) for GABHS and whether to begin antibiotic treatment prior to obtaining culture results. The throat culture should be used selectively when there are clinical (e.g., exudate, significant erythema, adenitis, and fever) or epidemiologic (e.g., exposure and epidemicity) factors to suggest streptococcal pharyngitis. As the clinical probability of GABHS increases, a positive culture is more likely to be a true positive rather than a streptococcal carrier. The decision to treat a patient with antibiotics is based on the rationale that penicillin treatment of GABHS pharyngitis prevents rheumatic fever and suppurative complications, as well as shortens the clinical course of pharyngitis. Antibiotic treatment is indicated in the child with a past history of rheumatic fever, the toxic-appearing child, the child with clinical scarlet fever, the child with symptoms suggesting an early peritonsillar abscess, or other situations in which there is a reasonably high likelihood of streptococcal disease or its sequelae. Many children presenting with sore throats will have signs and symptoms strongly predictive of not having GABHS and should not have diagnostic GABHS tests performed or be treated. In areas of the United States where rheumatic fever has increased, less selective criteria for diagnosing GABHS should be considered.

The streptococcal carrier poses a difficult diagnostic problem. Up to 50% of children symptomatic with sore throats and culture positive for GABHS do not have serologic evidence of streptococcal infection. These symptomatic carriers cannot be differentiated from true streptococcal infections by any readily available clinical test. Streptococcal carriers also may be asymptomatic. In practice, the symptomatic carrier is unrecognized as such and is treated with antibiotics; the asymptomatic carrier, when identified, also usually receives antibiotics. The failure rate of penicillin treatment is quite high for streptococcal carriers and, although rarely indicated, the combination of penicillin (either intramuscular or oral) plus rifampin has been shown to be more efficacious in eradication of pharyngeal carriage. Because of confusion over the carrier state, obtaining an additional culture after completing antibiotic treatment or obtaining cultures from close contacts of children found with GABHS is not routinely recommended. Carriers are at small risk for developing rheumatic fever.

Recommended treatment for GABHS pharyngitis is penicillin administered either orally or intramuscularly. Phenoxymethyl penicillin (penicillin V) 250 mg three or four times daily for 10 days is necessary to prevent rheumatic fever, although symptomatic improvement may be complete in 24 to 72 hours. In situations in which the risk of acute rheumatic fever is high and compliance is questionable, intramuscular benzathine penicillin G may be preferable to oral treatment. Current recommendations for rheumatic fever prophylaxis are 600,000 units of benzathine penicillin for patients weighing less than 60 lb and 1.2 million units for patients weighing more than 60 lb. The combination of 900,000 units benzathine penicillin and 300,000 units procaine penicillin is also acceptable. The physician must weigh the relative risks of the development of complications, either suppurative or nonsuppurative, following noncompliance with oral regimens against the discomfort and more serious allergic complications associated with intramuscular benzathine penicillin. Erythromycin (30–50 mg/kg/d) is an effective, inexpensive alternative antibiotic for the child allergic to penicillin.

Diphtheria is treated with equine antitoxin and penicillin or erythromycin to eradicate *C. diphtheriae*. The treatment of choice for tularemia is streptomycin or gentamicin.

Pharyngeal gonorrhea is treated preferably with ceftriaxone. For children weighing more than 100 lbs, ceftriaxone, 250 mg, is given intramuscularly and for children under 100 lbs, 125 mg given intramuscularly is appropriate (see Chap. 200, "Sexually Transmitted Diseases"). A serologic test for syphilis as well as an examination and culture for other sexually transmitted diseases is needed for the child or adolescent with oral gonorrhea. The social and psychological needs of the sexually abused child must also be addressed (see Chap. 20, "Child Abuse").

The symptoms of a sore throat can be treated with acetaminophen, lozenges, fluids to keep the throat moist, and salt water gargles alone or in combination. Many preparations of topical anesthetics such as the aqueous solution of lidocaine are available, but their efficacy in the young child is unproven. Their use should be avoided because of systemic reactions from their absorption and allergic sensitization.

INDICATIONS FOR HOSPITALIZATION OR REFERRAL

The child with uncomplicated pharyngitis is managed on an ambulatory basis. A child may occasionally be dehydrated or appear toxic and require treatment with intravenous fluids and parenteral antibiotics.

Peritonsillar abscess may complicate both GABHS and non-GABHS tonsillitis and requires surgical drainage and parenteral antibiotic therapy. Tonsillectomy is usually performed several weeks after the resolution of the acute infection, although some otolaryngologists prefer tonsillectomy during the acute phase. Retropharyngeal abscess is a potentially life-threatening infection and requires hospitalization for appropriate surgical drainage and intravenous antibiotic treatment.

Recurrent tonsillitis is the most frequent and controversial reason for which tonsillectomy is performed. A small group of children do indeed have a disproportionately high incidence of GABHS throat infections, and these children will have fewer infections after tonsillectomy. Whether this warrants the risks, complications, and costs of surgery requires a decision on an individual basis. Minimally, a physician should document by examination, not by patient or parental recall, that sore throats from GABHS are frequent (five or more per year), symptomatic (fever, erythema, exudate, adenitis), and costly (days lost from school or work, medical expenses) before considering tonsillectomy.

ANNOTATED BIBLIOGRAPHY

Denny FW: Current problems in managing streptococcal pharyngitis. J Pediatr 111:797–806, 1987. (Excellent discussion of carrier state, antimicrobial agents, rapid diagnosis and other bacterial causes of pharyngitis in the management of patients with GABHS pharyngitis.)

Gerber MA, Randolph MF, Demeo KK, Kaplan EL: Lack of impact of early antibiotic therapy for streptococcal pharyngitis on recurrence rates. J Pediatr 117:853–858, 1990. (Reviews serotyping of GABHS isolates to distinguish recurrences with the same serotype from new acquisitions with a different serotype.)

Kaplan EL, Hill HR: Return of rheumatic fever: Consequences, implications and needs. J Pediatr 111:244–246, 1987. (Editorial reviewing resurgence of acute rheumatic fever and the fact that outbreaks are not isolated; see also the article in the same issue by Congeni B, Rizzo C, Congeni J et al: Outbreak of acute rheumatic fever in northeast Ohio.)

Klein JO, Collins TL (eds): Proceedings of a symposium: Diagnosis of streptococcal pharyngitis. Pediatr Infect Dis J 8:811–837, 1989. (Update on the diagnosis of GABHS pharyngitis including clinical and epidemiologic factors, and use of throat culture and rapid tests; also addresses the issue of home screening for GABHS pharyngitis.)

Krober MS, Bass JW, Michels GN: Streptococcal pharyngitis: Placebo-controlled double-blind evaluation of clinical response to penicillin therapy. JAMA 253:1271–1274, 1985 (Does early treatment with penicillin favorably alter the clinical course of GABHS pharyngitis? This study says "Yes.".)

Levin RM, Grossman M, Jordan C et al: Streptococcal infection in children less than three years of age. Pediatr Infect Dis J 7:581–587, 1988. (Reports that classic presentation of streptococcosis in young children was not found but that with special culture techniques to isolate GABHS and serology, GABHS infection was found in 4.6% of young children, usually with pharyngitis, the common cold, or both.)

Marshall GS, Edwards KM: PFAPA syndrome. Pediatr Infect Dis J 8:658–659, 1989. (Concise review of the newly described syndrome of periodic fever, aphthous stomatitis, pharyngitis, and cervical adenitis.)

Pantell RH. Pharyngitis: Diagnosis and management. Pediatr Rev 3:35–39, 1981. (Excellent, detailed, and critical discussion of the cost and clinical effectiveness of various strategies for managing children with pharyngitis.)

Paradise JL, Bluestone CD, Bachman RZ et al: Efficacy of tonsillectomy for recurrent throat infection in severely affected children: Results of parallel randomized and nonrandomized clinical trials. N Engl J Med 310:674–683, 1984. (Important data that quantify the clinical benefits of tonsillectomy in a selected group of children.)

Parkhurst JB, San Joaquin VH: Tonsillopharyngeal tularemia—a reminder. Am J Dis Child 144:1070–1071, 1990. (Case report of tularemia pharyngitis with concise review of epidemiology, clinical presentation and treatment.)

82
Gingivostomatitis
Ilana Kraus

Gingivostomatitis is not a single disease. Rather, it is broadly divided into three entities that affect the oral mucosa: (1) *gingivitis* is an infection of the gingiva, the keratinized tissue between the teeth; (2) *gingivostomatitis* is an infection of both the gingiva and any other part of the oral mucosa; and (3) *stomatitis* is the term applied if lesions are in any part of the oral mucosa other than the gingiva.

PATHOPHYSIOLOGY AND CLINICAL PRESENTATION
Gingivitis

Gingivitis is a periodontal disease caused by bacterial plaque formation at the gingival margin. The bacterial overgrowth is noninvasive but causes local irritation resulting in a gingival inflammatory response.

Gingivitis affects over 50% of children. The term *adolescent gingivitis* is used when it arises in prepubertal and pubertal children, and it is believed that hormonal changes exacerbate this condition. On examination, the gingiva is red or bluish purple, having lost its pink appearance. The color change is due to the increased blood flow, with or without bleeding. The inflammatory response causes swelling of the gingiva. With progression, the sharp edges of the gums (papillae) become eroded and assume a stippled appearance. Minor mouth pain results, which is exacerbated by activities such as vigorous tooth brushing. A mild mouth odor (fetor oris) is frequently present.

Acute Necrotizing Ulcerative Gingivitis

Acute necrotizing ulcerative gingivitis (Vincent's infection, trench mouth) is believed to be caused by two bacterial organisms that are normal inhabitants of the oral flora: *Bacillus fusibacterium* and a spirochete, *Borrelia vincentii*. It is hypothesized that under certain conditions such as stress, severe malnutrition, or with excessive smoking, the local bacterial balance is altered, causing an overgrowth of these two organisms. This type of ulcerative gingivitis is rarely reported in young children in the United States and is more prevalent in adolescents and young adults.

In contrast to gingivitis, these bacteria invade the gingival mucosa. The inflammation begins at the interdental papillae, which becomes swollen and red, and progresses from the papillae to the gingival margins. A necrotic pseudomembranous exudate is formed, which eventually sloughs and leaves crater-like ulcers with a gray-white base and a linear red border.

Symptoms include severe pain, severe fetor oris, and a peculiar metallic taste. General malaise and decreased appetite are common. A mild fever and local lymphadenopathy may occur.

Acute Herpetic Gingivostomatitis

Acute herpetic gingivostomatitis is caused by herpes simplex virus (HSV), mainly type I. HSV is a DNA-containing virus and causes both primary and recurrent infections. The severity of primary infections may be inapparent or may range from extremely mild to extremely painful. After the primary infection, the virus becomes dormant but is reactivated in 20% to 40% of persons. Fever, stress, and sun exposure are frequent precipitants of viral reactivation. The most common form of recurrence is *herpes simplex labialis* (cold sore, fever blister), with lesions at the junction of the lips. Recurrences occasionally occur intraorally. Humans are the only known reservoir for the virus, and the disease is transmitted by close contact or through oral secretions. The incubation period is usually 3 to 4 days but may be up to 2 weeks. The virus is extremely prevalent: by puberty over 50% of adolescents will have antibodies to the virus, and this rate rises to 90% by adulthood. Infection occurs most commonly in children between 1 and 5 years of age.

Primary herpetic gingivostomatitis can present with the sudden prodrome of high fever, general malaise, refusal to eat or drink, and excessive drooling. Within 24 to 48 hours, vesicles appear on any part of the oral mucosa, but rarely on the lips and circumoral skin. The vesicles rupture early, leaving 2- to 10-mm ulcers that are covered by a yellow-gray membrane surrounded by an erythematous base. The ulcers may coalesce to form larger ulcers. The ulcers heal within 7 to 14 days without scarring. The pain usually subsides within 5 to 7 days, before complete healing occurs. Cervical (especially submaxillary and submental) lymphadenopathy is common.

Aphthous Stomatitis

Aphthous stomatitis, or aphthous ulcers, are recurrent oral ulcerations occurring most frequently on the labial or buccal mucosa, but they may appear anywhere within the oral mucosa. The etiology of this disease remains obscure. Local injury, stress, gluten sensitivity, allergy to chocolate and nuts, vitamin B_{12}, zinc, folate, or iron deficiencies, and the L form of *Streptococcus sanguinis* have all been implicated but are unproven. An autoimmune mechanism is currently believed to be the etiologic factor, but an autoantibody has not been found.

The disease is familial, and women are slightly more often affected than men. Peak onset is between 10 and 19 years of age. A burning sensation often heralds the lesion, after which a red macule appears. It progresses to form a shallow ulcer about 1 cm in diameter. Lesions are usually single, or in a cluster of up to four or five ulcers. They cause local discomfort but rarely systemic manifestations. The ulcers heal within 7 days and recurrence is the rule. If recurrence of aphthous ulcers is periodic (every 4 weeks) and persists for 5 to 8 days, it may be a manifestation of *cyclic neutropenia,* an obscure hematologic disorder in which cyclic maturational arrest of the granulocytes occur. A white blood cell count and differential count during recurrent attacks will establish the diagnosis.

DIFFERENTIAL DIAGNOSIS

Differential diagnoses usually arise only when intraoral vesicular lesions are present and HSV needs to be distinguished from other infections. Acute herpetic gingivostomatitis can be difficult to differentiate from other viral infections. *Herpangina,* caused by a coxsackievirus A, presents as small vesicular lesions that ulcerate in 2 to 3 days. It mainly affects children, causing a mild to high fever, malaise, and a sore throat. The lesions have a characteristic distribution that is the hallmark of the differential diagnosis. They are confined to the oropharynx (i.e., pharynx, tonsils, anterior tonsilar pillars, and soft palate). Healing is usually within 1 week. *Hand-foot-and-mouth disease,* also caused by coxsackievirus A, presents as vesicular lesions, most frequently on the tongue and buccal mucosa. General symptoms of mild fever, malaise, and mild lymphadenopathy are present. The buccal lesions are most often accompanied by a maculopapular and vesicular rash of the hands and feet. *Varicella* (chickenpox) may present as oral vesiculoulcerative lesions, which occur most commonly on the palate and resolve in 5 to 7 days. Skin lesions almost always precede the oral lesions and are diagnostic.

Aphthous stomatitis may sometimes be confused with herpetic gingivostomatitis. However, unlike HSV infection, they usually present as single or up to four lesions. Herpes most commonly affects the gingiva, whereas recurrent aphthous stomatitis rarely does.

Gingivitis and acute necrotizing ulcerative gingivitis are easily differentiated; gingivitis is a common disorder, whereas acute necrotizing ulcerative gingivitis is rare.

WORK-UP
History

A history of exposure to a person with gingivostomatitis should be sought. Since recurrent aphthous stomatitis is familial, inquiry should be made about a family history as well as the timing of recurrence. Because both gingivostomatitis and acute necrotizing ulcerative gingivitis are often secondary to stress and poor nutrition, these possibilities must be explored.

Physical Examination

The appearance, location, distribution, and number of lesions will often clarify the diagnosis. Lymphadenopathy may be present, and body rashes may be diagnostic.

Laboratory Tests

Occasionally, acute herpesvirus infection needs to be confirmed. A stained scraping of an ulcer reveals multinucleated giant cells with intranuclear inclusions. The herpesvirus can also be cultured or demonstrated by at least a fourfold increase in neutralizing antibody titers in acute and convalescent sera. If cyclic neutropenia is suspected, a complete white blood cell count and differential should be obtained every 2 to 3 days during recurrences.

MANAGEMENT

Gingivitis is best managed by a dentist or periodontist. Regular and proper oral hygiene is curative and prevents recurrence and should be reinforced by the physician. In acute necrotizing gingivostomatitis, the lesions should be promptly debrided (preferably by a dentist) and vigorous oral hygiene should be initiated. Oxygenating mouthwashes such as 3% hydrogen peroxide are effective in converting the anaerobic mouth condition to an aerobic environment. In severe cases, antibiotic therapy using penicillin or tetracycline, 250 mg four times a day is indicated. Metronidazole, 200 mg three times a day has been used with excellent results.

The dual goals in the treatment of acute herpetic gingivostomatitis are to prevent dehydration and control discomfort. Fluid intake to prevent dehydration must be encouraged. In the older child, local anesthetics such as 2% viscous lidocaine (Xylocaine), or Chloraseptic spray or lozenges containing benzocaine can be used. The parents, however, must be alerted to the danger of seizures from lidocaine and aspiration. In young children, a mixture of diphenhydramine (Benadryl) elixir (12.5 mg/tsp) with Kaopectate 1:1 may be used as either a mouth rinse or a paste to alleviate pain. Alcohol or other drying agents may be useful in drying and hence resolving skin lesions.

A child with active lesions should be temporarily excluded from day-care and school settings to protect other children. Older children with cold sores do not pose a great risk for spreading the infection, and thus they may attend school. Children who have eczema are at risk of developing *eczema herpeticum* and should be instructed to avoid contact with children with herpetic gingivostomatitis. Herpes gingivostomatitis in the immunocompetent child is not an approved indication for acyclovir, although the pediatrician may consider the use of oral acyclovir in a particularly se-

vere case for relief of pain and to avoid hospitalization for dehydration. Many authorities, however, recommend either intravenous or oral acyclovir in immunocompromised patients having HSV gingivostomatitis. The likelihood of therapeutic benefit is increased if acyclovir is used early in the infection. Some also recommend acyclovir treatment for atopic children to prevent eczema herpeticum. The dose for older children is 200 mg five times a day for 5 days. The occasional patient who suffers from severe recurrent herpes gingivostomatitis may benefit from chronic suppressive therapy (200 mg three times a day for 6 months). While topical acyclovir may be effective for primary herpes simplex labialis, it is not recommended because it is expensive and must be applied every 3 hours. Topical acyclovir is not effective for treating recurrent infections. Corticosteroids should not be used since they may disseminate the virus, and photodyes should be avoided because they may be carcinogens. Topical IDU and ARA-A are not effective in treating oral herpetic infections. A sun block applied to the lips may help prevent recurrent cold sores.

The treatment of aphthous stomatitis is aimed at symptomatic relief. Oral hygiene should be reinforced, and rinsing the mouth with hydrogen peroxide is recommended. Topical antibiotics such as 2% tetracycline mouthwash (250 mg capsule dissolved in 15-ml water) can be effective in reducing pain and promoting healing to avoid overgrowth of resistant opportunistic microorganisms. The rinse should be used sparingly and for short periods only. Topical corticosteroids are the most effective treatment. Their anti-inflammatory properties facilitate ulcer healing and should be used in the early stages of the disease to be most effective. Twenty-five-milligram pellets of hydrocortisone hemisuccinate or 0.1% triamcinolone paste are recommended. Stronger corticosteroid preparations should be avoided. Prolonged use of any corticosteroid should also be avoided because the oral mucosa is highly absorbent and adrenal suppression may result. Oral antibiotics should be prescribed for secondary bacterial infection.

INDICATIONS FOR HOSPITALIZATION

Young infants may occasionally refuse oral intake and will need intravenous rehydration therapy. An extension of herpetic stomatitis (e.g., encephalitis), a secondary bacterial infection, or a generalized herpetic infection is rare but, especially in young children, may cause the child to be toxic. Atopic children are at risk for eczema herpeticum. Hospitalization is often indicated for these severe infections.

ANNOTATED BIBLIOGRAPHY

Abrams RG, Jasell SD: Common oral and dental emergencies and problems. Pediatr Clin North Am 29:681–715, 1982. (Comprehensive discussion and nice illustrations of common conditions causing gingival pain.)

Blackman JA, Andersen RD, Healy A et al: Management of young children with recurrent herpes simplex skin lesions in special educational programs. Pediatr Infect Dis 4:221–224, 1985. (Good, sensible guidelines.)

Eversole LR: Clinical Outline of Oral Pathology: Diagnosis and Treatment. Philadelphia, Lea & Febiger, 1978. (Excellent illustrations and differential diagnosis.)

Hess GP, Walson PD: Seizures secondary to oral viscous lidocaine. Ann Emerg Med 17:725–727, 1988. (Discussion of lidocaine-induced seizures in two children.)

Perna JJ, Eskinazi DP: Treatment of oro-facial herpes simplex infections with acyclovir: A review. Oral Surg 65:689–692, 1988. (Discussion of clinical improvement with acyclovir, which inhibits HSV replication but has no effect on the latent viral state.)

Scully C: Orofacial herpes simplex virus infections: Current concepts in the epidemiology, pathogenesis, and treatment, and disorders in which the virus may be implicated. Oral Surg 68:701–710, 1989. (Good review.)

Spruance SL, Freeman DJ, Stewart JCB et al: The natural history of ultraviolet radiation–induced herpes simplex labialis and response to therapy with peroral and topical formulations of acyclovir. J Infect Dis 163:728–734, 1991. (Beneficial results from prophylactic and early oral treatment with acyclovir but not topical treatment.)

Wright JM, Taylor PP, Allen EP et al: A review of the oral manifestations of infections in pediatric patients. Pediatr Infect Dis 3:80–88, 1984. (Excellent elaboration of the differential diagnoses.)

83

Dentistry for the Pediatrician

Joan M. O'Connor

Most anomalies of the oral tissues are seen by the pediatrician before the child's first dental visit, which is usually at 2 to 3 years of age. Unfortunately, a large segment of the population has no dental care. Advances in dentistry, particularly in the fields of prevention and materials, have led to many questions from parents, which are frequently asked of pediatricians. The more common disorders of the mouth are outlined in this chapter and preventive recommendations for pediatric dentistry are reviewed.

SOFT TISSUE

The discussion of soft tissues includes disorders involving alveolar ridges, mucosa, the palate, and the floor of the mouth.

Eruption cysts are small, white, gray, or bluish translucent eruptions along the crest of the maxillary and mandibular ridges, probably resulting from remnants of the dental lamina. These cysts are usually shed shortly after birth.

Epstein's pearls are small, white, keratinized lesions found along the midpalatine raphe. Considered to be remnants of epithelial tissue trapped as the fetus grew, they are sometimes incorrectly referred to as natal teeth. They usually slough after birth.

In the older child, a bluish elevation of tissue is often seen in the molar region as a second primary molar or permanent first molar is about to erupt. This is known as an *eruption hematoma*. No treatment is necessary because the hematoma resolves when the tooth breaks through.

Congenital epulis of the newborn is an unusual benign, slow-growing, pedunculated tumor of the anterior maxillary (and less commonly mandibular) ridge. Ninety percent of these growths occur in female infants. Histologically, this disorder is similar to the granular cell myoblastoma. Surgical excision is the preferred treatment, and recurrence is rare.

Tumors of the intraoral accessory salivary glands occur frequently and are found throughout the oral cavity. Approximately one half of these tumors are malignant. The diagnosis is made by microscopic examination, but, clinically, a benign tumor is often nonulcerated, painless, and slow growing.

A *mucocele* is not a tumor, although it may resemble one. It is a common lesion of the lower lip, but it is not limited to that area. Because of the absence of salivary glands, it is not often seen on the attached gingiva or the anterior hard palate. A mucocele is believed to result from trauma that severs a minor salivary gland duct and causes the saliva to pool in the connective tissue. Since it does not contain an epithelial lining, it is not a true cyst. Superficial mucoceles appear bluish, whereas deeper ones may be pink because of the thickness of the overlying mucosa. It cannot be emptied by digital pressure, and the aspirant is sticky, clear, and viscous (which differentiates it from vascular lesions and superficial nonkeratotic cysts). An early mucoepidermoid tumor and mucinous adenocarcinoma must be ruled out. Thus, the clinician should inspect and palpate the base and the periphery of the site for induration, which might suggest a tumor rather than a mucocele. A complete excision and a pathologic examination is the preferred treatment.

A *ranula* is a mucocele of the tissue of the floor of the mouth. It often causes the tongue to be displaced forward and laterally. Surgical excision or marsupialization is recommended unless the size is so great that the displaced tongue causes obstruction. An emergency aspiration or incision and drainage is then necessary.

A *hemangioma* may be congenital or traumatic and may vary in size from a millimeter to several centimeters. It is often seen on the lips, buccal mucosa, and palate. As opposed to mucoceles and other cysts, it can blanch and empty with digital pressure. Blood can be aspirated with a fine needle. It is distinguished from an aneurysm and arteriovenous shunt by the absence of a pulse. Sclerosing agents, such as sodium psylliate or sodium morrhuate, used either singly or prior to surgical excision, are the preferred treatments.

THE TONGUE

Ankyloglossia (tongue tie) is a term given to any situation in which a short lingual frenum extending from the tongue to the floor of the mouth or lingual gingival tissue interferes with protrusion of the tongue. Despite some opinions to the contrary, it probably has no effect on speech or nursing in most cases. Thus, no treatment is warranted if the tongue can be protruded beyond the lips. If the tongue cannot be protruded, an evaluation of the functions of the tongue is necessary to determine if any treatment is required. True ankyloglossia results when the frenum is replaced by a thick fibrous band of tissue. When the gingiva is pulled from the lingual surface of the mandibular anterior teeth by either the result of the position of the attachment of the frenum or local inflammation, surgical repair is indicated.

Migratory glossitis (geographic tongue) is a common anomaly. It is characterized by red smooth areas resulting from desquamation of the keratin layers of papilla encircled by slightly elevated gray margins and is confined to epithelium. Two to four lesions usually occur at a time, and patterns may be altered daily. It usually only occurs in children, and its cause is unknown. No treatment is indicated.

Macroglossia may either be an idiopathic or a secondary condition. Lymphangioma and hemangioma are the two most common causes of macroglossia. In the tongue, a lymphangioma may present as a diffuse smooth or nodular enlargement. The enlargement is often unilateral. Its color is less blue than from a hemangioma, ranging from normal coloration to bluish, but it may be translucent. The aspirant is the distinguishing feature between the two lesions. Treatment is not necessary unless the tongue is sufficiently large to cause disfigurement or airway obstruction, in which case surgical excision is performed.

A transitory tongue enlargement is often caused by angioneurotic edema from an allergic reaction. The maintenance of the airway is important.

THE TEETH

An exception to the sequence depicted in Figure 83-1 is the eruption of a *natal* or *neonatal* tooth. About 85% are lower primary incisors rather than supernumerary teeth. A roentgenogram will determine the type of tooth. Most natal/neonatal teeth are hypermobile because of the inadequate root formation. If the tooth is so mobile that aspiration is feared, it should be removed. The removal is accomplished by gauze (to reduce the chance of losing the tooth due to the small, slippery nature of these teeth) with light finger pressure. This can be done by the pediatrician rather than referring the patient to a dentist; otherwise, the immature primary incisor will become more firm as the root develops.

A practical method of examining teeth is to divide the arches of the mouth at the midline and compare each tooth to its contralateral tooth in the arch. When examining a whole mouth, supernumerary or missing teeth are often overlooked because there is not the corresponding crowding or spacing present that might be expected; counting teeth minimizes this oversight. By looking for bilateral symmetry, teeth that have not erupted or exfoliated at approximately the same schedule as the corresponding contralateral tooth can be evaluated for pathology. If, for example, one permanent incisor has completely erupted and the corresponding incisor's predecessor has not loosened sufficiently for exfoliation, one might be suspicious of impaction, congenital absence, or the presence of a supernumerary tooth or odontoma. A referral should be made to a dentist if there is more than 6 months' difference between the eruption of corresponding teeth.

The congenital absence of teeth can be total (anodontia) or partial (oligodontia). *Anodontia* is rare and is often seen with hypotrichosis, anhidrosis, and asteatosis as a characteristic of ectodermal dysplasia. *Oligodontia* in the primary dentition is rare. It is more common in the permanent dentition. The most frequently missing teeth (in order of frequency) are the third molars, mandibular second bicuspids, maxillary lateral incisors, and maxillary second bicuspids; the absence may be unilateral or bilateral. Treatment depends on the space needs of the rest of the arch and the rate of root resorption of the primary tooth. If there is insufficient space for a normal-sized replacement to be made or if crowding exists elsewhere in the arch, orthodontic movement can reposition the teeth as necessary. Confirmation of congenitally absent teeth by roentgenograms allows for planning of proper treatment at the appropriate time.

The presence of a "double tooth" can be seen in either dentition, but it is more likely to be seen in the primary dentition. It is usually limited to anterior teeth. A double tooth is the result of either fusion or gemination. It either reduces the count (double tooth is counted as one) by one or results in the normal amount if the fusion is between a normal and a supernumerary tooth.

Some abnormalities observed on clinical examination, such as delayed eruption of a permanent incisor, a large space between the maxillary central incisors, severe labial positioning or rotation of an incisor, or prominent bulging of the alveolar ridge may be indicative of underlying pathology. The presence of unerupted supernumerary teeth, impacted teeth (normal teeth but diverging from the usual eruption path), or odontomas (calcified masses with some anatomic similarity to teeth) among the developing permanent teeth prevents normal eruption or alignment. Supernumerary teeth occur most commonly in the maxillary incisor region of the dentition, whereas impacted teeth are (in order of frequency) maxillary cuspids, central incisors, mandibular second bicuspids, and second molars. Odontomas can be discovered at any age or in any tooth-bearing area of the

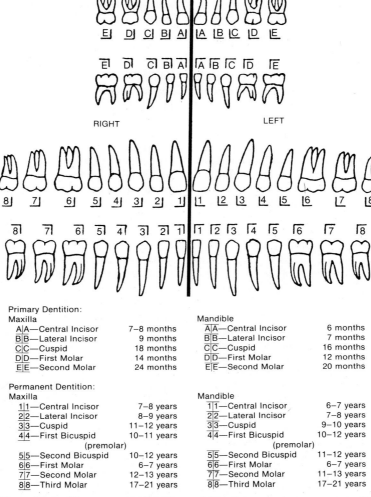

RIGHT   LEFT

Primary Dentition:

Maxilla			Mandible		
A|A—Central Incisor		7–8 months	A|A—Central Incisor		6 months
B|B—Lateral Incisor		9 months	B|B—Lateral Incisor		7 months
C|C—Cuspid		18 months	C|C—Cuspid		16 months
D|D—First Molar		14 months	D|D—First Molar		12 months
E|E—Second Molar		24 months	E|E—Second Molar		20 months

Permanent Dentition:

Maxilla			Mandible		
1|1—Central Incisor		7–8 years	1|1—Central Incisor		6–7 years
2|2—Lateral Incisor		8–9 years	2|2—Lateral Incisor		7–8 years
3|3—Cuspid		11–12 years	3|3—Cuspid		9–10 years
4|4—First Bicuspid		10–11 years	4|4—First Bicuspid		10–12 years
	(premolar)			(premolar)	
5|5—Second Bicuspid		10–12 years	5|5—Second Bicuspid		11–12 years
6|6—First Molar		6–7 years	6|6—First Molar		6–7 years
7|7—Second Molar		12–13 years	7|7—Second Molar		11–13 years
8|8—Third Molar		17–21 years	8|8—Third Molar		17–21 years

Figure 83-1. The names and locations of the primary and permanent dentition are depicted as well as their usual times of eruption.

mouth. The presence of any of these abnormalities is confirmed roentgenographically.

Surgical removal is the preferred treatment for supernumerary teeth and odontomas, whereas surgical exposure and orthodontic traction of the impacted tooth is used if its position is favorable for eruption.

Ankylosis of teeth is the abnormal bony fusion of dentin with bone. The ankylosed tooth is often identified as "submerging" because adjacent areas experience continued eruption and alveolar growth while the ankylosed area is static. The second primary molar is the most common tooth in which ankylosis occurs except for anterior teeth that have been traumatized. The treatment is varied depending on the severity. The tooth is often extracted, and a space maintainer is placed until the permanent tooth erupts.

An ectopic eruption of the permanent first molar, espe-

cially in the maxillary arch, is seen frequently. It is detected roentgenographically or clinically. The child will sometimes complain of pain in the area as the distal root is resorbed and oral fluids irritate the pulp. Many ectopic molars will correct spontaneously, but if the mesial edge is trapped, simple orthodontic intervention is recommended.

DENTAL CARIES

The incidence of dental caries has decreased considerably with the introduction of systemic and topical fluorides and fluoride toothpastes, earlier examination of children, the application of occlusal sealants, and increased dental health education. The main agents of caries production are streptococci (i.e., *S. mutans*, *S. sanguis*, and *S. salivarius*). The acids that demineralize enamel are derived from carbohydrate sources that have undergone microbial degradation. If enough acid is formed and remains in contact with the enamel, demineralization occurs and the caries process is initiated. Heredity may be a factor in determining resistance or susceptibility to caries, but the environmental factors learned from parents (hygiene and diet) are of much greater significance. The anatomy of the tooth, the degree of crowding, and the presence of appliances in the mouth are also factors in the caries process. The deep developmental pits and fissures on the occlusal (biting) surfaces of molars predispose them to carious lesions. Fluoride is effective in controlling smooth surface (i.e., those surfaces between the teeth in addition to the cheek and tongue sides of the tooth) caries but the chewing surface with its deep grooves receives little protection.

Occlusal sealants are organic polymers that bond to the surface of the enamel. It forms an impervious barrier to oral fluids long term. Clinical trials indicate that prolonged wear does occur with time but that resin tags in the enamel still provide protection. They are intended for teeth with deep developmental grooves. It is probably not cost effective to seal all primary molars. The greatest benefit comes from not having to cut into tooth structure as is done with amalgam restorations once caries is present. An amalgam restoration lasts only 8 to 10 years; at that point it must be replaced, which involves the removal of still more tooth structure. Since primary teeth may be lost before it would be necessary to replace the restoration, it may be argued to simply treat caries that develop in primary teeth and save the sealants for the permanent molars. (In addition, the primary molars usually have more shallow grooves, the material does not adhere as well to the enamel of primary teeth, and the primary molars are more accessible for good hygiene than the more posterior permanent molars.)

In March 1991, the Food and Drug Administration declared that "there is not valid data to demonstrate clinical harm to patients from amalgam or that having them removed will prevent adverse health effects or reverse the course of existing diseases." The National Institutes of Health has established panels to study this question further. Thus, existing restorations should, for the present, not be removed. Although amalgam has been the preferred restorative material for posterior teeth because of its strength and durability, newer composite materials are being developed and are suitable for small incipient caries seen in children. With the decreasing incidence of caries in children and the availability of alternative materials, amalgam may not be a concern in future generations.

Nursing bottle caries is the term used to identify the pattern of carious involvement of multiple teeth following prolonged nursing (either bottle or breast) at bedtime. When the child falls asleep, the liquid pools on the teeth because of the decreased salivary flow and diminished clearance from the mouth. Multiple maxillary incisors are usually involved, with occlusal surfaces of the first primary molars affected next most frequently. The mandibular incisors are rarely involved, probably because of the tongue's overlying position in nursing. By the time the second molars and cuspids erupt, the practice has usually been discontinued.

COMMON MALOCCLUSIONS

Anterior open bite is often associated with a thumb habit, tongue thrust, or abnormal tongue posture.

Because severe protrusion of maxillary anterior teeth renders teeth susceptible to fracture from trauma, early correction is often performed to minimize this risk.

Crossbite is the term applied to a malocclusion in which the maxillary tooth or teeth are positioned behind the mandibular in the anterior region or palatally in the posterior region. Crossbites are frequently seen in both the primary and mixed dentition and are quite varied according to severity. Single anterior tooth crossbites warrant immediate attention. When the teeth are closed, the maxillary incisor is trapped behind the opposing mandibular incisor(s) causing forward pressure on the mandibular incisor. As a result of this forward pressure, the gingiva often recedes from the front surface of the mandibular incisor. There is also a possibility of space loss on the maxillary arch as a result of drifting of the adjacent incisors into the space normally occupied by the maxillary tooth. The complete crossbite of all the incisors is indicative of a possible developing mandibular skeletal discrepancy. An evaluation regarding the extent of the problem and the timing of correction should be made by an orthodontist.

Posterior crossbites can be unilateral or bilateral. The treatment is an expansion of the width of the palate.

PERIODONTIUM

The most common gingival disorders are discussed in detail in Chapter 82.

Phenytoin (Dilantin)-induced gingivitis consists of generalized hyperplasia of the gingiva. Excellent oral hygiene should be stressed in children undergoing phenytoin therapy. Surgical removal of the excessive tissue is often done, but a recurrence is common.

Localized juvenile periodontitis is a disease that occurs in healthy pubertal patients and is characterized by severe and rapid bone loss. Particularly important is the fact that acute inflammatory gingival symptoms are absent. Treatment is best rendered by a specialist to try to minimize tooth loss as a result of the rapid bone loss. Tetracycline therapy has been used in some patients with varied success.

Gingival recession in children usually appears localized rather than generalized, as is the case in adults with advanced periodontal disease. Localized gingival recession is often seen along the labial surface of crowded mandibular incisors. This stripping of the gingiva from the root of the tooth results from pressure of the tooth against the buccal plate of bone or as the result of occlusal trauma. Toothbrush abrasion is another cause of gingival recession. Tooth brushing with a soft brush reduces this damage. Gingival grafting is necessary if the tissue loss is severe.

FLUORIDE

The usefulness of fluoride supplements to pregnant women who live in nonfluoridated areas has not been established, although no hazards have been discovered to contradict its use. However, studies suggest that the major effect of fluoride on the primary teeth is postnatally.

Fluoride supplements are recommended for nursing infants even in fluoridated areas because human milk contains such low levels of fluoride. Once the infant begins to drink water or formula made with fluoridated water, the fluoride should be discontinued.

Many studies show that fluoridated water reduces dental caries by 35% to 65%. In nonfluoridated areas or in areas where water is obtained from wells, it is recommended that daily supplements be given systemically (Table 83.1).

Many schools now have children participate in topical fluoride rinse programs (usually stannous or sodium fluoride). Such programs, along with semiannual topical application of acidulated phosphate fluoride at the dental visit and use of fluoridated toothpastes, have further decreased the caries rate in children. Care should be taken, however, to ensure that the fluoride given in schools is topical rather than systemic if water is fluoridated in the community or if fluoride supplements are already prescribed. If the water supply is not fluoridated, topical treatment may be used in conjunction with, but should not substitute for, systemic fluoride.

Topical fluoride rinses for children younger than 4 years of age should be administered carefully because the child may not have full control of swallowing reflexes.

The controversy of water fluoridation has resurfaced with a report by the National Toxicology Program that found that male rats developed a rare form of bone cancer from ingesting large amounts of fluoride. The Department of Health and Human Services released a report in February 1991 after a 9-month investigation and concluded that fluoride poses no detectable cancer risk for humans.

Table 83-1. Supplemental Fluoride Dosage Schedule*

	CONCENTRATION OF FLUORIDE IN DRINKING WATER		
AGE (YR)	*0–0.3 ppm*	*0.3–0.7 ppm*	*>0.7 ppm*
0–2	0.25 mg	0	0
2–3	0.5 mg	0.25 mg	0
3–16	1.0 mg	0.5 mg	0.25 mg

*2.2 mg sodium fluoride contains 1 mg fluoride

The incidence of *fluorosis* has increased in the past 40 years, which is an indication that total fluoride exposure may be more than necessary to prevent tooth decay.

COMMON QUESTIONS ASKED OF PEDIATRICIANS AND DENTISTS

Q. When should the child's first dental appointment be?

A. Two years old is the age recommended by the Academy of Pediatric Dentistry. At this age, usually an examination only is scheduled and the child is best held by the parent during the examination. An examination will reveal existing caries and eruption abnormalities and will provide an opportunity for oral hygiene instruction. At 3 years of age, a child is familiar with the routine, the dental office, and the staff and is able to participate in the examination, cleaning, and fluoride treatment.

Q. With the decreased incidence of tooth decay, how often should a child visit the dentist?

A. It is still recommended that a child be seen twice a year. In the preschool child, the personality development and changes are so rapid that a child who is seen only annually often finds the visit traumatic because he or she has forgotten the procedure; he or she does not remember the staff, and so forth. Once the permanent teeth begin to erupt, semiannual examinations allow interception of developing malocclusion at an early age.

Q. When should toothbrushing begin?

A. Cleaning of the teeth should begin as soon as teeth erupt. The parent should wipe the first teeth with a gauze before bedtime each day. A soft toothbrush can be used as early as tolerated. Once children are 2 to 3 years old, they should be allowed to brush their own teeth twice a day to encourage good hygiene habits, but at bedtime the toothbrushing should be completed by the parent. A child usually lacks manual dexterity to brush satisfactorily until he or she is almost 6 years old.

Q. When should toothpaste be used and what kind?

A. The greatest benefit of toothbrushing is the removal of plaque by the mechanical action of brushing. Toothpaste adds flavor, some abrasiveness for better cleaning, and fluoride for caries prevention. Toothpaste can be used once the child is mature enough not to ingest it. Any toothpaste with fluoride is recommended; the brand depends on preference. Some children do not like any flavor; it is probably wiser to forego toothpaste if brushing alone can be accomplished without a fight, rather than having every session be an ordeal.

Q. At what age should flossing start?

A. Rather than specifying a certain age, flossing should start when tight contact exists between teeth. If spaces are wide enough to allow access to all surfaces with a toothbrush, flossing is not necessary. A parent should floss for the child when indicated since children tend to lacerate their tissues.

Q. Is staining of teeth a permanent condition?

A. Extrinsic staining is usually of microbial origin except for that caused by oral iron preparations. Common stains are green (thought to be the result of chromogenic bacteria on the enamel surface); orange (often associated with poor hygiene); or black. Removal of these stains can be accomplished by the use of an abrasive pumice paste applied with rotary instruments.

Q. What is bruxism, and is treatment necessary?

A. Bruxism is an oral habit consisting of grinding or gnashing of the teeth, which occurs most often at night. Severe abrasion of the teeth (through both the enamel and the dentin layers) can occur. In the primary dentition no treatment is usually necessary, but if the habit continues and wear of the permanent teeth is observed, a plastic night guard can be used to lessen the damage to the teeth.

Q. At what age are braces applied to the teeth?

A. It is recommended that the occlusion should be evaluated at 7 years of age. Crossbites, ectopic eruptions, and severe incisor protrusions susceptible to fracture can be corrected at this age with limited treatment; attention can be directed toward correcting certain habits that contribute to malocclusions, such as thumb sucking and tongue thrust. Future spacing needs can be assessed, and future treatment can be planned. Most appliances for complete treatment are placed in the late mixed dentition stage.

Q. What are the major indications for braces?

A. Malocclusions that interfere with function such as anterior open bite, anterior and posterior crossbites, severe protrusion of incisors that make them susceptible to fracture, and those that are disfiguring causing emotional problems in development are the chief indications for orthodontic treatment.

Q. What is the role of thumb sucking in malocclusions? At what age, if any, are changes reversible?

A. Thumb sucking often results in protrusion of the maxillary incisors (sometimes accompanied by lingual inclination of the mandibular incisors) and anterior open bite (which is the more difficult malocclusion to correct). Many children suffer no effects to the dentition. However, thumb sucking may become a major family issue. Prior to the age of 4, efforts to reduce the habit are impractical because of the immaturity of the child and only result in increased stress for all concerned. As a child associates with other children in preschool programs, the habit usually stops (at least during the day). Some effects may be reversed if stopped by age 4.

Thus, it is at this age that a child should stop sucking on his or her thumb, finger, or a pacifier.

If damage is such that the habit should be stopped, several methods have proven somewhat effective. If the family agrees to not interfere, to stop any nagging, and to ignore the habit, a practitioner can often speak privately with the child and ask the child to keep a record and report progress made in decreasing the habit. Appliances can be made to serve only as a reminder to the child; these should preferably be removable, so that if it is emotionally necessary the child is still able to suck his or her thumb.

Q. Which causes more malocclusion: thumb sucking or a pacifier?

A. There is no proven answer to this question. The literature suggests that there is no difference between thumb/finger and pacifier sucking. Current belief is that orthodontic pacifiers are less likely to cause malocclusion and are probably the best option.

It should be remembered that many children with a sucking habit do not develop malocclusion. The force and direction of thumb or finger sucking varies greatly from child to child. More irregular malocclusions are seen with these than pacifier use, which can only fit in the mouth in one way. Malocclusion from both is corrected easily.

ANNOTATED BIBLIOGRAPHY

American Society of Dentistry for Children and The American Academy of Pedodontics. Pediatr Dent 5:89, 1983. (Good review of the use of pit and fissure sealants.)

Finn S: Clinical Pedodontics, 4th ed. Philadelphia, WB Saunders, 1973. (Good general pediatric dentistry textbook.)

Fluoridation. ADA News 22(5):1 and 22(7):1, 1991. (Interesting look at the political process in public health issues.)

Gellin M: The distribution of anomalies of primary anterior teeth and their effect on the permanent successors. Dent Clin North Am 28:69–80, 1972. (Detailed discussion of missing and supernumerary teeth in the primary dentition.)

Groenevald A et al: Fluoride in caries prevention: Is the effect pre-or post eruptive? J Dent Res 69:751–755, 1990. (Posteruptive.)

Marshall E: The fluoride debate: One more time. Science 247:276–277, 1990. (Good background of both sides of question.)

McDonald R, Avery D: Dentistry for the Child and Adolescent, 5th ed. St. Louis, CV Mosby, 1987. (Very detailed, well-written, and inclusive.)

O'Mullane DM: Future of water fluoridation. J Dent Res 69:756–759, 1990. (Traces the historical and political process of fluoride in the water system.)

Walker JD et al: A clinical review of preventive resin restoration. ASDC J Dent Child 57:257–259, 1990. (Good review of the use of sealants.)

Wood N, Gooz P: Differential Diagnosis of Oral Lesions. St. Louis, CV Mosby, 1975. (Excellent oral pathology textbook, especially in the differential diagnoses as well as in descriptions of pathology.)

84

Neck Masses

Basil J. Zitelli

The differential diagnosis of neck masses in children is extensive and includes congenital lesions, lymphadenopathy, and neoplastic disorders. Fortunately, most neck masses in children are benign inflammatory disorders, with malignancies comprising only about 10% of such masses in children admitted to the hospital.

CLINICAL ANATOMY AND PRESENTATION

Anatomically, two cervical triangles are formed by structures on each side of the neck. The anterior triangle extends from the mandible edge superiorly along the sternocleidomastoid muscle to the midline of the neck anteriorly. The posterior triangle is bounded by the sternocleidomastoid muscle, the distal two thirds of the clavicle, and the midline of the neck posteriorly. These triangles are important in the physical diagnosis of neck masses. Structures that can be palpated normally in the neck and are confused occasionally with pathologic processes include the angle of the mandible, the mastoid tip, the styloid process, the pyramidal lobe of the thyroid, the greater cornu of the thyroid, and the lateral processes of C2 and C6.

Certain historical and physical characteristics of common lesions may lead the clinician in the appropriate direction. Lesions present at birth suggest congenital cysts or anomalies. Congenital cysts, however, may become inflamed at a later time and may be confused easily with regional lymphadenitis. Inflammation as well as tenderness may be associated with lymphadenopathy and occasionally also malignancies. In general, lesions that progress slowly over several months are congenital and are frequently benign. A rapid growth over a few weeks, especially if inflammation is not present, suggests that a neoplastic process and malignancy must be considered. Risk factors associated with malignancies include the onset by 1 month of age, rapid and progressive growth, ulceration, a lesion fixed to or below the underlying fascia, and a lesion larger than 3 cm that is firm or hard. The older child may also exhibit symptoms of fevers, night sweats, and weight loss. Inflamed masses that become painful while eating suggest sialadenitis.

The location of the mass is important. Most masses in children lying anterior to the sternocleidomastoid muscle are benign. The exception to this rule is thyroid nodules; these should be suspected to be malignant until proven otherwise. Other malignancies are more likely to be found as a single mass in the posterior triangle or as multiple masses crossing into both the anterior and posterior triangles. Supraclavicular adenopathy is strongly associated with granulomatous or malignant disease in the mediastinum. Masses along the anterior border of the sternocleidomastoid muscle, especially if they are associated with a fistula that retracts with swallowing, are more likely to be branchial cleft anomalies.

COMMON CONGENITAL LESIONS OF THE NECK

Benign congenital lesions of the neck are almost always a thyroglossal duct cyst (72%), a branchial cleft cyst (24%), or a vascular malformation (4%) such as cystic hygroma or hemangioma.

Thyroglossal Duct Cyst

The most common congenital neck mass is the thyroglossal duct cyst, an embryologic remnant of the descent of the thyroid anlage from the base of the tongue. Most cysts and fistulas are detected before age 20. There is no sex or race predilection. Frequently, a fluctuant cystic mass ranging in size from 1 to 2 cm up to 5 to 6 cm is found in the midline just below the level of the hyoid bone. The mass may occasionally be lateral to the midline but anterior to the sternocleidomastoid muscle, making differentiation from branchial cleft cysts difficult. Other locations include the suprahyoid, suprasternal, transhyoid, and submental areas. When a sinus tract is present, drainage of mucoid material may occur and infection may lead to acute swelling and tenderness.

The mass is best examined when the neck is hyperextended. Characteristically, because of connections with the tongue, the cyst may rise with tongue protrusion and swallowing. Thyroglossal duct cysts usually do not transilluminate because of the overlying tissue and fascia.

Other diagnostic considerations include lingual thyroid, pyramidal lobe of the thyroid, sebaceous cyst, lipoma, and dermoid cyst. A failure of complete descent of the thyroid may lead to ectopic placement. This can be detected by noting absent thyroid tissue in the normal position on ultrasound examination. Sebaceous cysts do not move with tongue protrusion. Lipomas are usually more lobulated and softer than thyroglossal duct cysts, and dermoids are attached to the skin and move easily with it.

The treatment of thyroglossal duct cysts, sinuses, and fistulas consists of controlling infection with systemic antibiotics followed by complete surgical excision, which often includes resection of the midportion of the hyoid bone.

If dysgenic thyroid tissue is found in the cyst, thyroid function tests and a thyroid scan should be performed to examine for remaining thyroid tissue.

Branchial Cleft Defects

Defects of the branchial clefts may be formed from remnants of the branchial grooves and pouches being buried or failing to complete fusion. Branchial cleft anomalies may arise from any of the first four clefts. However, more than 95% of these defects arise from the second cleft, perhaps because it has the greatest depth and persists the longest. Defects of the second cleft are lateral and are usually recognized by age 30, although most are diagnosed in the early school-aged child before the age of 10. Bilateral defects occur in 2% of cases. Cysts are found approximately three times more frequently than fistulas. Although the cysts may vary in position, most are found in the carotid triangle and can be palpated anterior to the middle one third of the sternocleidomastoid muscle. The posterior border of the cyst is usually below the anterior margin of the sternocleidomastoid muscle. The mass is rounded, slightly movable, and, unless acutely infected, nontender. The mass may increase in size along with surrounding lymph nodes during periods of inflammation. Sinuses, when present, may open externally and are usually found as 2- to 3-mm slits anterior to the lower third of the sternocleidomastoid muscle. The fistula may also extend internally to open in the peritonsillar area. Skin appendages and sinuses coexist with branchial cleft cysts in 63% of cases, making diagnosis much easier.

The differential diagnosis includes lymphadenopathy, cystic hygroma, dermoid cyst, neurofibroma, aberrant thyroid, hemangioma, and lipoma. The fibrous tumor of congenital muscular torticollis can also be mistaken for a second cleft cyst. However, the mass in congenital muscular torticollis is within the belly of the sternocleidomastoid muscle (easily determined by cervical ultrasound examination) and there may be an associated head tilt with the head inclined to the affected side and the chin rotated to the opposite side. A complete examination of the ear, nose, throat, and nasopharynx is essential.

The treatment of branchial cleft cysts and fistulas is complete excision of the cyst and fistulous tract.

Vascular Lesions

Cystic hygromas (cavernous lymphangiomatous tissue) and hemangiomas comprise a small portion of benign congenital neck masses and are usually easily recognized. These vascular lesions are diffuse and easily compressible, and they often enlarge during a Valsalva maneuver. While cystic hygromas can be transilluminated, hemangiomas can be recognized by their more limited size and bluish hue of the overlying skin.

Cystic hygromas arise from lymphatic sacs that develop from mesenchymal tissue or from the jugular vein. These lesions may arise from within the anterior or posterior cervical triangle.

Nearly two thirds of these lesions are noted at birth, and 90% are diagnosed by the second birthday.

Cystic hygromas can compromise vital structures in the neck or enlarge secondary to hemorrhage or infection. Surgical excision may be difficult but remains the only effective

mode of therapy. Recurrence after removal of all grossly abnormal tissue is unlikely.

Hemangiomas may not be present visibly at birth but grow rapidly within the first year of life. Similar to cystic hygromas, hemangiomas can impinge on vital structures in the neck and can cause airway obstruction. Tumor growth usually ceases after the first birthday, and spontaneous regression usually occurs by 5 or 6 years. Therapy is not required except in cases of severe cosmetic deformities or interference of vital function, and the mass should be checked for spontaneous regression. Therapy, when necessary, may include prednisone or surgery.

LYMPHADENOPATHY

Palpable cervical lymph nodes are a common finding and may not represent an ongoing pathologic process. Nearly half of all 2-year-old children will normally have palpable cervical nodes. The percentage of children with palpable nodes increases with age as recurrent minor infections occur and the amount of lymphoid tissue increases in early childhood. *Lymphadenopathy* is usually defined as any nontender lymph node larger than 10 mm, except epitrochlear ($\geq$5 mm) and inguinal ($\geq$15 mm) nodes.

The evaluation of cervical adenopathy depends on a careful history and a detailed physical examination. The clinician should evaluate the location, size, shape, consistency, mobility, inflammation, suppuration, and skin discoloration. In addition, an examination for noncontiguous adenopathy and systemic disease should be included in the complete examination (See also Chap. 127, ''Lymphadenopathy'').

Viral Infections

Viral upper respiratory tract tract infections, by far, are the most common causes of enlarged cervical lymph nodes in children. The nodes are usually bilateral, discrete, oval, soft, and minimally tender. Most of the acute changes in the lymph node usually parallel the course of the respiratory infection or lag slightly by a few days. The size of the nodes, however, may not fully regress to their former size. One report demonstrated persistent adenopathy for 10 months after a herpesvirus infection. Besides the herpesviruses, adenoviruses and enteroviruses are commonly associated with cervical lymph node enlargement. In addition, Epstein-Barr virus infection may produce fever, malaise, and exudative tonsillopharyngitis, with localized cervical and often generalized lymphadenopathy including hepatosplenomegaly. The diagnosis of Epstein-Barr virus infection may be difficult, especially in the young child, because many preschoolers may not develop heterophil agglutinating antibodies. Twenty-seven to 91% of patients 2 to 5 years old with Epstein-Barr virus infection will be heterophil positive, whereas 53% to 94% of patients 6 to 10 years old and nearly 100% of older children will be positive. A definitive diagnosis can be made by measuring specific antibody titers to the viral capsid antigen and other viral components. Despite a typical mononucleosis-like illness, nearly half of patients will be Epstein-Barr virus negative. Cytomegalovirus infection, associated with lymphocytosis and atypical lymphocytes on peripheral blood smear, is a major cause of "Epstein-Barr virus negative" mononucleosis as are adenovirus and *Toxoplasma gondii*. Viral infections are usually self-limited and generally require no specific therapy.

Bacterial Infection

Lymphadenitis of the head and neck is most frequently secondary to infections to the upper respiratory tract, infections of the teeth and gingiva, or infections following trauma. *Staphylococcus aureus* and *Streptococcus pyogenes* cause between 40% and 80% of cases of acute unilateral cervical adenitis. Lymph nodes range from 2 to 6 cm and are tender with overlying warmth and erythema. Fluctuance may develop. Young infants, usually males between 3 and 7 weeks of age, may develop lymphadenitis associated with cellulitis, otitis media, and bacteremia; *S. aureus* and group B streptococci are the most common causative agents. Increasingly, anaerobic infections are being identified as causing acute lymphadenitis. Anaerobic organisms were recovered from 40% of needle aspirates in one series and were the sole organisms isolated in 20% of patients. Rarely, *Hemophilus influenzae* has been isolated from node aspirates as well. The treatment of bacterial lymphadenitis must account for a high percentage of penicillin-resistant *S. aureus*, and a semisynthetic penicillin, erythromycin, or cephalosporin should be used as initial therapy.

"Cold" Inflammatory Lymphadenitis

"Cold" inflammation (subacute or chronic inflammation) of the cervical nodes is frequently secondary to cat-scratch disease, atypical mycobacterial infection, or toxoplasmosis. Cat-scratch disease is a zoonotic infection following contact with a cat, a cat scratch, or a break in the skin with cat licks. A primary pustule develops 3 to 10 days after the scratch and may persist up to 8 weeks. In a small percentage of patients, the eye is the site of inoculum, resulting in conjunctivitis or an ocular granuloma with preauricular adenopathy. Impressive regional adenopathy develops about 2 weeks after inoculation but may not occur for nearly 7 weeks. Nodes are tender; they may occur in multiple sites (40% of cases); they may range from 1 to 8 cm; and they may persist 2 to 4 months and rarely up to 6 to 24 months. Lymph node biopsy typically demonstrates stellate granulomas and suppurative or caseous centers. The causative agent appears to be a small pleomorphic, gram-negative rod seen with Warthin-Starry silver impregnation stains of lymph node or pustular lesions. Trimethoprim-sulfamethoxazole has been reported to result in clinical improve-

ment. The aspiration of suppurative nodes is indicated. Rarely, surgical excision is necessary when the diagnosis is in doubt, or it may delay the diagnosis of a malignancy (see Chap. 207).

Atypical mycobacterial lymphadenitis predominately affects children 1 to 5 years of age, with its peak incidence in children 1 to 3 years of age. *Mycobacterium scrofulaceum* and *M. avium-intracellulare* are the most common offending organisms. Typically, the lymph node enlarges suddenly. The nodes are usually unilateral, in contrast to *M. tuberculosis* infections, which are usually bilateral. Minimal pain and tenderness are present, but no constitutional symptoms develop. Several nodes in an affected area may enlarge; they may become matted together and adhere to the overlying skin. Early skin changes consist of a neovascularization (rather than diffuse erythema) that progresses from pink to purplish red. The skin is not warm to the touch (hence "cold" inflammation). The skin becomes thinned and parchment-like, and eventually the node spontaneously suppurates after several months. Generalized adenopathy does not exist and chest roentgenograms are normal. A diagnosis may be difficult but is suggested if reaction to a 5-U dose of purified protein derivative (PPD)-tuberculin is between 5 and 10 mm of induration. A definitive diagnosis rests solely with isolation of the infecting organism. These infections have a low risk of communicability and generally do not respond to drug therapy alone. Most of the literature favors surgical excision of the infected nodes, although some physicians have favored a nonexcisional approach. Isoniazid and rifampin are recommended for *M. tuberculosis* infection.

Acquired *toxoplasmosis* most frequently presents as painless, asymptomatic cervical lymphadenopathy. Although nearly two thirds of patients have a single site of involvement, multiple sites, including the axillary and inguinal regions, may be infected. Patients with cervical adenopathy and *Toxoplasma* infection usually have posterior triangle involvement and no associated symptoms or only mild signs and symptoms such as fever, malaise, myalgia, sore throat, cough, and anorexia. Splenomegaly, palpable only a few centimeters below the costal margin, is usually transient. A generalized, nonpruritic, maculopapular rash most marked on the trunk and proximal extremities is also briefly visible. Patients may have leukocytosis with atypical lymphocytes and eosinophils on a peripheral smear. The diagnosis of an active infection is suggested by high titers to *Toxoplasma*, as measured by the Sabin-Feldman dye test. A definitive diagnosis rests with biopsy. No specific therapy is recommended for *Toxoplasma* lymphadenitis, although excision may be contemplated if the diagnosis is in doubt.

MALIGNANT TUMORS

Over 25% malignant tumors in children occur in the head and neck, and one of every seven children admitted with a neck mass will have a malignant tumor. For every six children with a malignant tumor of the head and neck, one will have an associated tumor of the nasopharynx. In contrast to adults who frequently develop carcinomas, tumors in children are of mesenchymal origin with lymphoid tumors predominating. The predominant tumor types are Hodgkin's disease, lymphosarcoma, rhabdomyosarcoma, fibrosarcoma, thyroid malignancies, neuroblastoma, and epidermoid carcinoma.

Age is a factor in the type of tumor that may be found. Children younger than 6 years of age most frequently have neuroblastoma, followed by lymphosarcoma, rhabdomyosarcoma, and Hodgkin's disease. In preadolescent children, Hodgkin's disease and lymphosarcoma occur with almost equal frequency whereas thyroid cancers and rhabdomyosarcomas follow. In adolescents, Hodgkin's disease is the most frequent malignant tumor of the head and neck.

Hodgkin's disease and lymphosarcoma comprise approximately two thirds of the malignant tumors of the head and neck in children. Although lymphosarcoma occurs approximately twice as frequently as Hodgkin's disease, a child with a neck mass has an equal chance of having either disease since Hodgkin's disease presents twice as frequently (80%) with a neck mass as does lymphosarcoma (40%). The mass of Hodgkin's disease is often painless, slowly enlarging, unilateral (80%), and firm. It is usually located in the upper one third of the neck, although if supraclavicular nodes are involved a mediastinal tumor is usually found as well. Approximately 6% of patients may present with preauricular adenopathy simulating parotid swelling or even cat-scratch disease. Usually children older than 5 years of age are afflicted with Hodgkin's disease and they have fewer extranodal sites of involvement compared with lymphosarcoma. In contrast, lymphosarcoma is more frequent in the younger patient, and extranodal sites such as the tonsils are up to four times more frequently involved than in Hodgkin's disease. Nodes are painless, rubbery, and discrete.

A rare benign condition that may confused with a lymphoid malignancy is sinus histiocytosis, a syndrome of massive, bilateral, painless cervical adenopathy usually occurring in blacks. Fever, leukocytosis with neutrophilia, elevated erythrocyte sedimentation rate, and diffuse hypergammaglobulinemia commonly occur. Adenopathy may persist for months to years before gradual spontaneous resolution occurs. Lymph nodes can be distinguished histologically from lymphomatous conditions. The cause is unknown, and the disease may recur.

Rhabdomyosarcoma accounts for about 10% of malignancies involving the head and neck and represents the most common solid tumor occurring in this region. It presents usually as a painless mass virtually at any site, and symptoms depend on the involved organ. The nasopharynx, middle ear, mastoid, and orbit are common sites of occurrence.

Fibrosarcoma and neurofibrosarcoma may present as a painless mass arising from the cheek, jaw, nose, or sinuses. They occur with half the frequency of rhabdomyosarcomas and have a low tendency to metastasize.

Thyroid nodules occur infrequently in children, but when they do, they have nearly an 80% chance of being malignant. This is particularly true if there is a history of radiation to the head or neck. Therefore, any thyroid nodule in a child should be considered malignant until proven otherwise. The nodules are generally midline or slightly lateral and are in close proximity to the thyroid gland. Most of the tumors are of the medullary or mixed papillary and follicular types. The prognosis in children with well-differentiated thyroid cancer after lobectomy and node dissection is far better than in other types of childhood cancer.

Although neuroblastoma is the most common solid tumor in childhood, it ranked sixth in frequency of malignancies involving the head and neck. Most neuroblastomas are metastatic from other sites and affect lymph nodes. A metastatic disease can be distinguished from a primary disease because neurologic signs are late occurrences as enlarged nodes impinge on neural structures. Primary neuroblastoma in the neck, on the other hand, has early onset of neurologic symptoms such as Horner syndrome.

Metastatic tumors to cervical nodes other than neuroblastoma must also be considered. They include the leukemias, thyroid malignancies, nasopharyngeal carcinoma, and other tumors that metastasize through lymphatic channels.

SYSTEMIC DISORDERS

Systemic disorders may have cervical adenopathy as part of generalized lymph node enlargement. Unusual cases of cervical lymphadenopathy include histoplasmosis and cryptococcosis, although more commonly these fungi cause primary pulmonary infections. Dissemination of these organisms, especially in immune-compromised hosts, may have generalized adenopathy as part of its clinical picture. Immune deficiency syndromes, including various forms of hypogammaglobulinemia, chronic granulomatous disease, hyper IgE syndrome, as well as the acquired immunodeficiency syndrome (AIDS) may be associated with enlarged lymph nodes. Progressive, generalized adenopathy, especially if associated with parotitis, should raise suspicions of human immunodeficiency virus infection in the infant (see Chap. 52).

Nodes may enlarge from chronic antigenic stimulation or primary infection, often with opportunistic organisms. Lymph node enlargement can also be found in association with hyperthyroidism. Sarcoidosis is virtually always accompanied by bilateral cervical node enlargement and may also include generalized adenopathy. Over 80% of patients will have scalene node involvement. Hilar adenopathy and other parenchymal changes on the chest roentgenogram can also be found. Autoimmune disorders such as systemic lupus erythematosus and juvenile rheumatoid arthritis often exhibit lymphadenopathy during active disease. Hemolytic anemias have occasionally been associated with recurrent, nontender enlarged nodes during bouts of hemolysis. Phenytoin administration has occasionally caused generalized adenopathy, usually preceded by other signs of hypersensitivity such as fever, rash, jaundice, and eosinophilia. Other drugs such as hydralazine and allopurinol have also been implicated in causing adenopathy. *Kawasaki* disease has cervical lymphadenopathy as part of its diagnostic criteria, although nodal enlargement may occur in only 50% of white patients. Other features of Kawasaki disease include prolonged fever; nonpurulent conjunctivitis; extremity changes with edema, erythema, or peeling of skin; rash; and oral mucosal involvement with strawberry tongue or dry and cracked lips. Although tularemia remains a rare cause of cervical adenopathy, the incidence of syphilis with its attendant generalized adenopathy is increasing in the pediatric population.

WORK-UP AND MANAGEMENT

A detailed history and physical examination is mandatory in the evaluation of every child with a neck mass and in most cases may be the only evaluation necessary. Laboratory examinations, if indicated, should be tailored to the individual case. Visual recognition is often sufficient to diagnose certain congenital lesions. It is not necessary to identify the causative agent in infectious lymphadenitis in all cases, especially when signs and symptoms are typical for viral adenopathy or if the patient responds to empiric antibiotic therapy when bacterial adenitis is suspected. Children who present with an unusual or persistent disease, or who have progression of symptoms, may require a further evaluation and perhaps an excisional biopsy. A thorough examination of the ears, nose, and throat, especially when a malignancy is suspected, is particularly important.

History should include onset and duration of symptoms; associated constitutional or systemic features; location; presence of pain or tenderness; overlying skin changes; exposure to animals such as cats, birds, farm animals, or wildlife; exposure to ill individuals; history of blood product usage or high-risk factors for human immunodeficiency virus infection; and drug or medication exposure.

Physical examination emphasizes the general state of health, including growth parameters and vital signs; location, size, color, and consistency of the mass; presence of acute inflammatory changes (warmth, erythema, tenderness or fluctuance); associated anatomic features such as sinus tracts, fistulas, or cartilage; fixation to skin or underlying fascia; matted nodes; and the presence of supraclavicular masses, generalized adenopathy, or hepatosplenomegaly.

If the mass presents shortly after birth, the clinician may examine the infant for a sinus or fistula that suggests a branchial cleft defect. If the lesion is soft, is spongy, and has a bluish hue, a hemangioma should be suspected, whereas a nondiscolored lesion that does not increase with a Valsalva maneuver may indicate a lymphangioma. Midline masses may indicate a thyroid mass or thyroglossal duct cyst. If the mass appears within the belly of the sternocleidomastoid muscle, neonatal torticollis is most likely.

Acute inflammatory lesions may be infected cysts, lymphadenitis, or sialoadenitis. Antibiotic therapy is warranted to calm acute inflammation and allow subsequent evaluation. Reinfection in the same site may indicate a cyst. The diagnosis is confirmed if a sinus or fistula tract is present.

Lymph node enlargement persisting more than 2 weeks without evidence of regression with antibiotic therapy leads the clinician along a different pathway. If inflammatory changes are present, a PPD test should be done and *Toxoplasma* titers can be obtained. If a history of exposure to cats and a primary lesion has been noted, a node aspirate, biopsy, or skin testing with cat-scratch antigen can be done to confirm the diagnosis. In the absence of inflammatory changes, drug effect, hyperthyroidism, autoimmune disorders, and human immunodeficiency virus infections can be considered. If the node lies in the supraclavicular fossa, evaluation should include PPD testing, a chest roentgenogram, and immediate biopsy since over one third of such nodes are malignant.

In general, a simple and directed laboratory evaluation provides the greatest yield. A complete blood cell count and differential, a heterophil test or titers to Epstein-Barr virus, cytomegalovirus, and *Toxoplasma* may be helpful when indicated. A chest roentgenogram may help determine mediastinal or pulmonary parenchymal disease. An aspiration of infected, fluctuant nodes will often identify the offending organism, and when coupled with antibiotics may be sufficient therapy for small abscesses. Large, fluctuant nodes usually require an incision and drainage. Node aspiration generally does not lead to a chronic draining fistula, except perhaps with inadequately treated infections or nodes chronically infected from mycobacteria, cat-scratch disease, or *Tularemia*. Acutely inflamed, fluctuant nodes rarely represent a tumor. Thus, there is almost no risk of spreading metastases by aspiration. Nodes minimally inflamed and fluctuant due to tumor necrosis may be aspirated by a direct approach that minimizes the length of the tract that may later have to be resected. A standardized 5-U PPD test may be helpful in identifying mycobacterial infections, and routine serologic data might help identify an underlying autoimmune disorder.

Ultrasound evaluation of neck masses yields characteristic appearances in thyroglossal duct cysts, neonatal torticollis, cystic hygroma, and adenopathy. It also aids in determining location, extent, and internal characteristics of the mass.

The clinician caring for a child with a neck mass is frequently confronted with the decision to biopsy a lesion or excise a node. Supraclavicular lymph nodes are associated with a malignancy or a granulomatous disease involving the mediastinum and should be biopsied early in the evaluation. Other clinical features suggesting serious disease leading to early biopsy include persistent fever or weight loss and fixation of the node to the skin and underlying tissues. An abnormal chest roentgenogram is strongly associated with a granulomatous disease or a malignant peripheral lympha-denopathy. Biopsies may yield specific diagnoses in 37% to 63% of cases. Approximately one in five patients with normal histology, reactive hyperplasia, or atypical inflam-mation will have a specific diagnosis identified on a subse-quent biopsy. In one series, patients who subsequently de-veloped lymphoma usually had the disease diagnosed within 8 months of the first biopsy. This strongly suggests that de-spite a nondiagnostic initial biopsy, patients who have a per-sistent disease or adenopathy should be monitored closely, and a second biopsy should be considered if the clinical picture changes.

ANNOTATED BIBLIOGRAPHY

Brook I: Aerobic and anaerobic bacteriology of cervical adenitis in children. Clin Pediatr 10:693–696, 1980. (Emphasizes the role of anaerobic organisms in infectious cervical adenitis; anaerobic or-ganisms were isolated in 38% of lymph node aspirates and were the sole pathogen isolated in 18%.)

Collipp PJ: Cat-scratch disease. Therapy with trimethoprim-sulfame-thoxazole. Am J Dis Child 146:397–399, 1992. (All 71 children with cat-scratch disease who were treated with TMP-SMX had ex-cellent results.)

Jaffe BF, Jaffe N: Head and neck tumors in children. Pediatrics 51:731–740, 1975. (Excellent review of 178 children with head and neck tumors presenting within a 10-year period.)

Kissane JM, Gephardt GN: Lymphadenopathy in childhood. Hum Pathol 5:431–439, 1974. (Retrospective review of 100 node bi-opsies, stating that 17% of patients with initial nondiagnostic bi-opsies eventually developed serious systemic disease.)

Knight PJ, Reiner CB: Superficial lumps in children: What, when, and why? Pediatrics 72:147–153, 1983. (Reviews the causes of pal-pable masses that were excised during an 11-year period and the criteria indicative of high risk for malignancies.)

Kraus R, Han BK, Babcock DS, Oestereich AE: Sonography of neck masses in children. AJR 146:609–613, 1986. (Reports on 49 pa-tients with neck masses evaluated by ultrasound, confirming the utility of this diagnostic method.)

Lake AM, Oski FA: Peripheral lymphadenopathy in childhood. Am J Dis Child 132:357–359, 1978. (Reviews a 10-year experience with excisional biopsy and emphasizes the need for continued follow-up.)

May M: Neck masses in children: Diagnosis and treatment. Pediatr Ann 5:517–535, 1976. (Superb comprehensive review of neck masses, with many pictures and tables.)

Saitz EW: Cervical lymphadenitis caused by atypical mycobacteria. Pediatr Clin North Am 28:823–839, 1981. (Excellent review of atypical mycobacterial adenitis including a nonexcisional approach to therapy.)

Torsiglieri AJ Jr, Tom LWC, Ross AJ III et al: Pediatric neck masses: Guidelines for evaluation. Int J Pediatr Otorhinolaryngol 16:199–210, 1988. (Review of 445 pediatric patients with neck masses coming to biopsy; excellent clinical summary, but slanted to pa-tients who underwent biopsy.)

Zuelzer WW, Kaplan J: The child with lymphadenopathy. Semin He-matol 12:323–334, 1975. (Classic review of both cervical and generalized lymphadenopathy in children.)

12

ENDOCRINOLOGIC PROBLEMS

85

Short Stature

Lynne L. Levitsky

Three of every 100 normal children are by definition at or below the third percentile for height. Most have either genetically programmed decreased adult height potential or delayed physiologic maturation. To be able to identify those children for whom short stature will persist into adult life, those children requiring medical therapy, and those children for whom discretionary therapy is potentially available, it is important to understand the pattern of normal and abnormal growth.

PATTERNS OF NORMAL GROWTH

The length and weight at birth depend on the sufficiency of intrauterine nutrition and blood gas exchange, as well as other poorly understood maternal and fetal factors. The growth rate in normal children in the first 2 postnatal years reflects the transition from the intrauterine to the intrinsic growth pattern. Growth rates in children with familial or "constitutional" short stature and those with delayed maturation may decrease precipitously. A period of stable growth at a lower percentile then ensues, with a gradually declining height velocity to levels as low as 3.7 cm/y in slow-growing boys and 4.2 cm/y in slow-growing girls for a short time just before puberty. The only interruption to that decline is the modest increase in height velocity between 6 and 8 years of age occasioned by the onset of adrenarche, the earliest increase in adrenal androgen production. When plotted on a standard growth curve, children are shown to maintain their growth along the same percentile lines from the ages of 2 to 3 years until the onset of puberty. Children who are delayed in puberty may appear to change growth percentiles at the time of normal puberty because they do not experience the sex steroid–induced pubertal growth spurt noted in the youngster with an average age at puberty. During puberty, children once again have accelerated growth, causing them to shift percentiles. The longer and more intense growth spurt in the boy leads to an average greater final height in males compared with females.

CLINICAL PRESENTATION

Three of every 100 children do not need an extensive laboratory evaluation because of small size. The decision to pursue an evaluation beyond the physical examination and history should be based on evidence of growth attenuation (growth rate less than the third percentile for age) or very short stature (height more than 3 SD below the mean for age) even if evidence for growth attenuation is not available. Rough figures used to define what is abnormal are growth rates of 5 cm/y or less before 5 years of age and of 4 cm/y or less between the ages of 5 and puberty.

DIFFERENTIAL DIAGNOSIS

Before birth, growth is affected by fetal pathology and by placental function. Children with placental dysfunction tend to be underweight compared with height (decreased ponderal index) and usually display catchup growth when removed from their detrimental intrauterine environment. Children with intrinsic fetal disorders (e.g., infection or exposure to drugs inhibiting cell replication) tend to be proportionately small and display other dysmorphic stigmata typical of these disorders. The capacity for postnatal growth is variable.

Postnatal growth depends on genetic endowment and environment. Normal genetic endowment may be associ-

ated with transient short stature if there is delayed maturation. The boy with delayed maturation is on the average
5 cm shorter than his early maturing peers by 5 years of age.
A multifactorial inheritance of familial short stature may
lead to short stature during childhood and decreased final
adult height. Abnormal genetic endowment often leads to
short stature. Disorders affecting bone and cartilage as well
as other disorders of multiple organ systems may adversely
affect growth. The major chromosomal abnormalities, with
the exception of the XYY syndrome and Klinefelter's syndrome, adversely affect growth. Genetic information on the
short arm of the X chromosome is necessary for the expression of normal height potential in girls.

Adequate nutrition is essential for good linear growth.
In affluent Western societies restricted intake leading to
poor linear growth may be related to food faddism, unusual
elimination diets, child abuse, or mechanical difficulties
in intake because of abnormalities of the oropharynx and
upper gastrointestinal tract. Malabsorption may cause decreased linear growth as may inborn errors of intermediary
metabolism that interfere with use of metabolic substrate.
(The influence of fad diets on growth is discussed in Chapter 15, Vegetarianism, and Chapter 188, Failure to Thrive,
offers a discussion complementary to this section.)

Some chronic illnesses many diminish appetite, inhibiting linear growth because of undernutrition. The mechanism of growth inhibition in other chronic illnesses is not
entirely understood. Inflammatory bowel disease may be
recognized because of growth inhibition before the onset
of clinically recognizable gastrointestinal signs and symptoms. Renal tubular acidosis may also produce asymptomatic growth failure. Many severely mentally retarded persons suffer from slow growth and short adult stature. In the
majority of cases the underlying insult producing the mental
retardation also affected cell multiplication and final height
potential. In some, the cause is an inability to take in adequate calories; and in others, disordered growth hormone
regulation has been implicated. Neuroendocrine dysfunction associated with delayed growth occurs in children with
deprivation dwarfism (psychosocial dwarfism or emotional
hypopituitarism). These are emotionally and sometimes
physically abused children with the clinical features of
slight underweight for height, potbellies, unusual eating and
gorging behaviors, large malabsorptive stools, and disturbed interpersonal relationships. When tested initially,
they manifest growth hormone deficiency and diminished
cortisol and thyroid hormone levels. After a brief period of
hospitalization or removal to a more favorable environment,
all neuroendocrine function returns to normal.

Drug therapies may affect growth rate. Both glucocorticoids and sex steroid analogues may affect ultimate
height. Glucocorticoids induce exogenous hypercortisol-
ism, antagonizing the peripheral effects of growth hormone.
Sex steroids initially stimulate growth, but by inducing premature epiphyseal function they may decrease the final adult

height. Drugs used for hyperactivity may act as appetite
suppressants and lead to a decrement in linear growth rate
in susceptible persons. They may also diminish linear
growth without a marked effect on weight.

A host of endocrine disorders can alter growth. *Hypothyroidism* is the most common acquired endocrine disease
of childhood after diabetes mellitus. It is associated with
remarkable growth arrest, a bone age that may be more
delayed than the height age, weight usually greater than
height, and, rarely, sexual precocity in females. The spectrum of growth hormone deficiency is presently being expanded. *Classic growth hormone* deficiency, both congenital and acquired, is diagnosed by deficient growth hormone
response to challenge by hypoglycemia, intravenous arginine, levodopa, or other stimuli. However, we now recognize slow-growing children with normal growth hormone
responses to these stimuli who may grow better with exogenous growth hormone and children with growth hormone
insensitivity (*Laron dwarfism*) who have normal or high
growth hormone responses but an inability to generate somatomedin C (insulin-like growth factor 1 [IGF-1]), the tissue mediator of growth hormone action. Furthermore, children may have partial growth hormone deficiency or
decreased growth hormone release over 24 hours but normal
growth hormone response to pharmacologic stimuli. These
disorders of growth hormone release may be transient or
permanent.

The first sign of excess cortisol production is a diminution in growth rate. Cortisol has an inhibitory effect on
growth even in physiologic amounts. Children with aldosterone deficiency and salt loss may have a decreased growth
rate or frank failure to thrive. Sexual precocity, except
when associated with hypothyroidism, initially induces rapid
growth. The high levels of sex steroids, however, leads to a
discordant advance in epiphyseal maturation and often to
short stature in adult life. Poorly controlled diabetes mellitus can have a deleterious effect on growth rate. Circulating
somatomedin inhibitors are generated in the insulin-deficient
state, and decreased levels of somatomedin C have been
reported.

WORK-UP

The laboratory evaluation of the patient with short stature
and growth failure can be appropriately directed and economically carried out only if preceded by a careful history
and physical examination.

History

The prenatal history is important in determining if intrauterine or intrapartum events have contributed to the growth
disorder. Children with intrauterine growth retardation may
have associated anomalies leading to continuing slow
growth and should not fail to have further evaluation just

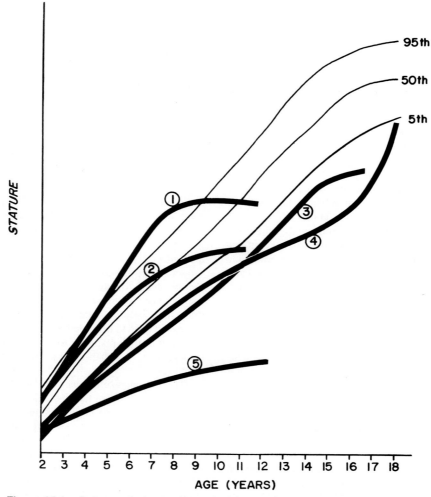

Figure 85-1. Patterns of abnormal growth: (1) sexual precocity with early epiphyseal fusion; (2) acquired growth failure (e.g., acquired hypothyroidism, renal disease, or glucocorticoid therapy); (3) genetic short stature; (4) delayed maturation; (5) congenital growth disorder (e.g., congenital hypopituitarism, achondroplasia, or cystinosis) (Adapted from Levitsky LL, Edidin DV: Growth disorders in children. Compr Ther 6:22-29, 1980)

because of inappropriately low birth weight for gestational age. A history of maternal medication use, illicit drug use, or alcohol abuse may define an etiology for the child's growth disorder. Perinatal difficulties such as breech presentation or intracranial hemorrhage may be associated with a hypothalamic pituitary disorder.

The growth pattern is important. Shifts from established growth curves after the first 2 to 3 years of life and until puberty suggest a pathologic etiology. When growth data are not available from physician's records, school records and clothing sizes may be used as an indicator of annual growth. The growth pattern of common disorders leading to short stature is graphically depicted in Figure 85-1. Physiologic maturation can be assessed in part by inquiry about

maturation of secondary dentition and age at onset of signs of puberty. Past illnesses, difficulty in feeding and dietary intake, unusual bowel habits, or other signs and symptoms of physical illness should be identified.

The family history is also important. Heights, weights, and ages at puberty of family members should be obtained. This serves a dual purpose: it supplies the physician with necessary diagnostic information and allows the family of the normal but slow-growing child the opportunity to review the familial nature of this phenomenon and gain reassurance through the review. A history of children with similar problems and of chronic illness or endocrine disease in other family members should be assessed.

A carefully obtained social history may point the way to

the diagnosis of psychosocial dwarfism or suggest the need for counseling because short stature has become a focal disruption in a child's life or in the family structure.

Physical Examination

Measurement of the child's height should not be carried out casually using an inaccurate office scale. The most accurate device is a carefully calibrated scale such as a Harpendon Stadiometer. However, careful measurement against a wall using a T-square with a built-in level is an adequate substitute. Length measurements should be recorded on the National Center for Health Statistics Charts until the age of 3 years. Height should be used thereafter. Standing height is always slightly less than length because of compression of intervertebral spaces in the standing position. Other measurements that can prove useful include head circumference, span, and lower segment in order to compute an upper/lower segment ratio. An abnormal head circumference might suggest a central nervous system disorder. Arm span should approximate height. A short arm span, measured fingertip to fingertip with the arms outstretched, might suggest a congenital disorder of bone or cartilage. The upper/lower segment ratio (lower segment measured from the top of the symphysis pubis to the heel is subtracted from height to obtain the upper segment) averages 1.7 at birth and decreases to 1 in the average white adult, reflecting a decreasing trunk to leg length ratio. If this ratio remains greater than 1, a disorder of bone or cartilage should be considered as a possible diagnosis. Severe untreated juvenile hypothyroidism is also associated with an increased upper/lower segment ratio.

The general physical examination should be taken as an opportunity to search for dysmorphic signs such as a high arched palate or unusual ears or hands. An assessment of adequacy of nutrition and general physical well-being should be made. Signs of chronic illness should be noted. Finally, physical maturation should be assessed by examining dental age and pubertal status. The Tanner rating system for pubertal maturation should be used in the initial assessment and follow-up.

Laboratory Tests

Minimum screening evaluation for children growing significantly below the third percentile or demonstrating growth attenuation should include a complete blood cell count, determination of erythrocyte sedimentation rate, thyroid function studies, and biochemistry screening to include electrolytes, carbon dioxide, blood urea nitrogen and creatinine, total protein, calcium, and phosphorus levels, a liver function test, and urinalysis with pH measurement. These screening studies will point to most occult chronic illnesses. A bone age roentgenogram permits the assessment of physiologic maturation and a prediction of adult height.

Growth arrest lines suggest a past illness or psychosocial dwarfism. In all short girls, a test for Turner syndrome should be obtained. Buccal smears may not be reliable and usually will not identify mosaic Turner syndrome. Levels of gonadotropins (luteinizing hormone and follicle-stimulating hormone) are clearly elevated in the presence of gonadal failure if the bone age is 11 or greater and may serve as a screening study after that time. The definitive study is an examination of chromosomal morphology. Rare girls with mosaic Turner syndrome may have normal peripheral blood chromosomes and elevated gonadotropins.

The somatomedin C assay (IGF-1) is useful as a screening device for growth hormone deficiency. Its limitations, however, must be recognized. Children younger than the age of 5 tend to have low somatomedin levels that cannot be clearly differentiated from children with growth hormone deficiency. Undernourished children tend to have low somatomedin C values. Some children with growth hormone deficiency have somatomedin C levels within the normal range. Randomly obtained plasma growth hormone levels do not serve a useful purpose because they are rarely elevated into a range that will permit differentiation of normal from growth hormone deficiency.

Most children with severe growth failure will offer clues from the history and physical examination as to which additional studies will be most productive. For instance, short girls with other clear stigmata of Turner syndrome might have chromosome analysis obtained immediately. The child with disproportionate measurements might undergo a skeletal roentgenographic examination to help with the diagnosis. A palpable thyroid gland might encourage the examiner to obtain antithyroid antibody titers. A history of urinary tract infection might provoke more investigation of the genitourary tract. Gastrointestinal symptoms or underweight might lead to an evaluation for malabsorption or inflammatory bowel disease.

TREATMENT

If the history, physical examination, and basic laboratory examination clearly delineate an etiology for short stature, management depends on the nature of the disorder. If no etiology can be ascertained, a period of 4 to 6 months of observation and remeasurement is often useful. Children with clear growth attenuation following such careful observation may then require further evaluation, including definitive studies of growth hormone release. Specific treatment of disorders of growth is often possible. However, most children seen with short stature do not have a pathophysiologic etiology. They suffer from familial short stature or delayed maturation or a combination of the two. Adjuvant medical therapy to enhance growth rate and final height is sometimes requested for these children. Often an open discussion of the issues with patient and family is satisfying to them and no further medical therapy is requested. In the boy with severely delayed maturation (no signs of puberty at 14 years) a short course of androgen therapy may be useful to improve self-esteem. Our usual treatment course is 75 mg of a depot testosterone preparation monthly for three doses. This causes the development of a small amount of pubic hair, some increase in phallic size, and a slight growth spurt. The growth rate often becomes subnormal for a period of several months after the effect of the last injection of testosterone dissipates. On rare occasions a second course of testosterone may be given several months later. This treatment schedule neither enhances nor decreases final height. Continued treatment with androgen likely would adversely affect final height and should be avoided.

The use of growth hormone to treat children with short stature is currently quite controversial because there is a limited pool of long-term data and the diagnosis of growth hormone deficiency has become muddled in recent years. Criteria for classic growth hormone deficiency were based up failure to respond to pharmacologic growth hormone stimuli (e.g., insulin hypoglycemia, arginine infusion, levodopa, clonidine) on two separate occasions, coupled with growth rate attenuation. In general, children with classic growth hormone deficiency, suspected because of associated findings or history, meet these criteria. Occasionally children who have had cranial irradiation, are clearly growth hormone deficient by growth rate criteria and if assessed by physiologic growth hormone release over an extended period may respond normally to pharmacologic growth hormone stimulation. On the other hand, growth hormone release over a 24-hour period may vary in the same person and may correlate with age and body mass as well as growth rate.

Children with a growth rate (not height) less than the third percentile for age and without other cause for diminished growth rate should have screening outpatient growth hormone testing. A number of provocative agents have been used. A blood sample for growth hormone obtained 1 hour after clonidine administration (100 μg/M^2 orally) may be used as a simple screening test. Clonidine may occasionally induce somnolence or hypotension even at this dose. Exercise has also been used as a standardized provocative test for growth hormone release but is somewhat less reliable as a stimulus. Other stimuli (insulin, arginine, levodopa sometimes with propranolol or estrogen potentiation) require more sampling and should probably not be used for initial screening. No growth hormone provocative test is effective in more than 90% of normal persons. Therefore, a single study demonstrating failure of growth hormone release is not conclusive.

Following stimulation, a value greater than 10 ng/ml analyzed by standard radioimmunoassay is considered normal. Values between 7 and 10 ng/ml have been considered evidence of partial growth hormone deficiency, and a response less than 7 ng/ml to two standard provocative tests is considered diagnostic of growth hormone deficiency.

Some newer assays for growth hormone have a lower range of normal values. The assay technique and normal range should therefore be noted.

Available biorecombinant growth hormone preparations differ in potency (units/mg). Growth hormone therapy may be begun at a dose of 0.5 units/kg/wk in growth hormone—deficient children. This dose is distributed into three or more injections per week. Growth hormone given daily seems more effective for long-term growth stimulation than three times weekly therapy. The growth rate usually slows after the first year of therapy. Increased dose or a change to daily injections may enhance the growth rate in later years. Growth rate, bone age, and thyroid function should be carefully followed in all children receiving growth hormone therapy. Children without classic growth hormone deficiency who respond to growth hormone therapy may also require increased growth hormone dose or injection frequency after the first year of therapy.

In otherwise normal children there is a general relationship between growth rate and physiologic growth hormone secretion. However, it is not clear that growth hormone therapy is required for normal adult height in every child with a period of low growth hormone secretion. Because of the confusion over the relationship between growth hormone secretion, growth rate, and response to growth hormone in the child who is not classically growth hormone deficient, it is probably reasonable at the present time to use a carefully obtained growth rate as an indicator of potential response to growth hormone, rather than invasive, complex, and expensive studies of growth hormone release over a 24-hour period.

It is wise to consider what is known about growth hormone therapy and growth disorders before developing an approach to the use of this potent pharmacologic agent. Growth hormone is clearly effective in improving the final height of children with classic growth hormone deficiency. Growth hormone therapy now seems to be effective in improving the final height of girls with Turner syndrome. There are no controlled data as to the effect on final height of growth hormone therapy for other conditions. However, children with excessive endogenous growth hormone secretion (gigantism) all grow excessively as long as they have not achieved epiphyseal fusion. Therefore, intuitively, it is likely that in most persons with open epiphyses, whatever the nature of the short stature, growth hormone therapy in pharmacologic dose could enhance growth rate and would improve final adult stature. However, recent authors have questioned whether growth hormone therapy disproportionately advances bone age or induces earlier puberty in individuals with an intact hypothalamic-gonadotropin-gonadal axis, thereby leading to a loss of some of this increased height expectation.

Aside from its cost, growth hormone has potential physical side effects that temper enthusiasm for its administration in extremely high dosage. High doses of growth hormone can induce "acromegaloid" changes in physical features. It is lipolytic and causes changes in body composition that may give normal short children an abnormal, excessively muscular appearance. A number of children receiving growth hormone have developed a slipped capital femoral epiphysis secondary to rapid growth. Growth hormone induces insulin resistance and may cause hyperglycemia or could lead to early induction of diabetes in susceptible persons. It may have specific effects on the immune system. Growth hormone receptors are on mononuclear cells, and there is a suspected, although weak, linkage of growth hormone therapy with leukemia. Persons with acromegaly may have a slightly greater chance of developing malignancies.

An expanded role for biosynthetic human growth hormone in the treatment of short stature is inevitable, even though the expense of such pharmacologic plastic surgery is presently exorbitant. However, the decision to use growth hormone outside of investigative trials in children who are not clearly growth hormone deficient must be weighed individually and be associated with criteria for use and criteria for discontinuation of therapy. Children with postcranial irradiation growth failure and Turner syndrome meet present objective criteria for growth hormone therapy. There does not seem to be a valid indication for growth hormone therapy in children with delayed maturation and prospects for adequate final height. There are no studies indicating that pharmacologic growth enhancement in these children, who will receive subcutaneous injections of growth hormone and repeated physician visits for many years, will lessen the emotional distress many feel during childhood and adolescence because of short stature and delayed puberty.

In children in whom final height prognosis is poor, the decision to begin growth hormone therapy should be conceived as a trial of efficacy, after the family has been carefully informed as to the potential for success and possible known and unknown adverse effects. Growth rate should be carefully monitored for at least 6 months. In children with growth attenuation and possible partial growth hormone deficiency, a growth hormone dose similar to that used in classic growth hormone deficiency (0.5 units/kg/wk administered three times per week or daily) is usually a sufficient trial. Growth hormone, in a dose higher than that used for classic growth hormone deficiency (0.6–0.8 units/kg/wk), can be administered for a period of 6 months, during which time growth rate is carefully monitored in children with Turner syndrome or other disorders clearly not growth hormone deficient. Addition of oxandrolone, a weak androgen, has improved growth in Turner syndrome. Criteria for continuing growth hormone therapy based on enhancement of growth rate (a 50% increase in growth rate, for instance) should be established in advance with the family, and if criteria are not met, growth hormone should be discontinued. A lesser increase in growth rate could also be a result of measurement error. In children with intrinsic bone or cartilage disorders, the effect of growth hormone on disordered bone growth (narrowing of cranial foramina or worsening of scoliosis) must be considered.

The ethical issues involved in treating every child in the third or fifth percentile with growth hormone, given the potential for both physical and psychological side effects, have been dealt with only partially to date. Furthermore, the economic repercussions of this decision are enormous. The role of growth hormone in the therapy of specific conditions associated with short stature will become more clear when the results of large scale trials are available, and the effect of growth hormone on final adult height, rather than growth rate, is known.

INDICATIONS FOR REFERRAL

Children growing steadily at a normal rate each year rarely require subspecialist evaluation. Children with growth attenuation always require a full evaluation of their disorder and referral to the appropriate subspecialist if the generalist pediatrician feels uncomfortable dealing with the management of the specific problem. At the present time, because of rapid changes in management and philosophy, growth hormone therapy should probably remain within the province of the endocrinologist.

PATIENT EDUCATION

The Human Growth Foundation, a national group composed of parents and friends of children with short stature, has educational materials available and can be a source of support for children with short stature and their families. The address of the national headquarters is 4607 Davidson Drive, Chevy Chase, MD 20815.

The Little People of America is an excellent resource organization for persons with very short stature. The address is Box 126, Owatonna, MI 55060.

Growing Up Small, by K.G. Pfieffer, makes good reading for families of children with short stature. The address of the publisher is Paul S. Eriksson, Middlebury, VT 05753.

ANNOTATED BIBLIOGRAPHY

Allen DB, Fost NC: Growth hormone therapy for short stature: Panacea or Pandora's box? J Pediatr 117: 16–21, 1990. (Presents cogent argument that there are no ethical reasons for limiting the use of growth hormone for the treatment of short stature.)

Bayley N, Pinneau SR: Tables for predicting adult height from skeletal age—revised for use with Greulich-Pyle Hand Standards. J Pediatr 40:423, 1952 (amended 41:371, 1952). (Easy-to-use height prediction tables that allow adult height predictions.)

Frasier SD, Lippe BM: Clinical Review 11: The rational use of growth hormone during childhood. J Clin Endocrinol Metab 71:269–273, 1990. (Critical review of indications for growth hormone therapy.)

Horner JM, Thorsson AV, Hintz RL: Growth deceleration patterns in children with constitutional short stature: An aid to diagnosis. Pediatrics 62:529, 1978. (Describes shifting growth patterns in the first several years of life.)

Lantos J, Siegler M, Cuttler L: Ethical issues in growth hormone therapy, JAMA 261: 102–104, 1989. (Presents cogent argument for limiting the use of growth hormone in the treatment of short stature.)

Smith DW: Growth and Its Disorders: Basics and Standards, Approach and Classifications, Growth Deficiency Disorders, Growth Excess Disorders and Obesity. Philadelphia, WB Saunders, 1977. (Classic reference work helpful in understanding normal growth patterns and disorders of growth.)

Tanner JM: Growth at Adolescence, 2nd ed. Oxford, Blackwell Scientific Publications, 1962. (Provides information on pubertal staging; for the generalist, the stages of puberty as defined by Tanner may be found in any standard pediatric endocrinology text.)

Tanner JM, Davies PSW: Clinical longitudinal standards for height and height velocity for North American children. J Pediatr 107:317–329, 1985. (Presents the gold standards for the determination of linear growth in North American children.)

Walker JM, Bond SA, Voss LD et al: Treatment of short normal children with growth hormone—a cautionary tale? Lancet 335:1331–1334, 1990. (Discussion of body composition changes in normal children receiving growth hormone.)

86

Diabetes Mellitus

Herbert Boerstling

Diabetes mellitus is a heterogeneous group of metabolic disorders with one common denominator—hyperglycemia, due to either absolute or relative insulin deficiency. It is the most common of the pediatric endocrine diseases, with a prevalence of 2:1000 children and an annual incidence of 16 new cases per 100,000 children.

Primary type I insulin-dependent diabetes mellitus (IDDM) is the major form of diabetes among children. It is an autoimmune disease that results in absolute insulin deficiency; all patients with IDDM must rely on insulin to control hyperglycemia and to prevent ketoacidosis. *Primary type II non-insulin-dependent diabetes mellitus* (NIDDM) is a group of disorders with carbohydrate intolerance due to relative or functional insulin deficiency. Patients with NIDDM are usually not insulin dependent nor prone to ketosis. Some obese adolescents may have this form of diabetes. Secondary diabetes mellitus occurs in patients with diminished pancreatic tissue or with other endocrine diseases that interfere with insulin action.

Primary type I insulin-dependent diabetes mellitus develops in persons who have the genetic predisposition (specific HLA antigens) and who may have suffered environ-

mental insults (e.g., viral infections or perhaps toxins) that trigger the progressive autoimmune destruction of the insulin-producing cells. Anti-islet cell or anti-insulin antibodies may be produced for years before the onset of overt diabetes mellitus.

PATHOPHYSIOLOGY

Insulin is an anabolic hormone released in bursts in response to food intake to promote glucose entry into cells and the synthesis of glycogen, lipid, and protein. During periods of fasting, insulin release decreases to a basal level. Counterregulatory hormones, such as epinephrine, glucagon, growth hormone, and cortisol are released to maintain blood glucose levels by increasing glucose production through glycogenolysis and gluconeogenesis, while enhancing fat breakdown to fatty acids and ketones for additional energy needs.

In diabetes mellitus, insulin deficiency limits glucose entry into cells and the body functions in the catabolic or fasting state. Decreased glucose utilization and unrestrained glucose production result in hyperglycemia and hyperosmolality. An osmotic diuresis results when the renal threshold of glucose reabsorption is exceeded ($\geq$160 mg/dL). Polyuria with loss of water, glucose, and electrolytes leads to dehydration and weight loss. Insulin deficiency also causes lipolysis, with hyperlipidemia and the conversion of free fatty acids to ketones, the cause of fruity breath. Urinary excretion of ketones causes further water and electrolyte loss, and metabolic acidosis occurs when the production of ketoacids exceeds excretion. Kussmaul respiration is an attempt to correct the acidosis. With increasing dehydration, hyperglycemia, hyperosmolality, and ketoacidosis, consciousness becomes progressively impaired and may lead to diabetic coma.

Chronic metabolic imbalance is the basis for the pathophysiology of long-term diabetic complications. Persistent hyperglycemia damages the microvasculature, partly due to glycosylation of vascular and basement membrane proteins, causing retinopathy and nephropathy. Joint contractures may be due to glycosylation of joint collagen and dermal proteins. Cataracts form when the sugar alcohol, sorbitol, accumulates in the lens. Neuropathy results from both microvascular damage and the accumulation of sorbitol in the myelin sheath. Macrovascular disease may be the result of glycosylation and elevated cholesterol and lipid levels.

CLINICAL PRESENTATION

Most children with diabetes are now diagnosed early in the course of the disease. They usually present with polyuria due to osmotic diuresis, polydipsia secondary to increased thirst from dehydration, and weight loss due to dehydration and calorie loss from glucosuria. Nocturnal enuresis may occur in a previously toilet-trained child. Fatigue, weakness, and listlessness are common complaints. Polyphagia is uncommon. The full-blown picture of severe diabetic ketoacidosis, with dehydration, Kussmaul respiration, fruity or acetone odor to the breath, and impaired consciousness, is now an uncommon presentation. Diabetic ketoacidosis may mimic an acute surgical abdomen.

DIFFERENTIAL DIAGNOSIS

Glucosuria without hyperglycemia occurs in benign renal glucosuria or in renal tubular disease. In the absence of hyperglycemia, polyuria and polydipsia suggest either diabetes insipidus or psychogenic polydipsia. Kussmaul respiration and metabolic acidosis without hyperglycemia or ketonuria occurs in salicylate poisoning. Children with Cushing's syndrome, pheochromocytoma, or acromegaly may present with hyperglycemia and glucosuria; however, the underlying endocrinopathy is usually apparent. Transient hyperglycemia may occur in children undergoing severe stress or trauma, including burns, or serious infections.

WORK-UP

A child presenting with any of the aforementioned symptoms should be tested for diabetes mellitus. Hyperglycemia confirms the diagnosis. Before initiating treatment, a complete blood cell count and differential should be obtained, along with evaluation of blood glucose, ketones, pH, glycosylated hemoglobin, electrolytes, blood urea nitrogen, and creatinine levels and urinalysis.

A newly diagnosed nonketoacidotic diabetic may be treated as an outpatient if the pediatrician has the expertise and the time to teach the principles of diabetes management and to carefully monitor the child when insulin treatment is begun. Otherwise the child should be referred to a pediatric endocrine service for care. A very young diabetic or a diabetic in moderate to severe ketoacidosis must be hospitalized.

MANAGEMENT

Successful treatment of a diabetic patient is dependent on effective initial education with periodic reassessment and update, a life-long learning process that empowers the patient and family to respond appropriately to the demands of diabetes care. Specific goals include an understanding of the cause of diabetes, the rationale for the use of the different types of insulin, the methods for home monitoring of diabetes, and the interrelationship between insulin, diet, and exercise on diabetes. Patients must learn to recognize and quickly treat the acute and subacute complications. Effort must be made to achieve the best possible care without risking serious reactions and with as few minor reactions as possible. With the proper knowledge and glucose control, the diabetic child should be able to attain normal growth and development and to forestall the long-term complications. Diabetics are also encouraged to wear Medic-Alert tags.

Table 86-1.   Key Characteristics of the Three Most Frequently Used Insulins

INSULIN NAME	INSULIN ACTIVITY (IN HOURS)		
	Onset	Peak	Duration
Short acting			
Regular	½	2–4	6–8
Intermediate			
NPH	2	4–12	24
Lente	2	8–10	24

To avoid reactions, meals and snacks must be consumed at intervals to coincide with these characteristics.

Insulin Regimen

Human insulin is recommended because of its lower incidence of insulin allergy, resistance, and lipoatrophy. The insulin is injected subcutaneously, rotating sites on the upper arms, thighs, buttocks, and abdomen to minimize lipohypertrophy.

A newly diagnosed diabetic, without ketoacidosis, may start with 0.25 unit of insulin per kilogram of body weight per day; a new diabetic with mild ketonuria may need 0.5 unit/kg/d. Established diabetics usually require 1.0 unit/kg/d. The insulin dose usually increases during adolescence to 1.25 to 1.50 units/kg/d and returns to 1.0 unit/kg/d after the pubertal growth spurt.

A twice-daily injection of a combination of intermediate-acting (either NPH or Lente) and short-acting (regular) insulins is recommended to approximate the physiologic insulin release in the nondiabetic state. The key characteristics of these insulins are outlined in Table 86-1. The ratio of intermediate to short-acting insulin is about 2:1, or two thirds NPH or Lente and one third regular insulin. Younger children may require less regular insulin. Two thirds of the total daily insulin is given before breakfast and the remaining one third is given before dinner. Careful adjustment of the insulin dose must be made in concert with response patterns documented by blood glucose tests over several days.

During the initial phase of treatment, about two thirds of the newly diagnosed diabetic children exhibit some recovery of beta cell function, resulting in significant decrease in their daily insulin dose to maintain normoglycemia. This "honeymoon" phase may last weeks to months, but eventually the autoimmune disease causes total destruction of beta cell function, resulting in complete dependence on exogenous insulin. Cyclosporine, an immunosuppressant, has been used with some success by research centers to preserve the residual insulin secretion and to prolong the "honeymoon" phase.

Monitoring of Diabetes Control

The semiquantitative double void urine test is unreliable and has been largely replaced by home blood glucose determinations. Home monitoring of blood glucose is reliable and acceptable to most children; it enables insulin doses to be adjusted to preprandial blood glucose, anticipated changes in activity or diet, and management of diabetes during illness. Those diabetics who rely on urine glucose monitoring are encouraged to change to blood glucose testing. Diabetics must check their urine for ketones whenever the blood glucose level is over 240 mg/dL and during illnesses.

For the school-aged child, the blood glucose target ranges are 80 to 120 mg/dL in the preprandial state and 80 to 180 mg/dL at other times. Because hypoglycemia can cause brain damage and learning disabilities, these ranges are relaxed to 90 to 140 mg/dL preprandially and 90 to 200 mg/dL postprandially for the preschool child.

The short-acting insulin administered before breakfast must be adjusted to bring the pre-lunch blood glucose level within the target range. If the blood glucose level before lunch is elevated, the morning regular insulin can be progressively increased by 1 to 2 units or up to 10% of the morning regular insulin dose every 3 to 4 days; if the blood glucose level is low, the regular insulin dose must be quickly reduced by a like amount daily to prevent hypoglycemic reactions. The morning intermediate insulin dose should be similarly titrated to bring the before-dinner blood glucose level to the target range. The regular insulin given before dinner regulates the blood glucose level at bedtime and should be be similarly adjusted. The before-dinner intermediate-acting insulin regulates the next morning's prebreakfast blood glucose level. This insulin dose must be adjusted carefully. The before-dinner intermediate insulin action peaks around 1 to 3 AM; excess dosage may precipitate hypoglycemia followed by rebound hyperglycemia and ketonuria—the *Somogyi reaction*. Patients may not be aware of hypoglycemic reactions during sleep; on awakening, they may complain of nightmares, night sweats, or headaches or may notice nocturnal enuresis. The treatment for the Somogyi reaction is to reduce the evening intermediate insulin dose in spite of the morning hyperglycemia and ketonuria. On the other hand, the elevated morning blood glucose level may be due to inadequate before-dinner insulin or to the *dawn phenomenon*—a rapid rise of blood glucose level after 2 to 4 AM due to the nocturnal surges of growth hormone and early morning surges of adrenocorticotropic hormone and cortisol that antagonize insulin action. Treatment is to increase the evening intermediate insulin dose. It may be necessary to do blood glucose tests between 1 and 3 AM and morning blood glucose and urine ketone tests to learn the cause of the morning hyperglycemia. Occasionally it is difficult to give the correct before-dinner intermediate insulin dose to avoid both the Somogyi reaction and to provide enough insulin to prevent the dawn phenomenon. Under such circumstances it may be necessary to split the evening insulin dose, give the regular insulin before dinner, and delay the intermediate insulin until bedtime.

Tight control within the target ranges may be hazardous and unrealistic for many diabetic children because of the increased potential for hypoglycemic reactions and a more restricted life-style. For some patients, a more realistic goal is to aim for the blood glucose level to be less than 180 mg/dL for young diabetics and less than 140 mg/dL for adolescent diabetics. Because insulin pumps have not been as successful in providing near-physiologic control, they cannot currently be recommended for routine use.

Nutrition

Balanced nutrition, with caloric intake appropriate for the age of the child and a consistent eating schedule are crucial for the management of diabetes. The child's adjustment to diabetes is facilitated when the entire family adopts this healthy eating regimen.

Children require approximately 1000 calories plus 100 per year of age daily. Of the total calories, 55% to 60% should be derived from carbohydrates, 30% from fats, and the remainder from proteins. Most of the carbohydrates should be complex carbohydrates, and food with refined or simple sugars should be minimized. High-fiber carbohydrates help to modulate glucose variation. The use of polyunsaturated fats such as margarine or vegetable oil should be encouraged, and substituting poultry, veal, and fish for red meat and eggs lowers the saturated fats and cholesterol.

The administration of the daily insulin doses assumes that meals and snacks are consumed at regular intervals to coincide with the onset and peak action of the two insulins. The daily eating pattern must be consistent in both time and content (total calories and carbohydrate content) of the meal and snack. Younger children usually have three meals and three snacks daily, with the total calories divided into 2/10 for breakfast, 2/10 for lunch, 3/10 for dinner, and 1/10 for each of the snacks at mid morning, mid afternoon, and bedtime. Older children usually omit the mid-morning snack; these calories may be added to their breakfast or lunch. To avoid middle of the night reactions, the bedtime snack must not be missed.

The diabetic's family should be referred to a nutritionist to learn the principles of balanced nutrition and food exchange. Food exchange allows flexibility in preparing meals and helps to minimize the dietary constraints.

Exercise

Exercise, whether unstructured play or competitive sports, should be encouraged. This not only promotes peer relationships and a personal sense of well-being but may also improve glucoregulation and lipid metabolism. It is easier for the diabetic to begin a daily exercise program if the entire family participates. The benefits of exercise outweigh the risks of hypoglycemic reactions that may occur during or after exercise. Hypoglycemia may result from increased insulin absorption in the exercising limb because of increased blood flow; insulin injection to the abdomen or buttocks may minimize this effect. Hypoglycemia may also be prevented if an additional carbohydrate exchange for every 30 minutes of exercise is consumed 30 minutes before exercising. If hypoglycemia occurs regularly with sports, the offending insulin dose may be reduced by 10% on sports days. It is important to inform coaches of the child's diabetes and to have glucose readily available to treat reactions.

Psychosocial Adjustment

The diagnosis of diabetes mellitus of a family member imposes strains and restrictions on the family as well as on the diabetic. Activities must be planned around meal or snack times within the constraints of insulin peak action. Fear of reactions and feelings of guilt contribute to overprotecting the diabetic child, which increases family stress with increased sibling rivalry and manipulation by the diabetic child. Adolescent diabetics are concerned with altered body image, regulated lifestyle, and peer acceptance, which often hinder good diabetes control.

The pediatrician must be patient and supportive and provide guidance. Counseling services must be made available to all diabetics and their families. Diabetes support groups help to foster understanding and adjustment to the disease. Diabetic camps help children adjust to the disease by learning self-care, recognizing that there are other children with diabetes, and realizing that they can live normal lives.

Management of Complications

Hypoglycemia is the most common acute complication. It occurs suddenly with rapid release of epinephrine in response to true hypoglycemia (blood glucose level less than 60 mg/dL) or to a rapid drop in blood glucose level but still in the normal range. Shakiness, sweating, and restlessness are common symptoms of the epinephrine response. Hunger, headache, confusion, coma, or seizure are signs of central nervous system glucopenia. If possible, hypoglycemia should be documented with a blood test and concentrated simple sugars, such as a nondietetic soft drink or candy, juice with additional sugar, or premade instant glucose, should be given. Glucagon, 0.5 mg for a child or 1.0 mg for an adolescent, should be given if the patient is unresponsive or unable to swallow. Since hypoglycemia is potentially life threatening, the cause of the reaction must be investigated and efforts made to prevent recurrence.

Ketoacidosis, a subacute complication, develops over a period of hours or days of persistent hyperglycemia resulting from inadequate insulin dose or to illness. Additional short-acting insulin is needed to correct hyperglycemia with moderate to high ketonuria. Between 5% to 10% of the total daily dose of insulin is administered in addition to the usual insulin dose for a child with moderate ketonuria; an additional 10 to 15% may be required for large ketonuria. Fluid intake should be encouraged to prevent dehydration. Addi-

tional short-acting insulin may be administered every 2 to 3 hours until the blood glucose level falls below 180 mg/dL. Urine ketones and blood glucose levels must be checked every 2 to 3 hours to monitor response and prevent reactions. Ketonuria resolves over a longer period of time. Additional calories may be provided to prevent hypoglycemia when the blood glucose level falls below 80 mg/dL. Ketoacidosis may be managed at home only if the pediatrician is readily accessible and if the family is cooperative and able to monitor the response to insulin. The diabetic must be evaluated if the clinical or laboratory data deteriorate.

Although there is no conclusive evidence that good diabetes control prevents long-term complications, there are ample data suggesting that poor control accelerates complications and that improved control decreases some of the existing complications. The pediatrician must provide the best care possible to delay or prevent the development of life-threatening chronic complications.

OFFICE FOLLOW-UP

The frequency of office visits depends on the needs of the diabetic child and/or family and the pediatrician's assessment of their knowledge of diabetes and its management. A stable, well-controlled diabetic may be followed every 3 months, with more frequent visits or telephone contact recommended for the new diabetic early in the course of diabetes management and for the less well managed diabetic.

Interval history with specific focus on the child and family's adjustment to the demands of diabetes at home and at school, including school performance and peer relationship, should be explored. The child's general health and sense of well-being should be assessed, as well as sleep patterns and nocturia. Insulin doses, injection sites and techniques, and glucose monitoring results must be carefully evaluated. Overall nutrition, including both content and timing of meals/snacks, is best assessed if the family provides a written 3-day dietary history. Reactions must be evaluated carefully and guidance provided to avoid recurrence. A review of systems should focus on illnesses that may interfere with diabetes control.

A thorough physical examination should be performed at each visit. Because height and weight are critical parameters in a diabetic child, growth charts must be accurately maintained. Particular attention should focus on blood pressure, peripheral pulses, fundoscopic examination, and neurologic examination, including deep tendon reflexes and sensory/vibratory examination. The thyroid and liver must be assessed. Hand and wrist joint mobility should be evaluated, looking for contractures (the prayer sign). Injection sites should be checked.

At the every-3-month visit, a glycosylated hemoglobin level should be obtained, since it provides an objective measurement of the quality of control over the preceding 2 to 3 months. Diabetes control is excellent if the glycosylated hemoglobin value is less than 8% (normal range, 6% to 9.5%). Control is good if the level is between 8 and 10%; control is fair if the level is between 10% and 12%. Any level over 12% is indicative of poor control; intensified efforts must be made to improve care.

Yearly laboratory studies should include urinalysis and blood tests for blood urea nitrogen, creatinine, cholesterol, triglycerides, and thyroid antibodies and thyroid stimulating hormone. Any proteinuria should prompt a 24-hour quantitative test for urine protein and creatinine clearance. An annual ophthalmologic visit is recommended.

INDICATIONS FOR REFERRAL AND ADMISSION

At any time, the primary care pediatrician may refer the diabetic child to an endocrinologist, especially if there is a problem with diabetes control, or to a mental health provider for counseling. A child with poor growth, recurrent significant reactions, and deteriorating glycosylated hemoglobin in spite of intensified efforts must be referred. A child with vomiting and diarrhea, dehydration, moderate to severe ketoacidosis, or an altered level of consciousness must be admitted for treatment.

ANNOTATED BIBLIOGRAPHY

Amiel SA et al: Impaired insulin action in puberty: A contributing factor to poor glycemic control in adolescent with diabetes. N Engl J Med 315:215, 1986. (Presents hypothesis that growth hormone may be one factor for the relative insulin resistance that occurs during puberty.)

Bougneres P-F et al: Limited duration of remission of insulin dependency in children with recent overt type 1 diabetes treated with low-dose cyclosporine. Diabetes 39:1264, 1990. (Report of a 2-year follow-up of children treated with cyclosporine at the onset of IDDM, with 65% achieving remission; however, the mean duration of remission was only a year, thus limiting wide-scale use of this immunosuppressant.)

Brink SJ et al: Insulin pump treatment in insulin-dependent diabetes mellitus: Children, adolescents, young adults. JAMA 255:617, 1986. (Discusses use of insulin pump in young diabetics and cites noncompliance with the increased demands of an intensive management program as an important factor to drop-out and complication rates, along with the high cost and meager improvement.)

Chase HP et al: Diabetes ketoacidosis in children and the role of outpatient management. Pediatr Rev 11:297, 1990. (Excellent review on the outpatient management of pediatric IDDM and inpatient care when necessary, with an update on the pathophysiology of ketoacidosis.)

Groth CG: Is diabetes mellitus an indication for pancreatic transplantation? Transplant Proc 21:2757, 1989. (Update on pancreatic transplantation as means of providing improved quality of life, where graft success rates have improved to 70–80%.)

MacLaren NK: How, when, and why to predict IDDM. Diabetes 37:1591, 1988. (Thought-provoking perspective on IDDM as a preventable disease with updates on the use of autoimmune studies to screen for IDDM and the use of immunosuppressants to delay the onset of the disease or induce or prolong remissions.)

Travis LB: An Instructional Aid on Insulin-Dependent Diabetes Mellitus. Galveston, TX, University of Texas Medical Branch, 1988. (Classic instructional aid for new diabetics and as a basis review with older diabetics.)

87

Gynecomastia

M. Joan Mansfield and Hal Landy

Gynecomastia is a common accompaniment of male puberty. About one half of normal boys develop subareolar breast enlargement averaging 2 to 2.5 cm in diameter in mid-puberty. This common type of physiologic self-limited pubertal gynecomastia is usually readily distinguished from gynecomastia occurring with primary testicular disorders, estrogen-producing tumors, liver dysfunction, or medications.

PATHOPHYSIOLOGY

Underlying all gynecomastia is an abnormality in the normal male ratio of androgens to estrogens, a relative excess of estrogens resulting in breast duct proliferation. Acini do not develop at the ends of the breast ducts in males because this requires the synergistic action of estrogen and progesterone. If hormonal stimulation is prolonged, fibrous tissue develops that will not regress when the hormonal imbalance is corrected. Several studies have found an androgen to estrogen ratio that is lower than normal. Lower free testosterone levels are also found in boys who develop pubertal gynecomastia. Excessive levels of estrogens created by peripheral conversion of adrenal androgens may also be a cause of pubertal gynecomastia. Since adrenarche precedes gonadarche, peripheral conversion of adrenal androgens to estrogens at a stage in puberty where testosterone production by the testis has not yet reached mature levels could result in a temporary relative estrogen excess. Prolactin levels have been found to be transiently elevated just prior to the onset of pubertal gynecomastia in longitudinal studies. This increase in prolactin appears to be secondary to estrogen excess and is not believed to be causally related to gynecomastia.

CLINICAL PRESENTATION

The average age at onset of physiologic pubertal gynecomastia is 13.2 ± 0.8 years. Gynecomastia may develop at genital Tanner stages II, III, or IV and usually lasts 12 to 18 months. Breast enlargement often begins unilaterally but usually becomes bilateral. Boys who develop pubertal gynecomastia tend to have an earlier onset of puberty and a lower body mass index (weight/height^2) than their peers. Pathologic gynecomastia may develop in the prepubertal, pubertal, or postpubertal male.

DIFFERENTIAL DIAGNOSIS

All causes of true gynecomastia share a common basis of a relative excess of estrogen. The source of this estrogen may be an excessive production by the testes or adrenal glands, excessive conversion of androgens to estrogens by extraglandular metabolism, or exposure to environmental estrogens. Gynecomastia that occurs in childhood prior to the normal time of puberty is rare. It is often pathologic and is usually accompanied by other evidence of precocious sexual development. Childhood gynecomastia may be caused by environmental exposure to topical or ingested estrogens or by estrogen-secreting tumors.

Leydig cell tumors of the testis secrete estrogen and can present as gynecomastia, which will be accompanied by precocious puberty if the tumor is present in childhood. Testicular development may be asymmetric, and a mass may be present, although in some cases, these tumors are too small to palpate. Human chorionic gonadotropin (hCG)-secreting germ cell tumors may present as gynecomastia and precocious puberty because both androgen and estrogen production by the testes is stimulated by hCG. Feminizing adrenal adenomas or carcinomas that secrete sex steroid hormones are another rare cause of gynecomastia in childhood.

Pathologic gynecomastia in the pubertal male may be due to any of the causes of gynecomastia in childhood but also may be caused by excessive peripheral conversion of androgens to estrogens, primary testicular disorders with or without chromosomal abnormalities, androgen resistance, liver dysfunction, or drugs.

Gynecomastia is a frequent presenting complaint in obese boys at puberty. Fatty tissue in the breast area may mimic true gynecomastia in many of these boys. True gynecomastia may also be more common in obese boys because of an excessive conversion of androgens to estrogens in adipose tissue.

Patients with suboptimal testicular function from various causes may present in puberty with gynecomastia. Altered testicular function can be associated with a chromosomal abnormality such as Klinefelter's syndrome (47, XXY), which occurs in 1 in every 400 males. One third of patients with Klinefelter's syndrome have gynecomastia. Elevated gonadotropins drive the hyperplastic testicular Leydig cells to secrete estrogen as well as androgens. Patients with Klinefelter's syndrome with gynecomastia have a risk of breast cancer similar to that of normal females, far in excess of that of normal males with or without gynecomastia.

If the patient with gynecomastia has incompletely masculinized genitalia with hypospadias or cryptorchism, he may have a chromosomal abnormality or the syndrome of androgen resistance. Patients with mixed gonadal dysgenesis or true hermaphroditism may develop gynecomastia during puberty. During puberty these patients develop breasts and may also have cyclic bleeding through a penile urethra or urogenital sinus. Patients with partial androgen resistance on the basis of decreased testosterone receptor function or 5α-reductase deficiency may also present as gynecomastia during puberty.

Causes of partial testicular failure resulting in gynecomastia with normal male karyotype include congenital anorchia (these patients may have testicular remnants that secrete some androgens and estrogens), damage from irradiation or chemotherapy, viral orchitis, and infiltrative lesions of the testis. Enzymatic defects in testosterone production, including some forms of adrenal enzyme insufficiency, are unusual causes of gynecomastia.

Prolactinomas are a rare cause of secondary hypogonadism in males. Excessive prolactin levels produced by a pituitary adenoma may suppress gonadotropin release and thus depress testicular function. Excessive prolactin may cause galactorrhea but does not directly stimulate breast tissue proliferation. Gynecomastia does not usually develop in males with prolactinomas.

Gynecomastia may occur in pubertal or postpubertal males with thyrotoxicosis (Graves' disease). Sex-steroid-binding globulin is increased in the presence of thyroid hormone excess, resulting in a decrease in the ratio of free biologically active testosterone to free estradiol. There is also an increase in the peripheral conversion of androgens to estrogens in hyperthyroidism. The diagnosis is usually clinically obvious with the presence of thyroid enlargement and symptoms of thyroid hormone excess.

Gynecomastia also occurs in patients with significant liver dysfunction, presumably caused by an alteration in sex steroid hormone metabolism. Breast enlargement occurs in some males recovering from starvation, perhaps due to temporary liver dysfunction. Gynecomastia can also be seen as the nutritional state improves during the treatment of a chronic illness associated with malnutrition.

Drugs that have been associated with gynecomastia include spironolactone, cimetidine, digitalis, metronidazole, and chemotherapeutic agents toxic to the testis. Spironolactone and cimetidine cause gynecomastia by interfering with the androgen receptor function. Heavy use of alcohol resulting in liver dysfunction may result in gynecomastia. There is some evidence that frequent use of marijuana may cause gynecomastia.

Tumors of the breast are an unusual cause of a breast mass in boys during childhood and adolescence. As in women, bloody nipple discharge, irregular fixed masses, and axillary adenopathy are suggestive of possible malignancy. Benign masses such as neurofibromas may be seen occasionally in the breast area in males and may be confused with gynecomastia.

WORK-UP

History

The age at onset of gynecomastia, its progression, and its duration should be determined. The relationship of breast enlargement to other pubertal events and the progression of puberty should be reviewed. A rapid progression of gynecomastia in the absence of testicular or genital enlargement or in the presence of testicular regression suggests an environmental or tumor source of estrogen. A family history of other males with marked gynecomastia suggests pubertal macromastia on a genetic basis.

Physical Examination

On physical examination, measurements of height, weight, arm span, and staging of sexual development with determination of testicular size and consistency are important. In addition, a testicular examination should be done looking for masses or asymmetry suggestive of a Leydig cell or other testicular tumors. Hypospadias and incomplete testicular descent suggest a syndrome of incomplete masculinization. The testes in fully developed males with Klinefelter's syndrome are small (2 to 2.5 cm in length) and firm due to the occurrence of tubular fibrosis. Early in pubertal development the testes of a patient with Klinefelter's syndrome may be difficult to differentiate from normal. The testes may also be small in other causes of hypogonadism. An evaluation of the breast enlargement should include a measurement of the dimensions of glandular tissue and areolae. Some obese patients may have *pseudogynecomastia,* which consists of smooth fatty tissue only. True glandular tissue has a more firm consistency and is palpable as a mobile symmetric mass embedded in fat underlying and extending out from under the areola. Gently squeezing the borders of the tissue together may cause a slight retraction of the nipple. Nipple discharge, fixed asymmetric masses, and axillary adenopathy should be sought. Signs of thyroid hormone excess as a cause of gynecomastia would include thyromegaly, rapid pulse, and diaphoresis. Evidence of liver dysfunction might include hepatomegaly, jaundice, or spider angiomas.

Laboratory Tests

Laboratory testing should be determined on the basis of the clinical presentation of the patient. If the patient is in mid-puberty with normal testicular volume for stage of development and has Tanner II breast development (less than 3 cm of glandular tissue), laboratory testing is usually not necessary since the patient has pubertal gynecomastia. If breast development has occurred in a prepubertal boy without genital changes or if genital abnormalities exist (small testes with penile enlargement, hypospadias, or incomplete testicular descent), the patient should be referred to an endocrinologist. A laboratory evaluation would include measurements of serum levels of luteinizing hormone, follicle-stimulating hormone, testosterone, and estradiol as a minimum and other sex steroid hormone metabolites if an adrenal abnormality is suspected. If the genitalia are abnormal or gonadotropin levels are elevated, a karyotype and buccal smear should be obtained. A serum β-hCG test can be included to rule out an hCG-producing tumor. If there is evidence of liver disease, liver function tests can be performed to evaluate hepatic dysfunction. Thyroid function tests should be done if there is a clinical suspicion of thyroid hormone excess. Thermography and testicular ultrasound examination can be useful in evaluating the patient suspected of having a testicular tumor too small to be definitely palpated. If there is a strong clinical suspicion of a feminizing adrenal tumor, an abdominal computed tomographic scan should be obtained.

MANAGEMENT

If the patient has physiologic pubertal gynecomastia, he can be reassured that transient breast enlargement is a normal part of male puberty and that it should resolve within 2 years. A follow-up at 6-month intervals is usually helpful to provide support and reassurance. Although most pubertal gynecomastia resolves spontaneously within 2 years, the patient with Tanner III or more breast development (more than 4 to 5 cm of breast tissue) is likely to be left with residual fibrous tissue even if the hormonal imbalance returns to normal. This patient may benefit from prompt referral for surgical correction. In counseling these boys, it is important to get a sense of the impact of the gynecomastia on the patient's lifestyle and self-image. A teenage boy will often refuse to go swimming, take off his shirt, or participate in school sports because of his concern about breast enlargement. In this case, if reassurance and support are insufficient, surgical referral may be appropriate. Medical approaches to the treatment of gynecomastia have included the use of antiestrogens (clomiphene), testolactone, and nonaromatizable androgens such as dihydrotestosterone. Although these medications can temporarily decrease breast tissue, they are not used routinely in pubertal gynecomastia.

INDICATIONS FOR REFERRAL

The patient should be referred to an endocrinologist for an evaluation of breast enlargement if gynecomastia begins in childhood or, after puberty is complete, if it persists beyond 2 years, if it is unusually prominent (Tanner III or more), or if it is accompanied by abnormal genital development.

ANNOTATED BIBLIOGRAPHY

Berkovitz GD, Guerami A, Brown TR et al: Familial gynecomastia with increased extraglandular aromatization of plasma carbon-19 steroids. J Clin Invest 75:176–769, 1985. (Increased extraglandular aromatase activity in familial macromastia.)

Biro FM, Lucky AW, Huster GA, Morrison JA: Hormonal studies and physical maturation in adolescent gynecomastia: J Pediatr 5:116:450–455, 1990. (Large prospective study of normal adolescent boys.)

Carlson HE: Gynecomastia. N Engl J Med 303:795–800, 1980. (General review of gynecomastia in all ages with an extensive list of references.)

Lee PA: The relationship of concentrations of serum hormones to pubertal gynecomastia. J Pediatr 86:212–215, 1975. (Longitudinal study of pubertal gynecomastia showing changes in estradiol and prolactin levels preceding the onset of breast enlargement.)

Moore DC, Schlaepfer LV, Paunier L, Sizonenko PC: Hormonal changes during puberty: V. Transient pubertal gynecomastia: Abnormal androgen-estrogen ratios. J Clin Endocrinol Metab 58:492–499, 1984. (Report of abnormal androstenedione to estrone ratios in pubertal gynecomastia.)

Wilson JD, Aiman J, MacDonald PC: The pathogenesis of gynecomastia. Adv Intern Med 25:1–32, 1980. (General review focusing on the endocrinology of gynecomastia.)

88

Precocious Puberty

M. Joan Mansfield and John F. Crigler, Jr.

Puberty is a series of interrelated hormonal, physical, and behavioral changes that transform the child into a fully grown adult capable of mature reproductive function. The first sign of female secondary sexual development is usually breast budding, which begins between the ages of 8 and 13 in 98.8% of American girls. The average age at onset of breast development in girls in the United States is 11 years, with peak height velocity being reached by 12 years and menarche at 12.7 years. Puberty occurs about 6 months earlier in black girls. In 98.8% of boys, secondary sexual development begins between the ages of 9 and 14. The first sign of development is testicular enlargement, which occurs at an average age of 11.5 years. Peak height velocity is attained at 14 years in boys, 2 years after the maximum height velocity in girls. Precocious puberty is defined as the onset of development 2.5 SD earlier than the mean age of entering puberty. By this definition, a girl who has breast development or pubic hair before age 8 or a boy with genital enlargement before age 9 has precocious secondary sexual development that should be evaluated.

PATHOPHYSIOLOGY

In normal children, the hypothalamic-pituitary-gonadal axis is active transiently in utero and in infancy, causing sex steroids to be produced by the gonads. Pulsatile hypothalamic secretion of gonadotropin-releasing hormone (GnRH) is then suppressed by the age of 6 months in boys and 2 to 4 years in girls and subsequently released from inhibition in late childhood, allowing puberty to proceed. The mechanism of this normal suppression and reactivation of GnRH secretion in childhood is not known.

Central precocious puberty is the result of premature secretion of GnRH by the hypothalamus activating the production and release of the pituitary gonadotropins luteinizing hormone (LH) and follicle-stimulating hormone (FSH) that cause the gonads to make sex steroids. In the case of idiopathic central precocious puberty, no specific cause for this shortened period of inhibition of GnRH secretion in childhood can be identified. Less commonly, central precocious puberty can be attributed to a central nervous system insult such as a local mass lesion, hydrocephalus, anoxic damage, head trauma, radiation, or infection that presumably damages inhibitory pathways in the hypothalamus. This is known as *neurogenic precocity.*

CLINICAL PRESENTATION

Premature sexual development is more common in girls than in boys. Although most girls have idiopathic central precocious puberty, most boys with premature sexual development have an identifiable cause of their precocity such as tumor, congenital adrenal hyperplasia, or familial gonadotropin-independent precocity.

In true precocious puberty, sexual maturation (breast development in girls and testicular and phallic enlargement in boys) is accompanied or preceded by an increase in the rate of linear growth and weight gain and by acceleration of skeletal maturation leading to premature epiphyseal fusion and a final adult height below genetic height potential. In girls, *pubarche* (the development of pubic hair), a white vaginal secretion (leukorrhea), and menarche may accompany or occasionally precede breast development. Ovulatory menstrual cycles have been documented as early as the first year of life, although cycles are more often anovulatory and irregular. Rarely, isolated vaginal bleeding may be the first sign of precocious puberty, although in these cases, local vaginal lesions as a cause of bleeding should be ruled out by direct visualization. Emotional lability, high energy levels, and increased appetite are symptoms of precocity often noted by parents. Patients with neurogenic precocity may have other neurologic symptoms and signs such as headaches with increased intracranial pressure, changes in vision, and seizures. Central precocity can occur in patients with neurofibromatosis, with or without identifiable central nervous system optic gliomas. Girls with acquired hypothyroidism occasionally present with early breast development that ceases to progress when the hypothyroidism is treated, suggesting that the activation of ovarian function is secondary to hypothyroidism.

DIFFERENTIAL DIAGNOSIS

The evaluation of a child with sexual precocity is directed toward separating the incomplete or self-limited forms of sexual development such as premature *thelarche* (breast development) or adrenarche from true precocious puberty and toward excluding the correctable and possibly life-endangering causes of precocity such as tumors and inborn errors of steroidogenesis.

There is a spectrum of intensity of precocious sexual development ranging from transient breast budding to complete central precocious puberty. The most common limited form of premature sexual development is premature thelarche. Breast enlargement, galactorrhea, or vaginal bleeding are not uncommon in the neonatal period in response to withdrawal of estrogens of fetoplacental origin. In addition, isolated breast development sometimes accompanied by white vaginal secretions may occur in girls younger than the age of 2 years in response to transient ovarian estrogen production possibly as a result of intermittent neuroendocrine-gonadal activity. This process is self-limited and is not associated with accelerated growth, progressive skeletal maturation, or pubic hair development.

Children occasionally have transient or intermittent precocious puberty in which secondary sexual development and acceleration of growth progress and then subside spontaneously. These episodes may recur.

A slowly progressive variant of precocious puberty exists in which breast development and skeletal maturation proceed very gradually and predicted adult height remains in the normal range.

Premature pubarche or sexual hair development before age 8 is not uncommon, particularly in black or Hispanic girls, and is usually associated with early maturation of androgen secretion by the adrenal gland (*adrenarche*). In the patient with premature adrenarche, linear growth and skeletal maturation are usually not significantly accelerated. Other evidence of adrenarche such as axillary hair or odor and acne, however, may be present.

The term *pseudoprecocity* is sometimes used to describe early sexual development that is not due to premature activation of the neuroendocrine-gonadal system. Autonomous ovarian cysts and androgen or estrogen-secreting tumors of the adrenals or gonads can cause premature sexual development without gonadotropins. In boys, untreated congenital adrenal hyperplasia may present as pseudoprecocity due to excessive adrenal androgen secretion. Similarly, premature pubarche without virilization can be seen in girls with the attenuated forms of congenital adrenal hyperplasia. Pseudoprecocity may also be caused by rare gonadotropin-

secreting tumors such as human chorionic gonadotropin (hCG)-secreting hepatoblastomas that activate steroid production by the gonads. Cases of precocious puberty in boys have been described in which testicular production of testosterone occurs in the absence of pituitary LH or FSH secretion. These boys often have a family history of precocious puberty limited to males. The mechanism of this gonadotropin-independent form of precocity is not understood, although a serum factor capable of stimulating testicular function has been identified in these patients. Similar gonadotropin-independent ovarian activity occurs in girls with McCune-Albright syndrome (bone cysts, pigmented lesions of the skin, and precocity).

WORK-UP

History

The sequence and time course of sexual development, growth acceleration, and behavioral changes should be reviewed carefully. Sex steroid–producing tumors often produce sudden, rapid sexual development, whereas idiopathic precocious puberty more closely approximates the timing of normal pubertal progression. The possibility of an external source of sex steroid hormones such as foods, cosmetics, or oral contraceptives should be investigated.

A past medical history should include a review of perinatal events that might have caused anoxic damage, a history of serious head trauma, congenital infection, meningitis or encephalitis, and central nervous system tumor or irradiation in the past. A history of neurologic symptoms such as seizures, headaches, or visual field defects should be sought.

Family history should include the timing of sexual development and final height in family members and family history of neurofibromatosis, congenital adrenal hyperplasia, or precocious puberty.

Physical Examination

On physical examination, measurements of height or length and weight should be made. Measurements of current and past growth data plotted on developmental charts for height and weight are valuable in determining the duration and extent of precocity. The skin should be examined for evidence of café-au-lait spots suggesting neurofibromatosis (multiple small brown macules with smooth edges) or McCune-Albright syndrome (one or more large brown macules with irregular borders). These lesions may emerge over time in the child who initially presents with precocity. Acne, axillary odor, or axillary hair suggests maturation of the adrenal gland. Hypothyroidism as a cause of precocity might be suggested by changes in hair or skin, enlargement of the thyroid, slowing of pulse, a growth chart showing a slowing of linear growth, and an even greater delay in skeletal maturation. A neurologic examination should include an assessment of the fundi and visual fields in addition to an assessment of development.

In the girl with premature development, the dimensions of areolae and glandular breast tissue should be measured and Tanner staging of the breasts and pubic hair recorded. The external genitalia should be examined for evidence of estrogenization. Under the influence of estrogen, the labia minora become mature and the vaginal mucosa becomes thicker and a paler pink, often with white secretions. Ovarian tumors often present as large abdominal masses in young children. A rectoabdominal examination with the child in frog-leg position is useful in the search for an ovarian mass. In the normal child, a button of cervical tissue can be felt in midline position. This may be larger than normal in the patient with precocious puberty as the uterus enlarges under the influence of estrogen. Masses that are not in the midline suggest ovarian tumors or cysts.

In boys, measurements of the dimensions of the testes and the midshaft diameter and stretched length of the penis can be helpful in documenting the progression of puberty. Testicular asymmetry or mass suggests a testicular tumor. Testes inappropriately small for the degree of phallic development are seen in boys with hCG-producing tumors or lesions of the adrenals (tumor or hyperplasia).

Heterosexual development, that is, gynecomastia in a male or virilization in a female (e.g., clitoromegaly, hirsutism, deepening of the voice) suggests the presence of a tumor that is secreting inappropriate sex steroids. Congenital adrenal hyperplasia usually presents with signs of virilization in a female.

LABORATORY TESTS AND INDICATIONS FOR REFERRAL

In the girl who has breast enlargement beyond early infancy in the absence of acceleration of growth or other evidence of precocity, a physical examination including growth measurements, measurements and staging of breast tissue, a rectoabdominal examination, and a roentgenogram of the left hand and wrist for bone age are usually sufficient initial procedures. A pelvic ultrasound examination may be done to rule out an ovarian mass lesion if the rectoabdominal examination is unsatisfactory. A vaginal smear obtained with a cotton swab and fixed immediately can be used to assess estrogen effect. Vaginal cells change from immature parabasal cells toward intermediate and finally to superficial squamous cells under the influence of estrogen. Since serum estradiol levels are often below the sensitivity of immunoassays in patients with precocious puberty, the vaginal maturation index is the most sensitive indicator of whether the child is in active puberty at the time of the examination. If the external genital examination and vaginal smear show little estrogen effect, and growth rate and bone age are normal, the patient can be followed at 3- to 6-month intervals

without further studies watching for progression of sexual development or acceleration of growth.

If the patient has accelerated growth with advancing bone age and progressive sexual development, she should be referred to a pediatric endocrinologist for a more complete evaluation of the cause of the precocity. Initial laboratory evaluation would include determination of LH, FSH, and estradiol values.

LH and FSH levels can be helpful in making the diagnosis of central precocious puberty or a gonadotropin-secreting tumor. However, gonadotropin pulses are often only secreted during sleep in early puberty, so that prepubertal LH and FSH values do not exclude an active hypothalamic-pituitary-gonadal axis. A GnRH stimulation test or nocturnal monitoring for gonadotropins can confirm the diagnosis of central precocity, but it is not necessary as an initial screening test.

A pelvic ultrasound examination can be done to investigate the possibility of an ovarian tumor or cyst. This procedure will often show multiple small ovarian cysts in patients with central precocious puberty; these are evidence of anovulatory ovarian activity. A single ovarian cyst is often found in the patient with McCune-Albright syndrome. These cysts often resolve spontaneously, sometimes recurring multiple times. If the diagnosis of McCune-Albright syndrome is suspected, a skeletal survey is necessary to search for bone lesions. A bone scan can sometimes detect cystic lesions of fibrous dysplasia not yet visible on roentgenograms.

If the child has evidence of central precocious puberty, cranial magnetic resonance imaging with gadolinium contrast should be obtained to rule out central nervous system tumor, mass lesion, or hydrocephalus. Small hypothalamic hamartomas may cause precocious puberty and can be seen with magnetic resonance imaging. Computed tomography is slightly less sensitive.

A boy who has genital enlargement should be referred to a pediatric endocrinologist without delay since there is a high probability of a specific cause of the precocity such as tumor or congenital adrenal hyperplasia. An initial examination would include a morning measurement of LH, FSH, hCG, and adrenal and gonadal sex steroid levels and a hand and wrist roentgenogram for bone age. A cranial magnetic resonance image with contrast enhancement should be obtained for any boy with central precocious puberty. If there is evidence of a testicular mass or asymmetry on the physical examination, a testicular biopsy or tumor removal should be undertaken. The diagnosis of congenital adrenal hyperplasia is made by serum hormonal analysis and sometimes includes a cosyntropin (Cortrosyn) stimulation test. If an adrenal tumor is strongly suspected, an abdominal computed tomographic scan is more useful in assessing the possibility of an adrenal mass than is adrenal ultrasound examination.

In the child who presents with premature pubic hair development without evidence of other premature sexual development, growth data should be plotted carefully and a bone age roentgenogram should be obtained. If the child has premature adrenarche, the bone age is generally appropriate for height. Pubarche with rapid acceleration of growth and skeletal maturation would suggest precocious puberty or an androgen-secreting lesion that should be evaluated by a pediatric endocrinologist. Clitoral enlargement is another indication of significant androgen excess deserving thorough investigation. In simple premature adrenarche, the dehydroepiandrosterone sulfate (DHEAS) level will be in the adrenarchal range (100 to 280 μg/dL) and other sex steroid hormone levels are normal for the stage of development. A normal dehydroepiandrosterone level for stage of development excludes an androgen secreting tumor. The attenuated form of congenital adrenal hyperplasia (21-hydroxylase deficiency) can be identified by an elevated early morning or adrenocorticotropic hormone–stimulated serum 17α-hydroxyprogesterone level. Other adrenal enzyme defects such as mild 3β-aldehydrogenase deficiency or 11-hydroxylase deficiency are best identified with an adrenocorticotropic hormone test.

MANAGEMENT

Medroxyprogesterone acetate (Depo-Provera) and cyproterone acetate have been used previously to suppress puberty in children with precocious sexual development. Both drugs produce incomplete suppression of gonadarche and, therefore, do not increase final height. Studies over the past 10 years have demonstrated that complete suppression of gonadarche can be achieved using long-acting agonist analogues of GnRH. These analogues are believed to paradoxically suppress the pituitary-gonadal axis by down-regulation of GnRH receptors of pituitary gonadotropins. In these investigations, GnRH analogues have been shown to completely suppress gonadotropin and gonadal sex steroid secretion when given in adequate doses by daily subcutaneous injection. Long-acting depot formulations of GnRH analogues can be given by intramuscular injection every 3 to 4 weeks. The suppression of gonadal activation by GnRH analogues appears to be specific, reversible, and safe. A halting or regression of breast development and a cessation of menses occur in girls and a regression in testicular size and muscular development occur in boys during GnRH analogue treatment. Patients have shown greater slowing of bone maturation than linear growth, thus increasing predicted adult height. There are now studies showing modest increases in final adult height in patients treated with GnRH analogues. Adrenarche is not blocked by GnRH analogue therapy so that pubic hair may progress in adrenarchal patients. GnRH analogue suppression of precocity offers the only means of treatment that can completely and selectively suppress puberty with the potential long-term benefit of restoring the genetic potential for adult stature. Patients who

are candidates for GnRH analogue therapy should be referred to a pediatric endocrinologist.

When sexual precocity is due to an organic lesion, initial treatment should be appropriate therapy for the lesion. Patients with congenital adrenal hyperplasia require treatment with glucocorticoids. Tumors of the adrenals and gonads, which are rare, can often be surgically removed, preserving as much normal tissue as possible.

If high levels of sex steroids have been present for a long time in a patient with pseudoprecocity from a tumor or congenital adrenal hyperplasia, central precocious puberty may develop following the elimination of the sex steroid source. Such patients as well as those with central nervous system tumors causing central precocity may be appropriate candidates for GnRH analogue therapy.

PATIENT AND PARENTAL EDUCATION

Parents of the child with premature thelarche or premature adrenarche may be reassured that the problem is self-limiting and has no long-term effects on growth and development. In the child with central precocious puberty, once a careful evaluation has excluded a tumor or other specific cause of precocity, the parents can be told that the puberty that the child is experiencing is a normal process except for its age at onset; thus, final sexual development and reproductive function should be normal, although adult height may be shorter than the child's genetic potential because of premature epiphyseal fusion. Best estimates of final adult height in children with precocity are obtained using the Bayley-Pinneau tables, with skeletal maturation determined using the Gruelich and Pyle atlas. It is important to know, however, that estimates of final height may decrease with the progression of sexual development because skeletal maturation advances more rapidly than linear growth.

In untreated persons, behavior and school problems may occur because of emotional lability and high-activity levels or poor self-image. Cognitive and psychological development are usually commensurate with chronologic age, not with physical appearance.

With the exception of familial gonadotropin-independent precocity in males and specific syndromes such as neurofibromatosis that are occasionally associated with precocity, other siblings or offspring of affected patients are not at increased risk for precocity.

ANNOTATED BIBLIOGRAPHY

Beopple PA, Mansfield MJ, Wierman ME et al: Use of a potent, long-acting agonist of gonadotropin releasing hormone in the treatment of precocious puberty. Endocr Rev 7:24–33, 1986. (Report of 5-year experience in 74 children.)

Gruelich WW, Pyle SI: Radiographic Atlas of Skeletal Development of the Hand and Wrist, 2nd ed. Stanford, CA, Stanford University Press, 1950–1959. (Includes the Bayley and Pinneau tables for height prediction.)

Hardin DS, Pescovitz OH: Central precocious puberty and its treatment with long acting GnRH analogs. Endocrinologist 1:163–169, 1991. (State of the art review.)

Styne DM, Grumbach MM: Puberty in the male and female: Its physiology and disorders. In Yen SSC, Yaffe R (eds): Reproductive Endocrinology, pp 313–384. Philadelphia, WB Saunders, 1986. (Very complete review of normal, precocious, and delayed puberty, including illustrations of Tanner staging.)

89

Delayed Puberty

M. Joan Mansfield and Hal Landy

Secondary sexual characteristics normally begin to develop between ages 8 and 13 in girls and ages 9 and 14 in boys. Breast budding is the first sign of development in 85% of girls followed by the development of sexual hair, then growth acceleration, and menarche, occurring at an average age of 12.7 years, after peak height velocity has passed. Some normal girls show sexual hair as the first sign of development. The first sign of development in boys is usually an enlargement of the testes to more than 2.4 cm in length (4 mL volume) at an average age of 11.5 years. This subtle physical change is followed by phallic enlargement, the development of pubic and axillary hair, and ultimately an increase in growth rate, with peak height velocity being reached about 2.5 years after the onset of testicular development. Boys normally complete testicular development in 3 ± 2 (SD) years. Girls reach menarche 2.3 ± 1 (SD) year after the onset of breast budding.

Delayed development is defined by the absence of breast budding by age 13 in girls or the lack of testicular enlargement by age 14 in boys, both 2.5 SD beyond the normal age at onset of these developmental changes. Alterations in the chronologic relationships of pubertal events, while not strictly delayed puberty, are also common causes for evaluation. These would include phallic enlargement in the absence of testicular enlargement in boys or the absence of menarche by age 16 or 4 years after the onset of breast development in girls.

PATHOPHYSIOLOGY

The physical changes of puberty are a response to rising levels of sex steroid hormones. In the normal sequence of events the rise in adrenal androgens known as *adrenarche* occurs by about age 8 and is followed several years later by an augmentation of hypothalamic gonadotropin-releasing hormone (GnRH) pulsations that trigger the synthesis and release of luteinizing hormone (LH) and follicle-stimulating hormone (FSH) from the pituitary. LH and FSH stimulate gonadal production of sex steroid hormones and development of germ cells. The absence of puberty may be the result of a failure at any point along the hypothalamic-pituitary-gonadal axis. The challenge of evaluating the child with delayed puberty is to differentiate between *constitutional delay of puberty,* that is, a normal variation in the tempo of development, and organic disease such as chronic illness, nutritional insufficiency, tumor, or primary endocrinopathy associated with delayed pubertal development.

CLINICAL PRESENTATION

Although delayed development occurs in both boys and girls, most patients who present for an evaluation of delayed development are high-school-aged boys who are concerned about their short stature as well as their lack of muscular and secondary sexual development, which put them at a disadvantage among their peers. Most of these boys have constitutionally delayed development; however, the clinical presentation of the patient with constitutional delay may be indistinguishable from that of the patient whose pubertal delay is the result of an organic lesion. Patients with constitutional delay of puberty have often been slow growers throughout childhood, with their growth curves following or being below the third percentile. Growth may slow even further as these children reach the age when puberty would normally occur, since growth velocity decreases in the absence of the normal sequence of hormonal changes that characterize adrenarche and gonadarche. Growth velocity increases into the normal range when these children enter puberty. Patients with constitutional delay may have a family history of delayed growth and development in relatives. Children with constitutional delay of puberty eventually enter puberty spontaneously. Although they have a longer time to grow before their epiphyses fuse, they tend to have a less exuberant growth spurt than earlier developers so that their final height is shorter than average.

DIFFERENTIAL DIAGNOSIS

Functional Causes of Delayed Puberty

Gonadotropin-releasing hormone secretion can be inhibited centrally by inadequate nutrition, chronic disease, environmental stress, intensive athletic training, hypothyroidism, and drugs such as opiates. Eating disorders associated with self-imposed restriction of caloric intake can delay or interrupt the progression of puberty. Although anorexia nervosa most typically develops in girls in mid-adolescence who have already entered puberty, young adolescent boys or girls who are dieting because of fear of obesity may present with the complaint of delayed development. Crohn's disease or celiac disease may also present as delayed development and poor growth as the major symptom. Since adolescence is normally a period of rapid growth and weight gain, failure to gain or small amounts of weight loss may be manifestations of significant nutritional inadequacy.

Hypothalamic Causes of Delayed Puberty

The ability of the hypothalamus to secrete GnRH may be damaged by local tumors (gliomas, germinomas, or craniopharyngiomas), infiltrative lesions such as central nervous system leukemia or histiocytosis, central nervous system irradiation, traumatic gliosis, or mass lesions such as brain abscesses or granulomas due to sarcoidosis or tuberculosis. Congenital defects in the ability to secrete GnRH (idiopathic hypogonadotropic hypogonadism) may be associated with midline facial defects or olfactory defects (Kallmann syndrome) and may be familial.

Pituitary Causes of Delayed Puberty

Puberty may not be initiated or may fail to proceed if the pituitary cannot respond to GnRH with LH and FSH production. This may be due to a pituitary tumor, selective impairment of gonadotrope function by hemochromatosis, or congenital or acquired hypopituitarism. Excessive prolactin production by a pituitary adenoma (prolactinoma) may halt or prevent puberty by interfering with gonadotropin production. Galactorrhea is present in only half of the patients with prolactinomas.

Gonadal Failure

If the gonads are unable to respond to LH and FSH, puberty will not proceed. The most common cause of gonadal failure is gonadal dysgenesis, which occurs in association with abnormalities of sex chromosomes (Turner syndrome). The gonads fail to develop and become rudimentary streaks. These patients are phenotypic females with normal female genitalia. They are classically short with a final height of less than 58 inches. Other identifying features of Turner syndrome are low-set ears, a webbed neck, a trident hairline, an increased carrying angle of the lower arms, and short fourth and fifth fingers and toes. Renal and cardiovascular congenital anomalies are common. Half of these patients have 45,X leukocyte karyotypes whereas the rest are mosaics with various X-chromosome abnormalities. Pure gonadal dysgenesis presents as absent puberty in patients with normal karyotype (46,XX or 46,XY), normal stature, and female phenotype. Males with Klinefelter's syndrome (47,XXY) may present with poorly progressing puberty caused by partial gonadal failure. Although they lack sperm production, their testes can make some testosterone when driven by high levels of gonadotropins (LH and FSH). In the 47,XXY patient with some pubertal development, the testes become small and firm. Gynecomastia and a eunuchoid body habitus are often present.

The causes of gonadal failure with normal karyotype include radiation, chemotherapy with certain agents such as cyclophosphamide, autoimmune oophoritis, or orchitis often in association with multiple endocrine abnormalities, viral orchitis or oophoritis, the resistant ovary syndrome, and gonadal failure associated with other diseases, such as congenital galactosemia in girls, ataxia telangiectasia, or sarcoidosis. Enzymatic defects, such as 17α-hydroxylase or 20,22-desmolase deficiency, that render the gonads unable to produce estrogens or androgens are another rare cause of primary gonadal failure. No cause for the gonadal failure can be found in some cases.

In males who are cryptorchid, the testes may fail to function, particularly if they remain intra-abdominal beyond infancy. Bilateral testicular torsion resulting in testicular destruction (anorchia) is another cause of gonadal failure in males. In the "vanishing testis syndrome," the testes are absent in a phenotypic male, presumably as the result of destruction in utero.

Primary amenorrhea with normal secondary sexual development may be caused by an anatomic abnormality of the reproductive tract such as an imperforate hymen, vaginal septum, or vaginal, cervical, or uterine agenesis. A person with a 46,XY karyotype who lacks the ability to respond to androgens (androgen resistance or insensitivity) presents as a phenotypic female with breast development and primary amenorrhea with an absent uterus and upper vagina.

WORK-UP

History

A detailed history and physical examination will help to focus and minimize the laboratory testing needed in the evaluation of the child with delayed development. The neonatal history should include previous maternal miscarriages and congenital lymphedema (Turner syndrome). The past medical history should focus on any history of chronic disease, congenital anomalies, previous surgery, radiation exposure, chemotherapy, or drug use.

Past growth measurements that are plotted on appropriate developmental charts for both height and weight are important in evaluating the child with delayed puberty. The overall pattern of growth and changes in that pattern often lead to a diagnosis. The child whose delayed puberty is associated with a nutritional deficiency due to an eating disorder, inflammatory bowel disease, or other chronic disease will show a greater decline in weight gain than in height. In contrast, the child who has delayed puberty on the basis of an endocrinopathy such as acquired hypothyroidism or gonadal dysgenesis will tend to have greater slowing of linear growth than of weight gain.

In the review of systems, special attention should be paid to weight changes, dieting, environmental stress, exercise and athletics, gastrointestinal symptoms, headaches, neurologic symptoms (including peripheral vision and ability to smell), and the symptoms suggestive of thyroid disease.

The family history should include the heights, weights, and timing of secondary sexual development and fertility of family members, a history of anosmia, and a history of endocrine disorders.

Physical Examination

The physical examination should include measurements of height and weight and vital signs. A search should be made for congenital anomalies, including midline facial defects. The patient should be examined for any evidence of secondary sexual development that may be quantified by Tanner staging of breasts and pubic hair in girls and genitalia and pubic hair in boys. Dimensions of areolae and any glandular breast tissue in girls can be measured as an indicator of past or present estrogen effect. In boys, measurements of the testicular volume or length and width, midshaft diameter, and stretched length of the penis are useful in assessing the presence and progression of sexual development. Pubic hair may be present, although the genitalia are prepubertal in a boy who has normal adrenarche but who lacks gonadal activation. Any evidence of heterosexual development, such as clitoromegaly or hirsuitism in girls or gynecomastia in boys should be noted.

The examination of the external genitalia in girls should focus on obvious congenital anomalies and an assessment of estrogen effect. A pale pink vaginal mucosa with white secretions indicates current estrogen exposure. A pelvic examination is not necessary as part of the initial evaluation of a girl with delayed secondary sexual development but should be done to rule out gynecologic congenital anomalies in the patient who has normal pubertal development but delayed menarche.

The neurologic examination should include visual fields by confrontation and olfactory testing.

Laboratory Tests

Initial laboratory studies include a complete blood cell count, erythrocyte sedimentation rate (helpful as a screening test for chronic illness such as inflammatory bowel disease), LH, and FSH, dehydroepiandrosterone sulfate, and testosterone or estradiol. A roentgenogram of the left hand and wrist for bone age is useful in assessing how much linear growth remains in the patient with short stature and delayed development. A predicted height can be obtained using the Bayley-Pinneau tables in the atlas of skeletal maturation by Gruelich and Pyle. The patient with constitutional delay will usually have an equal delay in height age and bone age.

LH and FSH determinations are only useful if they are elevated since early to mid pubertal levels during the day are indistinguishable from prepubertal levels. Elevated LH and FSH levels are suggestive of primary gonadal failure. If LH and FSH levels are elevated, a further laboratory evaluation would include leukocyte karyotyping in a search for a chromosomal abnormality. If the chromosomes are normal in the patient with gonadal failure, antigonadal antibody values may be obtained to look for autoimmune gonadal damage. Certain causes of ovarian failure such as the resistant ovary syndrome may reverse in time, offering some chance of fertility. A vaginal ultrasound examination or ovarian biopsy to document the presence or absence of follicles is usually postponed until adulthood when the patient wishes definitive information about her fertility.

In most patients with delayed puberty, the LH and FSH levels are in the normal prepubertal range. A further evaluation would then include determination of a prolactin level, thyroid function tests, a lateral skull roentgenogram, and if there is a suspicion of a central nervous system tumor, cranial magnetic resonance imaging or computed tomographic scan. If there is a question of multiple pituitary hormone defects, the patient may be referred to an endocrinologist for pharmacologic and physiologic tests of neuroendocrine functions.

Breast budding and vaginal maturation in girls and penile and testicular enlargement in boys are more sensitive indicators of neuroendocrine-gonadal function than a single daytime measurement of serum gonadotropin levels, estradiol, or testosterone. Testosterone or estradiol levels, however, may be valuable in following the patient whose puberty is not progressing normally by clinical assessment of growth and secondary sexual development.

The chief diagnostic challenge in the patient with pubertal delay is to distinguish between constitutional delay and true GnRH deficiency. No single test reliably separates patients with constitutional delay from those with idiopathic hypogonadotropic hypogonadism. The presence of midline facial defects, anosmia, cryptorchidism, or microphallus strongly suggests idiopathic hypogonadotropic hypogonadism; however, the diagnosis of idiopathic hypogonadotropic hypogonadism cannot be firmly established until the patient reaches the age of 18 years and is still prepubertal.

MANAGEMENT

Prior to age 14 in girls and age 16 in boys, if there is no evidence of underlying disease or neurologic abnormality and the initial evaluation reveals normal prepubertal hormonal levels, the patient can be seen at 6-month intervals for measurements of growth, assessment of pubertal status by physical examination, and reassurance if progression of secondary sexual development is evident. After the first signs of testicular or breast enlargement are observed, follow up at regular intervals is desirable to reassure the patient and parents that puberty is progressing. Since the testes begin to enlarge in males before increased testosterone production and associated increased growth velocity occur, support and guidance in dealing with the frustrations of delayed puberty are important even after there is evidence that secondary sexual development has begun.

If the evaluation reveals primary gonadal failure, cyclic estrogen and progestin therapy in girls or testosterone therapy in boys will be necessary. In girls, treatment with conjugated estrogens (Premarin) can be begun at a dose of 0.3 mg/d orally for the first year of treatment or until linear growth slows, and increased thereafter to 0.625 to 1.2 mg/d for the first 25 days of each month with 10 mg of medroxyprogesterone (Provera) added at days 13 to 25. The optimum dose of estrogen replacement for protection of bone density in adolescents remains to be established, but it appears to be higher than in menopausal women. Patients who have been on estrogen replacement for 4 to 5 years should have Papanicolaou smears regularly and should be referred to a gynecologist for an endometrial biopsy if irregular bleeding develops. The timing of initiation of sex steroid therapy to achieve maximum height depends on the patient's chronologic and skeletal age and current height velocity.

In boys with constitutional delay of puberty, 6-month courses of intramuscular injections of human chorionic gonadotropin (hCG) or testosterone enanthate can be used to initiate secondary sexual development. Exposure to hCG or testosterone may speed the onset of the patient's own puberty. Since sex steroids cause fusion of epiphyses, care must be taken in the timing and monitoring of these therapies so that final height is not compromised. These patients should therefore be referred to an endocrinologist for treatment. The timing of such intervention must take into account such complex issues as psychosocial stress, self-image, and school performance, which appear to be more affected by pubertal delay than by short stature alone. In both males and females whose delayed puberty is due to abnormalities in hypothalamic GnRH secretion that do not correct with time, fertility has been achieved in research programs using a small pump to deliver pulses of GnRH intravenously or subcutaneously for weeks or months. Some GnRH-deficient males will achieve spermatogenesis with hCG alone or in combination with human menopausal gonadotropin (hMG). Ovulation can also be induced by hMG and hCG in GnRH-deficient females.

PATIENT EDUCATION

Young adolescents are preoccupied with their physical appearance. Any variation from the normal timing of sexual development is a major source of embarrassment to them and evokes feelings of personal inadequacy. A review of a patient's progress in pubertal growth and sexual developmental charts can help to reassure him that growth is proceeding in a pattern that is normal for him. For patients who have a permanent defect in reproductive function, counseling and support from both the primary health care provider and medical specialist can be helpful in enabling the patient to establish a positive self-image of himself or herself as a capable adult. Further counseling by a mental health specialist may be necessary. Questions about fertility should be answered as they arise, with emphasis on the patient's ability to function normally as a marriage partner and as a parent of adopted children. Pregnancies have been achieved using in vitro fertilization with donor eggs in patients with ovarian failure.

ANNOTATED BIBLIOGRAPHY

Finkel DM, Phillips JL, Snyder PJ: Stimulation of spermatogenesis by gonadotropins in men with hypogonadotropic hypogonadism. N Engl J Med 313:651–655, 1985. (Describes the use of hCG and human menopausal gonadotropin to stimulate spermatogenesis in males with hypogonadotropic hypogonadism.)

Gruelich WW, Pyle SI: Radiographic Atlas of Skeletal Development of the Hand and Wrist, 2nd ed. Stanford, CA, Stanford University Press, 1950–1959. (Includes the Bayley and Pinneau tables for height prediction.)

Hoffman AR, Crowley WF Jr: Induction of puberty in men by long-term pulsatile administration of low-dose gonadotropin releasing hormone. N Engl J Med 307:1237–1241, 1982. (Report of induction of puberty using a portable pump to deliver intermittent GnRH in males with central hypogonadism.)

Rosenfield RL: Clinical review 6: Diagnosis and management of delayed puberty. J Clin Endocrinol Metab 70:559–562, 1990. (Succinct review with discussion of use of GnRH analogue stimulation tests to distinguish constitutional delay of puberty from idiopathic hypogonadotropic hypogonadism.)

Styne DM, Grumbach MM: Puberty in the male and female: Its physiology and disorders. In Yen SSC, Jaffe R (eds): Reproductive Endocrinology, pp 313–384. Philadelphia, WB Saunders, 1986. (Complete review of normal, precocious, and delayed puberty including Tanner staging and an extensive list of references.)

Tanner JM, Davies PSW: Clinical longitudinal standards for height and height velocity for North American children. J Pediatr 107:317–329, 1985. (Most useful in evaluating growth during puberty.)

13

Eye Problems

90

Visual Testing

Henry S. Metz

Visual testing is related directly to the age of the child being tested. As a rule, the younger the child, the more objective, the less subjective, and the less quantitative the test must be. It may not be possible to get the maximum amount of information desired about the visual system because of infancy, developmental delay, or the presence of coexisting motor or sensory handicaps. The aim of visual testing in a child should be to get as much information as possible. Visual testing devices offer no advantage over the considerably less expensive eye occluder and visual testing chart.

Visual acuity screening can, and should, be done on all children by the age of 3 to 3½ years. At an earlier age, behavioral clues, such as objection to occluding one eye during the cover test, should alert the pediatrician to investigate further or to refer the patient for evaluation by an ophthalmologist. A Snellen chart is adequate in older children.

I believe that a specific screening test for hyperopia (farsightedness) is unnecessary. Farsightedness often produces no problems and usually does not require treatment. Moderate to high hyperopia may manifest itself with esotropia and symptoms of "eye strain," which, in either case, would warrant a detailed examination.

VISUAL ACUITY

Observation. The examiner can often estimate a child's visual ability by observation. Does the child take an interest in his surroundings? Does the infant grasp for objects? Unsteady or wandering eye movements are a sign of subnormal vision. Parents can usually tell if their child sees well or behaves as if he or she has visual difficulty.

Observation of the pupillary response to light can also be useful. An active response indicates that light is able to reach the retina, the optic nerve is functioning, and the visual pathway is intact at least as far back as the posterior portion of the optic tract.

Fixation. Fixation with each eye can be determined using a colorful moving toy. A noisy toy can be used first to gain attention and a silent toy substituted later in the test. Central, steady, and maintained fixation suggests good vision, whereas unsteady fixation (e.g., nystagmus or wandering movements) suggests reduced vision.

Following. The ability to easily and smoothly follow an object of interest is evidence of at least moderate acuity. Caution should be used when interpreting the response of developmentally delayed youngsters to fixation and following tasks. They may have little interest and thus appear visually deficient, while in fact their visual system may be normal.

Optokinetic Nystagmus. An optokinetic drum or tape can be rotated horizontally or vertically before the child's eyes. Nystagmus elicited in response to this stimulus indicates that the stripes on the drum or squares on the tape can be seen. Although this is a gross estimation of vision, it is an objective measure and requires little cooperation or interest, while still providing useful information.

Allen Cards. Before children can recognize numbers, letters, or symbols they may be able to identify certain pictures. The Allen Cards have pictures of well-known items (e.g., telephone, tree, house) that can usually be recognized by 2½- to 3-year olds. The pictures are of equal size (the size of a 20/30 letter), and the examiner moves further and further away until the picture can no longer be identified

355

correctly. The farthest distance (in feet) that the card can be recognized correctly is the numerator of the acuity fraction with a denominator of 30 (e.g., 10/30). This not only provides a quantitative measure of acuity, but because the cards are often held closer than 20 feet from the child, maintains the youngster's interest in the test. The Allen Cards are easier than letter, number, or symbol charts, because the pictures are isolated and not on a line and therefore may result in a higher acuity score. Results with the Allen cards should not be equated exactly to the Snellen chart. It is most important to remember to compare the acuities between the two eyes.

HOTV, "E" or "C." The HOTV test requires the youngster to differentiate these four letters. Once this can be done, an acuity chart with these characters is used to test vision, usually at 10 feet or 20 feet. The child has a set of cards with these four letters, and he or she is asked to "match" the letter shown with one of the cards held by the examiner. The "E" or "C" requires the child to point his or her finger in the same direction as the "fingers" of the "E" or the opening of the "C" (up, down, left, right). This game can be taught by parents at home prior to the physician's examination. Charts or individual cards are available to measure vision with these figures.

Letters or Numbers. Once a child can read letters or numbers, acuity can easily be determined. Vision may normally be in the 20/30 or 20/40 range at age 3 or 4 and subjectively improves to 20/20 by the age of 6 or 7. Interest and cooperation are both necessary to obtain optimum visual acuity. A difference between eyes of two lines or more is as important as the absolute level of acuity.

More recently, the Bailey-Lovey chart has replaced the Snellen chart when more accurate measurements of visual acuity are required. These charts have the advantages of equal spacing between letters and lines of letters, an equal number of letters on each line, and equal difficulty of the letters among all the lines. The Bailey-Lovey charts are now standard for research studies (most appropriately) but have generally not found their way into pediatricians', or even ophthalmologists', offices. Thus, for clinical testing in a nonresearch setting, the Snellen chart remains the standard.

Visual Evoked Response and Preferential Looking (Teller Acuity Cards). Both visual evoked response and preferential looking tests are in the investigative stages but may provide an opportunity for a more quantitative visual evaluation within the first few months of life. In the visual evoked response (an objective test) technique, a flash or an alternating black and white checkerboard pattern is presented. The evoked electrical response from the visual cortex is computer averaged, and a tracing is produced that may be able to give information about acuity (without requiring fixation or accommodation for the flash stimulus). The absolute height of the tracing representing the electrical

response is less valuable than a significant difference in the tracing when both eyes are compared. When using the checkerboard stimulus, the child must pay attention to this target for the test to be useful, but it should produce more accurate results.

With preferential looking, the infant is presented with two disks, one gray and the other with a black and white striped pattern. The background luminance of each pattern is equal. In judging which disk the infant looks at, an estimate of acuity can be made as the stripe pattern is made thinner. The infant should be more interested in the striped pattern than the gray disk and is more likely to look at it if he or she can see it. This test is performed with the infant seated on a parent's lap approximately 3 feet from the target and one of the infant's eyes is covered. While one of the examiners changes the disk stripe size and the side on which the striped disk is presented (using a random presentation scheme), another tester, who cannot see on which side the striped disk has been placed (masked observer), observes the child to determine where he is looking. The smallest stripe size the infant looks at accurately is a measure of visual acuity. This is not the same as recognition acuity (as is Snellen acuity) but is a measure of edge recognition, a simpler task. Nevertheless, it is a measure of acuity in children at an age when it cannot easily be measured and provides valuable information when early acuity measurements are indicated. Although both the visual evoked response test and Teller Acuity Cards are not usually available in most ophthalmologists' practices, the tests can be obtained at many teaching centers and in some pediatric ophthalmologists' offices.

VISUAL FIELDS

Visual field testing provides a measure of peripheral vision, rather than central (foveomacular) vision. It cannot be performed in infants, although it may be estimated in young children and quantitated in older children. Visual field testing may be particularly useful in patients with suspected neurologic problems.

Threatening Gesture. A threatening gesture made by a hand or finger, approaching from the periphery, can give a gross indication if vision is present in one quadrant or one half of the visual field. This should be performed one eye at a time, with the other eye covered because visual fields of the two eyes overlap considerably. The gesture should not frighten the infant but provide only a momentary startle reaction.

Confrontation Fields. The child is asked to maintain fixation straight ahead (on the examiner's eye or nose or interesting fixation toy). The examiner then moves a finger in from the periphery, wiggles a finger, or asks the youngster to count the number of fingers being held up in a peripheral quadrant of the field, again keeping one eye covered. Although this is a qualitative test, quadrantic or hemianopic defects may be uncovered. This technique may be useful in children between the ages of 4 and 7.

Tangent Screen, Perimeter. Instrument testing of the visual fields provides quantitative, reproducible measurements. The tangent screen measures the central 30-degree field with the blind spot, while the perimeter provides information about the peripheral field, out to 70° to 75° temporally, with a less detailed blind spot. With young children (aged 7 to 8), fewer meridians should be investigated because the child may become fatigued and disinterested, providing unreliable responses. In children older than age 10, a more detailed examination is often possible.

To be performed successfully, computerized visual field testing requires long periods of attention. It may provide more accurate, reproducible results when performed in adults. Except for motivated teenagers, it should not be considered a procedure for most pediatric patients.

MUSCLE BALANCE

Misalignment of the visual axes, if monocular and not alternating, can cause unilateral reduction of central acuity (*amblyopia*). Therefore, methods to uncover strabismus are a valuable screening tool for visual acuity as well as for binocularity (see Chap. 97, "Amblyopia").

Observation. If the deviation is large (i.e., above 12 prism diopters [6°]), it can usually be noted by observation alone. An alternating form to strabismus will not result in amblyopia. An inturning of one eye (*esotropia*) is more common than an outward turn (*exotropia*). Infants with a flat nasal bridge and wide nasal epicanthal folds will often appear to be esotropic because less of the sclera (the white portion of the eye) shows on the nasal side of the eye than on the temporal side. These children can be shown to have straight eyes by other testing methods and are thus said to have "pseudostrabismus," without a true deviation. This appearance usually disappears with age. Amblyopia is not a problem in patients with pseudostrabismus, but one must be alert that children with a real esotropia can also have pseudoesotropia. Therefore, the pediatrician may not be able to rely on the infant's appearance alone.

Light Reflex. If the child is asked to fixate on a light held by the examiner, the reflex from the light will be seen on the cornea. When the eyes are straight, the reflex will be noted in the center, or just nasal to the center, of the pupil of each eye. With esotropia, the light reflex will be temporal to the pupillary center, and with exotropia, it will be more nasal to the center. Youngsters with "pseudostrabismus" will have central, symmetric pupillary light reflexes.

Cover Test. While the child is fixating on a target of interest, one eye is covered and the other eye is observed. If the eye does not move, the uncovered eye was straight. If it

does move, the uncovered eye shows a deviation. The cover test is performed on each eye separately. Any objection to covering one eye and not the opposite one suggests reduced vision (amblyopia).

Random Dot E. The random dot E is a test of binocularity by measuring stereo vision. Since some youngsters appreciate stereo targets easily while others do not, there is a relatively high false-positive response that makes the test of questionable acceptability. This test cannot usually be performed accurately in children younger than age 5 but may be useful in those older than age 7 or 8.

ANNOTATED BIBLIOGRAPHY

Scott WE, D'Agostino DD, Lennarson LW: Orthoptics and Ocular Examination Techniques. Baltimore, Williams & Wilkins, 1983. (Provides a good description of visual assessment methods and of various eye diseases in the pediatric patient, with an emphasis on strabismus.)

Wybar K, Taylor D: Pediatric Ophthalmology: Current Aspects. New York, Marcel Dekker, 1983. (Describes visual testing techniques in the pediatric patient as well as many ocular disorders of childhood and infancy.)

91

Visual Disturbances

Henry S. Metz

Young children who have eye diseases rarely complain. An abnormality can be determined by appearance or poor function. When only one eye is impaired, the child's activity and behavior may be normal. Only an examination of visual ability will uncover this problem.

Since one eye may have reduced vision while the other is normal, the eyes must be tested separately. An exception to this rule would be the patient who has latent nystagmus, which only becomes manifest when one eye is covered. With both eyes open, fixation is steady and acuity is improved.

An early diagnosis is important, since some conditions cannot be treated after a certain age. It is useful if children are examined by age 3. With a family history of eye disease (congenital cataracts, strabismus), an evaluation by 1 year of age is indicated.

PATHOPHYSIOLOGY

The eye functions much like a camera. Parallel rays of light from an image are refracted by the cornea. The light then passes through the aqueous humor in the anterior chamber and is refracted again by the lens. The light passes through the vitreous and stimulates the retina (inverted, as in a camera).

For the image to reach the retina undisturbed, the transparent media of the eye (i.e., cornea, aqueous humor, lens, vitreous) must be clear. Opacification (e.g., corneal scar, cataract, vitreous hemorrhage) will impair sight.

When the image is in focus in front of the retina, the picture on the retina will be blurred. The eye is *myopic* (nearsighted). This may be caused by a large eye or a strong optical focusing system (lens, cornea).

When the image is in focus behind the retina, the picture will also be unclear. The eye is *hyperopic* (farsighted). This may be caused by a small eye or a weak optical focusing system.

If the corneal front surface or the anterior curvature of the lens is not spherical (round), the image will not be in focus in a single plane and will, therefore, not be in focus on the plane of the retina, resulting in blurred vision. This is *astigmatism* and can exist alone or with myopia or hyperopia.

When the image reaches the retina, a signal is initiated that travels down the optic nerve, chiasm, and optic tracts to the geniculate body. There is hemidecussation of the nerve fibers in the chiasm as information from the temporal hemiretina remains ipsilateral while that from the nasal hemiretina crosses to the opposite side. Thus, unilateral visual field defects must be due to prechiasmal pathology. From the geniculate body, the signal goes to the optic radiations and then to the visual cortex in the occipital lobe. Chiasmal and postchiasmal lesions result in bilateral field abnormalities and may be hemianopic or quadrantanopic. As a rule, the more symmetric the field deficit, the more posterior the pathology.

CLINICAL PRESENTATION

Complaints

Young children often do not complain. If pain is a symptom, the youngster may rub the eye. If there is light sensitivity, increased tearing and avoidance of light or squinting may be noted. When the child is older, decreased vision or discomfort may be a complaint. It is not unusual for the first indication of subnormal acuity to be noted at a school examination.

Decreased Visual Acuity

During infancy, the best estimate of vision comes from behavioral observation. Are targets of interest (faces, toys) fixated steadily and followed? Is reaching observed for near objects? Does the child act as if his or her sight is normal? Specific tests can be performed as the child grows older (see Chap. 90). The Allen cards, HOTV test, "E" game, and Snellen charts are all useful to quantitate visual ability.

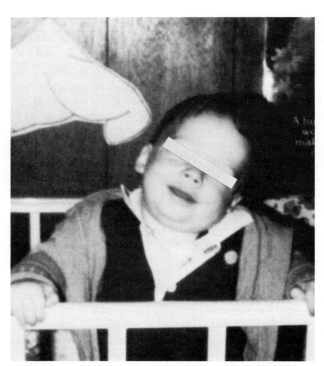

Figure 91-1.   Habit head tilt to the left shoulder caused by a right superior oblique muscle palsy.

Acuity should be essentially equal in each eye. An objection to covering one eye or a decreased performance on any of the aforementioned tests with one eye is abnormal. By age 3 or 4, acuity is usually at the 20/30 level, while at age 6, it has often reached 20/20. Squinting, which creates a pinhole aperture effect, suggests the presence of an uncorrected refractive error (most often myopia).

Abnormal Face or Head Position

A child holding his or her face or head in an abnormal position may indicate an eye problem because a head turn or chin tilt may improve visual acuity or correct diplopia. A superior oblique palsy might present as a head tilt to the opposite side (Fig. 91-1), whereas a lateral rectus palsy would cause a face turn to the same side as the palsy. Head tilts may also be caused by posterior fossa tumors (see also Chap. 134, "Torticollis").

A loss of corneal transparency reduces vision. Blood (hyphema) or white cells (hypopyon) in the anterior chamber can result from trauma or inflammation. A white pupil may be due to cataract, ocular tumor, persistent hyperplastic primary vitreous, or retrolental fibroplasia. A clear lens with loss of the normal "red reflex" from the fundus can be caused by vitreous opacification due to vitreous hemorrhage or infection.

Strabismus, which is a lack of parallel alignment of the visual axes, will often be noted if the angle of deviation is greater than 6 degrees (about 12 prism diopters). The turn may be inward (*esotropia*), outward (*exotropia*), upward (*hypertropia*), or downward (*hypotropia*). Upper eyelid ptosis may accompany strabismus in some patients or may be noted as an independent finding. A decreased range of ocular motility may be seen in some congenital conditions (Duane's or Brown's syndrome) or as a result of muscle palsy. True congenital sixth nerve palsy is rare in infancy. Abnormal or wandering eye movements (*nystagmus, opsoclonus*) suggest reduced vision.

Proptosis of the globe is often an indicator of an orbital tumor, since thyroid ophthalmopathy is infrequent in the pediatric age group. Orbital inflammatory disease and orbital cellulitis can also produce proptosis (see Chap. 95).

Conjunctival injection accompanied by discharge or tearing suggests conjunctivitis. If the engorgement of vessels is localized at the limbus (corneoscleral junction) with increased light sensitivity, iritis may be present. Corneal abrasions, foreign bodies, or ulcers also produce photophobia and foreign body sensation (see Chap. 93).

If the cornea is enlarged and hazy, congenital glaucoma should be considered, especially if this enlargement is accompanied by increased tearing and photophobia (see Chap. 98). When an enlarged cornea is clear, congenital megalocornea is a possible etiology. A small cornea is often seen with a small globe (micro-ophthalmia), and vision is usually subnormal.

The pupillary light response is usually a good indicator of optic nerve function. The lack of a brisk or equal direct response may indicate an optic nerve or optic tract lesion or, occasionally, an efferent defect involving the motor fibers of the third nerve to the pupillary sphincter.

Fundus abnormalities are best seen with the binocular, indirect ophthalmoscope. Optic nerve abnormalities, choroidal colobomas, retinal tumors, chorioretinitis, and retinopathy of prematurity should alert the practitioner to a need for further follow-up and care. Infants born prematurely with a birth weight of 1200 g or less have a much higher incidence of retinopathy of prematurity and should have a retinal examination by an ophthalmologist by 4 to 6 weeks of age.

DIFFERENTIAL DIAGNOSIS

Refractive Errors

Refractive errors are common, and vision can be improved by optical means (eyeglasses). When testing an older child, the trial of a pinhole aperture, which will improve acuity when the blur is due to refractive error, is a quick and easy method to rule out a more serious pathologic process.

Amblyopia

Amblyopia (lazy eye), reduced vision without an organic cause, can result from strabismus, anisometropia (and ametropia), or deprivation. *Strabismus* causes amblyopia when unilateral and not alternating. The lack of daily, foveal fixation of the strabismic eye leads to a decreased acuity. *Anisometropia*, an unequal refractive error in the two eyes, also reduces vision. It is due to a poorly focused image in one eye over time during early childhood. Anisometropia is usually only discovered on routine testing and does not present with symptoms or findings that would indicate a problem. *Deprivation* causes the most severe form of amblyopia and may be due to cataract, ptosis, corneal opacification, or vitreous hemorrhage. Prolonged, continuous therapeutic patching of one eye can also cause deprivation amblyopia (see Chap. 97), although it may be reversible.

Trauma

Blunt trauma will often lead to ecchymoses of the eyelids and subconjunctival hemorrhage. If the trauma is severe, a hyphema may result, the orbital floor may be fractured (with possible vertical diplopia and limitation of vertical gaze), and macular edema can be seen along with scattered retinal hemorrhages. Less severe trauma may include corneal abrasions and eyelid and corneal foreign bodies. These disorders are accompanied by increased tearing and conjunctival injection. Fluorescein staining generally demonstrates the defect.

Penetrating trauma is serious and threatens vision permanently. The anterior chamber may be collapsed and the globe filled with blood. Endophthalmitis secondary to infection is often catastrophic (see Chap. 99).

Infection and Inflammation

Superficial infections of the eyelids and conjunctiva usually present with conjunctival redness and discharge or crusting (see Chap. 93). External ocular infections may also be due to congenital nasolacrimal duct obstruction and usually present with excessive tearing as well as redness and discharge. Corneal infiltration or ulceration, appearing as a localized opacity, is more serious. *Iritis* is accompanied by perilimbal injection, light sensitivity, and, at times, reduced vision. Prolonged or recurrent anterior segment inflammation can lead to cataract formation and abnormal attachments of the iris to the lens (posterior synechia) and the angle of the anterior chamber (anterior synechia).

Chorioretinitis often appears as yellowish-white and may be accompanied by haze in the vitreous (vitritis). Long-standing, quiet foci are usually well circumscribed with a pigmented margin. White sclera shows through with localized areas of destruction of the retina and choroid. The causes include, but are not limited to, toxoplasmosis, lues, herpes simplex, toxocariasis, tuberculosis, and cytomegalic inclusion virus. Orbital cellulitis usually presents as proptosis, eyelid swelling, fever, and decreased ocular motility and, when severe, can be life threatening if cavernous sinus thrombosis develops (see Chap. 95).

Congenital Abnormalities

An *iris coloboma* is seen as a defect at the 6 o'clock position of the iris and, by itself, may cause no functional difficulties. When the iris coloboma is associated with a choroidal or optic disc coloboma there is a superior field defect and reduced vision if the macula is involved. *Aniridia* (absence of most of the iris) is associated with secondary glaucoma.

Congenital glaucoma may be noted soon after birth or in infancy. With increased intraocular pressure, the globe becomes enlarged and the cornea hazy. There is light sensitivity, increased tearing, and eventually optic nerve cupping.

Leukocoria (white pupil) has several causes. A congenital cataract will impair vision and will lead to deprivation amblyopia. The persistence of the hyperplastic primary vitreous will result in a white or gray pupillary reflex as will Coat's disease (an exudative retinopathy), retrolental fibroplasia (the end stage of cicatricial retinopathy of prematurity), retinoblastoma, a large choroidal coloboma, and nematode endophthalmitis (see Chap. 100).

Hypoplasia (or aplasia) of the optic nerve will cause reduced visual function. The optic nerve head will appear small, and a scleral ring may be seen around the disc. This ring should not be confused with the true nerve head.

Tumors

Retinoblastoma is the most common childhood ocular malignancy. It usually presents as leukocoria and strabismus (Fig. 91-2) but may appear as an endophthalmitis with hypopyon. Calcium is usually found on roentgenographic studies, and the family history may be positive.

Rhabdomyosarcoma is the most serious orbital tumor in the pediatric age group. It presents as sudden proptosis and decreased ocular motility and often progresses rapidly, not infrequently leading to death. When proptosis is noted, dermoid tumors, lymphangiomas, and cavernous hemangiomas of the orbit should also be considered.

Capillary hemangiomas of the eyelids are unsightly but generally improve with time. They become a problem when they are large enough to cover the visual axis, since deprivation amblyopia may result.

Vascular Diseases

The most common ocular vascular diseases of adults are diabetic retinopathy and hypertensive and arteriosclerotic vascular changes and are rarely seen in the pediatric population. *Retinopathy of prematurity* is common in infants with a birth weight under 1200 g, and it is almost invariably present with a birth weight under 1000 g. The peripheral retina is avascular, and a demarcation line or arteriovenous ridge may be noted. If progression occurs, extraretinal vascularization can lead to traction on the peripheral retina and, finally, a localized, then complete retinal detachment with cicatricial changes and blindness.

Central Nervous System Abnormalities

The physical examination of the eyes may not reveal any abnormalities, but visual acuity or visual field testing may reveal diminished functional ability. Field defects may be present and reduced acuity noted by behavioral clues or measurement. Wandering or jerky eye movements are evidence of decreased vision. Other neurologic abnormalities can accompany the visual dysfunction, and reduced corneal sensation, strabismus, limited ocular motility, and ptosis may be noted. An abnormal pupillary light reflex and optic atrophy are sometimes found. Papilledema is an indicator of increased intracranial pressure.

WORK-UP

History

A history should be obtained first, either from a parent or the patient, if the patient is sufficiently verbal and knowledgeable. Questions concerning the major complaint, the time of onset of symptoms, and the length of time and consistency of the problem should be asked. What has been the

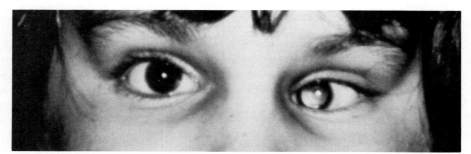

Figure 91-2. Retinoblastoma in the left eye. Leukocoria (white pupillary reflex) is present with a left estropia.

previous treatment and what was the response to this therapy? Is there a relevant family history? What is the general health of the child, and is any medication being used? Are there any known allergies?

Physical Examination

An examination should include an estimate or measurement of visual acuity. On external inspection, the following should be noted: the appearance of the eyelids, conjunctiva, and cornea; height and equality of the level of the upper eyelids; eyelid tumors or swelling; proptosis; injection of the conjunctiva; and localized or generalized changes in corneal transparency. The anterior chamber depth and clarity need to be evaluated. Pupillary shape, size, equality, and reaction to light are easy to examine. The muscle balance findings can be estimated by the light reflex and the cover test. Ocular rotations, using an interesting target, are important. Ophthalmoscopy requires pupillary dilation with a cycloplegic agent. The direct ophthalmoscope can provide a good look at the posterior pole of the fundus, including the optic disc, macula, surrounding vessels, and retina out to the equator. The binocular indirect ophthalmoscope provides an excellent view of the peripheral retina and an improved stereo view when eye movements are wandering or nystagmic.

Refraction needs to be performed by an ophthalmologist. Retinoscopy is a technique that measures the refractive error in an objective manner, whereas subjective refinement may be performed in older children. Automated refractors can also be used in children, although not easily in infancy.

A slit lamp biomicroscopic examination of the cornea, anterior chamber, and lens is useful to reveal pathologic problems not easily seen with unaided vision. It is especially helpful to identify flare (increased protein content) and cells (usually white blood cells) in the anterior chamber, which indicate ocular inflammation.

Intraocular pressure may be difficult to measure except in older, more cooperative children. It can be determined with a tonometer or estimated using finger palpation of the globe, although this latter method is not very accurate. The range of normal pressure is between 10 and 20 mm Hg.

Laboratory Tests

Radiographic studies, especially computerized tomography or magnetic resonance imaging can be useful in suspected central nervous system abnormalities, ocular tumors, trauma, and orbital cellulitis. Ultrasound studies are similarly useful and less expensive. A complete blood cell count, as well as various blood chemistries and a urinalysis can be helpful when systemic disease is a consideration. Culture and sensitivity testing are often not needed for conjunctivitis but are required in cases of corneal ulcer or endophthalmitis. The electroretinogram and electro-oculogram can provide specific information about retinal nerve cell layer and pigment epithelial cell layer function. The visual evoked response test can provide useful knowledge about optic nerve function and integrity of the visual cortex. Visual field testing is helpful with suspected neuro-ophthalmic disorders but can only be performed reliably in the older pediatric patient.

TREATMENT
Optical

The simplest, most frequently prescribed treatment for reduction in visual acuity is an optical correction. This is usually in the form of eyeglasses, although contact lenses have been used for specific problems (e.g., unilateral aphakia). A surgical technique called epikeratophakia, which involves sewing a preserved button of cornea on to the front surface of the child's cornea for optical purposes, has been tried but is often not successful. Myopia, hyperopia, astigmatism, and anisometropia are best treated with eyeglasses or contact lenses.

Patching

Patching treatment for strabismic and deprivation amblyopia remains the most successful modality. Some parents may erroneously believe that patching cures strabismus and that no further treatment will be necessary after the patch is removed. It is necessary to remind parents that patching only treats the amblyopia, not the deviation.

Anti-infective Agents

Superficial ocular infections can be treated by the topical application of antibiotics, either solution or ointment, to the eyelids and conjunctiva in patients with bacterial corneal ulcers or intraocular injection. The systemic route is useful for orbital cellulitis and endophthalmitis, and in cases of penetrating ocular trauma.

Topical antiviral agents are useful for herpes simplex keratitis. Topical corticosteroids should be avoided, since they can make the viral infection much worse. The local installation of antifungal agents can be helpful in culture-proven cases of fungal corneal ulcer.

Decongestants and Artificial Tears

Topical ocular decongestants are used for mild eye irritations or allergic reactions. Artificial tears assist the patient with dry eyes, although dry eyes are infrequent in children.

Corticosteroids

A mild concentration of a corticosteroid eye drop is helpful in allergic conjunctivitis that is not responsive to decongestants. Iritis requires the use of more potent topical preparations, usually with cycloplegic agents. Topical corticosteroids are contraindicated in herpes simplex keratitis, which often presents with a dendritic, branching pattern, enhanced by fluorescein staining.

An intralesional injection of corticosteroid can be used to treat large hemangiomas of the eyelid. Systemic corticosteroids are indicated for an orbital pseudotumor and may be prescribed in conjunction with antibiotics in cases of orbital cellulitis. They can also be helpful in thyroid ophthalmopathy in children. The prolonged use of corticosteroids (in topical or systemic form) can cause both cataract and glaucoma; thus, this medication should be used for specific indications and for the minimum amount of time required.

Surgery

Surgery to correct strabismus is the most common ophthalmologic procedure in the pediatric population. Since initial operation has a 70% to 75% success rate, it may have to be repeated. Cataracts that significantly interfere with vision require early surgery to prevent deprivation amblyopia. Penetrating trauma to the globe must be repaired immediately. Orbital fractures may be managed conservatively unless vision is disturbed (double vision, restriction of eye movements) or the fracture is so large that orbital contents slide into the maxillary antrum, resulting in enophthalmos. Ptosis surgery can be done prior to entering school, unless the ptosis is so severe that the visual axis is occluded causing deprivation amblyopia. Advanced retinoblastoma generally requires enucleation, although early cases and some patients with bilateral involvement have been successfully treated with external beam irradiation, cobalt plaques, and laser therapy. Cryotherapy of peripheral, avascular retina has been used successfully in progressing stages of retinopathy of prematurity. Orbital rhabdomyosarcoma requires orbital exenteration to prevent the spread of the tumor. Goniotomy and trabeculotomy have been successfully used to treat congenital glaucoma, although repeat surgery is not uncommon. Corneal transplant operations are occasionally done in children, and retinal detachment repair can be used when needed.

INDICATIONS FOR REFERRAL

Visual Acuity

When acuity is less than 20/30 in each eye or when there is a two line or more difference in acuity between eyes, a referral is indicated. In the infant or young or uncooperative child, poor fixation or objection to covering one eye more than the other suggests the need for a further evaluation.

Ocular Alignment and Movements

Strabismus, at any age, deserves referral, as does nystagmus. An inability to rotate one or both eyes normally should be investigated (see Chap. 96).

Pupil

Although small differences in pupil size may be physiologic, differences in response to light and accommodation are not. A pupil that is not round is unusual, although this is sometimes caused by congenital pupillary membranes, a benign condition. A loss of the red reflex demands immediate attention.

Tearing and Light Sensitivity

Increased tearing may indicate nasolacrimal duct obstruction or congenital glaucoma and deserves attention. Sensitivity to light can also be seen in congenital glaucoma but may suggest iritis. Both conditions benefit by early recognition and treatment (see Chap. 98).

Corneal Changes

Abnormally large or small corneas, or those with a conical shape (keratoconus), can degrade vision. Opacification and vascularization can similarly reduce acuity and deserve ophthalmologic referral.

Conjunctiva

An elevated or enlarging mass should be studied. Redness, discharge, and crusting suggest external infection. An attempt can be made to treat these findings with broad-spectrum, topical antibiotics. If no improvement is noted after a short time, an ophthalmologic opinion is useful.

Eyelids

Ptosis may be unilateral or bilateral. A referral is indicated, as it is for lumps of the eyelid (tumors, or chalazia), eyelid malposition (entropion—eyelid margin turned inward; ectropion—eyelid margin turned outward), or eyelid coloboma (see Chap. 94).

Vitreous

Opacity of the vitreous results in loss of the red reflex and reduced vision. It can be due to blood or inflammatory debris in the vitreous and requires ophthalmologic consultation. When blood is noted in the vitreous or retina, the possibility of child abuse should be considered.

Retina

Although scattered retinal hemorrhages may be noted after birth, they are usually transient. Chorioretinitis, coloboma, detachment, retinopathy of prematurity, a retinal mass, or a falciform fold should all be referred for ophthalmologic evaluation.

Optic Nerve

Optic atrophy as well as papilledema deserve both an oph-thalmologic as well as a neurologic evaluation. Aplastic or hypoplastic discs and cupping of the disc (especially if uni-lateral) require consultation.

Orbit

Proptosis may indicate an orbital tumor or orbital cellulitis. Both can be life threatening and may require the help of an ophthalmologist as well as a neurosurgeon, an otolaryngolo-gist, and an infectious disease consultant (see Chap. 95).

ANNOTATED BIBLIOGRAPHY

Gardiner PA: Vision in Children. New York, Appleton-Century-Crofts, 1982. (Good discussion of function and structure of visual system.)

Harley RD: Pediatric Ophthalmology, 2nd ed. Philadelphia, WB Saun-ders, 1983. (Encyclopedic work that is well-indexed and a good reference source on any ophthalmologic topic.)

Helveston EM, Ellis FD: Pediatric Ophthalmology Practice. St. Louis, CV Mosby, 1980. (Excellent use of photographs and line drawings with a good explanatory text.)

Metz HS, Rosenbaum A: Pediatric Ophthalmology—Medical Outline Series. Garden City, NY, Medical Examination Publishing Co, 1982. (Review of the major fields in pediatric ophthalmology for the pediatrician and family physician.)

Nelson LB, Brown GC, Arentsen JJ: Recognizing Patterns of Ocular Childhood Diseases. Thorofare, NJ, Slack & Co, 1985. (Good ba-sic outline of ocular disease patterns in children.)

92

Ophthalmia Neonatorum

Johan Zwaan

Any conjunctivitis in newborns during the first month of life is referred to as *ophthalmia neonatorum*. The inflammation may be chemically induced by the prophylactic use of silver nitrate eye drops, or it may be infectious. Staphylococci, *Chlamydia trachomatis,* and *Neisseria gonorrhoeae* are the more common agents involved; herpes simplex type 2 or various non-neisserial bacteria are less frequently found. (For related discussions but of a broader nature, see Chaps. 93, 196, and 200.)

PATHOPHYSIOLOGY

The administration of 1% silver nitrate in the conjunctival sac within 1 hour of birth to prevent venereal infection was first advocated by Credé in 1881. The chemical is only ac-tive against *N. gonorrhoeae* by binding to its surface protein and thus interfering with its metabolism. The compound needs to penetrate the microorganism to be effective. If ap-plication is delayed, or if a pregnant woman has a premature rupture of her membranes, bacteria may have time to invade the intact tissues of the neonatal eye and become inacces-sible to the silver nitrate solution; therefore, eradication may be incomplete. The compound is moderately irritating to the conjunctiva and often causes hyperemia and swelling. Leukocytes migrate into the tissues and the conjunctival sac, leading to a mild purulent discharge. The cornea can even develop a chemical keratitis with some permanent damage as a result. This is rare, unless the percentage of the silver nitrate solution exceeds the recommended 1%.

The infectious types of ophthalmia neonatorum are be-lieved to be the result of the passage of the newborn through an infected birth canal. The transfer of microorganisms to the ocular tissues of the newborn leads to conjunctivitis and occasionally keratitis.

Gonococcal ophthalmia is a hyperacute infection with a marked purulent exudate. If this infection is not treated promptly, membranes or pseudomembranes may develop. These are due to an outpouring of fibrinous exudate; con-densation of fibrin on the conjunctival surfaces may lead to the formation of a translucent pseudomembrane, which can obscure the conjunctiva and cornea. Occasionally, a true inflammatory membrane will form; attempts to remove the latter will leave a raw conjunctival surface. The gonococcal organisms can penetrate cells, including intact corneal epi-thelium, resulting in corneal ulceration. Gram negative diplococci located intracellularly in leukocytes are found on conjunctival smears. The almost universal use of routine prophylactic measures has made postnatal gonococcal con-junctivitis less frequent in the United States.

Chlamydia trachomatis is now the most common cause of conjunctivitis in the newborn. The inflammation is more moderate, and a papillary conjunctival reaction can be seen. Follicles, membranes or pseudomembranes, micropannus (superficial vascularization of the cornea), and corneal opacities, noted in adult trachoma, are unusual. Systemic involvement, however, is common and may consist of pneu-monia, otitis media, and rhinitis. Giemsa-stained conjunc-tival scrapings may show the presence of basophilic cyto-plasmic inclusion bodies in epithelial cells (see also Chaps. 93, 196, and 200). The yield of routine stains in infants is higher than in adults with the disease, and may be enhanced by immunofluorescent diagnostic tests.

Herpes simplex infections in the newborn are also be-lieved to be acquired during birth, although cases have been reported in which infection in utero was likely. This may occur by way of the transplacental route or across intact fetal membranes by way of the ascending route from the uterine cervix. Most cases are caused by type 2 herpes sim-plex; the oral strain, type 1, is found less commonly. With the increase in orogenital sex practices, the type of virus isolated can no longer be considered a useful criterion in the differentiation of in utero infection versus transmission from active lesions in the maternal birth canal. Herpes simplex infections in the newborn may be localized, involving the eye, skin, oral cavity, or central nervous system, or they may be disseminated. The ocular infection typically starts with conjunctival redness, swelling, and moderate discharge. Pseudomembranes may develop, and vesicles may be seen on the palpebral conjunctiva or skin of the eyelids. In almost half of the patients, the cornea will become involved. A punctate keratitis or a typical dendrite-shaped lesion may develop. Scrapings of the conjunctiva or cornea and smears from the vesicles show many mononucleated cells and, typically, giant multinucleated epithelial cells.

Nongonococcal bacterial infections may also be responsible for neonatal conjunctivitis. *Staphylococcus aureus* is commonly involved, but other microorganisms can cause infection. Of greatest concern are infections due to *N. meningitidis*; this organism can penetrate into the bloodstream through the intact conjunctiva and thus cause a systemic infection.

CLINICAL PRESENTATION

It should be stressed that the clinical manifestations of the various forms of ophthalmia neonatorum are not specific enough to allow an accurate diagnosis. Although the timing and the character of the signs are somewhat typical for each type of ophthalmia, there is considerable overlap and the physician should never rely only on clinical findings. Regardless of the causative agent, ophthalmia neonatorum is characterized by redness and chemosis (swelling) of the conjunctiva, edema of the eyelids, and discharge, which may be purulent. Thus, a full microbiologic evaluation is essential, particularly because conjunctivitis in a newborn should be considered an emergency until proven otherwise.

Chemical conjunctivitis is characterized by its rapid onset after birth (within 24 hours), its negative cultures, and its self-limiting nature. It disappears spontaneously in 3 to 5 days. The conjunctival injection is usually mild, but some lid edema and purulent discharge may be present. Permanent damage to the cornea is rare. The incidence of chemical ophthalmia is low and can be expected to decrease even more because of the increasingly frequent practice of using 0.5% erythromycin ointment instead of silver nitrate.

Inclusion conjunctivitis due to *C. trachomatis* becomes evident 5 to 12 days after birth, although occasionally it may occur as late as 3 to 4 weeks after birth. It is the leading cause of ophthalmia neonatorum (30%). The findings frequently involve only one eye. The inflammation is moderate, with mild conjunctival hyperemia and swelling, moderate lid swelling, and mucopurulent discharge. An inspection of the palpebral conjunctiva under magnification (slit lamp) may reveal a papillary reaction; other findings are rare. Chlamydial venereal infections are common and often asymptomatic.

The next most common neonatal conjunctivitis (about 15%) is due to *N. gonorrhoeae.* It starts 2 to 4 days postnatally, and the clinical findings are dramatic. There is a hyperacute conjunctivitis, with red and swollen conjunctiva and copious purulent discharge. Both eyes are usually involved. Pseudomembranes and membranes may form, and, because the organism can penetrate intact epithelial cells, superficial keratitis is common. Corneal ulceration and even perforation may develop rapidly if early and appropriate treatment is not instituted. The ulceration starts typically in the periphery and extends rapidly to a ring ulcer. The ulcer deepens and may cause perforation and then endophthalmitis. It is essential to realize that *N. meningitidis* conjunctivitis presents in a similar fashion. It can also penetrate intact tissues, and systemic dissemination can follow.

Staphylococcus aureus is responsible for about 10% of ophthalmia neonatorum. The conjunctivitis is similar to infection from *Neisseria,* but its onset is slightly later (from the third to seventh day). Other bacterial infections can start at any time.

Conjunctivitis caused by herpes simplex virus develops between 2 days and 2 weeks after birth. The conjunctival injection is moderately severe, and there is a mucopurulent discharge. The eyelids are swollen and red, and typical herpetic vesicles appear. Pseudomembranes may be present. Keratitis may follow the conjunctivitis in about half of the infants after 1 to 4 weeks. An inspection of the cornea under magnification, preferably by slit lamp, and after an application of fluorescein will reveal punctate staining or dendritic figures. Other parts of the eye can be involved; iritis and more generalized uveitis, chorioretinitis, and occasionally cataracts may be present.

DIFFERENTIAL DIAGNOSIS

A few conditions are occasionally mistaken for conjunctivitis. Subconjunctival hemorrhages, sometimes associated with birth, are bright red and diffusely spread through the tissue. There is no discharge, and they resolve in 1 to 2 weeks. Tearing and accumulation of some mucopurulent material at the nasal corner of the eye, because of nasolacrimal duct obstruction, usually do not develop until a few weeks after birth (see Chap. 98). The conjunctiva normally do not become injected. An exception may occur in the case of congenital dacryocystocele. This condition occurs when mucus accumulates in the lacrimal sac of newborns because of an obstruction. A bluish swelling is noted near the nasal corner of the eye. If the lacrimal sac does not drain spontaneously or by probing to relieve the obstruction, dacryocystitis may develop with tearing, purulent discharge, and conjunctivitis. The infection may occasionally spread and cause periorbital (preseptal) cellulitis (see Chap. 95). Congenital glaucoma presents initially with excessive tearing, photo-

Table 92-1. Average Time of Onset and Characteristics of the Most Common Causes of Ophthalmia Neonatorum

ETIOLOGY	ONSET (Days After Birth)	SEVERITY	NATURAL COURSE	FREQUENCY
Chlamydia trachomatis	5–12	Moderate	Chronic	Common
Neisseria gonorrhoeae	2–4	Severe	Rapid	Fairly common
Staphylococcus aureus	3–7	Severe	May resolve	Fairly common
Silver nitrate	<1	Mild	Self-limited	Common
Herpes simplex	2–15	Moderate	Progressive	Uncommon

phobia, and lid spasm. If the increased intraocular pressure persists, the cornea becomes hazy and its diameter enlarges. The conjunctiva, however, is generally not or only minimally hyperemic.

Although the diagnosis of ophthalmia neonatorum should be based on laboratory studies, the clinical findings and the timing of the infection may be helpful in the formulation of an initial impression. The essential characteristics are listed in Table 92-1, but to repeat, there is enough overlap so that they should not be relied on exclusively.

WORK-UP

Information should be obtained about the timing of the onset of the conjunctivitis. Because of the venereal origin of most of the cases of ophthalmia neonatorum, inquiries should be made about exposure to a maternal sexually transmitted disease.

Cultures should be obtained from the conjunctival sac on blood and Thayer-Martin or chocolate agar. Antibiotic sensitivity needs to be determined. Sugar fermentation tests may be necessary to distinguish *N. gonorrhoeae* and *N. meningitidis*. If indicated, viral cultures should be requested. *Chlamydia* may be diagnosed from McCoy cell cultures; direct immunofluorescence of cultures may expedite the diagnosis. Scrapings of the conjunctiva are done with a blunt platinum spatula, immediately transferred to glass slides, and fixed with 95% ethanol. Gram and Giemsa stains should be performed. The first is useful in the identification of bacteria, and the latter allows the characterization of the cellular infiltrate. Large numbers of neutrophils are typical for bacterial infections, while monocytes may be seen in viral conjunctivitis. Basophilic cytoplasmic inclusion bodies may be found in chlamydial ophthalmia neonatorum, and multinucleated giant cells are seen in herpetic infections. Immunofluorescence tests of the scrapings may be helpful, particularly for chlamydial infections.

TREATMENT

Chemical conjunctivitis does not require treatment. Irrigation of the conjunctival sac is not helpful and may make the eyes more irritated. Inclusion conjunctivitis is usually successfully treated with topical 10% sulfacetamide, erythromycin, or tetracycline ointment four times per day for 3 weeks. However, oral erythromycin is preferred because it has the added advantage of treating the nasopharyngeal colonization, which may cause reinfection, and of possibly preventing the chlamydial pneumonia syndrome. The newborn's mother and her sexual partner(s) need treatment as well. Oral tetracycline should not be used in newborns or nursing mothers because of deleterious effects on growing bones and teeth.

Because *N. gonorrhaeae* is now commonly penicillin-resistant, systemic or topical penicillin is no longer recommended. The cephalosporin Ceftriaxone, in a single daily intramuscular or intravenous dose of 25–50 mg/kg for 7 days, is the drug of choice. Spectinomycin may also be used if the organism is sensitive. Repeated lavage of the conjunctival sac with saline reduces the bacterial load and is helpful; topical treatment with antibiotics is not recommended. If gonococcal ophthalmia is suspected, the treatment should be started immediately without waiting for laboratory results.

Herpes simplex is treated with idoxuridine or vidarabine ointment four to five times daily for up to 3 weeks. In case of severe keratitis, cycloplegia may be necessary. Systemic acyclovir may reduce the risk for generalized *H. simplex* infection.

Non-neisserial bacterial ophthalmia neonatorum can be treated with erythromycin ointment four to six times daily. For gram-negative infections, gentamicin drops are chosen with the same frequency. *Hemophilus* is usually sensitive to tetracycline or erythromycin ointment. Mild bacterial conjunctivitis is self-limited, and saline washes may be adequate therapy. However, antibiotics will shorten the duration of the infection.

INDICATIONS FOR REFERRAL AND ADMISSION

Newborns with gonococcal conjunctivitis should be hospitalized for intravenous treatment and isolation. Other infections can usually be managed on an outpatient basis, unless a systemic infection is suspected. Proper precautionary measures should be taken to prevent the spread of the infection.

All these problems are best treated by a team effort, involving the pediatrician, the infectious disease specialist, and the ophthalmologist. An early consultation is recommended. Positively identified cases of venereal types of ophthalmia and of some other infections must be reported to the local or state health department. A referral to a community health nurse may be helpful.

ANNOTATED BIBLIOGRAPHY

Armstrong JH, Zacarias F, Rein MF: Ophthalmia neonatorum: A chart review. Pediatrics 57:884, 1976. (Summarizes findings in a large series of cases of ophthalmia neonatorum, with emphasis on the percentage distribution of etiologies.)

Haase DA, Nash RA, Nsanze H et al: Single-dose ceftriaxone therapy of gonococcal opthalmia neonatorum. Sex Transm Dis 13:53, 1986. (Describes currently recommended treatment for gonococcal ophthalmia.)

Hammerschlag MR, Cummings C, Roblin PM et al: Efficacy of neonatal ocular prophylaxis for the prevention of chlamydial and gonococcal conjunctivitis. N Engl J Med 320:769, 1989. (Discusses recommended prophylaxis for neonatal opthalmia.)

Hutchinson DS, Smith RE, Haughton PB: Congenital herpetic keratitis. Arch Ophthalmol 93:70, 1975. (Description of a patient with congenital herpes simplex conjunctivitis and keratitis, possibly acquired in utero; this report is accompanied by a review of the literature.)

Sandstrom KI, Bell AT, Chandler JW et al: Microbial causes of neonatal conjunctivitis. J Pediatr 105:706, 1984. (Reviews the causative factors in ophthalmia neonatorum.)

93

Conjunctivitis

Robert A. Catalano and Leonard B. Nelson

Conjunctival infections and inflammations are common in the pediatric population. Fortunately, few causes of conjunctivitis are severe enough to threaten vision. Therapy is often available to ameliorate symptoms and shorten the duration of clinical disease. Inappropriate therapy, however, can cause iatrogenic exacerbations and complications. This chapter will discuss the primary conjunctival disorders that occur in children. Ophthalmia neonatorum is discussed in Chapter 92, and eyelid infections are discussed in Chapter 94.

PATHOPHYSIOLOGY

The conjunctiva is a thin, transparent mucous membrane that covers the globe and inner surface of the eyelids. Conjunctival epithelium is nonkeratinized. Normal flora of the eyelid margins continually spills into the tears, helping to inhibit epithelial colonization by pathogenic organisms. The tears also contain lysozyme, lactoferrin, interferon, IgG, and secretory IgA. Conjunctival goblet cells produce mucin that entraps exogenous agents, including microorganisms. Langerhans' cells process antigens and initiate the immunologic reaction.

The first sign of conjunctival inflammation is hyperemia. The hyperemia may be localized under a foreign body or diffuse as in most conjunctivitis. Intraocular inflammations such as *uveitis* and *acute glaucoma* often cause hyperemia of the tissues of the globe itself with secondary dilatation of the overlying conjunctival vessels. It is important to ascertain the primary site of inflammation. The conjunctival vessels over the globe are fine and reticulated and bright red when inflamed. Vessels within the substance of the globe do not move with the conjunctiva; they tend to run radially from the cornea, and they are a darker violaceous color with intraocular inflammation.

Lymphatic tissue is normally present in the conjunctiva overlying the globe and in the fornix. In viral and chlamydial infections, lymphoid germinal centers termed *follicles* may become prominent. They are yellowish to grayish white, elevated, avascular nodules varying between 0.2 and 2.0 mm in diameter.

Inflammation of the conjunctiva lining the upper eyelid is seen as regular pinkish elevations termed *papillae*. They do not contain lymphoid germinal centers, and each usually has a central vessel, in contrast to the reticulated vascular supply seen at the base of follicles. They are usually smaller than follicles, except in vernal and giant papillary conjunctivitis, and are typically seen in atopic conditions.

The discharge seen in conjunctivitis is a mixture of transudated fluid, inflammatory cells, desquamated epithelial cells, mucin, and tears. Allergic and viral diseases usually have a watery discharge, whereas a purulent discharge is characteristic of an acute bacterial infection. In certain acute conjunctival reactions, the accumulation of fibrin and inflammatory cells can result in the formation of a pseudomembrane in the cul-de-sac. Pseudomembranes are easily removed by swabbing without inducing bleeding. More chronic conjunctival reactions can lead to adherence of the coagulin to the epithelium and the proliferation of blood vessels to form a true membrane that bleeds on scraping. Pseudomembranes and membranes are seen in bacterial (diphtheritic and streptococcal), viral (adenoviral), atopic (vernal), and chemical conjunctivitis as well as in the Stevens-Johnson syndrome.

CLINICAL PRESENTATION

Atopic Conjunctivitis

Allergic conjunctivitis is manifest by itching, redness, and swelling of the eyelids and conjunctiva (*chemosis*). It is chronic and recurrent and tends to wax and wane with or without treatment. Conjunctivitis associated with hay fever is an immediate type I hypersensitivity to air-borne antigens, resulting in mast cell degranulation and increased conjunctival vessel permeability.

Inflammation of the conjunctiva may also accompany *atopic dermatitis.* Conjunctival signs include chemosis, hyperemia, and papillae associated with itching. In some patients the conjunctiva may appear distinctly pale, smooth, or velvety. More typically, however, these patients are prone to develop crusting of the eyelid margins associated with a superimposed staphylococcal infection.

Giant papillary conjunctivitis is often caused by contact lenses, foreign bodies, and ocular prostheses. Giant papillae (larger than 1 mm) are seen in the conjunctiva lining the upper eyelid and are associated with erythema, mucus production, and itching.

Vernal conjunctivitis is a bilateral recurrent atopic eye disease occurring mostly in boys. The symptoms are usually worse in the spring and summer. Affected children may also suffer from asthma, eczema, or hay fever. Typically, the conjunctiva of the upper eyelids have large (5 to 8 mm) papillae and a cobblestone appearance. Over 80% of the children have itching and photophobia, and the child may pull a ropy, tenacious mucoid strand from under the upper eyelid several times a day. Poorly healing corneal ulcers may occur in more severe cases of vernal conjunctivitis.

Bacterial Conjunctivitis

Bacterial conjunctivitis is characterized by an acute purulent or mucopurulent discharge, foreign body sensation, and matting of the eyelashes. Between the ages of 3 months and 8 years, conjunctivitis due to *Staphylococcus aureus, Streptococcus pneumoniae,* and *Hemophilus* predominates. *S. aureus* shows no predilection for a seasonal or geographic location, whereas *S. pneumoniae* infection is typically seen in colder regions during the winter and *Hemophilus* infection occurs in warmer areas between May and October. *Hemophilus* is toxogenic and can be accompanied by patchy conjunctival hemorrhages. *Streptococcus pyogenes* is an infrequent cause of conjunctivitis, but the organism is invasive and is capable of causing a pseudomembrane.

Most acute bacterial conjunctivitis runs a self-limited course of approximately 10 days, but *Hemophilus* conjunctivitis occasionally can be part of a more ominous periorbital cellulitis (see Chap. 95). *Neisseria* is an aggressively invasive species most commonly seen in the newborn or in sexually active adolescents. It is characterized by a rapidly evolving, copiously exudative conjunctivitis associated with marked conjunctival and eyelid edema and can rapidly lead to corneal perforation and loss of the eye (see Chaps. 95, 196, and 200).

Viral Conjunctivitis

Viral conjunctivitis is characterized by a watery discharge, irritation, hyperemia, follicular response, and preauricular adenopathy. In children, adenovirus is the most common cause of *pharyngoconjunctival fever* and *epidemic keratoconjunctivitis.* An incubation period of 5 to 12 days is typical for both conditions. Pharyngoconjunctival fever is characterized by pharyngitis, fever, and follicular conjunctivitis and is self-limited, lasting 4 to 14 days. Epidemic keratoconjunctivitis often shows asymmetric involvement initially and runs a course of 7 to 14 days. It may be accompanied by petechial conjunctival hemorrhages and membrane formation. Severe cases of epidemic keratoconjunctivitis can involve the cornea with protracted symptoms of photophobia and decreased vision. Children remain infectious for as long as 14 days after the onset, and care is necessary to prevent the transmission of this highly contagious pathogen.

Herpes simplex virus infection usually occurs early in life. Primary ocular infection may be subclinical or may present as an acute unilateral follicular conjunctivitis with regional lymphadenopathy, with or without vesicular ulcerative lesions of the eyelids and corneal involvement. The initial infection is usually self-limited, but the virus remains latent in the trigeminal ganglion. A recurrent disease typically involves the cornea and is demonstrated by the staining of damaged epithelium by fluorescein dye, classically in a dendritiform pattern.

Molluscum contagiosum usually presents as an umbilicated lesion on the margin of the eyelid and rarely on the conjunctiva. The shedding of the virus onto the conjunctiva can lead to a chronic follicular conjunctivitis requiring surgical excision of the lesion.

Conjunctivitis is a common finding in childhood *rubella* and *rubeola,* occurring in up to 70%. It is noted concomitantly with the rash and is generally mild. Keratitis is said to occur in all children with measles but is symptomatic in only 50%.

Acute hemorrhagic conjunctivitis is a relatively recently described entity caused by enterovirus 70. It has been responsible for pandemics throughout both hemispheres in the past 15 years. Its incubation period is only 1 to 2 days, and the course is short with improvement starting on the third day. It is characterized by a watery discharge, preauricular adenopathy, chemosis, and subconjunctival hemorrhages ranging from small petechiae to large blotches. No serious sequelae have been reported.

Chlamydial Infections

Chlamydial organisms produce various disorders depending on the age of the affected person and subgroup involved. *Neonatal inclusion conjunctivitis* is discussed in Chapters 196 and 200. *"Adult" inclusion conjunctivitis* presents as an acute follicular reaction with a mucopurulent discharge in sexually active young adults. This often evolves into a chronic follicular conjunctivitis. It is associated with cervicitis and urethritis, and therefore systemic treatment is indicated. *Trachoma* is the result of repeated chlamydial infections transmitted by vectors with superimposed bacterial

Table 93-1. Differential Diagnosis of Red Eyes in Children

	CONJUNCTIVITIS	ACUTE GLAUCOMA	IRITIS
Vision	Normal	Markedly decreased	Decreased
Hyperemia	Superficial; brick-red color	Deep, circumcorneal violaceous color	
Phenylephrine	Blanches vessels	Deep vessels do not blanch	
Pain	Burning/itching	Severe pain	Moderate pain
Eyeball pressure	Normal	Elevated	Normal/reduced
Pupil	Normal	Mid-dilated/fixed	Small ± irregular
Cornea	Normal	Cloudy	Clear; ± precipitates on posterior surface

infections. In the early stages, trachoma and inclusion conjunctivitis are similar. In the later stages of trachoma, scaring of the conjunctiva becomes prominent, which leads to eyelid abnormalities and corneal damage.

DIFFERENTIAL DIAGNOSIS

Glaucoma and iritis are the two entities most important to differentiate from conjunctivitis. The distinguishing features of these conditions are noted in Table 93-1.

The prominent signs and symptoms found in the various forms of conjunctivitis are indicated in Table 93-2.

WORK-UP

History

It is important to ascertain whether a child with a red eye has visual impairment, photophobia, or pain, because these suggest more serious intraocular inflammation rather than conjunctivitis.

An acute conjunctivitis with significant purulent discharge is typical of bacterial infection. Itching is a prominent sign of allergy. Itching and photophobia in a child with a personal or family history of atopy and involvement during the summer with a ropy sticky discharge is typical of vernal conjunctivitis. A history of recent exposure to a person with "pink-eye" or upper respiratory tract infection is characteristic of viral disease. A chronic mucopurulent conjunctivitis in a sexually active adolescent suggests chlamydial infection. A recurrent painful red eye with apparent decreased vision and photophobia may indicate ocular herpetic disease.

Physical Examination

The physical examination includes characterizing the discharge, measuring the vision, and evaluating the clarity of the cornea. Preauricular involvement suggests viral infection. An examination with a hand-held magnifier under good illumination may demonstrate follicles or papillae. The phenylephrine test can be performed to determine the depth of the hyperemic vessels. Phenylephrine 2.5% eye drops will constrict conjunctival but not scleral or episcleral vessels. The hyperemia of conjunctivitis and secondary conjunctival reactions will be significantly blanched by phenylephrine administration, but the deeper hyperemic vasculature of intraocular inflammation will not. If there is a question of corneal involvement, the instillation of 1 drop of fluorescein dye and an examination with a Wood's lamp

Table 93-2. Differential Diagnosis of Childhood Conjunctivitis

	ATOPIC	BACTERIAL	VIRAL	CHLAMYDIAL
Discharge	C	Pur	C	Mu/Pur
Cell type	P/Eos	P	M	P/M
Itching	+	−	−	−
Lymphadenopathy	−	−	+	±
Injection	+	+ +	+	+
Hemorrhage	−	+ (H)	+ (A)(E)	−
Chemosis	+	+ +	±	±
Follicles	−	−	+	+
Papillae	+	±	−	±
Pseudomembrane	−	+ (S)	+ (A)	−

C, clear; Pur, purulent; Mu/Pur, mucopurulent; P, polymorphonuclear cells; Eos, eosinophils; M, mononuclear cells; H, *Hemophilus;*
A, adenovirus; E, enterovirus 70; S, *Streptococcus pyogenes*

should vividly show corneal involvement as a bright green defect.

Laboratory Tests

When the history and clinical findings are insufficient to render a confident diagnosis or when the infection is severe and recalcitrant to treatment, conjunctival cultures and scrapings are indicated. For bacterial infections, the most widely used media are blood and chocolate agar. Thayer-Martin medium is useful when *N. gonorrhoeae* is suspected, and thioglycolate is used to isolate microaerophilic species. Chlamydial cultures are available at many institutions. (*Note:* Wooden applicators should not be used because wood fibers inhibit chlamydial replication.) Viral cultures require special media and facilities and are generally not necessary for treatment. Immunofluorescent and immunoperoxidase techniques are available at some institutions for viral and chlamydial detection.

TREATMENT

Topical antibiotics are useful for bacterial infections. Sulfacetamide, erythromycin, and neomycin-polymyxin-bacitracin combinations are equally efficacious; however, children may develop an allergic reaction especially to neomycin. Corticosteroids are contraindicated in bacterial conjunctivitis.

Cold compresses and oral antihistamines are often helpful in reducing the itching present in allergic conjunctivitis. If the patient is still symptomatic, judicious use of topical antihistamines and vasoconstrictors may be beneficial. Sodium cromoglycolate 4% prevents the release of histamine and other biochemical mediators from mast cells and has been shown to be effective when used four times a day in conjunctivitis associated with hay fever.

Topical sodium cromoglycolate is also valuable for the prophylaxis and treatment of vernal conjunctivitis. Iced compresses, dark glasses, and oral antihistamines may also give significant relief. Topical opthalmic corticosteroids are effective but are associated with an increased incidence of cataracts and glaucoma. Desensitization to inhalant allergens and the surgical removal of papillae have not generally been found effective.

Viral conjunctivitis is often self-limited and generally does not require more than symptomatic treatment. If molluscum contagiosum is present on the eyelid margin, an excision of the lesion may be necessary to alleviate the conjunctivitis. A mild herpetic vesicular eruption of the eyelids without involvement of eyelid margins or conjunctiva requires no treatment. If vesicles are present on or near the eyelid margins, trifluridine 1% solution should be used six times per day until resolution. If conjunctival inflammation is present, the patient should be referred to an ophthalmologist for a corneal examination. Mild adenoviral conjunctivitis is self-limited and requires no therapy. Presently available ocular antiviral agents are not effective against adenovirus. Patients with adenovirus often have positive cultures for herpes simplex. Corticosteroids, therefore, should not routinely be used for epidemic keratoconjunctivitis. Herpes simplex keratitis may be made disastrously worse by the use of corticosteroids.

Chlamydial infections in children should be treated with a 2-week course of systemic erythromycin. Concomitant topical therapy is unnecessary. In neonatal infections the diagnosis of chlamydial conjunctivitis places the infant at high risk for the development of chlamydial pneumonia. Systemic therapy with erythromycin may also prevent pneumonia. Alternatively, erythromycin ointment four times a day for 3 weeks may be used.

INDICATIONS FOR REFERRAL OR ADMISSION

The pediatrician should be able to treat most cases of conjunctivitis. A referral to an ophthalmologist would be appropriate if the conjunctivitis is hyperacute or recalcitrant to treatment, or if intraocular inflammation cannot be ruled out.

Any ocular infection that involves the cornea or intraocular structures should be promptly referred to the ophthalmologist. Corneal ulcers usually require hospitalization and frequent application of enriched antibiotics or antifungal agents. Intraocular inflammation warrants a complete eye examination.

Although ophthalmic corticosteroid preparations are beneficial for many conditions, they are not without significant adverse effects. Corticosteroid-induced cataracts and glaucoma are well-recognized entities. If increased intraocular pressure persists in corticosteroid users, the optic nerve may be damaged, resulting in severe or total loss of vision. Corticosteroid use in the presence of herpes simplex infections can lead to disastrous corneal ulcers and a loss of the eye. For these reasons, ophthalmic corticosteroids should be used only by those persons specifically trained in recognizing and treating these complications. Any ocular condition severe enough to necessitate corticosteroid treatment should probably be best referred to an ophthalmologist.

BIBLIOGRAPHY

Beauchamp GR, Meisler DM: Disorders of the conjunctiva. In Nelson LB, Calhoun SC, Harley RD (eds): Pediatric Ophthalmology, 3rd ed. Philadelphia, WB Saunders, 1991.

Fedukowicz HB, Stenson S: External Infections of the Eye, 2nd ed. New York, Appleton-Century-Crofts, 1985.

Fraunfelder FT, Roy FH (eds): Current Ocular Therapy 2. Philadelphia, WB Saunders, 1985.

Jones BR: Allergic disease of the outer eye. Trans Ophthalmol Soc UK 91:441–447, 1971.

Matoba A: Ocular viral infections. Pediatr Infect Dis 3:358–366, 1984.

94

Styes and Chalazia

Johan Zwaan

Styes and chalazia are inflammations of the exocrine glands of the eyelids. These may be bacterial or granulomatous. The various glands involved are depicted in Figure 94-1. *Hordeolum* indicates any type of inflammatory papule of the eyelids. An *external hordeolum* or a *stye*, sometimes also called an *external chalazion*, is essentially a small abscess of the sweat glands or sebaceous glands associated with the eyelashes. Thus, it is located superficially at the margin of the eyelids. An *internal hordeolum* is an infection of a meibomian gland, a large sebaceous gland inside the tarsus of the eyelid. It is deeper in the eyelid and is usually larger than a stye. An *internal chalazion*, commonly referred to as a *chalazion*, is a sterile lipogranulomatous inflammation of a meibomian gland. A *pyogenic granuloma* is a mass on the conjunctival surface of the eyelid. This may develop when a chalazion points to this surface and breaks through it. It is granulation tissue that tends to enlarge fairly rapidly and is fragile.

PATHOPHYSIOLOGY

Hordeola are bacterial infections that are most commonly from staphylococci. They are abscesses with pus accumulating in the lumen of the involved glands. Histologically, they present the typical picture of an acute bacterial infection.

A chalazion is induced when the orifice of the meibomian gland is obstructed, preventing the excretion of the sebaceous product of the gland. The lipid material extravasates instead into the surrounding tarsal tissue and sets up a granulomatous foreign body reaction. Thus, the contents of a chalazion are usually sterile. There are many possible causes for the blockage such as dust, debris, or scarring from a previous infection or trauma. A chronic blepharitis or conjunctivitis may be the cause, with either the bacteria or the inflammatory response to them causing the obstruction. The pathologic appearance is that of a granulomatous reaction.

Pyogenic granulomas are fragile, highly vascularized masses, originating from the tarsal conjunctiva, where a chalazion has ruptured. Pyogenic granulomas consist of a loose accumulation of fibroblasts with many small blood vessels interspersed with lymphocytes and plasma cells.

CLINICAL PRESENTATION

External hordeola (styes, external chalazia) present as localized, discrete pustules on the front part of the eyelid margin, usually in association with a lash. They are red, swollen, and quite tender. The pain is proportional to the amount of swelling. Internal hordeola are abscesses of the meibomian glands and are located deeper in the eyelid, in the tarsus and away from the eyelid margin. Most point to the conjunctival side of the eyelid. When the eyelid is everted, the overlying conjunctiva is found to be red and elevated. Hordeola may extend occasionally in the opposite direction and point toward the skin. They may rupture spontaneously, releasing purulent material and granulomatous reaction products. Both types of hordeola may be complicated by cellulitis of the entire eyelid.

Chalazia are usually nontender, firm nodules within the tarsus. They can become fairly large and can fluctuate in size. Acute inflammatory signs are absent, except in rare cases when the process starts with a meibomianitis. Occasionally chalazia are large enough to press on the eyeball, inducing astigmatism that may cause some distortion of the vision.

Pyogenic granulomas occur on the conjunctival surface where a chalazion has broken through the surface. They tend to become larger fairly rapidly and may be visible over the edge of the eyelid. They are painless and fragile and are often pedunculated. Their appearance is somewhat reminiscent of a raspberry; they may bleed spontaneously.

DIFFERENTIAL DIAGNOSIS

The clinical presentation of all these lesions is typical; they can be distinguished by their location, the presence or absence of pain, and their appearance. If, in adults, a chalazion recurs repeatedly in the same location despite treatment by incision and curettage, a possible diagnosis of carcinoma of a meibomian gland needs to be considered. However, the occurrence of such a malignancy in the pediatric age group is rare (if it occurs at all).

MANAGEMENT

No work-up is required beyond clinical observation. If a child suffers repeated recurrences of styes, however, an immune deficiency may be present; occasionally, this is seen in anemia or diabetes mellitus. Bacterial cultures and determination of sensitivities are occasionally advisable in patients with recalcitrant blepharitis.

The treatment of external and internal hordeola is straightforward. The application of an ophthalmic antibacterial ointment, such as erythromycin or polysporin, into the conjunctival sac should be done four or five times daily. Warm compresses for several minutes a few times daily is helpful. Systemic antibiotics are rarely necessary and should only be used if there is cellulitis of the eyelid. The offending organism is almost always *Staphylococcus aureus*, and oral dicloxacillin, erythromycin, or cefaclor is usually effective. If the infection does not begin to resolve

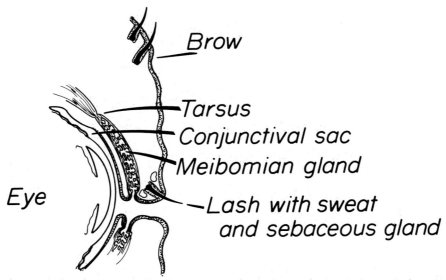

Figure 94-1. Schematic cross-section through the upper eyelid. The sebaceous and sweat glands associated with the lash are the sites of styes (*external hordeola*). The meibomian glands inside the tarsus can become infected, generally with *Staphylococcus aureus,* and then referred to as *internal hordeola.* Sterile lipogranulomatous inflammations are caused by an obstruction of the ostium of the glands at the posterior aspect of the lid margin and they are called *chalazia.*

in 48 hours, incision and drainage are indicated. This may be done under local anesthesia, but a brief general anesthesia is occasionally required for children.

Once the acute phase has passed, a recurrence may be prevented by good facial and eyelid hygiene. Daily use of warm compresses and scrubbing of the eyelids once or twice daily are beneficial. For the latter, a cotton-tipped applicator is wetted with very dilute baby shampoo (1 : 20) and is used to scrub the margin of the eyelid. The eyelids should, of course, be closed to prevent corneal irritation or abrasion.

Chalazia are treated in a similar fashion. With a combination of hot compresses and eyelid scrubs, followed by digital massage to stimulate drainage from the gland, many lesions will disappear during the course of 3 to 4 weeks, or will at least greatly improve. This is particularly true in the acute phase. Once the chalazion has become chronic, it will rarely subside with conservative measures. Incision and curettage become necessary. This is usually done from the conjunctival side of the eyelid. The eyelid is everted and a vertical incision is made through the conjunctiva into the cavity of the affected gland. This is followed by the removal of its contents, a curettage of the gland, and excision of the capsular wall. After the installation of an antibiotic ointment, a pressure patch is applied over the eye for a few hours. On occasion, the chalazion is approached from the skin side with a linear incision parallel to the eyelid margin. After removal of the chalazion, the skin may be sutured; no sutures are needed in the conjunctiva.

In some cases, an intralesional injection of a small amount of corticosteroids (0.2–1.0 mL of triamcinolone hexacetonide 20 mg/mL into and around the lesion) can be used to cure a chalazion. The injection should be done from the conjunctival side. An approach from the opposite side carries a small risk of penetration of the eye with consequent endophthalmitis. Pyogenic granulomas should be excised.

INDICATIONS FOR REFERRAL

If the stye does not improve after 48 hours of treatment with hot soaks and topical antibiotics, patients should be referred to the ophthalmologist for possible incision and drainage of the lesion.

Conservative treatment of a chalazion may be carried out for a few weeks before surgical therapy needs to be considered.

ANNOTATED BIBLIOGRAPHY

Jeffers JB, Bedrossian EH Jr: Medical and surgical treatment of chalazia. In Reinecke RD (ed): Ophthalmology Annual, vol 1, pp 97–116. East Norwalk, CT, Appleton-Century-Crofts, 1985. (Details the clinical appearance and, briefly, the pathology of various inflammations of the glands of the eyelids, including an extensive discussion of surgical and medical treatment.)

Pizzarello LD, Jakobiec FA, Hofeldt AJ et al: Intralesional corticosteroid therapy of chalazia. Am J Ophthalmol 85:818–821, 1978. (Describes how a corticosteroid injection of chalazia can cure as many as 90% of the lesions.)

95

Orbital Swelling and Infection

David J. Seidman and Leonard B. Nelson

The *orbit* is a bony cavity that has the approximate shape of a quadrilateral pyramid with its base directed forward and laterally. Because the orbit is a closed space, pathologic processes tend to present as *proptosis* (displacement of the eyeball forward), mass effect behind the eyelids, or inflammatory signs. A detailed discussion of all of the diseases producing swelling within the orbit is beyond the scope of this chapter. Therefore, a basic overview of conditions to consider when faced with a child who shows signs and symptoms of orbital swelling or inflammation is presented. Therapy is discussed for the more common infections; these are the conditions in which the pediatrician is most likely to have an active therapeutic role.

PATHOPHYSIOLOGY

The orbit is bordered medially by the nasal cavity and ethmoidal air cells, posteromedially by the sphenoidal sinus, superiorly by the frontal sinus and anterior cranial fossa, and inferiorly by the maxillary sinus. Anteriorly, the orbital septum separates the orbit from the subcutaneous and submuscular spaces of the eyelids. Categories of orbital disease in children include inflammation, vascular disorders, neoplasms, metabolic, and developmental anomalies.

CLINICAL PRESENTATION

In its most dramatic form, orbital disease may present with massive proptosis at birth. More commonly, it presents as a slowly enlarging mass in the orbit visible by way of mass effect behind the eyelids or by way of displacement of an eye away from the mass. More posterior masses may displace the eye forward and present as a progressive proptosis. Rapidly progressive proptosis, with or without inflammatory signs, is another clinical presentation that is frequently evident.

The conditions causing orbital swelling or inflammation are presented in Table 95-1.

Orbital Cellulitis

Orbital cellulitis, inflammation of the orbital contents, must be distinguished from *preseptal cellulitis,* which is inflammation of the subcutaneous tissues of the eyelids, brow, and forehead. In orbital cellulitis the infectious process extends posterior to the orbital septum. Most cases of orbital cellulitis result from the spread of infection from paranasal sinuses; the ethmoidal sinus is most commonly involved in

children. Other causes include puncture wounds that penetrate the orbital septum, surgical trauma within the orbit, *acute dacryocystitis* (infection of the lacrimal gland), extension from intracranial or dental infections, or seeding of the orbit by a bacteremia (most commonly *Hemophilus influenzae* type b).

Fever, eyelid edema, and rhinorrhea are the usual early signs of orbital cellulitis. Eyelid tenderness, warmth, and orbital pain follow. Conjunctival chemosis, decreased ability to move the eye, and proptosis occur later. As the infection progresses, congestion of retinal veins, chorioretinal striae, and increased intraocular pressure may occur. The damage to the ocular blood supply may lead to infarction of the retina and choroid. If uncontrolled, the infection can spread to the cavernous sinus, causing a cavernous sinus thrombosis, or intracranially, leading to empyema or brain abscess. The lack of response of the infection to adequate antibiotic therapy suggests the possibility that an orbital or subperiosteal abscess is present.

Dermoid Cyst

These choristomas are the most frequently encountered orbital tumors of childhood. They are nontender, circumscribed, rubbery masses most commonly located in the superior temporal quadrant of the orbit. More posteriorly located tumors may be present with proptosis, but without a clinically evident mass, with ptosis, or with restricted movement of the globe. If the cyst ruptures within the orbit, an inflammatory response to the released cyst contents may cause rapidly progressive proptosis and inflammatory signs similar to orbital cellulitis.

Capillary Hemangioma

Capillary hemangiomas occur during the first year of life. When the skin is involved, the lesion is commonly referred to as a *strawberry nevus.* An orbital hemangioma may be present with or without an associated hemangioma of the skin. In the absence of a skin lesion, an area of deep bluish discoloration underlying the eyelid skin, which increases in color when the child cries, may be a clue to the underlying *orbital hemangioma.* They are most common in the superonasal quadrant of the orbit. Approximately one third of such tumors are noted at birth; as the tumors increase in size during the first 6 months of life, 95% are noted. This tumor regresses spontaneously in 80% of children.

Nonspecific Orbital Inflammation (Orbital Pseudotumor)

Orbital pseudotumors are a group of idiopathic orbital inflammations with an acute or subacute clinical course. In the acute form there is a sudden onset of eyelid edema, erythema, chemosis, proptosis, and orbital pain. Inflammation of the intraocular tissues may also be present. The presentation may be much like orbital cellulitis.

Table 95-1. Differential Diagnosis of Orbital Swelling and Infection

MOST FREQUENT*	LESS FREQUENT
Dermoid cyst	Neurofibroma
Capillary hemangioma	Optic nerve glioma
Orbital cellulitis	Fibro-osseous tumors
Hemorrhage	Lymphangioma
Pseudotumor	Optic nerve meningioma
Hyperthyroidism	Histiocytosis X
Craniostenosis	Juvenile xanthogranuloma
Rhabdomyosarcoma	
Metastatic neuroblastoma	Meningoencephaloceles
	Microphthalmos with cyst
Leukemia—lymphoma	Teratoma
	Cavernous sinus thrombosis
	Metastatic Ewing's sarcoma

*The left-hand column represents the more frequent problems in an approximate order of frequency. Exact frequencies are difficult to obtain because most studies are biased by the nature of the referral center involved.

Rhabdomyosarcoma

Rhabdomyosarcoma is the most common primary orbital malignancy of children. The most common presentation is that of a unilateral proptosis, which increases rapidly. The disease may begin as a mass noted in the eyelid or the conjunctiva. The average age at onset is 7 to 8 years, although it may be congenital.

Hyperthyroidism

Girls are affected more commonly than boys in a ratio of 6:1. Although proptosis occurs, it is rarely of the degree seen in adults. Eyelid retraction is the most common early sign and is best appreciated on the initiation of downward gaze.

Metastatic Neuroblastoma

Between one third and one half of children with neuroblastoma will develop orbital metastasis. Less than 17% of cases of neuroblastoma will present initially in the orbit. Bilateral orbital metastases occur in more than one half of the patients. The orbital disease presents with proptosis and variable signs of orbital inflammation, which sometimes simulate acute cellulitis. Bilateral eyelid ecchymosis in the absence of trauma is characteristic.

Myeloid Leukemia

Myeloid leukemia may produce a localized infiltration of neoplastic cells in the orbit and, in this form, is referred to as *granulocytic sarcoma* or *chloroma*. The orbital signs often represent the initial presentation of the disease. The median age at presentation is 7 years.

Orbital Hemorrhage

A hemorrhage may occur secondary to birth trauma and forceps injuries, blood dyscrasias, scurvy, and vitamin K deficiency. Eyelid ecchymosis usually accompanies rapid proptosis. Hemorrhage into a preexisting vascular tumor, such as capillary hemangioma or lymphangioma, may cause a sudden rapid proptosis without ecchymosis.

DIFFERENTIAL DIAGNOSIS

Rapidly progressive inflammation of periorbital tissues and orbital contents is most commonly caused by bacterial orbital cellulitis. A distinction must be made from the more common preseptal cellulitis in which infection is limited to the subcutaneous and submuscular spaces of the eyelids, brow, and forehead. Proptosis, decreased eye movement, and pain on movement are *absent* in preseptal cellulitis.

Other causes of rapidly progressive proptosis with or without inflammatory signs include (1) nonspecific orbital inflammation (pseudotumor), (2) rhabdomyosarcoma, (3) metastatic neuroblastoma, (4) rupture of a dermoid cyst, and (5) hemorrhage into the orbit or into a preexisting hemangioma or lymphangioma. Orbital cellulitis, unlike the other conditions, usually causes fever and leukocytosis greater than 15,000 cells/mm^3.

The differential diagnosis of slowly progressive proptosis, stable proptosis, or orbital swelling involves the other diseases listed in the Table 95-1.

WORK-UP

History

The following is important in differentiating the causes of orbital disease: the age at which proptosis or swelling was first noticed; the rapidity with which the proptosis progressed; associated illness; a variation in proptosis from day to day or with crying or upper respiratory tract infections; a history of blunt or sharp trauma to the orbit; unilateral versus bilateral disease; a history of sinus disease; the presence of orbital pain or pain with movement of the eye; a change in the vision of either eye; and a general medical history.

Physical Examination

An examination should be made for the following: signs of inflammation (e.g., chemosis, eyelid edema, eyelid erythema, eyelid tenderness, or warmth); the direction in which the eye is displaced; resistance to gentle posterior displacement of the eye to displace the eye back into the orbit with palpation; pulsation of the eye; a bruit audible over the orbit; the status of extraocular movements; changes in the vision; a funduscopic examination including the optic nerve; and a general physical examination.

Laboratory Tests

Cultures are discussed under management. Plain roentgenograms will delineate orbital fractures and identify sinus disease associated with an orbital process (most commonly sinusitis associated with orbital cellulitis). Computed tomography has become the mainstay of radiographic orbital evaluation in differentiating severe preseptal from true orbital cellulitis and in detecting orbital tumors. A pathologic examination of biopsy specimens is also important in diagnosing orbital lesions. In children with rapidly progressive proptosis not consistent with orbital cellulitis, an early biopsy must be considered. If the orbital lesion is rhabdomyosarcoma, a biopsy specimen is required for the diagnosis and planning of therapy.

MANAGEMENT

Preseptal Cellulitis

The most common pathogens in preseptal cellulitis are *Staphylococcus aureus, Streptococcus pyogenes,* and in children younger than 5 years of age, *Hemophilus influenzae* type b. *H. influenzae* produces a characteristic blue-purple eyelid discoloration. Anaerobes are less common, and clostridia must be considered in cellulitis associated with dirty wounds. The conjunctiva and any purulent wound drainage should be Gram stained and cultured. If a fluctuant abscess is present, drainage should be performed near the lateral superior orbital rim. In a less severe infection, oral antibiotic therapy with a penicillinase-resistant penicillin or a cephalosporin is acceptable. The Gram stain should be used as a guide to an appropriate antibiotic choice. If the Gram stain is unavailable or uninformative, penicillin G and a penicillinase-resistant penicillin should be administered. In children younger than 5 years of age ampicillin (or amoxicillin) should be used in place of penicillin G. If ampicillin resistance is common, cefaclor or chloramphenicol may be considered. Intravenous therapy should be considered if the infection does not respond to oral antibiotics, if extensive eyelid edema develops, or if signs of orbital cellulitis develop.

Orbital Cellulitis Secondary to Sinusitis

In orbital cellulitis, a Gram stain identification of organisms and a culture may be difficult unless purulent material can be found on the nasal or nasopharyngeal mucosa. If available, this material should be cultured and a smear prepared for a Gram stain. Intravenous antibiotic therapy is then guided by Gram stain results. The most common organisms are *Staphylococcus aureus, Streptococcus pyogenes, Strep-*

tococcus pneumoniae, anaerobes, and, in children younger than 5 years of age, *H. influenzae* type b. Intravenous penicillin G and a penicillinase-resistant penicillin or a third-generation cephalosporin as a single therapy are therefore treatments of choice in the absence of Gram stain information. In children younger than 5 years of age, ampicillin is substituted for penicillin. Sinus decongestion with nasal spray or oral decongestants should also be attempted. Surgical drainage of sinuses is reserved for those infections that do not respond promptly to antibiotics. The presence of an orbital abscess indicates the need for surgical drainage within the orbit.

A discussion of the management of other orbital processes is beyond the scope of this chapter, and the reader is referred to the bibliography.

INDICATIONS FOR REFERRAL AND HOSPITALIZATION

Children with orbital swelling or infection should be managed by an ophthalmologist together with the pediatrician. An orbital biopsy is best performed by an ophthalmologist who has experience in orbital surgery. In situations in which the sinuses are involved, an otorhinolaryngologist should be consulted.

Children with severe preseptal cellulitis or orbital cellulitis should be hospitalized for intravenous treatment with antibiotics, and their ocular and neurologic status should be closely monitored. In other cases of rapidly progressive proptosis, hospitalization should be considered. The decision is based on an evaluation of the immediate risk to the visual system and central nervous system along with contemplated diagnostic and therapeutic approaches. This decision is best made in consultation with an ophthalmologist.

ANNOTATED BIBLIOGRAPHY

Hornblass A, Herschorn BJ, Stern K, Grimes C: Orbital abscess. Surv Ophthalmol 29:169, 1984.

Jones DB, Steinkuller PG: Microbial preseptal and orbital cellulitis. In Tasman W, Jaeger EA (eds): Duane's Clinical Ophthalmology, vol 4, chap 25. Philadelphia, JB Lippincott, 1989. (Broad coverage of diagnosis and treatment, with specific recommendations.)

Jones IS, Jakobiec FA, Nolan BT: Patient examination and introduction to orbital disease. In Duane TD, Jaeger EA (eds): Clinical Ophthalmology, vol 2, chap 21. Philadelphia, Harper & Row, 1985. (Clinically relevant discussion of orbital anatomy, an orbital physical examination, and a review of the literature concerning the frequency of various orbital lesions in childhood.)

Kennerdel JS, Dresner SC: The nonspecific orbital inflammatory syndromes. Surv Ophthalmol 29:93, 1984. (Discussion of the various forms and therapy of orbital pseudotumor.)

Macy JI, Mandelbaum SH, Minckler DS: Orbital cellulitis. Ophthalmology 87:1309, 1980. (Detailed case report demonstrating the approach to differential diagnosis and management in an 11-year-old child initially believed to have rhabdomyosarcoma.)

Nicholson DH, Green WR: Ocular tumors in children. In Nelson CB, Calhoun JH, Harley RD (eds): Pediatric Ophthalmology, 3rd ed. Philadelphia, WB Saunders, 1991. (Includes a discussion of orbital tumors of childhood along with a discussion of other causes of proptosis.)

Weiss A, Friendly D, Eglin K et al: Bacterial periorbital and orbital cellulitis in childhood. Ophthalmology 90:195, 1983. (Retrospective review of the clinical features, microbiology, and therapy for 137 children with orbital cellulitis.)

96

Strabismus

Johan Zwaan

Strabismus is a misalignment of the eyes, resulting in a deviation of the visual axis so that they do not meet at the object being looked at. When one eye is turned in relative to the other one, it is called *esotropia* ("crossed eyes"). In *exotropia* or "wall-eyes" one eye is turned out, while a vertical deviation is a *hypertropia* or *hypotropia*. A *tropia* is an overt turn of the eye, whereas a *phoria* is latent and only becomes obvious when the fusion of the images between the eyes is disrupted.

There is a major difference between young children and adults in their reactions to strabismus. Adults have diplopia if their eyes become misaligned. In children, on the other hand, the visual system of the brain is still immature and amenable to changes. The image from the deviating eye is suppressed, leading to a loss of depth perception. If this situation persists, the visual acuity of the affected eye will decrease, which is termed *amblyopia*. It is important to realize that amblyopia will not occur as long as both eyes are being used alternatingly, with no significant preference for the use of either eye.

The terms *strabismus* and *amblyopia* or *"lazy eye"* are often confused. The first represents a deviation of the eyes with no meaning attached concerning possible changes in visual acuity. The second indicates a decrease in visual acuity, which may be due to strabismus or to other causes, such as a cataract or a large difference in refractive error between the two eyes (see Chap. 97 for a complete discussion on amblyopia).

WORK-UP

History

The history should include the time of onset of strabismus and, if appropriate, a documentation of trauma and diplopia. An inquiry should be made regarding a familial occurrence of strabismus.

Physical Examination

A detailed eye examination, including a dilated fundus examination and cycloplegic refraction or retinoscopy, is essential.

Computed tomographic scans and roentgenograms are indicated if neurologic disease is suspected or if the strabismus is acquired following trauma.

The most useful tool for initial strabismus screening is a small penlight. The light or a small toy is moved in all cardinal directions of gaze, and the child is enticed to follow it with his or her eyes to determine if any restrictions of gaze are present.

Next, while the child looks at the light, the corneal light reflex is noted. The image of the light should be in the center of the pupil in both eyes, if the eyes are aligned. If one eye is turning, the image of the light will be displaced, nasally for an exotropia and temporally for an esotropia. One can even attempt to estimate the amount of the turn. Each millimeter of deviation corresponds to roughly 15 diopters. Thus, because the radius of the cornea is 5 to 6 mm, an esotropia of around 45 diopters is present if the corneal light reflex is found halfway between the center and the edge of the cornea.

In the cover-uncover test, the child is made to fixate on an object for several seconds. This may be a mechanical toy or a cartoon at "distance" (a standard distance of 20 ft) or a hand-held puppet nearby. The examiner now occludes one of the child's eyes and observes possible movements of the opposite one. If the latter has to move out to take up fixation, it is esotropic. Similarly, if the eye has to move in, an exotropia is present. By placing one hand on the head of the child and thus restraining it somewhat, one can conveniently use the thumb as an occluder. The cover-uncover test should be repeated for the other eye. The alternate cover test is designed to demonstrate latent deviations or phorias. The occluder (thumb) is moved rapidly between the two eyes to prevent use of the eyes together (binocular fusion). This tends to bring out latent deviations, and any movement of the eye being uncovered indicates a phoria.

TYPES OF STRABISMUS

In most cases of strabismus, the underlying pathogenic mechanism is unknown. The central control mechanisms are probably disturbed, but the exact problem has not been pinpointed. It is more likely that these mechanisms are involved in children with cerebral palsy, trisomy 21, and other conditions involving the central nervous system. These groups have significantly higher incidences of strabismus than the general pediatric population. Nevertheless, subtle changes of the extraocular muscles themselves cannot be excluded. The pathophysiology is easier to understand in patients with paralytic strabismus or with strabismus caused by mechanical restrictions.

Pseudostrabismus is often confused with congenital esotropia. The eyes appear to turn in, but in reality they are perfectly aligned. This false impression is created by the presence of prominent epicanthal lidfolds in many infants, which cover up some of the nasal sclera. Thus, the eye seems to be closer to the nose than it really is. Use of the corneal light reflex test or the cover-uncover test makes it easy to differentiate the pseudo-form from real esotropia. With growth of the nasal bridge, the epicanthal folds become less pronounced and the "strabismus" goes away. This occurrence has given rise to the myth that esotropia may resolve spontaneously. This is not the case.

Occasionally, the optical and anatomic centers of the pupil do not coincide. Thus, the corneal light reflex is seen nasally, yet on the cover test the eye does not move at all. This effect, known as a *positive angle kappa,* can be quite deceiving. It may be particularly pronounced in infants with *retinopathy of prematurity,* formerly known as retrolental fibroplasia or toxoplasmosis chorioretinitis, in which the macula has been "dragged" temporally due to scarring.

Secondary strabismus can follow various eye diseases. A cataract, a large anisometropia (a difference in refractive error), particularly high myopia in one eye, or a scar in the macula can first present as strabismus, usually esotropia. Next to leukocoria, esotropia is the most common presenting sign in retinoblastoma. Thus, all children with strabismus should undergo a detailed eye examination including a dilated fundus examination.

Congenital, or preferably *infantile, esotropia* becomes noticeable 1 to 2 months postnatally. Typically, an alternating esotropia will be present and, if the turn is large, the infant tends to cross fixate or look across the nose with the right eye to see to the left and vice versa. If no other problems are found, surgery is the preferred treatment. The timing of the intervention is controversial. Some ophthalmologists prefer to operate when the infant is about 6 months old; others wait until 1 or even 2 years after birth.

In *accommodative esotropia,* the turn is related to accommodation. *Accommodation* is the adjustment of lens power to focus on objects. Normal eyes use this mechanism for near vision, and, when the mechanism is activated, convergence or turning in of both eyes also occurs. Hyperopes need to accommodate more than average, and the eyes may converge inappropriately, thus leading to esotropia. The same effect happens when the convergence response is too large for the amount of accommodation required. Thus, the ideal treatment consists of eliminating the need to accommodate. A resolution of the esotropia should follow, and, indeed, this is often the case. After a full correction of hyperopia with eyeglasses or the prescription of bifocal lenses, the eyes may become perfectly straight. If the deviation has existed for a while, a complete resolution may not be obtained with eyeglasses and strabismus surgery may be needed. Strong miotic drops, such as echothiophate or isoflurophate, can occasionally be used to reduce the accom-

modation. Long-term use is not recommended because of the potential for significant side effects. Both are potent cholinesterase inhibitors with sustained activity. If children on these medications require surgery, succinylcholine should be avoided or given with extreme caution to prevent cardiovascular or respiratory collapse.

Exotropia can be *intermittent* or *constant.* In the intermittent type, visual functions usually develop normally. Unless the eye deviates frequently, no treatment is necessary, although some ophthalmologists do recommend surgery. Constant exotropia can lead to amblyopia, which should be treated first, usually by patching; surgery can be performed later. Interestingly, children with exotropia are often photophobic and tend to squint or close the affected eye in bright light. This may be the first sign noted by parents.

Brown's syndrome is an example of strabismus caused by a mechanical restriction. Brown's syndrome may be congenital or traumatic. The superior oblique tendon either is short or is prevented from moving freely in its sheath at the trochlea. As a result, poor elevation is present on adduction of the eye and the eye may even dip down on going in, while elevation temporally may be normal. The child usually finds a head position in which he or she can use both eyes together, thus preserving binocular vision. Unless a vertical deviation is present in primary gaze, surgery is not necessary.

In *Duane's syndrome,* the lateral rectus is not innervated by the sixth cranial nerve but by the third cranial nerve. Abduction beyond the midline does not occur, and when the eye is adducted, both medial and lateral rectus muscles contract. This pulls the eye back into the orbit, and, as a result, the lid fissure becomes narrower on adduction. Again, head turning may be present as a compensatory mechanism and binocular vision is possible. Surgery may be done if an esotropia is present or if the head turn is cosmetically objectionable.

Trauma is the most common cause of an acquired or congenital palsy. If a palsy is of recent onset, a neurologic work-up is recommended to exclude brain tumor, cerebrovascular anomalies, meningitis, or hydrocephalus. A computed tomographic scan is helpful. A relatively benign form of palsy can follow a viral infection, such as a cold. These often resolve spontaneously, but in the meantime patching may be necessary to alleviate diplopia and to prevent amblyopia. Strabismus surgery may be needed if the deviation persists for several months.

Third cranial nerve palsies may be congenital. They are characterized by a reduced adduction, elevation, and depression of the eye. Thus, the involved eye is exotropic and hypotropic. In addition, the upper eyelid is ptotic. The pupil may be dilated, and accommodation may be impaired. Amblyopia is quite common in the congenital variety of third cranial nerve palsy. If the palsy is acquired at a later age, severe diplopia is present, unless the ptotic eyelid acts as a patch, obscuring the visual axis of the involved eye. Acquired third cranial nerve palsies may be due to trauma or, less frequently in children, to central nervous system abnormalities. Surgery will give a partial correction only; the goal is to have the eyes straight in the primary position with as large a range of motion as possible. The patient has to learn to adjust to the lack of eye motility by moving the head.

A *sixth cranial nerve palsy* may occasionally be present at birth. It results in a large esotropia with an inability to abduct the eye beyond the midline.

A *fourth cranial nerve palsy* is compensated for by tilting the head to eliminate a vertical deviation. Visual development may be normal. The palsy is not infrequently confused with torticollis because of the head tilt, and an attempt may be made to correct the latter with a brace, exercises, or even surgery. With the loss of the compensatory head tilt, the eyes are no longer aligned and amblyopia or a loss of binocularity may be the result (see also Chap. 134, "Torticollis"). In addition to the congenital form, the condition may be acquired, generally following trauma, and diplopia will be present. Mild forms may clear spontaneously, but if the deviation is large, surgery is helpful.

INDICATIONS FOR REFERRAL

All children with suspected strabismus should be referred for detailed eye examinations, if only to exclude retinoblastoma and other causes of secondary strabismus. Moreover, the treatment of strabismus is so specialized that it is best left to the pediatric ophthalmologist. Strabismus, in particular infantile esotropia, will not clear spontaneously, and an early evaluation and treatment are essential for the prevention of vision loss due to amblyopia.

ANNOTATED BIBLIOGRAPHY

Von Noorden GK: Binocular Vision and Ocular Motility. St. Louis, CV Mosby, 1985. (Provides a thorough discussion of all aspects of strabismus and amblyopia.)

97
Amblyopia

Johan Zwaan

Amblyopia is a significant decrease in visual acuity caused by interruption of normal visual development during a critical period in the first few years of life. The interruption occurs when there is no maintained, sharply focused image at the fovea of the retina. The cause for the poor im-

age—opacities in the optical pathway, deviation of the eye, or poor focus due to high refractive errors—seems less important than the age at onset, the severity of the disturbing factor, and its duration. A large difference in visual acuity between the two eyes is particularly amblyopiogenic.

Classic definitions of amblyopia state that the loss in vision is not associated with structural changes. This is incorrect because there is always some abnormality of the eyes or adnexa that predisposes the child to the development of amblyopia.

Amblyopia may affect up to 5% of the population. The condition is potentially reversible when diagnosed early enough within the window of visual development that, depending somewhat on the cause of amblyopia, is no later than 7 years of age. Even though usually only one eye is affected and the child is therefore only marginally handicapped, aggressive treatment of amblyopia is warranted, if only to provide the patient with a "spare" eye.

PATHOPHYSIOLOGY

Information on morphologic abnormalities of the human brain in amblyopia is limited. Based on animal studies, however, it is likely that the numerous potential causes for amblyopia (Table 97-1) all have similar effects on the lateral geniculate body and the visual cortex. Experimental eyelid closure, strabismus, and anisometropia are accompanied by shrinkage of cells in those parts of the lateral geniculate body that are connected with the deprived eye. In strabismus this shrinkage may be limited to the binocularly innervated cells of the lateral geniculate body, but in other types of amblyopia all relevant parts of the lateral geniculate body are involved, particularly those that receive input exclusively from the deprived eye.

Table 97-1. Causes of Amblyopia

TYPE	CAUSE
Unilateral	
Suppression	Strabismus Esotropia Exotropia (rarely)
Poor focus	Anisometropia Hyperopia (common) High myopia

Visual deprivation	Dense cataract
	Vitreous hemorrhage
	Opaque cornea
	Eyelid closure (complete)
	  Ptosis (rarely)
	  Capillary hemangioma

Bilateral	
Visual deprivation	Bilateral cataracts High bilateral hyperopia Motor-type nystagmus

Electrophysiologic findings correlate with the anatomic ones: recordings from striate neurons are normal, when driven from the normal eye, but few neurons respond to the amblyopic eye. These anatomic and physiologic changes in the afferent visual system can only be induced if the amblyopiogenic stimulus is applied during the restricted period when the visual centers of the brain are still differentiating.

Two basic mechanisms have been proposed. The first holds that a lack of proper retinal stimulation from visual deprivation leads to developmental arrest of the visual system or to atrophy of preexisting connections. The second theory proposes that abnormal binocular interactions are responsible. There is evidence to believe that both mechanisms may be important.

In *strabismus*, the foveal image seen by the fixating eye corresponds to an image on the peripheral retina of the deviated eye. The conflicting information coming in from the turning eye is suppressed at the cortical level. If there is an asymmetry in the strabismus with one eye being preferred over the other, *this will lead to amblyopia*. In congenital esotropia this is usually not the case. The eyes are used alternatingly and vision is frequently excellent and equal in both eyes.

In *anisometropia* (the two eyes have an unequal refractive status), the risk for amblyopia is much higher for the most farsighted (hyperopic) eye. Unless the myopia is extreme, it is much less prone to be associated with amblyopia.

Bilateral high hyperopia is often associated with amblyopia. The eyes cannot maintain the constant accommodation needed to focus on objects at whatever distance they are located; the resulting blurred image is amblyopiogenic.

Dense congenital cataracts or other opacities in the ocular media interfere with image formation. This bilateral, equal visual deprivation causes a permanent loss of normal corticoretinal connections, if the problem is not remedied very early in life. Infants have to undergo cataract removal and appropriate optical correction before the age of 2 months to avoid permanent reductions in vision. Surgery in an older child may be technically successful, yet not yield better than 20/200 vision (which is considered legal blindness in most states). In addition, nystagmus will usually develop, which by itself can further reduce the vision.

CLINICAL PRESENTATION AND DIFFERENTIAL DIAGNOSIS

Any time that the vision is bilaterally less than anticipated for the age of the child or when there is an acuity difference between the eyes, amblyopia should be suspected. Organic reasons for the reduced vision need to be excluded. Optic nerve hypoplasia, abnormalities of the retina such as retinitis pigmentosa, and cortical blindness all result in reduced or lost vision, but the clinical history and examination usually reveal these diagnoses. *Amblyopia is a diagnosis of exclusion.* If potential amblyopiogenic factors such as refractive errors and cataracts have been corrected and the vision is still reduced, the assumption is that amblyopia is present.

There are certain indicators that make this conclusion more likely. Children with amblyopia do better when their vision is tested with single, isolated letters or figures than with the rows of symbols of the standard visual acuity charts. Amblyopes are more sensitive to the "interaction" between adjacent figures on a row, which makes them more difficult to recognize. This is known as the *crowding phenomenon*. If "functional" reduction in vision is suspected, the use of neutral density filters can be elucidating. First, a filter is found that is sufficiently dense to reduce the visual acuity of the normal eye from 20/20 to 20/40. The same filter in front of a truly, "organically" amblyopic eye will often remarkably reduce the acuity. This is not true for functional amblyopia, in which the filter will have little influence, if any.

WORK-UP

Although a good history is helpful in excluding causes for reduced vision other than amblyopia, the diagnosis can only be made after a detailed eye examination and after correction of the deficiencies, which this examination reveals. Thus, more than one visit is commonly needed to establish amblyopia. For example, if astigmatism is found as a possible cause for reduced vision, amblyopia cannot be diagnosed with certainty until after the child has been fitted with eyeglasses correcting the refractive error and the vision is remeasured and found still to be reduced.

The cornerstone of the examination rests on obtaining reliable visual acuity for each eye separately, which in children can be difficult. The measurement needs to be adapted for their age, using Allen figures or E-game in lieu of the Snellen chart if necessary (see Chap. 90). The examiner has to be skilled and quick to maintain the child's attention and has to be certain that the child does not "peek" with the other eye. If the child is very young, clinical judgment is very important. Fixation pattern (is it central, steady, and maintained?) or patterns of ocular preference may be the only information available to establish the presence of amblyopia.

Motility examination, refraction (or more commonly retinoscopy), and anterior segment and dilated fundus examinations are required to find possible causes for the amblyopia.

Laboratory tests, such as visually evoked responses, electroretinography, or computed tomography and magnetic resonance imaging can be helpful in excluding organic causes for reduced vision. The visual evoked response may demonstrate asymmetries in response found in amblyopia.

TREATMENT

The principles for the treatment of amblyopia are simple. First, the underlying cause for the amblyopia needs to be recognized and treated. For example, if a cataract prevents the formation of a sharp image, surgery is usually necessary to clear the optical media. This procedure must be followed by optical correction of the resulting iatrogenic aphakia with a contact lens or eyeglasses. Less commonly, an intraocular lens implant or epikeratophakia, in which a donor corneal button is sutured on top of the existing cornea, may be used. A cloudy cornea may require a transplant or, if the opacity is related to increased intraocular pressure, glaucoma needs to be controlled. A large refractive error or significant anisometropia has to be neutralized with eyeglasses.

The second component of the treatment program consists of penalization of the preferred, stronger eye. This is usually done by occlusion therapy. Patching of the good eye may by itself induce amblyopia, and patients undergoing this treatment need to be observed carefully. Generally, full-time patching should not be done for longer than 1 week of occlusion for each year of age without checking visual acuities. The duration of patching required to obtain a reversal of the amblyopia increases with age.

INDICATIONS FOR REFERRAL

All children with a visual acuity of less than 20/40 or with a difference in acuity between the two eyes should be referred to an ophthalmologist. Patients with cataracts or strabismus, and those with a positive family history for these problems or for amblyopia, should also be seen by a (pediatric) ophthalmologist. Amblyopia requires close medical attention for at least the period in which the brain is sensitive to the development of amblyopia and during the period in which amblyopia therapy can be effective. Because of the need for frequent detailed eye examinations to monitor the treatment, the pediatric ophthalmologist is the clinician of choice for children with amblyopia.

ANNOTATED BIBLIOGRAPHY

Simons K: Visual acuity norms in young children. Surv Ophthalmol 28:84–92, 1983. (Reviews the visual acuities to be expected for children at different ages and the methods, including screening techniques, suited for the measurement of acuity in the pediatric population.)

Von Noorden GK: Amblyopia: A multidisciplinary approach. Invest Ophthalmol 26:1704–1716, 1985. (Extensive review of the basic and clinical evidence underlying current thinking about the pathogenesis of amblyopia.)

Von Noorden GK: Binocular Vision and Ocular Motility, 4th ed. St. Louis, CV Mosby, 1991. (Clearly written and comprehensive review of amblyopia and strabismus.)

Wiesel T, Hubel D: Effects of visual deprivation on morphology and physiology of cells in the cat's lateral geniculate body. J Neurophysiol 26:578–585, 1963. (One of a classic series of papers establishing the significance of a critical time period in the normal development of the visual system.)

98

Tearing

William P. Boger, III

Tearing (or epiphora) is a common presenting symptom in both the pediatrician's and ophthalmologist's offices. Tearing may be due to the overproduction of tears or to a blockage of the lacrimal drainage apparatus. An excessive production of tears (e.g., due to a corneal foreign body or other corneal irritation) needs to be differentiated from an obstruction in the nasolacrimal draining apparatus. The most common cause of nasolacrimal duct obstruction is a congenital anomaly.

PATHOPHYSIOLOGY

The watery component of tears is produced by the accessory lacrimal glands in the subconjunctival tissues of the eyelids and also by the lacrimal gland, which is both within and under the lateral portion of the upper eyelid. The movements of the eyelids distribute the tears over the surface of the eye, thus cleaning the cornea, and the movements of the eyelids also "pump" tears into the lacrimal drainage apparatus. At the medial aspect of each eyelid margin, close to the nose, there is a small opening or punctum. The puncta of the upper and lower eyelids connect to the canaliculi, which join in the common canaliculus, which, in turn, enters the nasolacrimal sac. The nasolacrimal sac sits in a bony fossa in the side of the nose, and the nasolacrimal duct passes down a bony channel to open into the nostril under the inferior turbinate. The most common congenital anomaly of this system is an obstruction at the lower end of the nasolacrimal duct, which prevents tears from passing into the nostril. Tears and mucus accumulate in the nasolacrimal sac, and recurrent infections occur because of this stagnation.

CLINICAL PRESENTATION

Characteristic of congenital nasolacrimal duct obstruction is a teary eye with discharge but with no conjunctival injection or photophobia. Many newborns have a brief chemical conjunctivitis following the instillation of silver nitrate at birth, and it is therefore usually difficult to be sure if a newborn has nasolacrimal duct obstruction until he or she tears persistently and develops recurrent episodes of discharge during the early months of life. Discharge on the lashes or lashes stuck together in the morning but with the conjunctiva white and uninjected is characteristic of congenital nasolacrimal duct obstruction. Episodes of true conjunctivitis (discharge and conjunctival injection) may occur secondary to the nasolacrimal duct obstruction. The presence of a discharge and a recurrent infection indicate that the obstruction is low in the lacrimal drainage apparatus. If the obstruction is higher at the level of the puncta or canaliculi, the youngster will tear but will not have thick discharge or crusting.

DIFFERENTIAL DIAGNOSIS

In developing a differential diagnosis, important considerations include the age of the youngster, the presence or absence of a concomitant red eye, the character of any discharge on the lashes or in the tear film, the presence or absence of photophobia, and the presence or absence of soft tissue involvement around the eye.

Congenital Nasolacrimal Duct Obstruction

Tearing that is intermittently or constantly present from birth is most likely caused by a congenital nasolacrimal duct obstruction. Symptoms of congenital nasolacrimal duct obstruction usually are noted in the first few weeks of life. The amount of secretions tends to vary from day to day. There is no swelling of eyelids, and the conjunctiva is not injected. Firm pressure over the medial canthus results in reflux of matter from the puncta. In an older infant who suddenly acquires tearing, an overproduction of tearing (from a corneal foreign body, for example) is suggested rather than an obstruction of the nasolacrimal duct.

Tearing With a Red Eye

The differential diagnosis of tearing with a red eye includes the multiple causes of conjunctivitis (see Chap. 93) as well as corneal problems (*keratitis*) and intraocular inflammation (*iritis*). In contrast to conjunctivitis, keratitis and iritis tend to produce photophobia in addition to a red and teary eye. The nature of the injection can also be used as a differentiating characteristic. In both keratitis and iritis, the injection will be most intense around the cornea (ciliary injection) and least intense in the fornices. The red eye of conjunctivitis, in contrast, will be most intense in the fornices and least prominent near the cornea. With keratitis and iritis, tearing will occur but usually with little discharge.

A mild conjunctivitis secondary to silver nitrate *Credé* prophylaxis is common. Unfortunately, parents are sometimes inappropriately reassured over the telephone during the first week of their newborn's life when, in fact, their newborn is developing a serious infection. Gonococcal infection must be suspected and eliminated in all cases of purulent conjunctivitis in the first few days of life. Because *Neisseria gonorrhoeae* can rapidly penetrate the cornea, gonococcal conjunctivitis presents an urgent situation (see Chap. 92).

Chlamydial conjunctivitis usually begins 5 to 12 days after birth, and differentiation from gonococcal disease can be difficult. The diagnosis is made by seeing cytoplasmic inclusions on a Giemsa stain of conjunctival scrapings. Culture techniques have only recently become available and require special media. Silver nitrate prophylaxis is ineffective against *chlamydia*. A long-term follow-up has indicated that poorly treated newborns may develop a trachoma-like corneal pannus or corneal vascularization, which can be prevented by appropriate topical antibiotic therapy. The newborn should receive topical sulfonamide, erythromycin, or tetracycline ophthalmic ointment four times a day for 3 weeks, oral erythromycin, or both (see Chaps. 92, 93 and 200).

Mild nonspecific conjunctivitis is so common and generally responds so readily to a topical antibiotic preparation that a routine culture of this condition is not necessary. A culture may be helpful if there is something unusual about the conjunctivitis, or if it is severe. An associated preauricular node suggests a viral or chlamydial etiology. Erythromycin ophthalmic ointment four times a day for at least 5 days is a satisfactory initial regimen. Follow-up should be in 3 days if the conjunctivitis is not significantly improved or in 5 days if it is not completely resolved.

Itching is a prominent feature of an injected watery eye with *allergic conjunctivitis* and is common in youngsters who have allergic disorders such as hayfever and asthma. Allergic conjunctivitis may also occur in a youngster who does not have such a strong history of systemic allergies.

An extreme allergic response in the conjunctiva occurs in *vernal conjunctivitis,* with papillary nodules forming on the tarsal surface of the upper eyelids, and in "limbal" vernal conjunctivitis in which nodules form at the corneoscleral junction. Vernal conjunctivitis of the upper eyelid may produce such prominent, firm nodules that the roughened eyelid surface scratches the cornea continually. Topical corticosteroids can dramatically reduce the size of the allergic nodules and make the patient comfortable. Because corticosteroid eye drops may produce cataracts and glaucoma and may worsen corneal epithelial infections with herpes simplex, these drugs should be prescribed only by an ophthalmologist.

Tearing With Photophobia

Keratitis and iritis must be considered. The most important causes of *keratitis* in children include the following:

- *Infantile glaucoma* (congenital glaucoma)—It is crucial to make this diagnosis early in life before vision has been irreparably damaged or lost. It is important to maintain a high index of suspicion and to consider it routinely in the differential diagnosis of ocular problems of childhood, particularly in the newborn with tearing.

  Tearing, photophobia, cloudy cornea, and corneal enlargement in one or both eyes are the classic signs of infantile glaucoma. These signs may be present at birth (truly congenital); they may develop in the newborn period; or they may develop in the first few years of life (thus the term *infantile* is more appropriate). Only one sign may be present initially, and it is important not to wait for the full constellation before undertaking a complete evaluation for glaucoma. After 2 years of age, the corneas generally do not enlarge, even if the intraocular pressure is elevated. In the childhood years, the configuration of the optic nerve cupping and asymmetry between the cupping in the two eyes is the principal early sign of glaucoma for the nonophthalmic physician.

- *Corneal foreign body*—Corneal foreign bodies should be removed promptly. They are painful, and significant delays increase the chance of a secondary infection. Metallic foreign bodies that have been on the cornea for a time will often leave a "rust ring" after the major foreign body has been removed.
- *Herpes simplex*—Herpes simplex may present initially only on the eyelids. It may affect the eyelid margins and eyelashes (herpetic marginal blepharitis), or it may affect both the conjunctiva and the cornea (herpetic keratoconjunctivitis). Herpes simplex is a serious cause of blindness in the United States because of its tendency to leave scars in the cornea. Topical corticosteroids may significantly worsen the course of corneal epithelial infection with herpes simplex and thus they must be avoided.
- *Ultraviolet keratitis*—The cornea absorbs ultraviolet irradiation and may be injured by sunlamp burns, arc welding flashes, or excessive ultraviolet exposure from any source (e.g., snow blindness). Characteristically, intense corneal pain develops approximately 6 hours after the exposure. Visual acuity is diminished (by corneal epithelial irregularity), and many fine punctate lesions of the cornea may be detected by fluorescein staining and a close examination with magnification. Topical erythromycin ophthalmic ointment, tight eye patches for 24 hours, and systemic analgesics are appropriate therapy.
- *Contact lens problems*—Contact lenses have become popular and their use is widespread. Contact lens problems bear consideration in the differential diagnosis of tearing in older children. Corneal abrasions caused by contact lenses may become secondarily infected and, if ulcerations develop, may threaten vision.

A red eye with little or no discharge may be the result of *acute iritis* rather than conjunctivitis. The pupil may be somewhat smaller in the eye with iritis if the process is unilateral. For the primary care physician, the differentiation between iritis and keratitis rests on the examination of the cornea. With no apparent corneal pathology, iritis is the likely diagnosis. Since definitive diagnosis and management depend on a slit lamp examination, patients who might have iritis should be referred to the ophthalmologist.

Tearing With Significant Swelling and Erythema in the Soft Tissues Around the Eye

Congenital nasolacrimal duct obstruction may also be the underlying etiology for a severe infection of the nasolacri-

mal sac (*dacryocystitis*). Dacryocystitis presents as a red and tender swelling over the medial aspect of the eyelids on the side of the nose. The child may be severely ill. This presentation of acute dacryocystitis needs to be *differentiated* from orbital cellulitis and periorbital cellulitis.

Orbital cellulitis denotes the infection of tissues behind the orbital septum with involvement of the retrobulbar structures producing proptosis, chemosis, limitation of the eye movement, and possibly reduction of vision. The orbit is usually infected from a contiguous structure, often an infected sinus. This is a life-threatening condition and requires emergency treatment because infection may spread posteriorly to the cavernous sinus.

Periorbital cellulitis is a facial cellulitis that involves the eyelids, and it may produce an alarming swelling and closure of the eyelids. The eye itself, however, retains full range of movement; it is not proptotic, and it has good visual acuity and normal pupillary reactions. Parenteral antibiotics are indicated for periorbital cellulitis (see Chap. 95 for a more complete discussion).

WORK-UP

An etiologic diagnosis of tearing can usually be made by the pediatrician in the office on the basis of a history and physical examination with careful consideration to the aforementioned differential points.

History

Congenital nasolacrimal duct obstruction alone characteristically does not present with a red eye or photophobia and has an intermittent history from birth. Tearing and discharge may remit spontaneously in one eye, while the other eye may continue to shows signs of nasolacrimal duct obstructions.

Physical Examination

The presence of a nasolacrimal duct obstruction can be confirmed by digital pressure on the nasolacrimal sac. If the nasolacrimal duct is obstructed, tears and mucus accumulation in the distended nasolacrimal sac will reflux out the canaliculi and puncta. This maneuver not only confirms the diagnosis of a nasolacrimal duct obstruction but can also occasionally be curative. Not infrequently, firm pressure over the nasolacrimal sac may result in a "popping" sensation with a release of tears and mucus into the nostril, thus relieving the nasolacrimal duct obstruction.

Laboratory Tests

Under most circumstances, the low-grade infection accompanying nasolacrimal duct obstruction can be treated satisfactorily with pressure over the nasolacrimal sac and topical antibiotic ointments (or drops). If the infection is particularly severe and is resistant to a change of antibiotics, or if a dacryocystitis exists, culturing the discharge and antibiotic sensitivity testing may be helpful.

TREATMENT

Eighty to 90% of youngsters who have congenital nasolacrimal duct obstruction will experience remittance of the obstruction spontaneously during the first 9 to 12 months of life. It becomes increasingly rare for the nasolacrimal duct obstruction to remit spontaneously after 1 year of age. The parents should be taught how to provide compression over the nasolacrimal sac, and they should continue this treatment at home to keep the sac empty. During the first 6 to 9 months, it is best to prescribe direct pressure over the nasolacrimal sac (four times a day initially and then as frequently as necessary to keep the sac empty of mucoid material) and to prescribe antibiotic ointment (e.g., erythromycin ophthalmic ointment). The treatment is directed toward avoiding infection and minimizing stagnation. Topical antibiotic therapy should be started at the first sign of infection (e.g., crusting or discharge on the lashes) without waiting for a full-blown conjunctivitis to develop. Many parents find it easier to instill antibiotic eye drops as opposed to eye ointment, but the blinking mechanism is so vigorous in youngsters that the antibiotic eye drops are quickly washed away. Because the ointment lingers longer, it is generally more effective. If the infection cannot be controlled with a particular eye drop, the pediatrician should not only change the antibiotic to one with a different spectrum, but he or she should also consider changing to an ointment rather than a drop.

It is helpful for each pediatrician to discuss nasolacrimal duct obstruction with the ophthalmologist or pediatric ophthalmologist who will be examining the child when a referral is made. There is a consensus that nasolacrimal duct obstruction can be relieved in most cases by probing and irrigating the nasolacrimal duct. Although there is no controversy within ophthalmic circles with regard to the efficacy of probing, there is some variation in the recommended timing of the probing and irrigation. Some ophthalmologists, if presented with a family unhappy with a child who has a purulent, recurrently infected eye, probe at presentation regardless of age. Other ophthalmologists note that 80% to 90% of youngsters with nasolacrimal duct obstruction will experience spontaneous remittance by 9 months of life if they are treated with "massage" and antibiotics. If the discharge is minimized so that the only evidence of the nasolacrimal duct obstruction is excessive clear tearing without discharge and if the parents understand their options with regard to the timing of the probing, it would be reasonable for the pediatrician to keep the problem under surveillance until 8 or 9 months of age. It is helpful for the ophthalmologist to have the opportunity to review the options again with the parents; and if the nasolacrimal duct obstruction does not remit spontaneously, a probing and irrigation can be scheduled around the first birthday.

An advantage of probing early is that youngsters are smaller and therefore weaker and require less restraint for probings done in the office. Most ophthalmologists who do office probings will tend to probe children early, whereas most ophthalmologists who wait 9 to 12 months to see if the problem will remit spontaneously tend to use a rapid-acting general anesthetic on an outpatient basis for the probing in the older child. Because endotracheal intubation is not required, the procedure can be done under "mask" anesthesia in an ambulatory surgery unit. Most youngsters with nasolacrimal duct obstruction are symptomatically improved after the initial probing, but if tearing persists, another probing is indicated. If several probings have failed, the situation is unusual and perhaps a nasolacrimal duct intubation with Silastic tubing or a dacryocystorhinostomy may be required. Nasolacrimal duct obstruction in the context of craniofacial malformation or trauma to the midfacial region are settings in which these more complicated procedures are often required. It is distinctly unusual for a youngster with a normal facial structure to fail to respond to multiple probings.

Dacryocystitis should be treated with systemic antibiotics. Once the infection is cleared, the obstruction and cause of the problem may be relieved by a probing of the nasolacrimal duct. Acute dacryocystitis at any age or congenital dacryocele noted in the newborn period should be referred to the ophthalmologist as soon as the situation is recognized or even suspected.

To relieve *allergic conjunctivitis,* mild vasoconstricting agents such as naphazoline can be given topically as eye drops. These agents should not, however, be used on a continual basis. Systemic antihistamines may be helpful, although their efficacy is controversial. Topical vasoconstrictors and topical antihistamines generally do not result in a dramatic improvement. Cromolyn eye drops are more effective than the topical vasoconstrictors and topical antihistamines.

Many superficial *corneal foreign bodies* can be brushed away with a cotton-tipped applicator or a blunt spatula after a drop of local anesthetic (e.g., 0.5% proparacaine) is placed in the eye. A cotton-tipped applicator may carry away more corneal epithelium and therefore leave a larger corneal abrasion, but since a cotton-tipped applicator is blunt, many physicians feel comfortable using it around the eye. A sharp needle is needed to remove embedded material. Any sharp object brought close to the eye should be kept tangential to the cornea and not perpendicular to it to avoid a tragedy if the youngster should suddenly get loose from restraints or if someone accidentally strikes the physician's arm or hand. A large rust ring may retard satisfactory healing. Patients with rust rings and patients with deeply embedded corneal foreign bodies in the central cornea involving the visual axis should be referred to an ophthalmologist. Once the foreign body is removed, the remaining defect is treated like a corneal abrasion with antibiotic ointment and a tight eye patch.

If the classic branching dendritic form of an active corneal herpetic ulcer is seen with fluorescein staining, an ophthalmologist should be consulted. If the child is known to have previously had ocular herpes simplex or if it is suspected, it is best to let an ophthalmologist evaluate and treat a new episode of red eye. Although not helpful when placed topically on skin lesions, the antiviral agents idoxuridine (Stoxil), vidarabine (Vira-A), and trifluridine (Viroptic) can be helpful when used topically on active corneal lesions from herpes simplex.

ANNOTATED BIBLIOGRAPHY

El-Mansoury J, Calhoun JH, Nelson LB, Harley RD: Results of late probing of congenital nasolacrimal duct obstruction. Ophthalmology 93:1052–1054, 1986. (Report of 104 patients with 138 blocked nasolacrimal ducts who underwent probing of nasolacrimal duct obstruction after the age of 13 months; 129 (93%) were free of symptoms after the first probing.)

Ogawa GSH, Gonnering RS: Congenital nasolacrimal duct obstruction. J Pediatr 119:12–17, 1991. (Good current review recommending referral to an ophthalmologist by no later than 12 months of age for nasolacrimal duct obstruction.)

Paul TO: Medical management of congenital nasolacrimal duct obstruction. J Pediatr Ophthalmol Strabismus 22(2):68–70, 1985. (Report of 55 infants with 62 obstructed nasolacrimal ducts who were followed prospectively using medical treatment; 89% of the nasolacrimal ducts (55/62) opened without surgical probing in the first 16 months of life.)

Petersen RA, Robb RM: The natural course of congenital obstruction of the nasolacrimal duct. J Pediatr Ophthalmol Strabismus 15(2):246–250, 1978. (Report of 50 infants with 65 blocked nasolacrimal ducts who were followed prospectively with medical treatment for 8 to 13 months; 58 ducts in 54 patients opened spontaneously without probing.)

Robb RM: Probing and irrigation for congenital nasolacrimal duct obstruction. Arch Ophthalmol 104:378–379, 1986. (Primary probing continued to be an effective treatment well after 2 years of age and was successful in two 5-year-old patients.)

99

Acute Eye Trauma

Johan Zwaan

Accidents involving children's eyes are common and can be frightening to patient, parent, and physician. Even relatively minor injuries, such as corneal abrasions that can be expected to heal without any sequelae, may be accompanied by severe pain and decreased vision. It is essential that a complete examination of the eye be performed to distinguish major from minor injuries because the initial impression can be deceiving. For example, it may appear that a pellet from a BB gun has only caused a laceration of the eyelid. The pellet may, however, have penetrated into the orbit, resulting in severe damage to the posterior aspect of the eye or to the optic nerve.

WORK-UP

A detailed history should be obtained while the initial evaluation and treatment are in progress. This should include the nature and the time of the injury, the possible administration of first aid, current symptoms, and previous eye history such as the wearing of eyeglasses. In chemical burns it is important to ascertain the nature of the chemical involved. Tetanus immunization should be current. If there is a possibility that the child needs an examination under anesthesia or surgery, the child should not be allowed to eat or drink. The time of the last oral intake should be noted.

Care should be taken not to make the injury worse. If a penetrating wound is present, a slight pressure on the eye may lead to extrusion of intraocular tissues, with disastrous consequences. If such an injury is suspected, no attempt at a detailed examination should be made. The eye should be covered with a shield, such as a cone shaped from a piece of carton or the top of a can, which rests on the orbital bone surrounding the eye, without touching the eye itself, and the child should be referred immediately to the care of an ophthalmologist. Indeed, even though a referral may lead to a delay in the evaluation and treatment, there is no harm in this as long as the delay is moderate. One exception to this is chemical burns, which constitute a real emergency and have to be treated without any delay.

If the child has eye pain, the examination is made easier by the instillation of a topical anesthetic. As the drops take effect, blepharospasm will diminish and the patient will become more comfortable and cooperative.

An attempt should be made to record the patient's visual acuity. If no formal vision chart is available or if the child is too young to comprehend letters, a test can be improvised using readily available objects, words, or pictures in magazines. It is very reassuring if it can be established that the child can see.

The eyelids and the periorbital area should be inspected for hemorrhage, swelling, lacerations, and position. The ability to open and close the eyes needs to be established. The orbital rim should be palpated for discontinuities of the bones or masses. Tenderness should be noted.

An inspection of the eyes requires opening of the eyelids. The lids need to be separated if this is not done voluntarily. It is essential to do this without exerting any pressure on the eye. One can rest the proximal parts of the fingers on the orbital rim and use the tips to gently retract the eyelids. A penlight illuminating the eye from the side is helpful. If lacerations of the cornea or conjunctiva or prolapse of intraocular tissues is obvious, or if the pupil has a pear shape (indicating a possible prolapse), the examination should be stopped and the patient should be referred to an ophthalmologist. Otherwise, fluorescein can be applied to the eye, preferably with a dry strip rather than in solution, to check for abrasions. The use of a blue light or Wood's lamp and magnifying loupes is helpful. Defects of the iris or blood in the anterior chamber may be present.

Pupillary reactions, asymmetry, and shape should be noted. The motility of the eyes should be checked by having the child follow a small object or light.

A fundus examination requires dilatation of the pupils. Changes in the media, such as cataracts or vitreous hemorrhage, may interfere, but one should attempt to at least document the status of the optic disc, macula, and retinal vasculature. Retinal hemorrhages or edema and occasionally foreign bodies may be noted. The inspection of the periphery of the retina requires the use of the indirect ophthalmoscope and is commonly left for the ophthalmologist.

If there is any question of orbital fractures or intraocular or orbital foreign bodies, appropriate roentgenograms should be ordered.

CHEMICAL BURNS

Chemical burns to the eye constitute a true emergency; seconds literally do count. Acids, bleach, and similar products tend to coagulate the superficial tissues of the eye, which prevents further penetration into deeper layers. These burns are somewhat self-limiting and tend to heal better and leave less scarring. On the other hand, alkalis (e.g., oven and toilet bowl cleaners, lye, or ammonia) combine with tissue lipids and cause softening. Thus, they continue to penetrate into the tissues and cause progressive damage. The cornea and even the iris and lens may show severe involvement. Organic solvents and fluids such as gasoline can cause severe conjunctivitis and keratitis, but the damage is usually superficial.

In all cases, immediate irrigation of the eye should be performed using a gentle but steady stream of saline or water for 20 to 30 minutes, or even longer in the case of alkali burns. The eyelids need to be held apart, if necessary with retractors, and topical anesthetics may be applied.

After the initial flushing the child should be referred to the care of an ophthalmologist. The eye should not be patched during the transport to allow more chemicals to be washed out by the tearing of the eyes. In alkali burns, it is advisable to continue the eye irrigation during the transfer to the referral facility.

THERMAL BURNS

Because of protective reflexes, the eye itself is rarely burned, although occasionally a cinder, part of a match, or a cigarette may hit the cornea or conjunctiva. The resulting burn is usually superficial and often heals with little or no scarring. The treatment is the same as that for a corneal abrasion. Burns of the eyelids may be small and require the application of only an antibiotic ointment until healed. Saline-soaked dressings should be applied if the burns are large. If eyelid closure is incomplete because of the destruction of tissue or edema, the eye must be protected from drying out by the use of artificial tears, protective ointments, or even suturing together of the upper and lower eyelids (tarsorrhaphy).

ULTRAVIOLET BURNS

Exposure to light from sunlamps or welding, or to ultraviolet light reflecting from snow or sand, can cause a superficial keratitis. Typically, severe pain develops several hours after the exposure in combination with blurred vision, photophobia, and a scratchy foreign body sensation. Prophylactic antibiotic ointment and a patch are applied. Systemic analgesics may be needed for intense pain. Fortunately, the cornea almost always heals without sequelae in 1 to 2 days.

EYELID INJURIES

Contusions of the eyelids are common and result in swelling and ecchymosis. Their resolution can be expedited by the use of cold compresses. It is not unusual for a "black eye" to spread after a few days, even across the nose bridge to involve the contralateral eye. Thus, the location of the hemorrhage may not correspond to the site of the original injury. Orbital fractures and retrobulbar hemorrhages should be excluded.

Ptosis of the upper eyelid may be reflective, to protect the eye, or may be due to swelling or hemorrhage within the lid tissue or to hemorrhage within the levator muscle. A spontaneous resolution is the rule but may not be the case when oculomotor nerve damage or dehiscense of the levator muscle has occurred (see also Chap. 158, "Ptosis").

Superficial lacerations of the lids can be repaired by the nonophthalmologist with the use of local anesthesia. If they are small, Steri-strips may allow adequate closure. Large or full-thickness lacerations, particularly those involving the lid margin or the medial area where the lacrimal drainage system is located, are best repaired in an operating room by the ophthalmologist. If orbital fat is noticed in the wound, the orbital septum has been involved and the risk for orbital cellulitis increases; prophylactic use of systemic antibiotics should be considered.

ORBITAL FRACTURES

Roentgenograms need to be ordered on all patients who may have an orbital fracture. The most typical of these is a *blowout fracture*. When the orbit is hit with a blunt, large object such as a tennis ball, the compression of the orbital contents increases the intraorbital pressure, which in turn blows out the weakest part of the orbital wall (i.e., the floor). This may lead to a prolapse of tissue, including the inferior extraocular muscles, into the maxillary sinus. The eye may be enophthalmic, and vertical diplopia can occur because of the entrapment of the inferior rectus muscle, edema, or hemorrhage. The diplopia will often resolve spontaneously, and, unless severe enophthalmia is present, surgery may not be needed. It can certainly be postponed for 1 to 2 weeks to allow resorption of edema or hemorrhage.

CONJUNCTIVAL INJURIES

Subconjunctival hemorrhages can appear frightening, but they are often caused by minimal trauma or may even be spontaneous. They absorb in 1 to 2 weeks. A more serious underlying injury needs to be excluded and, if spontaneous subconjunctival hemorrhages appear repeatedly, work-up for a bleeding disorder is indicated.

Conjunctival lacerations by themselves are not very important, and they rarely require suturing. However, they may indicate a penetrating injury to the eye, and surgical exploration is warranted if the laceration is large or if there are other indications for possible penetrating trauma.

Chemosis or edema of the conjunctiva may be the result of insect stings. Cold packs to reduce the swelling and perhaps oral antihistamines are helpful. Swelling accompanying other ocular or orbital trauma may indicate a serious injury.

CORNEA

Corneal abrasions are common. The loss of corneal surface epithelium exposes the free endings of the corneal nerve fibers, causing severe pain. Copious tearing and blepharospasm are usually present, and a secondary iritis may cause a ciliary spasm and miosis. The examination is facilitated by the use of topical anesthetic drops, which give dramatic relief. Large abrasions may be seen with a penlight; more subtle ones require the use of fluorescein. One should look for foreign bodies, particularly in the conjunctival cul-de-sac and under the upper eyelid, which must be everted. Foreign bodies may be removed with a cotton-tipped applicator or by irrigation. If the foreign body adheres strongly, gentle scraping with a disposable injection needle or the use of a dental bur may be needed. This is best done by an ophthalmologist with the help of a slit lamp. A short-acting cycloplegic is applied, followed by an antibiotic ointment and a tight patch. The latter should be left until the next day. After the removal of the patch, a topical antibiotic may be continued three to four times daily for a few days. Abrasions and foreign body injuries generally heal without significant scarring.

If a *corneal laceration* is found, the child should be kept quiet, using sedation if necessary, until the injury can be evaluated in the operating room. The eye should be covered with a shield to avoid pressure on the eye.

ANTERIOR CHAMBER

When the eye is hit with sufficient energy to cause a tear in a small ciliary blood vessel, bleeding into the anterior chamber (i.e., a *hyphema*) results. Most hemorrhages are small and layer out inferiorly. The blood is absorbed in a few days. If the hyphema is large or if there is a rebleeding and the absorption takes longer, blood staining of the cornea or glaucoma may occur. All patients with hyphemas should be referred to the ophthalmologist because of the risk of rebleeding and associated complications. A small hyphema is treated with rest; some physicians prescribe topical cycloplegics or corticosteroids, others give no medications at all except for sedatives. The usefulness of antifibrinolytic drugs has been established. A large persisting hyphema may require surgical evacuation to prevent complications.

An intraocular infection following injury or a sterile inflammation may lead to the accumulation of pus in the anterior chamber, called a *hypopyon*. The material should be aspirated and sent for culture.

IRIS

Tears or holes in the iris may result from a penetrating trauma. Blunt injury can lead to iris sphincter rupture or to dialysis of the iris. A spastic miosis can occur even with no direct injury to the iris.

Traumatic iritis, which may follow a relatively minor injury, can only be diagnosed with certainty with a slit lamp, demonstrating the presence of leukocytes and serum proteins ("flare") in the anterior chamber. Clinically, its presence can be suspected if the child complains of photophobia and the pupil is found to be sluggishly reactive and often somewhat dilated. The accompanying injection tends to be centered immediately around the cornea and is known as a "ciliary flush." Iritis is treated with cycloplegics and topical corticosteroids.

TRAUMATIC CATARACT

Both blunt and penetrating trauma can result in the opacification of the lens. The cataract may develop rapidly or may develop after a significant delay. Less commonly, the lens may become dislocated if its suspensory ligaments are ruptured, resulting in its edge being visible in the pupil. Fragments of lens may cause an inflammatory response, causing lens-induced uveitis. In all these situations, surgery to remove the lens usually becomes necessary, unless a cataract does not interfere significantly with vision.

OPTIC NERVE

Contusion injuries of the optic nerve range from swelling of the optic nerve head, similar to papilledema, to a complete avulsion. Ironically, in the latter, the optic disc at first may appear normal in the presence of a severe visual deficit. The finding of a Marcus Gunn pupil is diagnostic, with the degree of the afferent pupillary defect related to the degree of optic nerve damage.

POSTERIOR SEGMENT TRAUMA

The compression and decompression of the eye caused by a blunt force generates shearing forces between the coats of the eye and the vitreous. This may result in various injuries. A rupture of blood vessels may lead to a vitreous hemorrhage. A retinal tear appears as a circumferential posterior retinal break in the area where the posterior vitreous base has been detached. Similarly, an anterior tear may occur along the anterior vitreous base near the ora serrata. Both may lead to retinal detachments. More localized traction may result in a macular hole or retinal tears elsewhere, which can progress to detachments. Choroidal ruptures are usually curvilinear and concentric to the disc. If such a rupture involves the macula, a permanent visual impairment results. Retinal edema (*commotio retinae*) is visible as a whitish discoloration of the retina. The accompanying decrease of vision is temporary. Intraretinal and preretinal hemorrhages generally resolve with little or no sequelae.

A penetrating trauma is equally varied. Treatment depends on the type of injury. If the damage is so severe that the salvage of the eye or of vision is unlikely, enucleation may have to be performed. Two possible complications of penetrating wounds are bacterial endophthalmitis and sympathetic ophthalmia.

In *endophthalmitis*, the signs and symptoms are more severe than one would anticipate on the basis of the trauma alone. Pain, conjunctival edema and injection, and anterior chamber and vitreous reaction are all much greater than expected. The media may loose their clarity. All penetrating injuries should be treated prophylactically with intravenous and topical antibiotics for at least 5 days. If evidence of infection is present, this regimen should be supplemented with periocular injections of antibiotics, vitrectomy, and an intravitreal injection of antibiotics.

Sympathetic ophthalmia is caused by an autoimmune reaction to retinal or uveal pigment antigens, secondary to injury to one eye. It results in a bilateral granulomatous inflammation, thus involving the originally noninjured eye. If left untreated, sympathetic ophthalmia will cause blindness of the nontraumatized eye. Initial symptoms are those of iritis, with a disproportionate decrease in visual acuity. If the injured eye is enucleated within 2 weeks of being injured, sympathetic ophthalmia will probably not occur. Once the inflammation has started, systemic corticosteroids or even immunosuppressants are needed to save the eye.

ANNOTATED BIBLIOGRAPHY

Crawford JS: Eye injuries in children. In Transactions of New Orleans Academy of Ophthalmology: Pediatric Ophthalmology and Strabismus, p 327. New York, Raven Press, 1986. (Reviews the mechanisms of traumatic eye injuries, including sympathetic ophthalmia and endophthalmitis.)

100

Leukocoria

Johan Zwaan

When parents report that their infant has a "white pupil" or a "cat's eye," or when the pediatrician finds such an abnormality, serious concern should be raised. Leukocoria almost always indicates a major eye disease such as a retinoblastoma. In leukocoria, the normally bright red reflex of light bouncing back from the fundus is greatly diminished or entirely absent. A white mass or a whitish reflex may be noted in the pupil.

PATHOPHYSIOLOGY

Abnormalities of the lens, the vitreous, or the retina or combinations of these may be responsible for the presence of leukocoria.

Any opacity of the lens may be termed a *cataract,* although the term is usually reserved for opacities that are dense and large enough to interfere with vision. They may be unilateral or bilateral, and they involve all or part of the lens. The cause of the opacification is often poorly understood. Cataracts involving only one eye are usually nonhereditary and are believed to be due to an abnormal developmental event. Bilateral cataracts are frequently hereditary or may be part of a generalized embryopathy, such as those related to a maternal infection during pregnancy, primarily rubella. In children with disturbances of carbohydrate metabolism, such as galactosemia, galactose kinase deficiency, or diabetes mellitus, sugar alcohols may accumulate within the lens cells. This increases the osmolarity of the cytoplasm, which draws water into the cells and causes the cells to swell, thus inducing cataract formation.

Persistent hyperplastic primary vitreous is a developmental anomaly involving the vitreous as well as the lens and retina. The eye is frequently also microphthalmic. The condition is usually unilateral and sporadic. A dense white vitreous membrane or plaque is attached to the posterior aspect of the lens, and blood vessels may be seen within the membrane. The membrane exerts traction and may pull the ciliary processes centrally behind the lens, where they are visible as a darkly pigmented fringe. The same mechanism can lead to retinal detachment. The cause for the anomaly is not known.

Any abnormality of the retina in which part of it is altered enough to cause the reflection of light from it to be white rather than orange or red can present as leukocoria.

Medullated nerve fibers consist of patches of retina in which the normally unmyelinated axons of the nerve fiber layer have become myelinated. They are occasionally confused with retinal tumors, but they are entirely benign. The cause for the myelination is unknown.

Chorioretinal colobomas are the result of a failure of the closure of the choroidal fissure early in embryonic development. Their location is always inferonasal from the optic disc, the position of the choroidal fissure on the embryonic optic stalk. They consist of white or yellowish areas of sclera not covered, as is the case normally, by retina and choroid.

The most feared cause of leukocoria is *retinoblastoma*. This potentially lethal tumor, responsible for about 1% of tumor deaths in children up to the age of 15 years, is due to a somatic mutation in about two thirds of patients and to autosomal dominant inheritance in the remainder. The prognosis depends on the stage at which the tumor is diagnosed. Fortunately its frequency is rare; approximately 300 new cases are diagnosed annually in the United States.

Congenital chorioretinitis due to toxoplasmosis, cytomegalic inclusion disease, or herpes simplex virus infection usually results in chorioretinal scars. These appear as irregular white lesions, often with some pigment mottling and with a hyperpigmented border. It is assumed that, in most cases, the infection is inactive or subclinical at the time of birth. Severe systemic abnormalities, especially involving the central nervous system, may be present.

Retinal *toxocariasis* is caused by ingestion of the eggs of *Toxocara canis* or, less commonly, *Toxocara catis*. This leads to visceral larva migrans, which may affect the eye. The infestation can present as a vitreous abscess, a lesion of the posterior pole, or an inflammatory mass in the periphery of the retina with secondary vitreoretinal membranes. The lesion may be confused with retinoblastoma. It is rare for both the eye and visceral organs to be infected.

A total *retinal detachment* may lead to leukocoria. The detachment is the result of a separation of the outer layers of the retina from the retinal pigment epithelium, with subretinal fluid accumulating between the layers. Retinal detachment may be found at birth as a congenital anomaly. More commonly, it is due to a break in the retina, which allows fluid to enter the subretinal space (rhegmatogenous detachment), to traction by vitreoretinal membranes (traction detachment), or to a build-up of subretinal fluid, when exudation exceeds absorption (exudative detachment). All three mechanisms may occur in children. Breaks in the retina are commonly the result of trauma, and child abuse should be suspected. Other causes are myopia, aphakia following cataract removal, and retinopathy of prematurity. Traction detachments can occur in diabetes mellitus, sickle cell retinopathy, and retrolental fibroplasia. Exudative retinal detachments may accompany retinoblastoma and other retinal neoplasms, uveitis, and Coats' disease.

Coats' disease is characterized by vascular dilatations on the surface of the retina and hard exudates, which progress to exudative detachments. If the disease is not treated, total retinal detachment will follow and will eventually atrophy the eye. The disease is sporadic, occurs more in males than in females, and generally affects only one eye.

Retinopathy of prematurity, previously known as *retrolental fibroplasia,* can progress to total retinal detachment and thus give the appearance of a white pupil. Retinopathy of prematurity occurs most frequently in premature infants who have been treated with supplemental oxygen, but it can also occur in full-term infants or in infants who have not received oxygen. The peripheral retinal vessels are not fully developed at the end of gestation, more so on the temporal side of the retina than on the nasal side. The normal process of vasculogenesis is arrested by injury, presumably linked to oxygen exposure. A ridge of mesenchyme develops, which forms an abrupt border between the vascularized and the avascular retina. Differentiation eventually resumes in this tissue, and the abnormal structure regresses in about 90% of the infants. In about 10%, neovascularization occurs and the primitive cells break through the internal limiting membrane of the retina and grow into the vitreous, along the surface of the retina. This leads to fibrovascular membrane proliferation and finally to traction retinal detachment.

CLINICAL PRESENTATION AND DIFFERENTIAL DIAGNOSIS

Leukocoria is found in such a diversity of eye abnormalities that only a detailed eye examination allows a differential diagnosis to be made. In addition to a white pupil, reduced visual acuity may be present and the eyes may be misaligned; esotropia is found more commonly than exotropia.

The lens opacities characteristic of both cataracts and persistent hypoplastic primary vitreous are located immediately behind the plane of the iris. They may be dense and large enough to prevent any view of the fundus. Persistent hypoplastic primary vitreous is present if blood vessels or ciliary processes are seen in association with the lens opacity.

A long-standing vitreous hemorrhage (e.g., from trauma, diabetes, or sickle cell disease) shows up as a yellowish discoloration behind the lens.

Medullated nerve fibers have a fluffy cotton-like appearance and often fan out from the optic nerve, following the normal course of the retinal nerve fibers. Patches may be found some distance away from the optic disc. Retinal blood vessels tend to weave in and out of the areas of myelination. Except for enlargement of the normal blind spot or the presence of additional scotomas, there is usually little, if any, effect on vision.

Colobomas present as more or less round areas of white sclera, which are fairly sharply defined and which often have a hyperpigmented border. They vary in size and are located in the inferonasal fundus, although they may be large enough to include the optic nerve or the bulk of the retina. Iris colobomas may be seen and, if the anomaly is large, microphthalmia is common. The effects on visual acuity are related directly to the extent of the lesion(s) and may range from scotomas that are small and difficult to detect to severe visual loss.

The presentation of toxocariasis and retinoblastoma is similar, with a white mass (or masses) found in the retina and occasionally in the vitreous. Indeed, the differentiation is sometimes not possible based on clinical findings and may not be made until after the enucleation of the eye. The presence of calcium detected by computed tomography or ultrasound examination is typical, but not pathognomonic, for retinoblastoma.

The scars of chorioretinitis are difficult to differentiate, although the ones caused by toxoplasmosis tend to be more pigmented than those due to herpes or cytomegalovirus. All of these may be associated with an overlying vitreous reaction. The differential diagnosis is usually based on systemic and laboratory findings.

Retinal detachments need to be distinguished on the basis of careful indirect ophthalmoscopy. The presence of abnormal blood vessels and exudates point to Coats' disease; tears or holes in the retina are typical for rhegmatogenous detachments. The age of the child at the time of the appearance of the abnormality may be helpful in making a diagnosis. A congenital detachment is obviously present at birth. Detachments due to retinopathy of prematurity tend to occur within the first year of life, although they may develop later. Coats' disease is not manifest until the child is several years old.

WORK-UP

History

A careful gestational history should be taken, including a possible exposure of the mother to infectious disease during pregnancy. Genital herpes simplex and risk factors for infection with *Toxocara* or *Toxoplasma* (from exposure to household pets or from eating poorly cooked meat) need to be documented. A history of prematurity or trauma and the age of the child at the time of discovery of leukocoria may yield important clues. The occurrence in family members of eye problems associated with leukocoria may allow an early tentative diagnosis.

Physical Examination

A detailed eye examination is essential. This requires that the pupil be dilated with mydriatics. In addition, the eyelids should be kept open, if necessary by the use of eyelid retractors. The head should be immobilized, preferably voluntarily or otherwise by holding the head or wrapping the child. An adequate examination often requires the use of general anesthesia. Generally, this examination is best done by a (pediatric) ophthalmologist. Ultrasound examination and computed tomography are useful, particularly when the ocular media are sufficiently opaque to prevent a good view of the fundus.

Laboratory Tests

Laboratory tests need to be tailored to the suspected diagnosis. A routine urinalysis may reveal glucosuria or galactosuria, which is evidence of a disturbance of carbohydrate metabolism, sometimes responsible for cataractogenesis. Blood chemistry may show elevated serum glucose levels (in diabetic cataracts) or hypocalcemia, which occasionally causes cataracts. An enzymatic analysis of erythrocytes and serum allows a specific diagnosis of abnormalities of galactose metabolism. A *Toxoplasma,* rubella, cytomegalovirus, herpesvirus (TORCH) screen is helpful for the differential diagnosis of infantile cataract and chorioretinitis. If a white mass is present in the retina or vitreous and retinoblastoma or *Toxocara* is suspected, an enzyme-linked immunosorbent assay for the latter is available. Chromosome analysis, including prophase banding, may be helpful in cases of retinoblastoma due to a chromosome deletion. With the isolation of the gene, whose absence may be responsible for the development of retinoblastoma, a more specific test for this disease, possibly allowing prenatal diagnosis, is available for a limited group of patients. Spinal taps and bone marrow examinations should be performed on patients with retinoblastoma to exclude metastases. Colobomas can also be associated with chromosome anomalies.

TREATMENT

The treatment of the disorders underlying the presence of leukocoria obviously differs depending on the particular disorder. Medullated nerve fibers and colobomas usually require no treatment; exceptions depend on what associated findings are present.

Cataracts and persistent hypoplastic primary vitreous are treated by lensectomy, sometimes in combination with vitrectomy, if they are dense enough to interfere with the formation of a sharp image on the retina. This needs to be done on an urgent basis to prevent the development of deprivation amblyopia. Even more important than the surgical therapy is a rigorous and aggressive follow-up treatment (e.g., optical correction of the resulting aphakia and antiamblyopia treatment). Without these, the visual results will be as bad as if the cataract surgery had not taken place at all.

Active chorioretinitis may require appropriate antimicrobial therapy. Toxoplasmosis is treated with a combination of pyrimethamine and sulfonamides, together with folinic acid to prevent platelet depression caused by the first medication. Corticosteroids are occasionally used. Systemic antiviral medications are available for chorioretinitis caused by herpes simplex. Cytomegalovirus infection may be treated by intravitreal injection.

The treatment of retinoblastoma depends on the stage of

the disease. Advanced cases require enucleation to prevent metastatic disease. If both eyes are involved, an attempt will be made to save the less involved eye. Photocoagulation, cryotherapy, and irradiation are common treatment modalities. Chemotherapy is indicated when the tumor has become extraocular, although these cases are almost always fatal. A periodic follow-up with examinations with the patient under anesthesia is essential because new tumors may arise in the retina several years after the original diagnosis. Additionally, it has been shown that patients with the genetic type of retinoblastoma have a high incidence of secondary tumors later in life, particularly osteogenic sarcoma of the orbit.

Early diagnosis of retinopathy of prematurity and treatment with cryotherapy is imperative. Once retinal detachment has occurred, the prognosis becomes very poor.

Retinal detachments, including those of retinopathy of prematurity and Coats' disease, are treated surgically, usually with scleral buckle procedures and often in combination with vitrectomy. No specific therapy is available for *Toxocara* infection; depending on the extent of involvement, infected eyes may be enucleated.

INDICATIONS FOR REFERRAL

All patients with a white pupil should be referred on an urgent basis. Many of the disorders causing leukocoria need to be treated rapidly to prevent an irrevocable decrease of vision. Retinoblastoma can be life threatening.

ANNOTATED BIBLIOGRAPHY

Beller R, Hoyt CS, Marg E et al: Good visual function after neonatal surgery for congenital monocular cataracts. Am J Ophthalmol 91:559, 1981. (Indicates that excellent visual results are possible with early cataract surgery and rigorous antiamblyopia therapy.)

Catalano JD: Leukocoria, the differential diagnosis of a white pupil. Pediatr Ann 12:499, 1983. (Good review of the causes of leukocoria.)

Cryotherapy for Retinopathy of Prematurity Cooperative Group: Multicenter trial of cryotherapy for retinopathy of prematurity: Three-month outcome. Arch Ophthalmol 108:195, 1990. (Describes the results of a national multicenter study of cryotherapy for retinopathy of prematurity, concluding that an unfavorable outcome is significantly less frequent for eyes receiving cryotherapy.)

Flynn JT: Retrolental fibroplasia: Update. In Transactions of the New Orleans Academy of Ophthalmology: Pediatric Ophthalmology and Strabismus, p 293. New York, Raven Press, 1986. (Excellent review of retinopathy of prematurity.)

Metz HS, Rosenbaum AL: Pediatric Ophthalmology. New York, Medical Examination Publishing Co, 1982. (Contains good reviews of pediatric cataracts and retinal problems in addition to other topics.)

14

GASTROINTESTINAL PROBLEMS

Ronald E. Kleinman, Section Editor

101

Vomiting

Harland S. Winter

Vomiting is a common occurrence in infancy and childhood. To identify a possible cause for this symptom, a complete history and a thorough physical examination are more helpful than laboratory studies. The reason for vomiting may be as simple as overfeeding, but several disease entities may be involved. Most frequently, treatment is directed at controlling the symptom until a cause is identified.

PATHOPHYSIOLOGY

Vomiting should be differentiated from regurgitation, rumination, and retching. *Regurgitation* is an effortless expulsion of gastric contents, usually occurring in infancy. *Rumination* is the regurgitation of ingested food, which is then rechewed and reswallowed. Some clinicians believe that it represents self-stimulatory behavior and that it may reflect a psychological disturbance. *Rumination* may also be associated with esophagitis, but somatic and psychological components may both play a role. In severe situations, a dramatic weight loss with marasmus may result. In contrast, vomiting and retching are active processes in which a strong contraction of the abdominal muscles leads to increased intra-abdominal pressure and elevation of the diaphragm into the thorax. *Retching* involves voluntary attempts to empty the stomach and uses thoracic musculature, whereas vomiting is more passive and results from compression of abdominal musculature. With vomiting, the pyloric sphincter contracts and the cardia rises and opens so that the gastric contents are ejected forcefully by the high intra-abdominal pressure. During the abdominal

contraction, no active contractions are noted in the esophagus. After several seconds, peristaltic activity starts in the upper esophagus, clearing its contents into the stomach. The esophageal sphincter closes after this secondary wave. Emesis is mediated by the vomiting center in the reticular brain formation. The afferent nerves most frequently come from the gastrointestinal tract or from the chemoreceptor trigger zone located on the floor of the fourth ventricle, but other receptors are located in the pharynx, heart, bile ducts, and respiratory tract. (This may explain the association of vomiting with biliary tract disease or pneumonia.) Efferent fibers use the sympathetic, vagal, and phrenic nerve pathways. From a clinical viewpoint, decibels distinguish vomiting from retching; retching is loud, whereas vomiting is relatively silent.

CLINICAL PRESENTATION

Specific aspects of the clinical presentation should be sought to establish the cause of vomiting. Causes of vomiting in infancy may be identified by seeking information about diet and previous medication that may be related to an intolerance of a specific food or drug. A history of weight loss increases the possibility of an organic lesion or a chronic problem, whereas an excessive weight gain may indicate overfeeding. Information on the quality and quantity of the vomitus should be obtained because it is useful in localizing the source of the problem. The presence of bile suggests an obstruction distal to the duodenum. Undigested food may be found in disorders affecting the esophagus, such as achalasia or stricture. Mucus is often noted in infants with feeding problems or pylorospasm. Blood or hematemesis usually indicates mucosal ulceration of the esophagus, stomach, or duodenum. The relationship of vomiting to meals may help to define the cause. Early morning vomiting before eating is observed frequently in patients with intracranial hypertension (it is usually projectile) or in metabolic diseases. Vomiting that occurs when a meal is finished suggests psychological disorders or peptic ulcer. In peptic disease, vomiting frequently relieves the pain in contrast to pancreatic or biliary tract disorders in which symptoms may persist after emesis. Associated symptoms such as fever, diarrhea, jaundice, dysphagia, head trauma, or pain must be identified.

DIFFERENTIAL DIAGNOSIS

Patients may vomit for several reasons. These include inflammation of the mucosa of the gastrointestinal tract (e.g., gastroenteritis), stretching of an organ or membrane (e.g., bowel obstruction or otitis media), vestibular reflex (e.g., seasickness), stimulation of the chemoreceptor trigger zone (e.g., radiation therapy or metabolic disorders such as diabetes mellitus or salt-losing adrenogenital syndrome), and increased intracranial pressure (e.g., brain tumor). In the newborn, nonsurgical causes may have presentations similar to problems requiring surgical intervention. In addition to pyloric stenosis, it is especially necessary to identify other anatomic congenital or acquired causes of vomiting. Abdominal distention associated with the absence of passage of meconium suggests either atresia or intestinal stenosis. If bilious vomiting is present, the obstruction is below the ampulla of Vater. *Bilious emesis in a newborn must be evaluated immediately*, and one should assume a bowel obstruction until the appropriate diagnostic studies are performed. Meconium ileus on a plain film may imply cystic fibrosis. Abdominal distention may be absent with a partial obstruction, as seen with an intestinal diaphragm, because fluid and gas may pass through the lesion. Intermittent vomiting is usual in malrotation of the bowel with midgut volvulus. Although in older children abdominal pain is often evident initially, it may resolve as the bowel undergoes ischemic necrosis. In the newborn, bilious emesis may be the only clinical manifestation of a midgut volvulus with malrotation. The patient may have a limited time of relative well-being before presenting in septic shock. Vomiting in a healthy-appearing infant suggests a dietary protein intolerance, but the diagnosis can only be established after other etiologies have been eliminated. Immaturity of the lower esophageal sphincter usually causes regurgitation, which to some observers may be viewed as forceful emesis. Formula improperly prepared can result in emesis. Swallowed blood from an excoriation on the mother's breast may result in hematemesis because blood is an irritant to the child's gastrointestinal tract. The birth history may provide important clues regarding the cause of vomiting. A difficult delivery may be associated with vomiting due to cerebral ischemia, cerebral edema, or intracranial hemorrhage.

As a manifestation of systemic disease, vomiting may be associated with a fever in acute infections or with delayed development and seizures in either meningitis, hydrocephalus, subdural effusion, or inborn errors of metabolism (e.g., salt-losing adrenogenital syndrome). Other clinical features are helpful in reducing the diagnostic possibilities.

Diarrhea is often associated with vomiting in gastroenteritis. When fever is present, otitis media, pneumonia, and urinary tract infections are possible. Jaundice suggests hepatitis or biliary tract obstruction, as noted with cholelithiasis or choledocholithiasis.

Abdominal pain associated with emesis may be due to appendicitis, volvulus, or intussusception. If the pain is intermittent and colicky or if an abdominal mass is palpable, one should consider an intussusception and perform a diagnostic as well as potentially therapeutic barium enema.

Migraine, abdominal epilepsy, or intracranial tumors may present predominantly with vomiting but are usually also associated with a headache or seizure activity. Diabetic ketoacidosis often is accompanied by a history of polyphagia and weight loss. The causes for cyclic vomiting may be multifactorial, but the recurrent attacks are usually associated with headache, fever, and abdominal pain. Persistent vomiting progressing to a stuporous state suggests progressive hepatic failure, as witnessed in Reye syndrome. Some patients, however, may have a mild course without neurologic sequelae. Many of the children with "mild Reye syndrome" have been identified as having the metabolic disorder medium-chain acetyl-CoA dehydrogenase deficiency.

The relationship of emesis to drug therapy should be considered. Theophylline and erythromycin commonly cause vomiting. Radiation therapy and most drugs used for treatment of malignancy cause vomiting. Agents such as *cis*-platinum, nitrogen mustard, dactinomycin, and cyclophosphamide may cause more emesis than agents such as doxorubicin and methotrexate, and radiation therapy (see the display, Causes of Vomiting).

Causes of Vomiting

INFANCY

Overfeeding
Gastroesophageal reflux
Soy/milk protein intolerance
Sepsis
Pyloric stenosis
Intestinal obstruction
Malrotation
Subdural effusion
Metabolic disorder
Adrenal insufficiency
Neurologic damage

Otitis media
Diabetes mellitus
Increased intracranial pressure
Meningitis
Appendicitis
Hepatitis
Reye syndrome
Intussusception
Migraine
Abdominal epilepsy
Ketotic hypoglycemia
Drug intolerance/toxicity

CHILDHOOD (in addition to those listed above)

Gastroenteritis
Peptic ulcer disease
Pneumonia

ADOLESCENCE (in addition to those listed above)

Anorexia nervosa
Bulimia
Pregnancy

A discussion of the differential diagnosis of vomiting would be incomplete if psychological problems were not mentioned. Anorexia nervosa and bulimia must remain at the top of the list in the adolescent population and should be considered while an organic lesion is being sought. An adolescent with an unplanned pregnancy may first seek help because of vomiting. In all situations, the physician must be aware of and sensitive to the significant issues for each age group.

WORK-UP

History

The evaluation of the vomiting patient is guided by the age of the child. In the neonatal period, special attention should be given to the type, amount, and method of feeding; the quantity and quality of vomitus (bilious, undigested food, blood); the child's hunger; the timing of vomiting with respect to the meals; and the concurrence of dysphagia, abdominal pain, or diarrhea. A family history of dietary protein intolerance may be relevant. Drugs prescribed prior to delivery may be important. The growth curve frequently helps to separate functional disorders from organic lesions. A history of fever or head trauma must be sought. Inquiry must also be made about seizures and abnormal movements. After the neonatal period, additional historical data such as the presence of headache, polydipsia, polyuria, muscle weakness, or drug ingestion may be more relevant. If the child has lost weight, evidence for inflammation and some determination about body image should be ascertained.

Physical Examination

Since vomiting has so many causes, the physical examination should be complete and should include an evaluation of each organ system, vital signs, and assessment of the state of hydration.

In the infant, observation of the abdomen may reveal abdominal distention associated with hyperperistaltic waves. A pyloric tumor may be palpable, especially if the examination is performed immediately following a bout of emesis. A neurologic examination may reveal focal findings, delayed neurologic development, seizure activity, hypotonia, or papilledema. Signs of infection may include rales or bulging tympanic membranes. In older children, a thorough abdominal examination will include palpation in the right lower quadrant for guarding or rebound, which suggests appendicitis or inflammatory bowel disease.

Laboratory Tests

Aided by the clinical work-up, diagnostic laboratory studies should help identify the etiology of vomiting. An Apt test in suckling infants who vomit blood can prove that the blood was swallowed from the mother's breast. In the in-fant, barium enema examination may reveal a large bowel obstruction, whereas an upper gastrointestinal series may demonstrate esophageal stricture, intestinal stenosis or atresia, duodenal webs, pyloric stenosis, or malrotation. Abdominal ultrasound examination can be beneficial in establishing the diagnosis of pyloric stenosis and thus avoiding a roentgenographic study. The plain film of the abdomen with an upright roentgenogram will guide the clinician in deciding whether to examine first the lower bowel or the upper bowel. As discussed in Chapter 102, the pH probe is the best way to identify pathologic reflux. A work-up for sepsis, including a complete blood cell count with differential, urinalysis, and cultures of blood, stool, and spinal fluid should be performed in any child believed to have a systemic illness. Liver function tests and determination of serum glucose, ammonia, and electrolytes levels may be appropriate along with organic and amino acids if hepatic or metabolic disease is suspected. Results of immunologic studies such as IgE and radioallergosorbent testing to casein, β-lactoglobulin, or soy are usually normal even in infants with confirmed intolerance. As yet, no reliable diagnostic laboratory test can confirm suspected protein intolerance. In those children suspected of having a neurologic disease, an electroencephalogram, computed tomography, or specialized neurologic testing may be necessary. A pregnancy test may be indicated in the ovulating female.

Laboratory studies must also be used to evaluate the complications of emesis. Acutely, three major metabolic consequences occur in association with dehydration. Potassium deficiency is caused by both a decreased food intake and a loss in the vomitus. Second, alkalosis results because of a loss of hydrogen ion, an accumulation of H^+ intracellularly, and a contraction of the extracellular fluid due to sodium depletion. Third, sodium depletion results from a loss of sodium in vomitus. Chronic complications of vomiting include metabolic disorders, aspiration pneumonia, or Mallory-Weiss syndrome in which bleeding is due to a tear at the gastroesophageal junction. In these conditions, chest roentgenograms or upper endoscopy may be useful for diagnostic purposes.

TREATMENT AND MANAGEMENT

Every pediatrician receives telephone calls from a parent concerned about a child who is vomiting. *Any child with emesis plus colicky abdominal pain should be evaluated immediately.* Generally, if vomiting or fever has persisted for over 24 hours, the child should be examined. If the problem has started recently, the clinician should try to assess the level of dehydration. When did the child last urinate? What is the state of consciousness and activity? Are mucous membranes moist? If the child can tolerate small sips of fluid, an attempt should be made at oral rehydration. If all oral feedings are refused, the child should be evaluated by the physician. An electrolyte solution (e.g., Pedialyte or Gatorade) is optimal, but if this is not available a decarbonated soft drink, jello, or tea can be used for a limited period. An attempt should be made to provide both sodium and potassium. Should the child continue to vomit, have any changes in state of consciousness, persist with a fever, or show signs of dehydration, then he or she should be examined.

Corticosteroid therapy may be life saving if adrenal insufficiency is suspected. If an anatomic abnormality is found, surgery may be necessary, with the exception of an intussusception, in which a barium enema may be both diagnostic and therapeutic. In general, no standardized approach exists for the management of vomiting because therapy depends on an identifiable etiology. One exception to this principle is the management of vomiting associated with chemotherapy. Although more severe than vomiting from acute causes, some of the treatment used for *chemotherapy-induced emesis* can be applied to other causes. Preparation of the child to anticipate vomiting after chemotherapy is important, but one must be careful not to place emesis basins or foods with strong aromas near the patient. These agents can act as triggers to induce vomiting. A prophylactic treatment is most helpful. If anxiety is a factor, diazepam or lorazepam may be beneficial. If vestibular symptoms are prominent, dimenhydrinate, diphenhydramine, or transdermal scopolamine may be beneficial. Sucking on candy or auditory distractions may reduce sensory triggers.

Drug therapy should be initiated prior to chemotherapy. Thiethylperazine (Torecan) is one of the most effective phenothiazines and is available in a tablet, suppository, or injectable formulation. If given intravenously, it should be administered over 60 minutes to decrease extrapyramidal side effects. Diphenhydramine (Benadryl) may be given concomitantly to avoid the central nervous system side effects of the phenothiazines and also to provide additional sedation. Perphenazine (Trilafon) is another phenothiazine that can be administered either intravenously or orally. Prochlorperazine (Compazine) and Promethazine (Phenergan) are safest to use in children younger than the age of 5 years, but they have little antiemetic effect. Their main benefit probably results from the sedation.

Other antiemetic therapeutic agents may have a role in the refractory patient. Metoclopramide (Reglan) seems to work well in the patient receiving *cis*-platinum or other chemotherapeutic agents. If should be administered with diphenhydramine to decrease extrapyramidal side effects. Cannabinoid derivatives have been shown to be beneficial. Benzquinamide (Emete-con) is a nonphenothiazine that is slightly better than a placebo in controlling emesis. For the severely ill patient, high-dose corticosteroids or intravenous pentobarbitol (Nembutal) sedation may be required for symptomatic relief.

INDICATIONS FOR REFERRAL OR ADMISSION

An indication for admission of a vomiting patient is either for a diagnostic evaluation or acute therapy for one of the following complications: a metabolic abnormality, an aspiration, gastrointestinal bleeding, or moderate to severe dehydration. A young child with mild dehydration and continued vomiting may also warrant hospitalization. An identified underlying problem may prompt a consultation to the appropriate subspecialist.

ANNOTATED BIBLIOGRAPHY

Arthur RJ et al: Barium meal examination of infants under four months of age presenting with vomiting: A review of 100 cases. Pediatr Radiol 14:84–86, 1984. (Assessment of infants with regurgitation from a radiologic perspective.)

Dodge JA: Vomiting and regurgitation. In Walker WA, Durie PR, Hamilton JR et al (eds): Pediatric Gastrointestinal Disease, pp 32–41. Philadelphia, BC Decker, Inc, 1991. (Current comprehensive review.)

Fordtran JS: Vomiting, pp 127–143. In: Gastrointestinal Disease: Pathophysiology and Management. Philadelphia, WB Saunders, 1975. (Pathophysiology of vomiting, its etiology in infancy and childhood, metabolic consequences.)

Hanson JS, McCallum R: The diagnosis and management of nausea and vomiting: A review. Am J Gastroenterol 3:210, 1985. (Review of the causes of vomiting and nausea.)

Lichtenstein PK, Heubi JE, Daugherty CC et al: Grade I Reye's syndrome: Frequent cause of vomiting and liver dysfunction after varicella and upper respiratory tract infection. N Engl J Med 309:133–139, 1983. (Mild Reye, and how it may be caused by medium-chain acetyl dehydrogenase deficiency.)

Sallan SE, Cronin CM: Adverse effects of treatment. In DeVita V, Hellman S, Rosenberg S (eds): Cancer—Principles and Practice of Oncology, pp 2008–2013. Philadelphia, JB Lippincott, 1982. (Discussion of the management of emesis in patients with malignancy.)

102

Gastroesophageal Reflux

Tien-Lan Chang and Harland S. Winter

Gastroesophageal reflux is defined as the effortless return of stomach contents into the esophagus. In adults, this phenomenon may cause irritation of the lower esophagus and may produce the pain sensation that is commonly referred to as "heartburn." In the pediatric age group, especially in infants, vomiting is the most common manifestation of gastroesophageal reflux. Since there are many causes of vomiting, it is important for the pediatric practitioner to establish a differential diagnosis for each patient and to proceed with the appropriate evaluation before embarking on a specific therapy.

Gastroesophageal reflux is recognized as a common occurrence of infancy. In one report of 1100 infants studied in the first 5 days of life, 18% had forceful vomiting and

38.5% had mild spitting or regurgitation. Reflux, however, does not constitute a problem unless complications develop, and the vomiting is frequently not even brought to the attention of the pediatrician. Most infants with reflux improve with age; however, infants who persist in having reflux after weaning to solid foods are more likely to have pathologic gastroesophageal reflux and the potential of sequelae.

PATHOPHYSIOLOGY

In the normal esophagus, food is propelled by primary peristaltic contractions down to the stomach. The lower esophageal sphincter, which is a high pressure zone above the gastroesophageal junction, relaxes to allow the passage of the food bolus and contracts again after it passes. In adults, the lower esophageal sphincter serves as a barrier against reflux, but other mechanical factors including an intra-abdominal segment of lower esophagus, an acute esophago-gastric angle, and the phrenoesophageal membrane are also important in preventing regurgitation. The esophagogastric angle is obtuse in the infant and therefore the child primarily relies on the intrinsic lower esophageal sphincter pressure to prevent reflux. A low lower esophageal sphincter pressure, however, may not be the most important mechanism for reflux. Simultaneous recordings of esophageal pH and lower esophageal sphincter pressure in adults and children have shown that reflux occurs most frequently in association with transient relaxation of lower esophageal sphincter or with an increase in the intra-abdominal pressure. Only a small percentage of children had spontaneous reflux in association with a low basal lower esophageal sphincter pressure. Hiatus hernia most commonly is a result of chronic reflux with shortening of the esophagus. Its clinical significance in children, however, is unclear.

CLINICAL MANIFESTATIONS

In young infants, vomiting or regurgitation is the major symptom of reflux. It is usually effortless, but may also be forceful, and is often present in the first week of life. Reflux happens frequently after feeding, but it may occur in sleep. In some infants with pathologic reflux, vomiting or regurgitation may not be evident. Hyperirritability, refusal of feeding, or poor weight gain may be the only signs in some; whereas guaiac-positive stools, hematemesis, or recurrent respiratory infections will lead to the suspicion of gastroesophageal reflux in others. Older children with asthma may also have gastroesophageal reflux, and some may have clinical improvement when reflux is controlled. However, gastroesophageal reflux as a cause of asthma has not been established. Patients with apnea and near-miss sudden infant death syndrome (SIDS) may also have a significant incidence of reflux. In one study, reflux was found in 55 of 58 "near-miss" infants. However, because other risk factors are also found in these patients and because reflux is so common in this age group, a definite cause-and-effect rela-

tionship between gastroesophageal reflux and apnea or SIDS remains difficult to establish. For example, fewer than one half of patients with alleged gastroesophageal reflux–related respiratory symptoms had symptoms witnessed during the 18- to 24-hour esophageal pH study.

DIFFERENTIAL DIAGNOSIS

Although vomiting or regurgitation is the major symptom of gastroesophageal reflux, there are many other causes of vomiting. For example, patients with anatomic obstruction, such as pyloric stenosis, achalasia, antral or esophageal web, malrotation, and mass lesions of the abdomen, may have a subtle onset of vomiting indistinguishable from that of gastroesophageal reflux; their course, however, is unrelenting and progressive. Patients with acute otitis media, urinary tract infection, or viral or bacterial gastroenteritis often have a fever or diarrhea. The vomiting is distinguishable from gastroesophageal reflux by the abrupt onset, the usually limited course, and the abnormal physical or laboratory findings. Milk or soy protein intolerance may cause diarrhea as well as vomiting indistinguishable from gastroesophageal reflux. The stools may be grossly blood streaked secondary to the mucosal inflammatory response in the rectum, but the emesis is usually not grossly bloody. A diagnosis of an allergic cause is supported by the presence of eosinophils in the biopsy specimens of the stomach or rectum and by the resolution of symptoms on an elimination diet. Confirmation of the diagnosis rests on a recurrence of symptoms following a rechallenge of the suspected substance. Eosinophilic gastroenteritis, an allergic process in which the allergies are unknown, may present with vomiting. Metabolic acidosis secondary to an inborn error of metabolism or to ingestion of a toxic substance should be considered in evaluating any child presenting with vomiting. Increased intracranial pressure from head injury, brain tumor, obstructive hydrocephalus, or Reye syndrome may present subtly as intermittent vomiting. A careful neurologic examination should help in ruling out this group of diseases. Other possible causes of vomiting in pediatric patients that should be easily differentiated from gastroesophageal reflux by their clinical presentations include obstructive uropathy, hepatobiliary disease, and pancreatitis.

WORK-UP

A complete history and physical examination should eliminate many of the possible causes of vomiting (see Chap. 101).

History

The history should include significant events around birth, such as prematurity and perinatal stress, which might predispose to central nervous system injury. A history of apnea and the use of medications such as theophylline should be sought. The onset, frequency, and forcefulness of vomiting may be helpful in diagnosing an anatomic abnormality since gastroesophageal reflux would be an unlikely cause in a child who starts to vomit at several months of age. A review of systems should include symptoms such as headache, abdominal pain, dyspnea, fever, diarrhea, and urinary difficulty.

Physical Examination

A complete physical examination emphasizing growth parameters, neurologic development, and an abdominal examination should be performed. A child whose only symptom is regurgitation and who has grown well, has normal developmental milestones, and has a normal physical examination can be followed prospectively. If the child has any of the complications that suggest pathologic reflux such as failure to thrive, gastrointestinal bleeding (anemia or blood per rectum), or recurrent respiratory illness, further studies are then necessary.

Laboratory Tests

Laboratory studies should include a complete blood cell count, differential, stool sampling for occult blood, urinalysis, and capillary pH or serum bicarbonate determination. An upper gastrointestinal series may be indicated to eliminate anatomic abnormalities. The esophageal pH probe study is the most sensitive test for gastroesophageal reflux. It involves placing a probe by way of the nares into the distal esophagus at a point calculated to be 87% of the distance from the nares to the lower esophageal sphincter. The pH probe is connected to a monitor that records change in esophageal pH over time. A reflux episode is defined as a drop in pH to less than 4. Polygraphic monitoring of chest movement, nasal air movement, oxygen saturation heart rate, and esophageal pH monitoring may be helpful in patients with respiratory symptoms possibly related to reflux. Technetium-99m scintiscanning involves a feeding containing the radioisotope and may detect reflux into the esophagus and aspiration of the isotope into the lungs. In addition, it can provide a quantitative measurement of gastric emptying rate. Esophageal manometry has been helpful in providing probable explanations for the pathogenesis of gastroesophageal reflux and reflux esophagitis in that it may reveal a low lower esophageal sphincter pressure or poor propagation of esophageal contractions. It cannot assess the frequency and the duration of reflux, which are provided by the esophageal pH probe study. The role of esophageal manometry is mainly limited to preoperative evaluation of patients who have failed medical therapy and who are candidates for surgical management of gastroesophageal reflux. Patients who have poor esophageal motility may not do well with a fundoplication because the procedure may restrict the flow of material from the esophagus. Upper endoscopy allows direct visualization of the esophagus, stomach, and duodenum. It provides visual evidence of severe inflammation or ulceration of the esophagus and guides the biopsy, but it is often inaccurate in diagnosing mild or moderate esophagitis. An esophageal biopsy provides documentation of hyperplasia of the basal zone of epithelium, increased height of the papillae, and presence of intraepithelial eosinophils or neutrophils.

TREATMENT

For a young infant who has vomiting or regurgitation as the only manifestation of gastroesophageal reflux, the medical therapy should consist of frequent small feedings, burping after each feeding, and placing the infant prone, on an inclined surface at 30 degrees. The semi-upright position allows gravity to work against reflux. The prone position has been demonstrated radiologically to keep the gastroesophageal junction in a superior position relative to the liquid contents of the stomach. This postural treatment reduces the frequency and duration of reflux in comparison to other body positions. Contrary to previous teaching, it has been shown that placing the infant supine, semi-upright in the infant seat actually leads to more reflux compared with the prone position. Thickened feedings have been part of antireflux therapy since the 1950s and may be beneficial when used in conjunction with postural treatment; however, proof of its effectiveness has not been established. The small but frequent feedings are advocated to provide adequate nutrition and reduce the possibility of overdistending the stomach. Since reflux in most infants will resolve, either because of neuromuscular maturation, transition to a more solid diet, adoption of a more upright posture with age, or a combination of these factors, further studies and treatment for gastroesophageal reflux are not necessary unless the symptoms persist beyond 1½ years of age.

INDICATIONS FOR REFERRAL

For children with possible complications of gastroesophageal reflux, and for children with vomiting persisting beyond 1½ years of age, a full diagnostic evaluation should be undertaken in consultation with a pediatric gastroenterologist. After ruling out other possibilities and establishing reflux as the diagnosis, medical management should be directed at both reflux and its complications. Several antireflux medications are now available. Bethanechol, a cholinergic agonist, increases lower esophageal sphincter tone and esophageal motility. It has been shown to decrease both reflux frequency and duration in the fasted state and to improve weight gain in patients failing to thrive secondary to reflux. Metoclopramide also increases lower esophageal sphincter tone, improves esophageal motility, and enhances gastric emptying. Its major drawbacks are central nervous system and extrapyramidal side effects, including dystonia and tardive dyskinesia. Domperidone is a new drug under investigation with purported absence of the neurologic side effects of metoclopramide. These medications are best taken 30 minutes prior to a meal. Cisapride, which is available in Europe, is another prokinetic agent that may be effective in reducing symptoms of reflux.

Cimetidine or antacids are used for patients with esophagitis. Children younger than 6 months of age who are treated with aluminum-containing antacids may be at increased risk for developing aluminum toxicity. If long-term therapy is prescribed, the physician should be aware of this complication. Patients who have esophagitis and ongoing reflux should be monitored because *Barrett's esophagus,* a metaplastic lesion in which the squamous epithelium is replaced by columnar epithelium, and stricture may develop as complications. Patients with failure to thrive have been treated with supplemental nasogastric tube feeding at night, but this therapy may exacerbate the reflux. A repeat esophageal *p*H probe study or an esophageal biopsy may help to assess the effectiveness of therapy if the patient fails to show clinical improvement after a 4- to 8-week course of therapy. Although controlled studies have shown a steady improvement in weight gain and decreased reflux in treated patients, studies of long-term results are inconclusive.

SURGICAL TREATMENT

Before antireflux drugs were available, surgery was the only option when patients failed to respond to postural therapy and small frequent feedings. Two types of operations have been used. The gastropexy procedure involves pulling down the lower esophagus into the abdomen and anchoring the stomach either to the median arcuate ligament or to the anterior abdominal wall. The fundoplication procedure involves pulling down the lower esophagus and wrapping it either completely or partially with the fundus of the stomach. Nissen fundoplication is now the most widely used procedure. A gastrostomy for feeding may be needed in patients who swallow poorly and who are at risk for aspiration. In uncontrolled studies, the success of the operation in eliminating reflux and in improving growth has been over 90%. Success in eliminating respiratory symptoms is only 77%. Patients who have an incomplete resolution of respiratory problems are more likely to have other associated disorders, such as mental retardation, seizures, congenital heart disease, repaired tracheoesophageal fistula with or without esophageal atresia, and disorders of the laryngotracheobronchial tree. It is possible that, in some of these patients, respiratory symptoms are not due to reflux but are instead related to associated disorders. In patients whose reflux is controlled on medical treatment, but whose respiratory symptoms remain unaltered, surgery may not be beneficial. Surgical complications are common and include paraesophageal hernia, small bowel obstruction, pneumonia, malalignment of the wrap, and wound infections. Some authors advocate surgery in patients with coexistent apnea and gastroesophageal reflux, citing favorable statistics in the literature. In our opinion, a strong correlation between

symptom and gastroesophageal reflux should be sought for each patient prior to surgical intervention. Without this evidence, a medical trial should be given.

It is hoped that, by following this approach and appropriately educating parents, much of the formula changes and use of antispasmodic agents, which are currently used widely for "spitting," will be avoided.

ANNOTATED BIBLIOGRAPHY

Carre IJ: The natural history of the partial thoracic stomach (hiatus hernia) in children. Arch Dis Child 34:344–353, 1959. (Classic study of a particular group of patients with gastroesophageal reflux.)

Jeffrey HE, Rahilly P, Read DJ: Multiple causes of asphyxia in infants at high risk for sudden infant death. Arch Dis Child 58:92–100, 1983. (Among other potential mechanisms of asphyxia, reflux is found in 55 of 58 "near-miss" infants.)

Meyers WF, Roberts CC, Johnson DG, Herbst JJ: Value of tests for evaluation of gastroesophageal reflux in children. J Pediatr Surg 20:515–520, 1985. (Comparison of the tests in sensitivity and specificity for gastroesophageal reflux.)

Orenstein SR, Whitington PF, Orenstein DM: The infant seat as treatment for gastroesophageal reflux. N Engl J Med 309:760–763, 1983. (Study on the effect of position on gastroesophageal reflux.)

Pearl RH, Robie DK, Ein SH et al: Complications of gastroesophageal antireflux surgery in neurologically impaired versus neurologically normal children. J Pediatr Surg 25:1169–1173, 1990. (Neurologically impaired children have a failure complication rate from fundoplication that is much higher than that found in neurologically normal infants.)

Tsou VM, Young RM, Hart MH, Vanderhoof JA: Elevated plasma aluminum levels in normal infants receiving antacids containing aluminum. Pediatrics 87:148–151, 1991. (Infants younger than 6 months of age may be at risk for aluminum toxicity when taking aluminum-containing antacids.)

Werlin SL, Dodds WJ, Hogan WJ et al: Mechanisms of gastroesophageal reflux in children. J Pediatr 97:244–249, 1980. (Manometric study of reflux that parallels the study in adults.)

Winter HS, Madara JL, Stafford RJ et al: Intraepithelial eosinophils: A new diagnostic criterion for reflux esophagitis. Gastroenterology 83:818–823, 1982. (Presence of esophageal intraepithelial eosinophils correlated with abnormal acid clearance determined by esophageal *p*H probe monitoring.)

103
Acute Abdominal Pain
Samuel N. Nurko

It is the frequent and often difficult task of the pediatrician to evaluate a child with sudden onset of severe abdominal pain. The differential diagnosis is large, but the pediatrician's first obligation is to decide whether a true emergency—whether surgical or medical—exists.

Appendicitis, usually the parents' major concern, must also be a primary concern of the physician. In the absence of acute abdominal signs and symptoms, time is available to observe and cautiously approach diagnosis and therapy.

PATHOPHYSIOLOGY

Abdominal pain results from a complex series of physiologic processes that often make the pain difficult for the patient and the physician to interpret. However, clues to the disease process may be provided by the location and character of the pain.

In general, visceral pain is dull and diffuse whereas parietal pain is sharp and localized. Visceral pain fibers are located in the muscular wall of hollow viscera and the capsule of solid viscera. Many organs have common innervation with a low concentration of nerve endings, leading to poor localization of pain. The location is sensed in the path of innervation and is almost always midline. Pain from the liver, pancreas, biliary tree, stomach, and upper small bowel is generally felt in the epigastrium. The distal small bowel, cecum, appendix, and ascending colon send pain signals to the periumbilical region. The distal intestine, urinary tract, and pelvic organs are sensed in the suprapubic area. Visceral nerves are stimulated by tension and stretching rather than cutting, tearing, or crushing. Tissue congestion and inflammation tend to sensitize nerve endings and lower their threshold to stimuli. The exact mechanism by which tissue inflammation and ischemia cause visceral pain is unclear.

Parietal pain, on the other hand, is mediated by stimuli such as acute inflammation, in the parietal peritoneum. The sensation is usually more intense and is much better localized because of the greater concentration of nerve endings in the skin. Lateralization of a process is usually possible. Referred pain has many of the characteristics of parietal pain but is felt in remote areas enervated by the same nerves as the affected organ. Pain is referred when visceral stimuli become overwhelming.

CLINICAL PRESENTATION

Acute abdominal pain is a presenting feature of many diseases. The most important are conditions that will deteriorate rapidly without surgical intervention. They must be quickly differentiated from nonsurgical problems. Unfortunately, many signs and symptoms are found in both surgical and nonsurgical patients with equal frequency. It is difficult to define diagnostic criteria that are disease specific.

It should be emphasized that a careful history and physical examination (including a rectal examination) are mandatory because they provide important information regarding the diagnosis and enable the pediatrician to arrive at a correct assessment in the majority of the cases. Yet, in some instances and despite a careful evaluation, the diagnostic dilemma is often resolved only after laparotomy.

An abdomen with findings that suggest surgery will be needed is referred to as an *acute abdomen*. Generalizations can be made that will aid in the diagnosis. Symptoms are usually progressive, and abdominal pain and tenderness are typically well localized, often with rebound. Nausea, vomiting, and anorexia are associated but nonspecific symptoms. It is characteristic of an acute abdomen that pain precedes the onset of vomiting. The onset of pain simultaneously with, or after, vomiting suggests gastroenteritis. A moderate temperature elevation is common but may also be seen in nonsurgical diseases. Acute pain that is steady for more than 6 hours is usually surgical. Repeat examinations at intervals by the same observer are often the most helpful method of identifying an acute abdomen. The goal is to intervene surgically before a ruptured viscus, intra-abdominal bleeding, or strangulation ischemia develops.

The character of a pain can sometimes be used to distinguish between diseases. A duodenal ulcer is often described as burning or gnawing; intestinal obstruction as crampy; and acute appendicitis as achy. The significance of intensity is difficult to evaluate except at its extremes. The perception of painful stimuli can be modified by both central and peripheral neurologic processes. Psychological and emotional factors may also affect how pain is sensed by a person.

DIFFERENTIAL DIAGNOSIS

In evaluating a child with acute abdominal pain, it is necessary to decide from the beginning if the problem is medical or surgical.

Appendicitis is the most common disease requiring surgery in childhood. The true incidence is unknown, but it is estimated that between 7% and 12% of a population will develop appendicitis at some time during their lives. It may occur at any age, but it is most common in the teenage and young adult years. Appendicitis is much less common in children younger than 2 years of age (less than 1% of all cases of appendicitis) and is rare in those younger than 1 year of age. The classic presentation is periumbilical crampy pain progressing to constant right lower quadrant pain in a child with fever, anorexia, vomiting, and leukocytosis. The process typically evolves steadily over 12 hours. Thus, repeat examinations at 4 to 6 hours intervals often clarify uncertain diagnoses. Atypical presentations are common, particularly in the younger age groups where rupture found at the time of surgery has been reported in 40% to 65%. An infant with appendicitis may present with only irritability, discomfort on movement, and flexed hips; and if his inflamed appendix is retrocecal, there may be no abdominal wall tenderness. It may hurt to cry so the child may be silent even though he or she is in pain. Appendicitis must be considered in any ill-looking child with a changing abdominal examination and no obvious alternative cause.

A perforated viscus, an obstruction with strangulation, and a ruptured ectopic pregnancy are common surgical emergencies of the abdomen in childhood and must also be identified as quickly as possible. Other causes of acute abdominal pain are likely to evolve more slowly, allowing time for observation and evaluation.

Conditions that most often mimic an acute surgical abdomen are gastroenteritis, urinary tract infection, and mesenteric adenitis. *Gastroenteritis* may present as severe abdominal pain, which is usually diffuse and crampy but may mimic the more localized symptoms of appendicitis. Profuse diarrhea commonly differentiates gastroenteritis from appendicitis, but diarrhea is seen in about 15% of patients with appendicitis, probably caused by irritation of the colon by the inflamed appendix. Headache, fever, and chills early in the course tend to favor a viral process.

Infections of the urinary tract may also present with severe abdominal pain and tenderness. High fever and chills point toward pain from this cause. Acute pyelonephritis may be present without symptoms of dysuria. Differentiation from appendicitis can be difficult because an inflamed pelvic appendix may cause urinary frequency and urgency. Pyuria is a common finding in appendicitis and other diffuse intra-abdominal processes.

Mesenteric adenitis is found in approximately 11% of children treated surgically for appendicitis. Mesenteric adenitis is a diagnosis made at laparotomy and generally cannot be differentiated from appendicitis until surgery is performed. Primary peritonitis is another diagnosis that may be made at laparotomy. However, because this is more common in a child who has other chronic illnesses such as leukemia in remission or nephrotic syndrome, a diagnostic paracentesis prior to surgery may be helpful. If the patient has gram-positive diplococci or if the fluid is nonpurulent (in contrast, fluid from secondary peritonitis is usually grossly purulent with organisms present), treatment with intravenous antibiotics and watchful waiting may be the preferred treatment. Some cases of primary peritonitis are caused by gram-negative rods, and, if found, a paracentesis would not be helpful in differentiating primary from secondary (i.e., from a ruptured viscus) peritonitis. Therefore, in that situation, a laparotomy should be carried out expeditiously.

Intussusception is one of the most common causes of abdominal pain in infancy. Severe colicky pain that is paroxysmal and sometimes manifested only by screaming in the very young patient alternating with quiescent periods with or without vomiting is intussusception until proven otherwise. The pain is usually periumbilical and more severe than that caused by gastroenteritis. The classic presentation includes a right upper quadrant mass (70% of cases) and currant jelly stools (60%), which are, however, a late finding. Early, kidney-ureter-bladder and upright films of the abdomen may appear normal. A barium enema frequently reduces idiopathic intussusception and should be performed on an emergency basis, but only within the first 24 hours of presentation. Surgical reduction is necessary when peritonitis has developed, a pathologic lead point has been identified, or radiologic reduction has been unsuccessful.

Meckel's diverticulum can occur at any age but is also most common in children younger than 2 years of age. It usually presents as painless rectal bleeding but rarely becomes inflamed and mimics appendicitis. Meckel's diverticulum may serve as a lead point for intussusception and may occasionally perforate.

Several other conditions that present as acute abdominal pain are common in infancy. Incarcerated hernias do not have to be strangulated to cause symptoms. An incarcerated hernia will cause abdominal pain, and a tender mass will be noted over the area of the external ring. Another cause of lower abdominal pain in boys is testicular torsion, although the usual presentation is scrotal pain (see Chap. 118). Hirschsprung's disease may cause an intermittent obstruction from retained feces and may progress to enterocolitis and perforation. Obstructive symptoms early in life may represent midgut volvulus. These patients are often too young to express abdominal pain. Thus, an infant who has been perfectly healthy and suddenly develops a refusal to eat, bile stain vomiting, obstipation, and abdominal distention should have a midgut volvulus secondary to malrotation ruled out immediately. Trauma and child abuse must also always be considered.

Other gastrointestinal diseases that present as acute abdominal pain include peptic ulcer disease, biliary tract disease, *Yersinia* enterocolitis, and, less commonly, pancreatitis, inflammatory bowel disease, and gastrointestinal tumors. Peptic ulcer disease can be seen in any age group but is most easily recognized when the child is verbal and can localize the pain and its relation to meals. In infancy, vomiting may be the only symptom. Pancreatitis presents as a steady epigastric pain that often radiates to the back. The diagnosis is difficult and is confirmed by laboratory and radiologic means. Cholecystitis may present as right upper quadrant or epigastric pain. Cholangitis is usually associated with jaundice. Crohn's disease during an acute flare may resemble appendicitis. However, patients usually present for an elective rather than emergent evaluation because of the chronicity of the disease. *Yersinia* enterocolitis may also be confused with appendicitis because fever, vomiting, and abdominal tenderness may overshadow diarrhea. A diagnosis can be made by appropriate stool culture.

Many common causes of acute abdominal pain are not diseases of the gastrointestinal tract. Pneumonia (particularly of the right lower lobe) is a frequently overlooked etiology. No child should be taken to surgery without an evaluation of the chest for pneumonia. An examination of the lower lobes is probably the most useful role of the plain abdominal film in evaluating a child for appendicitis. Streptococcal pharyngitis and tonsillitis may also be associated with abdominal pain and fever.

Symptoms of diabetic ketoacidosis include severe abdominal pain, nausea, vomiting, and anorexia. Many newly diagnosed diabetics present mimicking appendicitis. Caution must be used with known diabetics who may develop diabetic ketoacidosis secondary to true appendicitis. Acute rheumatic fever may present with fever and abdominal pain in its early stages. Henoch-Schönlein purpura presents with gastrointestinal symptoms before the characteristic rash in 18% of patients. Hemophilia, hemolytic uremic syndrome, and sickle cell disease are other hematologic diseases that can have severe abdominal pain. Children with leukemia may have abdominal pain secondary to their disease. The development of acute appendicitis becomes a serious problem in a child who has leukemia or another immunosuppressed state. Continuing immunosuppressive therapy may mask a serious underlying abdominal illness. These children should be seen early in the course of their ailment, and surgery should also be performed early.

Gynecologic disorders commonly present with acute abdominal pain in adolescent girls. Pelvic inflammatory disease can be difficult to differentiate from appendicitis. Nausea and vomiting tend to be more common in appendicitis. The symptoms of pelvic inflammatory disease usually last longer at presentation and may often begin within 1 week of menses. There may be a prior history of venereal disease. Physical findings that differentiate pelvic inflammatory disease are bilateral adnexal tenderness, bilateral peritoneal signs, and cervical motion tenderness (see Chap. 121). Ectopic pregnancy, pelvic endometriosis, corpus luteal hematoma, ovarian cyst, chronic salpingitis, and mittelschmerz must also be considered.

A rare cause of acute abdominal pain is hepatic porphyria. A first attack may consist of fever, vomiting, and epigastric or right iliac fossa pain. Symptoms rarely begin before adolescence. A diagnosis is made by finding porphyrins in the urine and stool. Pain from renal and ureteral calculi is usually in the costovertebral angle area. When the stone migrates, the location of the pain may be expressed anywhere along this path and may extend down into the genital area.

WORK-UP

Identification of an acute abdomen is the priority in children presenting with acute abdominal pain. Reliable predictors of surgically correctable disease are localized pain, the pattern of migratory pain classically described in appendicitis, rebound tenderness on examination, and elevated polymorphonuclear leukocyte count. A diagnosis must be based on a careful history and physical examination.

History

A large number of acute abdominal conditions can be diagnosed by considering carefully the history of onset. The age of the patient is important because certain conditions occur only within particular age groups. For example, acute intussusception rarely occurs in children older than 2 years of age. A detailed history is essential to determine the timing, location, and character of the pain. The child with peritonitis will typically complain of pain exacerbated by coughing, jumping, or jiggling. However, if the peritonitis has

been present for a while and is walled off, the child may manifest a sense of well-being. The child with appendicitis will sometimes not be able to climb stairs or stand up straight. It should be noted whether vomiting is present and whether it preceded or followed the onset of pain. Diarrhea and urinary tract symptoms are less specific but may be important. It is crucial to identify a history of predisposing disease such as diabetes, sickle cell disease, hemophilia, inflammatory bowel disease, pancreatitis, venereal disease, pelvic inflammatory disease, pregnancy, recurrent pneumonia, or urinary tract infection. Previous abdominal surgery and trauma are important considerations, and any suggestion of child abuse must be pursued.

Physical Examination

During a complete physical examination, including a rectal and pelvic examination, the physician must look for signs of peritonitis or localized tenderness. Inconclusive examinations should be repeated by the same physician in 4 to 6 hours to rule out progressive disease. Signs of acute fluid or blood loss into the abdomen require immediate surgery. A right upper quadrant mass suggests intussusception. The chest should be examined for signs of pneumonia. The inguinal and femoral areas should be inspected for evidence of an incarcerated hernia and testicular torsion.

A precise knowledge of anatomy is important. This starts with those structures that are the least variable in their position—the voluntary muscles and cerebrospinal nerves. Their examination is important because they can be irritated directly or reflexly by inflammatory changes in the intraabdominal organs (e.g., diaphragmatic rigidity in cases of a subphrenic abscess, psoas irritation in appendicitis, or obturator internus problems in pelvic inflammation). The distribution of the segmental nerves is also important. For example, loin pain occurs with testicular radiation and shoulder pain with diaphragmatic irritation.

Just as knowledge of anatomy is important in the evaluation of inflammatory lesions, a precise knowledge of physiology is useful in the evaluation of obstructive lesions. A large array of abdominal pathology arises in tubes whose walls are composed mainly of smooth muscle, and it is important to remember that these abdominal viscera are not sensitive to stimuli such as crushing, cutting, or tearing. The pain arises from stretching, distention, or excessive contraction against an obstruction

Laboratory Tests

The laboratory evaluation must include a complete blood cell count with differential and urinalysis. Polymorphonuclear blood cell count is commonly elevated in appendicitis and other surgical emergencies. An elevated total white blood cell count is found in many surgical and nonsurgical diseases and thus is less useful. A urinalysis is essential to rule out pyelonephritis, renal calculi, hemolytic-uremic syndrome or Henoch-Schönlein purpura. Some red or white blood cells may, however, be seen in children with appendicitis. Glycosuria is an important finding suggesting that the patient has diabetes.

A radiologic evaluation should be dictated by individual presentation. Plain films are helpful in identifying intestinal obstruction, free intra-abdominal air, and pneumonia. The search for a rare calcified appendicolith does not warrant the use of an abdominal series in any child suspected of having appendicitis. Barium enemas are not diagnostic for appendicitis but may be therapeutic for intussusception. Ultrasound examination and intravenous pyelography are reserved for special circumstances and are usually unnecessary in the routine evaluation of acute abdominal pain.

However, abdominal/pelvic ultrasound examination is particularly useful when biliary, pancreatic, or gynecologic/obstetric problems are suspected or to evaluate for complications of appendicitis.

MANAGEMENT AND INDICATIONS FOR REFERRAL

A surgical exploration is indicated in any child with an acute abdomen and progressive signs of deterioration for which there is no satisfactory explanation. In children with suspected appendicitis, prolonged observation and repetition of laboratory studies serve only to increase the risk of perforation. The morbidity associated with a perforated appendix remains higher than that associated with simple appendicitis, despite modern antibiotic therapy. Expectant therapy for appendicitis is not indicated, and a referral to a pediatric surgeon should be made immediately when an acute abdomen is suspected. Sedatives and analgesics should be withheld until the surgeon's first examination. Subsequently, sedation may relieve discomfort and actually improve the abdominal examination.

A suspected ruptured ectopic pregnancy must be referred to a gynecologist or surgeon immediately. A referral for a pelvic examination may be indicated in adolescent girls with acute abdominal pain in whom a proper examination has not been possible and when the diagnosis is unclear.

Intussusception must be reduced as soon as possible with a barium enema. A delay may lead to a loss of bowel due to ischemia. A pediatric surgeon should be consulted quickly if the radiologist is unable to reduce the intussusception or if there are signs of peritonitis.

The prognosis for a child with an acute abdomen is excellent if the condition is treated appropriately. Overdiagnosis of appendicitis is common in most surgical practices. Fifteen to 20% of patients (30% of adolescent girls) presenting with right lower quadrant pain have a normal appendix at surgery. The 15% morbidity associated with a negative laparotomy is accepted in an attempt to avoid the complications of a perforated appendix and peritonitis.

Therapy for acute abdominal pain of nonsurgical origin varies depending on the patient's diagnosis. A follow-up is essential to ensure that acute symptoms do not become chronic complaints.

ANNOTATED BIBLIOGRAPHY

Bongard F, Landers DV, Lewis F: Differential diagnosis of appendicitis and pelvic inflammatory disease. Am J Surg 150:90–96, 1985. (Discussion of the differential diagnosis between appendicitis and pelvic inflammatory disease.)

Cheung LY, Ballinger WF: Manifestations and diagnosis of gastrointestinal diseases. In Hardy JD (ed): Textbook of Surgery, 2nd ed, p 460. Philadelphia, JB Lippincott, 1988. (Good overview.)

Hatch EI: The acute abdomen in children. Pediatr Clin North Am 32:1151–1164, 1985. (Discussion of appendicitis and its differential diagnosis.)

Karp MP, Caldorola VA, Cooney DR et al: The avoidable excesses in the management of perforated appendicitis in children. J Pediatr Surg 21:506–510, 1986. (Discussion of alternatives in the surgical care of appendicitis.)

Nauta RJ, Magnant C: Observation vs. operation for abdominal pain in the right lower quadrant: Roles of the clinical exam and the leukocyte count. Am J Surg 151:746–748, 1986. (Good discussion of evaluation.)

Silen W (ed): Cope's Early Diagnosis of the Acute Abdomen, 17th ed. London, Oxford University Press, 1987. (Classic book of the acute abdomen.)

104
Recurrent Abdominal Pain
Samuel N. Nurko

Recurrent abdominal pain is one of the most common and challenging symptoms encountered in the practice of general pediatrics; and in a gastroenterologic subspecialty clinic, it represents one of the most frequently made diagnoses. Recurrent abdominal pain is usually defined as three or more episodes of pain occurring over 3 months severe enough to interfere with routine activity. It has been estimated that even though from 10% to 18% of school-age children suffer from recurrent abdominal pain, a diagnosable "organic" pathology can only be found in less than 10%. The physician must balance the fear of missing a treatable diagnosis against clinical wisdom that suggests a low likelihood of organic disease. Even though emotional factors are often identified to help explain the attacks, recurrent abdominal pain remains a serious disease with a potential for long-term morbidity. In this chapter the focus is on the diagnosis of the functional type of recurrent abdominal pain, with emphasis on "organic" causes in the differential diagnosis. The therapy must be compassionate, redirecting the patient's focus of attention with reassurance and support.

PATHOPHYSIOLOGY

When no "organic" cause is found, environmental and psychosocial stresses are hypothesized to cause the pain. Commonly, children with recurrent abdominal pain have parents who also complain of chronic abdominal pain, possibly suggesting a genetic influence. More likely, however, abdominal pain is a means of communicating to each other that an underlying problem exists. Patients commonly exhibit "internalizing" behavior characterized by anxiety, mild depression, withdrawal, and low self-esteem. This behavior is fostered within a family structure characterized by maternal depression, overprotectiveness, rigidity, and lack of conflict resolution.

Stress associated with school and social performance, emotional conflicts brought on by development and changing maturity, and the real or threatened loss of a friend or family are frequent in the histories of children with recurrent abdominal pain. An illness may reveal a vulnerability that had previously remained hidden. Symptoms that may have been very real at first may continue supported by secondary gain. The extreme concern of either the parents or the physician serves only to reinforce the symptoms.

It is unclear why these children respond to these stresses by complaining of abdominal pain. Most children do not. Some children may be more sensitive to painful body signals, a sensitivity that may be genetically or environmentally determined. On the other hand, the signals may be sensed normally, but stress may accentuate pains that might otherwise go unnoticed. Pain may even be the result of a malfunction of a normal physiologic process. Hyperactivity of the autonomic nervous system, noted in many children with recurrent abdominal pain, may cause pain by altering intestinal motility. Constipation, giardiasis, and lactose intolerance also alter motility and stimulate the stretch receptors that cause pain. Each has been suggested as a cause of recurrent abdominal pain, but an inconsistent response to therapy has made it clear that many factors must be involved. It is possible, then, that recurrent abdominal pain represents an alteration in intestinal motor activity as a result of the effect of a heterogeneous group of physical and psychosocial stressful stimuli on a susceptible patient.

CLINICAL PRESENTATION

Recurrent abdominal pain typically presents in children 5 to 10 years old, although the diagnosis can be considered in children between the ages of 3 and 16 years. It is more common in girls than in boys. The incidence is greater in women, particularly in the later years. Onset of symptoms after the age of 14 is rare and most consistent with the diagnosis of the *irritable bowel syndrome*. If the child is younger than 4 years, a more thorough work-up is necessary. Children with recurrent abdominal pain often appear relatively unconcerned about their problem.

Patients usually complain of a dull, colicky, periumbilical pain that is intermittent on a daily basis with a complete recovery in between episodes. In more than half the patients, each episode lasts less than 1 hour, and less than 3 hours in another 40%. Clustering of pain episodes lasting several weeks to months has been described. Continuous pain is rare, occurring in less than 10% of children.

The pain is rarely focal, and localization away from the umbilicus should suggest another diagnosis. The characterization of the pain is usually described in vague terms, and no distinct association between the pain and eating, position, or time of day can be found. Behavior patterns and daily activities are interrupted by the episodes but do not always seem consistent with the severity of the pain. Abdominal pain does not awaken the patient from sleep, but it may interfere with the ability of the patient to fall asleep. Associated symptoms may include a low-grade temperature, pallor, headache, and vomiting. Constipation is also often seen. One of these associated symptoms may occur in up to 50% to 70% of cases. Over-the-counter medications, such as antacids and anticholinergics, do not alleviate the pain. Complex rituals including application of hot packs, careful repositioning, and gentle rubbing by a parent are the sole providers of relief.

WORK-UP

An evaluation of the child with recurrent abdominal pain must be carefully organized from the start. A haphazard approach will destroy the family's confidence in accepting the physician's diagnosis and recommendations. Unnecessary diagnostic tests and referrals may only reinforce the already problematic symptoms.

It should be made clear early on that there is a low likelihood of finding an organic etiology and that there is no physical danger to the child. This idea is often difficult for the family to accept because the symptoms are so upsetting. The possibility that the symptoms are stress related and that counseling may be an important part of therapy should be introduced early to all patients with recurrent abdominal pain. The physician must communicate an understanding that the symptoms are real and he or she must reassure the patient that complaints will not be ignored.

History

The initial detailed history must rule out suspicion of an underlying organic illness and look for evidence of emotional stress or behavior problems. Routine questions including the onset, character, duration, and location of pain should be asked. Aggravating and relieving factors should be sought. A nutritional history will often help characterize the nature of the complaint. Gastrointestinal symptoms, including bowel pattern, must be examined for changes. Several commonly used medications, such as tetracycline and erythromycin, can cause abdominal pain. Constant attention must be paid to the possibility of a hidden agenda throughout the interview.

Key points to look for in the history are pain that awakens the patient from sleep, pain focal in nature and referred to areas away from the umbilicus, persistent fever, weight loss or growth failure, bilious vomiting, gastrointestinal bleeding, or urinary tract symptoms. Each suggests that the cause of the pain is more likely organic and that the diagnostic approach should be modified.

In his classic monograph, Apley described several emotional factors commonly identified in patients with recurrent abdominal pain: marital discord between parents, rigid or demanding parenting styles, a detached father, an ill or depressed mother, school problems, and a perfectionist personality in the child. A death in the family or an important upcoming examination may be elicited in the history. It is important to note the interaction between patient and parents during the interview. Commonly, the child will be eager to talk and relatively unconcerned. Conflict within the family is commonly denied. The home environment tends to discourage the child's independence.

A family history is often positive for relatives with abdominal pain. Personal issues concerning drug abuse, sexual activity, and pregnancy must be discussed privately with the child. Time should be spent focusing on the patient's friends, interests, and goals. Behavioral or emotional problems may be more obvious in this context.

Physical Examination

The physical examination is usually unremarkable, but it must be thorough to help rule out organic disease. Emphasis is on overall impression of "wellness," growth pattern, hepatomegaly or splenomegaly, blood pressure, abdominal tenderness, abdominal masses (particularly in the right lower quadrant), costovertebral pain, perianal pathology, skin alterations, joint swelling, and neurologic examination. A rectal examination should be performed and stool tested for occult blood.

The patient rarely has abdominal pain during his or her initial examination. It is useful to reexamine the patient during an attack. Physical findings and signs will not usually match the severity of the complaints. Remember that a diagnosis of recurrent abdominal pain does not preclude the onset of a new acute disease. Both the history and physical examination must be reviewed at each contact, with close attention to changes from previous examinations.

Laboratory Tests

Laboratory tests should be kept to a minimum. The initial tests that need to be performed are shown in Table 104-1. Depending on the above results, and the history and physical examination, other tests may be necessary. It is important to remember that extensive testing may only serve to entrench the symptoms by supporting a secondary gain or some other emotional etiology.

Less than 5% of all cases will have an organic lesion if

Table 104-1. Laboratory work-up

Initial Screening Tests
Complete blood cell count with differential and reticulocytes
Erythrocyte sedimentation rate
Total protein and albumin
Urinalysis and urine culture
Stool guaiac
Stool for ova and parasites

Additional Tests
These should be performed only if indicated by the history, findings on physical examination, or screening laboratory tests

Lactose breath test
Liver function tests
Pancreatic amylase and lipase
Serum electrolytes, blood urea nitrogen, and creatinine
Abdominal ultrasound
Upper gastrointestinal series with small bowel follow-through
Barium enema
Intravenous pyelogram
Esophagogastroduodenoscopy
Colonoscopy
Electroencephalography
Other (e.g., porphyrins, lead)

symptoms suggestive of organic illness are not also present. If initial screening tests are negative, further testing with an upper gastrointestinal series, esophagoduodenoscopy, or barium enema are rarely helpful. However, if symptoms or screening tests suggest an organic etiology for the pain, the diagnostic evaluation should depend on the specific presentation.

DIFFERENTIAL DIAGNOSIS

Even though most children with recurrent abdominal pain do not have an organic pathology, there are many diseases that can present as chronic abdominal pain (Table 104-2). Most can be suspected after a careful history and examination or if there are abnormalities in the initial screening tests.

The first step in the diagnosis of recurrent abdominal pain is to verify that the symptoms are chronic. Acute abdominal pain is discussed in Chapter 103. Recurrent abdominal pain can be distinguished from most other causes of chronic abdominal pain that present as signs and symptoms of organic disease. An ill-looking child or a child with persistent fever, weight loss, growth failure, or anemia suggests that recurrent abdominal pain is not the correct diagnosis. Focal abdominal tenderness, pain that awakens a child at night, bilious vomiting, hematemesis, hematochezia, or melena suggest a gastrointestinal etiology. *Urinary tract disease* is the most common organic cause of recurrent abdominal pain and must be considered even without symptoms of dysuria and frequency.

Peptic ulcer disease needs to be considered when evaluating a child with recurrent abdominal pain. Abdominal pain is the presenting symptom in up to 55% of children

Table 104-2. Organic Causes of Abdominal Pain

Gastrointestinal	Extraintestinal
Peptic ulcer disease	*Renal*
Gastroesophageal reflux	Urinary tract infections
Constipation	Ureteropelvic junction
Lactose intolerance	obstruction
Inflammatory bowel disease	Renal calculus
Pancreatitis	
Cholecystitis and	*Gynecologic Problems*
cholelithiasis	Teratomas
Intermittent volvulus	Pregnancy
Appendiceal colic	Pelvic inflammatory disease
Intermittent small bowel	Dysmenorrhea
obstruction	
Infections (parasites, bacteria)	*Other*
	Hernias
	Lead intoxication
	Abdominal epilepsy
	Porphyrias
	Musculoskeletal disorders
	Conversion reactions
	Substance abuse

with this disease, and the pain may be atypical of the classic descriptions of ulcer pain. Ulcer disease should be suspected if there is a positive family history; if the pain is epigastric, associated with meals, present at night, or awakens the child; and if there is associated vomiting, weight loss, or signs of gastrointestinal blood loss. It has even been suggested that an ulcer should always be excluded in an adolescent before a diagnosis of recurrent abdominal pain is made.

Adolescents present their own special problems. Dramatic behavioral changes associated with abdominal pain should raise the suspicion of substance abuse. A sexual history is essential in each postpubertal patient because concern over pregnancy, venereal disease, or homosexuality may cause a healthy-appearing child to complain of pain. Adolescent girls may have a higher incidence of organic disease because of gynecologic disorders. Mittelschmerz, endometriosis, and pelvic inflammatory disease must always be considered.

Lactose and sorbitol intolerance should always be considered in the presence of diarrhea, bloating, and increased flatulence. Controversy exists, however, as to the exact role that carbohydrate malabsorption plays in the majority of children with recurrent abdominal pain.

Diagnoses difficult to distinguish from recurrent abdominal pain based on symptoms alone are giardiasis and constipation. Remember that a positive diagnosis does not eliminate concurrent psychosomatic illness and that treatment often fails to relieve the symptoms. Early Crohn's disease may present as recurrent abdominal pain but is unlikely in the absence of growth failure, anemia, and blood in the stool. Henoch-Schönlein purpura (HSP), celiac disease, and *Yersinia* enterocolitis most commonly present as an acute disease but may each mimic recurrent abdominal pain. Pancreatitis can be chronic but should be differentiated on the

basis of presentation. Meckel's diverticulum and intestinal duplications almost never present with pain. Causes of abdominal pain that are often forgotten include lead poisoning, abdominal epilepsy, osteomyelitis of the spine, psoas abscess, and abdominal, inguinal, and femoral hernias. Each must be considered as the evaluation progresses.

MANAGEMENT

Primary care physicians are usually the first professionals involved in treating children with recurrent abdominal pain. Commonly, their approach is to exclude organic disease rather than to make a positive diagnosis of "nonorganic" abdominal pain. By the time the child is referred to a gastroenterologist, 50% will have had the pain from 1 to 5 years, and the specialist usually confronts very frustrated parents who have not been reassured by all the negative tests. It is therefore very important that if a diagnosis of nonorganic recurrent abdominal pain is made that it be communicated to the parents as a positive, and not a negative, diagnosis.

The treatment of recurrent abdominal pain is based on the reassurance that no serious organic disease exists and that the child is in no physical danger. The discussions with the family should emphasize that recurrent abdominal pain is common and that many possible causes exist. Stressful events and emotional issues should be identified as possible contributory factors. Counseling should be initiated to help the child and family deal with symptoms that may not immediately disappear. Normalization of life-style, including an immediate return to school and a de-emphasis of pain episodes, is essential. A plan for follow-up and support by the physician should be outlined clearly so that the patient and family do not feel abandoned. If an organic cause for the pain is found, treatment should, of course, be begun.

Lactose-intolerant patients should receive a lactose-free diet for 2 weeks as a therapeutic trial. If there is a positive response, this should be continued for longer periods; depending on the symptoms, small quantities of milk may be added later. The use of high-fiber diets has been advocated for the treatment of irritable bowel syndrome in adults, and this may also be beneficial for the treatment of children with recurrent abdominal pain, particularly those with constipation. The empiric use of antacids and H_2 blockers has been advocated by some while the diagnostic work-up is in progress, but there are pitfalls to this approach. Even in the presence of well-documented peptic ulcer disease a positive response with symptom elimination may take some time, and there may also be a strong placebo effect. If a good response is obtained, and there are no signs of severe illness, then a complete course of medication should be given and further work-up reserved if symptoms recur.

Other medications are not indicated for the treatment of recurrent abdominal pain. Sedatives and analgesics may be dangerous and may lead to either psychological or physiologic dependence. Antispasmodics offer no consistent help and may even aggravate the symptoms. Placebos will serve only to undermine the trust on which the physician–patient relationship and, therefore, recurrent abdominal pain therapy is based.

INDICATIONS FOR REFERRAL

A referral should rarely be necessary for children with recurrent abdominal pain. If the rapport between the physician and patient is good, the parents usually will not insist on looking to other physicians for other answers. A specialist may be needed when other signs or symptoms of organic illness are present.

A surgeon offers little help unless an acute abdominal problem is suspected. Chronic appendicitis should not be considered a cause of recurrent abdominal pain. Appendectomy usually fails to relieve symptoms. An exploratory laparotomy without persistent fever, focal tenderness, palpable mass, or obstructive symptoms is not indicated.

Peptic ulcer disease is often considered when evaluating a child with chronic abdominal pain. Classic symptoms of epigastric pain at night and during fasting that is relieved by food may or may not be present. A referral to a gastroenterologist for an upper gastrointestinal series or an esophago-duodenoscopy should be considered only in the case of classic symptoms, a strong family history, night pain, weight loss, persistent vomiting, an abnormal complete blood cell count, or stool positive for occult blood. The gastroenterologist may also offer a lactose breath hydrogen test for the diagnosis of lactose intolerance. In practice, a lactose breath hydrogen test gives no better diagnosis than a lactose-free diet trial.

Abdominal epilepsy is an often mentioned but uncommon cause of intermittent abdominal pain. It should be suspected only when pain is associated with an impairment of consciousness and postictal symptoms. A referral to a neurologist for an electroencephalogram is then indicated. This is a difficult diagnosis to make and will depend on an abnormal electroencephalogram during an episode of abdominal pain.

Evaluation by a child psychiatrist or psychologist should be undertaken if there is a clear conversion reaction, depression and anxiety, or maladaptive family behavior.

Hospitalization should only be necessary when the emotional environment at home has deteriorated so that observation in a neutral environment is deemed necessary. Because symptoms disappear in up to 50% of children who are hospitalized and hospitalization will reinforce the perception of the severity of the "illness," hospitalization is not usually recommended. If the child is admitted, a second opinion may be indicated to support the primary physician's diagnosis and management plan. The patient and family must not expect a battery of new tests. The opportunity to observe the patient alone and during an episode of pain should be taken. The length of hospital stay should be minimized to avoid fostering a dependence on the illness.

The treatment of the patient and family as a single unit is the key to success in recurrent abdominal pain. The family must understand and believe that a problem exists even if the definitive etiology of the pain cannot be found. Despite all the reassurance and understanding that the physician can offer, symptoms of abdominal pain are likely to persist, or change somatic form, as the child moves into adulthood. Recurrent abdominal pain is a signal that all is not well and deserves immediate intervention and often long-term care.

ANNOTATED BIBLIOGRAPHY

Apley J: The Child with Abdominal Pain, 2nd ed. Oxford, Blackwell Scientific Publications, 1975. (Classic monograph.)

Apley J, Hale B: Children with recurrent abdominal pain: How do they grow up? Br Med J 3:7, 1973. (Follow-up of a classic study looking at the effect of supportive therapy.)

Farrell MK: Abdominal pain. Pediatrics (Suppl) 74:955–957, 1984. (Good discussion of clinical features and counseling component of therapy.)

Feldman W, McGrath P, Hodgson C et al: The use of dietary fiber in the management of simple, childhood, idiopathic, recurrent abdominal pain. Am J Dis Child 130:1216–1218, 1985. (Use of a simple treatment.)

Levine MD, Rappaport LA: Recurrent abdominal pain in school children: The loneliness of the long-distance physician. Pediatr Clin North Am 31:969–991, 1984. (Excellent discussion of causes of recurrent abdominal pain.)

Middleton AW, Banning A: Recurrent abdominal pain in children. Aust Fam Physician 13:426–427, 1984. (Brief practical approach with emphasis on the emotional makeup of the family.)

Pineiro-Carrero VM, Andres JM, Davis RH et al: Abnormal gastro-duodenal motility in children and adolescents with recurrent functional abdominal pain. J Pediatr 113:820–825, 1988. (Description of some physiological intestinal alterations in this disorder.)

Tomamasa T, Hsu JY, Shigeta M et al: Statistical analysis of symptoms and signs in pediatric patients with peptic ulcer. J Pediatr Gastroenterol Nutr 5:711–715, 1986. (Highlight of "alarm" symptoms that suggest the presence of peptic ulcer disease.)

105

Acute Diarrhea

Samuel N. Nurko

Diarrheal disease continues to be one of the primary causes of morbidity and mortality in the third world. Although diarrheal disease in the United States is not such an overwhelming problem, in children younger than 2 years old, up to 20% of acute care visits to large metropolitan hospitals are related to diarrheal illness. Moreover, the incidence of hospital admissions for children younger than 1 year old is approximately 8 cases per 1000, and diarrhea accounts for as much as 10% of the potentially preventable deaths in children in the United States.

Diarrhea can be defined as an excessive loss of fluids and electrolytes in the stool. Any daily fecal loss exceeding 200 mL/m^2 is considered excessive. In infants, losses exceeding 20 mL/kg are considered significant. The transport of water across the intestinal mucosa is passive, and consideration of the pathophysiology of any type of diarrhea must center on the net transport of glucose, sodium, chloride, and amino acids that are the major determinants of intestinal water absorption.

PATHOPHYSIOLOGY

There are five mechanisms of diarrheal production:

1. *Osmotic*—This condition occurs when osmotically active particles are present in the intestinal lumen. Examples include the dumping syndrome, lactase deficiency, and overfeeding.
2. *Secretory diarrhea*—This condition results from the inhibition of ion absorption or stimulation of ion secretion. Examples are the secretory diarrheas that occur secondary to bacterial exotoxins or diarrheas secondary to substances produced by the body that activate secretion, such as gastrin in the Zollinger-Ellison syndrome.
3. *Deletion or inhibition of a normal active ion absorptive process*—This can be congenital, such as in the case of congenital chloridorrhea, or acquired, such as in bile salt deficiency and pancreatic enzyme deficiencies.
4. *Inflammation*—This is usually secondary to a decrease in the anatomic or functional areas, such as occurs in mucosal diseases like celiac sprue, after bacterial invasion, or after bowel resection.
5. *Abnormal intestinal motility*—Abnormally reduced peristalsis may allow bacterial overgrowth; rapid motility may reduce contact time between the small bowel mucosa and its contents.

CLINICAL PRESENTATION AND DIFFERENTIAL DIAGNOSIS

Acute diarrhea is usually a self-limited illness lasting a few days to a week. Persistent diarrhea typically persists longer than 2 weeks and may be associated with malabsorption, malnutrition, or both (see Chap. 106). Almost all acute diarrhea in children is caused by intestinal infections or food intolerance, although it can also be secondary to an infection outside the bowel, such as in the urinary or respiratory tracts. Other possibilities include food poisoning, inflammatory disorders (e.g., inflammatory bowel disease, hemolytic uremic syndrome, Henoch-Schönlein purpura), and iatrogenic causes (e.g., antibiotics, laxatives). The most common infectious agents that cause enteric infections vary worldwide and consist of viruses, bacteria, or parasites. In addition to the commonly associated pathogens (e.g., rotavirus), in recent years new pathogens have been associated with the development of acute diarrhea in normal hosts. These have included *Cryptosporidium, Aeromonas,* and other agents (Table 105-1). The identification of the causative agent in an episode of acute diarrhea may facilitate proper therapy. The presence of specific clinical manifestations alone is not pathognomonic of any causative agent, although certain symptoms suggest specific causes. For example, bacterial organisms that invade the mucosa often cause fever, and if the colon is primarily involved, abdominal pain, tenesmus, fecal urgency, and stools with blood and mucus (e.g., *Salmonella, Shigella,* and *Campylobacter*). Patients with secretory diarrhea have abdominal cramps with the passage of a low to a moderate number of large volume stools (e.g., cholera and enterotoxigenic *Escherichia coli*).

WORK-UP

History

It is important to obtain a thorough dietary record (e.g., breast-feeding, formulas), and changes in the diet should be correlated with stool frequency and form. A history of other family members with gastrointestinal complaints, travel or origin from areas where there is contamination of the water system, endemic infections, time spent in day care, or foods recently ingested are also important.

Inquiry should be made regarding previous growth, appreciating the fact that the failure to gain weight is usually secondary to hypocaloric intake. A family history should inquire about relatives with chronic diarrhea, cystic fibrosis, celiac sprue, inflammatory bowel disease, or other chronic conditions. The number, consistency, odor, and presence of blood or mucus of stools and other associated symptoms, particularly fever, vomiting, or abdominal cramps, should be described. Short incubation (less than 24 hours), short duration (less than 24 hours) illnesses are usually due to the ingestion of a preformed toxin. If the duration is several days, infection with an agent that produced enterotoxin or invasion is likely. The number of wet diapers and their dampness in the preceding 6- to 8-hour period is useful to gauge hydration.

Physical Examination

The physical examination should focus initially on the hydration status of the patient, after having rapidly assessed the airway and ventilation. Vital signs, particularly blood pressure and heart rate, should be monitored. Skin turgor, moistness of mucosal membranes, and tearing are useful. Weight/age and height/age should be determined to assess the nutritional status, and a careful abdominal and rectal examination should then be performed. A complete physical examination is mandatory to ensure that the symptoms are not a manifestation of either an extraintestinal

Table 105-1.   Causes of Acute Infectious Diarrhea

AGENTS	PATHOLOGIC/ PHYSIOLOGIC Toxic	Invasive	INCUBATION	AGE	DIARRHEA	DYSEN-TERY	BLOOD	FECAL WHITE BLOOD CELLS
Viral								
Rotavirus	0	Villous blunting	2–3 days	< 5 years; peaks 2 years	Watery	0	0	12%
Norwalk virus	0	+	1–3 days	All	46%	0	0	0
Bacterial								
Campylobacter fetus ss. *jejunum*	0	+ +	2–11 days	Any: epidemic 1–5 years 10–29 years	Initially watery	+ +	90%	85%
Salmonella	0	+ +	8–48 hours	Any	Foul-smelling mucous, loose	+	80%	75%
Shigella	+	+ +	36–72 hours	Any: peaks 2–10 years	Odorless, Mucous	+ +	+ +	84%
Escherichia coli								
Enterotoxigenic	+ +	0	24–48 hours	Any: peaks < 1 year	Profuse, watery	0	0	0
Enteroinvasive	0	+ +	46–72 hours	Any	Watery-mucoid	+ +	+	85%
Enteropathogenic	0 or +	0	24–48 hours	< 1 year	Watery-severe	+	0	0
Yersinia	+	+	4–10 days	Any: peaks 2 years	Watery	+	10%	10%–50%
Aeromonas hidrophilia	+ +	Rare	?	Highest in < 3 years	Watery	25%	Rare	—
Clostridium difficile	+	—	5–10 days	All	Profuse watery	—	+ +	50%
Parasitic								
Giardia	0	Duodenum	10–21 days	Any: peaks 4 years	Loose, watery foul-smelling	0	0	0
Amebiasis	—	+ +	7–21 days	All	Mucous, small amounts	+ +	+ +	85%–100%
Cryptosporidium	—	±	1–7 days	All	Profuse watery	—	—	—

infection (e.g., otitis) or a systemic disease (e.g., hemolytic uremic syndrome) and to determine if there is systemic toxicity.

Laboratory Tests

In the child with uncomplicated diarrhea and no evidence of dehydration or toxicity, an extensive evaluation is not appropriate. However, in the toxic, dehydrated patient, additional studies may assist in determining the etiology, the hydration status, and the presumptive need for specific therapy.

The examination of the stool is the single most important step in defining the diarrheal illness. It should be observed for color, consistency, odor, and the presence or absence of blood or mucus. A stool with a yeasty or acidic odor suggests carbohydrate malabsorption; a purulent odor suggests colitis. The stool pH should be obtained, and a pH less than 6 suggests carbohydrate malabsorption. A Clinitest should be performed, remembering that certain baby formulas (e.g., Nursoy) have nonreducing sugars, so that the stool needs to be hydrolyzed with hydrochloric acid before the Clinitest is performed. The presence or absence of blood should also be determined; it is more commonly found in colitic infections. An examination of the stool for fecal leukocytes is another method to narrow the diagnostic possibilities (see Table 105-1).

A culture of the stool should usually be reserved for

ABDOMINAL PAIN	FEVER	VOMITING	EXTRAINTESTINAL	SEASON	DURATION UNTREATED	ROUTE	OTHER
Mild	50%–75%	90%	Upper respiratory tract in 50%; dehydration	Winter	5–6 days	Fecal-oral; respiratory	Diagnosis by enzyme-linked immunosorbent assay
Mild	Rare	75%	0	0	1–3 days	Fecal-oral	Explosive; epidemic nature
Severe in 60%	80%	30%	Seizures; hemolytic-uremic syndrome; dehydration (all rare); failure to thrive	All year but peak in July	2–7 days	Fecal-oral; food and water; person to person	Relapse 20%; neonatal transmission; chronic diarrhea; failure to thrive
Moderate	75%	Usual	meningitis; osteomyelitis; failure to thrive	Warm	3–7 days	Animal or human source; food; fecal or oral	Infants at risk for invasive disease; increased risk in sickle-cell disease
Severe	50%–70%	Rare	Seizures in 12%–45%; Occasional bacteremia	Warm	7–14 days	Fecal; oral; rarely food	Common in day-care centers; dehydration rare
Crampy	20%; Low Grade	Common	Dehydration	Summer	3–10 days	Oral-fecal; food and water	Leading cause of travelers' diarrhea
Moderate	Common	0	0	?	?	Oral-fecal; food	Diagnosis by guinea pig test
Mild to 0	20%	Common	Severe dehydration	Fall	7–14 days	Oral-fecal; person to person	Epidemics in nurseries
Crampy 60%	50%–80%	40%	Mesenteric adenitis; arthritis; septicemia	Winter	14–21 days	Food; animals; oral-fecal	Chronic diarrhea can occur; may mimic appendicitis; serologic evaluation useful in epidemics
Mild	Rare	Young children	Rarely Sepsis; Liver	Summer peak	< 7 days; 25% up to 4 weeks	Drinking water	Geographic differences in symptoms; may cause travelers' diarrhea; diagnosed by trophozoites in fresh specimen
Moderate	Frequent	Frequent	Acute abdomen (uncommon)	0	Stops when antibiotics are stopped	—	Diagnosed by toxin measurement; Clostridium difficile common in normal newborns after antibiotic use
Crampy	0	Common	Growth retardation; synovitis	0	4–6 weeks	Person to person: water; food; cross species	Frequent in day-care centers; sprue-like syndrome
Moderate to severe	Rare self-limited	Rare	Liver abscess	0	< 7 days	Food	Fulminant colitis; ameba can present as acute diarrhea only
Moderate	Frequent	Frequent	In immunodeficient patients	0	48 hours–3 weeks	Fecal-oral Oral-fecal	Dehydration common; animal contact; rarely chronic

those patients in whom the results will alter the therapeutic plan. It should be performed in all children younger than 1 year old who are toxic, children with severe dehydration, as well as those with underlying hemoglobinopathies or immunocompromised states. Patients with fever and bloody diarrhea have a higher positive yield when a bacterial culture is obtained.

If many members are in the same family or day care, or if a family member is a food handler, cultures are indicated for epidemiologic reasons. The enzyme-linked immunosorbent assay (ELISA) for rotavirus may be useful in selected cases. Specialized facilities are necessary to identify enteropathogenic *Escherichia coli,* enterotoxigenic *E. coli,* and the invasive strains, and the test should be done in evaluat-

ing epidemics. Ova and parasitic examinations should be reserved for patients in whom there are suggestive epidemiologic and clinical data (e.g., areas where parasites are frequent, particularly in afebrile patients with bloody diarrhea), bacterial cultures are repeatedly negative, or the diarrhea lasts more than 1 week.

The value of a proctosigmoidoscopy with biopsy in patients with acute diarrhea is limited. It should be performed when pseudomembranous colitis is suspected, or in ill patients who have an underlying chronic illness or are immunosuppressed (e.g., patients with the acquired immunodeficiency syndrome). It is also indicated in patients with negative cultures and persistent symptoms, especially bloody diarrhea.

Table 105-2. Specific Treatment for Infectious Diarrhea

AGENT	INDICATIONS	TREATMENT	ALTERNATIVES	COMMENTS
Campylobacter	Gastroenteritis	None		Erythromycin does not change clinical course. It decreases Campylobacter excretion.
	Severe symptoms	Erythromycin, 40 mg/kg q6h for 5–7 days	Clindamycin, 300 mg q6h; tetracycline, 250 mg q6h for 5 days	
	Sepsis	Gentamicin, 5 mg/kg q8h for 2 weeks, or chloramphenicol, 75 mg/kg/d q6h for 2 weeks		
Salmonella	Carrier	None		
	Acute gastroenteritis	None		Concern that antibiotics may prolong the carrier state
	Bacteremia or enteric fever	Ampicillin, 200 mg/kg/d q4h for 2 weeks or Chloramphenicol, 75 mg/kg/d IV or PO q6h for 2 weeks	Trimethoprim/ sulfamethoxazole TMP, 10 mg/kg/d SMX, 50 mg/kg/d q12h for 2 weeks	
	Disseminated infection	Same, but for 4–6 weeks		
	Children < 3 mo with acute gastroenteritis and children with failure to thrive	Same for 2 weeks		
Shigella	All patients if symptomatic when diagnosis is made	Trimethoprim-sulfamethoxazole TMP, 10 mg/kg/d SMX, 50 mg/kg/d q12h per 5 days or Ampicillin, 100 mg/kg q6h for 5 days	Tetracycline in adults 7.5 g orally in one dose	Antibiotics promptly control the infection.
	Asymptomatic carriers	Treat as above if in day care or to prevent spread between family members		
Escherichia coli				
Enteropathogenic	Life-threatening infection; nursery epidemic	Neomycin, 30 mg/kg q8h for 5 days	Colistin	No controlled trials
Enterotoxigenic	Gastroenteritis	Probably none		For prevention of diarrhea doxycycline has been recommended.
Enteroinvasive	Same as shigellosis	Probably none		
Yersinia	Gastroenteritis	None		
	Sepsis	Gentamicin, 5 mg/kg q8h	Chloramphenicol, 75 mg/kg q6h	
Aeromonas	Severe diarrhea	Trimethoprim-sulfamethoxazole TMP, 10 mg/kg/d SMX, 50 mg/kg/d q12h for 7 days		Usually self-limited
	Chronic diarrhea			
	Inmunocompromised host			
Clostridium difficile	Severe colitis	Discontinue initial antibiotic Vancomycin, 500 mg/1.73 m² q6h	Metronidazole, 15–30 mg/kg q8h Bacitracin, 2000 U/kg/d q6h	Most infections stop when the initial antibiotic is stopped. Vancomycin is very expensive.
Giardia	All symptomatic cases	Quinacrine, 6 mg/kg q8h for 7 days or Metronidazole, 15 mg/kg q8h for 7 days	Furazolidone, 5 mg/kg q6h for 7 days	Concerns about carcinogenesis
Entamoeba histolytica	Proctocolitis	Metronidazole, 15–30 mg/kg q8h for 5–10 days If trophozoites persist, diiodohydroxyquin, 30–40 mg/kg/d for 20 days	Secnidazole Tinidazole Dehydroemetine, 1.5 mg/kg/d IM for 5 days	Repeat sigmoidoscopy after treatment A liver abscess may develop, so close F/U is necessary

TREATMENT

The therapy for acute diarrhea may be divided into two components: specific therapy, if available (antibiotics for certain infections) (Table 105-2), and empiric (supportive) therapy.

Antibiotics are sometimes given to children with acute diarrhea. It has to be remembered that most episodes of diarrhea are self-limited and that the indications for their use are limited. In general, they should be restricted to septic infants, to patients with cholera, shigellosis, or typhoid, to infants younger than 3 months old with salmonellosis, to patients with infections with *Clostridium difficile,* and to patients with amebiasis or giardiasis.

Irrespective of the specific etiology of the diarrhea, if diarrheal losses of body water and electrolytes continue without adequate replacement, increasing dehydration, acidosis, cardiovascular collapse, and death will ensue. Infants, and children with underlying conditions (e.g., cystic fibrosis, diuretic therapy) are more susceptible to dehydration. The objective of the therapy should be the restoration or maintenance of adequate hydration and electrolyte balance, the avoidance of measures that could prolong the course of the disease, and the maintenance or restoration of the patient's nutritional status. The initial management must ensure that the patient's condition is stable, and, if not, initial steps should be taken to stabilize the patient.

A wide variety of nonspecific antidiarrheal agents are available. The most widely used are adsorbents (e.g., kaolin and pectin, bismuth subsalicylate, attapulgite) and those that have an antimotility effect (e.g., tincture of opium, diphenoxylate with atropine, loperamide). Many are available as over-the-counter preparations and even though they may be beneficial, they do not generally change the final outcome of the diarrheal episode. Of all the agents, three (loperamide, bismuth subsalicylate, and attapulgite) have shown in limited studies to be potentially effective as an adjunct in the treatment of acute diarrhea in children, but more information and larger studies are needed to confirm their efficacy and safety. It has to be stressed that (1) most episodes of acute diarrhea are self-limited and the prevention of dehydration and later malnutrition are the most important aspects of treatment and (2) some of the antidiarrheal agents may have potentially serious side effects, particularly in infants and patients with high fevers and dysentery. At present it can be said that none of the studied nonspecific antidiarrheal drugs have shown to be of sufficient benefit and safety to justify their routine use in the management of acute diarrheal episodes in infants and children.

The advent of intravenous rehydration represented an important step in management of severe diarrhea. Traditionally the rehydration of ill children with acute diarrhea has been accomplished by hospitalizing infants and administering intravenous fluid therapy, while fasting the patients for variable periods of time. After adequate rehydration is achieved, variable types of "clear liquids" or oral rehydration solutions (which are usually hyperosmolar; Table 105-3) are then administered and intravenous fluids are slowly weaned. Then a period of "bowel rest" is prescribed for 24

Table 105-3. Comparison of Solutions Used in Oral Rehydration

	SODIUM (mEq/L)	POTASSIUM (mEq/L)	CHLORIDE (mEq/L)	BASE (mmol/L)	GLUCOSE (mmol/L	OSMO-LALITY
Stool Losses						
Normal	22	50	21	?		
Enterotoxigenic *Escherichia coli*/Rotavirus	30–65	18–60	26–55	5		
Cholera	90–120	30	85–120	10		
Solutions						
Rehydration:						
WHO-UNICEF Oral Rehydration Salts	90	20	80	10	111	310
Rehydralyte	75	20	65	10	140	305
Maintenance:						
Infalyte	50	20	40	10	111	270
Lytren	50	25	45	10	111	290
Ricelyte	50	25	45	34	*	200
Pedialyte	45	20	35	10	140	250
Resol	50	20	50	11	111	270
Clear Liquids:						
Cola	2	0.1	2	13	730	750
Gingerale	3	1	2	4	500	540
Apple juice	3	28	30	0	690	730
Chicken broth	250	8	250	0	0	450
Tea	0	0	0	0	0	5
Gatorade	23.5	2.5	17	3	222	330

*30 g of rice syrup solids, which forms glucose when digested.

Adapted from Avery ME et al: Oral therapy for acute diarrhea. N Engl J Med 323:891–894, 1990 to 48 hours, and formula (usually lactose-free, one-fourth to one-half strength advancing to full strength) and later other foodstuffs (e.g., BRAT [*b*anana, *r*ice, *a*pplesauce, *t*oast] diet) are usually introduced slowly over 2 to 5 days. In the less severely ill children the use of "clear liquids" and no food or milk are the common practice. This "conventional therapy" is still widely used in many American hospitals, but fortunately this approach is changing.

There are other (usually better) alternatives for the treatment of dehydration in children with diarrhea. It has been shown all over the world, including the United States, that oral rehydration is an effective way to treat acute diarrheal illness. More than a decade ago the United Nations International Children's Emergency Fund (UNICEF) and the World Health Organization (WHO) incorporated oral rehydration as the cornerstone of their child-survival efforts and recommended its widespread implementation as an effective, simple and inexpensive therapy for dehydration in infants and children. It is worth mentioning that it does not require the use of sophisticated equipment, and it can be administered and supervised by nonprofessional staff. In the past decade it has been shown all over the world that oral rehydration therapy is effective in the treatment of children with mild, moderate, and severe dehydration and for maintenance therapy, independent of the type, etiology, or sodium content of the stool in the different diarrheal illnesses.

Oral rehydration therapy is based on the physiologic observation that there is a coupled intestinal transport of glucose and sodium, with active absorption of the former in the small bowel promoting the absorption of the latter, and, more importantly, that this mechanism is intact during the episodes of acute diarrhea.

The WHO UNICEF formula contains sodium, 90 mEq/L, potassium, 20 mEq/L, bicarbonate, 30 mEq/L, chloride, 80 mEq/L, and glucose, 111 mM (2%), with an osmolarity of 331 mOsm/L (see Table 105-3). This can be achieved by adding 20 g of glucose/L, 3.5 g/L of sodium chloride, 1.5 g/L of potassium chloride, and either 2.9 g/L of trisodium citrate or 2.5 g/L of sodium bicarbonate. In the United States, a variety of premixed solutions of glucose, electrolytes, and water are available, and they all have compositions approximating that of the WHO formula (see Table 105-3). Although data are preliminary, rice-based oral rehydration solutions appear to be more effective than glucose-based oral rehydration solutions in reducing the rate of stool loss and in shortening the duration of diarrhea.

In 1985, the American Academy of Pediatrics (AAP) Committee on Nutrition endorsed the use of oral fluid therapy and post-treatment feeding. As is shown in Table 105-4, the AAP recommends a carbohydrate–sodium ratio of less than 2:1 and a rehydration solution with 75 to 90 mEq/L of sodium and a maintenance solution with 40 to 60 mEq/L of sodium.

Oral rehydration is successful in 95% to 98% of patients and intravenous therapy is usually required in only 2% to 5% of cases. It has been shown repeatedly that vomiting is

Table 105-4. Recommendations Made by the Committee on Nutrition of the American Academy of Pediatrics

Glucose electrolyte solutions:
    Rehydration: 75–90 mEq/L of sodium
    Maintenance: 40–60 mEq/L of sodium

Carbohydrate to sodium ratio should be less than 2:1
Rehydration solutions can be used to provide maintenance fluids when given with breast milk, water, or low-carbohydrate juice

Feeding should be reintroduced in the first 24 hours
    Initial foods may include the following:
        Infants: Breast milk, diluted formula or milk
        Older patients: Rice cereal, bananas, potatoes, other non-lactose carbohydrate-rich foods

Adapted from Snyder JD: Use and misuse of oral therapy for diarrhea: Comparison of US practices with American Academy of Pediatrics recommendations. Pediatrics 87:28–33, 1991, and from American Academy of Pediatrics, Committee on Nutrition: Use of oral fluid therapy and posttreatment feeding following enteritis in children in a developed country. Pediatrics 75:358–361, 1985.

not a contraindication for using oral rehydration solutions. Oral therapy usually fails in patients who have high rates of stool loss (i.e., over 10 mL/kg/h). Periorbital edema has been described transiently in 6% to 25% of hospitalized children who are being treated with oral rehydration; it is usually self-limited, resolves when the volume of oral rehydration solution is decreased, and has not been associated with either hypernatremia or untoward consequences. The WHO oral rehydration solution formula has also been used in the treatment of hypernatremic dehydration and, although a modified "slow" method has been employed successfully, further studies are necessary before oral rehydration can be recommended for this purpose. (For a more extensive discussion of dehydration, see Chap 189.)

The approach to diarrhea by most pediatricians in the United States and elsewhere consists of a variable period of fasting. The main arguments advanced for limited fasting are avoidance of the consequences of malabsorption, namely, acidosis, excessive fluid losses, depletion of the bile acid pool, and possible mucosal injury from unabsorbed foods. Advocates of continued feeding suggest that this practice will prevent insufficient intake of protein and calories, maintain or stimulate repair of the intestinal mucosa, and sustain breast-feeding. Studies that address the impact of early feeding show that if early feedings are introduced, the outcome is favorable.

The available data show that the introduction of appropriate early feedings is beneficial and that it may reduce stool output and frequency and hasten recovery, with improvement in the nutritional outcome. Rice, corn, potatoes, wheat, and other staple foods have been demonstrated to be well-tolerated.

It is difficult to make dietary recommendations with complete confidence. Nevertheless, until a definitive causal relationship between early dietary therapy and chronic malabsorption or food allergy can be established, the only aspects of early feeding during acute diarrhea that are proven to be potentially harmful are excessive fluid loss and increased malabsorption, particularly secondary to carbohydrate intolerance. Since those complications can easily be monitored clinically and stool characteristics can be closely followed, reintroduction of foods immediately after rehydration is recommended. Breast-feeding should be continued once rehydration is completed. Children who are fully weaned should receive their usual diet, and it is usually suggested to first try small amounts of the regular formula that the child usually takes, reserving the lactose-free formulas for those children who show a clinical intolerance to lactose. The consumption of foods should also be encouraged. Generally, the child should determine the amount of food to be consumed, and food should not be forced on unwilling, anorectic infants; however, food should be offered to the hungry infant despite ongoing diarrhea. Once diarrhea subsides, extra food should be available to enable a recovery of any nutritional deficit caused by the acute illness.

INDICATIONS FOR ADMISSION

All patients with circulatory insufficiency (10% to 15% dehydration), inability to drink, alteration in consciousness, and intractable vomiting should be initially rehydrated with parenteral fluids. They should be admitted to the hospital and, as soon as they are stable, should complete rehydration orally. Toxic-appearing patients as well as those in which the family is unable to precisely follow the oral rehydration guidelines should also be admitted.

ANNOTATED BIBLIOGRAPHY

Avery ME, Snyder JD: Oral therapy for acute diarrhea: The underused simple solution. N Engl J Med 88:891–894, 1990. (Discussion on the use and importance of oral rehydration.)

Barkin R: Acute infectious diarrheal disease in children. J Emerg Med 3:1, 1985. (Good review of etiology.)

Davidson GP, Goodwin D, Robb TA: Incidence and duration of lactose malabsorption in children hospitalized with acute enteritis: Study in a well-nourished urban population. J Pediatr 105:587, 1984. (Prospective study of the natural history.)

Farthing MJ, Keusch GT: Enteric Infections: Mechanism, Manifestations and Management. New York, Raven Press, 1988. (Excellent and authoritative review on all aspects.)

Kotloff KL, Wasserman SS, Steciak JY: Acute diarrhea in Baltimore children attending an outpatient clinic. Pediatr Infect Dis 7: 753–759, 1988. (Study on the etiology in an urban area.)

Lifshitz F (ed): Management of acute diarrheal disease. J Pediatr 118(suppl):S25–S109, 1991. (Emphasizes aspects of rehydration and early feeding.)

Santosham M, Foster S, Reed R et al: Role of soy-based, lactose-free formula during treatment of acute diarrhea. Pediatrics 76:292, 1985. (Compares early feedings with traditional therapy.)

Snyder JD: Use and misuse of oral therapy for diarrhea: Comparison of U.S. practices with American Academy of Pediatrics Recom-

mendations. Pediatrics 87: 28–33, 1991. (Study on the actual use of oral rehydration in United States' hospitals.)

Symposium on the management of acute diarrhea. Am J Med 88 (suppl 6A), 1990. (Up-to-date review on the nonspecific and specific treatments of acute diarrhea.)

106

Malabsorption Syndrome and Chronic Diarrhea

Wayne I. Lencer

Pediatricians often consider malabsorption in the differential diagnosis of several common childhood syndromes, such as failure to thrive, short stature, or chronic diarrhea. Malabsorption can be defined as a failure to digest or absorb dietary nutrients. It is a manifestation of a disease and not a specific entity. The clinical syndrome ranges from those children with obviously large foul-smelling stools or chronic diarrhea and growth failure to nearly asymptomatic children with laboratory evidence of a nutritional deficiency. Practically, then, malabsorption should be considered in any patient who has a nutritional deficiency unexplained by dietary factors.

PATHOPHYSIOLOGY

All nutrients have three broad phases of digestion and absorption. The intraluminal phase comprises events that occur within the lumen of the gut. These are most sensitive to disturbances in the pancreatic and biliary functions. The intestinal phase defines those events that occur at the enterocyte surface or within the cell and are sensitive to disturbances of the intestinal mucosa itself. The removal phase refers to the transport of nutrients from the enterocyte to other organs for metabolism or storage.

The digestive processes of the intraluminal phase act to solubilize lipids in water and begin the breakdown of starch and protein. Pancreatic secretions handle the bulk of intraluminal digestion. Dietary lipids, however, require the additional presence of bile acids and thus a normally functioning liver, biliary tract, and terminal ileum. (Bile acids are reabsorbed at the terminal ileum and recycled.) Ninety percent of ingested lipids are in the form of triglyceride. These are hydrolyzed at a basic pH to free fatty acid and monoglyceride by the combination of pancreatic colipase, lipase, and bile salts. When above the critical micellar concentration, bile salts solubilize the fatty products of triglyceride hydrolysis by forming micelles. Micelles carry fatty acids and glycerol with fat-soluble vitamins and cholesterol to the enterocyte surface. Defects in these intraluminal processes tend to produce considerable fat malabsorption.

The pancreas also secretes critical enzymes for the digestion of starch and proteins. Amylase hydrolyzes amylopectin (starch) to maltose, maltotriose, or À-limit dextrans. Similarly, trypsin (activated by enterokinase at the mucosal surface) acting with carboxypeptidase and elastase (activated in turn by trypsin) hydrolyzes protein to free amino acids and short-chain peptides. The products of both starch and protein digestion move to the enterocyte surface by diffusion.

The intestinal phase begins at the brush border and includes intracellular processing of dietary lipids and proteins. This phase completes the digestion and absorption of carbohydrates and proteins and serves to package lipids in a soluble form suitable for the systemic circulation.

Lipids diffuse passively through the cell membrane. The enterocyte then re-forms triglyceride from absorbed fatty acids and monoglycerides, adding phospholipids, apoproteins, and cholesterol to make chylomicrons. The transport of chylomicrons into the lymphatics requires the specific apoprotein β-lipoprotein.

Lactase, sucrase-isomaltase, and glucoamylase contained in the brush border of the enterocyte further hydrolyze maltotriose, maltose, α-limit dextrans, and ingested disaccharides (sucrose and lactose) to their component monosaccharides (glucose, galactose, and fructose). Hydrolysis of lactose to galactose and glucose by the brush border enzyme lactase is the rate-limiting step.

Transport of dietary nutrients across the intestinal epithelium probably occurs by two general mechanisms: transcellular and paracellular transport.

Monosaccharides are transported into the cell by specific membrane proteins in either a sodium-coupled process (glucose and galactose) or by facilitated diffusion (fructose). Small peptides are transported intact through the cell membrane on carrier proteins or are further hydrolyzed to free amino acids by brush border enzymes where other carrier proteins facilitate their absorption. Absorbed peptides are hydrolyzed within the cytosol to free amino acids. These, together with absorbed free amino acids, diffuse into the portal circulation.

Recent evidence shows that small dietary nutrients are also transported across the epithelium by permeating tight junctions in a process called solvent drag.

Defects of the intestinal phase, although almost always causing carbohydrate malabsorption, may or may not produce fat malabsorption. The degree of steatorrhea depends on the extent of mucosal injury. Viral gastroenteritis, for example, characteristically causes patchy mucosal injury that may not damage enough mucosa to cause fatty stools, whereas celiac disease causes diffuse damage and almost always steatorrhea.

The removal phase acts to carry products of absorption to the systemic circulation and is affected by diseases of the portal and lymphatic circulation.

CLINICAL PRESENTATION

The clinical presentation of malabsorption is as varied as the disease entities that cause it. Classic signs of gastrointestinal tract dysfunction such as chronic diarrhea, the passage of frequent, large, pale, oily, and foul-smelling stools, increased flatus, abdominal distention, or possibly increased appetite may or may not be obvious. A combination of dietary and psychosocial factors causes most nutritional deficiencies in childhood. A nutritional deficiency may, in turn, cause malabsorption. The dietary history plays a critical role in distinguishing undernutrition from malabsorption. In uncertain cases of growth failure, catch-up growth after a clinical trial of adequate nutrition in a controlled environment indicates a normal gastrointestinal tract.

Growth failure is the most common sign of a nutritional deficiency in childhood and the most common presentation of malabsorption. Early detection of growth failure depends on growth monitoring. Plots of weight against height on standard curves (from the National Center for Health Statistics) provide early evidence of growth failure often before other clinical signs are evident. Plots of height against age or of height velocity will show stunting due to chronic nutritional deficiency. Other measures of nutritional status such as skinfold thickness correlate highly with anthropomorphic measurements and assess lean body mass (see also Chaps. 12 and 188).

Lactose malabsorption is the most common cause of malabsorption in a general pediatric practice due to the normal ontogenic decline in lactase expression. Classic symptoms include persistent diarrhea after infectious diarrhea (so-called secondary lactase deficiency), bloating, abdominal distention, and pain.

Malabsorption can present with signs of vitamin deficiency. Diseases causing defects in the intestinal phase processes will cause a deficiency of water-soluble vitamins and minerals such as folic acid, vitamin B_{12}, iron, and other B vitamins. Pallor, fatigue, or dizziness due to anemia, cheilosis, glossitis, dermatitis, and peripheral neuropathy may be presenting signs of a malabsorption syndrome. Defects in either pancreatic or biliary processes commonly cause deficiency of the fat-soluble vitamins A, D, E, and K. This may produce hyperkeratosis of skin (vitamin A), ecchymosis and hematuria (vitamin K), and tetany, bone pain, or rickets (vitamin D).

A nutritional deficiency in older children may present as delayed puberty.

Symptoms and signs of the underlying disease process often dominate the clinical picture. For example, children who have cystic fibrosis or an immunodeficiency may present with a chronic cough or a recurrent pulmonary infection. Those who have hepatic disease may have cirrhosis and its complications, and those who have inflammatory bowel disease may present with abdominal pain. The clinical picture in those cases suggests its own diagnostic strategy. Those children with vague symptoms or nonspecific signs such as persistent loose stools, short stature, or growth failure will benefit from a carefully done nutritional assessment, documentation of nutritional deficiency, and consideration of malabsorption in those children in whom dietary or social causes of undernutrition are not found.

DIFFERENTIAL DIAGNOSIS

The differential diagnosis of malabsorption in pathophysiologic groups is listed in the display, Selected Differential Diagnosis of Malabsorption.

Of these disorders, acute and chronic infection, giardiasis, postinfectious enteritis, allergic enteritis, celiac disease, and cystic fibrosis are the most common diseases affecting children. Newborns have physiologic steatorrhea resulting from decreased bile acid pools and decreased pancreatic function. This developmentally "normal" malabsorption must be differentiated from disease in the very young child.

WORK-UP

History and Physical Examination

The diagnostic approach depends heavily on the clinical presentation. Clinical malabsorption in the neonatal period warrants aggressive diagnosis, treatment, and early referral. In infants and older children, the dietary history will identify most cases of nutritional deficiency due to undernutrition. Temporal associations between symptoms and the introduction of various nutrients such as cow's milk, sucrose, or gluten-containing grains suggest food sensitivity, enzyme deficiencies, or celiac disease, respectively. Symptoms of systemic disorders associated with malnutrition, a history of abdominal surgery, or recent or past travel should be sought. The physical examination may reveal evidence of a nutritional deficiency. The height and weight plotted accurately on appropriate growth curves will identify growth failure. Sexual development should be noted. The thickness of subcutaneous tissue, skin elasticity, and muscle wasting in the buttocks, thighs, and arms may indicate a recent loss of weight. Dry, fine, easily pulled out hair can be seen in protein-deficiency states. The abdomen might be distended or locally tender. Other signs of nutritional deficiency previously mentioned may be present.

Laboratory Tests

Occult blood in the stool indicates damage to the intestinal mucosa. The presence of polymorphonuclear leukocytes occurs with inflammatory diseases. Cultures will investigate infectious causes. Three fresh stool samples examined for ova and parasites will detect between 50% and 80% of those children with giardiasis. A fresh liquid stool sample with *p*H less than 5.5 and reducing substances indicates sugar malabsorption. Hemoglobin and hematocrit determinations, urinalysis, and sweat tests should be done routinely. A bone

Selected Differential Diagnosis of Malabsorption

Intraluminal phase abnormalities
   Cystic fibrosis
   Chronic pancreatitis
Malnutrition
Decreased conjugated bile acids
   Liver production and excretion
      Neonatal hepatitis
      Biliary atresia: intrahepatic and extrahepatic
      Acute and chronic active hepatitis
      Disease of the biliary tract
      Cirrhosis
      Fat malabsorption in the premature infant
   Intestinal factors
      Short bowel syndrome
      Bacterial overgrowth
         Blind loop
         Fistula
         Strictures—regional enteritis
Abnormalities of the intestinal phase
   Mucosal diseases
      Infection, bacterial or viral
      Infestations
         Giardia lamblia
         Fish tapeworm
         Hookworm
      Malnutrition
      Drugs: methotrexate, antibiotics
      Crohn's disease
      Chronic ulcerative colitis
      Cow's milk intolerance and soy protein intolerance
      Secondary disaccharidase deficiency
      Hirschsprung's disease with enterocolitis
      Celiac disease
   Circulatory disturbances
      Cirrhosis
      Congestive heart failure
   Abnormal structural makeup of gastrointestinal tract
   Selective inborn absorptive defects
   Endocrine disease
Defective delivery phase
   Intestinal lymphangiectasis
   Congestive heart failure
   Regional enteritis with lymphangiectasis
   Lymphoma
   Abetalipoproteinemia
Miscellaneous
   Renal insufficiency
   Immunity defects
   Maternal deprivation
   Collagen disease
   Intractable diarrhea of early infancy

Adapted from Silverman A, Roy CC (eds): Pediatric Clinical Gastroenterology. St. Louis, CV Mosby, 1983.

age test will assess growth potential and may show osteomalacia or rickets. Complete blood cell count, differential, determination of mean corpuscular volume, total protein/albumin, calcium, phosphate, alkaline phosphatase, ferritin, and folate, and liver function tests may be useful if abnormal.

In uncertain cases, the pediatrician may want direct evidence of malabsorption before proceeding with a further work-up or a small bowel biopsy. Unfortunately, the serum carotene value depends heavily on dietary intake and, when reduced, does not reliably reflect the absorptive function. To demonstrate malabsorption, the D-xylose absorption and 72-hour quantitative fecal fat collection are the most useful tests. Neither test, however, is highly sensitive. Some children with normal D-xylose and fat collection will require a further work-up, including a small bowel biopsy, unless a specific diagnosis has been made by other means such as in cystic fibrosis.

D-Xylose is absorbed by diffusion and on the same transport protein as glucose but with much less affinity. Its absorption reflects the available mucosal surface area and therefore the mucosal function. An oral dose of 14.5 g/M^2 followed by a 60-minute blood level will give a 20-mg/dL rise or greater in normal persons.

Fat absorption requires normal function in all phases of digestion and absorption. This makes the 72-hour fat collection the most sensitive test for malabsorption. A positive qualitative Sudan stain for stool fat, however, precludes the need to collect a 72-hour stool sample. For at least 2 days before and throughout the 72-hour collection, the child must take a normal diet high in fats. Parents keep a dietary diary to quantitate fat intake. The diet diary may demonstrate inadequate nutrition, which was previously unsuspected. The amount of fat excreted in stool is normally less than 10% of intake. Beware of falsely "normal" tests from inadequate stool collection. Attempts should be made to collect all stool excreted during the collection period.

Although an abnormal 72-hour fat collection may reflect a defect in any phase of absorption or digestion, an abnormal D-xylose suggests that the defect lies in the intestinal phase. The tests supplement each other and direct further investigations. For example, a normal D-xylose and abnormal fat suggest a defect in the intraluminal processes such as pancreatic insufficiency, small bowel overgrowth, or liver disease. An abnormal D-xylose with a normal 72-hour fat collection indicates intestinal phase dysfunction such as in celiac disease or postinfectious enteritis. Abnormal tests in either case are indications for referral and consideration of small bowel biopsy. Again, the sensitivity of the tests (80%) means normal results do not necessarily rule out malabsorption. Children with nutritional deficiency *unexplained by dietary factors* should be referred to a pediatric gastroenterologist for a small bowel biopsy. Normal tests, however, in those children with nonspecific symptoms but without nutritional deficiency do *not* support further investigation unless other signs develop.

A small bowel biopsy can be done safely (mortality rate less than 0.001% to 0.0001%) and with little trauma to child and family. The small bowel biopsy, however, does not establish a specific diagnosis in every case of malabsorption. Biopsies will reliably diagnose diseases that affect the mucosa diffusely and are likely to require treatment, such as celiac disease.

Diseases that produce patchy mucosal lesions, such as postinfectious enteritis and milk allergic enteropathies, are, with few exceptions in the pediatric practice, transient and resolve with time. In many children, then, a normal small bowel biopsy may be followed by a period of watchful waiting. It is not recommended to place children on a gluten-free diet without a biopsy confirmation of celiac disease. The empiric treatment of children suspected of celiac disease causes undue hardship for many more families who do not have celiac disease than benefits those who do.

Secondary lactose malabsorption is the most common malabsorption diagnosis encountered by the practicing physician. Lactose and sucrose hydrogen breath tests demonstrate a lactase or a sucrose-isomaltase deficiency with a sensitivity of 80%. An increase in breath H$_2$ of more than 10 to 20 ppm above baseline value indicates fermentation of nonabsorbed carbohydrate. Falsely normal results occur in 2% to 20% of individuals and may be due to recent antibiotic treatment or to the lack of hydrogen-producing flora. Small bowel overgrowth often causes an abnormal lactulose breath test. Upper gastrointestinal and small bowel follow-through barium studies may show changes characteristic of malabsorption or anatomic defects. Sigmoidoscopy and biopsy can confirm ulcerative colitis and Crohn's disease. None of these, however, are appropriate screening tests, and they should be used only later in the work-up with specific aims in mind.

TREATMENT

A specific diagnosis dictates specific treatment in diseases causing malabsorption as in other syndromes. Several general principles, however, can help in management. Elemental formulas containing monosaccharides, small peptides, and medium chain triglycerides (MCT) oil circumvent many steps of normal digestion and absorption, and can be used successfully in most children with malabsorption syndromes. Hydrolyzed proteins and MCTs are soluble in water and do not require bile salts or pancreatic enzymes. In children with severe fat malabsorption, such as cystic fibrosis or chronic liver disease, water-soluble forms of vitamins A, D, K, and E at double doses should replace their fat-soluble counterparts. Formulas containing monosaccharides do not require fragile brush border enzymes such as lactase. Finally, total parenteral nutrition can be used when enteral feedings of elemental diets fail.

Although discussed in greater detail in Chapter 105, the treatment of common diarrhea warrants mention here. Postinfectious enteritis explains most cases of malabsorption seen by the practicing pediatrician and is the set up for the development of intractable diarrhea. The avoidance of morbidity from diarrhea depends largely on feeding practices. For almost all cases of dehydration due to diarrhea, oral rehydration solutions, such as the World Health Organization (WHO) oral rehydration solution, will rehydrate the child, correct acidosis, and improve appetite. As soon as rehydration is achieved and in those children not initially dehydrated, feedings of breast milk, or one-half to full-strength formula or a diet supplemented with electrolyte solutions and free water, can and should be offered immediately. The diet is advanced in strength as the infant's appetite improves. Minor changes in stool volume or consistency bear little meaning. Lactose need not routinely be restricted following acute infectious diarrhea. Breast milk is usually very well-tolerated throughout the diarrheal illness. Since sucrase and isomaltase are linked membrane enzymes, the use of sucrose-free, corn syrup formulas makes little sense. This strategy will achieve a positive nutrient and fluid balance in almost all cases of diarrhea.

ANNOTATED BIBLIOGRAPHY

Friedman HI, Nylund B: Intestinal fat digestion, absorption and transport. Am J Clin Nutr 33:1139–1180, 1980. (Excellent review of digestive physiology that supplements the pathophysiology discussed.)

Gray GM: Carbohydrate digestion and absorption. N Engl J Med 292:1125, 1975. (Excellent review of digestive physiology that supplements the pathophysiology discussed.)

Silverman A, Roy CC (eds): Pediatric Clinical Gastroenterology, chap. 10. St. Louis, CV Mosby, 1983. (Discussion of malabsorption from the pediatric perspective.)

Pappenheimer JR, Reiss KE: Contribution of solvent drag in the absorption of nutrients in the small intestine. J Membr Biol 100:123–136, 1987.

Saavedra JM, Perman JA: Current concepts in lactose malabsorption and intolerance. Annu Rev Nutr 9:475–502, 1989. (Excellent review of lactose malabsorption.)

Schmitz J: Malabsorption. In Walker WA, Durie PR, Hamilton JR et al (eds): Pediatric Gastrointestinal Disease. Philadelphia, BC Decker, 1991. (Comprehensive discussion of pathophysiology and clinical presentation.)

107

Inflammatory Bowel Disease

Esther Jacobowitz Israel

Inflammatory bowel disease (IBD) constitutes an increasingly large proportion of chronic intestinal disease in the pediatric age group. It has an overall incidence of 4 to 6 cases per 1000 and a prevalence of 40 to 100 per 100,000. The peak age at onset is between 10 and 30 years, and 20% of all patients are younger than 20 years old.

PATHOPHYSIOLOGY

The pathogenesis of IBD (Crohn's disease and ulcerative colitis) remains unknown. It is likely that Crohn's disease and ulcerative colitis are separate disorders that share some clinical features and do not share a common cause. Several etiologies have been proposed for both, including heredity, environment and diet, immunologic aberrations, and ineffective mucosal integrity. Supporting the environmental theory is the higher incidence of Crohn's disease in specific areas of the world, including Northern Europe and North America, and a greater prevalence in urban areas. Dietary intake of fiber and fat may play a role, and a history of breast feeding during infancy may confer a degree of protection. Psychological stress has also been implicated in relapses of established disease. Over the years numerous infectious agents have been proposed as the cause of IBD, but Koch's postulates have yet to be fulfilled for any agent. The clustering of cases according to family, race, and ethnicity supports the role of genetic factors in the etiology of IBD. The incidence rate of IBD in the Jewish population is three to six times that in the general population, and 20% to 40% of children with IBD have a first-degree relative with the disease. There is an association of ankylosing spondylitis and HLA-B27 with IBD, but there is no specific tissue type consistently associated with the disease.

An impaired intestinal mucosal barrier that allows for increased antigenic exposure to the gastrointestinal immune system has also been proposed as an etiologic factor in IBD. There are data to suggest that mucosal integrity is impaired in Crohn's disease, including frequent findings of elevated levels of antibodies specific for cow's milk protein, enteric bacterial products, and intestinal proteins. Healthy relatives of patients with IBD have also been noted to have impaired intestinal epithelial integrity. Whether impaired mucosal barrier function is a consequence of inflammation or is implicated in the etiology of the disease is unknown. Impaired epithelial integrity does not appear to occur in ulcerative colitis.

Immunologic processes appear to be centrally involved in the pathogenesis of IBD. Crohn's disease and ulcerative colitis are marked by chronic activation of the intestinal immune system. Since many similarities to other inflammatory disorders such as arthritis exist, IBD is considered by some to be an autoimmune disease in which components of the intestinal immune system mount a response against intestinal epithelial cells. It has also been suggested that IBD occurs in persons who cannot develop tolerance for normal intestinal antigens, leading to unregulated activation of the gut immune system and chronic inflammation. Since immune responses are governed genetically, this ultimately reflects an inherited defect.

Thus, Crohn's disease and ulcerative colitis appear to have a polygenic basis, probably influenced by environmental factors.

CLINICAL PRESENTATION

The clinical presentation of ulcerative colitis and particularly Crohn's disease in children may be insidious. Some of

Table 107-1.   Differential Diagnosis Between Ulcerative Colitis and Crohn's Disease

FEATURE	CROHN'S DISEASE	ULCERATIVE COLITIS
Rectal bleeding	Rare	Common
Diarrhea	Moderate/absent	Very common
Abdominal pain	Almost always	Less frequent
Weight loss	Severe	Moderate
Growth retardation	Common	Less common
Extraintestinal signs	Less common	Common
Small bowel involvement		
Extensive	10%	Never
Distal ileum	90%	Never
Colon	75%	100%
Rectum	50%	95%
Anus	85%	5%
Distribution of lesions	Segmental	Continuous
Pathologic changes	Focal transmural ± granulomas	Diffuse mucosal

the differences in presentation are noted in Table 107-1. Abdominal pain is almost always a feature of Crohn's disease, whereas diarrhea, hematochezia, and tenesmus are present more frequently in ulcerative colitis. Growth failure and weight loss can occur in both diseases, although are more common in Crohn's disease. Extraintestinal manifestations including skin lesions (erythema nodosum and pyoderma gangrenosum), arthralgias and arthritis, and liver disease (sclerosis cholangitis, biliary cirrhosis) occur primarily in patients with colonic disease (either Crohn's colitis or chronic ulcerative colitis).

DIFFERENTIAL DIAGNOSIS

The causes of abdominal pain in children are numerous and include peptic ulcer disease, esophagitis, renal disease, pancreatitis, appendicitis, and intussusception. Bloody diarrhea, on the other hand, is less common, and infectious agents must always be excluded. Ischemic colitis associated with Henoch-Schönlein purpura and hemolytic uremic syndrome should be considered. In the patient with evidence of extensive inflammation, weight loss, and abdominal pain, lymphoma should also be suspected.

WORK-UP

History

Abdominal pain, weight loss, and bloody diarrhea are the major clues to the presence of IBD. Specific questions regarding symptoms related to the extraintestinal manifesta-

tions of IBD are particularly relevant and include a history of mouth ulcers, arthralgias, recurrent fevers, and eye or liver problems. The nature, timing, and location of the abdominal pain are extremely important. Abdominal pain in the right lower quadrant related to food intake is common in Crohn's disease; a history of nausea and vomiting suggests small intestinal narrowing secondary to the disease. The symptom of anorexia is often present, perhaps being secondary to postprandial discomfort. The pain in ulcerative colitis is usually lower abdominal and left sided. Fatigue and a past history of anemia are frequently present. Growth charts are extremely helpful since there is often a falloff in the height percentile over several years that helps distinguish chronic IBD from a more acute process. Known exposures to family members, friends, and schoolmates with similar symptoms are clues to an infectious process rather than IBD. Because of the hereditary features of IBD, a family history should routinely be taken.

Physical Examination

A thorough physical examination should be performed in any patient being evaluated for abdominal pain, hematochezia, or weight loss. This begins with vital signs sometimes detecting orthostasis, and growth measurements, since 10% to 30% of children with IBD present with short stature. Examination of the skin may show jaundice or a rash, most notably erythema nodosum or pyoderma gangrenosum, representing some of the extraintestinal manifestations of the disease. Scleral icterus or iritis may be seen, and ulcerations may be noted in the mouth, again due to the systemic nature of the disease. A flow murmur secondary to anemia may be heard, and hepatomegaly can be present. The extremities may show clubbing, arthritis, or edema secondary to hypoalbuminemia. The abdominal examination may be normal or more commonly show tenderness. Often in Crohn's disease the tenderness is localized in the right lower quadrant from inflammation in the terminal ileum. Tenderness on the left side and on rectal examination is more typical of colonic disease. In ulcerative colitis, the rectal examination will show gross blood and mucus, while occult blood is noted in more proximal disease. Perirectal disease with perianal fistulas, tags, and abscesses are seen in Crohn's disease. Pubertal development is often delayed.

Laboratory Evaluation

Unfortunately there is no one test that diagnoses IBD, and therefore the diagnosis depends on a combination of assessments, including laboratory evaluation. A complete blood cell count often shows leukocytosis and anemia. Signs of inflammation, with elevation in the acute phase reactants, are usually seen in IBD, although some patients may have a normal erythrocyte sedimentation rate, white blood cell count, and platelet count. Serum total protein and albumin may be low because of undernutrition and protein losing enteropathy. Hepatic transaminase and bilirubin values may be elevated when the patient has hepatic extraintestinal manifestations of IBD. Stool specimens should be examined for leukocytes, blood, and bacterial pathogens, including *Clostridium difficile* and toxigenic strains of *Escherichia coli.* Ultimately, radiologic and endoscopic examinations of the gastrointestinal tract help to confirm the diagnosis. Upper gastrointestinal contrast roentgenograms with small bowel follow-through are essential to define the small bowel disease in the distal parts of the small intestine, which occurs in 90% of patients with Crohn's disease. In Crohn's disease, lesions can occur from the esophagus to the anus with intervening normal areas (skip areas). Thirty percent of biopsy samples taken during endoscopy of a patient with Crohn's disease will show granulomas on histologic examination.

Chronic ulcerative colitis causes a continuous lesion from the rectosigmoid area up to the nonaffected area, seen on colonoscopy or barium enema. A barium enema should be avoided in cases of severe colitis because of the risk of perforation. On occasion the barium enema examination may look entirely normal, while colonoscopic examination with biopsy demonstrates the chronic and acute inflammatory changes of ulcerative colitis.

TREATMENT

The treatment for IBD is primarily directed toward decreasing the inflammation. An additional important goal of therapy in children is nutritional rehabilitation and restoration of normal growth.

The various categories of pharmacologic agents used to manage IBD derive from the theories of its pathogenesis. Thus, anti-inflammatory agents, immunomodulators and immunosuppressants, and antimicrobials are used, systemically and locally, in different combinations. The mainstay of medical therapy is oral corticosteroids, at a dose of 2 mg/kg up to a maximum of 40 to 60 mg/d. As the signs and symptoms of inflammation subside, the corticosteroid (prednisone) dose is tapered, since there is no evidence that continuous administration in the absence of active disease prevents relapses. Alternate-day corticosteroid therapy has been shown to be effective and also decreases the side effects related to corticosteroid therapy, such as fluid retention, acne, striae, weight gain, cataracts, bone demineralization, and growth retardation. Topical corticosteroids (suppositories or enemas) are also used in patients with ulcerative colitis limited to the distal colon. Newer corticosteroid preparations are being developed that have little effect on endogenous cortisol production, cause fewer side effects, but still have a profound suppressive effect on IBD.

If the patient has colonic disease (Crohn's colitis or chronic ulcerative colitis), sulfasalazine is added to the medical regimen or is used as primary therapy in patients with mild ulcerative colitis. Originally used in the 1930s for treatment of rheumatoid arthritis, sulfasalazine was found to be more effective in the management of colitis. Only partially absorbed in the small intestine, the diazo bond of sulfasalazine is reduced in the colon by indigenous bacteria and the active moiety, 5-acetyl salicylic acid (5-ASA) is released but poorly absorbed, acting locally as an anti-inflammatory agent. In recent years, local treatment with 5-ASA enemas has been effective in distal colitis and oral 5-ASA agents have been developed as an alternative to sulfasalazine for sulfa-sensitive patients.

Immunomodulatory agents have also been used to manage Crohn's disease. The purine antagonists, 6-mercaptopurine and azathioprine, can be helpful in obtaining a remission when used in conjunction with corticosteroids, allowing for tapering of the corticosteroid dose. They are also helpful in the management of patients with Crohn's disease and enteric fistulas. Since it may take up to 9 months to see a beneficial effect with these drugs, they are not helpful in managing acute complications. Other immunosuppressants that have shown recent promise in the management of refractory IBD are cyclosporin A and methotrexate, although their efficacy remains controversial.

Antibiotics have also been used to treat patients with IBD. Metronidazole has been used successfully to manage Crohn's colitis, fistulas, and the perianal complications of Crohn's disease.

In recent years, the leukotrienes have been implicated as important mediators of the inflammatory response, and therefore leukotriene antagonists are being studied as agents in the management of IBD.

The beneficial use of total parenteral nutrition and elemental enteral diets as primary treatment for acute Crohn's disease and as adjunctive treatment for complications such as subacute obstruction, perianal fissures, enteric fistulas, and growth failure has been documented. The elemental enteral formulations available are relatively unpalatable so they may need to be provided as a constant night-time nasogastric infusion, although some patients are able to drink their required amount. The major limitations with this management protocol are patient compliance and a relatively rapid relapse rate, about 4 to 6 months.

In addition to the effect on disease activity and its intestinal complications, there may be numerous nutritional and metabolic imbalances in IBD. Many of these problems are related to the diseased ileum, which is particularly important in the digestive, absorptive, metabolic, and nutritional activities of the gastrointestinal system. Ileal disease or resection and disease in the upper intestine can be associated with diminished or absent absorption of vitamin B_{12}, bile acids, lactose intolerance, protein-losing enteropathy, diminished absorption of trace metals such as zinc, calcium, and magnesium, fat malabsorption, and defective absorption of vitamin D metabolites. The administration of cholestyramine to bind bile acids can minimize the diarrhea associated with this malabsorption and loss of enterohepatic circulation. Supplementation with zinc, vitamin B_{12}, iron, and folate is often necessary.

Finally, when pharmacologic and nutritional therapy fail to bring about an adequate remission of the disease process or its complications, surgical options need to be considered. A total colectomy in patients with chronic ulcerative colitis is curative. However, there is no cure for Crohn's disease, and surgery always needs to be cautiously approached because of the risks of repeated intestinal resections and the potential establishment of a short gut and its attendant complications.

ANNOTATED BIBLIOGRAPHY

Greenstein AJ, Janowitz MD, Sachar DB: The extraintestinal complications of Crohn's disease and ulcerative colitis: A study of 700 patients. Medicine 55:401–408, 1976. (Retrospective review analyzing the pattern and incidence of the extraintestinal manifestations of IBD.)

Grenberger N: Indications for surgery in inflammatory bowel disease: A gastroenterologist's opinion. In Kirsner JB, Shorter RG (eds): Inflammatory Bowel Disease, 3rd ed, p 529. Philadelphia, Lea & Febiger, 1988. (Rational conservative approach to the consideration of surgery in IBD.)

Levine MD, Rappaport LA: Recurrent abdominal pain in school children: The loneliness of the long-distance physician. Pediatr Clin North Am 31:969–991, 1984. (Excellent approach to the evaluation of the patient with recurrent abdominal pain, a very small percentage of whom have IBD.)

MacDermott RP, Stenson WF: Alterations of the immune system in ulcerative colitis and Crohn's disease. Adv Immunol 42:285–328, 1988. (Review of the immunologic changes seen in IBD that may be involved in the pathogenesis of the disease.)

Markowitz J, Daum F, Aiges M et al: Perianal disease in children and adolescents with Crohn's disease. Gastroenterology 86:829–834, 1984. (Review of the scope and characteristics of perianal disease in childhood Crohn's disease.)

Peppercorn MA: Advances in drug therapy for inflammatory bowel disease. Ann Intern Med 112:50–60, 1990. (Recent advances in drug therapy for IBD and the effectiveness of the newer agents.)

Rosenthal SR, Snyder JD, Hendricks KM, Walker WA: Growth failure and inflammatory bowel disease: Approach to treatment of a complicated adolescent problem. Pediatrics 72:481–490, 1983. (Presents a review of studies that document that growth failure is primarily a result of undernutrition and a plan to overcome growth failure with nutritional reconstitution.)

Seidman, EG: Nutritional management of inflammatory bowel disease. Gastroenterol Clin North Am 17:129–155, 1989. (Review of the role of nutritional therapy as primary and adjunctive therapy of IBD.)

Verhave M, Winter HS, Grand RJ: Azathioprine in the treatment of children with inflammatory bowel disease. J Pediatr 117:809–814, 1990. (Prospective study of immunosuppressive therapy in IBD in children showing its efficacy as an adjunctive agent.)

108
Constipation

James H. Berman

Constipation is, in many ways, a paradigm for pediatric disease. It represents a complex interaction of parental and cultural expectations, development, gastrointestinal physiology, and nutritional factors. Any potential diagnosis and its attendant therapy must be discussed in the context of this interaction. Constipation has been estimated to account for 4% of all pediatric office visits. These figures do not include most patients with transient symptoms who do not seek medical attention.

DEFINITION

The first task of the pediatrician is to determine what the parent or patient means by the term *constipation*. Constipation may be defined as an intestinal dysfunction in which the bowels are difficult or painful to evacuate. This rather broad definition will serve to reassure many parents whose children are asymptomatic although their stooling patterns do not meet some cultural or parental expectations. Defining a frequency of stooling that is abnormal is difficult because of the great influence of dietary and environmental factors. Various population surveys in adults have established a range of three times a day to three times a week. Infants taking various feedings exhibit a similar range of stooling frequency to that of adults. Defining difficulty in passing a bowel movement is more subjective and thus even more difficult to quantify than stool frequency. It is easy to recognize that the passage of pellet-like hard stools is abnormal, but the passage of a soft stool that requires considerable straining may be more difficult to classify. In the infant and toddler age groups, parents often mistake the normal passage of stool (face turning red and pulling up legs) or even straining to withhold stool as a symptom of constipation. Stools flowing around a fecal impaction may be diarrheal.

WORK-UP

Fortunately, despite the high incidence of constipation, few patients with constipation have a significant organic abnormality. However, a careful history and physical examination may elicit complaints that raise more alarm. *Functional constipation* (no definite organic etiology) should not interfere with normal growth and development. Failure to thrive, particularly when associated with constipation, may occur in patients with Hirschsprung's disease, celiac disease, and various metabolic disturbances. Developmental delay and neuromuscular disorders can often present as constipation. Moderate to tense abdominal distention rarely occurs in functional constipation but is often noted in patients with obstructive processes, celiac disease, and Hirschsprung's disease. In the absence of an anal fissure, the presence of blood is of concern, although colitis, neoplasm, or an obstructing polyp are rare in childhood. Colicky abdominal pain may occur in functional constipation, especially while straining for stools, but abdominal tenderness is usually absent. Vomiting is not usually reported in patients with functional constipation. Excessive milk intake, anticholinergic drugs, lead toxicity, cathartic abuse, narcotics, and aluminum-based antacids can produce constipation. Iron-containing vitamin preparations can give rise to constipation. There is no evidence that iron-fortified infant formulas produce constipation, and they are important in the prevention of iron deficiency. Finally, constipation as a cause for fever, seizures, upper respiratory tract infections, otitis, or psychosis is probably more of a myth than a reality.

The presence of constipation in the newborn is always worrisome. More than 90% of infants will have their first stool within 24 hours after birth. Abdominal distention and vomiting are signs of functional or anatomic obstruction. Intestinal atresias and stenoses as well as meconium ileus may first present as constipation. An abdominal roentgenogram demonstrates an obstructive gas pattern and air–fluid levels. Functional ileus is usually associated with ill infants, those of low birth weight, and infants with respiratory distress. The presence of hypoactive bowel sounds, distention, and feeding intolerance makes functional ileus difficult to differentiate from an anatomic obstruction. The abdominal roentgenogram may show diffuse dilatation of the bowel, and there are generally no air–fluid levels.

Hirschsprung's disease (congenital aganglionic megacolon) merits special mention. It represents the most common cause of neonatal abdominal obstruction and is the organic cause commonly considered in the evaluation of constipation at any age. Although increasing awareness of the disease has produced earlier diagnosis, one third of all cases remain undiagnosed until after 3 months of age and 15% to 25% of cases are not diagnosed until after 5 years of age. The diagnosis of Hirschsprung's disease may be delayed in those cases involving only a short segment of the colon. An early diagnosis may reduce the incidence of enterocolitis (high mortality) and spare patients the morbidity of chronic constipation. Newborns who fail to pass stool in the first 48 hours of life, or who pass a meconium plug, should be observed closely. If stooling problems persist, an investigation with a mucosal rectal biopsy and a barium enema is indicated. Infants and older children in whom Hirschsprung's disease is suspected may be first screened with rectal manometry.

Infants may be bothered by the discomfort of passing a stool through an *anal fissure.* Congenital hypothyroidism, renal tubular acidosis, hypercalcemia, and diabetes insipidus are rare causes of constipation. The association of a developmental delay or sacral anomalies with constipation is suspicious for neuromuscular disorders or myelodysplasia.

The second year of life is marked by an increasing variety of foods in the child's diet and the gradual acquisition of a conscious control over defecation. Parents maintain an expectation that their offspring will soon be free of diapers, an event with implications for parental life-style as well as the child's development. Unfortunately, the low-fiber toddler diet and the complex process of toilet training can make this time of life troubled by constipation. As with other newly discovered skills in this age group, the toddler with some control over defecation may choose to withhold a stool. The reason may be that he finds it uncomfortable to pass or as a gesture of independence. The parent often complains that the child will grimace and strain and then pass a small amount of stool. Other children may pass giant bowel movements infrequently. The child can spend long, unproductive sessions on the toilet. Parents often interpret these symptoms as intestinal blockage when, paradoxically, the child is actually withholding stool. The presence of an anal fissure, which produces pain on defecation, makes the child's desire to withhold a stool understandable. Emotional stresses, such as the birth of a sibling, inconsistent or coercive toilet training, or separation from parents may also lead to withholding of stool.

Minor illnesses can produce changes in bowel patterns through several mechanisms. Febrile illness, anorexia, and vomiting produce a mild dehydration provoking constipation. Some variation in gastrointestinal motility has been suggested as a possible mechanism. Finally, decreased dietary fiber intake during the period of illness contributes to the constipation. Rarely, bacterial enteric pathogens, such as *Salmonella,* may present as fever and constipation rather than the more typical diarrhea. Once again, the presence of abdominal pain, distention, and vomiting with constipation are worrisome signs. Intussusception, volvulus, or previously undiagnosed Hirschsprung's disease are all possible in the toddler age group.

Older children have a more varied diet and display other mechanisms for exerting control over their environment. Constipation may still be a problem in this age group. In fact, encopresis, or fecal soiling, may occur in 1% to 2% of first graders. Encopresis, as defined by the passage of stool outside the toilet after 4 years of age, is associated with a high psychological morbidity (see Chap. 34).

Children with mental retardation, neuromuscular disorders, or those with surgically corrected Hirschsprung's disease may continue having difficulty passing stools. The school bathroom is a frightening or embarrassing place for many children, who thus defer having a bowel movement for many hours. Active social schedules may also contribute to producing a back-up of stool in the distal colon. The consumption of "junk food," characteristically low in fiber, further aggravates the problem. As mentioned earlier, it is not uncommon for a child with Hirschsprung's disease to escape diagnosis until school age or later. In addition, acquired hypothyroidism, intestinal tumors, or even inflammatory bowel disease may present as constipation. Finally, urinary tract infections are not uncommonly associated with constipation. Patients with recurrent urinary tract infections should be questioned about their bowel habits.

TREATMENT

The treatment of constipation should be tailored to the individual patient. The mechanisms responsible for normal variations in stooling pattern should be explained to parents as completely as possible. Written information or diagrams are often helpful. By coping with parental and societal expectations, counseling may be the only therapy required. Parents should be cautioned that although they and the pediatrician remain concerned about the child's health, an excessive vigilance over the child's stooling and toileting behavior diminish the child's feelings of autonomy and increase the tension over what should be a normal physiologic process. At an extreme, such attention may even aggravate the constipation. The parents and child should be aware that the treatment of constipation and encopresis requires long-term, consistent intervention and follow-up. A concrete treatment plan and measurable goals to be attained aid greatly in this process. A general rule of thumb is that the constipation will take as long to reverse as the time the child has had the constipation before treatment.

Constipation during infancy generally responds to increasing the fluid intake. Osmotic agents such as Karo syrup (5 to 15 mL/8-oz bottle) or malt soup extract (Maltsupex [Wallace], 1 to 4 tablespoons per day) have also been used. Glycerin suppositories act locally to stimulate the passage of stool.

Dietary fiber is a complex mixture of compounds including cellulose, hemicellulose, mucilages, gums, pectin, and lignins. These substances vary in their water-holding properties and effects on bacterial fermentation. Fiber has attracted much attention for its hypocholesterolemic effects and possible role in the prevention of colon and other cancers. Several national panels have advocated an increase in the intake of dietary fiber for adults. Recommendations for children have been more guarded. Concerns have been raised that a high-fiber diet may alter the mineral balance in children, but there are little clinical data to support this objection. Unfortunately, the high-fiber legumes and whole-grain products do not traditionally appeal to a child's palate. A household survey conducted by the United States Department of Agriculture showed that a significant percentage of children consume less than the recommended daily allowance for fruits, vegetables, and cereals. Some parental education regarding the benefits of increasing fiber intake for the whole family may help alter these findings. Fiber may be conveniently added to the diet through the use of whole-grain breads. Legumes such as peas and beans are good sources of fiber and are an enjoyable snack when eaten frozen, directly from the package. They are often more popular in soups than as a standard vegetable side dish. Peanut butter, citrus fruits, apples, and bananas are also good sources of fiber. The water-soluble fiber in the latter two is often exploited to firm up loose stools following acute gastroenteritis. This does *not* mean that the foods are constipating. Crude bran (tasteless) may be added to prepared and baked foods at 1 to 2 teaspoons per serving. Diced prunes, dates, and raisins are less objectionable when added to cookies or sprinkled over cereal. High-fiber cereals (9 g/serving) are also useful. Although the caloric density of most fiber-rich foods is low, the child benefits from a higher intake of vitamins A and C and a reduced intake of refined sugar. These benefits appeal to many parents. The alteration in caloric density of the food can be minimized by including nuts and legumes in the diet. Commercially prepared fiber preparations of psyllium seeds or polycarbophil (Fibercon [Lederle]; Fiberall [Ciba Consumer]; Citrucel [Lakeside]) are frequently beneficial as a supplement in older children. Although adequate fluids should be taken with fiber products, no more than 32 oz of milk or formula should be consumed daily.

Stool softeners, like dioctyl sodium sulfosuccinate (Colace [Mead Johnson]) are surface active agents increasing the penetration of stool by water. They also have some effect on gastrointestinal motor and secretory functions. These agents are useful in treating simple constipation or in aiding in maintaining soft stools while weaning the patient from mineral oil. They may be most useful in the child with developmental disability who requires chronic stool softening without the side effects of mineral oil. Doses of 5 to 10 mg/kg/d may be required.

Lactulose (Cephulac [Merrell Dow]) is a nonabsorbed carbohydrate that loosens stool by producing an osmotic load in the colon. Although it is a safe and effective stool softener, its use may be limited by its cost.

Cathartic laxatives are rarely indicated in childhood. Bisacodyl (Dulcolax [Boehringer]) may be useful in the evacuation of stool during the initial therapy for chronic constipation. Frequent use of cathartic laxatives may cause significant fluid and electrolyte disturbances, colonic mucosal changes, and laxative dependence.

Mineral oil (liquid petrolatum) is a hydrocarbon mixture that produces a loose, frothy stool. Although not especially palatable, it can be mixed with chocolate syrup or blenderized with fruit juice and ice cubes to make an appealing cocktail. Several flavored mineral oils are available, but some of these also contain cathartics. Doses as low as 1 to 2 teaspoons may be effective in relieving constipation, but much larger doses are generally required for chronic constipation and encopresis. One tablespoon for each 15 kg given twice daily is a good initial dose. The dose may then be increased by 0.5 tablespoon (7.5 mL) every other day until the stools produced are loose, but not runny. These stools are difficult to withhold and should eliminate straining. The passage of mineral oil through the rectum can cause unpleasant anal irritation and is generally a sign that the dose is too low, with leakage occurring around impacted stool. Small amounts of mineral oil are absorbed systemically, producing deposits in the liver, spleen, lymph nodes, and other tissues. Although these findings may not be clinically significant, adults chronically taking mineral oil have been reported to have, on liver biopsy, lesions resembling chronic hepatitis. Recent evidence has shown that mineral oil does not have a significant impact on fat-soluble vitamin absorption. Routine vitamin supplementation is therefore not required. Although reports of lipoid pneumonia following the aspiration of mineral oil are uncommon, its use in infants, children with severe gastroesophageal reflux, or in those with significant neurologic impairment is contraindicated. Mineral oil doses should not be given just before bedtime.

Chronic Constipation and Encopresis

Therapy for chronic constipation or encopresis requires counseling and the flexible use of the aforementioned medications, since there is no universally effective remedy. Although there is considerable controversy surrounding different treatment protocols, most methods include the following aspects: First, promote normal attitudes toward bowel function as mentioned earlier. Second, assess the degree of fecal retention and remove retained feces. Third, reeducate the bowel toward normal function, and, finally, emphasize the importance of frequent follow-up. An objective assessment of the degree of fecal retention may be achieved through physical findings (the presence or absence of a left lower quadrant mass) or an abdominal plain roentgenogram revealing the amount of feces within the colon. Serial studies can then be employed to measure progress. The reaccumulation of retained stool is frequently associated with treatment failures. Because of an overlap with the normal population, a measurement of intestinal transit time is probably not helpful. Changes in rectal manometric data with treatment are, at the moment, not a clinically proven method for following patient progress or as a prognostic tool (see also Chap. 34).

Removing retained feces from the colon is an important first step in reestablishing normal bowel function. Although enemas are an effective method of evacuating the colon, they represent a significant loss of control for the child, are often uncomfortable, and may produce fluid and electrolyte disturbances. Recently, balanced electrolyte colonic lavage solutions (CoLytely, Braintree; Colyte, Reed, and Carnick) have been developed. They cleanse the bowel by producing an osmotic diarrhea, but have no significant effect on water or electrolyte balance. Large volumes of solution should be ingested for effective evacuation. A school-aged child should drink 2 L of solution each day on 2 consecutive days. If the salty taste of the solutions or the volume required

makes compliance difficult, the entire 4-L dose can be given through a small nasogastric feeding tube in the office at a rate of 750–1000 mL/h. Nausea and bloating may occur, but vomiting is unusual. Hospitalization is occasionally required for "clean-out" when a dysfunctional family situation precludes good compliance with the program.

Reeducation of bowel habits involves several components. The *maintenance* of soft stool ensures the ease of passage and decreases withholding. Mineral oil effectively produces the appropriate stool softness. The dose should be increased slowly until the stools are loose, but not runny; rarely are more than 4 oz/d required if the initial clean-out was effective. Since this therapy represents some loss of control on the part of the child, a simultaneous process of enlisting the patient's help in the treatment plan is important. A comparison of bowel training with athletic training is useful. Many treatment protocols include reward systems such as a star chart. The goals to be achieved should be attainable and easily measured (e.g., four stools in the toilet = one red star; four red stars = one new toy). The reward should be for producing a stool in the toilet, not the absence of soiling. All of the child's caretakers should administer the system consistently. Toileting at specific times, when the chances of successful stooling are better, is beneficial. These times include mornings and 1 hour after meals. The possibility of needing to toilet at an inopportune moment (e.g., at school or in a shopping mall) is thus also minimized. Teachers should be aware that the child may need to make an emergency visit to the toilet.

INDICATIONS FOR REFERRAL

Biofeedback techniques employing rectal manometry have thus far not proven more effective than conventional therapy, but they may benefit individual patients. Because some children with refractory constipation have Hirschsprung's disease, treatment failures should be assessed with rectal manometry or rectal biopsy before continuing the treatment. Family noncompliance and psychological dysfunction are the leading causes of treatment failures. A psychiatric referral can prove helpful in children with major social or family dysfunction. Older children may be particularly bothered by the embarrassment, loss of self-esteem, and social isolation associated with soiling in their clothes.

ANNOTATED BIBLIOGRAPHY

Abrahamian FP, Lloyd-Still JD: Chronic constipation in childhood: Longitudinal study of 186 patients. J Pediatr Gastroenterol Nutr 3:460, 1984. (Review of manometric data and response to treatment.)

Arhan P, Devroede G et al: Idiopathic disorders of fecal continence in children. Pediatrics 71:774, 1983. (Reports that many patients date the onset of constipation from infancy.)

Barness LA, Dallman PR et al: Plant fiber intake in the pediatric diet. Pediatrics 67:572, 1981. (AAP Nutrition Committee recommendations.)

Clayden GS, Lawson JN: Investigation and management of longstanding constipation in children. Arch Dis Child 51:918, 1976. (Useful management techniques for chronic constipation.)

Cummings JH: Constipation, dietary fibre and the control of large bowel function. Postgrad Med J 60:811, 1984. (Review of intestinal effects of dietary fiber.)

Kleinhaus S, Boley SJ et al: Hirschsprung's disease: A survey of Members of the Surgical Section of the American Academy of Pediatrics. J Pediatr Surg 14:588, 1979. (Documents incidence of enterocolitis and missed diagnosis in a large series of patients.)

Levine MD: The schoolchild with encopresis. Pediatr Rev 2:285, 1981. (Good review of approach to chronic constipation and encopresis.)

Weaver LH: Bowel habit from birth to old age. Gastroenteral Nutr 7:637–640, 1988. (Demonstrates normal variation in bowel habits for each age group.)

109

Hepatomegaly

Tien-Lan Chang and Ronald E. Kleinman

The etiology of hepatomegaly is often determined by a complete history, a physical examination, and a few laboratory tests. However, because of the many possible causes of an enlarged liver or spleen and the potential need for specialized testing, a systematic approach is useful in differentiating the diagnosis.

DEFINITION

Hepatomegaly means enlargement of the liver. In adults, enlargement of the liver is often first appreciated by palpation of the liver edge below the right costal margin. In normal children, especially in infants, the liver edge is frequently palpable below the costal margin and therefore cannot by itself be considered an abnormal finding. It has also been shown that there is no correlation between the vertical span (by radiography) of the liver and the liver edge (by palpation) below the costal margin. An accurate estimation of the liver size is best made clinically by percussion of the upper border and palpation of the lower border of the liver at the right midclavicular line. The liver span, obtained by this method, for normal newborns is 5.9 ± 0.7 cm and for older normal children, 6.5 cm $+ 0.022 \times$ age. Eleven centimeters is the upper limit of normal for children 5 to 12 years of age. Measurements in different planes by ultrasound, nuclear scan, or computed tomography will provide an accurate assessment of the liver volume. Confirmation of hepatomegaly by one or another imaging study is important because a misinterpretation of the liver size may lead to an unnecessary diagnostic evaluation and anxiety in the patient and parents. For example, Riedel's lobe is a tongue-like projection of the right lobe that increases the liver span but does not necessarily cause an increase in the total volume of the liver.

PATHOPHYSIOLOGY, CLINICAL PRESENTATION, AND DIFFERENTIAL DIAGNOSIS

Although the classification of diffuse versus focal processes is somewhat artificial because there are clearly disorders that produce discrete lesions found diffusely throughout the liver, we have found this to be a useful approach to the differential diagnosis of hepatomegaly.

Diffuse Enlargement of the Liver

A diffuse enlargement of the liver occurs either as a result of the excessive storage of nutrients or their metabolites or as a result of an accumulation or proliferation of red or white blood cells or macrophages.

Amyloidosis with storage of the amyloid protein in the liver rarely occurs in childhood, whether primary or secondary. In contrast, systemic α_1-antitrypsin deficiency is one of the most common causes of chronic liver disease in childhood. The periodic acid–Schiff (PAS)-positive, diastase-resistant material, which is immunologically identical with α_1-antitrypsin, accumulates in hepatocytes. A mononuclear cell infiltrate in portal areas also contributes to the hepatomegaly. Although patients who have this disorder may be asymptomatic, some may present either with neonatal jaundice or later in childhood with cirrhosis and its complications or with chronic lung disease.

An accumulation of fat in hepatocytes is seen in malnutrition, diabetes mellitus, cystic fibrosis, obesity, Reye syndrome, Wolman's disease, cholesterol ester storage disease, glucocorticoid use, and during the course of parenteral nutrition. Although fatty change is usually found diffusely throughout the liver, focal fatty metamorphosis can also occur in association with the conditions already mentioned and should be considered in the differential diagnosis of focal lesions of the liver. Fatty metamorphosis associated with hepatocellular injury occurs in drug-induced hepatitis (e.g., tetracycline) and metabolic disorders (e.g., hereditary fructose intolerance, galactosemia, tyrosinemia, α_1-antitrypsin deficiency and Wilson's disease). The storage of lipid in reticuloendothelial cells is seen in Gaucher's disease (glucocerebrosidosis), Niemann-Pick disease (sphingomyelinosis), and lipoprotein lipase deficiency.

Carbohydrate accumulates in the liver in two groups of inherited metabolic disorders: glycogen storage diseases and mucopolysaccharidoses. Depending on the enzyme deficiency, the clinical presentation may be different for patients with a glycogen storage disease. In contrast, patients with mucopolysaccharidoses usually share certain clinical features that permit a provisional diagnosis. These include short stature, stiff joints, corneal clouding, deafness, hirsuitism, upper airway narrowing (resulting in respiratory insufficiency), nerve root compression, and a gradual mental deterioration.

Patients with infantile GM_1 gangliosidosis (β-galactosidase deficiency) have an increased accumulation of both glycolipids (GM_1 ganglioside) and mucopolysaccharides in the liver, other visceral organs, and the nervous system. These patients are hypotonic in the neonatal period and developmentally delayed thereafter. Hepatomegaly is often evident by 6 months of age.

In addition to cellular enlargement, the various types of cells within the liver may increase in number. A cellular increase resulting in hepatomegaly most commonly comes from inflammatory infiltrates, which may be due to infectious, immunologic, metabolic, or toxic causes. Along with an increase in the inflammatory cells, there may also be Kupffer cell hyperplasia as part of the reaction to injury (see Chap. 110). Periportal inflammation and ductular proliferation can also be seen in obstructive biliary diseases (e.g., biliary atresia). Malignant cellular infiltrates can occur with lymphomas, leukemias, and reticuloendothelioses (e.g., histiocytosis X). Residual extramedullary hematopoiesis can occur in normal full-term neonatal livers in the first few days of life. This fetal function may be "recalled" in conditions in which the marrow space is occupied by malignant cells or metabolic products (e.g., cystinosis, oxalosis) and in erythroblastosis fetalis, in which the marrow erythropoiesis is inadequate to meet the demands that result from increased hemolysis.

An accumulation of blood in the liver, or hepatic congestion, is due to postsinusoidal obstruction of the portosystemic blood flow. The obstruction may occur at different levels, and the principal diseases causing the obstruction include right-sided heart failure, inferior vena cava or hepatic vein obstruction (Budd-Chiari syndrome), and veno-occlusive disease. Severe lung disease (cor pulmonale), congenital heart disease, pericardial effusion, and certain cardiomyopathies are the main reasons for right-sided heart failure. The causes of hepatic vein thrombosis include oral contraceptives, tumorous compression or invasion of the hepatic vein or inferior vena cava, and a congenital web at the hepatic vein–inferior vena cava junction. Veno-occlusive disease is most often associated with chemotherapy and radiation therapy in patients with malignancies. Ascites is a frequent accompanying sign with all types of veno-occlusive disease.

Focal Disorders of the Liver

Diseases that produce focal or multifocal lesions in the liver can be classified as tumors, cysts, granulomas, or abscesses.

Primary malignant liver tumors in pediatric patients include hepatoblastoma, hepatocellular carcinoma, and em-

bryonal sarcoma. Some patients with these tumors may complain of weakness, anorexia, or vomiting, but frequently these patients present with an abdominal mass with no other symptoms or complaints. Hepatoblastoma is usually clinically apparent and diagnosed before the infant is 18 months of age, whereas hepatocellular carcinoma and embryonal sarcoma are generally diagnosed in childhood. The prognosis for survival with hepatoblastoma is better than for hepatocellular carcinoma because it is less likely to have metastasized at the time of diagnosis and is more often resectable. The most common metastatic tumors in the liver in childhood are Wilms' tumor and neuroblastoma. The clinical presentation of patients with these tumors often cannot be distinguished from that of primary hepatic tumors.

Nonmalignant tumors of the liver include adenomas, focal nodular hyperplasia, hamartomas, and vascular tumors. Cavernous hemangioma is the most common type of benign tumors in adults and children. Hemangioendothelioma is usually diagnosed before 1 year of age. Most of the vascular tumors regress with age, and some tumors grow for a time before regressing. Some patients may develop high-output heart failure, and some patients may have a syndrome of thrombocytopenia, anemia, and delayed clotting resembling disseminated intravascular coagulopathy (Kasabach-Merritt syndrome).

The other benign tumors are all rare. Patients who have glycogen storage diseases and those using oral contraceptives are at increased risk for developing adenomas. Some authors consider adenomas to be premalignant because of reports of patients with adenomas who subsequently died of hepatocarcinoma.

Cystic diseases of the liver include congenital hepatic fibrosis and intrahepatic bile duct ectasia (Caroli's disease). Congenital hepatic fibrosis is characterized by broad bands of connective tissue in a portal and periportal distribution, with multiple dysmorphic bile ducts lying within these bands. The liver involvement may be either complete or partial. The disease is virtually always associated with renal disease. Major causes of morbidity and mortality in these patients are renal insufficiency, cholangitis, and problems related to portal hypertension. Intrahepatic bile duct ectasia (Caroli's disease) may be complicated by cholangitis and gallstone formation. Other cystic lesions include benign solitary cyst, hydatid cyst (from infection by *Echinococcus*), cyst from trauma or infarction, and cysts associated with certain rare congenital malformations.

Hepatic granulomas can occur with several infectious agents, including *Mycobacterium* (tuberculosis and leprosy), *Brucella, Salmonella, Leptospira, Actinomyces, Blastomyces, Histoplasma, Cryptococcus, Coccidioides, Plasmodium* (malaria), *Leishmania, Toxoplasma, Schistosoma, Fasciola, Cysticercus, Toxocara,* and *Ascaris.* Noninfectious causes include berylliosis, sarcoidosis, and certain drugs such as carbamazepine.

A hepatic abscess may originate from hematogenous

dissemination, by direct extension of infection from the biliary tract, or from a contiguous site of infection. In infants and young children, the hematogenous spread of systemic infection is the most common mechanism, occurring in patients with compromised host defense mechanisms. In older children and young adults, trauma and amebae are the major causes of hepatic abscesses.

Splenomegaly

The spleen may be enlarged alone or often in association with hepatomegaly, hence its importance in the differential diagnosis of liver disease. The liver may be shrunken, in patients with cirrhosis with the result that the enlarged spleen is the first evidence of liver disease discovered during a physical examination. The major mechanisms responsible for splenomegaly are portal hypertension, lipid storage, lymphohistiocytic proliferation (e.g., histiocytosis X, Epstein-Barr virus infection), sequestration (e.g., immune hemolytic anemia), extramedullary hematopoiesis, and infiltration by hematologic malignancies. Portal hypertension can be suprahepatic, intrahepatic, or prehepatic. Suprahepatic causes have already been discussed (i.e., Budd-Chiari syndrome). Intrahepatic causes include any chronic liver disease leading to cirrhosis, congenital hepatic fibrosis, noncirrhotic regenerative hyperplasia, hereditary telangiectasis, and hepatoportal sclerosis. Prehepatic causes of portal vein obstruction include cavernous transformation of the portal vein and portal vein thrombosis. Although the pathogenesis of cavernous transformation of the portal vein is unknown, umbilical vein catheterization and omphalitis have been reported as possible risk factors. (See Chap 128, for a more complete discussion.)

WORK-UP

History and Physical Examination

The history and physical examination provide the initial screening to eliminate many of the unlikely causes of hepatomegaly and provide clues to the diagnosis. This history should include age at onset, associated symptoms (e.g., nausea, vomiting, fever, anorexia, weight loss), duration of symptoms, environmental exposure to toxins (including drugs), exposure to persons with infections, travel to areas endemic with certain parasitic infections, and family history of inherited diseases. Growth and development should be noted in both a history and a physical examination because failure to thrive is often an indication of a chronic metabolic or nutritional disorder. Perhaps the most helpful clues are obtained from an examination of the skin and eyes in addition to the abdominal examination. Cutaneous manifestations of liver disease include jaundice, spider angiomas, excoriations, and caput medusae. Easy bruising suggests a clotting problem. Cutaneous vascular nevi may point to the presence of hemangiomas in the liver. Possible eye findings include cataracts, macular spots, and Kayser-Fleischer

rings. The liver should be palpated for tenderness, degree of firmness, smoothness, and nodularity. A pedunculated mass arising from the liver surface may be either an adenoma or focal nodular hyperplasia. Both the left and right lobes should be examined, because in cirrhosis the right lobe may be normal or small whereas the left lobe is compensatorily enlarged, and in the case of hepatic tumors there may be asymmetric involvement of the lobes. The left side of the abdomen should be palpated for splenic enlargement. The enlargement of other organs and masses and the presence of ascites should be ascertained.

Laboratory Tests

The first screening tests should include a complete blood cell count, differential, platelet count, sedimentation rate, and liver function tests, such as evaluation of prothrombin time, albumin, total protein, bilirubin, serum glutamic oxaloacetic transaminase, serum glutamic pyruvic transaminase, and alkaline phosphatase. Hematologic disorders may be suggested by anemia, thrombocytopenia, or an abnormal blood smear. A bone marrow examination is usually helpful in their diagnosis. Liver function tests, however, are not helpful in the diagnosis of primary malignant liver tumors, and cirrhotic patients may have only mild changes. Abnormal blood sugar, cholesterol, and triglyceride values, although nonspecific, may suggest a metabolic basis for hepatomegaly in conjunction with other laboratory tests. Based on one's clinical suspicion, other more specific tests can be ordered, such as α_1-antitrypsin and α-fetoprotein values (for liver tumors), serum ceruloplasmin, copper, and 24-hour urine copper values (for Wilson's disease), and serologic studies for infectious diseases.

Imaging Studies

Several imaging studies are now available that not only distinguish focal from diffuse processes but also may provide information about the nature of the lesions. A plain roentgenogram of the abdomen can indicate the size of the organs as well as any calcified lesions (e.g., neuroblastoma, hydatid cyst). Ultrasound examination and computed tomography provide information regarding the size and homogeneity of the liver. Ultrasound examination is less expensive, more easily performed, and requires little patient preparation, whereas computed tomography is slightly more sensitive in detecting focal lesions and fluid collections. An intravenous pyelogram following hepatic imaging can identify the presence of the primary tumor and its relation to the kidney (renal or suprarenal).

Radionuclide scans provide different information depending on the agents used. Technetium-99m sulfur coloid is extracted by reticuloendothelial cells so that any disturbance in the structure of the liver will cause a nonhomogeneous picture. The ^{99m}Tc IDA derivatives are taken up by the hepatocytes and excreted into bile and are useful in the diagnosis of cholestatic disorders. A delay in hepatic imaging may also indicate significant hepatocellular dysfunction. Gallium-67 is concentrated by a tumor or an abscess. When the scans are used in combination with other studies (e.g., arteriography), the type of focal lesions can often be determined prior to the tissue diagnosis. For example, a *cold* spot on the sulfur colloid scan due to an adenoma will be normal on the ^{99m}Tc IDA scan and will be highlighted on an arteriogram, whereas an abscess will be *cold* on the sulfur colloid and ^{99m}Tc IDA scans but *hot* on the gallium scan.

Magnetic resonance imaging may be used for studying both diffuse and focal disorders. Compared with computed tomography, it is superior in soft tissue contrast discrimination and in identifying and defining vascular structures such as vascular tumors, cavernous transformation of the portal vein, and collateral veins associated with portal hypertension. Its main disadvantage lies in the prolonged imaging time, which leads to less sharp images because of respiratory motion.

Invasive Studies

A liver biopsy is sometimes necessary for making a diagnosis as well as for assessing the severity of the disease. In many cases a closed percutaneous needle biopsy will be sufficient for histologic, biochemical, and infectious disease studies. However, a closed biopsy may be hazardous with vascular tumors and is therefore contraindicated. An open liver biopsy, with or without arteriography, is necessary for the diagnosis of solid tumors of the liver. Cholangiography, either endoscopic or intraoperative, may also help to distinguish the nature of the lesion.

INDICATIONS FOR REFERRAL AND TREATMENT

The most common cause of hepatomegaly is acute hepatitis of viral etiology. The majority of patients (90%) will recover without sequelae and need not be referred. All other patients with abnormalities in liver function and patients with splenomegaly with or without hepatomegaly will often be referred for an evaluation.

Patients with fulminant hepatic failure of any cause, as evidenced by a high bilirubin values and a prolonged prothrombin time greater than two times normal, should be cared for in a tertiary hospital setting. In those cases in which a tumor is suspected, the evaluation is best done in a setting where surgical support is available. For many of the metabolic diseases, a multidisciplinary approach is needed for both evaluation and management.

ANNOTATED BIBLIOGRAPHY

Alvarez F, Bernard O, Brunelle F et al: Congenital hepatic fibrosis in children. J Pediatr 99:370–375, 1981. (Report of correct clinical diagnosis based on clinical, biologic, and radiologic criteria.)

McDonald GB, Sharma P, Matthews DE et al: Veno-occlusive disease of the liver after bone marrow transplantation: Diagnosis, incidence and predisposing factors. Hepatology 4:116–122, 1984. (Review of this iatrogenic problem.)

Pereyra R, Andrassy RJ, Mahour GH: Management of massive hepatic hemangiomas in infants and children: A review of 13 cases. Pediatrics 70:254–258, 1982. (Report of 30% mortality in a small group of patients.)

Reiff MI, Osborn LM: Clinical estimation of liver size in newborn infants. Pediatrics 71:46–48, 1983. (Report of measurement by percussion/palpation that correlated poorly with palpation of the liver edge.)

Silberstein EB, Gilbert LA, Pu MY: Comparative efficacy of radionuclide, ultrasound and computer tomographic liver imaging for hepatic metastases. Curr Concepts Diagn Nucl Med 2(3):3–9, 1985. (Concise review with several good references.)

Stark DD, Felder RC, Wittenberg J et al: Magnetic resonance imaging of cavernous hemangioma of the liver: Tissue specific characterization. Am J Radiol 145:213–222, 1985. (States that magnetic resonance imaging has a 90% accuracy in the diagnosis of hemangiomas, better than any other imaging study.)

Younoszai MK, Mueller S: Clinical assessment of liver size in normal children. Clin Pediatr 14:378–381, 1975. (Reports normal range of liver size for children 5 to 12 years of age.)

110
Hepatitis
Glenn T. Furuta and Colette Deslandres-Leduc

Viral infections are the most frequent cause of hepatitis in patients younger than 20 years old. In one study, 32% of reported cases of hepatitis in this age group were caused by hepatitis A virus (HAV), 10.3% were caused by hepatitis B virus (HBV), and 13.1% were labeled non-A, non-B hepatitis (hepatitis C, D, E). Other causes of hepatitis in infants, children, and adolescents include a wide spectrum of metabolic, toxic, ischemic, and immunologic disorders (see also Chap. 195).

PATHOPHYSIOLOGY

Regardless of the mechanism leading to hepatocellular injury, one of the consequences is a loss of the selective permeability of the cellular membrane with spilling of aspartate aminotransferase and alanine aminotransferase into the systemic circulation. An impaired clearance of unconjugated bilirubin from serum occurs because of a diminished uptake of bilirubin into the hepatocyte, impaired intracellular binding, and decreased conjugation. Unconjugated bilirubin then accumulates in the circulation, producing icterus. High levels of free indirect serum bilirubin in the perinatal period may cause kernicterus. The excretion of conjugated bilirubin is also altered and a "regurgitation" of water-soluble conjugated bilirubin into the circulation causes icterus and dark, tea-colored urine. Clay-colored or pale stools occur because of a decrease or an absence of pigments that originate from both the diet and the bile.

With almost total hepatocyte dysfunction, a compromise of liver synthetic function becomes clinically apparent. Hepatocytes synthesize factors I (fibrinogen), II (prothrombin), V, VII, IX, and X. Factors II, VII, IX, and X require vitamin K for formation and are the most sensitive to hepatocellular disease. The prothrombin time closely reflects hepatic synthetic function because it depends on factors II, V, VII, and X. The partial thromboplastin time will also be affected, but to a lesser degree. The liver also plays a major role in glucose homeostasis; thus, hypoglycemia may occur with massive hepatocellular necrosis. Albumin synthesis also diminishes with the loss of hepatocyte function. Severe hypoalbuminemia as well as decreased hepatic degradation of aldosterone contribute to the accumulation of ascites and peripheral edema.

The pathophysiology of hepatic encephalopathy is still uncertain and probably multifactorial. This neuropsychiatric syndrome is widely believed to have a metabolic basis. The various "toxins" incriminated in the development of hepatic encephalopathy include ammonia, short-chain fatty acids, mercaptans, neural inhibition from γ-aminobutyric acid, and false neurotransmitters.

CLINICAL PRESENTATION

The prodrome of acute viral hepatitis consists of malaise, fatigue, anorexia, nausea, vomiting, low-grade fever, and abdominal pain. In 5% to 15% of cases, a triad of symptoms (*Caroli's triad*) similar to serum sickness occurs, consisting of headaches, rash, and arthralgias. Although more commonly reported with HBV, this is also noted with HAV and non-A, non-B hepatitis. A "flulike syndrome" can also occur with headache, fever, and myalgia.

An icteric phase often follows the prodrome and is characterized by dark urine, pale, clay-colored stools, and jaundice. With the onset of jaundice some symptoms abate whereas others worsen. The fever, arthralgias, and headaches typically disappear. Jaundice usually peaks within 5 to 10 days. Its duration varies from a few days to 6 to 7 months (an average of 1 to 3 weeks). As the jaundice increases, the other symptoms of liver disease intensify. Anorexia, fatigue, and weight loss may be severe. The first signs of recovery include the disappearance of nausea and vomiting with the return of appetite. Malaise, usually the first symptom to appear, is also the last to resolve.

Hepatitis can also present in a fulminant manner with signs of overt hepatic failure such as coagulopathy, ascites, and encephalopathy. The alteration of mental status is an early feature of fulminant hepatitis. It usually takes the form of increasing somnolence and confusion, although some patients will show agitation, violent behavior, and frank delirium. A progression to coma occurs rapidly.

Most children with viral hepatitis are asymptomatic. Indeed, in studies conducted in day-care centers only 4% to 16% of young children suspected of transmitting HAV to an older family member had symptoms of hepatitis, whereas a larger proportion of adults with HAV were symptomatic. Most HBV infections are also asymptomatic. Finally, hepatitis may be anicteric and may present only as nonspecific symptoms of anorexia, asthenia, and weight loss or in some cases as unexplained joint symptoms, colitis, and erythema nodosum.

DIFFERENTIAL DIAGNOSIS

Most cases of hepatitis are generally of viral origin. During the neonatal period, hepatitis presents as different clinical and pathologic findings and is therefore discussed separately.

Neonatal Hepatitis

In 1977, Danks and associates reported on 105 patients with neonatal hepatitis and described an incidence of 1:8000 live births. Intrauterine infections were responsible for approximately 20% of the cases: 12% cytomegalovirus (CMV), 2% toxoplasmosis, and 6% others (e.g., rubella, *Treponema pallidum* infection, and enterovirus infection). α_1-antitrypsin deficiency was found in 11% to 15% of the patients and galactosemia occurred in 5% of the patients. The etiology of the hepatitis in the remaining 50% to 60% of the cases was unknown. Other known causes of neonatal hepatitis include the TORCH syndrome and HBV, adenovirus, varicella, *Listeria monocytogenes,* other infectious agents, and the metabolic disorders fructosemia and tyrosinemia. The term *neonatal hepatitis* may be used to describe all cases of "hepatitis" in newborns or may be restricted to the clinical situation in which no definable cause is found for a newborn who suffers from prolonged cholestasis, who is younger than 2 months of age, and whose liver biopsy specimen displays giant cells. Such infants are more likely to be male, premature, or small for gestational age and have a positive family history (15%) for neonatal hepatitis. The mortality rate has been reported to be as high as 30%.

Postneonatal Period

Hepatitis A virus is the most frequent causal agent of hepatitis and has an incubation period of 2 to 4 weeks. It is transmitted by the oral-fecal route, predominantly by contaminated food such as shellfish or other foods washed in contaminated water. The virus can also be disseminated by food handlers responsible for the terminal preparation of food before serving. Toddlers in day-care centers are most susceptible to acquiring HAV because of the difficulty in maintaining good oral-fecal hygiene in this setting. Fortunately, children younger than 2 years of age are usually asymptomatic with HAV. Chronic hepatitis does not develop after the acute illness of HAV, although a small number of all patients will develop fulminant hepatitis. The estimated fatality rate from HAV is 0.14%. Reports suggest that while the incidence of HAV is declining, the incidence of HBV is increasing.

Hepatitis B has an incubation period of 3 to 10 weeks. It is transmitted through numerous body fluids, including blood, saliva, tears, sweat, nasopharyngeal secretions, urine, genital secretions, and possibly human milk. In the pediatric age group, most cases are acquired through the nonparenteral route. HBV causes less than 10% of blood-transfusion hepatitis. Unlike HAV, HBV may induce a carrier state, which in the United States is estimated to occur in 0.1% to 0.5% of the general population. The chronic carrier rate is much higher in other parts of the world. In China, for example, 5% to 15% of the population is infected. A patient is considered a chronic carrier when hepatitis B surface antigen (HBsAg) is present in the serum for more than 6 months. The likelihood of developing the carrier state varies inversely with age. Seventy to 90% of infants born to mothers positive for HBeAg and HBsAg will become infected, and up to 90% of these infected infants will become HBV carriers, whereas only 6% to 10% of acutely infected adults become carriers. Chronic carriers may be healthy or may have chronic hepatitis that may evolve to cirrhosis. Chronic HBV and the carrier state have also been associated with hepatocellular carcinoma.

Most of the *non-A, non-B hepatitis* infections are caused by hepatitis C and hepatitis E viruses. *Hepatitis C* may account for up to 85% of non-A, non-B hepatitis in the United States. It is transmitted primarily through parenteral exposure such as intravenous drug use and blood transfusion. About half the cases result in chronic hepatitis, and approximately half of those patients with chronic hepatitis develop cirrhosis. Hepatitis C is also strongly associated with hepatocellular carcinoma. The *hepatitis E* virus is enterically transmitted and is mainly found in Third World countries. Its course is similar to hepatitis A, and a chronic form has not yet been reported. *Hepatitis D* (the delta agent) is only seen with hepatitis B infection.

The delta agent is a distinct virus from HBV but requires HBV infection for its own replication. Thus, it will only occur in patients who are HBsAg carriers. It can cause either an acute or a chronic hepatitis. Its transmission is similar to that of HBV.

Among the other viral causes of hepatitis, mononucleosis (caused by Epstein-Barr virus) and CMV should be considered. Jaundice is uncommon in mononucleosis, but biochemical abnormalities demonstrating hepatocellular disease will occur in 25% to 50% of the cases. Cytomegalovirus may produce a mononucleosis-like syndrome and is a common cause of subclinical hepatitis after transfusion. CMV has been isolated from the white blood cells of 5% of healthy blood donors. CMV, herpes simplex, and varicella zoster can induce a severe and fulminant hepatitis in immunocompromised patients. Rubella, rubeola, mumps, and varicella zoster can cause mild elevations of serum aminotransferase activity in otherwise healthy patients.

Once viral hepatitis has been excluded, metabolic, ischemic, immunologic, and drug-induced causes of hepatitis need to be considered. In the school-aged and particularly the adolescent population, Wilson's disease, also known as hepatolenticular degeneration, must be included in the differential diagnosis of acute hepatitis. It is characterized by a deficiency in ceruloplasmin and abnormal deposition of copper in various tissues, including the liver, kidneys, central nervous system, and cornea (*Kayser-Fleischer rings*). Wilson's disease can present as an acute fulminant hepatitis and thus mimic acute viral hepatitis. It can also present as chronic active hepatitis and cirrhosis. If left untreated, it progresses to cirrhosis and degenerative central nervous system disease.

Sickle cell disease can cause a *sickle cell hepatopathy* because of hepatic ischemia. The disorder is characterized by abdominal pain, malaise, nausea, and jaundice with markedly elevated serum aminotransferases. Thus, in a population already at risk for acquiring viral hepatitis because of numerous transfusions, the differential diagnosis of hepatitis is even more difficult.

Included among the immunologic disorders that may present as an acute viral hepatitis are systemic lupus erythematous, juvenile rheumatoid arthritis, ulcerative colitis, and Crohn's disease.

Several drugs commonly prescribed for pediatric patients have been associated with hepatitis or hepatocellular necrosis: aspirin, acetaminophen (at toxic levels), cimetidine, indomethacin, ketoconazole, methotrexate, phenytoin, valproic acid, and tetracyclines must be mentioned. Aspirin has been epidemiologically linked to Reye syndrome, although the pathogenesis and cause are poorly understood. Reye syndrome is characterized by an acute noninfectious encephalopathy and noninflammatory fatty infiltration of several organs, particularly the liver and the kidneys. It can present as acute fulminant hepatitis. An association has also been reported with influenza B virus and varicella.

WORK-UP

History

A complete history in a patient with suspected hepatitis will include the character of the illness and its chronicity, including the duration, onset, and possible recurrence of jaundice. Information should also be obtained about possible predisposing conditions for acquiring hepatitis. Some of these antecedents are contact with other persons infected with hepatitis, travel in a developing country, shellfish ingestion, alcohol ingestion, illicit intravenous-drug abuse, blood-product transfusions, homosexual practice, medications, day-care attendance or residence in other institutional settings, and a family history of liver disease and cirrhosis.

Physical Examination

Icterus is first seen in the sclera and will become apparent when the bilirubin is over 2.5 mg/dL. Hepatomegaly and pain on percussion over the liver may be more obvious in acute hepatitis than in cirrhosis, in which the liver appears firm and may be smaller than normal. Other signs to look for include ascites, spider hemangiomas, collateral circulation over the abdomen, and splenomegaly. An examination of the skin in children suffering acute HBV infection may reveal the Gianotti-Crosti syndrome (a papular acrodermatitis). The eye examination may reveal the typical Kayser-Fleischer ring of Wilson's disease. Petechiae and mucosal bleeding reflect a coagulopathy. The extremities may reveal clubbing in patients with long-standing disease. Finally, in fulminant hepatitis or decompensated chronic liver disease the patient will manifest hepatic encephalopathy, which is characterized by asterixis and *fetor hepaticus*. Fetor hepaticus is the most specific sign of hepatic encephalopathy. It is described as a sweetish, slightly fecal smell.

Laboratory Tests

Chemical confirmation of hepatitis is provided by the measurement of alanine aminotransferase (SGPT), aspartate aminotransferase (SGOT), bilirubin, and alkaline phosphatase. The first indication of hepatocellular injury is an increase in aspartate aminotransferase and alanine aminotransferase levels. In a fulminant hepatitis, the rise in aminotransferase levels may be missed. The serum bilirubin value will variably be elevated, and the increase may involve both the direct and indirect fractions. Serum alkaline phosphatase and 5′ nucleotidase are usually only mildly elevated. With major hepatocellular dysfunction, the prothrombin time will increase ($\geq$ 2 seconds more than normal) as will blood ammonia.

Serologic markers of infection establish the diagnosis of hepatitis A and B. *IgM anti-HAV* is present following acute infection with hepatitis A virus and is the most useful antibody to diagnose acute HAV. IgM anti-HBcAg along with HBsAg in serum reflect acute infection with hepatitis B. With the appearance of clinical symptoms HBsAg, HBeAg, and HBV-DNA titers peak. HBsAg and HBV-DNA correlate with infectivity. Delta agent and anti-delta antibodies should also be searched for in an HBsAg-positive patient. Hepatitis C serology is now available; hepatitis E serology is presently available only in research centers.

In a newborn, *Toxoplasma,* rubella, cytomegalovirus, herpesvirus (TORCH) and syphilis antibody titers, serum and urine amino acids, serum electrophoresis, Pi typing of $\dot{A}_1$-antitrypsin, and examination of urine for reducing substances should be done. The urine may be negative for reducing substances if the patient is not ingesting enough of them and a determination of specific cellular enzyme levels will then be necessary. Positive reducing substances can be secondary to a variety of medications. Older patients should be tested for Wilson's disease by obtaining a serum ceruloplasmin level and a 24-hour urine collection for copper. A test for mononucleosis and a toxin screening test should be included in the evaluation of a teenager with hepatitis.

TREATMENT AND MANAGEMENT

Therapy for viral hepatitis is directed at minimizing the complications. Control of coagulopathy and bleeding may be obtained with the injection of vitamin K and plasma infusions. Hypoglycemia is managed by constant glucose infusion, and ascites is treated by restricting salt intake to 10 mEq/m^2/d of sodium and limiting fluid intake to 1500 mL/m^2/d. Therapy focused at regulating ammonia balance is often effective in treating hepatic encephalopathy. This includes decreasing the dietary intake of protein to 0.5 g/kg/d (to decrease ammonia production) and decreasing the absorption of ammonia from the gastrointestinal tract using lactulose and neomycin. Lactulose at a starting dose of 15 mL orally three times a day will act as a cathartic and will also reduce the stool *p*H to less than 5.5, thus trapping ammonia in an acid milieu with conversion to the less diffusible ammonium. Neomycin acts by sterilizing the bowel, thus decreasing the bacterial conversion of protein to ammonia. There may be some benefit from using these two agents together initially and then discontinuing one after 24 to 48 hours.

A specific treatment should be applied when a metabolic, immunologic, or drug-induced cause of the hepatitis is identified. Penicillamine, for example, will bind excess copper present in Wilson's disease and may reverse the hepatic and central nervous system disease. In drug-related hepatic injury, the offending drug must be stopped and supportive care administered.

PREVENTION

Prophylactic measures exist to prevent HAV and HBV. Preexposure prophylaxis for hepatitis A for patients who plan to travel to developing countries includes a single dose of immunoglobulin (from 0.02 to 0.06 mL/kg depending on the length of travel). If a patient has been exposed to HAV, he should receive the immunoglobulin within 2 weeks following exposure as a single dose of 0.02 mL/kg. Preexposure prophylaxis of HBV is administered with the hepatitis B vaccine. The following groups are at higher risks for acquiring HBV and should be protected by the vaccine: selected health care workers, clients and staff of institutions for the mentally retarded, patients on hemodialysis, homosexuals, illicit drug abusers, chronic recipients of blood products, household and sexual contacts of HBV carriers, and international travelers. Hepatitis B vaccine is administered in three doses, with the second and third dose given 1 and 6 months, respectively, after the first dose. Children younger than the age of 10 should receive 10 μg/dose (0.5 mL); older children should receive 20 μg/dose (1 mL).

Once the patient has been exposed to HBV he should receive both the hepatitis B immune globulin (HBIG) and the vaccine. The most frequent pediatric indication for postexposure prophylaxis is for the newborn born to an HbsAg-positive mother. Such infants should receive 0.5 mL of hepatitis B immune globulin intramuscularly and 10 μg of hepatitis B vaccine intramuscularly within 12 hours of birth. Follow-up booster doses of vaccine are given at 1 and 6 months of age. It is now recommended that all infants in the United States be vaccinated against hepatitis B. (See Chap. 14 for an expanded discussion on hepatitis B vaccination.)

Immune globulin is not effective in prophylaxis against hepatitis C and E viruses. Interferon therapy for chronic hepatitis C infection is being investigated.)

INDICATIONS FOR REFERRAL

If the biochemical evaluations of the patient with hepatitis is not helpful in making the diagnosis, a percutaneous liver biopsy should be performed. Abnormal aminotransferase values over a 3- to 6-month period should prompt the pediatrician to refer the patient for a liver biopsy. This will help clarify the degree of chronicity of the disease process and determine the need for more aggressive treatment.

ANNOTATED BIBLIOGRAPHY

Balistreri WF: Viral hepatitis. Pediatr Clin North Am 35:375–407, 1988. (Thorough review of the common viral causes of hepatitis.)

Centers for Disease Control: Recommendations for protection against viral hepatitis. MMWR 39:1–27, 1990. (Update on preexposure and postexposure prophylactic measures against hepatitis.)

Danks DM, Campbell PE, Jack I et al: Studies of the etiology of neonatal hepatitis and biliary atresia. Arch Dis Child 52:360–367, 1977. (Review of 105 patients with neonatal hepatitis.)

Dick MC, Mowat AP: Hepatitis syndrome in infancy: An epidemiological survey with 10-year follow up. Arch Dis Child 60:512–516, 1985. (Provides follow-up information on 54 patients.)

Hadler SC, Webster HM, Erken JJ et al: Hepatitis A in day care centers: A community wide assessment. N Engl J Med 302:1222–1227, 1980. (Review of HAV epidemiology in relation to day-care centers.)

Hepatitis. Semin Pediatr Gastroenterol Nutr 2(2), 1991. (Current discussions of highlights of the different types of viral hepatitis.)

Jones EA: Hepatic encephalopathy: An update. Viewpoints Dig Dis 18:1–6, 1986. (Review of toxins incriminated in hepatic encephalopathy.)

Ludwig J, Axelsen R: Drug effects on the liver: An updated tabular compilation of drugs and drug-related hepatic disease. Dig Dis Sci 28:651–666, 1983. (Excellent tabulation of adverse effects of drugs on human liver.)

Steven CE: Perinatal hepatitis B virus infection: Screening pregnant women and protection of the infant. Ann Intern Med 107:412, 1987. (Summary of important factors in hepatitis B screening and vaccination.)

111
Gastrointestinal Hemorrhage
Victor L. Fox

Gastrointestinal bleeding is a common problem in pediatric practice. The passage of red blood in a child is sufficiently alarming to lead to immediate parental and medical attention. Reports of dark brown emesis or black stool always deserve further investigation to confirm the presence or absence of blood. In addition, stool should always be tested for occult blood whenever iron-deficient anemia is noted. Patients presenting with massive hemorrhage require immediate stabilization before further diagnostic evaluation is pursued. Limited laboratory studies are necessary. Efficient use of complementary endoscopic and radiologic techniques will, in most cases, complete the diagnostic evaluation. Most bleeding is controlled by medical therapy. The causes of bleeding are numerous and may be characterized partially by localization to the upper or lower gastrointestinal tract. The ligament of Treitz serves by convention as the dividing line between the upper and lower tracts.

In this chapter gastrointestinal bleeding without respect to localization is discussed first and then upper and lower gastrointestinal bleeding are considered separately.

WORK-UP
History and Physical Examination

The characterization of the presenting hemorrhage is essential in the initial history. The description of color, consistency, and site of emerging blood may suggest the etiology and actual site of bleeding. *Hematemesis* refers to vomiting of either fresh blood or coffee-ground–like material representing hematin. The presentation of hematemesis may overlap with hemoptysis (coughing blood) particularly when bleeding arises from a site in the nasopharynx or proximal subglottic region or when secondary aspiration of blood occurs. Bleeding from sites proximal to the ligament of Treitz frequently presents as hematemesis. *Melena* refers to dark, tarry, or sticky stool representing blood from either the upper gastrointestinal tract or the small intestine. *Hematochezia* is the passage of fresh blood through the rectum. This occurs with bleeding from the colon or rectum. It may rarely occur with brisk upper gastrointestinal hemorrhage and accelerated intestinal transit as seen in newborns. Delayed transit may allow proximal colonic hemorrhage to present as melena rather than hematochezia. Currant jelly stool characterizes a mixture of blood and mucus seen with ischemic or inflammatory lesions such as intestinal intussusception or acute colitis. Maroon stool describes a mixture of red and dark blood seen with bleeding from the distal small bowel or proximal colon. Formed stool with streaks or flecks of red blood along its surface generally indicates a bleeding fissure or other anorectal lesions.

Additional pertinent historical information includes significant underlying medical disorders such as chronic liver disease, use of medications such as aspirin or nonsteroidal anti-inflammatory preparations, and associated complaints such as vomiting, gastroesophageal reflux, abdominal pain, tenesmus, constipation, diarrhea, arthralgia, weight loss, or growth delay. The past medical history may reveal neonatal umbilical catheterization or a severe episode of dehydration predisposing the patient to portal vein thrombosis. A pertinent family history includes hereditary coagulopathies, familial polyposes, peptic ulcer disease, inflammatory bowel disease, Ehlers-Danlos syndrome, and telangiectasia.

Whereas vital signs provide immediate information regarding the severity of the hemorrhage, a careful examination of the nose, oropharynx, skin, abdomen, and anorectal area provides important clues to etiology. One should look for bruising, unusual pigmented lesions seen in Peutz-Jeghers syndrome and in blue rubber bleb nevus syndrome, spider nevi seen in chronic liver disease, telangiectasia seen in Osler-Weber-Rendu disease, skin hyperelasticity seen in Ehlers-Danlos syndrome, and soft tissue or bone tumors suggesting Gardner's syndrome. Liver disease or portal hypertension may be manifest as jaundice, ascites, prominent abdominal venous pattern (caput medusae), hepatosplenomegaly, or splenomegaly alone. Fissures and anorectal fistulas are often evident on careful visual inspection of the anus. Juvenile polyps are most often found in the sigmoid colon or rectum and may on occasion be palpated on digital rectal examination.

Laboratory Tests

Few laboratory studies are necessary in the initial evaluation of a child with suspected gastrointestinal bleeding (see the display, Recommended Laboratory Studies for Gastrointestinal Bleeding). The confirmation of blood in stool or emesis is foremost. Various food and chemical substances (e.g., red tomatoes, beets, red food coloring, gelatin, fruit juices, chocolate, blueberries and cranberries, iron, and bismuth subsalicylate [Pepto-Bismol]) may resemble blood in the stool or gastric contents. Hemoccult paper may be used to detect occult blood in stool. This test uses guaiac (a colorless phenol) in combination with hemoglobin to yield a blue-colored quinone.

False-negative results may occur with a dried specimen or recent vitamin C ingestion. False-positive guaiac results may occur with the ingestion of red meat or uncooked peroxidase-rich vegetables (e.g., horseradish) and elemental iron.

The HemoQuant, which is more sensitive and more specific than Hemoccult, converts heme to porphyrins that are assayed fluorometrically. It offers the advantage of quanti-

Recommended Laboratory Studies for Gastrointestinal Bleeding

Guaiac test (or suitable alternative)
Hematocrit
Red blood cell indices
Reticulocyte and platelet count
White blood cell and differential cell count
Prothrombin and partial thromboplastin time
Bilirubin
SGOT and SGPT
Alkaline phosphatase
Urinalysis*
Blood urea nitrogen and serum creatinine*

*If hemolytic-uremic syndrome is suspected.

fying minute amounts of blood loss in stool. Gastric fluid may be tested by Hemoccult although sensitivity is poor at pH less than 3. The test, called Gastroccult, reportedly detects blood in gastric fluid more reliably because its sensitivity is not affected by changes in pH. In the case of gastrointestinal bleeding in the newborn, fetal hemoglobin should be distinguished from adult maternal hemoglobin. Both the Apt and the Kleinhauer tests distinguish fetal from adult hemoglobin on the basis of greater resistance of fetal hemoglobin to pH-related alteration. In the case of a nursing infant, direct inspection of the mother's nipples for inflammation or bleeding often reveals the source of bleeding.

Plain roentgenograms of the abdomen are of limited diagnostic value. Supine and upright views of the abdomen are only indicated when there is a suspicion of intestinal obstruction, perforation, or abdominal mass.

STABILIZATION AND TRIAGE

Patients who present with a history of mild to moderate upper gastrointestinal tract bleeding and evidence of blood on nasogastric aspirate require hospitalization for at least 24 to 48 hours for close observation and diagnostic evaluation. Rectal bleeding, depending on the severity of presentation and associated signs and symptoms, may not require immediate hospitalization. Further diagnostic evaluation can often be performed in an outpatient setting.

The patient who presents with a massive upper or lower gastrointestinal hemorrhage requires emergency supportive care and immediate diagnostic evaluation. Vital signs should be followed at 15-minute intervals. A nasogastric tube is placed to determine whether bleeding is proximal to the ligament of Treitz. The nasogastric tube should be left in place to assess ongoing losses. Direct aspiration from a preexisting gastrostomy tube is not always reliable, especially when the patient is in a supine position. An aspirate negative for blood does not exclude the possibility of an upper gastrointestinal tract source. The bleeding may have stopped, or it may arise from the duodenum and flow distally away from the tube. The presence of blood-free bile in the nasogastric aspirate more confidently excludes the possibility of ongoing bleeding proximal to the ligament of Treitz. Saline lavage should be employed when bleeding is active to more effectively remove clots and blood. Iced saline lavage offers only questionable therapeutic benefit by stimulating local vasoconstriction and should be discouraged. Coagulation may improve at more physiologic temperatures. Furthermore, care must be taken with the young infant to avoid hypothermia. Cooling may result in even greater mucosal susceptibility to stress and ulceration.

A short, large-bore venous catheter should be placed for intravascular volume replacement. Isosmotic solutions such as normal saline or Ringer's lactate solution are initially sufficient, followed by appropriate blood products. Immediate transport to a tertiary facility should be arranged once the patient's condition has been stabilized.

UPPER GASTROINTESTINAL TRACT BLEEDING

The diagnostic possibilities of upper gastrointestinal tract bleeding must be considered with respect to the patient's age (Table 111-1).

Bleeding in the newborn period may result from causes unique to this period of life, such as complications of the birthing process or those of premature birth. When endoscopic evaluation is performed, the cause of upper gastrointestinal tract bleeding in children younger than 12 months of age can usually be determined.

The newborn may swallow maternal blood while emerging from the birth canal or may later ingest small amounts of blood while nursing from an inflamed and bleeding breast nipple. Gastritis or ulcers may occur in the sick ("stressed") term or premature newborn. The etiologic role

of gastric hypersecretion and circulating newborn or maternal gastrin levels has not been well studied. Coagulopathy associated with infection and resulting in prolonged clotting times or a reduction in platelet number may result in acute hemorrhage. Since the introduction of prophylactic vitamin K administration shortly after birth, the incidence of so-called hemorrhagic disease of the newborn has declined substantially. Infants who have a deficient dietary intake of vitamin K, fat malabsorption, altered bowel flora due to use of antibiotics, and are breast fed are at greater risk for this disease.

Beyond the first month of life, inflammatory and erosive mucosal lesions predominate as the cause of upper gastrointestinal tract bleeding. One retrospective study by Cox and Ament reviewed upper gastrointestinal tract bleeding in 68 patients ranging in age from younger than 1 year to 18 years. The five most common causes, in descending order of frequency, were duodenal ulcer (20%), gastric ulcer (18%), esophagitis (15%), gastritis (13%), and varices (10%).

Factors suspected of contributing to the development of erosive mucosal lesions include stress from surgery, burns, or increased intracranial pressure, pathologic hypersecretion of gastric acid, and injury or disruption of the mucosal barrier by ischemia/hypoxia, bile acids, antiprostaglandin drugs such as salicylates, and infection. Reports have implicated a *Campylobacter*-like organism recently named *Helicobacter pylori* in the pathogenesis of acid-peptic gastric and duodenal disease. Upper gastrointestinal and probably lower gastrointestinal hemorrhage occur in adolescent long-distance runners. Esophagitis occurs typically in the setting of chronic gastroesophageal reflux and delayed acid clearance from the distal esophagus. Infectious agents such as cytomegalovirus and *Candida albicans* may also cause severe ulcerating or erosive esophagitis in the immunocompromised host.

Forceful vomiting and retching at any age can lead to superficial mucosal laceration at the gastroesophageal junction followed by bleeding and is known as the *Mallory-Weiss* syndrome. A careful endoscopic examination may identify this lesion.

Gastric or esophageal varices arise from *portal vein hypertension*. This may be due to intrahepatic or extrahepatic causes. Cirrhosis represents the cause of 75% to 90% of all pediatric cases of portal hypertension. Congenital hepatic fibrosis followed by various infiltrative diseases, hereditary telangiectasia (Rendu-Osler-Weber disease), and schistosomiasis should also be considered. Extrahepatic causes of portal hypertension include prehepatic portal vein obstruction and the Budd-Chiari syndrome. Varices resulting from any of the above rarely present clinically with bleeding before 1 year of age. Variceal bleeding, however, should always be considered in the differential diagnosis of an upper gastrointestinal tract hemorrhage because the treatment and prognosis markedly differ from that of the more common mucosal lesions.

Table 111-1. Common Causes of Upper Gastrointestinal Hemorrhage

NEWBORN (BIRTH–1 MO)	INFANCY-ADOLESCENCE
Swallowed maternal blood	Gastritis
Gastritis	Esophagitis
Esophagitis	
Ulcer (gastric or duodenal)	Ulcer
Coagulopathy associated with infection	Mallory-Weiss syndrome
	Varices
Vascular malformation	Gastrointestinal duplication
Hemorrhagic disease (vitamin K deficiency)	Vascular malformation
	Polyps
	Coagulopathy
	Hemobilia

WORK-UP

Following the stabilization and localization of bleeding to the upper gastrointestinal tract, a decision must be made for the timing and type of further diagnostic evaluation. Endoscopy is more sensitive and more specific than barium contrast radiologic studies in the identification of bleeding lesions. The sensitivity of endoscopy approaches 90%. Contrast radiography identifies approximately 50% of lesions. Air contrast barium studies enhance the sensitivity for superficial mucosal lesions but still fall short of endoscopy. Some studies indicate that duodenal ulcers may be detected equally by contrast radiography and endoscopy. Contrast studies offer the advantages of a noninvasive, easily administered and readily available test. The disadvantages include comparatively lower sensitivity, inability to distinguish innocent from active lesions in the case of coexistent varices and gastritis or ulcer, and potential interference with subsequent nuclear medicine imaging. Endoscopy permits optimal detection with visual and biopsy confirmation and potential therapeutic intervention, such as electrocoagulation, thermocoagulation (heater probe), sclerotherapy, or polypectomy. Endoscopy involves the risk of an invasive procedure accompanied by drug-induced sedation. Additionally, an endoscopist skilled in pediatric procedures is not always readily accessible.

The indications for early endoscopy remain controversial. Studies in adults have shown no significant difference in outcome between patients who were or were not studied by early endoscopy. Endoscopy is recommended for children with persistent or recurrent bleeding, with suspected variceal bleeding, and with severe hemorrhage where there is urgency in making a specific diagnosis.

Angiography may be necessary in the rare instance that brisk bleeding obscures endoscopic visualization of the bleeding site. A bleeding rate in excess of 0.5 to 1 mL/min is required for adequate angiographic visualization of the bleeding site. Angiography is particularly useful in the assessment of portal hypertension and variceal bleeding and in the detection of biliary tract hemorrhage (hemobilia) or vascular malformations.

MANAGEMENT

Medical therapy for erosive mucosal lesions is directed toward acid reduction or neutralization. Antacids alone are indicated for patients with ongoing hemorrhage. Alternating solutions containing magnesium and aluminum hydroxides are delivered in 0.5 to 1 mL/kg doses every 1 to 2 hours to maintain gastric pH greater than 5. Histamine-receptor antagonists such as cimetidine offer no proven additional benefit in the setting of active bleeding. Antacids are more effective than cimetidine in both consistently elevating gastric pH and preventing acute hemorrhage in critically ill patients.

The histamine-receptor antagonists cimetidine and ranitidine play an important role in the chronic outpatient treatment of duodenal ulcer. Pharmacologic reports recommend cimetidine in a dosage of 20 to 30 mg/kg/d administered in six divided doses and ranitidine in a dosage of 1.25 to 1.9 mg/kg/d administered in two divided doses. Outpatient therapy with antacids or H_2 blockers generally extends for 4 to 6 weeks to permit adequate healing.

More aggressive management of bleeding lesions includes electrocoagulation, thermocoagulation, laser therapy, vasopressin infusion, embolization, and surgical resection or devascularization.

Variceal hemorrhage is managed acutely with intravenous vasopressin starting with 0.002 to 0.005 U/kg/min. Balloon tamponade using a Sengstaken-Blakemore tube is deferred whenever possible to avoid serious complications of it use (i.e., esophageal rupture). Sclerotherapy has been performed successfully in increasing numbers of children. This may be employed for both acute and prophylactic management. Endoscopic varix ligation or banding has also been performed successfully in pediatric patients. Other prophylactic management has included the use of propranolol. Intractable variceal bleeding may require embolization, surgical devascularization, or portosystemic vascular shunting.

LOWER GASTROINTESTINAL TRACT HEMORRHAGE

As in upper gastrointestinal tract hemorrhage, the causes of lower gastrointestinal tract hemorrhage must be considered with respect to the patient's age (Table 111-2). Swallowed maternal blood represents the most common cause of neonatal blood loss in the stool. *Anal fissures,* often subtle on examination, are perhaps the next most frequent source of rectal bleeding in the newborn. This problem, suspected to arise from local trauma caused by the passage of frequent or hard stool, remains the most common cause of insignificant rectal blood loss in all age groups, with the exception of adulthood. It is then replaced by another form of anorectal disease, hemorrhoids, which is uncommon in childhood. *Necrotizing enterocolitis,* a condition typically arising in the premature newborn and multifactorial in etiology, may be heralded by the presence of small amounts of blood in the stool. Intestinal malrotation with midgut volvulus together with necrotizing enterocolitis represent catastrophic ischemic events that generally present as small amounts of rectal blood loss. Whereas the latter occurs characteristically in the neonatal period, the former has been described in all ages, usually in association with intense pain and vomiting. *Cow's milk protein* or *soy protein hypersensitivity* may present as acute colitis with hematochezia. This occurs typically in the first 3 to 4 months of age and rarely beyond age 1 year.

After anal fissure, *enterocolitis* represents the next most common cause of rectal bleeding in all pediatric age groups.

Table 111-2. Common Causes of Lower Gastrointestinal Hemorrhage

NEWBORN (BIRTH–1 MO)	INFANT (1 MO–1 Y)	CHILDHOOD (1–12 Y)	ADOLESCENT (>12 Y)
Swallowed maternal blood	Anal fissure	Anal fissure	Anal fissure
Anal fissure	Upper gastrointestinal hemorrhage	Juvenile polyp	Idiopathic inflammatory bowel disease
Upper gastrointestinal hemorrhage	Intussusception	Intussusception	Upper gastrointestinal hemorrhage
Cow's milk or soy protein allergy	Meckel's diverticulum	Meckel's diverticulum	Infectious diarrhea
Necrotizing enterocolitis	Infectious diarrhea	Infectious diarrhea	Meckel's diverticulum
Midgut volvulus	Milk protein allergy	Upper gastrointestinal hemorrhage	Hemolytic-uremic syndrome
Coagulopathy		Hemolytic-uremic syndrome	Henoch-Schönlein purpura
		Henoch-Schönlein purpura	Angiodysplasia
		Idiopathic inflammatory bowel disease	

The typical presentation includes diarrhea and variably fever, cramping abdominal pain, and vomiting. Bacterial pathogens include *Salmonella, Shigella, Campylobacter, Yersinia enterocolitica,* and *Clostridium difficile.* A cytotoxin-producing serotype of *Escherichia coli* (0157:H7) has been reported to cause sporadic cases of hemorrhagic colitis, including that seen with hemolytic-uremic syndrome. *Neisseria gonorrhoeae* causes a proctitis that may present as hemorrhagic exudate. Patients who have an unusual exposure or travel history and immunocompromised patients are at risk for less commonly found viral and parasitic pathogens. These include cytomegalovirus, herpes simplex virus, and *Entamoeba histolytica.*

Intussusception occurs most frequently between 3 months and 3 years of age. The typical clinical presentation includes abdominal distention and pain, vomiting, palpable abdominal mass in approximately two thirds of patients, and passage of mucoid bloody stool, often described as currant jelly stool. Bleeding is rarely massive and may be occult. In contrast, bleeding from *Meckel's diverticulum* generally occurs in the absence of significant pain, although large amounts of blood in the intestine may result in cramping discomfort. The blood loss can be massive. Bleeding follows ulceration of ectopic gastric mucosa in both Meckel's diverticulum and intestinal duplication.

Juvenile polyps represent a common source of rectal bleeding in childhood. They are benign hamartomatous lesions with a rich vascular supply. A digital rectal examination will identify 20% to 30% of these lesions. Bleeding is typically bright red, small in amount, and painless. The natural history is one of involution by late adolescence. Bleeding may occur in association with the passage of tissue representing an involuting, sloughed polyp. Various polyposis syndromes may present as bleeding. Histopathology, inheritance pattern, and associated lesions further identify the specific entity. A more detailed description of polyposis syndromes exceeds the scope of this discussion.

Hemolytic-uremic syndrome and *Henoch-Schönlein purpura* represent two multiorgan system, vasculitic disease entities of uncertain etiology. Both occur in childhood and are often associated with rectal bleeding. Hemolytic-uremic syndrome is characterized by the findings of microangiopathic hemolytic anemia, thrombocytopenia, and acute renal failure. Clinical symptoms of gastroenteritis with abdominal pain, vomiting, and diarrhea (often bloody) frequently precede the illness. Acute colitis occurs in approximately 50% of cases. If colitis does not precede the illness, it may occur concomitantly. The colitis may result from a documented bacterial enteropathogen or may be idiopathic, mimicking the presentation of an ulcerative colitis. Intestinal perforation due to ischemia has been reported. Henoch-Schönlein purpura characteristically produces an urticarial rash on the buttocks and lower extremities that progresses to papular purpuric lesions. Skin edema and large-joint arthralgia frequently occur. More serious complications involve renal disease (40%) and gastrointestinal symptoms (50% to 70%). Abdominal pain, vomiting, and both upper and lower gastrointestinal tract hemorrhage have been reported. The small intestine is primarily affected, with findings resembling those of regional ileitis. Massive intestinal bleeding has been reported, although guaiac-positive stool or minor gross blood loss is more the rule.

Idiopathic inflammatory bowel disease (IBD) must always be considered in the older child or adolescent presenting with rectal bleeding. Fulminant hemorrhagic colitis can occur with either ulcerative colitis or Crohn's disease. Although ileitis commonly results in occult blood loss, it does not generally cause significant gross rectal bleeding (see Chap. 107 for a complete discussion).

Rare causes of lower gastrointestinal tract hemorrhage

include various vascular lesions. Intestinal hemangiomas may exist alone or in association with neonatal hemangiomatosis, the blue rubber bleb nevus syndrome, and Turner syndrome. Turner syndrome may also be complicated by telangiectasia or abnormal serosal vessels. Bleeding telangiectatic lesions commonly located in the stomach are characteristically seen in patients with Osler-Weber-Rendu disease.

Patients with Ehlers-Danlos syndrome may present with rectal bleeding, presumably due to friable intestinal mucosa and anal tissue.

WORK-UP

The child's age, history of illness, and specific findings on physical examination or laboratory evaluation will narrow the differential diagnosis.

Anal fissure can be excluded by a careful examination of slightly everted anal mucosal folds. A nasogastric aspirate is then obtained to exclude the upper gastrointestinal tract source. Wright's stain of the stool is used to identify inflammatory cells, particularly polymorphonuclear leukocytes. The presence of inflammatory cells limits the diagnosis to causes of acute colitis. The patient's clinical status generally allows time for a careful exclusion of infectious etiologies before more invasive testing is pursued. Appropriate bacterial cultures, and when indicated, serologic testing, viral cultures, and fresh stool for ova and parasite examination and for *C. difficile* toxin assay should be obtained as soon as possible.

Rigid or flexible proctosigmoidoscopy is a valuable tool early in the diagnostic evaluation. Proctosigmoidoscopy and biopsy combined with external anal examination will establish the source of rectal bleeding in more than 50% of cases. A flexible endoscopy provides the additional therapeutic option of polypectomy at the time of diagnosis. In the absence of distal findings on sigmoidoscopy, an air contrast barium enema should be performed to look for more proximally located polyps or other mucosal or submucosal lesions. The findings on barium enema examination may help direct a complete colonoscopic examination. Skilled endoscopists may prefer to proceed directly to colonoscopy rather than obtain a prior contrast study. A barium enema is a useful diagnostic and therapeutic tool in the evaluation for suspected intussusception. This study must be performed cautiously when ischemia is suspected to avoid the complication of perforation. When the character of the hemorrhage suggests a bleeding Meckel diverticulum or intestinal duplication, a technetium pertechnetate scan should be performed prior to barium studies. An injection with pentagastrin may enhance the sensitivity of the scan. Residual barium may interfere with radioisotope detection. ^{99m}p3Tc-pertechnetate is selectively concentrated in gastric mucosa; this tissue is present ectopically in up to 50% of Meckel's diverticula.

When bleeding is brisk or continuous, the site of bleeding must be established as quickly and accurately as possible. ^{99m}Tc-labeled red blood cell scintigraphy represents a sensitive, noninvasive test that should be performed prior to angiography. Selective angiography can then be directed by the scintigraphic findings. Angiography provides precise vascular anatomic detail and the nonoperative therapeutic approach of embolization.

MANAGEMENT

Therapy is often supportive and directed toward the underlying disorder, such as a coagulopathy or infection. It may simply require the removal of an antigenic stimulus as in milk-protein–induced colitis. Anal fissures usually heal in response to therapy for underlying constipation (when present) and local wound care. A combination of stool softener, sitz baths, and locally applied hydrocortisone-containing cream or ointment is often successful. Corticosteroids have been used to treat gastrointestinal involvement of Henoch-Schönlein purpura, although insufficiently controlled prospective data fuel controversy over this therapy. Corticosteroids have proven beneficial in the treatment of Crohn's and idiopathic ulcerative colitis. Ischemic lesions are generally treated supportively. Surgery may be employed to explore and remove gross anatomic lesions compromising blood flow or to remove segments of transmurally infarcted or perforated bowel. Surgery is obviously required for the removal of a Meckel diverticulum or ulcerated intestinal duplication. Flexible endoscopy is now used safely and routinely for polypectomy in pediatric patients. Innovations in endoscopic therapy such as electrocoagulation and laser therapy have not been evaluated for routine use in children. Successful transcatheter embolization has been reported in only a few pediatric patients. The overall safety and the rate of success is difficult to estimate.

ANNOTATED BIBLIOGRAPHY

Chang MH, Wang TH, Hsu JY et al: Endoscopic examination of the upper gastrointestinal tract in infancy. Gastrointest Endosc 29:15, 1983. (Large series of endoscopic findings in patients younger than 1 year old presenting with upper gastrointestinal tract bleeding.)

Cox K, Ament ME: Upper gastrointestinal bleeding in children and adolescents. Pediatrics 63:408, 1979. (Retrospective review of upper gastrointestinal tract hemorrhage in 68 patients emphasizing reliability of endoscopic findings.)

Gryboski JD, Walker WA: Gastrointestinal bleeding. In Gastrointestinal Problems in the Infant, pp 85–121. Philadelphia, WB Saunders, 1983. (Comprehensive discussion of gastrointestinal bleeding in infancy, including an extensive bibliography.)

Hyams JS, Leichtner AM, Schwartz AN: Recent advances in diagnosis and treatment of gastrointestinal hemorrhage in infants and children. J Pediatr 106:1, 1985. (Discussion of recent diagnostic and treatment modalities.)

Lloyd CW, Martin WJ, Taylor BD, Hauser AR: Pharmacokinetics and pharmacodynamics of cimetidine and metabolites in critically ill children. J Pediatr 107:295, 1985. (One of few studies examining kinetics and activity of this drug in children.)

Meyerovitz MF, Fellows KE: Angiography in gastrointestinal bleeding in children. AJR 143:837, 1984. (Retrospective review of angiographic studies in 27 patients with focus placed on indications and diagnostic and therapeutic efficacy.)

Nickerson HJ, Holubets MC, Weiler BR et al: Causes of iron deficiency in adolescent athletes. J Pediatr 114:657, 1989. (Gastrointestinal source of blood loss identified predominantly in female runners.)

Oldham KT, Lobe TE: Gastrointestinal hemorrhage in children. Pediatr Clin North Am 32:1247, 1985. (Review with surgical orientation.)

Parik N, Sebring ES, Polesky HF: Evaluation of bloody gastric fluid from newborn infants. J Pediatr 94:967, 1979. (Comparison of Kleihauer and Apt tests applied to gastric fluid, including notation of pitfalls of both tests.)

Tuggle DW, Bennet KG, Scott J, Tunell WP: Intravenous vasopressin and gastrointestinal hemorrhage in children. J Pediatr Surg 23:627, 1988. (First study to evaluate dosage in pediatric patients.)

15

GENITOURINARY PROBLEMS

112

Urinary Tract Infections

Jerold C. Woodhead

Host factors and bacterial virulence factors combine to cause urinary tract infection (UTI) and consequent renal damage. Most infection-related renal damage occurs during infancy and early childhood. Timely identification of acute infection, appropriate treatment, detection of patients at risk for renal scarring, and prevention of recurrent infection can greatly reduce the risk of an adverse outcome.

PATHOPHYSIOLOGY

Infection may occur at any point in the urinary tract from urethral meatus to renal parenchyma. In the newborn period, boys develop UTIs more frequently than girls. Beyond the newborn period, most UTIs occur in girls. Ascending bacterial infection has been identified as the most common mechanism by which UTIs develop in both boys and girls. *Escherichia coli* causes almost 90% of first infections and 75% to 80% of recurrent infections. Other less common causative organisms include klebsiella species, proteus species, and enterococci, although any bacterial species may cause infection. *Staphylococcus saprophyticus* causes the dysuria-pyuria syndrome in adult women (and probably also in adolescent girls), as do *Chlamydia, Trichomonas,* and viruses.

HOST FACTORS

Host factors that promote UTI include female sex, vesicoureteral reflux (VUR), urinary tract obstruction, consti-

pation, and poor perineal hygiene. Uncircumcised males have an increased risk for UTI during infancy. Breast-fed infants may have a lower rate of UTI than formula-fed infants. The inflammatory response to infection causes tissue damage and scarring.

Vesicoureteral reflux is the major structural abnormality associated with UTI and renal damage, occurring in as many as one third of all children with UTI. Up to 50% of children younger than 5 years of age who have UTI *and* fever also have VUR. VUR appears to be less common among black children than among white children. Over 80% of children younger than the age of 5 years who have recurrent UTI and persistent VUR develop renal scarring. New renal scars may develop, however, in older children. Approximately 25% of end-stage renal disease in childhood results from damage caused by infection in structurally abnormal urinary tracts.

Vesicoureteral reflux results from incompetence of the functional sphincter at the vesicoureteral junction and allows direct transmission of organisms in bladder urine to the kidney. The combination of increased pressure, infection, and the inflammatory response results in pyelonephritis with scarring and eventual loss of renal function. VUR occurs in families, in some cases having an autosomal dominant inheritance pattern. VUR may also result from trauma to the vesicoureteral junction (e.g., calculi), abnormal neurologic control of the bladder (e.g., meningomyelocele), dysfunctional voiding (bladder dyssynergia), and obstruction such as posterior urethral valves or ureteroceles. Infection itself causes inflammation and edema of the vesicoureteral junction and alters ureteral peristalsis. This results in transient, low-grade reflux that resolves promptly with effective antibiotic treatment.

The inflammatory response to infection mediates most tissue damage and scarring. When organisms reach the renal parenchyma, host defense mechanisms promote granulocyte mobilization to the site of infection. Granulocyte aggregations may cause local ischemia, which damages tissue. In addition, phagocytosis releases substances from granulocytes (including superoxide, hydrogen peroxide, hydroxyl radical, singlet oxygen, and myeloperoxidase) that destroy bacteria but also cause tissue damage with resultant scarring.

The relationship between circumcision and UTI has received recent emphasis. Accumulated evidence suggests that, because bacterial adherence factors may be more important in UTI pathogenesis than hematogenous infection, circumcision may reduce the risk of UTI in infant boys. P-fimbriated strains of *E. coli* and *Proteus,* which adhere tightly to epithelium of the urinary tract, most commonly cause these infections. Infants may be colonized at birth from maternal flora or in the postnatal period from family members or other persons. In Europe, where newborn circumcision is uncommon, approximately 1% of boys will develop symptomatic UTI. In the United States several surveys have demonstrated a substantially higher risk of UTI among uncircumcised infants than among those circumcised in the newborn period. These data have been cited by many in the United States to support arguments in favor of routine newborn circumcision, although a cause-and-effect relationship has not been proven. (For a discussion on potential risks and benefits of routine circumcision, see Chapter 9.)

Bacterial Virulence Factors

Bacterial virulence factors, especially those that promote adherence of bacteria to either bladder mucus or to the epithelium of the urinary tract have an important role in the pathogenesis of UTI. A number of substances elaborated by bacteria also promote infection and tissue damage. Endotoxin causes reduced ureteral peristalsis with resultant obstruction to urine flow; hemolysins damage the urinary tract during the course of infection.

Adherence to epithelial cells and mucus is promoted by bacterial structures called fimbriae. Two types have association with UTI: type 1 fimbriae and P-type fimbriae. Bacteria with type 1 fimbriae attach to glycoproteins in bladder mucus and commonly cause cystitis but generally do not cause pyelonephritis, unless VUR allows them access to the upper tracts. P-fimbriated *E. coli,* on the other hand, have a strong association with pyelonephritis. They adhere tightly to the epithelium of foreskin and other urinary tract structures, which prevents "wash out" by urine flow and allows bacteria to ascend to the upper tracts in the absence of reflux. Unfortunately, no test available for use in the physician's office can assist in identification of "uropathogenic" organisms.

CLINICAL PRESENTATION

Clinical clues vary with age. Infants typically present with fever, irritability, and other signs of systemic illness, including failure to thrive, vomiting, and diarrhea. In addition, signs of bladder obstruction such as abdominal distention, weak or threadlike urinary stream, infrequent voiding, and discolored or malodorous urine may accompany signs of sepsis. The younger the infant, the more likely are sepsis and structural abnormalities associated with, or causative of, UTI. Toddlers may complain of abdominal discomfort and have fever, altered voiding pattern, and malodorous urine. Preschool children may complain of voiding discomfort, or they may develop recurrent enuresis, in addition to fever and abdominal or flank pain. School-age children and adolescents typically have "classic" signs and symptoms (i.e., dysuria, frequency, urgency, abdominal or flank pain, and fever). Diagnosis is most difficult in infancy and early childhood because clinical clues are nonspecific.

Differential Diagnosis

Fever occurs commonly with UTI, especially before 1 year of age, but fever as the *only* sign of UTI is not common. However, recurrent fever without an obvious cause in an infant should prompt consideration of UTI. Vomiting, diarrhea, and failure to thrive may accompany metabolic, gastrointestinal, cardiovascular, and neurologic disorders, as well as urinary infection.

Dysuria, frequency, urgency, and hesitancy occur with urethral and bladder mucosal irritation from infectious, chemical, or physical causes (see Chap. 113). These symptoms, associated with a urine culture having 10^2 to 10^4 colonies/mL, occur in adult women and probably in adolescent girls with the *dysuria-pyuria syndrome.* Sexual abuse must also be considered in children with traumatic or sexually transmitted infectious causes of dysuria.

Abdominal pain associated with UTI must be distinguished from appendicitis, pelvic abscess and pelvic inflammatory disease, all of which may also cause dysuria and pyuria. A vaginal discharge may accompany sexually transmitted diseases. UTI may also be related to intercourse. Constipation predisposes to UTI and also causes abdominal pain, dysuria, and urinary incontinence.

WORK-UP

Urine Collection

Contamination of voided urine occurs commonly, particularly if urine bags are used to obtain specimens from infants and young children. Even adult women have a contamination rate of 20% to 30% for "clean catch" voided urine. Despite meticulous technique, *bagged urine has an unacceptably high rate of contamination.* Culture results from bagged urine have validity only if reported as *"no growth."*

Midstream voided urine specimens provide acceptable samples for urinalysis and culture if a child can void on request. A girl should have her perineum and labia cleaned gently with water and mild soap; a boy should have his penis cleaned (with the foreskin retracted if uncircumcised). *Do not use antiseptic soaps or solutions* because, if not completely rinsed off before voiding, they may sterilize or reduce the colony count of the urine specimen. Do not attempt to "sterilize" the urethral meatus. Cultures of voided urine with more than 5×10^4 colonies/mm^3 in an asymptomatic patient or with 10^3 to 10^4 colonies/mL in a symptomatic patient may indicate infection, but only when confirmed by repeat culture.

Catheterization of the bladder with a sterile, small-gauge, straight catheter provides urine specimens with minimal risk of contamination and minimal patient discomfort. A sterile No. 5 French feeding tube may be used to catheterize newborns and young infants. Complications of catheterization may be minimized by restricting use of the procedure to those infants and children with symptoms and signs that suggest a high likelihood of UTI. Sterile technique further reduces the risk of introducing infection into an uninfected urinary tract. Growth of more than 10^2 colonies/mL indicates infection. Catheterization combines reliability with low levels of patient risk and discomfort.

Suprapubic aspiration of the bladder provides urine samples with low likelihood of contamination. This safe, easily learned technique may be performed on patients of any age, but practical considerations restrict its use to young infants. Complications, including "dry taps" and hematuria, may be reduced with careful attention to technique, but the procedure does cause discomfort to the infant and, often, a great deal of anxiety for some parents. Urine obtained from a suprapubic aspiration should have no growth on culture; *any growth signifies infection.* No other method of urine collection offers as much diagnostic certainty.

Urinalysis

Traditional urinalysis has a time-honored role but limited usefulness in the diagnosis of UTI. Urine concentration, centrifugation speed and duration, and volume of sediment examined may affect microscopic quantification of pyuria, hematuria and bacteriuria. In addition, urine culture may be positive in the absence of pyuria, and urinary leukocytes may originate from causes other than infection. Protein concentration determined by dipstick may be elevated falsely by alkaline urine pH or may be reduced falsely by dilute urine. Infants may have apparently normal urinalysis despite positive culture.

Examination of *uncentrifuged* urine for bacteria and leukocytes may prove useful in office evaluation of patients with suspected UTI. Bacteria seen on a sample of uncentrifuged urine have a correlation of approximately 80% with a urine culture having more than 10^5 colonies/mL; the correlation increases to 95% when bacteria are identified on Gram stain. Use of a hemacytometer further aids in the detection and quantification of both bacteria and leukocytes,

eliminates the need to stain urine sediment, and offers the same correlation with positive cultures as bacteria detected by Gram stain. More than 10 leukocytes/mm^3 in uncentrifuged urine examined with a hemacytometer correlates strongly with cultures having more than 10^5 colonies/mL. Lower colony counts in the dysuria-pyuria syndrome have a strong correlation with more than 8 leukocytes/mm^3.

Chemical Tests

Tests designed to detect bacteriuria include nitrite dipsticks, tetrazolium reduction, and catalase and endotoxin detection. The leukocyte esterase test detects pyuria but should not be used to decide on the need for urine culture.

The nitrite dipstick has the most clinical utility. Based on the conversion of urinary nitrate to nitrite by certain strains of bacteria, the dipstick detects nitrite colorimetrically. False-positive results occur rarely, but false-negative results are common. The test can be performed reliably *only* on a first voided morning urine specimen, since time is required for the conversion to nitrate to nitrite; it *cannot* be used for infants or for children with enuresis. The causes of false-negative nitrite tests include inadequate incubation time, infection with bacteria that do not reduce nitrate, and low dietary nitrate. The nitrite test has its major use as a screening tool to detect recurrent infection in high-risk populations. A positive test should prompt urine culture. Used properly, the test may be performed at home by parents.

Urine Culture

A UTI cannot be diagnosed without urine culture, but physicians often forego cultures because of high cost, specimen handling problems, and slow reporting of results by hospital and commercial laboratories. However, cultures may be done in the office with either the standard culture methods or the commercially available "dipslide" technique (e.g., Uricult). Both provide equivalent reliability, lower cost, more timely results, and less inconvenience than cultures done in an outside laboratory. Dipslides are especially convenient. They do not require additional equipment or laboratory assistants and may even be incubated overnight at room temperature. Differential growth on the two media that coat the slide allows preliminary bacterial identification, and comparison of bacterial growth to pictorial standards allows estimation of colony count. When needed, subculture from the slide by a microbiology laboratory allows precise bacterial identification and antibiotic susceptibility testing.

Proper handling of urine specimens reduces the risk of erroneous culture results. Optimally, urine should be cultured immediately after collection, but practicality often dictates a delay from collection to culture. Doubling time for urinary pathogens may be as short as 20 minutes at room temperature, while growth stops at 4°C. Immediate refrigeration of urine specimens prevents bacterial overgrowth from contaminants and permits reliable colony counts when urine is later cultured.

Bacterial identification and determination of antibiotic susceptibilities are *not necessary in most uncomplicated UTIs*. Both require the services of a hospital or commercial laboratory, add specimen handling problems, and increase cost. Because most UTIs are caused by *E. coli* sensitive to commonly used antibiotics, *rapid clinical response to treatment and a negative culture 2 to 4 days after initiation of treatment* serve the same ends as sensitivity testing. However, any patient with systemic toxicity at initial presentation or who fails to respond promptly to treatment should have a urine sample sent to a laboratory for bacterial identification and antibiotic susceptibility testing.

MANAGEMENT

Antibiotic Treatment

Oral antibiotics effective against *E. coli* are listed in Table 112-1 along with the appropriate dose and dosing interval. All produce a high concentration of antibiotic in the urine and rapidly eradicate sensitive organisms. Choice of antibiotic depends on the child's past history of adverse reactions, both allergic and nonallergic (e.g., severe diarrhea), plus the dosing frequency and cost. Taste of some antibiotic suspensions, particularly generic forms, may reduce acceptability.

Treatment for 10 days suffices; longer therapy offers no advantage. However, in uncomplicated infections in adolescents, shorter regimens may improve compliance and may reduce inconvenience, side effects, and cost, while providing therapeutic results comparable to longer therapy (Table 112-2). Single-dose therapy may be used for adolescent girls with uncomplicated UTI, but 3-day treatment with trimethoprim-sulfamethoxazole may be more effective. Single dose and short course therapy has *not* been proven effective

Table 112-1. Antibiotic Treatment of Urinary Tract Infections: Standard 10-Day Therapy for Acute Infection

ANTIBIOTIC	DOSE AND FREQUENCY	REMARKS
Amoxicillin	15 mg/kg tid	
Amoxicillin + clavulanate	15 mg/kgA + 7.5 mg/kgC tid	
Ampicillin	10–15 mg/kg qid	Fasting
Cefixime	8 mg/kg once daily	
Cephalexin	6–12 mg/kg qid	
Nitrofurantoin	1–2 mg/kg qid	age > 1 mo
Sulfisoxazole	40 mg/kg qid	age > 2 mo
Tetracycline	250 mg/dose qid	age > 8 y
Trimethoprim + sulfamethoxazole	4 mg/kgT + 20 mg/kgS bid	age > 2 mo

Table 112-2. Antibiotic Treatment of Urinary Tract Infections: Short Therapy for Adolescents with Uncomplicated Acute Infection

ANTIBIOTIC	DOSE AND FREQUENCY	DURATION
Amoxicillin	2–3 g	One dose
Sulfisoxazole	1 g	One dose
Trimethoprim + sulfamethoxazole	2 double-strength tablets *or* 1 double-strength tablet bid	One dose 3 days

for infants and children and cannot be recommended. Infants with high fever and UTI or those for whom sepsis is a consideration should be managed in hospital with parenteral antibiotics, as should any child or adolescent with symptomatic pyelonephritis.

FOLLOW-UP

Documentation of Treatment Effectiveness and Recurrent UTI

Urine should be recultured 2 to 3 days after the start of standard 10-day therapy or 3 to 4 days after completion of short-course therapy. Sterile urine demonstrates antibiotic effectiveness. If urine is not sterile, or if the patient remains symptomatic, another urine specimen should be submitted for bacterial identification and susceptibility testing and a broad-spectrum antibiotic should be prescribed. Urine should be recultured 3 days later to confirm antibiotic effectiveness. Once infection has been eradicated, screening for recurrent infection should be done in 1 month (or just before the radiologic evaluation). Further cultures every 3 months for 1 year and then yearly for 2 to 3 years will suffice to screen for recurrent infection. Obviously, fever or other signs of UTI mandate urine culture at any time. Dipslide cultures are ideal for follow-up. Nitrite dipsticks may replace screening urine culture for children who have achieved bladder control; a positive test should be confirmed with culture.

Identification of Structural Abnormalities

Vesicoureteral Reflux. The most reliable technique to identify VUR is the voiding cystourethrogram (VCUG). *All children younger than 3 years of age should have evaluation of the urinary tract to detect VUR after the first documented UTI.* In addition, *boys at any age* should have VCUG performed after the *first* infection. Girls older than 3 years with systemic toxicity suggestive of pyelonephritis (e.g., fever, flank pain), recurrent UTI (especially if accompanied by poor growth, hypertension or reduced renal function), or failure of infection to respond promptly to therapy also have a high likelihood of VUR and should be studied

Table 112-3. Antibiotic Treatment of Urinary Tract Infections: Prophylactic Antibiotics to Prevent Recurrent Infection

ANTIBIOTIC	DOSE AND FREQUENCY	REMARKS
Nitrofurantoin	1–2 mg/kg bid	Age > 2 mo
Trimethoprim + sulfamethoxazole	2 mg/kgT + 10 mg/kgS qd *or* 1 mg/kgT + 5 mg/kgS bid	No wetting Bedwetting
Methenamine	18 mg/kg qid 500 mg/dose qid 1 g/dose qid	Age < 6 y Age 6–12 y Age > 12 y; must keep urine pH ≤ 5.5

with VCUG. The optimal time to obtain a VCUG is 4 to 6 weeks after completion of treatment of the acute infection. Low-dose prophylactic antibiotics (Table 112-3) will reduce the likelihood of recurrent infection until VCUG can be completed.

The appearance of the urinary tract on the VCUG is used to grade reflux. In low-grade reflux, contrast material is detected in the ureter and may reach up to the renal pelvis with no or minimal distention (grades I, II, and III in the International Reflux Grading scheme). High-grade reflux describes obvious distention of ureters and renal pelvis and may include gross hydronephrosis (grades IV and V). The more severe the reflux, the lower the likelihood of spontaneous resolution and normal renal function.

The radionuclide cystogram is another procedure that allows identification of VUR. It has the advantage of lower radiation exposure than that associated with VCUG. However, this technique provides less detail and requires specialized equipment and physician expertise, which are often not readily available. The radionuclide cystogram may have its greatest use in monitoring low-grade VUR for spontaneous resolution.

Renal Structure. Evaluation of renal structure is also important in children who have UTIs. Excretory urography (i.e., intravenous pyelography [IVP]) provides both structural and functional information but requires intravenous infusion of contrast material. Ultrasound examination has replaced the IVP in many cases as the preferred procedure, even though it provides only structural information and requires expertise on the part of the radiologist for interpretation. On balance, the lack of invasiveness and the reduced risks and discomfort favor ultrasound examination over IVP as the procedure of choice for initial structural evaluation. However, if the VCUG demonstrates VUR, especially of high grade, the IVP is the preferred test because it more precisely delineates structure. The ultrasound examination may have a role in screening family members if there is concern about familial VUR: As a general rule, an infant born to parents known to have VUR, or whose sibling has VUR, should have a screening ultrasound done to look for

urinary tract dilatation. Detection of a dilated urinary tract should prompt more complete evaluation, including VCUG. The child with pyelonephritis or signs of urinary tract obstruction should undergo renal ultrasonography during the early phases of treatment. If an IVP is necessary, it should be delayed until infection has been controlled with antibiotic therapy and acute toxicity and fever have resolved.

MANAGEMENT OF REFLUX

Whenever VUR has been diagnosed, it must be followed assiduously. In general, yearly evaluation of VUR, with either VCUG or radionuclide cystogram, and monitoring of renal growth, with renal ultrasound or IVP, should continue as long as VUR persists. Low-grade VUR resolves spontaneously in almost 80% of cases and urologic evaluation is *unnecessary* unless VUR is complicated by poor growth, hypertension, or reduced renal function. Higher grades of reflux do not spontaneously resolve and indicate more severe urinary tract damage. Patients with high grade VUR should have urologic evaluation, preferably by a pediatric urologist, and almost always require cystoscopy and ureteral reimplantations. Surgical management of high-grade VUR generally stops reflux but cannot reverse preexisting renal damage.

Prevention of Recurrent Infection

Prevention of recurrent infection in patients with VUR greatly reduces the risk of renal scarring. This requires continuous prophylactic antibiotic therapy (see Table 112-3) until VUR ceases, whether spontaneously or after urologic surgery. Methenamine may be useful for prophylaxis of patients who are allergic to antibiotics, but large quantities of cranberry juice or vitamin C must be ingested to acidify urine to *p*H 5.5. This therapy is difficult to maintain for long periods.

Some children with normal urinary tract structure have recurrent infection. Antibiotic prophylaxis (usually given for 6 months) will prevent recurrence and reduce the morbidity associated with UTI. Prophylaxis also alters bacterial fimbriae to reduce bacterial adherence and, hence, pathogenicity.

Teaching a child the proper wiping technique after bowel movement may reduce fecal contamination in the vaginal introitus and urethra. Similarly, control of constipation and associated encopresis will reduce perineal soiling and allow normal bladder sphincter function.

INDICATIONS FOR REFERRAL OR HOSPITALIZATION

All infants and children with symptomatic pyelonephritis, sepsis, or obstructive uropathy should be hospitalized. Infants with obstructive signs (e.g., midline lower abdominal distention; flank mass; infrequent or prolonged voiding; weak, dribbling, or "threadlike" urinary stream; or ballooning of the penile urethra) must be evaluated by a pediatric urologist, as should any child who has severe VUR. In addition, children who have any degree of VUR along with hypertension, growth retardation, reduced renal function, anemia, or other structural renal abnormalities should also have urologic evaluation.

PATIENT EDUCATION

Parents must understand the consequences of UTIs, the need for timely and comprehensive management, and the importance of compliance with treatment plans. Many adults experience UTI as a minor annoyance and assume that the same holds true for infants and children. Physicians should avoid terms such as *cystitis* or *bladder infection* because they may lessen the importance of UTI in the minds of parents.

ANNOTATED BIBLIOGRAPHY

Crain EF, Gershel JC: Urinary tract infections in febrile infants younger than 8 weeks of age. Pediatrics 86:363–376, 1990. (UTIs were identified in 75% of febrile infants less than 8 weeks old. Fifty percent had "normal" urinalysis despite positive urine culture. Uncircumcised males had an increased risk of UTI. Urine culture is mandatory in the evaluation of febrile infants.)

Hellerstein S, Wald ER, Winberg J et al: Consensus: Roentgenographic evaluation of children with urinary tract infections. Pediatr Infect Dis 3:291–293, 1984. (Recommends evaluation of first UTI in girls younger than age 3 and in boys at any age.)

Herzog LW: Urinary tract infections and circumcision: A case control study. Am J Dis Child 143:348–50, 1989. (Reports that uncircumcised male infants had a significantly higher likelihood of UTI than circumcised infants.)

Johnson CE, Shurin PA, Marchant CD et al: Identification of children requiring radiologic evaluation for urinary infection. Pediatr Infect Dis 4:656–663, 1985. (Discusses the radiologic evaluation of UTI and presents results of a prospective study designed to identify markers for children at risk for renal damage.)

Jones KV, Asscher AW: Urinary tract infection and vesicoureteral reflux. In Edelman CM Jr (ed): Pediatric Kidney Disease, 2nd ed, pp 1943–1991. Boston, Little, Brown, 1992. (Comprehensive overview of UTI, epidemiology, pathophysiology, diagnosis, management, and complications.)

Lebowitz RL: Pediatric uroradiology. Pediatr Clin North Am 32:1353–1362, 1985. (Discusses the techniques available for evaluation of the urinary tract, describes each technique, and provides guidelines for their use.)

Roberts JA: Pathogenesis of nonobstructive urinary tract infections in children. J Urol 144 (part 2):475–479, 1990. (Discusses bacterial virulence factors including type 1 and P-fimbriae and relates the inflammatory response to infection-associated renal scarring.)

Smellie JM, Willems CED: Vesico-ureteric reflux: Recent research and its effect upon clinical practice. In Catto GRD (ed): Urinary Tract Infection (New Clinical Applications, Nephrology), pp 39–85. Boston, Kluwer Academic Publishers, 1989. (Review of pathophysiology, diagnosis, consequences and management of VUR.)

Todd JK: Diagnosis of urinary tract infections. Pediatr Infect Dis 1:126–131, 1982. (Describes techniques that can be used in the office laboratory to diagnose UTI.)

113
Dysuria and Frequency

*Roopa S. Hashimoto and
Jerold C. Woodhead*

Dysuria refers to painful micturition, and *frequency* is an increase in the number of voidings with or without increased urinary volume. Both occur commonly in children and adolescents. Accompanying symptoms are common and include urgency, hesitancy, and urinary incontinence.

PATHOPHYSIOLOGY

Any process that irritates the mucosa of the bladder or urethra may result in dysuria, including infection, trauma, and mechanical or chemical irritation. Pain receptors in the bladder are sensitive to distention and strong contractions. Inflamed or irritated perineal and vaginal tissue may be further irritated during urination with accompanying pain.

Frequency may result from various causes, the most common one is increased fluid intake. In urinary tract infection, frequency results from bladder mucosal inflammation and bladder spasm. The bladder capacity is decreased by pain associated with inflammation. Excitement and stress may raise intravesical pressure and relax the detrusor muscle, thus prompting urination. Cold weather may also lead to an increased frequency and volume of urination because vasoconstriction of the peripheral circulation increases the rate of urine production.

CLINICAL PRESENTATION

The clinical presentation of dysuria and frequency varies with age and etiology. Normally, infants and toddlers void 6 to 30 times per day, 3- to 5-year olds void 8 to 14 times per day, 5- to 8-year olds void 6 to 12 times per day, and 8- to 14-year olds void 6 to 8 times per day. In infants younger than 6 months of age, micturition is started at a critical bladder volume of about 30 mL. This volume is increased to 60 mL by 1 year of age and to 100 mL by 2 years of age. Dysuria and frequency may be difficult to identify in infancy but may be suspected if parents note crying associated with voiding or diaper dermatitis resistant to treatment. During infancy, *circumcised* boys may be at increased risk of urethral meatal irritation with associated dysuria, whereas *uncircumcised* boys have an increased risk of urinary tract infections. The infant with urinary tract infection may have dysuria along with malodorous urine, failure to thrive, or signs of systemic infection. Toddlers may have dysuria noted only because of changes in voiding habits, signs of urinary tract infection, or a perineal rash and irritation. Older children and adolescents have the ability to complain of pain with urination; urinary frequency and other associated symptoms are also more evident. "Classic" signs and symptoms of urinary tract infection predominate in this age group. Sexually active adolescents with dysuria may have sexually transmitted infection. Dysuria may also be the presenting complaint in sexual abuse. Urethral prolapse presents with a painful, purple, mulberry-like mass in the perineum associated with dysuria or urinary retention.

DIFFERENTIAL DIAGNOSIS

Common infectious causes of dysuria or frequency include bacterial infection of the urinary tract (see Chap. 112), viral hemorrhagic cystitis, gonococcal and nongonococcal urethritis, herpes simplex or varicella lesions in the periurethral region, candidal dermatitis, and vulvovaginitis (see Chap. 119). All of these may cause the *dysuria-pyuria syndrome,* which has been identified in adult women and probably occurs in adolescent girls, especially those who are sexually active. Patients who have this syndrome have voiding symptoms and pyuria but no signs of systemic illness. Urine cultures are sterile or have low colony counts of *Escherichia coli* or *Staphylococcus saprophyticus,* although other gram-negative and positive organisms occasionally cause the syndrome. Because the dysuria-pyuria syndrome has been formally described only for adult women, its diagnosis should be made carefully, if at all, and only in adolescent girls who have urine cultures with colony counts in the range of 10^2 to 10^4/mL or who have sterile urine and vulvovaginitis.

Trauma and irritation commonly cause dysuria. Falls, masturbation, and sexual abuse may traumatize periurethral and perineal tissues and produce painful urination. Toddlers may insert foreign bodies into the vagina or urethra. Irritant dermatitis from urine, or soap and bleach residue in diapers, may cause dysuria, as can chemical urethritis from bubble bath, soap, or deodorants. Other causes include urethral meatal ulceration (usually in circumcised boys), urethral stricture resulting from trauma, urinary calculi (usually associated with hematuria), and pinworm infestation.

Miscellaneous causes of dysuria or frequency include appendicitis with a pelvic abscess, bladder outlet obstruction, Reiter disease, urethral prolapse, drugs, renal tuberculosis, prostatitis, and pollakiuria (i.e., frequency caused by stress or excitement). Dysuria plus urinary retention may be caused by the ingestion of various drugs, including amitriptyline, chlordiazepoxide, imipramine, or isoniazid. Frequency may result from the ingestion of antihistamines, carbamazepine, demeclocycline, fenfluramine, and excess vitamin D. Girls with group A β-hemolytic streptococcal pharyngitis may develop streptococcal vaginitis, which

causes dysuria and perineal discomfort. Encopresis presumably causes frequency because fecal impaction reduces bladder capacity and also promotes relaxation of the urethral sphincter. In addition, constant fecal soiling predisposes to urinary tract infection.

WORK-UP

History

History alone often identifies the etiology of dysuria and frequency and avoids an excessive work-up. Chills, fever, and signs and symptoms compatible with urinary tract infection point to an infectious cause, although dysuria without a systemic illness may also be caused by an infection of the urinary tract.

A preceding viral illness followed by the acute onset of painful, frequent, bloody urination suggests *hemorrhagic cystitis.* The physician should ask about a history of recurrent herpes lesions or recent infection with varicella. A history of vaginal discharge along with dysuria and frequency in the pubertal girl suggests sexually transmitted diseases such as *Neisseria gonorrhoeae, Trichomonas, Chlamydia,* or *Candida* infection (See Chap. 200). Similar symptoms in a prepubertal girl suggest sexual abuse. Night crying in young girls may point to irritation caused by pinworm migration from the rectum to the vagina or urethra. The physician should ask about trauma, including falls, masturbation, foreign body insertion into the urethra or vagina, and sexual abuse. A description of a weak urinary stream or a history of constant dribbling may provide clues that lead to the diagnosis of bladder outlet obstruction or bladder diverticula.

An inquiry should be made about medications (both prescription and over-the-counter) and illicit drug ingestion. The use of detergents, soaps, bubble bath, or deodorants may not be mentioned by parents unless specifically asked about. Information about bowel habits including constipation, soiling, and the method used by young girls to wipe themselves after bowel movements often proves valuable in the search for the etiology of dysuria. Causes of acute and chronic emotional stress should be sought when *pollakiuria* is suspected. This syndrome occurs in previously toilet-trained children who have a sudden onset of daytime urinary frequency without incontinence. With normal urinalysis, further work-up is not required unless incontinence becomes a problem or urinary tract infection is documented.

Physical Examination

The physical examination of a child with frequency and dysuria should be thorough. Inspection may reveal abdominal distention, rashes or evidence of perineal trauma, urethral lesions, or vaginal discharge. Vaginal examination will allow the identification of a foreign body, vaginitis, or trauma. Abdominal masses may be of renal, bladder, or bowel origin. Pain with palpation or percussion of the bladder or kidneys points to urinary tract infection. Rectal examination may disclose impacted feces or a tender pelvic abscess. Observation of the urinary stream may reveal abnormalities such as spraying or dribbling. Listening to the sound of the urinary stream may be more practical with girls.

Laboratory Tests

The most important tests in the laboratory evaluation of dysuria and frequency are urinalysis and culture of an appropriately collected specimen. At all ages, if infection appears likely, catheterization of the bladder provides the specimen with the least likelihood of contamination. Suprapubic bladder aspiration carries the risk of hematuria, which may confuse the diagnostic process. If analysis of midstream voided urine from an older child or adolescent identifies bacteriuria, pyuria, hematuria, or a positive culture, optimal (although not mandatory) management includes one or more repeat urine evaluations to confirm the abnormality. (Culture criteria for the diagnosis of urinary tract infection are discussed in Chapter 112.) Voided urine that is persistently sterile or has low colony counts despite voiding symptoms may signal the dysuria-pyuria syndrome, but, as mentioned, this diagnosis should be made cautiously.

Pyuria is most reliably detected in uncentrifuged urine examined with the aid of a hemocytometer. When a counting chamber is used, urine with more than or equal to 8 white blood cells/mm^3 has a high association with the dysuria-pyuria syndrome; more than 10 white blood cells/mm^3 correlates strongly with urine culture of more than 10^5 colonies/mL. Pyuria may also be identified in centrifuged urine, but sources of error are numerous, and quantification of pyuria is much less certain than with the hemocytometer.

A suspicion of sexually transmitted infection mandates cultures for gonorrhea from the urethra, vagina, cervix, rectum, and oropharynx, depending on the patient's age and clinical history. A chlamydial culture may not be available to the office-based physician. A wet mount examination of vaginal discharge may demonstrate trichomonas. Potassium hydroxide prep and culture may aid in the identification of candida.

If pinworms are suspected, a transparent tape test should be done during the office visit and examined for pinworm ova. If negative, parents should be taught the technique and sent home with slides to be done on 3 separate days early in the morning before the child arises or when night crying occurs.

Streptococcal vaginitis is identified by culture.

TREATMENT

With adequate therapy, dysuria and frequency caused by urinary tract infection resolve rapidly. Except in adolescents who fit the clinical description of the dysuria-pyuria syndrome, infection of the urinary tract accompanied by dysuria should be treated according to standard regimens (see Chap. 112). In adult women and probably in adolescent girls, the dysuria-pyuria syndrome represents bacterial infection of the urinary tract in a high proportion of cases. Single-dose antibiotic therapy is known to be effective for *adult* women with this syndrome (amoxicillin, 2 or 3 g orally; sulfisoxazole, 1 g orally; or trimethoprim-sulfamethoxazole, one or two double-strength tablets orally). Efficacy of single-dose antibiotic therapy for adolescents has *not* been well studied. One study showed that a 3-day treatment with trimethoprim-sulfamethoxazole (one double-strength tablet twice daily) was more effective than single-dose treatment with this antibiotic when urine culture had more than 10^5 colonies/mL. A short course of therapy (single-dose or 3-day) is not recommended in infants and children.

Dysuria associated with sexually transmitted diseases at any age responds to treatment for the specific infection. Sexually active adolescents with urethritis or vaginitis caused by *Chlamydia* may be treated with doxycycline (100 mg twice daily for 10 days), tetracycline (500 mg four times a day for 10 days), or erythromycin (500 mg four times a day for 7 days). Erythromycin at this high a dose may be accompanied by an unacceptable rate of gastrointestinal side effects. *N. gonorrhoeae, Trichomonas,* and *Candida* infections should be treated according to standard practice (see Chap. 200).

Pinworm infestation responds to a single 100-mg dose of mebendazole, but pruritus and dysuria may persist for several days. Physical or chemical irritation of the urethra or perineum decreases with the removal of the offending irritant and by the use of sitz baths in warm water for 20 to 30 minutes, three or four times daily. Hydroxyzine may reduce the itching of varicella. If analgesia is desired, acetaminophen (10 mg/kg/dose) or phenazopyridine (100 mg/dose) may alleviate pain. Aspirin (10 mg/kg/dose) may be used if the child does not have varicella or influenza.

INDICATIONS FOR REFERRAL OR HOSPITALIZATION

Dysuria associated with pyelonephritis may require management in the hospital. Children who have evidence of bladder obstruction, urethral prolapse, abnormal urinary stream, or urethral trauma need a urologic evaluation. Sexually abused children may need hospitalization for protective reasons and *must* be referred to social services. The child who has pollakiuria may require a referral to a psychologist.

ANNOTATED BIBLIOGRAPHY

Asnes RS, Mones RL: Pollakiuria. Pediatrics 52:615–617, 1973. (Report of four cases with a discussion on the differential diagnosis of increased frequency of urination.)

Bauer SB, Retik AB, et al: The unstable bladder of childhood. Urol Clin North Am 7:321–336, 1980. (Report of 110 children with symptoms of lower urinary tract dysfunction.)

Green M: Pediatric Diagnosis, pp 407–409. Philadelphia, WB Saunders, 1992. (Discussion of urinary frequency, oliguria, polyuria, the urinary stream, and incontinence, including an outline of the the signs and symptoms of each complaint.)

Hellerstein S: Urinary Tract Infections in Children, pp 96–104. Chicago, Year Book Medical Publishers, 1982. (Review of the causes, diagnosis, and treatment of frequency and dysuria in patients who do not have bacteriuria.)

Hjalmas K: Urodynamics in normal infants and children. Scand J Urol Nephrol Suppl 114:20–27, 1988. (Discussion of urodynamics in infants and children, including the development of lower urinary tract function, urodynamic indications, techniques, variables, and diagnostic value.)

Koammaroff AL: Acute dysuria in women. N Engl J Med 310:368–375, 1984. (Reviews the causes and treatment of dysuria in adult women and provides an updated definition of "positive" urine culture.)

Koff SA, Byard MA: The daytime urinary frequency syndrome of childhood. J Urol 140:1280–1281, 1988. (Retrospective review of 43 completely toilet-trained children who suddenly developed isolated daytime urinary frequency.)

Mazeman E, Foissac MC: Urologic pain in pediatric practice. Probl Urol 3:336–345, 1989. (Reviews pathologic, physiologic, and clinical features of pain in pediatric urology and discusses treatment.)

Schmitt BD: Daytime wetting (diurnal enuresis). Pediatr Clin North Am 29:9–20, 1982. (Excellent review of the causes of daytime wetting, including a section on daytime frequency as well as an appendix with instructions for the parent.)

Zoubek J, Bloom DA, Sedman AB: Extraordinary urinary frequency. Pediatrics 85:1112–1114, 1990. (Report of 46 children with isolated urinary frequency. Discusses the importance of a careful history, physical examination, and urinalysis. In the absence of findings, no treatment is necessary.)

114

Hematuria

Craig B. Langman

The appearance of macroscopic blood in the urine is one of the most frightening signs that occurs to parents and patients, although it may not portend serious disease. Alternatively, the presence of microscopic hematuria, a potentially grave sign of serious renal pathology, is often treated lightly by the physician and parent/patient. In this chapter the chronic, serious disorders associated with hematuria are separated from the disorders that may be self-limited, re-versible, preventable, or, if chronic, nonthreatening to normal renal function.

PATHOPHYSIOLOGY

Red blood cells may enter the urinary tract from the level of the glomerulus to the urethral meatus and may result in either macroscopic or microscopic hematuria. Therefore, the mere presence of isolated red blood cells in the random urinalysis may not be helpful in the determination of where bleeding in the urinary tract is occurring.

The presence of blood in the urinary space is, in itself, not painful; therefore, the occurrence of painful hematuria should alert the clinician to search for an underlying cause in which hematuria also occurs.

Glomerular inflammation presumably damages the capillary basement membrane so that a diapedesis of red blood cells ensues. If the exit of red blood cells into the urinary space is brisk, gross hematuria may result in the characteristic brownish red color of the urine. However, if the leak of red blood cells is slower, only microscopic hematuria will be manifest. Interestingly, the degree of glomerular inflammation (assessed either pathologically or clinically) does not correlate with the presence of gross hematuria. There are no studies to document that red blood cell excretion is constant for any particular degree of glomerular inflammation, and thus several urine specimens should be examined to determine the presence or absence of red blood cells.

Red blood cells that enter the urinary stream below the level of the nephron unit (glomerulus and tubules) are more likely to manifest as gross hematuria, although again the severity of such lesions does not correlate with actual red blood cell excretion rates.

DETECTION

Children quickly learn that the color of normal urine is not red or brown. Thus, children as young as 3 years of age may report gross hematuria to their parents or at least be able to give a historical reply to its presence when asked by the clinician. Gross hematuria often appears the color of tea, presumably because of the breakdown of heme pigments present in the hemoglobin of red blood cells.

Microscopic hematuria is easily detected in the random urinalysis with the use of the common "dipstick" examination or with a direct microscopic examination of the urinary sediment. The "dipstick" evaluation for the detection of blood relies on a chemical reaction (orthotoluidine oxidation) that detects the presence of heme pigment. The test is exquisitely sensitive, so that only 5 to 10 red blood cells per high power field (HPF) may cause a positive reaction. On direct microscopic examination of the urinary sediment, 3 to 5 red blood cells/HPF may be viewed as normal in the pediatric population.

DIFFERENTIAL DIAGNOSIS

Pseudohematuria

The clinician must remain aware of the false-positive findings of "hematuria" by the dipstick examination; therefore, all positive readings should be followed by the direct microscopic examination of the urinary sediment to document the degree of red blood cell excretion. Because the chemical reaction in the dipstick detects heme pigments, other heme-containing proteins in the urine will give a false-positive reaction. The most common interfering heme pigment comes from myoglobin. *Myoglobinuria,* which may be either benign (after strenuous exercise) or indicative of more severe systemic pathology (e.g., muscle trauma, child abuse or viral myositis), will therefore cause a false-positive reaction; however, severe myoglobinuria may itself cause a glomerular lesion and lead to red blood cells in the urine. This latter situation should be apparent from the clinical history and the physical examination. Myoglobin may be detected in the urine by a myoglobin-specific electrophoretic assay.

Free hemoglobin in the urine (hemoglobinuria) will also give a positive dipstick examination. Although hemoglobinuria may be seen clinically during transfusion reactions or after severe burn injuries, exogenous chemicals are more common causes of the disorder. These include several toxic compounds (e.g., chloroform, oxalic acid, potassium chlorate) found in household agents and compounds toxic only to patients with glucose-6-phosphate dehydrogenase deficiency, such as sulfonamides and fava beans.

Exogenous substances may produce a dark brown or red urine, although red blood cell excretion is normal. Such substances include the aniline dyes used for coloring candy, the naturally occurring pigments of berries (elderberry and blackberry), and phenolphthalein, used in laxative preparations.

Lastly, the ingestion of several drinks containing chemical coloring agents may cause the presence of bright red urine. However, the dipstick and microscopic examination will reveal the absence of red blood cells. It is also important to remember that this clinical situation may simulate the coloring of *melena or hematochezia.*

The dipstick may occasionally be positive for blood although the microscopic examination is negative. This may be artifactual, because the exposure of red blood cells to dilute urine will produce hypotonic cell lysis. Thus, an examination of a freshly prepared urinary sediment will substantially reduce the likelihood of this phenomenon.

Newborns may have a pinkish color to their urine as the result of a large amount of urate excretion. This is easily confirmed by the presence of typical urate crystals on microscopic examination of the urinary sediment. However, red blood cell excretion is normal in this transient condition. *Serratia* urinary infections may produce a pinkish tinge to the urine.

Extrarenal Hematuria

It is uncommon for urinary bleeding to be the sole manifestation of systemic bleeding disorders. However, it is common to see gross and microscopic hematuria when there is a systemic disturbance in the hemostatic process. Thus, blood in the urine has been seen with thrombocytopenia, disseminated intravascular coagulation (apart from true renal pathology, which may coexist), and in specific coagulation factor disorders (inherited and acquired).

Glomerular Hematuria

The pathognomonic finding of glomerular hematuria is red blood cell casts in the urinary sediment. Casts are formed from red blood cells embedded in a proteinaceous matrix, which has a distinct three-dimensional character under the microscope. Glomerular hematuria may be divided into acute nephritic, chronic nephritic, and nephrotic conditions.

Acute glomerulonephritis may be part of a systemic process, as in systemic lupus erythematosus, Henoch-Schönlein purpura, or hemolytic-uremic syndrome, or be isolated to the kidney, as in post-streptococcal glomerulonephritis. Generally, significant proteinuria is also present. The hematuria may be gross or microscopic.

Chronic glomerulonephritis associated with hematuria as the presenting complaint includes two important entities, Berger's disease and hereditary nephritis. *Berger's disease* is a chronic, relapsing cause of recurrent gross and microscopic hematuria and often, proteinuria. This entity, which is characterized pathologically by the presence of IgG–IgA immune complexes in the glomerular mesangium, is often precipitated by an innocent viral infection or strenuous physical exertion. The prognosis is uniformly good in children who present without an elevated serum creatinine level or nephrotic range proteinuria. *Hereditary nephritis* comprises many inherited glomerular disorders, the best known of which is Alport's syndrome, in which a hearing loss is an important feature. A careful family history is important because affected family members may only show microscopic hematuria in the early phases of the disease. Although gross hematuria is seen frequently in adult patients with polycystic kidney disease, it is not common in children with that disease.

Childhood nephrosis, in which minimal change nephrotic syndrome represents the most common histologic variety, has microscopic hematuria associated with it in approximately 20% of cases. However, the other histologic varieties of childhood nephrosis have a higher prevalence of hematuria. The presence of either hypertension or azotemia and hematuria, in the context of childhood nephrosis, should alert the clinician to the presence of a lesion other than minimal change. (See also Chaps. 115 and 193.)

Renal vascular disorders may also be associated with hematuria. Both renal vein thrombosis and renal arterial embolus/thrombus formation have associated gross or microscopic hematuria.

The clinical history and physical examination should point to one of these possible diagnoses in which hematuria is a frequent, but not isolated, finding.

Interstitial-Tubular Hematuria

Although any tubulointerstitial disorder may be associated with microscopic hematuria, the most important condition seen clinically is that of *idiopathic hypercalciuria*. This inherited disorder in which excessive urinary calcium excretion occurs has been associated with the presence of gross and microscopic hematuria. It may be detected by the finding of an elevated urinary calcium to creatinine ratio from randomly obtained urine (values >0.18 are abnormal) and the demonstration of an increased 24-hour excretion of calcium (to >4 mg/kg). Except for several cases of Berger's disease, no other renal lesions likely coexist with this cause of hematuria. Hematuria in idiopathic hypercalciuria is commonly recurrent but rarely painful as would occur if a renal stone were causing hematuria.

Extrarenal Hematuria

The entry of red blood cells into the urine beyond the tubulointerstitial area of the kidney may be the result of an abnormality in the collecting system (renal pelvis), the ureter, the bladder, and the urethra. These disorders more commonly result in bright red, rather than brownish, gross hematuria; however, either may occur in a particular patient with extrarenal hematuria. Phase contract microscopy of the urine may differentiate glomerular hematuria with the typical deformed red blood cell from extrarenal hematuria, with the lack of red blood cell shape change.

Anatomic dilatation of the renal pelvis, seen in ureteropelvic junction obstruction, is associated with hematuria and, occasionally, proteinuria. This lesion may be silent until hematuria is discovered after otherwise innocent abdominal (or flank) blunt trauma. Diseases in which hydroureter is present (e.g., reflux nephropathy) are commonly associated with hematuria.

Another important cause of hematuria secondary to dilatation of the pelvis is *Wilms' tumor*. This common mesodermal tumor of childhood is generally associated with an abdominal mass and, possibly, systemic arterial hypertension.

Unilateral ureteral bleeding is seen commonly in patients with either sickle trait or sickle disease hemoglobinopathies. The exact mechanism of the ureteral bleeding is unknown but may involve altered vascular integrity as the result of reduced oxygen tension in the renal papillae, collecting system, and ureter. Gross hematuria is the most common presentation of this condition and should be suspected in any individual with these hemoglobinopathies.

Bladder inflammation that results in hematuria is generally related to the presence of a urinary tract infection. Although a bacterial infection is the most common etiology, *viral cystitis* (especially adenoviral cystitis) is associated with painless gross hematuria. Other anatomic lesions of the bladder may also be associated with hematuria, although other clinical manifestations may predominate. (See also Chap. 113.)

Isolated ureteral inflammation, as seen in tuberculosis, is an uncommon cause of hematuria. Urethral inflammation as a cause of hematuria is rare in the first decade of life but assumes greater clinical importance in the teenager in whom sexually acquired nongonococcal urethritis is a relatively common cause of hematuria and dysuria. Frequent masturbation in men may be associated with hematuria, presumably on the basis of urethral irritation. Foreign bodies and self-induced injection of water placed in the urethra commonly produce a purulent discharge, with hematuria as often a minor component of the clinical picture. Urethroprostatitis may be associated with significant hematuria in childhood. Meatal ulceration in circumcised newborns is a special situation that may cause gross hematuria.

Renal Trauma

Minor blunt trauma to the renal fossae or abdomen may be associated with microscopic hematuria. Generally, this is the result of a small renal contusion, but, rarely, it may be the result of significant lesions of the renal vascular or collecting systems. However, the absence of hematuria after significant trauma should not be interpreted as evidence of a lack of renal trauma; complete rupture of the kidney may not be associated with any abnormalities of the urinalysis unless the contralateral kidney is also (less severely) damaged.

Miscellaneous Causes of Hematuria

Essential hematuria is a diagnosis of exclusion, in which microscopic hematuria is not associated with any demonstrable pathology. However, because many more patients with microscopic hematuria are evaluated for the presence of idiopathic hypercalciuria, the diagnosis of essential hematuria is seldom made in the pediatric population. Familial hematuria is closely allied to both of these conditions. There is no progression to chronic renal insufficiency in either condition. *Papillary necrosis* may present with gross or microscopic hematuria. This disorder is seen in children with sickle cell trait and anemia, and severe and chronic pyelonephritis and is secondary to chronic analgesic abuse (including acetaminophen, phenacetin, and aspirin). The condition may be associated with flank pain. On rare occasions, frank papillae or fragments can be seen in the urine.

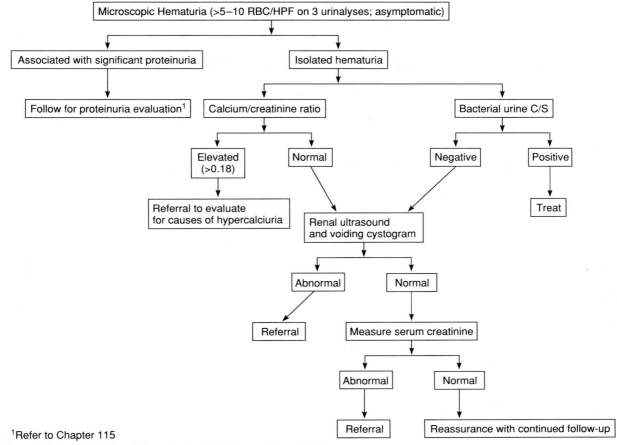

Microscopic Hematuria (>5–10 RBC/HPF on 3 urinalyses; asymptomatic)

Associated with significant proteinuria

Isolated hematuria

Follow for proteinuria evaluation[1]

Calcium/creatinine ratio

Bacterial urine C/S

Elevated (>0.18)

Normal

Negative

Positive

Referral to evaluate for causes of hypercalciuria

Renal ultrasound and voiding cystogram

Treat

Abnormal

Normal

Referral

Measure serum creatinine

Abnormal

Normal

Referral

Reassurance with continued follow-up

[1]Refer to Chapter 115

Figure 114-1.   Evaluation of the patient with microscopic hematuria.

DIAGNOSTIC EVALUATION AND INDICATIONS FOR REFERRAL

A logical approach to the evaluation of a child with hematuria may be based on the initial presentations of microscopic hematuria or painless or painful gross hematuria, as suggested in the algorithms in Figures 114-1 and 114-2. The demonstration of a single urinalysis with an abnormal red blood cell excretion (>5 red blood cells/HPF) in an asymptomatic child should be repeated two to three more times in 7 to 14 days. The evaluation should proceed if three such urinalyses demonstrate hematuria. If subsequent urinalyses fail to demonstrate hematuria, the clinician is advised to recheck the urine in 1 month's time and, if still normal, again in 6 months, before assigning a benign outcome to the initial finding.

If only isolated microscopic hematuria is demonstrated in the absence of a bacterial urinary infection, an evaluation for hypercalciuria is suggested. If that evaluation is normal, and the hematuria is persistent, formal anatomic studies with renal ultrasound examination and voiding cystourethrography are suggested. At this time, serum renal function should be evaluated by the measurement of serum creatinine concentration. If all evaluations are normal, and the hematuria persists, a diagnosis of essential hematuria may be made.

If the child presents with painful gross hematuria, the clinician is encouraged to obtain a computed tomographic scan or magnetic resonance image of the kidney once the child is well hydrated. Consultation is almost always required for the child with painful gross hematuria. Alternatively, if painless gross hematuria occurs, and the patient is without a disorder in which hemoglobin S is present, a consultation is again suggested in pediatric nephrology if proteinuria is present and in pediatric urology if proteinuria is absent. It is also important to document the level and site of bleeding in the patient with a sickle hemoglobinopathy, and the guidance of pediatric urologists is helpful in this regard. (See Fig. 114-2 for indications for admission to the hospital.)

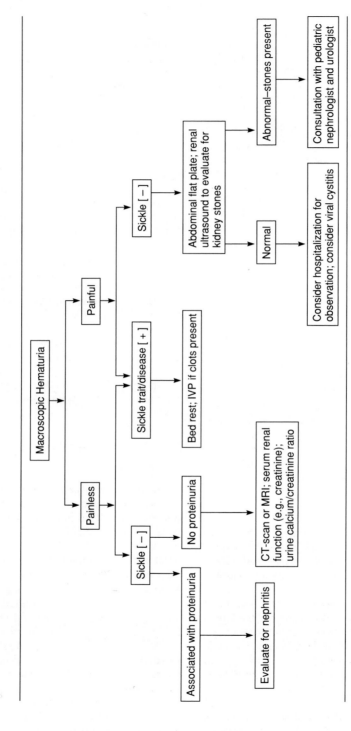

Figure 114-2. Evaluation of the patient with macroscopic hematuria.

ANNOTATED BIBLIOGRAPHY

Northway JD: Hematuria in children. J Pediatr 78:381–396, 1971. (Gives an excellent clinical and common sense approach to the evaluation of children with hematuria of diverse origin.)

Pardo V, Berian MG, Levi DF, Strauss J: Benign primary hematuria. Am J Med 67:817–822, 1979. (Convincing pathologic evidence of the benign nature of hematuria in the absence of a positive evaluation.)

Vehaskari VM, Rapola J, Koskimies O et al: Microscopic hematuria in schoolchildren: Epidemiology and clinicopathologic evaluation. J Pediatr 95:676–684, 1979. (Report of almost 9000 children between 8 and 15 years of age who were screened for hematuria, only 1% of whom had increased red cell excretion in two or more urinalyses; importantly, coexisting proteinuria alone was associated with important abnormalities on renal biopsy. Their conclusion is important to remember: low-grade hematuria, without other findings referable to the kidneys, probably represents the upper range of the physiologic variation in red cell excretion.)

115

Proteinuria

Craig B. Langman

Proteinuria is one of the most common abnormalities discovered on a routine urinalysis. It may be accompanied by other signs and symptoms of parenchymal renal disease, or it may occur as the sole manifestation of an underlying nephropathy. It may also be found in various benign or self-limited conditions that carry a uniformly good prognosis. The differentiation by the clinician of a disease state from a benign condition may be a difficult task. This chapter presents an approach to determine the etiology of proteinuria.

PATHOPHYSIOLOGY

Healthy children may excrete up to 4 mg/M^2/h of protein. Normal adults may excrete up to 150 mg/24 h. This protein consists of 40% albumin, 40% tissue proteins derived from the kidney and other urinary structures, 15% immunoglobulins, and 5% other plasma proteins.

The glomerulus normally provides a barrier to the leak of proteins into the urine when the molecular size is 40,000 or less and in a charge-specific manner to exclude anionic species such as albumin. In proteinuric states the normal steric hindrance and charge selectivity of the glomerulus may be altered so that an increased amount of protein is deposited in the urine and exceeds the tubular capacity for reabsorption.

The tubular portion of the nephron is primarily responsible for the reabsorption of small molecular proteins, such as α_2-protein, β_2-microglobulin, and smaller γ-globulins.

The presumed mechanism for tubular proteinuria is the ineffective reabsorption of normally filtered proteins, although experimental and clinical evidence is scarce.

DETECTION

A commonly employed method of detection of protein in the urine is that of the citrate-buffered tetrabromophenol colorimetric ("dipstick") test. This test depends on urinary protein, especially albumin, to alter a pH-sensitive dye, resulting in the characteristic deepening green appearance of the dipstick with an increasing amount of proteinuria. This test is termed *qualitative,* since the "amount" of protein detected on the dipstick is greatly affected by the specific gravity of the urine that is tested. Thus, normal amounts of urine protein may be read as positive if the urine is highly concentrated; similarly, abnormal amounts of urine protein may not be detected if the urine is sufficiently dilute. False-positive urine samples may occur if the sample is excessively alkaline.

A semiquantitative test to detect the abnormal excretion of protein is the ratio of urinary protein to creatinine, both of which are determined biochemically. Normal values in children are less than 0.1 but may be affected by altered patterns of creatinine excretion.

The most accurate method to measure urinary protein excretion is by a timed urine collection of usually 12 or 24 hours. The adequacy of such a collection may be independently assessed by the level of creatinine excretion, which should be at least 10 to 15 mg/kg/24 h. Protein excretion less than 4 mg/M^2/h is normal, and higher values are abnormal.

DIFFERENTIAL DIAGNOSIS

Pseudoproteinuria

There are several situations in which the clinician may find that the dipstick is positive for protein but quantitation reveals no proteinuria. Patients receiving semisynthetic penicillins excrete a breakdown product in their urine that reacts in a false-positive manner with the reagent on the dipstick. Additionally, benzalkonium chloride (Zephiran) and some radiocontrast agents will also cause a false-positive reaction on the dipstick.

Other Benign Conditions in Which Proteinuria Occurs

There are three major entities in this category, and renal function remains normal in a long-term follow-up evaluation. The first of these conditions may account for as much as 25% to 30% of proteinuria on random, in-office urinalyses and is termed *orthostatic proteinuria.* The child excretes abnormal amounts of urinary protein (>4 mg/M^2/h) when in the upright position but excretes normal amounts of protein when in the recumbent position. This is easily diagnosed by using two timed urine collections; that is, one from the recumbent position and one from the standing position. One protocol to document orthostatic proteinuria is the collection of the first morning voided specimen after the patient has emptied the bladder at bedtime the night before and has remained asleep in bed during the period of collection. The standing sample is a collection of urine following that first voided specimen for the remainder of the day and including the bedtime voided specimen that night. It is therefore essential to document *normal* protein excretion in the "recumbent" specimen. Greater than 50-year follow-up of patients with orthostatic proteinuria has documented normal renal function in all patients in whom renal function was normal at the outset.

The other entity of altered protein excretion that has a benign outlook is *exercise-induced proteinuria*. This entity is commonly seen in healthy adolescents and also carries an excellent prognosis. One method to detect this entity involves having the patient void, run up and down stairs for several minutes, and then void again. Commonly, the first voided urine specimen is negative and the post-exercise urine specimen is strongly positive for protein.

The outlook of *fever-induced proteinuria* is also excellent. Any febrile state may be accompanied by proteinuria, presumably resulting from an increased glomerular filtration rate. This proteinuria immediately disappears when the fever abates.

Proteinuria of Renal Origin

Documentation of other causes of an abnormal amount of protein is indicative of significant renal pathology. Proteinuria is usually classified as either glomerular or tubular, depending on the site of entry of the protein into the urine. Several clinical pictures may be differentiated in each type of proteinuria. Protein excretion rates that are less than 40 mg/M^2/h are compatible with proteinuria of either type, but greater amounts of proteinuria occur with glomerular protein leakage only.

The major clinical syndromes in which glomerular proteinuria occurs may be divided into three entities: (1) acute nephritic syndrome, (2) nephrosis, or (3) chronic renal insufficiency.

The *acute nephritic syndrome* is associated with hematuria (occasionally macroscopic) and often with red blood cell casts in the urine. Systemic hypertension and edema may be present on physical examination, and mild azotemia may be present in the blood. In contrast, 85% of children from 2 to 10 years of age who have nephrosis have a urine specimen that only contains protein in amounts greater than 40 mg/M^2/h. The other components of the syndrome include hypoalbuminemia and edema, often with accompanying hyperlipidemia. However, 20% of these patients may also have associated microscopic hematuria. Patients with chronic renal insufficiency, in addition to glomerular pro-

teinuria, often have a telescoped urine sediment that consists of casts of acute and chronic nature. Hypertension is common, and azotemia is present. Growth failure may also be manifest. (For further discussion of edema, see Chapter 193.)

Many systemic diseases have associated glomerular proteinuria. The most common in children include poststreptococcal glomerulonephritis, Henoch-Schönlein purpura, nephritis, and systemic lupus erythematosus. Essential hypertension is distinctly uncommon as the cause of proteinuria in a hypertensive child and should alert the clinician to other underlying renal pathology. Diseases intrinsic to the kidney that result in glomerular proteinuria include Berger's (IgA) nephropathy, hereditary nephritis (of which Alport's syndrome is one example), and the variants of childhood nephrosis (focal glomerulosclerosis, membranous nephropathy, and membranoproliferative glomerulonephritis).

Lastly, diabetes mellitus is a frequent cause of fixed proteinuria when the disease has been present for more than 10 years. However, children with diabetes younger than 10 years of age may have exercise-induced proteinuria as an early manifestation of diabetic nephropathy, and it carries a worse prognosis only in this group of patients.

Tubulointerstitial diseases resulting in proteinuria on the urinalysis may be subdivided into acute or chronic in nature. Acute interstitial nephritis is usually secondary to immunologic disorders, drug hypersensitivity, or infections. Drug hypersensitivity or reactions may also have accompanying hematuria and eosinophiluria; eosinophilia may rarely be present as well. A fever and a rash may also be present. Drugs commonly associated with acute interstitial inflammation include antibiotics, especially the β-lactam classes and nonsteroidal anti-inflammatory drugs.

Immunologic disorders, including collagen vascular diseases that cause interstitial nephritis and proteinuria, are generally associated with elevated serum γ-globulins or cryoglobulins.

The tubular proteinuria that occurs in pyelonephritis generally resolves when the infection is eradicated. The persistence of proteinuria is usually indicative of a structural abnormality, an indolent infection, or a stone. Chronic interstitial diseases are commonly the result of infections, drugs, poisonings with heavy metals, or genetic diseases or are of an immunologic nature.

Urinary tract malformations, especially any form of obstructive uropathy, and ureteral reflux without obstructive uropathy may also be associated with proteinuria. In a few cases, this proteinuria may reflect the earliest detectable abnormalities. It is, therefore, recommended to document normal genitourinary structure in the child who has proteinuria at the time of a bacterial urinary tract infection.

Chronic tubulointerstitial diseases may be associated with blood electrolyte abnormalities, and these electrolyte changes in combination with the finding of proteinuria may be the clue to the presence of the underlying nephropathy. The electrolyte abnormalities commonly take the form of an acidosis; if proximal in origin, hypokalemia is present, and if distal in origin, hyperkalemia occurs. In addition, the inability to concentrate the urine (fixed isosthenuria) may also be observed. If an inability to concentrate the urine is suspected, a water deprivation test *should not* be performed without clinical observation because of the risk of significant dehydration.

WORK-UP

Figure 115-1 depicts an easy, cost-effective way to evaluate a child with proteinuria found on routine urinalysis. If the urine specific gravity is reflective of urinary concentration (specific gravity >1.020) and trace or 1+ protein is found on dipstick testing, the physician can reassure the patient of the likely benign nature of the finding. If a dipstick reading

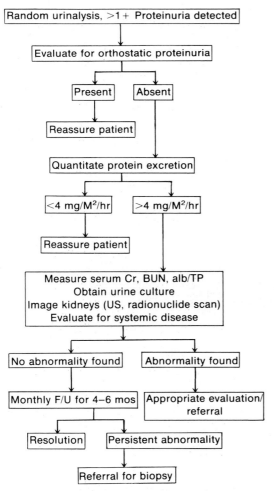

Figure 115-1. Algorithm for evaluation of proteinuria. (*Cr,* creatinine; *BUN,* blood urea nitrogen; *Alb,* albumin; *TP,* total protein; *US,* ultrasound)

of more than 1+ is found, orthostatic proteinuria should be evaluated as the cause and, if documented, the patient should again be reassured. If testing reveals recumbent proteinuria, then a formal quantitation of urine protein excretion should be undertaken. There is no role in the usual clinical setting for fractionation of urine protein into albumin, globulins, and so forth, because most children excrete, almost exclusively, only albumin. If significant proteinuria is demonstrated (>4 mg M^2/h), an appropriate history, physical examination, and laboratory investigation (see Fig. 115-1) should be planned, remembering the major clinical syndromes of proteinuria mentioned earlier.

INDICATIONS FOR REFERRAL

An abnormality, in addition to the significant proteinuria, demands a further evaluation or referral. If proteinuria is the sole abnormality and persists for 4 to 6 months on monthly follow-up visits, a referral to a pediatric nephrologist is warranted for eventual renal biopsy. This will allow a histologic diagnosis that may also have prognostic implications.

ANNOTATED BIBLIOGRAPHY

Milteny M: Urinary protein excretion in healthy children. Clin Nephrol 12:216–221, 1979. (Comprehensive study of the constituents of proteinuria in children, including newborns.)

Springberg PS, Garrett LE, Thompson AL et al: Fixed and reproducible orthostatic proteinuria: Results of a 20-year follow-up study. Ann Intern Med 97:516–519, 1982. (Report of 64 patients initially studied as adolescents and restudied 20 years later who remained free of functional renal impairment.)

West CD: Asymptomatic hematuria and proteinuria in children: Causes and appropriate diagnostic studies. Pediatrics 89:173–182, 1976. (Classic paper by one of the best clinicians of pediatric nephrology.)

116

Groin Hernias and Hydroceles

Robert P. Foglia

A mass in the groin or scrotum of a child is a relatively common pediatric problem. The embryology, anatomy, pathophysiology, evaluation, and management of the child with a hernia or hydrocele are reviewed in this chapter.

EMBRYOLOGY, ANATOMY, AND PATHOPHYSIOLOGY

Late in the first trimester of fetal development, a diverticulum of the peritoneum develops bilaterally at the level of the internal ring and extends in the male toward the scrotum.

Beginning at about the seventh month of gestation, the testis, which early in gestation had migrated to the inguinal canal, begins to descend through the inguinal canal into the scrotum. As the testis descends, the diverticulum of the peritoneal lining, the *processus vaginalis,* descends with the testis. Normally, shortly after birth, the processus vaginalis begins to close. This leaves only the most distal portion of the processus, the tunica vaginalis that surrounds the testis, patent. The major factor in the development of a hernia or hydrocele in a child is the continued patency of the processus vaginalis. At the time of birth in full-term male infants, the testes will be fully descended in 95% of infants.

Inguinal hernia is divided into two types: *indirect* or *direct*. The indirect inguinal hernia constitutes almost all of groin hernias in children younger than 3 years of age. It is caused by a lack of obliteration of the patent processus vaginalis and is thus a congenital hernia. As the child increases intra-abdominal pressure, either with crying or straining, a portion of the abdominal viscera may enter the hernia sac at the internal inguinal ring and then descends partially or completely through the inguinal canal and into the scrotum. Whether a bulge appears only in the groin, or both in the groin and the scrotum, depends on whether the processus vaginalis or hernia sac is only partly patent or fully patent into the scrotum. If a child has a large indirect inguinal hernia, the constant pressure from the abdominal viscera in the hernia sac at the level of the internal inguinal ring can gradually widen this area from the ring medially. This can create an acquired direct inguinal hernia along with the congenital indirect inguinal hernia. In contrast, as the child becomes older, the incidence of direct inguinal hernias increases. The direct hernia is usually acquired, and bowel contents can protrude into the inguinal canal through the weakened floor. A *femoral hernia* is rare in children, having an incidence in several series of only 0.2%. In a femoral hernia, the defect is inferior to the inguinal ligament and is medial to the femoral vein.

The difference between a hernia and a hydrocele is the contents of the processus. If the neck of the processus at the internal inguinal ring is wide enough to allow abdominal viscera to enter, and if abdominal viscera are present in the sac, then this is a *hernia*. If only fluid is present in the processus and if abdominal viscera have never been noted in the processus, this is a *hydrocele*. In the female, the equivalent of the processus vaginalis is the canal of Nuck; it contains the round ligament as it descends to the labia majorum. The small intestine is the most common structure found in a hernia sac in a boy. In the female, the hernia is more likely to contain the ovary and fallopian tube.

The presence of a patent processus vaginalis does not necessarily mean the child has or will develop a hernia or hydrocele. Although the processus is closed in most children within the first several months of life, it has been shown in adults who died with no clinical evidence of a groin hernia that 20% had a patent processus vaginalis.

INCIDENCE

Approximately 2% of boys will develop inguinal hernias. The incidence increases in progressively more premature infants and ranges from 13% to 30%. Hernias are 6 to 15 times more common in boys than girls, but in children younger than 1 year of age this gender disparity is less pronounced. Over one third of all hernias will be diagnosed before 6 months of age, and one half will be diagnosed before the child's first birthday.

Ten to 15% of children, especially those younger than 1 year of age, will have clinically apparent bilateral hernias. If only one hernia is present, it is twice as likely to be on the right side. Children with conditions that increase intra-abdominal pressure, such as ventriculoperitoneal shunts, ascites, or bronchopulmonary dysplasia, have a higher incidence of hernias. Children with connective tissue disorders such as Ehlers-Danlos syndrome and the acid mucopolysaccharidoses (Hurler-Hunter complex) also have an increased incidence of hernias.

CLINICAL PRESENTATION AND DIFFERENTIAL DIAGNOSIS

The most common finding is that the parent sees a "bulge" or "lump" in the child's groin or scrotum. The mass may be present transiently, it may come and go, or it may be present constantly. The pediatrician's major objective is to determine what caused the "bulge." The differential diagnosis includes inguinal hernia, hydrocele, undescended testis, retractile testis, inguinal lymphadenopathy or abscess, and femoral hernia. Except with incarceration and strangulation, a hernia usually occurs without pain. (See Chap. 118 for a discussion of the causes of genital pain.)

An accurate description by the parents as to where they saw the lump or bulge is helpful in making the correct diagnosis. If it were present in the inguinal region or in the inguinal region and scrotum, it is likely to be a hernia; if there was a transient swelling in the scrotum alone, it may be a hydrocele. A key point is that an inguinal hernia causes a "lump" or "mass" above the inguinal ligament.

An understanding of the anatomy of the inguinal canal is also helpful in making the clinical diagnosis. The examination for a hernia begins first with an inspection to determine if there is asymmetry and to see if an obvious mass is present. The examiner should ascertain if the testes are in their normal position because an undescended or retractile testis can appear as a groin mass. The child with lymphadenopathy or an inguinal abscess may have evidence of a recent infection, such as tenderness, a fever, or leukocytosis. The mass caused by infection is usually not directly over the inguinal canal, and it feels matted and more firm than the abdominal viscera found in a hernia. Erythema and tenderness over the inguinal region may be present with both lymphadenopathy and with a hernia having incarcerated bowel and a compromised blood supply. The findings in the child with a hernia are a sausage-shaped mass originating at the internal inguinal ring and extending a variable distance down the inguinal canal. If the processus is patent completely, the herniated viscera may extend all the way into the scrotum. A femoral hernia presents as a mass more medial than the usual hernia and may be seen as a mass high in the proximal thigh, which increases in size as the patient increases intra-abdominal pressure.

If the hernia is not identifiable, it may be helpful to have the child increase intra-abdominal pressure (e.g., crying, straining, or Valsalva maneuver) in an attempt to have the hernia protrude. A hydrocele can often be differentiated from a hernia by a history and physical examination. The parent of the child with a hydrocele will describe the boy's scrotum as being normal sized when he awakens but that during the day it increases in size. If the mass is only in the scrotum with no mass palpable above the pubis and has been present for a relatively long time (over 8 hours) and if the child does not have abdominal distention, has not vomited, and is not fussy, this is more likely to be a hydrocele than an incarcerated hernia. The ability to transilluminate a scrotal mass does not help differentiate a hernia from a hydrocele because an incarcerated bowel loop in a newborn easily transilluminates, as does a hydrocele. Attempted aspiration of a "probable" hydrocele should not be considered because an erroneous diagnosis may lead to tragic consequences. In contrast, palpating the proximal extent of the mass may be helpful. Hydroceles will often be limited to the scrotum alone. If the examiner can palpate the pubic ramus and the cord structures exiting at the external inguinal ring and does not feel a bowel loop, then it is unlikely that the scrotal mass is a hernia. A rectal examination can be helpful in the child younger than 1 year of age. The examiner carries out a bimanual examination with one finger in the rectum and with the other hand palpates the lower abdomen. If there is no loop of bowel intervening at the pubic ramus, it is unlikely that the mass is an incarcerated hernia. The use of an abdominal roentgenogram is also helpful because if air is present below the inguinal ligament, this is indicative of a hernia. However, if an incarcerated bowel loop below the inguinal ligament is fluid filled, this may give a false impression of no hernia.

DIAGNOSTIC STUDIES

Herniography

It is possible to inject contrast material into the peritoneal cavity and outline a patent processus vaginalis or hernia sac if one is present. In especially problematic cases, this technique is helpful but there are several caveats involved with its use. It is an invasive procedure and carries a small but finite risk of injury to the bowel. If a patent processus is outlined, this may not constitute an indication for an operation because a patent processus is not prima facie evidence

for a hernia. If there is an incarcerated hernia, a herniogram may give a false-negative picture because no peritoneal fluid can flow down into the processus owing to the bowel loop incarcerated at the inguinal ring preventing any contrast material from passing into the hernia sac.

Ultrasound Examination

Ultrasound examination of the inguinal region and scrotum offers an excellent method to evaluate the presence of a suspected irreducible inguinal hernia. It can differentiate a hydrocele with peritoneal fluid from a true hernia with a bowel loop present in a hernia sac either in the inguinal region or in the scrotum. It is noninvasive, can be repeated, and can identify one or multiple loops of bowel. Furthermore, it identifies abdominal visceral structures (i.e., intestine or ovary) in the inguinal canal and not simply the presence of a patent processus vaginalis. Ultrasound examination in most instances has become the study of choice if the diagnosis of an irreducible hernia is questioned.

MANAGEMENT

An inguinal hernia requires operative repair. It does not resolve spontaneously, and there is no role for a truss in its management. The major risk associated with an inguinal hernia is incarceration. Approximately two thirds of all incarcerated hernias occur in children younger than 1 year of age. If the child has an easily reducible hernia, an operative correction should be scheduled at the earliest convenience. The exception to this recommendation is the premature infant. Because of the increased risk of postanesthetic respiratory problems, if the hernia is easily reducible, an elective operation may be deferred until the infant is at least 42 weeks' total gestational age. This notwithstanding, others have advocated operative repair shortly after the hernia is diagnosed. The basis for this recommendation is that these infants often have chronic lung disease and have increased abdominal pressure. By waiting a number of weeks before operative repair, the infant may convert an indirect inguinal hernia into a hernia with both direct and indirect components where the entire floor of the canal is opened. These hernias are more difficult to repair and have an increased risk of recurrence. Also, these premature infants would stay in the nursery postoperatively and not be discharged home. Therefore, any increased risk of anesthesia could be closely monitored postoperatively.

If the hernia cannot be easily reduced, the first step in management consists of reduction; otherwise, this may lead to strangulation of the bowel, especially in males. In females, an incarcerated hernia often contains an ovary or a fallopian tube and there is less risk of strangulation.

The child with an incarcerated hernia is usually fussy, and if the bowel has been incarcerated for more than 4 to 6 hours, the abdomen will often be distended. Ninety-five percent of incarcerated hernias can be reduced. This is done by exerting steady constant pressure on the most distal portion of the hernia contents in the direction of the internal ring with one hand. Dorsal force is then directed with the other hand at the level of the internal ring. Usually with merely maintaining steady pressure, some of the air is displaced from the incarcerated loop of bowel into the adjacent bowel proximal to the neck of the hernia. The remainder of the bowel usually then promptly reduces. If the bowel remains incarcerated, sedating the infant with meperidine (Demerol) or chloral hydrate, and trying again usually works. The use of ice packs over the incarcerated bowel has not been found to be helpful and will upset the child; therefore, this practice is contraindicated.

If the hernia reduces easily, the child may go home and elective repair should be scheduled within 1 to 2 weeks. If, however, there has been difficulty in reducing the hernia, the child should be admitted to the hospital, maintained at NPO, and have an intravenous line started. The child's abdomen should be examined over the next 8 hours to evaluate for evidence of bowel ischemia. Operative repair should then be performed 24 to 48 hours later after the edema has resolved. If the hernia cannot be reduced, or if any aspect of the diagnosis and immediate management is questioned, emergency operative repair is indicated.

OPERATIVE REPAIR

Inguinal hernia repair can easily be performed on an outpatient basis. The child comes into the outpatient area in the morning, is operated on, and is usually discharged within 2 to 3 hours. The exceptions to this practice are children with significant congenital heart disease, lung disease, or a history of apnea, or children who were born prematurely and are younger than 6 months old. These children have a higher risk of postoperative respiratory problems, and as a rule it is preferable to have these children admitted and observed during the night following surgery.

The hernia repair is performed under general anesthesia and consists of an incision made in a skin crease, dissection down to the inguinal canal, identification of the hernia sac, freeing it from the cord structures to the level of the internal ring, and then high ligation of the sac. The distal portion of the sac should be left wide open or excised. If there is evidence of weakness of the floor of the inguinal canal or if the internal ring is wide open, the floor of the inguinal canal is reinforced. The use of a local anesthetic, such as bupivacaine, to block the ilioinguinal nerve and sensory dermatomes offers good pain relief for up to 12 hours. Likewise, a caudal anesthetic gives excellent pain relief during and after the procedure. When the child is examined again in the office, the parents will often comment how the following day their child acted as though he was never operated on. The use of a spinal anesthetic in certain high-risk patients, especially infants with chronic lung disease, has en-

joyed good success. It has been shown to decrease the risk of respiratory complications in infants with a prior history of apnea.

Hydroceles in children younger than 1 year of age do not require an operation because over half of these will resolve spontaneously with the obliteration of the patent processus. Operative repair is recommended if the hydrocele is so large that it is uncomfortable for the child or if the hydrocele is still present in a child older than 1 year of age. If abdominal viscera are seen at any time in the inguinal canal or scrotum, then the child now has a true hernia and not only a hydrocele, and operative repair is indicated.

CONTRALATERAL EXPLORATION

Much debate has centered about the question of exploration of the opposite asymptomatic side when a symptomatic hernia is being repaired on the other side. In children younger than 1 year of age, there is a 40% to 50% likelihood of a hernia being present on the opposite side even if none is seen clinically. A second hernia also appears more commonly in females. Therefore, a reasonable course is to explore the contralateral asymptomatic side in children younger than 1 year of age.

COMPLICATIONS

The major preoperative complication is incarceration leading to bowel obstruction and, potentially, strangulation of the bowel. If the bowel cannot be reduced manually, emergency herniorrhaphy is required. An inspection of the bowel at operation allows the assessment of its viability; and, in some cases, resection of the affected bowel must be done. Testicular compromise has also been found to occur secondary to venous obstruction by the incarcerated hernia. The vas deferens is quite small in infants, and there is a small risk of injury to this delicate structure during herniorrhaphy. In the female, the fallopian tube or ovary is often in the hernia sac and injury may occur to these structures unless care is taken prior to the removal of the sac.

The chance of recurrence of a hernia is small and is usually considered secondary to not having performed a high ligation of the hernia sac at the level of the internal inguinal ring. Alternatively, the child may return with a direct component of an inguinal hernia after a high ligation of an indirect hernia has been performed.

ANNOTATED BIBLIOGRAPHY

Harper RG, Garcia A, Sia C: Inguinal hernia: A common problem of premature infants weighing 1000 grams or less at birth. Pediatrics 56:112, 1975. (Excellent review.)

Holder TM, Ashcraft KW: Groin hernias and hydroceles. In Holder TM, Ashcraft KW (eds): Textbook of Pediatric Surgery, p 594. Philadelphia, WB Saunders, 1980. (Easily readable and excellent reference.)

Moss RL, Hatch EI: Inguinal hernia repair in early infancy. Am J Surg 161:596–599, 1991. (Review of 384 infants younger than 2 months of age who underwent successful hernia repair.)

Rowe MI, Clatworthy HW: Incarcerated and strangulated hernias in children. Arch Surg 101:136, 1970. (Review of 2764 patients with inguinal hernias.)

Rowe MI, Lloyd DA: Pediatric Surgery, pp 779–793. Chicago, Year Book Medical Publishers, 1986. (Comprehensive review.)

Steward DJ: Preterm infants are more prone to complications following minor surgery than are term infants. Anesthesiology 56:304, 1982. (Excellent discussion of postoperative respiratory problems in infants after hernia repair.)

117

Undescended Testes

Robert P. Foglia

Cryptorchidism, a word derived from the Greek *cryptos* (hidden) and *orchis* (testis), is the general term used to define all forms of undescended testes. This is not an uncommon problem and causes considerable anxiety and concern for parents and patients.

EMBRYOLOGY

The development of the testis in the embryo begins in the abdomen. Testicular descent starts in the seventh fetal month, and over the subsequent weeks the testis progresses through the inguinal canal, out of the external ring, and into the scrotum. This descent is guided by the gubernaculum, a muscular cord that extends between the scrotum and testis.

Testicular descent is influenced by the presence of gonadotropic and androgenic hormones during fetal development. The failure of the testes to descend into the scrotum during fetal life may, in part, be related to either a lack of these hormones or the inability of the testes to respond to them. Despite this, there is no clear evidence to suggest that a cryptorchid testis with mechanical obstruction to its descent will further descend in response to exogenous or endogenous hormones.

DIFFERENTIAL DIAGNOSIS

Several types of undescended testes should be distinguished because pathophysiology and treatment are different.

Anorchia, the complete absence of a testis, can occur on infrequent occasions. It is more common on the right side, and the ipsilateral scrotum is underdeveloped. Because of their common embryologic background, agenesis of the kidney and ureter may occur in association with an absent testis.

The *true undescended testis* has undergone an arrest of its descent along its normal route to the scrotum. Approximately 3% of male term newborns and 20% of premature male infants have undescended testes at birth. By 1 year of age, over 80% of all cryptorchid tests at birth are in the scrotum. Of those testes not in the scrotum at 1 year of age, approximately one third are merely retractile so that a true undescended testis occurs in approximately 0.4% of males. About 14% of boys with cryptorchidism come from families with members who have had this condition. Approximately 65% of children with an undescended testis will have a hernia sac associated with the testis and cord structures.

A retractile testis is a physiologic variation of normal and is the result of an overactive cremasteric muscular reflex and incomplete attachment of the testis to the scrotum by the gubernaculum. This results in the testis being held in a higher position during periods of muscular stimulation such as with activity or in a cold environment. The retractile testis is often bilateral. As the child gets older, the testis becomes larger and the cremasteric reflex becomes less active so that the previously retractile testis remains in the scrotum.

The examination of the child with a suspected undescended testis is begun by first ensuring that the room is warm and that the examiner's hands are not cold. The scrotum should be inspected because with a cryptorchid testis the scrotum is usually not fully developed on the affected side. When the child is relaxed and in a supine position, the examiner's hand is then swept from the anterior-superior iliac spine over the inguinal canal and toward the pubis in an attempt to palpate a testis. This procedure should be done several times; and, if unsuccessful, it should also be done with the child in a cross-legged, squatting, and standing position. Eighty-five percent of testes not in the scrotum will be located in this manner. The position, consistency, and size of the testis should be noted both in comparison to the contralateral testis and to the testes of boys of similar age.

If the testis is not in the scrotum, several possibilities exist. It may be truly undescended, having suffered an arrest to its descent. The true undescended testis may be in the inguinal canal or may be in an intra-abdominal location (and not palpable). Most undescended testes are caused by a mechanical factor, a hernia sac, or a shortened spermatic artery not allowing the testis to descend into the scrotum. Alternatively, the testis may be in an ectopic position having descended through the inguinal canal, passed through the external ring, but then having come to rest in a position in the superficial inguinal space, thigh, or perineum. Another possibility is that it is a retractile testis. If a testis can be palpated in the inguinal canal or in a position over the pubis and with manipulation can be brought down into the scrotum, then this, by definition, is a retractile testis. It is important to distinguish a retractile testis from an undescended testis because the former will function normally, will descend as the cremasteric reflex lessens, and does not require operative treatment.

The undescended testis may have become arrested in its descent, may have undergone an in utero torsion, or may be a dysgenetic testis. A careful examination of the testis at the time of operation is essential because the markedly atrophic testis should be excised; likewise, a testis that appears abnormal should be biopsied.

It is a common misconception that an undescended testis will spontaneously descend during or after puberty. This is probably due to observation of this phenomenon in patients with retractile testes. There is no evidence to suggest that pubescent changes, either hormonal or growth related, will cause the migration of a true undescended testis into the scrotum.

COMPLICATIONS OF CRYPTORCHIDISM

Spermatogenesis

Failure of the testis to descend into the scrotum leaves it subject to a body temperature of 1.5°C to 2.5°C higher than that of the scrotum. This may severely retard the normal maturation of the gonad. Testicular growth begins at birth and proceeds continuously. Studies of testicular biopsy specimens show that cryptorchid testes have a normal morphology and germ cell content during the first 2 years of life. However, after this time, there is a significant decrease in germ cell content and tubular growth, progressive degenerative changes, and significant dysmorphic features developing in the undescended testis of the 2- to 5-year old. Furthermore, it has been suggested that autoantibodies may be produced by the cryptorchid testis that may cause degenerative changes in the opposite normally descended testis. Thus, an untreated undescended testis may result in the inability of one or both gonads to produce normal mature sperm.

Malignancy

There is abundant literature concerning the relationship of cryptorchidism and testicular malignancy. Three to 12% of testicular tumors develop in a cryptorchid testis. This indicates that the chance of developing a testicular malignancy is approximately 40 times higher in an undescended testis than in a normal testis. The chance of malignancy occurring is almost five times higher in an intra-abdominal testis when compared with an inguinal testis. Most testicular tumors are of germ cell origin, thus raising the question of the relationship between dysgenesis in the cryptorchid testis and its possible differentiation into a testicular malignancy. Several studies have also shown an increased incidence of malignant degeneration of the contralateral normally positioned scrotal testis. This may be due to dysgenetic features or may be secondary to hormonal influences by the cryptorchid testis.

The length of time a testis is subjected to an abnormal environment appears to influence its potential for malignancy. The most common age at which a testicular tumor is diagnosed is at 25 to 30 years, and this is why pediatricians rarely see or hear of a testicular tumor developing in one of their patients who has an undescended testis. The age of the child at the time of operation appears to be important. In one review, the authors found that of all patients who subsequently developed a testicular malignancy after an orchidopexy, only 3% of these children were younger than 10 years of age at the time of orchidopexy.

If the degree of degenerative change is related to the incidence of malignancy, then it would follow that orchidopexy should be performed sooner rather than later. The undescended testis is also significantly more difficult to examine and monitor for the development of abnormalities.

Other complications of undescended testes include the greater vulnerability to trauma, hernia, the higher incidence of gonadal loss resulting from a torsion, and, finally, the anxiety and embarrassment expressed by both patients and parents, especially over the possibility of sterility. Therefore, a recommendation for treating the undescended testis should be made for the child who has this condition and who is older than 1 year of age.

TREATMENT

The goal of treatment is to bring the testis into a low scrotal position. Two methods have been used: hormonal and operative.

Hormonal Method

During embryologic development, testicular descent appears to be strongly influenced by the hypothalamic-pituitary axis. Because of this, both human chorionic gonadotropic (hCG) and gonadotropin releasing hormone (GnRH) have been used to treat cryptorchidism. The parenteral use of hCG has been associated with a 15% to 40% rate of successful testicular descent, and the use of GnRH has been associated with a success rate of 50% to 80%. Much conjecture has centered on the efficacy of hormonal therapy because many of the studies have not been well controlled. This is especially true in regard to defining whether the patient had a retractile testis or an undescended testis. One double-blind study resulted in a 19% testicular descent rate with GnRH and only a 6% success rate with hCG. This study carefully excluded boys with retractile testes, which was probably a major factor in the results. When patients with a retractile testis are excluded, most cases of undescended testes are limited by mechanical factors, such as a hernia or a shortened spermatic artery; thus, the rationale for hormonal therapy is not convincing. In selected cases, however, such as when a testis is not palpable, hormonal therapy can be helpful. It causes an enlargement of the testis and may cause partial testicular descent. Both of these effects can make the subsequent orchidopexy easier.

Operative Method

Orchidopexy consists of the translocation of the testis from its anomalous position to a normal position in the scrotum by means of correcting the mechanical factors limiting its descent. The procedure is usually on an outpatient basis and is performed through an inguinal incision. It is accomplished by freeing the spermatic vessels and cord from the frequently present hernia sac. Often, this allows sufficient length on the cord structures to bring the testis into the scrotum. If further length is needed, opening the floor of the inguinal canal and changing the course of the cord structures medially through the floor of the inguinal canal achieves sufficient length to bring the testis into the scrotum without tension on the vessels. In some patients, especially those with the testis high in the inguinal canal, the spermatic vessels must be mobilized in the retroperitoneum through the inguinal incision to gain the appropriate length to bring the testis into the scrotum in a tension-free manner. A small pocket is then made in a dependent position in the scrotum between the skin and dartos layer (a *dartos pouch*) to hold the testis in place.

At exploration, if the testis appears normal and is not intra-abdominal, it can usually be brought down into the scrotum without difficulty. The identification of a markedly atrophic or abnormal testis suggests that the testis had undergone an in utero torsion or that it is dysgenetic. In this circumstance, the removal of the testis should be done because the risk of a subsequent malignant degeneration in that testis is higher than the probability of normal spermatogenesis and testosterone production from the testis.

If no testis is identified, and there are no spermatic vessels and vas deferens present, a retroperitoneal exploration is necessary to exclude the possibility of an intra-abdominal testis. The use of laparoscopy may be a helpful adjunct to the evaluation of these patients. It has also been suggested that because of the high risk of malignancy in an untreated cryptorchid testis, an orchiectomy should be performed for an intra-abdominal testis in postpubertal boys.

Orchidopexy can be carried out at any age, but it appears that elective repair after 1 year of age is most sensible. Almost all boys with an undescended testis at birth will undergo spontaneous descent, if it is to occur, before their first birthday. Histologic evidence shows dysmorphic features in cryptorchid testes after the age of 2 to 3 years. As noted previously, there appears to be some relationship between the length of time the testis was in an abnormal position and the subsequent development of a testicular malignancy, even after orchidopexy. The success rate after orchidopexy is measured longitudinally by the rate of fertility in these patients, and it is 80% to 90%.

COMPLICATIONS

When performed by experienced surgeons, orchidopexy has a low rate of complications. Most complications are related to injury to the delicate blood supply to the testis or vas deferens, either by torsion or by undue tension during the procedure. A testis placed in the scrotum will infrequently retract back into the inguinal canal. Since the floor of the inguinal canal is reconstructed following the mobilization of the cord structures, there is a potential for the development of a direct inguinal hernia, but this is an unusual occurrence.

ANNOTATED BIBLIOGRAPHY

Cendron M, Keating MA, Huff DS et al: Cryptorchidism, orchiopexy and infertility: A critical long-term retrospective analysis. J Urol 142:559–562, 1989. (Report of a long-term follow-up of patients who underwent orchidopexy between 1950 and 1960 showing an 87% incidence of fertility after correction of a unilateral undescended testis and 33% in patients with a history of bilateral undescended testis.)

Fonkalsrud EW: The undescended testis. In Welch JK, Randolph JG, Ravitch MM et al (eds): Pediatric Surgery, 4th ed. Chicago, Year Book Medical Publishers, 1986. (Excellent overview and reference.)

Hadziselimovic F: Treatment of cryptorchidism with GnRH. Urol Clin North Am 9:413, 1982. (Written by one of the experts on the subject of hormonal therapy for undescended testes.)

Martin DC: Malignancy and the undescended testis. In Fonkalsrud EW, Mengel W (eds): The Undescended Testis, pp 144–156. Chicago, Year Book Medical Publishers, 1981. (Good review of the incidence of malignancy in this group of patients.)

Mengel W, Hienz HA, Sippe WG: Studies on cryptorchidism: A comparison of histologic findings in the germinal epithelium before and after the second year of life. J Pediatr Surg 9:445, 1974. (Report of dysmorphic features occurring in an undescended testis in early childhood.)

Rajfer J, Handelsman DJ, Swerdloff RS et al: Hormonal therapy of cryptorchidism: A randomized double-blind study comparing human chorionic gonadotropin and gonadotropin-releasing hormone. N Engl J Med 314:466–470, 1986. (Results of a study that carefully excluded boys with retractile testes and found a relatively low success rate with hormonal therapy.)

118

Genital Pain

Daniel P. Ryan and
Daniel P. Doody

The most common genital problems encountered in children are discussed in this chapter. Sexual abuse is a related problem and is discussed separately in Chapter 20. Although the differences between boys and girls are obvious there are often similarities in many of these processes. The chief complaint of pain or a problem "down there" is common, encompassing the region from the lower abdomen to the inguinal areas and the genitalia. The clinician must also be aware that referred pain originating in the retroperitoneum, from the genitourinary tract, or from within the abdomen may be the actual source of the pain in the inguinal or genital area. Conversely, when vague abdominal pain is the primary complaint, the origin of the pain may be from the inguinal or genital areas.

PENILE PAIN

The primary complaint of penile pain by a young boy raises a wide spectrum of possible etiologies. These range from urinary tract infection to underlying psychologic problems to sexual abuse. Although the clinician needs to consider the differential diagnosis, problems can often be identified with a good history and physical examination. Many complaints arise from the foreskin in uncircumcised males that are not present in those who are circumcised. Phimosis, paraphimosis, penile foreskin adhesions, and balanitis are common sources of complaints (see also Chap. 9).

An apparent *phimosis* is universally present in the newborn with narrowing of the preputial opening. However, it nearly always resolves by 5 years of age. Some children, who have suffered some inflammation or infection resulting in scarring of the foreskin, will develop a true phimosis in which the foreskin cannot be retracted over the glans. This phimosis can be the primary cause of many problems involving the foreskin, including the potentially dangerous condition of paraphimosis. In *paraphimosis,* the tight constricting ring of the phimosis is pulled past the coronal sulcus of the glans penis. This encircling band leads to lymphatic obstruction, worsening swelling, and eventually venous obstruction with potential tissue loss.

Many children who present with this difficulty are in their early teenage years and are quite uncomfortable by the time they seek medical advice. Since the etiology of paraphimosis is the forceful retraction of the prepuce, it is often associated with masturbation or sexual abuse, and the child is reluctant to bring the problem to parenteral or medical attention early in its course. In a late presentation, usually the glans and the foreskin are impressively swollen. If manual reduction is not possible in the office or emergency department, a surgical release of the constricting band by a dorsal slit in the foreskin under local anesthesia is the most rapid way to resolve the acute problem. Circumcision is the definitive treatment but is often not advised in the acute situation until the edema resolves.

Balanitis (infection of the foreskin) and *balanoposthitis* (infection of the foreskin and the glans penis) are other problems often seen in children with phimosis. The infection is usually attributed to poor local hygiene since the area under the foreskin cannot be well-cleaned. The causative bacteria are most often skin flora but occasionally are due to gram-negative organisms. Warm soaks in the bathtub along with a course of oral antibiotics will usually resolve the problem. Not all episodes of balanitis are associated with phimosis, so observation and instruction for good local hygiene are recommended. If a phimosis becomes apparent over the ensuing 6 months, circumcision is indicated.

Penile foreskin adhesions are usually asymptomatic and present difficulties only with the development of balanitis or, rarely, with painful erections in older children. Soft adhesions between the glans and the foreskin are normal in the small child, and these attachments often release spontaneously with time. Good local hygiene is provided by gently retracting the foreskin and cleaning the area. Occasionally, thickened adhesions develop if the foreskin is prematurely and forcibly retracted. Separating the adhesions without a circumcision is usually an inadequate treatment option. To prevent adhesions from reforming following forcible retraction, the glans and prepuce must be cleaned and lubricated shortly after the retraction. However, the child is usually too tender for most parents to do an adequate job. A circumcision is often required for definitive treatment and should be recommended.

Urethral meatal stenosis is an infrequent problem in the circumcised male. It is presumed that the toxic contents of the diaper contribute to meatal stenosis because this problem is rarely seen in uncircumcised boys. The suspected etiology is an inflammatory reaction or superficial infection related to diaper rashes that causes scarring at the urethral meatus. These children may present with dysuria, straining, and painful urination. Most often the parents are alerted to the problem when they notice how long it takes these children to empty their bladders. The treatment of meatal stenosis is either dilatation or a formal meatoplasty performed under anesthesia. Unless a urinary tract infection has been documented, radiologic investigations are not necessary.

Trauma to the penis is an uncommon problem, but lacerations from zippers and direct trauma from accidents must be evaluated gently and carefully. The history is sometimes vague and may raise suspicion of physical or sexual abuse. Lacerations of the penis from local trauma can be treated as any other open wound. However, because of the sensitive nature of the area, these injuries often require general anesthesia for repair.

An unusual but distressing problem is *priapism*. In this condition, the penis becomes uncontrollably engorged for a prolonged period of time because of defective venous drainage of the corpora. It may be idiopathic, but it is most commonly associated with sickle cell disease in adolescents, often as a form of sickle crisis. Priapism can also be caused by leukemia, trauma, tumors, or encircling foreign bodies. Treatment is surgical for the idiopathic condition but supportive if an underlying cause is identified. If the pain is persistent, urologic evaluation is urgently indicated because delay in treatment may result in loss of erectile function.

Foreign bodies of the urethra are unusual but do occur in children. They do not necessarily indicate that these children have been abused because the foreign bodies are most often placed by the child. It is usually an older child who presents with these problems, and occasionally this may be a manifestation of underlying psychological difficulties.

Finally, penile pain can be referred from a primary source in either the bladder or the prostate. *Prostatitis* is uncommon in children unless there is an associated malformation of the urinary tract.

THE ACUTE SCROTUM

Scrotal and testicular pain are common complaints in children presenting for urgent evaluation. The diagnostic problem presented by the acute scrotum is one that continues to confound clinicians. Unfortunately, in many of these patients, there is no perfect test other than scrotal exploration to be absolutely certain about the diagnosis. A good history and physical examination, however, will reveal the source of pathology in a large percentage of cases. Judicious use of Doppler ultrasound and testicular scanning can be useful in certain cases, although "normal" results do not always rule out the diagnosis of testicular torsion. Many of these children are evaluated in the emergency department and do not require hospitalization. The major diagnostic categories include hernias, hydroceles, hemorrhage into a testicular tumor, trauma, epididymitis or orchitis, testicular torsion, or torsion of a testicular remnant.

Acute scrotal or testicular pain and swelling are the presenting complaints in the conditions mentioned earlier. Acute expansion of a hydrocele often brings a patient to medical attention. Neonatal hydroceles represent fluid that has been trapped in the processus vaginalis as the connection with the abdomen has closed, and observation will allow the vast majority of these lesions to resolve without surgery by 1 year of age. The presence of an associated inguinal hernia or the ability to express the fluid out of the hydrocele into the abdomen with manual compression (communicating hydrocele) indicates surgical repair is needed. In an otherwise healthy, older child, trauma, infection, inflammation, and tumor growth can lead to the development of a hydrocele, although most frequently the etiology of these hydroceles is idiopathic. In the absence of pain or tenderness, elective surgery for the hydrocele is indicated to rule out a concomitant hernia.

The distinction between a hydrocele and a scrotal extension of an inguinal hernia should be made on physical examination. Palpation of a normal spermatic cord above the area of swelling is reassuring that a hernia has not come through the internal inguinal ring. If the cord is thickened, a rectal examination with palpation of the internal inguinal ring will often give the correct diagnosis. Incarcerated inguinal hernias, even without symptoms of bowel obstruction, can lead to compromise of the spermatic vessels with subsequent testicular atrophy in up to 15% of cases. Thus, if this diagnosis is suspected, urgent surgical exploration is indicated. Transillumination can be misleading, particularly in an infant, as a fluid-filled loop of intestine may appear the same as a hydrocele on examination. (See Chap. 116 for a more complete discussion on groin hernias and hydroceles.)

Acute torsion of the testis can occur at any age, but the peak incidence is at 14 years. Two thirds of patients are adolescents, but another cluster occurs in the newborn period. The complaint of testicular pain must always be taken seriously if loss of the testis is to be averted. Patients operated on within 6 hours of the onset of symptoms have a 90% testicular salvage rate. Very few testes will survive when torsion has lasted longer than 24 hours. Unfortunately, the onset of symptoms and their progression over time are not specific and a large degree of clinical overlap is found with testicular torsion, torsion of an appendix testis, and the inflammatory conditions of epididymitis and orchitis.

Torsion of the testis occurs when the normal fixation of the testis is absent or abnormal. Normally the epididymis is fixed posteriorly by the mesorchium and is in close approximation to the testis. The tunica vaginalis incompletely surrounds the testis; and if the mesorchium is absent, as in the "bell clapper" deformity, torsion may occur within the tunica (intravaginal torsion). Adolescent torsion of the testis is almost always associated with the bell clapper deformity, and there is a 70% chance the contralateral testis has the same anatomic defect. The cremasteric muscle has been implicated in a causal role because testicular torsion is often associated with sporting events or occurs shortly after awakening from sleep. When the testis undergoes torsion, the lymphatic drainage and the venous outflow are initially occluded. With progressive swelling or further twisting, the arterial inflow is lost and the tissue will undergo ischemic necrosis. In neonatal torsion or torsion of an undescended testis, the testis is poorly fixed within the scrotum and the entire cord and tunica vaginalis may twist, the so-called "extravaginal torsion."

Pain in the testis is the presenting symptom in 80% of patients. The pain usually starts acutely but gradually and progressively worsens over a few hours. Nearly 20% of the patients can relate a history of minor trauma, and one third have had prior episodes of similar but transient pain that may indicate intermittent torsion. The severity of pain is variable and may not be related to the degree or duration of the torsion. Swelling of the scrotum gradually develops and is followed by erythema and warmth. In many cases, associated symptoms include nausea, vomiting, or a poorly defined visceral pain.

Physical examination of children with torsion of the testis is usually diagnostic. These children look ill and anxious while moving little. The ipsilateral scrotum is often edematous, erythematous, and warm. The entire testis is enlarged, usually elevated, and in a "transverse lie." The testis is exquisitely painful, and the spermatic cord above the testis is also thickened and usually tender. Doppler ultrasound examination in the emergency department or office can be helpful if one can find the testicular artery within the spermatic cord, follow it down to the testis, and identify an abrupt loss of flow. The ultrasound examination can be misleading in inexperienced hands since the surrounding inflammation may falsely signal flow. Even with an experienced observer, the estimated accuracy of the Doppler examination is only 70%.

The clinical diagnosis of testicular torsion is often not obvious. If any doubt exists, scrotal exploration is indicated. Delay in surgery will only increase the risk of loss of the testis. The role of nuclear medicine scans is to reassure the clinician that torsion does *not* exist in patients who are suspected of having other scrotal problems, and these tests should not be used to confirm a suspected testicular torsion.

The *appendix testis* and *appendix epididymis* are vestigial tissues ranging in size from 1 to 6 mm across, often with a pedunculated attachment to the testis or epididymis. This small stalk is the anatomic etiology for torsion and subsequent infarction of the appendage. Torsion of an appendix testis may present as exactly the same complaints as torsion of the entire testis. Close questioning usually shows that the symptoms have gradually developed over the course of a few days rather than a few hours. Boys with torsion of an appendix testis tend to be embarrassed, active, and alert, compared with those with torsion of the entire testis. Associated gastrointestinal symptoms are usually absent. Erythema and edema of the scrotum are less marked, and the tenderness can usually be localized to the area of the appendix testis or epididymis, while the main body of the testis remains nontender. The physical finding of the "blue dot" sign is confirmatory and diagnostic. If a blood flow scan is obtained, it will show normal or increased flow to the symptomatic testis, indicating surrounding inflammation.

Surgery is not always indicated if the diagnosis is torsion of the appendix testis. The natural history of the infarcted appendage is for it to undergo necrosis with resolution of the symptoms in 2 to 5 days. Symptomatic treatment with nonsteroidal anti-inflammatory medications may provide relief. In cases in which the diagnosis is in doubt or if pain is persistent and severe, surgical exploration and excision of the infarcted tissue will result in both prompt relief of symptoms and confirmation of the diagnosis.

Inflammatory conditions within the scrotum also present with testicular pain and swelling similar to that of torsion. True bacterial orchitis is rare, and these boys often look toxic and have a high fever in association with their primary complaint of testicular pain and swelling. *Orchitis* associated with viral parotitis (mumps) is the most common cause. The onset of pain is sudden and often difficult to distinguish from torsion. The entire testis is swollen and tender while the overlying scrotum is warm, erythematous, and tender, often with associated painful inguinal lymphadenopathy. Microhematuria may be present with mumps orchitis. The testicular blood flow scan will show increased

flow to the affected side. If an abscess is present within the testis, a central nonperfused area may be seen.

Epididymitis is a common diagnosis in older patients who present with scrotal pain. In the sexually active boy, the diagnosis is often evident on physical examination. Tenderness of the epididymis and along the vas deferens without specific swelling or tenderness of the testis is often present. Specific questioning regarding symptoms of urethritis and sexual activity and rectal examination to detect prostatitis are indicated. Treatment should consist of antibiotics to cover sexually transmitted diseases after cultures are obtained and counseling the patient regarding identification of partners at risk. (See also Chap. 200 for a complete discussion of sexually transmitted diseases.)

Unfortunately, many children are diagnosed as having "epididymitis" who do not have clear symptoms and findings. Boys who complain of pain in the testis and have associated tenderness of the epididymis without sexual contact or history with physical findings of torsion of the appendix testis fall into the category of "epididymitis." Usually the urinalysis is normal and a testicular blood flow scan is normal. With the lack of a specific diagnosis, inflammation of the epididymis is diagnosed. Many of these children have a single episode that does not recur, but a few will have an abnormality of the urinary tract and may return with pyelonephritis at a later date. If true epididymitis is suspected in a young patient, a voiding cystourethrogram is indicated.

Testicular tumors may present as sudden swelling and pain. The child may have noticed a gradual enlargement of the testis over the preceding weeks and then the appearance of acute symptoms, often associated with minor trauma. Hemorrhage into a small nonpalpable tumor may lead to these symptoms. A reactive hydrocele may be present. Often there is little, if any, associated inflammation or pain unless intraparenchymal hemorrhage has occurred. Testicular ultrasound is very helpful in making the diagnosis.

Direct trauma to the testis can cause severe symptoms. The testis is usually mobile enough to avoid being crushed, but the testis can be caught against the pubis and rupture. In the case of ruptured testis, the scrotum is massively swollen and ecchymotic. The testis is very tender, and its borders are often indistinct on palpation. Ultrasound examination can identify fractures of the testis, and exploration is indicated to repair the testis and evacuate the hematoma. If a testicular fracture is not found, symptomatic treatment with scrotal support, warm sitz baths, and analgesics is indicated. With massive pelvic and scrotal trauma, an associated rupture of the bladder or urethra should be evaluated with a retrograde urethrogram and cystogram.

GENITAL PAIN IN FEMALES

Complaints from young girls about genital pain are much less common than in boys. The most likely cause is an inguinal hernia, which may present as a bulge primarily within the labia. Hydroceles along the canal of Nuck can also present acutely and need to be differentiated from an incarcerated inguinal hernia. Incarceration of the ovary must be treated urgently because vascular compromise and torsion have been reported. Inguinal hernias in girls occur at one tenth the incidence seen in boys (see also Chap. 116). Careful physical examination will often reveal the rare patient with *testicular feminization syndrome* presenting as a hernia or a palpable gonad in the inguinal canal.

Foreign bodies of the vagina are a common source of problems in school-age girls, usually resulting in symptoms of vaginal discharge and itching. Unfortunately, sexually transmitted diseases now occur in nearly all age groups, and appropriate cultures and evaluations are necessary. Tumors of the genitourinary tract can present as the same symptoms and, following appropriate radiologic imaging studies, examination under anesthesia may be necessary to fully evalu-

ate the problem. Imperforate hymen may present as cyclic abdominal pain and primary amenorrhea in an older child who is otherwise developing normally.

ANNOTATED BIBLIOGRAPHY

Knight PJ, Vassy LE: The diagnosis and treatment of the acute scrotum in children and adolescents. Ann Surg 200:664, 1984. (Excellent review of complaints presenting as acute scrotal pain in children, their diagnosis, and treatment.)

Leape LL: Torsion of the testis. In Welch KJ, Randolph JG, Ravitch MM et al (eds): Pediatric Surgery, 4th ed, vol 2, pp 1330–1335. Chicago, Year Book Medical Publishers, 1986. (Concise discussion of torsion of the testis, appendix testis, and epididymitis.)

Sacknoff EJ, Dretler SP: Urologic emergencies. In Wilkins EW Jr. (ed): MGH Textbook of Emergency Medicine, pp 446–472. Baltimore, Williams & Wilkins, 1978. (Classic chapter dealing with adult urologic problems that often overlap with adolescent urologic problems.)

16

GYNECOLOGIC PROBLEMS

119

Vulvovaginitis

Deborah E. Smith and
Jacob A. Lohr

Complaints of vulvar itching, soreness, or vaginal discharge are common throughout childhood and adolescence. Etiology, possible diagnoses, and appropriate management depend somewhat on the age of the patient. In younger girls, a knowledge of the anatomy of prepubertal genitalia and a consideration of daily living habits are as important as an understanding of vaginal microbiology. Infections do occur in this age group, but they predominate in adolescents, particularly after the onset of sexual activity. A more detailed discussion of the common sexually transmitted causes of vulvovaginitis is found in Chap. 200, and pelvic inflammatory diseases are discussed in Chap. 121.

PREPUBERTAL VULVOVAGINITIS

Pathophysiology

A *physiologic leukorrhea* is common in the female newborn. This is a mucous vaginal discharge that may be tinged with blood. It is caused by intrauterine maternal estrogen stimulation of the vaginal mucosa and a withdrawal at delivery. The leukorrhea gradually resolves within 2 to 3 weeks.

The prepubertal child is particularly susceptible to vulvovaginitis, and indeed this occurs in almost all girls at some stage. Without estrogen stimulation, the vaginal mucosa is thin, shiny, red, and atrophic. Vaginal secretions, which are minimal, have a neutral *p*H. The vagina is relatively close to the anus, and the preadolescent vulva lacks the protection of thick labia and pubic hair. In addition,

once the child is out of diapers, toileting is less closely supervised and wiping techniques are usually suboptimal. Thus, contamination of the vagina with bowel flora can be expected, with or without symptoms of vulvovaginitis. Normal prepubertal vaginal flora include diphtheroids, *Staphylococcus epidermidis*, α-hemolytic streptococci, and lactobacilli. *Escherichia coli* is frequently present and in one series was isolated from the vaginal secretions of 90% of girls younger than 3 years of age. It is less common with increasing age.

Clinical Presentation and Differential Diagnosis

Typical complaints include vulvar redness with discomfort such as itching, burning, or a discharge. The presentation is often late, and chronic excoriation may lead to superinfection.

Vulvar inflammation is frequently caused by suboptimal hygiene and by chronic abrasion from masturbation, contact with play equipment, or sitting in sand boxes. A chemical irritation may arise from the use of harsh soaps or bubble baths. The equivalent of diaper dermatitis can be associated with the wearing of tight-fitting nylon underpants, tights, jeans, or leotards, particularly in hot weather and in overweight girls. Nonspecific vulvovaginitis is also associated with pinworm infestation causing perianal pruritus; scratching leads to perineal excoriation and secondary vulvitis. An adult pinworm may occasionally migrate to the vagina, giving rise to a discharge. A vaginal discharge with or without vulvitis can also be caused by a foreign body.

Specific infections are associated with vulvovaginitis in the prepubertal child. In this age group, infection with *Neisseria gonorrhoeae* or with *Chlamydia trachomatis* presents as a vulvovaginitis rather than a cervicitis. When gonorrhea is diagnosed by culture, this is considered as specific evidence of child sexual abuse. The same is true for a diagnosis of vaginal chlamydia infection in the child who is older than 3 years old; perinatal transmission is a possible etiology in

462

infants and toddlers. Vulvovaginitis can also be caused by trichomonas infection and genital warts (condyloma acuminata). Again, child sexual abuse is a likely etiology; however, nonsexual contact is also possible. Other specific infections include group A *β-hemolytic streptococcus* and yeast (*Candida albicans*).

Upper respiratory tract infections and systemic diseases such as chickenpox, scarlet fever, and measles can cause a vaginitis. Vulvovaginitis may also be related to an ectopic ureter, a pelvic abscess, or a fistula. Finally, some skin conditions including atopic dermatitis, seborrhea, or psoriasis may have an associated vulvitis.

Work-Up

History. Details of the presenting symptoms must be noted, including the chronicity and a description of any discharge (e.g., quantity, color, or odor). A malodorous discharge is typically associated with a vaginal foreign body such as retained toilet tissue, or, much more rarely, with a *Shigella* vaginitis or a necrotic tumor. Blood-stained discharge is also typical of a vaginal foreign body; other possible causes include trauma from play (e.g., bike riding or playground equipment), sexual abuse, vulvar irritation secondary to pruritus or masturbation or, rarely, a tumor. A copious, purulent discharge or a thin mucoid discharge is caused by streptococcal infections, and a greenish discharge is more typical of trichomoniasis, gonorrhea, chlamydia, or a foreign body. The child should be asked to demonstrate her toileting technique for wiping. A review of systems is useful, noting any history of recent illnesses such as otitis media or streptococcal pharyngitis in the child or mother or use of antibiotics predisposing to a yeast infection. The physician must also consider asking directly about the possibility of sexual abuse or potential contact with infected adults.

Physical Examination. The physical examination starts with the general observation of the child and her clothing. A full examination is needed with particular attention to a genital inspection. This can be done with the child supine in the frogleg position. She may assist with spreading apart her labia. A knee-to-chest position also allows an excellent view of the vagina and frequently the cervix, which is particularly useful when a foreign body is suspected. To assume the knee-to-chest position, the child is instructed to kneel and then lie forward onto her chest and folded arms, keeping her bottom up. An otoscope may be used for vaginoscopy. A rectal examination may be used to palpate a foreign body and to check for normal pelvic anatomy.

Laboratory Tests. Tests are indicated when a vaginal discharge is present, and particularly if it is persistent. Since urethral colonization may occur, a urinalysis should be done to look for white blood cells, trichomonads, or yeast. Vaginal secretions are collected using a Dacron- or cotton-tipped applicator moistened with nonbacteriostatic saline or aspirated with a sterile medicine dropper. Wet preparations with

normal saline and with 10% potassium hydroxide may confirm the urine findings, showing white blood cells, trichomonads, or yeast. The presence of yeast is relatively uncommon; if yeast organisms are found, glycosuria should be ruled out. Gram stains of vaginal secretions may be useful; however, the finding of gram-negative intracellular diplococci is only suggestive of *N. gonorrhoeae* infection; of note, normal vaginal flora include nongonococcal neisseria species. Finally, specimens should be sent for culture, including media for gonorrhea and anaerobes. A chlamydia test should be included, ideally a culture. However, the cost may be prohibitive. Of the other chlamydia tests available, the DNA probe is quite sensitive; if positive results are obtained the diagnosis must then be confirmed with a culture. A syphilis test should be done if sexual abuse is suspected, and particularly if there is a diagnosis of *N. gonorrhoeae, C. trachomatis, Trichomonas,* or genital warts. Under these circumstances, tests for human immunodeficiency virus and hepatitis B virus should also be considered. The Scotch tape test for pinworms may be useful; if this is the likely cause, the mother should also check the child's anus at night for adult pinworms.

Treatment

General hygiene measures will improve symptoms and should be encouraged. These include good toileting techniques (wiping gently from front to back), use of white cotton underpants and loose-fitting clothes, and avoidance of bubble baths and other irritants. Sitz baths are useful twice or three times a day in plain warm water for 10 to 15 minutes. The genitalia should be washed with a soft cloth with or without a mild soap and patted dry or air dried if possible.

The majority of cases (up to 85%) will have a nonspecific etiology, with cultures growing gram-negative organisms such as *Escherichia coli* or normal flora. Topical application of a diaper cream once or twice daily may be sufficient to lessen the symptoms and to allow healing. The child may apply the cream to the vulvar area, with parental supervision.

Hydrocortisone cream 1% can be used for one or two treatments. For a persistent vulvovaginitis lasting 3 to 4 weeks, local application of an antibacterial cream at night may be useful (e.g., AVC cream, Vagitrol, Sultrin). An alternative is a broad-spectrum oral antibiotic (ampicillin, 50 mg/kg/d divided into four doses, or a cephalosporin such as cefaclor, 20–40 mg/kg/d divided into two or three doses) for 10 to 14 days. If symptoms continue, an estrogen cream (e.g., Premarin) will thicken the vulvar epithelium, making it more resistant to infection. This cream should be prescribed for local use every night for a maximum of 2 to 3 weeks and then every other night for an additional 2 weeks. Caution is needed because systemic absorption may cause irreversible vulvar hyperpigmentation and also breast tenderness, which is reversible.

Some patients present with an acute severe edematous

vulvitis. Appropriate management includes 15-minute sitz baths every 4 hours. Baking soda or saline may be added to the water, but soap should be avoided. Air drying is preferable. Witch hazel pads (Tucks) rather than toilet paper should be used for wiping. Within 2 to 3 days, symptoms should improve, and baths can then be alternated with the application of calamine lotion. For a more pruritic vulvitis, local applications of 1% hydrocortisone cream may be used.

Specific infections should be treated appropriately in addition to the general measures as listed above. *Enterobius vermicularis* (pinworm) infestations are treated with mebendazole (Vermox), one 100-mg tablet for children of all ages, with repeat therapy 2 weeks later. *Neisseria gonorrhoeae* vaginitis in children weighing less than 4.5 kg is treated with a single intramuscular dose of either ceftriaxone, 125 mg, or spectinomycin, 40 mg/kg. *Chlamydia trachomatis* vaginitis is treated with erythromycin, 30 to 50 mg/kg/d divided into three or four doses per 24 hours, for 10 days. In children older than 9 years old and weighing less than 45 kg, *Chlamydia trachomonas* vaginitis can be treated with tetracycline, 20–50 mg/kg/d divided into four daily doses for 7 days, or with doxycycline, 5 mg/kg/d divided into twice-daily doses. Trichomonas infection is treated with metronidazole (Flagyl), 10 to 30 mg/kg/d up to 250 mg three times a day orally for 5 to 7 days. An alternative is 1 g as a single oral dose. In children weighing more than 45 kg, *N. gonorrhoeae,* chlamydia, and trichomonas infections are treated with adult regimens (see later). Streptococcal vaginitis (group A β-hemolytic streptococcus or *Streptococcus pneumoniae*) is treated with penicillin, 125 to 250 mg orally three or four times a day for 10 days, or with erythromycin, 30 to 50 mg/kg/d divided into three of four doses for 10 days. The maximum dose is 250 mg three times a day. Vulvovaginitis caused by *Candida albicans* can be managed with nystatin cream (or ointment if the lesions are dry) applied locally to the vulva three times a day for 2 weeks. Alternatives are miconazole 2% (Monistat) or clotrimazole 1% (Gyne-Lotrimin, Mycelex) creams. Persistent yeast infections may require treatment with nystatin, 100,000 units/mL, 1 ml orally four times a day, in addition to topical therapy. Various treatment options exist for condylomata acuminata. These include local cryotherapy with liquid nitrogen, topical application of trichloracetic acid (80%–90%), or topical use of podophyllin (10%–25%) in compound tincture of benzoin. After podophyllin application, the genitalia must be washed in 1 to 2 hours. Subsequent symptoms of burning and soreness can be managed with lidocaine 2% jelly or with petroleum jelly. Repeated treatments may be needed at weekly intervals; referral should be considered if the lesions are extensive or difficult to treat. (For a more complete discussion on the treatment of sexually transmitted diseases, see Chap. 200.)

Long-term complications of vulvovaginitis depend on the specific etiology. It is thought that *labial adhesions* may result from chronic vulvar irritation, leading to erosion of the labial epithelium and subsequent adhesions. Labial adhesions frequently occur between the ages of 6 months to 6 years. Mild cases require no treatment; with increasing estrogen levels at puberty, the labia will separate. More extensive adhesions may occlude the vaginal orifice, impairing drainage of secretions and even of urine. Under no circumstances should forceful separation be used. Not only is this traumatic to the child, but there is also a high incidence of recurrence of the adhesions. An estrogen-containing cream such as Premarin should be applied twice a day for 2 weeks, and then nightly for an additional 1 to 2 weeks. The cream should be rubbed into the adhered area while gently separating the labia. Nightly applications of a bland ointment (e.g., K-Y jelly or A and D ointment) should then be continued for several months to prevent the re-formation of the adhesions. This treatment can be extended for 1 year if there is a history of previous treatment failures.

Indications for Referral

Occasionally, when the diagnosis is unclear or the symptoms are resistant to appropriate therapy, a referral should be made. Referral is usually indicated when there is any suggestion of sexual abuse (see Chap. 20).

ADOLESCENT VULVOVAGINITIS

Pathophysiology

The most common cause of discharge in the adolescent age group is a noninfectious *physiologic leukorrhea*. This is a milky-white discharge that represents the shedding of the vaginal cells and endocervical mucus. It may start months before menarche. Once the menstrual cycle is established, the discharge shows cyclic changes, being profuse and watery at mid cycle and stickier and scantier in the second half of the cycle. Leukorrhea is diagnosed by direct inspection. A wet preparation with normal saline will show epithelial cells only. The treatment consists mainly of reassurance and improved general hygiene as described earlier. Occasionally pads may be useful. Tampon use should be restricted to menses only to minimize the risks of developing toxic shock syndrome. Daily tampon use can also be associated with vaginal ulceration.

The pattern of normal flora found in the adolescent vagina depends entirely on whether the adolescent has been sexually active. Before the onset of sexual activity, the normal flora closely resemble that found in the prepubertal child, with the addition of *Gardnerella vaginalis*. Vaginal colonization and infection in the sexually active adolescent show patterns similar to adults, varying somewhat in different groups studied. Organisms can include *N. gonorrhea,* aerobic and anaerobic streptococcus spp, staphylococcus spp, lactobacillus spp, mycoplasma spp, *Ureaplasma urealyticum, C. trachomatis, Trichomonas vaginalis* and candida spp.

Clinical Presentation

Complaints vary and include a vaginal discharge, localized lesions, nonspecific irritation, and the *urethral syndrome* characterized by dysuria, urinary frequency, and pyuria (see Chap. 113). Although these latter findings are characteristic of urinary tract infections, in the sexually active population vulvovaginitis is the first consideration.

Work-Up

History. As with the prepubertal child, a history of the presenting symptoms is needed. These may include dyspareunia and pelvic pain. Symptoms may have been present for many months, since adolescents typically present late because of denial, embarrassment, or even fear of the examination. The physician should inquire about underlying disorders such as diabetes and recent or current medications (e.g., antibiotics or birth control pills) since these agents predispose to candidal vaginitis. It is vital to know if the adolescent is sexually active or if there is a history of assault. Frequently, however, the patient may not be willing to share this information. Multiple infections may coexist, and details of previous treatments or treatment failures are useful.

Physical Examination. In most cases, the physical examination must include a pelvic examination in addition to careful inspection of the genitalia. Single-digit palpation of the vagina is helpful in locating the cervix and in preparing the adolescent for the insertion of the speculum. The Huffman speculum is particularly useful because it has long, slim blades and can be inserted comfortably into most young adolescents. A bimanual examination should complete the physical assessment, noting particularly any areas of tenderness on palpation.

Laboratory Tests. Wet preparations with normal saline and 10% potassium hydroxide are made of any discharge,

looking for the presence of trichomonads, clue cells (suggestive of *Gardnerella vaginalis*), numerous bacteria or yeast hyphae. Gram stains are not useful. A sample should be sent for *N. gonorrhoeae* culture, and a chlamydia test (preferably a culture if available but more usually a fluorescent antibody screening test or a DNA probe test) is mandatory. Syphilis serology is needed, particularly if ulcerations or condylomata are found. A Papanicolaou smear is also necessary in adolescents with condylomata. In a previously undiagnosed case of genital blistering or ulceration, a viral culture should be sent to confirm suspected herpes infection. In all adolescents with diagnosed sexually transmitted diseases, a test for human immunodeficiency virus and a hepatitis screening test should be considered.

Differential Diagnosis and Treatment

Leukorrhea is the main noninfectious cause of vulvovaginal symptoms. The details of the presentation, diagnosis, and management were outlined earlier. The treatment of all vulvovaginal complaints should include good hygiene. Also seen in this age group is a nonspecific bacterial overgrowth causing a copious discharge. This diagnosis is suggested by the wet preparations and by subsequent negative test results. Treatment is with a topical antibiotic cream such as triple sulfa cream or AVC vaginal cream used twice daily for 2 weeks. Other noninfectious causes of vulvovaginal symptoms should be considered. An allergic reaction may be associated with perfumed soaps and douches, or with contraceptive creams. Skin disorders such as atopic or seborrheic dermatitis or psoriasis may involve the vulvar region. The treatment is similar to that for lesions elsewhere on the skin. Psychosomatic vulvovaginitis has also been described.

More common are certain specific infectious etiologies: these are listed with appropriate therapy in Table 119-1. More extensive discussions of treatment are found in Chap- *(Text continues on p. 467)*

Table 119-1. Vulvovaginitis in Adolescents

CLINICAL PREPARATION	CAUSE	SOURCE	DIAGNOSIS	TREATMENT
Milky discharge	Leukorrhea	Physiologic	History; saline wet preparation: epithelial cells	Reassurance, general hygiene
Profuse nonspecific yellow discharge	Bacterial overgrowth	Antibiotic use; poor hygiene; contamination with bowel flora after anal intercourse	History; saline wet preparation: multiple bacteria, white blood cell	Triple sulfa cream or AVC cream bid × 2 weeks. Hygiene
Foul-smelling discharge: bloody or purulent	Foreign body (usually retained tampon)		History and pelvic with speculum examination	Remove cause; irrigate vagina with warm water; general hygiene
Urethral syndrome; mucopurulent discharge	*Chlamydia trachomatis*	Sexual contact	Culture, fluorescent antibody screen, DNA probe	Doxycycline, 100 mg PO bid × 7 days; erythromycin 50 mg, PO qid × 7 days; treat contacts

(continued)

Table 119-1.   Vulvovaginitis in Adolescents (*continued*)

CLINICAL PREPARATION	CAUSE	SOURCE	DIAGNOSIS	TREATMENT
Mucopurulent discharge	*Neisseria gonorrhoeae*	Sexual contact	Culture	Ceftriaxone, 250 mg, IM once, *or* spectinomycin, 2 g, IM single dose *and* doxycycline, 100 mg, PO bid × 7 days
White "cottage cheese" discharge; pruritus; dysuria	*Candida albicans*	Not usually sexually transmitted Predisposing factors: diabetes mellitus, birth control pills, antibiotic use, corticosteroids, pregnancy, obesity, tight clothing	Potassium hydroxide preparation: budding pseudohyphae	Miconazole vaginal cream q hs × 7 nights *or* clotrimazole, 200-mg tablet per vaginum qhs × 3 nights
Yellow-green frothy discharge; vulvitis; ectropion; strawberry cervix	*Trichomonas vaginalis*	Usually sexual contact	Saline wet preparation: dancing flagellated organisms	Metronidazole (Flagyl), 1.5–2 g, PO single dose *or* metronidazole, 250 mg, PO tid × 7 days; for persistent infections, rule out reinfection; treat contacts; *note:* Flagyl has Antabuse effect
Profuse gray-white discharge; strong fishlike odor	*Gardnerella vaginalis*	Normal flora *or* sexual contact?	Vaginal pH > 4.5; saline wet prep: clue cells (i.e., large epithelial cells coated with refractile bacteria)	Metronidazole, 500 mg, PO bid × 7 days; treat contacts if recurrent symptoms
Pruritis, dysuria, dyspareunia	Genital warts; human papilloma virus	Direct contact, usually sexual	Inspection; rule out secondary syphilis with serology; Papanicolaou smear	Treat any coexisting vaginitis; cryotherapy with liquid nitrogen; trichloroacetic acid 80%–90% applied directly and repeated weekly as needed; podophyllin 10%–25% in tincture of benzoin applied directly, washed off 2–4 hours later, and repeated weekly as needed; treatment may cause burning that can be relieved with sitz baths or topical anesthetic jelly; cautery with laser therapy
Pain, pruritus, dysuria, urethral or vaginal discharge; vesicles; dyspareunia; systemic symptoms	Genital herpes simplex	Sexual transmission	Inspection; viral culture; Wright's stain of scraped lesion base: multinucleated giant cells with inclusions	Symptomatic relief: sitz baths, topical anesthetic gel; for initial infection, acyclovir, 200 mg, 5 times a day × 7–10 days may be used. This does not prevent recurrences. This drug is not recommended during pregnancy
Pruritis, crabs, nits (eggs on pubic hair)	Pediculosis pubis	Physical contact not necessarily sexual; infested clothing	Inspection	1% lindane (Kwell) shampoo single application: thorough washing of clothing; repeat in 1 week if needed
Bumps, vulvar papules	Folliculitis, *Staphylococcus aureus* or *Streptococcus pyogenes*		Inspection	Warm sitz baths bid–tid; topical antibacterial cream; oral antibiotics for extensive acute infection (e.g., erythromycin, cephalexin)

ter 200. It should be noted that while some infections only cause a localized disease, others have significant long-term sequelae. *N. gonorrhoeae* and *C. trachomatis* infections are associated with chronic abdominal pain, pelvic inflammatory disease, and infertility. Herpes genitalis is almost always recurrent, and symptoms can be debilitating; in some patients, it causes a serious psychosexual disturbance. Condylomata acuminata are caused by human papillomavirus; some strains are associated with cervical carcinoma. Candidal vulvovaginitis is frequently a chronic intermittent problem that can be troublesome. Finally, of particular concern to the pediatrician are those vaginal infections that may be passed to the newborn during delivery. These include herpes, gonorrhea, chlamydial infection, and condylomata. (For discussion of these conditions, see Chaps. 196 and 200.)

ANNOTATED BIBLIOGRAPHY

Altchek A: Vulvovaginitis, vulvar skin disease and pelvic inflammatory disease. Pediatr Clin North Am 28:397–432, 1981. (Provides great detail on numerous conditions.)

Bacon JL: Pediatric vulvovaginitis. Adolesc Pediatr Gynecol 2:86–93, 1989. (Excellent up-to-date review.)

Centers for Disease Control: STD treatment guidelines. MMWR 8 (No. S-8), 1989. (Current guidelines for the treatment of sexually transmitted diseases.)

Emans SJ, Goldstein DP: Pediatric and Adolescent Gynecology, 3rd ed. Boston, Little, Brown & Co, 1990. (Best textbook available; excellent general resource.)

Martien K, Emans SJ: Treatment of common genital infections in adolescents. J Adolesc Health Care 8:129–136, 1987. (Broad discussion of appropriate treatments including costs.)

120

Menstrual Problems

Odette Pinsonneault

Abnormal vaginal bleeding and dysmenorrhea are common gynecologic complaints during adolescence. These symptoms may be a tremendous source of anxiety for the young patient and her parents and should never be disregarded. Although adolescent menstrual problems, in most cases, have a dysfunctional origin, a thorough evaluation is essential to rule out an organic pathology.

Most of the time, abnormal menstrual patterns are *dysfunctional uterine bleeding* (i.e., unrelated to anatomic lesions of the uterus) and self-correct with the establishment of ovulatory menstrual cycles. In some instances, however, the bleeding problem requires therapy because of an excessive blood loss in amount, duration, or frequency, or secondary anemia. Abnormal menstrual bleeding may also reflect an underlying gynecologic or systemic disease.

In adolescents, primary dysmenorrhea is the leading etiology of menstrual pain. The possibility of a pelvic pathologic process should, however, be kept in mind. The early diagnosis and treatment of these conditions may save reproductive function.

ABNORMAL MENSTRUAL BLEEDING

Pathophysiology

The first postmenarchal years are frequently characterized by anovulatory menstrual cycles because the immature hypothalamic-pituitary-ovarian axis has not yet developed the positive estrogen feedback that is essential to obtain the mid-cycle luteinizing hormone (LH) surge and ovulation. Accordingly, the endometrium is subjected to continuous estrogenic stimulation, unopposed by the growth-limiting and stabilizing effect of progesterone (which should be secreted by the corpus luteum after ovulation). The endometrium, therefore, becomes thickened to such a point that it cannot sustain its integrity and suffers superficial breakages. Consequently, menses are likely to be irregular, prolonged, and excessive.

Clinical Presentation

Dysfunctional uterine bleeding may present as a wide variety of clinical pictures, ranging from minor deviations from the normal menstrual cycle to life-threatening hemorrhages.

The most clinically significant presentation is *acute menorrhagia,* which is characterized by heavy vaginal bleeding lasting for many days or even weeks. This occurs, most often, after a long episode of amenorrhea and sometimes with the first menstrual period. In this situation, the adolescent may be severely anemic or hypovolemic and requires emergency therapy. Since acute menorrhagia results from anovulatory menstrual cycles, dysmenorrhea is not a characteristic feature, although the uterus contracting to expel blood clots may cause painful cramps.

Recurrent hypermenorrhea, defined as self-limiting but excessive menstrual bleeding, either in amount or duration, and occurring more or less regularly, is also frequent in the adolescent. It is always difficult to accurately estimate blood loss. In general, menstrual bleeding exceeding 7 days in duration, or the use of more than 20 moderately soaked pads or tampons per period, or more than 6 well-soaked pads or tampons in any particular day, is considered to be excessive. Recurrent hypermenorrhea may also cause secondary anemia.

Polymenorrhea, or short menstrual cycles, is another frequent occurrence in adolescents. When interpreting this complaint, the physician should obtain a detailed history, because several young patients calculate their menstrual cycles from the last day of a period to the first day of the next one. Menstrual cycles less than 21 days (from the first day of a period to the first day of the next) are abnormally short; they may lead to anemia or interfere with the quality of life.

Oligomenorrhea (defined as menstrual cycles longer than 40 days) is also a common menstrual irregularity secondary to the physiologic anovulation in the perimenarchal patient. It does not usually cause distress, unless associated with excessive bleeding. A persistence of oligomenorrhea 3 to 4 years after menarche or any evidence of androgen excess should be investigated because it may be the manifestation of an endocrine dysfunction.

Differential Diagnosis

Although dysfunctional uterine bleeding is the most frequent etiology of menstrual abnormalities in the adolescent, all other causes should be ruled out.

In the patient with severe or prolonged vaginal bleeding, the differential diagnosis includes *pregnancy-related complications* (i.e., spontaneous abortion, ectopic pregnancy, complications of pregnancy termination procedures, and gestational trophoblastic diseases). Some *local conditions* affecting the genital tract such as vaginal, cervical, uterine, and estrogen-secreting ovarian tumors, congenital anomalies of the uterus and vagina associated with partial obstruction of the menstrual flow, pelvic inflammatory disease, the presence of an intrauterine contraceptive device, traumatic lesions of the lower genital tract, and intravaginal foreign bodies should be excluded. Many *systemic diseases* may be responsible for menorrhagia, principally blood dyscrasias (e.g., coagulation defects, leukemia, iron deficiency), endocrine disorders (hypothyroidism/hyperthyroidism, diabetes mellitus, adrenal diseases), and debilitating diseases (e.g., renal and hepatic diseases, inflammatory bowel diseases, tuberculosis).

Work-Up

History. A complete medical history should be obtained for every patient with abnormal vaginal bleeding. A detailed menstrual history, including age at menarche, length of cycles, duration of flow dysmenorrhea, and estimation of blood loss (e.g., pads count, blood clots), often points to the diagnosis or may reveal that there is no problem at all. A notion of habitual dysmenorrhea is suggestive of ovulatory cycles and makes the diagnosis of an organic pathologic process more likely. A thorough endocrine questionnaire, including galactorrhea, hirsutism, symptoms of thyroid dysfunction, and diabetes mellitus, is essential. The adolescent should be questioned, in a nonjudgmental manner, about sexual activity, contraception, and the possibility of pregnancy. In the patient with acute vaginal bleeding or recurrent hypermenorrhea, the history of a prior hemor-

rhage (gynecologic and nongynecologic) or easy bruising should be sought. Ten percent of females with a coagulation defect present with excessive menstrual bleeding as the first symptom of their blood disorder.

Physical Examination. During the physical examination, the physician should look for signs of hypovolemia or anemia. Abdominal palpation rules out masses and peritoneal signs. A complete pelvic examination should be performed, including a speculum visualization of the vagina and cervix, and a bimanual palpation of the internal genital structures. In the young teenager with only mild symptoms, the speculum examination can be deferred, provided the uterus and adnexa are normal by rectoabdominal palpation. Tanner stages of pubertal development should be recorded, as well as any evidence of androgen excess or other endocrine dysfunction.

Laboratory Tests. In the patient with acute menorrhagia or recurrent hypermenorrhea, a complete blood cell count including platelets, should be obtained. In the presence of a normal or only slightly decreased hematocrit, an elevated reticulocyte count may help to confirm an excessive blood loss. Coagulation studies (prothrombin time, partial thromboplastin time, bleeding time), as well as thyroid function tests, blood glucose determination, and cervical cultures are also indicated. A serum β-human chorionic gonadotropin or another highly sensitive pregnancy test should be performed for every patient, even when she denies sexual activity, because adolescents do not easily volunteer this information, especially during a crisis situation. In the patient with a long-standing history of irregular menses, evaluation of follicle-stimulating hormone, luteinizing hormone, and prolactin values is necessary to rule out endocrine pathologies. A pelvic ultrasound examination may be useful to further define an enlarged uterus or adnexal masses, but if the pelvic examination is normal, this ultrasound examination does not need to be performed in every case.

Management

Therapy for menstrual abnormalities depends on the severity of the bleeding aberration. When there are only *minor deviations from the normal menstrual cycle,* the best management is reassurance and observation for spontaneous establishment of ovulatory cycles. The patient should be encouraged to keep a menstrual calendar that will make future evaluation easier.

In the patient with *acute menorrhagia,* the treatment consists of combined hormonal therapy and blood replacement as necessary. High doses of estrogen will heal endometrial bleeding sites and rapidly stop the hemorrhage. At the same time, progestational agents need to be given to induce endometrial stability. The most practical method to achieve both of these goals is the administration of oral contraceptives containing high doses of estrogen and progestin.

Preparations containing 100 μg of ethinyl estradiol and 2 mg of norethindrone (Ortho Novum, 2 mg, or Norinyl, 2 mg) can be used with the following regimen: one tablet every 4 hours until the bleeding stops or decreases appreciably (24 to 36 hours); then, one tablet every 6 hours for 24 hours, one tablet three times a day for 48 hours, and one tablet twice daily for 15 days. Since these commercial preparations are not available in all pediatric hospitals' pharmacies, it is useful to know that two tablets of Ortho Novum 1/50 or Norinyl 1/50 are equivalent to one tablet of Ortho Novum or Norinyl, 2 mg. Many other similar therapeutic regimens have been described and work equally well. In the presence of profuse bleeding, intravenous administration of conjugated estrogens, Premarin, 25 mg, every 4 hours for three to six doses, may be added to the treatment to accelerate endometrial hemostasis.

After the completion of this initial treatment, the patient will have withdrawal bleeding and should then be kept under progestational therapy for 3 months, using low dose oral contraceptives (<50 μg of estrogen). This progestational influence allows the endometrium to recover its normal height.

A failure of hormonal therapy to control the hemorrhage within 24 to 36 hours is an indication for dilatation and curettage. This surgical approach is necessary in 20% to 30% of cases and is usually curative.

Further therapy is intended to prevent a recurrence because, if anovulation persists, an hyperplastic endometrium is likely to rebuild. In the sexually active adolescent, low-dose oral contraceptives are continued. When contraception is not a concern, medroxyprogesterone acetate (Provera), 10 mg/d for 10 days, is given every 6 to 8 weeks if spontaneous menses do not occur. This type of therapy has the advantage of not suppressing the hypothalamic-pituitary-ovarian axis and, therefore, does not interfere with the establishment of ovulatory cycles.

Recurrent hypermenorrhea can be treated with low-dose oral contraceptives when concomitant birth control is needed. Medroxyprogesterone acetate, 10 mg/d from day 16 to day 25 of each cycle, or according to a calendar-month schedule, may also be given to induce the formation of a progestational endometrium and withdrawal bleeding. Prostaglandin synthetase inhibitors, prescribed as for the treatment of primary dysmenorrhea, may be used to reduce the blood flow.

Polymenorrhea is best treated by the administration of medroxyprogesterone acetate, 5 or 10 mg/d from the 16th to the 25th days of each cycle. In the presence of very short cycles (<18 days), the medication is given from day 11 to day 25. This will maintain endometrial stability and prevent premature shedding. Oral contraceptives are also an acceptable therapeutic alternative.

Hormonal therapy for adolescent dysfunctional uterine bleeding is continued for 3 to 6 months, and the patient is then observed for a recurrence.

Indications for Referral or Admission

Profuse bleeding, signs of hypovolemia, a hematocrit lower than 28%, unreliability, and an unclear diagnosis are indications for hospitalization. Patients in whom an organic pathology is suspected and those not responding to the usual hormonal therapy should be referred to a gynecologist for further investigation and treatment.

DYSMENORRHEA

Pathophysiology

Most adolescents experiencing menstrual pain have primary dysmenorrhea, which means that there is no organic cause responsible for the symptoms. The most accepted pathophysiologic explanation for primary dysmenorrhea is an exaggerated production of endometrial prostaglandins, resulting in increased myometrial contractions, uterine ischemia, and sensitization of pain nerve terminals. Since falling progesterone levels, secondary to corpus luteum regression, initiate prostaglandin biosynthesis, primary dysmenorrhea occurs on the basis of ovulatory menstrual cycles.

Clinical Presentation

Primary dysmenorrhea usually begins 6 months to 2 years after menarche with the establishment of ovulatory menstrual cycles. The symptoms vary from mild discomfort to agonizing pain and are described as lower midabdominal cramps. Radiation of pain to the lower back, labia majora, and inner thighs is frequent. Accompanying systemic symptoms such as nausea, vomiting, headache, fatigue, nervousness, and dizziness are common. Pain usually begins within the few hours preceding or following the initiation of the menstrual flow and lasts for less than 2 days.

Differential Diagnosis

Endometriosis is probably the most frequent organic cause of dysmenorrhea. This disease is often subtle in the adolescent and does not always present as the classic physical findings. The diagnosis of endometriosis should be suspected whenever there is no response to the usual therapy of primary dysmenorrhea or when the pelvic examination reveals adnexal or uterosacral tenderness. Endometriosis should always be confirmed laparoscopically before undertaking therapy.

Acute and chronic pelvic inflammatory disease may be responsible for dysmenorrhea. In this situation, symptoms are mediated by increased prostaglandin production secondary to the inflammatory reaction. The presence of an *intrauterine contraceptive device* is frequently a cause of menstrual pain. Increased prostaglandin secretion associated with the intrauterine device–induced sterile endometrial inflammation is responsible for the cramping (see also Chap. 121).

Obstructing malformations of the reproductive tract, such as a blind uterine horn or an obstructed hemivagina, may occasionally be a source of dysmenorrhea. These anomalies cause menstrual blood to accumulate above the obstruction and secondary endometriosis. An examination in these patients often reveals a vaginal or pelvic mass.

Finally, in some patients, a *psychogenic* etiology is present. Dysmenorrhea may reflect familial, social, scholastic, and sexual maladjustment or may be used as a pretext to obtain narcotic prescriptions.

Work-Up

History. A complete menstrual history should be obtained, with special attention to the time elapsed between menarche and the onset of dysmenorrhea. The pain should be defined in terms of its timing in relation to the beginning of the flow, location, radiation, duration, accompanying symptoms, severity and degree of disability experienced by the adolescent. Prior treatments and their efficacy should be discussed. A thorough psychosocial and familial assessment may give a clue to a psychogenic etiology. The patient should be questioned about sexual activity, because it will influence the choice of therapy. The complaint of dysmenorrhea in adolescents also frequently masks a request for birth control.

Physical Examination. Both a general physical examination and a complete pelvic examination are essential. Most of the time, it will be normal, but it is the only means to detect evidence of organic disease. Bimanual rectovaginal palpation to rule out uterosacral nodularities or tenderness should be performed in every patient. However, because of the early stage of the disease, the examination in adolescents with endometriosis is frequently normal. The speculum examination may be deferred in the young, mildly dysmenorrheic teenager.

Laboratory Tests. Laboratory tests are not necessary when the clinical evaluation suggests primary dysmenorrhea. When pelvic inflammatory disease is a possibility, a complete blood cell count and erythrocyte sedimentation rate should be obtained. A pelvic ultrasound examination is performed to define pelvic masses or when congenital anomalies are suspected. Laparoscopy is the only reliable method of diagnosing endometriosis and chronic pelvic inflammatory disease.

Management

The treatment of primary dysmenorrhea is based on its severity. In the patient with only mild discomfort, reassurance and analgesics, such as aspirin or acetaminophen, may be all that is necessary. When the intensity of symptoms indicates more specific therapy, either prostaglandin synthetase

Table 120-1. Treatment of Primary Dysmenorrhea With Prostaglandin Synthetase Inhibitors

DRUG	DOSAGE
Ibuprofen (Motrin)	400–600 mg q6h
Naproxen (Naprosyn)	250–375 mg q8–12h
Naproxen sodium (Anaprox)	550 mg, then 275 mg q6h
Mefenamic acid (Ponstel, Ponstan)	500 mg, then 250–500 mg q6h

inhibitors or oral contraceptives may be used, the choice depending on the birth control need.

Prostaglandin synthetase inhibitors produce effective relief of primary dysmenorrhea in 75% to 90% of patients. Since these agents need to be taken only for the usual duration of symptoms and also because of their low incidence of side effects, this therapeutic approach is usually well accepted by the patient. The most commonly used regimens are summarized in Table 120-1. They are all equally effective, although some patients may have a good response to one agent and not to another.

The medication should be started at the onset of menstrual bleeding and continued for the usual duration of symptoms. In patients in whom cramping precedes the flow, therapy may be initiated 24 to 48 hours before menses or, if cycles are not predictable, at the first sign of discomfort. Frequent follow-up visits or telephone contacts, to adjust the dosage or change the medication, ensure the best compliance and results. Prostaglandin synthetase inhibitors may also prove useful in the treatment of intrauterine device–induced dysmenorrhea.

Prescription of oral contraceptives as for birth control is a good therapeutic alternative for the sexually active adolescent or when prostaglandin synthetase inhibitors fail to relieve primary dysmenorrhea. Oral contraceptives are effective in 90% of cases. In some instances, combined therapy with both prostaglandin synthetase inhibitors and oral contraceptives is necessary to obtain painless menses.

Indications for Referral

Whenever an organic etiology of dysmenorrhea is suspected, the adolescent should be referred for evaluation of the need for laparoscopy or other diagnostic tests. A delay in the diagnosis and treatment of endometriosis or obstructing malformations of the reproductive tract may compromise future fertility.

ANNOTATED BIBLIOGRAPHY

Abnormal Menstrual Bleeding

Claessens EA: Adolescent dysfunctional uterine bleeding. Contemp Obstet Gynecol Can 5(3):7–13, 1988. (Excellent concise review of the pathophysiology, diagnosis, and treatment of adolescent dysfunctional uterine bleeding.)

Pelvic Inflammatory Disease

Emans SJH, Goldstein DP: Pediatric and Adolescent Gynecology, pp 219–234. Boston, Little, Brown & Co, 1990. (Comprehensive chapter on the evaluation and management of menstrual irregularities in adolescents.)

Jaffe SB, Jewelewicz R: Dysfunctional uterine bleeding in the pediatric and adolescent patient. Adolesc Pediatr Gynecol 4(2):62–69, 1991. (Good review of the pathophysiology, differential diagnosis, and therapy for dysfunction uterine bleeding that also includes a discussion of premenarchal vaginal bleeding.)

Pinsonneault O, Goldstein DP: Gynecologic disorders in adolescents: II. Dysfunctional uterine bleeding and breast masses. Female Patient 10(12):41–44, 1985. (Discussion of the differential diagnosis and management of adolescent dysfunctional uterine bleeding.)

Dysmenorrhea

Altcheck A: Dysmenorrhea in the young patient. Female Patient 8(9):36/7–36/28, 1983. (Discussion of the evaluation and treatment of adolescent dysmenorrhea.)

Dawood MY: Dysmenorrhea. Clin Obstet Gynecol 25:719–727, 1983. (Good review of the role of prostaglandins in primary and secondary dysmenorrhea.)

Emans SJH, Goldstein DP: Pediatric and Adolescent Gynecology, pp 291–299. Boston, Little, Brown & Co, 1990. (Clear and concise discussion of the management of the dysmenorrheic adolescent.)

Pinsonneault O, Goldstein DP: Gynecologic disorders in adolescents: I. Pain syndromes. Female Patient 10(11):21–27, 1985. (Discussion of the differential diagnosis and management of dysmenorrhea and chronic pelvic pain in adolescents.)

Smith RP: Primary dysmenorrhea and the adolescent patient. Adolesc Pediatr Gynecol 1(1):23–30, 1988. (Comprehensive review of the mode of action and use of nonsteroidal anti-inflammatory drugs in the treatment of primary dysmenorrhea.)

121
Pelvic Inflammatory Disease

Jean Brodnax

Pelvic inflammatory disease (PID) is the clinical syndrome resulting from the ascending spread of microorganisms from the vagina and endocervix to the endometrium, fallopian tubes, or contiguous structures. It is one of the most serious complications of sexually transmitted diseases (STDs). (For a discussion on sexually transmitted diseases, see Chapter 200.)

Pelvic inflammatory disease is diagnosed at the highest rate during the teenage years. The younger the sexually active female, the greater is her risk of developing PID. The risk is 1:8 for sexually active 15-year-old girls and decreases to approximately 1:80 for sexually active 24-year-old women. Of the 1 million women in the United States treated each year for PID, 70% are younger than 25 years of age. There has been a slight decrease in the overall incidence of PID, but the rate for the adolescent female continues to increase. Although PID occurs more frequently among nonwhite adolescents, the recent increase in adolescent PID is mainly attributed to the increase in PID among white adolescents.

Pelvic inflammatory disease has many medical consequences, with infertility being the most important. The risk of infertility is 11% after one episode, 34% after two episodes, and 54% after three or more episodes. Other medical sequelae include tubo-ovarian abscess, ectopic pregnancy, chronic pelvic pain, dyspareunia, and repeated episodes of PID.

Since PID occurs so frequently in adolescents and may impact on the reproductive futures of these generally healthy young women, it is crucial that the practicing pediatrician be able to recognize and appropriately treat this potentially devastating disease.

PATHOPHYSIOLOGY

It is postulated that adolescents are more prone to PID because of the high incidence of STDs in this age group; immature immune systems that increase susceptibility to ascending infections; larger zones of cervical ectopy that predispose to *Chlamydia trachomatis* and *Neisseria gonorrhoeae* infections; and thinner cervical mucus resulting from the relative estrogen dominance of this age group.

Other general risk factors include use of intrauterine devices, a previous history of PID or gonococcal disease, and multiple sexual partners. The risk is decreased with oral contraceptive use (as is the severity of the disease if PID does develop), which is believed to result from less permeable cervical mucus and a decreased menstrual flow. PID risk is also decreased with barrier forms of contraception and probably with the spermicide nonoxynol-9.

Chlamydia trachomatis (cultured from the cervix in 25% to 40% of patients) and *N. gonorrhoeae* (cultured from the cervix in 20% to 40% of patients) are the most common organisms associated with PID in adolescents. *N. gonorrhoeae* is more commonly isolated in the first episode than in subsequent episodes. Endogenous aerobic and anaerobic bacteria are less commonly associated organisms and include *Mycoplasma* species, coliforms, *Gardnerella vaginalis*, group B *Streptococcus*, *Hemophilus influenza*, *Bacteroides* species, *Peptococcus*, and *Peptostreptococcus*. It is important to note that PID is often a polymicrobial infection and that organisms isolated from the upper genital tract by laparoscopy or culdocentesis do not necessarily correlate with those recovered from cervical cultures alone. (*N. gonorrhoeae* and *C. trachomatis* may "pave the way" for other ascending pathogens; however, aerobic and anaerobic organisms may initiate PID without antecedent *N. gonorrhoeae* or *C. trachomatis* infection.)

Ten to 17% of women who have endocervical gonococcal infection will develop PID. The most susceptible time is during or immediately after menses; it is believed to be secondary to the loss of the protective cervical mucus plug during menses and to the excellent culture medium of blood. In addition, the endometrium normally provides local protection against bacteria, which is lost when sloughed.

Neisseria gonorrhoeae probably produces salpingitis by direct upward extension from the cervix, causing cell destruction that results in a purulent exudate. When PID damages a fallopian tube, it may become scarred and lose its protective cilial lining, thus predisposing the tube to subsequent episodes of PID. If the bacteria extends to the ovaries, a tubo-ovarian abscess may result. If pus escapes into the peritoneum, peritonitis will develop.

Ten to 30% of women with endocervical chlamydial infection will develop PID. *C. trachomatis* also produces PID by direct upward extension from the endocervix, also usually associated with menses. In contrast to the gonococcus, which limits itself to the mucosal surface of the tube, *C. trachomatis* and other facultative and anaerobic bacteria may cause infection below the basement membrane in the subepithelial connective tissue and muscularis and serosal surfaces, thus increasing the likelihood of permanent tubal damage. In addition, chlamydia may remain in the fallopian tubes for months or years following an initial infection, causing progressive tubal damage.

The presence of an intrauterine device may cause PID by interference with local host defense mechanisms. Tailed devices may serve as conduits for the ascent of bacteria into the endometrial cavity. If attached to sperm or trichomonads, bacteria may also be transported into the upper genital tract.

CLINICAL PRESENTATION

The clinical presentation of PID is highly variable. Laparoscopic studies have shown that relying on the presence of the "classic" triad of lower abdominal pain, evidence of genital tract infection, and pelvic tenderness on bimanual examination to make a clinical diagnosis of PID will result in many erroneous, as well as missed, diagnoses. Diagnostic accuracy is increased with the addition of other findings. Table 121-1 lists the common signs, symptoms, and criteria for PID.

Lower abdominal pain is the most frequent complaint of patients who have PID. It may be absent in up to 5% of patients who have disease verified by laparoscopy. The length and intensity of the pain may be affected by the causative organism. Patients with gonococcal PID tend to have severe abdominal pain of rapid onset within a few days of menses. The pain of chlamydial PID may be so insidious that many women who have tubal obstruction and evidence

Table 121-1. Criteria for the Diagnosis of Acute Pelvic Inflammatory Disease

All three of the following should be present:
- Lower abdominal tenderness
- Cervical motion tenderness
- Adnexal tenderness (may be unilateral)

plus

One of the following should be present:
- Temperature >100.4°F (38°C)
- White blood cell count >10,500/mm³
- Purulent material obtained by culdocentesis
- A inflammatory mass present on bimanual pelvic examination and/or ultrasound examination
- Erythrocyte sedimentation rate >15 mm/h
- Evidence of the presence of *Neisseria gonorrhoeae* and/or *Chlamydia trachomatis* in the endocervix by either Gram stain (gram-negative intracellular diplococci) or monoclonal antibody for *C. trachomatis*
- Presence of >5 white blood cells per oil-immersion field on Gram's stain of endocervical discharge

of chlamydial infection have no recollection of ever having experienced pelvic pain. Patients with nongonococcal, nonchlamydial PID also tend to have mild to moderate pelvic pain. A sexually active adolescent with pleuritic, right upper quadrant pain, with or without evidence of PID, may have the *Fitz-Hugh-Curtis syndrome*. This is a perihepatitis (inflammation of the liver capsule), usually associated with gonorrheal or chlamydial disease.

Vaginal discharge of recent onset is present in 75% of patients with gonococcal or chlamydial PID. It is less common in nongonococcal, nonchlamydial PID.

Intermenstrual bleeding due to endometriosis occurs in 40% of patients. Fever is noted in less than one half of patients. Dysuria and frequency may occur in a small proportion of women. Patients with severe disease may experience nausea and vomiting.

DIFFERENTIAL DIAGNOSIS

The differential diagnosis of PID includes acute appendicitis, acute pyelonephritis, twisted ovarian cyst, ruptured corpus luteum cyst, ectopic pregnancy, endometriosis, gastroenteritis, and vaginitis. In acute appendicitis, pain is unilateral and the sedimentation rate is usually normal with an elevated white blood cell count and left shift, whereas in PID pain is usually bilateral and the sedimentation rate is usually elevated with a normal white blood cell count. In acute pyelonephritis, costovertebral angle tenderness is usually present and urinary symptoms may be the chief complaint. A twisted ovarian cyst, bleeding corpus luteum cyst, or unruptured ectopic pregnancy typically cause unilateral pain and tenderness, and white blood cells are not present on a normal saline preparation of cervical secretions. A ruptured ectopic pregnancy commonly causes acute hypotension, tachycardia, and falling hematocrit. Endometriosis is an infrequent diagnosis in adolescents and is manifested typically by cyclic, rather than constant, pelvic pain. In gastroenteritis, abdominal pain and tenderness are diffuse and vomiting or diarrhea usually dominate the clinical picture. Lower abdominal pain may be seen in simple vaginitis, but true adnexal tenderness is rare. Many of these diagnoses may be made by laparoscopy in patients clinically diagnosed as having PID.

WORK-UP

History

A history obtained from the patient should include questions about onset, duration, location, and intensity of abdominal pain; presence and character of vaginal discharge or bleeding; and systemic symptoms such as fever, nausea, or vomiting. One should elicit a sexual history, inquiring specifically about the number of sexual partners and type of sexual practices. Other important information includes timing of the last menstrual cycle, contraceptive history, and previous episodes of STDs or PID.

It must be stressed that a heavy reliance on symptoms may lead to a misdiagnosis because the clinical picture in PID is so variable and nonspecific.

Physical Examination

A complete physical examination should be done on any patient with suspected PID, not only to look for possible associated conditions (such as gonococcal pharyngitis, arthritis, rash, or right upper quadrant tenderness) but also to rule out other diagnoses.

In patients with PID, the abdominal examination usually reveals bilateral lower quadrant tenderness without an associated mass. Rebound tenderness will be present if the inflammation has extended to the peritoneal surface. Right upper quadrant tenderness, with or without signs of PID, is present in perihepatitis.

On speculum examination of the vagina and cervix, a thick endocervical discharge is present in most cases of gonococcal and chlamydial PID. On bimanual examination, cervical motion tenderness and uterine and adnexal tenderness are present. The adnexal tenderness is most commonly bilateral, although one side may be more tender than the other. Adnexal fullness or swelling may be felt, but a true tubo-ovarian abscess is present in only 15% to 20% of cases.

Laboratory Tests

Routine hematologic blood tests have limited diagnostic value in PID. The white blood cell count and hematocrit are usually normal. The sedimentation rate is elevated above 15 mm/h in only 75% of women; thus, a normal value does not rule out the diagnosis.

A microscopic examination of cervical secretions is frequently helpful. Increased numbers of white blood cells (5 cells or more per high-power field) are almost always seen on a normal saline wet preparation and are diagnostic of cervicitis. Absence of white blood cells in cervical or vaginal secretions should lead to consideration of diagnoses other than PID. Gram stain may show gram-negative intracellular diplococci in gonococcal PID, but it is positive in only two thirds of women with positive gonococcal cultures of the cervix.

Cultures of cervical secretions for *N. gonorrhoeae* should be taken. Rapid diagnostic tests to identify chlamydia in cervical secretions are available. In women, the chlamydiazyme enzyme immunoassay is 98% to 100% sensitive and 91% to 95% specific when compared with the gold standard chlamydial culture. Culture is generally not available to the office practitioner.

A sensitive pregnancy test should be done to rule out an ectopic pregnancy. Pelvic ultrasound examination may prove useful in the diagnosis of PID since it may be abnormal (showing adnexal enlargement or a tubo-ovarian abscess) in up to 85% of adolescents with a clinical diagnosis of PID. The diagnosis of tubo-ovarian abscess may warrant more prolonged treatment, better anaerobic antibiotic coverage, and possibly surgery. Pelvic ultrasound examination may also be used to follow patients clinically for response to treatment.

The aforementioned laboratory work may be helpful but alone is not diagnostic of PID. Laparoscopy, which is the only absolute way to make the diagnosis, is impractical in most cases.

MANAGEMENT

The goals of treatment in PID are the acute relief of discomfort and the prevention of infertility and other chronic sequelae.

The antibiotic treatment of PID is far from an exact science, largely because it is caused by multiple organisms. Treatment should include coverage for *N. gonorrhoeae* (including penicillinase-producing strains), *C. trachomatis*, and the mixed aerobic and anaerobic genital flora. There is currently much controversy over the best choice of drug or drugs to treat this broad spectrum of organisms.

Table 121-2 shows the Centers for Disease Control's 1991 recommendations for inpatient and outpatient treatment of PID. Notable changes from prior recommendations include the following:

1. Inclusion of cefotetan (given every 12 hours) as an alternative drug to cefoxitin (given every 12 hours) for inpatient use
2. Substitution of other cephalosporins for cefoxitin and cefotetan, based on their activity against involved organisms
3. Discontinuation of the sole use of oral antibiotics (penicillin G or ampicillin/amoxicillin) for outpatient ther-

Table 121-2. Summary of 1991 Guidelines for Treatment of Pelvic Inflammatory Disease

Inpatients

Regimen A
Cefoxitin (2 g IV q6h)
or
Cefotetan* (2 g IV q12h)
    plus
Doxycycline (100 mg PO or IV q12h)
After Discharge:
Doxycycline (100 mg PO twice daily to complete a total of 10–14 days of therapy)

Regimen B
Clindamycin (900 mg IV q8h)
    plus
Gentamicin (2.0 mg/kg as IV loading dose followed by 1.5 mg/kg IV q8h in patients with normal renal function)
After Discharge:
Doxycycline (100 mg PO twice daily to complete a total of 10–14 days of therapy)[†]

Outpatients
Cefoxitin[‡] (2 g IM)
or
Ceftriaxone (250 mg IM)
    plus
Doxycycline (100 mg PO twice daily for 10–14 days)

---

*Other cephalosporins (e.g., ceftizoxime, cefotaxime, and ceftriaxone), which provide adequate coverage against gonococci and other facultative gram-negative aerobic and anaerobic bacteria, may be given in appropriate doses.

[†]Continuation of clindamycin (450 mg PO, 4 times daily, for a total of 10–14 d) may be considered as an alternative.

[‡]Probenecid (1 gm PO is given with each of these regimens except ceftraixone).

---

apy due to the nationwide prevalence of penicillinase-producing *N. gonorrhoeae*

4. Allowance for the use of oral doxycycline initially in inpatient therapy since blood levels are equal for orally and intravenously administered doxycycline.

The current recommendations for treating PID are listed in Table 2. There are other aspects of these treatment regiments to bear in mind. The clindamycin/gentamicin combination is not very active against *N. gonorrhoeae*. Clindamycin is active against *C. trachomatis* in vitro, but there is some question about its clinical efficacy. Ceftriaxone does not have very good activity against anaerobes.

Other treatment options are being explored in the search for a single-agent antibiotic regimen to treat PID. The combination of a penicillin plus a β-lactamase inhibitor may provide the appropriate antimicrobial spectrum of activity to treat PID. Possibilities include ampicillin/sulbactam, ticarcillin/clavulanate, and amoxicillin/clavulanate. However, penicillin may not be efficacious in treating *Chlamydia*. In addition, there is a high incidence of adverse reactions, usually gastrointestinal, when the oral forms of the above drugs are used.

Ciprofloxacin, a new quinolone, has been compared with the combination of clindamycin plus an aminoglycoside in several recent studies. Clinical cure rates have been high with ciprofloxacin, but the treatment of mucosal *C. trachomatis* infections appears inadequate. In addition, ciprofloxacin has limited activity against anaerobes.

Thus, the clinician must decide which regimen to use, based on probable organisms involved, compliance of the patient, severity of illness, and cost. Sicker patients should receive aggressive parenteral therapy.

Patients who have suspected tubo-ovarian abscesses should be hospitalized and managed with parenteral antibiotics for 48 to 72 hours. If no improvement occurs by that time, surgical exploration should be considered, not only in an attempt to preserve fertility but also to prevent rupture. A ruptured tubo-ovarian abscess is a surgical emergency.

All outpatients with PID should be reevaluated in 48 to 72 hours to assess improvement, and again after the completion of antibiotic therapy. Patients with PID should be counseled on STDs. Their partner should be examined for evidence of STDs and treated presumptively for 7 to 10 days with an antibiotic, such as doxycycline, which treats both *N. gonorrhoeae* and *C. trachomatis*.

INDICATIONS FOR REFERRAL OR ADMISSION

Any primary care provider who suspects a diagnosis of PID in an adolescent and feels unsure of, or uncomfortable with, the diagnosis, should refer the patient immediately to an adolescent or gynecologic specialist.

About 75% of patients with PID are treated on an outpatient basis. Indications for hospitalization include the following:

- Possibly all adolescents
- Temperature greater than 101.3°F (38.5°C)
- Patient acutely ill and appearing toxic
- Noncompliance with, or failure to respond, to an outpatient regimen
- Pregnancy
- Presence of pelvic or tubo-ovarian abscess
- Clinical signs of peritonitis
- Strong suspicion of a surgical problem in the differential diagnosis

ANNOTATED BIBLIOGRAPHY

Centers for Disease Control: PID: Guidelines for prevention and management. MMWR 40(RR-5):1, 1991. (Good public health perspective of the magnitude of the problem.)

Emans SJH, Goldstein DP: Pediatric and Adolescent Gynecology, 3rd edition. Boston, Little, Brown & Co, 1990. (Up-to-date, detailed discussion of pelvic inflammatory disease in the adolescent.)

Golden N, Neuhoff S, Cohen H: Pelvic inflammatory disease in adolescents. J Pediatr 114:138, 1989. (Emphasizes frequency of tubo-ovarian abscess and usefulness of ultrasound in the adolescent with pelvic inflammatory disease.)

Peterson H, Galaid E, Zenilman J: Pelvic inflammatory disease: Review of treatment options. Rev Infect Dis 12(suppl 6):S656, 1990. (Excellent up-to-date review of various options in the treatment of pelvic inflammatory disease, explaining advantages and disadvantages of each therapeutic regimen.)

Shafer M, Sweet R: Pelvic inflammatory disease in adolescent females. Pediatr Clin North Am 36(3):513, 1989. (Well-organized review of pelvic inflammatory disease in the adolescent.)

Sweet R: Pelvic inflammatory disease and infertility in women. Infect Dis Clin North Am 1(1):199, 1987. (Includes detailed discussion of sequelae of pelvic inflammatory disease.)

17

HEMATOLOGIC PROBLEMS

Orah S. Platt, *Section Editor*

122

Anemia

Orah S. Platt

There are four common office scenarios that the pediatrician is faced with when evaluating a child for anemia. The most common occurs when the healthy youngster who comes for a routine well-child visit is found to have a slightly low hematocrit as part of a standard office screening procedure. The second is when a child is brought in by a parent who suspects anemia because the child seems pale, sluggish, or is a "picky eater." The third is the child who is found to have an abnormal complete blood cell count (CBC) in the orderly process of being evaluated for failure to thrive, recurrent infections, chronic diarrhea, or other chronic conditions. The least common is the child who is brought in with a rather nonspecific complaint who is obviously seriously ill, is extremely pale, is possibly jaundiced, and needs immediate emergency evaluation and management.

The common laboratory measurements that "define" anemia are the hematocrit and hemoglobin. In general, these measurements vary directly and can, therefore, be used interchangeably, knowing that the hematocrit value is usually approximately three times the hemoglobin value. Clinicians are usually more comfortable with one of these measurements than the other. In this chapter, *hematocrit* rather than *hemoglobin* will be used.

PATHOPHYSIOLOGY

Anemia can be strictly defined as having an hematocrit below the "lower limit of normal" for age. From a functional point of view, *anemia* means not having enough oxygen-carrying capacity in the blood for a person to conduct his or her normal activities. The combination of these two definitions frees the practitioner from solely using published (and highly variable) "normal" values and allows room for clinical judgment. For example, two 7-year olds come into the office the same day. One is in for a routine examination before going off to camp: his hematocrit is 34%. The other child has cystic fibrosis, mainly with chronic lung disease, and she is having more trouble keeping up with her classmates. Her hematocrit is 37%. Comparing these two children clinically, the one with the higher hematocrit is the one who needs to be evaluated for anemia.

A person can only become anemic in three ways: (1) by not producing red blood cells efficiently (ineffective production or hypoplasia), (2) by having red blood cells that survive for a relatively short time in the circulation (hemolysis), or (3) by bleeding. These three categories have their characteristic presentations and differential diagnoses.

CLINICAL PRESENTATION

Hypoplastic or ineffective-production anemias are common and develop gradually over long periods of time. Because of the luxury of time these patients can make the physiologic adjustments that can result in their tolerating extremely low hematocrits with apparent equanimity. The classic example is the iron-deficient "milk baby" who, at 16 months of age, is astonishingly pale yet perfectly comfortable with an hematocrit of 15%. These patients are usually tachycardic with loud systolic murmurs, and they rarely show any other physical findings.

Children who have hemolytic anemias generally fall into two categories: acute and chronic. *Acute hemolysis* is rare but dramatic in presentation. These are usually children who do not have a prior history of anemia and who suddenly become profoundly anemic and jaundiced, sometimes passing wine-colored urine. An example of this situation typically occurs in May when little boys with glucose-6-phosphate deficiency ingest moth balls while their parents gather up the family's winter clothes. These children have not had time to gradually make physiologic adjustments to their low hematocrit and they become symptomatic with tachycardia, lethargy, sometimes with congestive heart failure, or liver or splenic enlargement.

Chronic hemolysis usually presents as a mild to moderate anemia in a child who has periodically had episodes of mild icterus or frank jaundice. These children are typically well-compensated with mild tachycardia, systolic murmurs, and often liver or spleen enlargement. These children are sometimes so well-compensated hematologically that the diagnosis is made as part of a work-up for jaundice, splenomegaly, or gallstones, and not anemia. The most important chronic hemolytic anemia to diagnose early is sickle cell anemia (see Chap. 123).

Bleeding also occurs in acute and chronic forms. Acute bleeding is obviously not usually a difficult clinical diagnosis to make unless the blood is hidden in a cryptic space, such as a psoas muscle, or in a cryptic patient, such as a teenager who denies blood in the stool. In addition to the usual tachycardia, systolic murmurs, and pallor, these patients may have postural hypotension. Chronic bleeding can be difficult to ferret out. Most of these patients will be more anemic from the iron deficiency that results from the loss of red blood cells than from the loss of the red blood cells themselves.

DIFFERENTIAL DIAGNOSIS

The hypoplastic or ineffective-production anemias can be caused by a long list of common and rare disorders. The single most common cause of anemia in children is *iron deficiency*. Less common are the various thalassemia syndromes, drugs such as chloramphenicol, folic acid deficiency, and chronic diseases such as tuberculosis, juvenile rheumatoid arthritis, and liver, renal, or thyroid disease. Rare disorders include the acquired and congenital bone marrow failure syndromes, leukemias, and malignancies, as well as metabolic disorders including vitamin B_{12} deficiency syndromes.

Acute fulminant hemolytic anemias are rare but usually arise in boys with glucose-6-phosphate deficiency who are exposed to oxidants (e.g., fava beans, antimalarials, or some viruses); patients with acute infections associated with autoantibody production (e.g., infectious mononucleosis, *Mycoplasma* pneumonia); and patients with other acute infections that lyse red blood cells by various methods (e.g., *Hemophilus influenzae, Clostridium,* and malaria). Rarely will hemolysis be the most prominent feature of the hemolytic-uremic syndrome.

Chronic hemolytic anemias in children are usually either inherited hemoglobinopathies such as sickle cell disease or inherited red blood cell membrane disorders such as heredi-

tary spherocytosis. Rarely, red blood cell enzyme deficiencies, such as pyruvate kinase deficiency, or chronic autoimmune hemolytic anemias are encountered.

Blood loss is discussed in detail in other chapters that deal with specific problems such as gastrointestinal bleeding (see Chap. 111), hematuria (see Chap. 114), and menorrhagia (see Chap. 120).

WORK-UP

History

The history is an important aspect is the work-up of an anemic child. A family history should include information on the national heritage of parents and grandparents, other family members with anemias, splenectomy, jaundice, early gallbladder disease, sickle cell trait, or thalassemia trait (minor or Mediterranean anemia). The child's nutritional history should be reviewed in detail (as well as the mother's if she is nursing the infant). The child's past medical history and a review of systems is important with special attention to episodes of jaundice (including the newborn period), extremity pain, possible sites of blood loss, recent infections, exposures, drugs, or travel.

Physical Examination

A comprehensive physical examination can be helpful in evaluating an anemic child. Plotted growth parameters, vital signs, and a general assessment will help establish chronicity and a level of concern. A quick survey for the following findings can be helpful: pallor, jaundice, petechiae, bruises, frontal bossing, adenopathy, murmurs and signs of congestive failure, organomegaly, and congenital anomalies.

Laboratory Tests

First decide if the patient really warrants an anemia evaluation based on published norms and your clinical judgment. If so, the laboratory examination begins simply with a CBC, reticulocyte count, and examination of the peripheral smear. If the patient is anemic, the next step is to note the mean corpuscular volume (MCV) (or mean corpuscular hemoglobin concentration [MCH], which varies with MCV). If this information is not available, note if the smear is hypochromic and microcytic.

If the child is microcytic, it is likely that he or she has iron deficiency. The best test for iron deficiency is a therapeutic trial. If the results of the iron trial are good, the next step is to determine the cause of the iron deficiency. This may simply be a matter of reviewing the nutritional or blood loss history, or it may need to be pursued more vigorously, for example, with stool examination. In young children, since the possibility of coexisting lead poisoning should not be overlooked, a lead level is indicated. If the therapeutic trial is equivocal, or if compliance is questioned, iron studies such as total iron binding capacity, serum iron, and ferritin may be helpful. Each of these tests, however, has its own idiosyncrasies and may not always yield a perfectly satisfying answer. If the office is equipped with an hematocrit centrifuge, a visual inspection of the spun plasma can give useful information. The plasma normally has a slight straw color. In iron deficiency, this color fades and the plasma appears colorless like water. In hemolytic anemias, the plasma will be bright yellow, and in some fulminant acute cases it will be brown.

If the child is microcytic but not iron deficient, he or she probably has a thalassemia syndrome, especially if the family is of Mediterranean, Asian, or African heritage. The next step is to examine the blood of the parents. If one of the parents is also mildly anemic and microcytic, the diagnosis is fairly secure, and no further evaluation is necessary. If both parents are microcytic and are planning to have more children, this diagnosis needs to be pursued more fully with hemoglobin electrophoresis and possibly gene mapping to determine whether they are at risk of producing a child with thalassemia major and whether they would benefit from genetic counseling. Hemoglobin electrophoresis will identify a patient with β-thalassemia trait as having an elevated hemoglobin A_2 level. Patients with α-thalassemia trait have normal hemoglobin electrophoresis patterns and can be definitively diagnosed only by gene mapping.

If the child has a normal MCV and a high reticulocyte count, a careful examination of the smear may be helpful. Elongated sickle forms, target cells, and fragmented cells suggest a sickle syndrome and warrant a hemoglobin electrophoresis. A predominance of spherocytes could mean hereditary spherocytosis or an autoimmune hemolytic anemia. An examination of the parents' CBC and smear, a Coombs test, and an osmotic fragility test will usually be diagnostic. Elliptocytes usually mean hereditary elliptocytosis, although this is almost never associated with much hemolysis. Normal morphology and no parent with reticulocyte elevation should suggest a careful search for bleeding.

If the anemic child has a normal or slightly elevated MCV and a low reticulocyte count, a blood urea nitrogen and creatinine determination, liver function tests, and thyroid studies may detect an underlying chronic disease.

TREATMENT

The treatment of the anemic child depends on the cause of the anemia. The most common anemia treated in the office is iron deficiency anemia. This deficiency is corrected by treating the underlying cause of the anemia (e.g., altering the diet, treating the ulcerative colitis, purging the parasites) and providing a supplementation to rebuild the iron stores. This can usually be accomplished orally by treating with 2 to 6 mg/kg/d of elemental iron for 3 to 6 months depending on the degree of deficiency and the daily dose of iron. A

gastrointestinal disturbance may result in poor compliance. Many patients would rather be on a lower dose for a longer time than endure the gastrointestinal symptoms. Heme iron in the form of meat is probably the best tolerated iron preparation. Parenteral iron is reserved for the rare patient who is unable to comply with conventional therapy or who has an abnormal iron absorption.

Thalassemia trait does not require treatment. Patient and parental education, however, is important. The emphasis is on the potential genetic implications and on the remarkable resemblance between thalassemia trait and iron deficiency and the fact that iron therapy is not indicated.

Hereditary spherocytosis is usually treated (except in mild cases) by elective splenectomy after 5 or 6 years of age. This therapy effectively eliminates the anemia and the risk of gallstones but carries with it the potential risk of overwhelming bacterial sepsis. Parental and patient education is critical in the care of the splenectomized patient and in understanding the genetic implications of the disease.

The treatment of sickle cell disease is discussed in Chapter 123.

INDICATIONS FOR REFERRAL OR ADMISSION

The same general guidelines pertaining to admitting critically ill children apply to children who have anemia. Children with congestive failure, hypotension, and profuse bleeding obviously need to be in the hospital. In addition, even relatively comfortable children with low hematocrits need to be hospitalized until the diagnosis is clarified; then, with appropriate therapy even with a low hematocrit, they can be managed as outpatients.

The following is a list of disturbing features in children with anemia that warrant an early discussion with a hematologist: neutropenia, thrombocytopenia, myeloblasts or other immature myeloid elements, nucleated red blood cells, elevated MCV without reticulocytosis, positive Coombs' test, congenital anomalies, unexplained failure to thrive, unexplained fevers, and bone pain.

ANNOTATED BIBLIOGRAPHY

Abshire TC, Reeves JD: Anemia of acute inflammation in children. J Pediatr 103:868–871, 1983. (Delineation and explanation of this anemia commonly seen in children hospitalized with inflammatory diseases.)

Addrigo JE, Hurst D, Lubin BH: Congenital hemolytic anemia. Pediatr Rev 6:201–208, 1985. (Clinical and laboratory approach to the child with hemolytic anemia.)

Groopman J: Management of the hematologic complications of human immunodeficiency virus infection. Rev Infect Dis 12:931—937, 1990. (Excellent review of AIDS-associated hematologic findings.)

Miller DR: Anemias: General considerations. In Miller DR, Brehner RI, McMillan CW (eds): Blood Diseases of Infancy and Childhood, 5th ed, pp 97–114. St. Louis, CV Mosby, 1984. (Detailed overview of the problem including an excellent discussion of etiologic and morphologic classifications of the anemias, as well as an understandable explanation of appropriate laboratory tests used in diagnosis.)

Reeves JD: Iron supplementation in infancy. Pediatr Rev 8:177–184, 1986. (Complete summary of the clinical problems and issues of iron deficiency.)

123

Sickle Cell Anemia

Orah S. Platt

A single sickle gene is carried by about 10% of African Americans. These asymptomatic persons with sickle trait have no significant medical problems, and their identification is important only in terms of genetic counseling. The clinically important homozygous sickle state—sickle cell anemia—is emphasized in this chapter. Other less common sickle syndromes such as hemoglobin SC disease and sickle cell thalassemia are briefly discussed.

PATHOPHYSIOLOGY

Children who have sickle cell anemia produce no normal hemoglobin A; instead, they synthesize sickle hemoglobin (hemoglobin S), a variant of hemoglobin A that contains valine (an amino acid that decreases protein solubility in water) instead of glutamic acid (an amino acid that promotes protein solubility in water). This single amino acid substitution does not interfere with the oxygen transport properties. Normally, hemoglobin in the red blood cell stays dissolved even in the extremes of the body's pO_2, pH, temperature, and osmolarity. In contrast, hemoglobin S has a tendency to come out of solution—polymerize at low pO_2, low pH, low temperature, and increased osmolarity. This polymerization reaction damages the red blood cell and causes a chronic hemolytic anemia. Additionally, if this reaction occurs in small vessels, ischemia or infarction of the particular tissue may ensue. The clinical picture of sickle cell anemia is a combination of chronic hemolytic anemia and ischemia.

CLINICAL PRESENTATION

The sickle mutation is located in the β gene, a gene that only becomes active in the later stages of gestation. Since the fetal hemoglobin gene is unaffected, infants who have sickle cell anemia are born without anemia and without the vaso-occlusive problems that are characteristic of the disease. (However, the disease can, and should, be diagnosed in the newborn period to provide appropriate care even be-

fore the disease is clinically apparent.) Symptoms usually begin to emerge as the production of hemoglobin S increases in the third and fourth months of life. On routine examination, although these infants have normal growth and development, they may be noted to be pale and somewhat jaundiced and have splenomegaly. These findings are extremely variable; they may be subtle, and they may easily go unnoticed. It is not unusual for this chronic hemolytic anemia to go undiagnosed for a few years if the blood is not examined. The hemolytic anemia is a chronic and permanent feature of the disease, which is present whether or not the patient experiences acute vaso-occlusive episodes. The physiologic adjustments to this anemia are remarkable, and therefore the anemia is usually well tolerated. These children are generally "healthy" and happy; they are able to participate fully in academic and athletic programs; and they are only periodically and unpredictably stricken by vaso-occlusive episodes.

The most common first acute presentation of the vaso-occlusive tendency of the disease is the *hand-foot syndrome*. These cranky infants present with swollen, tender, hot hand(s) or foot (feet), often a low-grade fever, and leukocytosis. If the child is not known to have sickle cell anemia, a mistaken diagnosis of trauma is common. These irritable children with ischemia of their bones respond well to oral hydration and analgesics; there is no specific therapy. The episode rarely lasts more than a few days and essentially always resolves without permanent morbidity.

As the child gets older, bone ischemia is less likely to be accompanied by signs of inflammation. These "painful crises" present as varying degrees of pain (usually in bone, but sometimes as diffuse abdominal or chest pain) with varying degrees of fever or leukocytosis. Most of these painful episodes can be managed at home by experienced parents, with oral hydration, rest, and analgesics. These children may require hospitalization for parenteral analgesics and hydration.

Although painful crises are the most common of the acute presentations of sickle cell anemia, the most dangerous presentation is infection. The major cause of death in children with sickle cell anemia under 5 years of age is overwhelming pneumococcal sepsis. Despite splenomegaly, these children have functional asplenia with all the risks associated with splenectomy at an early age. This frequently fatal complication may present in the context of an unimpressive febrile illness. The early diagnosis of sickle cell anemia is geared to the prevention and early recognition and treatment of this complication.

DIFFERENTIAL DIAGNOSIS

Sickle cell anemia is in the differential diagnosis of any black or Hispanic infant whose parents either have or do not know whether they have sickle trait, and any black or Hispanic child with a chronic hemolytic anemia. The hemoglobin electrophoresis makes the definitive diagnosis. In infancy, the hemoglobin electrophoresis reveals only hemoglobin S and hemoglobin F; no hemoglobin A is present. In older children and adults there is little hemoglobin F and a predominance of hemoglobin S; there is no hemoglobin A. Other sickle syndromes that are associated with some degree of hemolytic anemia and vaso-occlusion are hemoglobin SC disease and sickle cell thalassemia. These syndromes can also be diagnosed on the basis of the hemoglobin electrophoresis, although in some cases of sickle cell thalassemia family testing may need to be done for clarification.

WORK-UP

History

Because of efficient community-based screening programs that focus on genetic counseling and education of persons with sickle cell trait, family histories may provide important information on the presence of the sickle gene in the family. In older children, the review of systems including questions about jaundice, bone pain, or abdominal pain may be helpful. However, it must be kept in mind that a negative history of symptoms does not exclude sickle cell anemia because there is a wide variation in clinical severity with some patients not experiencing symptoms until late in life.

Physical Examination

The newborn with sickle cell anemia has an entirely normal physical examination. By 4 months of age, slight pallor and icterus may be apparent. By 1 year of age the child usually has splenomegaly although, as noted earlier, this enlarged spleen is no longer functional. Splenomegaly usually disappears by 5 years of age because the spleen undergoes its process of autoinfarction. Height and weight are usually normal during the first 5 to 7 years of life, although the weight is usually below typical normal values thereafter. Signs of puberty are delayed 3 to 4 years in both boys and girls. As described in Chapter 122, the response to chronic anemia usually involves some degree of tachycardia, tachypnea, and cardiomegaly, often with loud systolic ejection murmurs.

Laboratory Tests

Newborn screening of cord blood is an efficient and effective method of identifying infants with sickle cell anemia so they can be started on penicillin prophylaxis as soon as possible. If screening results are unavailable, the pediatrician should re-screen by performing hemoglobin electrophoresis. By about 1 year of age, the child with sickle cell anemia has developed the classic complete blood cell count findings including hematocrit in the 20s, reticulocyte count in the

20s, normal mean corpuscular volume, white blood cell count in the teens, and an elevated platelet count. The peripheral smear shows fragmented cells, long crescent-shaped irreversible sickled cells, target cells, Howell-Jolly bodies, and an occasional nucleated red blood cell. The indirect bilirubin value and lactate dehydrogenase value are elevated. The sickle cell preparation is positive (as is that of the patient's sickle trait parents), and the hemoglobin electrophoresis pattern is classic with a predominance of hemoglobin S and no hemoglobin A. These findings are present regardless of whether the patient is experiencing a "crisis."

TREATMENT

Children with sickle cell disease must receive routine health maintenance, including the standard immunizations. These children need to be seen every few months to monitor baseline laboratory data (e.g., complete blood cell count, reticulocyte count) and intercurrent events. Prophylactic penicillin (125 mg orally twice daily) should be given for the first 5 years of life. In addition, these children should receive pneumococcal vaccine at 2 years of age. Supplemental folic acid (1 mg/d) is particularly useful for children with little fresh green vegetables in their diets. Most importantly, the family should be aware of the importance of seeking medical attention for even "trivial" illnesses. The threat of pneumococcal sepsis is so serious in children younger than 5 years of age that all complaints of fever, poor feeding, irritability, and so forth should be evaluated in person rather than by telephone.

INDICATIONS FOR REFERRAL OR ADMISSION

The following is a list of acute problems that require emergency admission or referral: fever—to rule out sepsis; pneumonia; splenic sequestration crisis—lower than usual hematocrit with larger than usual spleen; aplastic crisis—lower than usual hematocrit with lower than usual reticulocyte count; severe painful crisis; stroke, seizures, or extraordinary headache; visual disturbances; and priapism. The following chronic conditions merit consultation: persistent hip pain; leg ulcers; deteriorating liver, renal, pulmonary, or cardiac function; and pregnancy or contraception issues.

ANNOTATED BIBLIOGRAPHY

Charache S, Dover GJ et al: Hydroxyurea-induced augmentation of fetal hemoglobin production in patients with sickle cell anemia. Blood 69:109–116, 1987. (Clinical application of a drug used to modify the course of sickle cell anemia by augmenting the production of hemoglobin F.)

Cole TB, Smith SJ, Buchanan GB: Hematologic alterations during acute infection in children with sickle cell disease. Pediatr Infect Dis J 6:454–457, 1987. (Clinical study that illustrates the relative uselessness of white blood cell counts or band counts in diagnosing infection in children with sickle cell anemia.)

Embury SH: The clinical pathophysiology of sickle cell disease. Ann Rev Med 37:361–376, 1986. (Excellent discussion.)

Gaston MH et al: Prophylaxis with oral penicillin in children with sickle cell anemia: A randomized trial. N Engl J Med 314:1593–1599, 1986. (Randomized double-blind placebo-controlled clinical trial showing efficacy of penicillin prophylaxis in sickle cell anemia.)

Serjeant GR: Sickle Cell Disease. New York, Oxford University Press, 1985. (Extensively documented yet clearly written and easily readable clinically oriented work covering genetics, prenatal diagnosis, complications, and therapies for the sickle cell syndromes.)

124
Bleeding Disorders in Newborns
Orah S. Platt

One of the most anxiety-provoking clinical situations that pediatricians face is the bleeding newborn. Fortunately, most of these bleeding disorders can be quickly diagnosed using a few basic laboratory tests and they can be managed in a relatively straightforward manner. "Sick" infants bleed as a consequence of their underlying illness (e.g., sepsis and hypoxia) and usually require vigorous support with blood products as well as aggressive therapy for the underlying disorder. In contrast, apparently "healthy" infants who bleed usually have primary defects of coagulation that are either hereditary or immune-mediated. Therapy for these infants is aimed at correcting the specific coagulation defect.

PATHOPHYSIOLOGY

The hemostatic pathways that protect older children and adults from bleeding also apply to the newborn. The basic components are platelets and soluble coagulation factors. In newborns as well as in adults, platelets adhere to damaged endothelium and undergo a release reaction that causes the formation of a platelet plug. The soluble coagulation factors react in a relatively orderly cascade and organize fibrin into a tight clot.

Although there are no significant qualitative differences between clotting in adults and newborns, there are some quantitative differences that must be kept in mind when interpreting laboratory data. The most important quantitative differences result from a relative deficiency of the vitamin K–dependent coagulation factors: factors II, VII, IX, and X. Because deficiencies of factor II (prothrombin) and factor X prolong both the prothrombin time (PT) and the par-

tial thromboplastin time (PTT), factor VII deficiency prolongs the PT, and factor IX deficiency prolongs the PTT, it is easy to understand why normal newborns have prolonged PT and PTT (up to a few seconds over normal for PT and 10 to 15 seconds over normal for the PTT, depending on the individual laboratory norms). In term infants treated with vitamin K at birth, the PT usually approaches adult norms in the first week, while the PTT may take weeks to reach adult values. In preterm infants, the time to achieve normal values is longer.

CLINICAL PRESENTATION

Many normal infants with no coagulation abnormalities are born with petechiae or bruises that result from a difficult labor or delivery. These are essentially healthy newborns whose bleeding symptoms are limited locally to traumatized tissue and do not persist. Interestingly, most infants born with inherited coagulation disorders, such as hemophilia, do not have any spontaneous bleeding problems and are frequently not diagnosed until later in life. However, when these infants are traumatized, significant soft tissue bleeding can occur (e.g., a massive subgaleal hematoma following a difficult delivery). Other infants have been diagnosed following prolonged bleeding at circumcision, although many boys with hemophilia have been inadvertently circumcised during the newborn period without complication.

Oozing from venipuncture sites, showering petechiae, and bloody urine or stools are common in critically ill infants with sepsis, prematurity, hypoxia, necrotizing enterocolitis, and the other serious systemic diseases of newborns. In these infants, bleeding is a complication of the underlying disorder and usually represents a complex combination of plasma factor deficiency and thrombocytopenia, usually either on the basis of consumption, defective production, or both. In contrast, when apparently healthy infants have extensive and evolving petechiae and mucous membrane bleeding, the diagnosis is usually immune-mediated thrombocytopenia.

DIFFERENTIAL DIAGNOSIS

The differential diagnosis of bleeding disorders differs in apparently sick and apparently healthy infants. In critically ill newborns, the likely causes of bleeding are disseminated intravascular coagulation (DIC), peripheral platelet consumption, factor deficiencies associated with liver disease, accidental heparinization, and compromised vascular integrity.

Healthy newborns bleed from local trauma, immune thrombocytopenia, maternal aspirin ingestion, vitamin K deficiency, hereditary clotting factor deficiency, or rarely from decreased platelet production syndromes (thrombocytopenia absent radii [TAR] syndrome, Fanconi's anemia, Wiskott-Aldrich syndrome).

WORK-UP

History

A newborn's past medical history is obviously short. In this case the history focuses on the family and particularly on the mother. A detailed listing of the mother's drug history is crucial. Of particular interest is ingestion of aspirin in the immediate prepartum period. Coumarin is not given to pregnant mothers since it is associated with fetal malformations as well as neonatal bleeding complications. Heparin, on the other hand, can be safely used in pregnancy as it does not cross the placenta.

The mother's medical history is important. Were there any previously affected pregnancies? Does or did the mother have idiopathic thrombocytopenic purpura, lupus, or any other chronic disease associated with defects in immune regulation? Does the mother or any other family member have any bleeding tendency (e.g., menorrhagia, prolonged nosebleeds, bleeding after dental extraction, bleeding after surgery, and hemarthroses)?

Physical Examination

A thorough physical examination will define the clinical nature of the bleeding and will categorize the infant as belonging to either the "sick" or "healthy" groups. Classically, bleeding from thrombocytopenia results in small superficial ecchymoses, sprays of petechiae, and oozing from mucosal surfaces, conjunctivae, retinas, kidneys, or the central nervous system. Soluble coagulation factor deficiencies tend to cause more soft tissue bleeding, umbilical stump bleeding, and prolonged bleeding following surgical procedures.

The upper extremity abnormalities of the TAR syndrome result in a seriously shortened and deformed arm—not just a subtle radiographic finding. Fanconi's anemia, a rare disorder itself, rarely presents with thrombocytopenia at birth. The physical anomalies of this syndrome vary considerably from patient to patient; and although hand and thumb abnormalities are classic findings, they are not always present. Other anomalies that can be associated with this syndrome include congenital cardiac malformations, abnormal kidney position or shape, and microcephaly.

Laboratory Tests

The only laboratory tests that will be needed to evaluate most bleeding newborns are the platelet count, PT, and PTT. These tests need to be interpreted in the context of the normal values for age and degree of prematurity as well as for the possibility for laboratory error.

Platelet Count. The normal platelet count for a newborn is the same as for an adult: greater than or equal to $150,000/mm^3$. However, thrombocytopenia is unlikely to be the primary cause of bleeding unless the platelet count is lower than $50,000/mm^3$. Most automated complete blood cell count machines measure platelet count directly. A fast esti-

mate of platelet count can be done by examining the peripheral smear, multiplying the number of platelets per high-power field by 15,000. For example, about 10 platelets per high power field is roughly a normal platelet count of $150,000/mm^3$. The platelet count may be seriously underestimated if the smear is made from a difficult heel stick because the natural tendency of the platelets is to adhere to the cut heel and not to flow onto the glass slide. In the newborn with thrombocytopenia, it is essential to measure the mother's platelet count.

PT and PTT. These tests measure all of the important clotting proteins except factor XIII. As mentioned earlier, both the PT and PTT are affected by vitamin K deficiency and need to be age corrected. The major pitfalls in obtaining an accurate PT and PTT are too little plasma in the citrated collection tube and too much tissue trauma and time in performing the venipuncture. In an infant whose hematocrit is over 60%, the sample must be collected in a special tube with half the citrate removed. Care must be taken to do a quick and trauma-free venipuncture to avoid contaminating the needle with tissue thromboplastin. Another source of error is contamination of the sample with heparin from an intravenous line.

TREATMENT

The treatment of bleeding newborns obviously depends on the clinical situation and the overall clinical impression and results of screening laboratory data.

Sick Newborns

Decreased Platelets, Increased PT, and PTT. These infants generally have DIC secondary to sepsis, acidosis, hypoxia, and so forth. The major therapy is aimed at treating the underlying condition. Blood product support includes the use of fresh frozen plasma and platelets. These infants typically need a unit of platelets every 12 to 24 hours as well as 10 to 15 mL/kg fresh frozen plasma. In severe cases in which patients continue to bleed despite aggressive replacement, exchange transfusions are sometimes helpful. Heparin therapy is not advised in infants whose major clinical problem is hemorrhage. However, if the DIC is associated with thrombosis (e.g., necrosing digits or skin) heparin therapy is useful.

Decreased Platelets, Normal PT, and PTT. These sick infants usually have platelet consumption without disseminated coagulation. As for the infants with frank DIC, the treatment is aimed at the underlying disorder. These infants usually require frequent platelet transfusions to maintain a relatively safe platelet count of over $50,000/mm^3$.

Normal Platelets, Increased PT, and PTT. These infants are likely to have compromised liver synthesis of coagulation proteins. Typically, these infants also have low albumin levels, sometimes even in the presence of normal transaminase levels. Although parenteral vitamin K should continue to be supplied, plasma infusions are critical to maintain normal hemostasis. The half-lives of some of the coagulation proteins are quite short (hours), and thus infusions need to be repeated frequently in cases of severe liver dysfunction.

Normal Platelets, PT, and PTT. These are compromised infants who have serious intracranial or pulmonary hemorrhage even though they have no demonstrable clotting abnormality. It is postulated that such gravely ill infants have compromised vascular integrity and poor tissue support as a result of their underlying disorder. In this setting, blood component therapy is not likely to make a significant clinical difference.

Healthy Newborns

Decreased Platelets, Normal PT, and PTT. When a vigorous healthy term infant presents with isolated thrombocytopenia, the most likely diagnosis is immune thrombocytopenia. This is a passively acquired disorder in which antiplatelet antibody passes from the mother to the infant in utero. There are two major classes of immune platelet destruction in newborns: isoimmune thrombocytopenia and immune thrombocytopenia due to maternal idiopathic thrombocytopenic purpura.

Isoimmune thrombocytopenia is analogous to Rh incompatibility. The mother has a normal platelet count but is lacking a platelet antigen (usually PLA-1) that is present on the infant's platelets. Fetal platelets enter into the maternal circulation early in the pregnancy and have caused her to produce an antibody that crosses the placenta and destroys the infant's (but not her) platelets. Although most fetuses and infants tolerate their thrombocytopenia very well, some do suffer severe and possibly fatal hemorrhages just before or after delivery. Since most hospitals are not organized to provide emergency platelet antigen testing, the diagnosis of isoimmune thrombocytopenia rests on clinical grounds. Therapy for these infants with platelet counts less than 50,000/mm^3 or with bleeding symptoms consists of a unit of carefully washed maternal platelets, intravenous γ-globulin (1 g/kg/d), prednisone (1–2 mg/kg/d), and a random unit of platelets if platelets from the mother are not available.

Maternal idiopathic thrombocytopenic purpura is an autoimmune disease of the mother in which she produces an antibody that cross reacts with all platelets. The mother is usually thrombocytopenic, but some mothers are able to compensate for the increased platelet destruction and thus have normal platelet counts despite the presence of antiplatelet antibody in the plasma. Symptomatic or severely thrombocytopenic infants of mothers with idiopathic thrombocytopenic purpura should be treated with intravenous γ-globulin, random platelets, and prednisone. If bleeding persists, and the platelet count is unsupportable, exchange transfusion should be performed.

Normal Platelets, Prolonged PT, and PTT. These findings are associated with the *classic hemorrhagic disease of the newborn—vitamin K deficiency.* The routine use of parenteral vitamin K in the delivery room has essentially eliminated this disease. However, some infants are overlooked (especially if there is an emergency at delivery or if the child is not born in a hospital) and become profoundly vitamin K deficient over the first few days of life. Bleeding, if it occurs, usually appears on about the fourth day of life. The treatment involves administration of vitamin K and, if necessary, fresh frozen plasma.

Normal Platelet Count, Normal PT, and Prolonged PTT. This coagulation pattern usually indicates an inherited plasma factor deficiency. In a boy, the likely diagnoses are the X-linked factor VIII or factor IX deficiencies or the autosomal dominant Von Willebrand's disease. In a girl, Von Willebrand's disease is the most likely. As mentioned previously, these disorders rarely cause significant bleeding problems in newborns unless there is trauma. Therapy is usually unnecessary, but in the case of serious bleeding, fresh frozen plasma should be used.

Normal Platelets, PT, and PTT. Hemorrhages in most healthy infants with normal coagulation screening tests are likely due to local trauma or vascular anomalies. Inherited platelet abnormalities are rare, but maternal aspirin ingestion may result in a transient neonatal platelet disorder. If the infant is symptomatic, a platelet transfusion will be necessary. Factor XIII deficiency is a rare condition that results in delayed localized bleeding (e.g., 1 or 2 days following circumcision or from a dry umbilical stump). This factor deficiency can be diagnosed by measuring the specific factor and treated with fresh frozen plasma.

INDICATIONS FOR REFERRAL

Depending on the capabilities of the local nursery, many newborns with bleeding disorders will need to be referred for intensive care management. Interpretation of coagulation data may require consultation, especially if specific factor analyses are required. The management of pregnant women at high risk for delivering infants with bleeding problems should be coordinated with an obstetrician, pediatrician, neonatologist, and hematologist.

ANNOTATED BIBLIOGRAPHY

Avery GB: Neonatology—Pathophysiology and Management of the Newborn, 3rd ed. Philadelphia, JB Lippincott, 1987. (Provides information on almost any topic pertaining to bleeding disorders in the newborns.)

Beardsley DS: Immune thrombocytopenia in the perinatal period. Semin Perinatol 14:368–373, 1990. (Excellent review of recent diagnostic and therapeutic advances in immune thrombocytopenia in newborns.)

Buchanan GR: Coagulation disorders in the neonate. Pediatr Clin North Am 33:203–220, 1986. (Well-presented overview of the pathophysiology and laboratory tests to evaluate bleeding disorders in the newborn.)

Glader BE (ed): Perinatal haematology. Clin Haematol 7(1), 1978. (Provides information on almost any topic pertaining to bleeding disorders in the newborn.)

Oski F, Naiman JL: Hematologic Problems in the Newborn, 3rd ed. Philadelphia, WB Saunders, 1982.

Zipursky A (ed): Perinatal hematology. Clin Perinatol 2(2), 1984. (Provides information on almost any topic pertaining to bleeding disorders in the newborn.)

125

Bleeding Problems in Older Children

Orah S. Platt

Bleeding is one of the most common reasons for referring a child to a hematologist. The symptoms are dramatic, the differential diagnosis is worrisome, and parental anxiety is high.

PATHOPHYSIOLOGY

Platelets are the first line of defense against bleeding. With a breech of vascular integrity, platelets adhere to the damaged endothelium and cause other platelets to aggregate at the local site. Once the primary platelet plug is in place, the soluble coagulation proteins of the plasma respond in organized classical cascade and stabilize the plug to become a firm fibrin clot.

When the platelet count is reduced below approximately 50,000/mm³, small capillary lesions (petechiae) appear and the skin and mucous membranes become more vulnerable to minor trauma.

Normally the megakaryocytes in the bone marrow produce enough platelets to maintain the count above 150,000/mm³. A normal platelet lasts for about 5 days in the peripheral circulation. Thrombocytopenia results if the platelet survival time is reduced to hours or minutes. Under these circumstances, the platelets are usually larger in size than normal (indicating a population of young platelets) and numerous megakaryocytes appear in the marrow. On the other hand, if the marrow is affected by toxin, infiltration, or congenital defect, production will drop and thrombocytopenia will develop. These platelets tend to be small and the marrow may be infiltrated with tumor cells, storage cells, and so forth or else have diminished numbers of megakaryocytes. Since megakaryocytic quantitation is not reliable, it is sometimes necessary to give radiolabeled platelets and determine their survival to determine whether thrombocytopenia is due to increased destruction or decreased production.

CLINICAL PRESENTATION

"Platelet-type" bleeding presents as a mild to severe bleeding tendency characterized by petechiae, mucous membrane bleeding (e.g., from the nose, gastrointestinal tract, genitourinary tract, retina, central nervous system), bleeding from superficial cuts, or superficial skin hemorrhages. Menstrual bleeding can be profuse. In contrast, the soluble coagulation factor deficiencies typically present as hemarthroses of soft tissue and deep muscle hemorrhages.

DIFFERENTIAL DIAGNOSIS

In the child with "platelet-type" bleeding, there are four major diagnostic possibilities: (1) thrombocytopenia, (2) platelet dysfunction, (3) diffuse vasculitis, and (4) von Willebrand's disease. Although more than one of these possibilities may occur at the same time, in general, a platelet count will distinguish between thrombocytopenia and the others.

In otherwise healthy children with the acute onset of isolated thrombocytopenia—the most common diagnosis is idiopathic thrombocytopenic purpura. The major diagnosis to exclude is acute lymphocytic leukemia. In sick, febrile children, the major diagnosis to consider first is meningococcemia.

In the patient with documented thrombocytopenia, the major diagnostic considerations are conveniently classified as either an increased destruction or a decreased production. The thrombocytopenias that result from increased peripheral destruction can be antibody mediated (e.g., idiopathic thrombocytopenic purpura, drug-induced), coincident with localized consumption (e.g., vascular malformation, hemolytic-uremic syndrome, vasculitis) or disseminated intravascular coagulation (DIC), associated with hypersplenism or toxin (e.g., drug, infection).

The hypoproduction thrombocytopenias include infiltrative disease including leukemia, storage diseases, and granulomatous diseases. Acquired or drug-induced aplastic anemia as well as the constitutional bone marrow failure syndromes (e.g., thrombocytopenia absent radii [TAR] syndrome, Fanconi's anemia) are possibilities.

For the child with a hemarthrosis or large soft tissue hemorrhage, the possibilities include one of the hemophilias (factor VIII or IX deficiency in boys; other, less common deficiencies in either sex). Hemarthrosis is unusual in von Willebrand's disease.

Von Willebrand's disease, usually inherited as an autosomal disorder, results in a defective glycoprotein (the von Willebrand factor) responsible for adhesion of platelets to subendothelial surfaces.

It should always be kept in mind that bleeding may not be a hematologic problem but rather a manifestation of child abuse. When purpura presents in a healthy appearing child with a normal hematologic profile, one must also consider the possibility that it is factitious. *Factitious purpura* may be self-induced or caused by someone else. A clue to this diagnosis is its unusual shape or position. These lesions may also result from cupping and coin rubbing.

WORK-UP

History

The history should include a family history of bleeding or platelet disorders. A complete drug and toxin exposure history is important. The timing, distribution, and nature of the bleeding will determine the severity and the degree of chronicity. Fever or other signs of infection may indicate disseminated infection. Systemic symptoms of weight loss, sweating, or bone pain suggest the possibility of bone marrow disease.

Physical Examination

Growth parameters, vital signs, and general assessment will help in establishing the chronicity and the level of concern. The following findings should be noted: pallor, jaundice, petechiae, peripheral thromboses, bruises, fundal hemorrhages, lymphadenopathy, hepatomegaly or splenomegaly, congenital anomalies, and hemarthroses.

Laboratory Tests

Begin with a complete blood cell count (including a platelet count and an examination of the peripheral smear), a prothrombin time (PT), and a partial thromboplastin time (PTT). If everything except the platelet count is absolutely normal, the child is likely to have idiopathic thrombocytopenic purpura. Most clinicians would favor performing a bone marrow aspirate to exclude leukemia at this stage. The techniques for measuring antiplatelet antibody vary and are frequently not helpful in establishing a diagnosis of idiopathic thrombocytopenic purpura in children. *Idiopathic thrombocytopenic purpura is a clinical diagnosis and does not rest on any single diagnostic test, including the bone marrow examination and platelet antibody test.*

If the PT and PTT are elevated in association with thrombocytopenia, the patient is likely to have DIC and must have cultures taken immediately to facilitate therapy.

A prolonged PTT and/or PT without thrombocytopenia suggests the possibility of a coagulation factor deficiency.

Laboratory diagnosis of von Willebrand's disease may be difficult because abnormalities are variable and even individual patients may have variability in their own bleeding profile. The platelet count is normal, whereas the bleeding time and PTT will usually be abnormal.

If the peripheral smear shows fragmented red blood cells, thrombocytopenia, but normal PT and PTT, the he-molytic-uremic syndrome is a possibility. Blood urea nitrogen and creatinine values should be evaluated.

The diagnosis of diseases such as leukemia and storage diseases require expert help and special bone marrow examinations.

TREATMENT

In most pediatric practices, idiopathic thrombocytopenic purpura is the most common acute bleeding disorder that can be treated on an outpatient basis. If the platelet count is greater than $50,000/mm^3$ and the child is not bleeding, he or she should avoid contact sports and ingestion of aspirin and notify the pediatrician of any bleeding episode. In the patient with less than 50,000 platelets/mm^3 who is symptomatic (and has had a bone marrow examination to rule out leukemia), a short course of prednisone (2 mg/kg/d for 10 days, then tapering of the dosage over 10 days) will usually decrease the bleeding tendency even though the platelet count may not change very much or have a sustained elevation. Under special circumstances such as thrombocytopenia presenting in association with varicella, intravenous γ-globulin therapy can be lifesaving. A small proportion ($<25\%$) of children with idiopathic thrombocytopenic purpura are refractory to standard outpatient management and eventually require splenectomy.

If severe bleeding occurs from von Willebrand's disease (e.g., postoperatively), consultation with a hematologist is critical. Some patients may respond to infusions of desmopressin acetate (DDAVP), whereas others will require factor VIII concentrates that are not monoclonal-antibody purified. Ideally, patients with this disorder should be identified preoperatively and undergo a desmopressin challenge test. Most patients have a mild to moderate form of the disease and do not require therapy unless they need surgery, such as for tonsillectomy. Epistaxis, the most frequent manifestation, is treated with local measures (see Chap. 79).

INDICATIONS FOR REFERRAL OR ADMISSION

Any febrile child with thrombocytopenia and petechiae (with or without elevated PT and PTT) should be hospitalized and treated for presumed sepsis. Children with any of the following complicating features should be evaluated in consultation with a hematologist: symptomatic or prolonged thrombocytopenia, neutropenia, myeloblasts on smear, anemia, bone pain, or congenital anomalies.

The sorting out of factor deficiencies usually require the input of a hematologist. The laboratory evaluation is in evolution, and the interpretation of laboratory tests can be difficult. Once a diagnosis of specific factor deficiency is made, the primary pediatrician should work with the hematologist in planning a chronic treatment program with shared responsibilities. Likewise, patients with severe von Willebrand's disease as well as those patients scheduled to undergo operative procedures should be referred to a hematologist. A nephrologist will be helpful in managing the hemolytic-uremic syndrome.

ANNOTATED BIBLIOGRAPHY

Bussel JB. Schulman I et al: Intravenous use of gamma globulin in the treatment of chronic immune thrombocytopenic purpura as a means to defer splenectomy. J Pediatr 103:651–654, 1983. (Describes the beneficial responses of 9 of 12 children with chronic idiothrombocytopenic purpura treated with intravenous γ-globulin.)

Castle V, Andrew M, Kelton J et al: Frequency and mechanisms of neonatal thrombocytopenia. J Pediatr 108:749–755, 1986. (Incidence and etiology data on neonatal thrombocytopenia in a study population of 807 infants admitted to an intensive care unit.)

Naiman J: Disorders of platelets. In Oski FO, Naiman JL (eds): Hematologic Problems in the Newborn, pp 183–215. Philadelphia, WB Saunders, 1982. (Complete discussion of neonatal thrombocytopenia emphasizing diagnosis and management.)

Ruggeria ZM, Zimmerman TS: von Willebrand factor and von Willebrand disease. Blood 70:895–904, 1987. (Good discussion of this disorder.)

Stuart MJ, McKenna R: Diseases of coagulation: The platelet and vasculature. In Nathan DG, Oski FO (eds): Hematology of Infancy and Childhood, pp 1234–1286. Philadelphia, WB Saunders, 1980. (Exhaustive discussion of thrombocytopenia in the pediatric population emphasizing pathophysiology.)

126

Neutropenia

Orah S. Platt

The normal absolute neutrophil count (i.e., mature plus immature neutrophils) varies widely between 1000 and 8000 cells/mm³, depending on age and race. In general, whites have higher neutrophil counts than blacks, and children younger than 10 years of age have lower neutrophil counts than adults. As a rule of thumb, the lower limit of normal neutrophil count is 1500 in white children and 1000 in black children.

Most cases of neutropenia are discovered in the process of evaluating the white blood cell count of a child with an acute febrile illness. Less frequently, neutropenia is identified as an incidental finding in healthy children who have a routine complete blood cell count (CBC). The pediatrician rarely finds neutropenia where he or she expects it—in a patient with recurrent bacterial infections.

PATHOPHYSIOLOGY

Neutrophils are produced in the bone marrow, where they progress from the stem cell stage to the mature neutrophil stage in about 2 weeks. The marrow itself is a reservoir of mature neutrophils that eventually leave to enter the peripheral circulation either to marginate along vessel walls or be swept up with the flowing red cells. The neutrophil has a brief life span of a few hours in the circulation. The control of neutrophil production and distribution is not completely understood but involves a complex interplay between cellular and humoral factors. Neutropenia can be caused by faulty production or maturation in the marrow, increased margination or sequestration in the reticuloendothelial system, or peripheral destruction. The clinical distinction between decreased production and increased peripheral destruction of neutrophils is difficult. There is no neutrophil equivalent of the reticulocyte, nor is there a neutrophil survival test.

The major functions of the neutrophil are to recognize, chase, engulf, and kill bacteria. The major clinical consequence of neutropenia is serious bacterial infection, a complication that is rarely encountered unless the neutrophil count is less than 500 cells/mm³.

CLINICAL PRESENTATION

Although many patients with neutropenia are entirely asymptomatic, there is a pattern of infection that should arouse the pediatrician's suspicion of neutropenia. The tissues most often infected in children with neutropenia are the vulnerable portals of entry of bacteria. These sites are the mouth, skin, lungs, and perianal areas. Gingival and oral mucosal lesions are common and can be the most painful and distressing complication of chronic neutropenia. Recurrent skin abscesses are also seen in patients with neutropenia, although the most common cause of this type of infection is repetitive exposure to *Staphylococcus aureus* in a relatively unhygienic environment. In those rare patients with cyclic neutropenia, a clear-cut pattern of recurrent infections every 2 to 3 weeks is classic.

DIFFERENTIAL DIAGNOSIS

Healthy Children

Infection. Probably the most common cause of isolated neutropenia in otherwise healthy children is infection. The mechanism can be complex—a combination of decreased production (by toxin, antibody, or direct invasion), increased margination (in active reticuloendothelium or infected tissues), and increased peripheral destruction (antibody, drug, or toxin mediated). This type of neutropenia occurs in both viral and bacterial infections. The diagnosis is usually made by observing the resolution of the neutropenia as the infection subsides.

Toxins. Although environmental toxins such as heavy metals, organic compounds, and ionizing radiation can cause neutropenia, the most likely suspects are drugs. Drug reactions causing neutropenia can be direct toxic effects of the drug, hypersensitivity reactions, or antibody mediated. Some of the drugs that have been implicated in neutropenia that are commonly used by pediatricians are trimethoprim-sulfamethoxazole, chloramphenicol, and oxacillin. In most cases the etiology of neutropenia cannot be determined precisely, especially because an intercurrent infection is usually present. However, it is always prudent to stop all medications (even over-the-counter drugs) when neutropenia is present.

Antibody Mediated. As mentioned earlier, drugs and infections have been implicated in provoking antibody-mediated neutropenia. Such premature destruction of neutrophils or their marrow precursors has also been described in children with chronic autoimmune disorders and immunodeficiencies. An occasional case of isoimmune neutropenia in newborns has also been described. These diagnoses are difficult to make because of the technical problems involved in determining and interpreting the presence of antineutrophil antibody.

III Children With Prolonged Neutropenia

Congenital Bone Marrow Failure Syndromes. Although not usually present at birth, some rare congenital bone marrow failure syndromes may present with isolated neutropenia. Where neutrophils are still present (albeit in small numbers) the morphology is often abnormal, with decreased lobulation or dysmorphic granules. These syndromes include Kostman's syndrome, Fanconi's anemia, Schwachman-Diamond syndrome, cartilage-hair hypoplasia, Chédiak-Higashi syndrome, and dyskeratosis congenita. Many of these syndromes have characteristic congenital abnormalities, bone marrow findings, and chromosomal abnormalities.

Immune Disorders. Many of the congenital immunodeficiencies, including the various dysgammaglobulinemias and agammaglobulinemias, are associated with various degrees of neutropenia. The mechanisms can involve both peripheral destruction and decreased production. Interestingly, in some cases, the neutropenia improves with the administration of replacement γ-globulin.

Metabolic Disorders. Several aminoacidurias have been associated with neutropenia. In many of these cases there is megaloblastic maturation reminiscent of vitamin B_{12} or folic acid deficiencies, which can also cause neutropenia in children.

WORK-UP

History

It is important to obtain a comprehensive family and personal history in evaluating the child with neutropenia. The nature and timing of infections in the child and in the family are critical information. Any history of bone morrow failure or chronic blood disorder in the family can be helpful clues, as can be a history of drug or environmental exposure.

Physical Examination

A complete physical examination is necessary in evaluating the child with neutropenia. Plotting of growth parameters and noting any congenital anomalies are important in establishing chronicity and in pointing to some of the congenital syndromes. The examination should include a careful inspection of the mouth, lungs, skin, and perianal areas and palpation of the liver and spleen.

Laboratory Tests

The laboratory evaluation of the child with neutropenia begins with a CBC and an examination of the peripheral smear. Special attention should be paid to the mean corpuscular volume (if increased, one should suspect bone marrow failure or megaloblastosis) and to the morphology of the neutrophil (lobulation pattern, granule morphology). If there is no associated anemia, thrombocytopenia, or neutrophil dysmorphology, and the child appears well, the CBC can be followed two times a week for approximately 6 weeks to determine chronicity and possible cyclicity. If the neu tropenia persists, quantitation of immunoglobulins should be done.

TREATMENT

Well Child With Incidental Neutropenia

Well children with incidental neutropenia must have all drugs stopped and must be checked carefully with twice-weekly CBCs until resolution of the disorder or referral. Parents must be educated that all illnesses and fever must be reported at once.

Fever and Neutropenia

Children with neutropenia and fever are a high-risk group for fulminant sepsis. All children with fever and neutropenia should have a careful physical examination, CBC, cultures, and chest roentgenogram. Any infection must be treated vigorously. A close and careful observation must be maintained if no sign of infection is found. For those patients with absolute granulocyte counts less than $500/mm^3$, parenteral broad-spectrum antibiotics should be administered.

Chronic Neutropenia

No specific therapy is available in most cases of chronic neutropenia. Bone marrow transplantation and growth factor therapy can be used under certain circumstances. Most patients, however, will be managed in a supportive fashion, with particular attention to oral, skin, and perianal hygiene, as well as prophylactic antibiotics in severe cases.

INDICATIONS FOR REFERRAL OR ADMISSION

Sorting out the cause of neutropenia can be a difficult and discouraging task. In an otherwise healthy child, the neutropenia can be monitored twice weekly for approximately 6 weeks after all drugs have been stopped. If the neutropenia has not resolved, a quantitative measurement of serum immunoglobulins may point to an associated immunodeficiency. This result would warrant a referral to an immunologist. However, if the immunoglobulin levels are normal, if a decrease in any other cell lines appears, if there is evidence of failure to thrive, or if there are associated anomalies, the patient should be further evaluated in consultation with a hematologist.

Any febrile or infected child with less than 500 neutrophils/mm³, regardless of the cause of neutropenia, should be hospitalized for extensive culturing and administration of broad-spectrum antibiotic coverage.

ANNOTATED BIBLIOGRAPHY

deAlarcon PA, Goldberg J, Nelson DA, Stockman JA: Chronic neutropenia: Diagnostic approach and prognosis. Am J Pediatr Hematol Oncol 5(1):3–9, 1983. (Detailed discussion of the work-up of the child with chronic neutropenia and a diagnostic approach of differentiating benign and serious forms of these disorders; good bibliography.)

Jonsson OG, Buchanan GR: Chronic neutropenia during childhood, a 13-year experience in a single institution. Am J Dis Child 145:232–235, 1991. (Excellent recent review.)

Lange RD, Jones JB: Cyclic neutropenia. Am J Pediatr Hematol Oncol 4:363–367, 1981. (Excellent review of the clinical manifestations of cyclic neutropenia and its management.)

Oski FO: Neutropenia in children. Pediatr Rev 3:108–112, 1981. (Succinct overview of etiologies, differential diagnoses, normal values, and diagnostic work-up of childhood neutropenia.)

Rogers ZR, Bergstrom SK, Amylon MD et al: Reduced neutrophil counts in children with erythroblastopenia of childhood. J Pediatr 115:746–748, 1989. (Reminder that neutropenia may complicate transient erythroblastopenia of childhood.)

Sadowitz PD, Oski FO: Differences in polymorphonuclear cell counts between healthy white and black infants: Response to meningitis. Pediatrics 72:405–407, 1983. (Demonstrates the differences in neutrophil counts in both healthy and ill black children and white children.)

127

Lymphadenopathy

Orah S. Platt

Almost every child in a typical pediatric practice eventually appears with enlarged lymph nodes. The cervical and inguinal nodes are most commonly involved. Most of these children are simply reacting normally to new environmental antigens and require little more than a limited physical examination. An outline to the approach to the evaluation of the child who has lymphadenopathy is presented here. Cervical lymphadenopathy and other neck masses are discussed in Chapter 84.

Most "normal" palpable lymph nodes are discrete, freely mobile, nontender, and less than 3 mm; these are the nodes commonly referred to as "shotty." There is no uniform definition of lymphadenopathy. It is variously defined as having a diameter of greater than 10 to 25 mm.

PATHOPHYSIOLOGY

The lymph nodes provide the optimum setting for the education and function of lymphocytes of all types. Here, antigens are presented, recognized, and responded to. This process frequently involves lymphocyte proliferation, a reaction that can cause a node to enlarge. Pathologists describe this as *reactive hyperplasia*. This is the situation in most children who have adenopathy in the setting of uncomplicated viral or bacterial illnesses. The node itself sometimes becomes infected, enlarges, and becomes exquisitely tender because it is acutely invaded by neutrophils. Lymph node enlargement can also occur when the node is invaded and destroyed architecturally by malignant cells.

CLINICAL PRESENTATION

Lymphadenopathy is usually a straightforward diagnosis presenting as a mass in a node-bearing region. Since most of these areas are easily accessible to examining fingers and eyes, masses are usually apparent. Rarely, non–lymph node masses appear in these regions and can be confusing. Some of these masses include developmental anomalies such as thyroglossal duct cysts (see Chap. 84). Other masses that can masquerade as nodes include tumors or infections of bone or soft tissue and vascular anomalies. Enlarged nodes in the mediastinum and along the aorta become symptomatic when they impinge on other structures and require various radiographic techniques to be delineated.

A supraclavicular node is especially worrisome since it suggests a malignancy. This may be the "sentinel" node of Hodgkin's disease. Rapidly enlarging, fixed, matted, or hard nodes are fortunately uncommon but are disturbing because they also suggest a malignancy.

DIFFERENTIAL DIAGNOSIS

Since there are so many causes of lymphadenopathy, it is convenient to classify the differential diagnosis into groups. Lymphadenopathy may be generalized or regionalized, and location provides a clue to its etiology. Generalized lymphadenopathy suggests systemic disease. Infection is most common, but the differential diagnosis includes a long list of other conditions such as malignancy and collagen vascular disease. Occipital lymphadenopathy is almost always secondary to a scalp infection, and epitrochlear nodes are often present in cat-scratch disease (see Chap. 207); these are examples of how location of regional nodes may suggest a diagnosis.

Generalized Adenopathy with Fever

When generalized adenopathy with fever is present it usually represents the classic infectious diseases of childhood including cytomegalovirus infection, mononucleosis, chickenpox, rubella, measles, toxoplasmosis, and enterovirus infection. Acute acquired immunodeficiency syndrome and Kawasaki disease should also be considered. These diseases are diagnosed based on their clinical presentation, epidemiology, clinical course, and corroborating laboratory findings.

Generalized Adenopathy Without Fever

Although a low-grade fever may be present, children with generalized adenopathy without fever generally do not appear to have an acute infectious disease. They may have a hypersensitivity reaction such as drug allergy, collagen vascular disease such as juvenile rheumatoid arthritis, or neoplasm such as leukemia or lymphoma.

Localized Adenopathy With Fever

Children with localized adenopathy and fever usually have a localized infection with enlargement of the appropriate draining node or nodes. Viral upper respiratory tract infections account for many of these nodes, although bacteria such as staphylococci and streptococci are common pathogens. The more immunocompromised the host, the greater the possibilities of unusual microorganisms become.

Localized Adenopathy Without Fever

Although children with localized adenopathy without fever may have a rather indolent infection without an obvious local lesion, they are at risk for malignancy such as lymphoma, Hodgkin's disease, or leukemia.

WORK-UP

History

The history should clarify how long the lesion has been present and whether it was associated with any obvious infection. It is important to note if there have been significant systemic features such as weight loss, failure to gain weight, night sweats, and fatigue. Unusual exposure to animals, ingestion of unpasteurized milk, or travel to exotic regions should also be investigated.

Physical Examination

Growth parameters, vital signs, and a general assessment will help in establishing the chronicity and level of concern.

All the node-bearing areas and liver and spleen should be examined, with the size, texture, and tenderness noted. For localized adenopathy, a detailed examination of the appropriate draining region should be done to find the possible source of infection. At the same time, pallor, jaundice, petechiae, or excessive bruises should be noted.

Laboratory Tests

Most children will not require any laboratory studies when adenopathy is found, because the cause is usually obvious. For persistent or particularly worrisome adenopathy, a good initial screening would include a complete blood cell count with differential and platelet count, an erythrocyte sedimentation rate, a mono spot test, a purified protein derivative (PPD), and a chest roentgenogram.

TREATMENT

Most cases of adenopathy are part of a self-limited disease process that requires no treatment. Next in frequency are other common bacterial infections that are either primary, such as lymphadenitis, or secondary to (or associated with) other infections, such as pharyngitis, otitis media, or skin infections, which are easily treated with broad-spectrum oral antibiotics. Penicillin may be used if *Streptococcus* is the likely pathogen. Otherwise, amoxicillin, dicloxacillin, erythromycin, or cephalosporins offer better coverage for other organisms such as staphylococci. Rarely, unusual infections, malignancies, or chronic diseases will require sophisticated diagnostic tests and treatment. The dilemma for the pediatrician is how long to follow an entirely healthy child who has enlarged nodes without an obvious diagnosis.

INDICATIONS FOR REFERRAL OR ADMISSION

The child with an infectious etiology who appears toxic, a child who is immunocompromised, a newborn, or a child in whom the infection is progressing despite outpatient management should be hospitalized and receive parenteral antibiotics.

Ultimately, sorting out the etiology of lymphadenopathy hinges on the lymph node biopsy. Children with the following characteristics should be referred for consultation, and then a decision can be made regarding the need for hospitalization:

- Persistent (usually longer than 2 months) undiagnosed adenopathy
- Enlarging or matted, nontender adenopathy
- Association with worrisome signs and symptoms such as weight loss, failure to thrive, bone pain, sweating during the night, and hepatosplenomegaly
- Association with abnormality in complete blood cell count, purified protein derivative test, or chest roentgenogram
- Association with fever of unknown etiology

It is frequently helpful to consult either an oncologist or an infectious disease specialist (depending on the clinical intuition of the pediatrician) rather than going directly to the surgeon for a biopsy. The medical specialist will be able to work with the surgeon to facilitate the special culturing and handling of the specimen in the pathology laboratory.

ANNOTATED BIBLIOGRAPHY

Altman AJ (ed): Pediatric oncology. Pediatr Clin North Am 32(3), 1985. (Good collection of articles describing the most common childhood cancers having associated peripheral lymphadenopathy.)

Hicks RV, Melish ME: Kawasaki syndrome. Pediatr Clinic North Am 33:1151–1176, 1986. (Comprehensive discussion of this multisystemic disease in which cervical lymphadenopathy is one of the six major diagnostic criteria.)

Knight PJ, Mulne AF, Vassy LE: When is lymph node biopsy indicated in children with enlarged peripheral nodes? Pediatrics 69:391–396, 1982. (Presents guidelines for performing a diagnostic biopsy.)

Knight PJ, Reiner CB: Superficial lumps in children: What, when, and why? Pediatrics 72:147–153, 1983. (Good discussion as to which lumps ought to be regarded as worrisome.)

Lake AM, Oski FA: Peripheral lymphadenopathy in childhood. Am J Dis Child 132:357–359, 1978. (Reviews their 10-year experience with excisional biopsy to determine if clinical features are predictive of histologic diagnosis.)

Marcy SM: Infections of lymph nodes of the head and neck. Pediatr Infect Dis 2:397–405, 1983. (Practical and comprehensive.)

128

Splenomegaly

A. Stephen Dubansky

The spleen is normally palpable in 10% of the pediatric population. Twenty to 30% of healthy newborns, 10% of normal 1-year olds, and 1% to 3% of healthy 18-year olds may have spleens palpable approximately 1 cm below the left costal margin. Pathologic splenomegaly is a relatively uncommon problem. However, when it occurs, splenomegaly can represent a puzzling diagnostic problem and a source of great concern.

PATHOPHYSIOLOGY

The spleen, a major reticuloendothelial organ, consists of masses of lymphocytes, plasma cells, and macrophages (white pulp) associated with an extensive network of Billroth's cords and sinusoids (red pulp). The spleen acts as a filter, a reservoir, an important producer of humoral proteins, and an organ of erythropoiesis.

The normal spleen removes damaged, antibody- or complement-coated, and senescent blood cells from the circulation. It serves as a filter for intravenous particulate antigens. The spleen is a reservoir for one third of the body's platelets. Additionally, the spleen normally contains 25 to 50 mL of blood, as well as plasma proteins such as factor VIII. When enlarged for any reason, the reservoir's capacity of platelets, red blood cells, and white blood cells may increase, resulting in decreases in any or all of these cell lines. The spleen has the primary role in producing antibody to intravenous particulate antigen. It is a major site of synthesis of IgM, properdin, and tuftsin, a polypeptide that stimulates neutrophil chemotaxis. When the child is afflicted by disorders such as thalassemia major or osteopetrosis, the spleen may serve as a site of extramedullary hematopoiesis.

CLINICAL PRESENTATION

First, the enlarged spleen must be differentiated from other left upper-quadrant masses. Confusion occasionally arises when differentiating splenomegaly from nephromegaly (e.g., Wilms' tumor). However, careful palpation reveals that the spleen's upper extent is lost under the left costal margin, and its tip moves caudally during inspiration. A massively enlarged left hepatic lobe may sometimes be confused with an enlarged spleen. Percussion will assist in differentiating the spleen from a floating rib. Commonly, pulmonary hyperinflation and flattening of the diaphragms as seen in reactive airway disease or bronchiolitis may allow the physician to feel an otherwise normal-sized spleen. In differentiating the normal and the pathologically enlarged spleen, one must remember that the spleen may be palpated 1 to 2 cm below the costal margin in a healthy child. Pathologic spleens may also be that size, but they are commonly firm or tender to palpation.

Splenomegaly may develop suddenly or gradually. The spleen may increase, decrease, or remain unchanged in size. The child may be free of any obvious systemic symptoms or may appear acutely or chronically ill. These varying modes of presentation will help clarify the cause of the enlargement. It is most important to differentiate the acutely and transiently enlarged spleen of a viral infection from the chronic splenomegaly that requires further examination and definition.

DIFFERENTIAL DIAGNOSIS

The list of possible diagnoses is long and is composed of common, unusual, and frankly esoteric disorders (see the display, Causes of Splenomegaly). The causes have been grouped in the following categories: infectious, immunologic, congestive, hematologic, malignant, metabolic, and miscellaneous. A detailed discussion of the various possibilities is beyond the scope of this text. The emphasis will be placed instead on a meticulous and thorough history and physical examination and on the minimal laboratory testing usually sufficient to uncover the appropriate diagnostic category if not the specifically responsible disease.

Causes of Splenomegaly

INFECTIOUS

Viral
   Mononucleosis
   Rubella
   Rubeola
   Cytomegalovirus infection
   Herpes virus infection
   Coxsackie virus infection
   Human immunodeficiency virus infection
Bacterial
   Subacute bacterial endocarditis
   Sepsis
   Splenic abscess
   Tuberculosis
   Salmonellosis
   Congenital syphilis
   Tularemia
Fungal
   Histoplasmosis
   Coccidiomycosis
   Protozoal
      Malaria
      Toxoplasmosis
   Parasitic
      Schistosomiasis
      Trypanosomiasis
      Visceral larva migrans
   Rickettsial
      Rocky Mountain spotted fever

IMMUNOLOGIC—INFLAMMATORY

Juvenile rheumatoid arthritis
Systemic lupus erythematosus
Serum sickness
Chronic granulomatous disease
Drug-induced pseudolymphoma (phenytoin)
Rheumatic fever

HEMATOLOGIC

Sickle hemoglobinopathy
Thalassemia major
Hereditary red blood cell membrane disorder
Hereditary red blood cell enzyme disorder
Rh and ABO diseases
Autoimmune hemolytic anemia
Iron deficiency anemia
Osteopetrosis

CONGESTIVE

Portal vein obstruction
Budd-Chiari syndrome
Congestive heart failure
Hemochromatosis
Pericarditis
Chronic hepatitis
Wilson's disease
Cystic fibrosis
Biliary atresia
Sarcoidosis

METABOLIC

Tay-Sachs disease
Gaucher's disease
Niemann-Pick disease
Metachromatic leukodystrophy
Hyperlipoproteinemia, type I
Gangliosidoses
Galactosemia
Wolman's disease
Fructose intolerance

MALIGNANT

Leukemia
Lymphoma, Hodgkin's and non-Hodgkin's
Langerhans cell histiocytosis

MISCELLANEOUS

Idiopathic—normal variant
Splenic trauma
Hemangioma
Hamartoma
Cyst
Fibroma
Lymphangioma
Amyloidosis
Hyperthyroidism

WORK-UP

History

A careful neonatal history may reveal omphalitis or umbilical vein catheterization compatible with a subsequent portal vein thrombosis. Did the mother have an unexplained infection or rash during pregnancy indicating congenital infection (e.g., TORCH syndrome)? A social history may reveal travel to endemic areas of malaria or travel to areas of, or exposure to persons with, typhoid fever, tuberculosis, histoplasmosis, or coccidioidomycosis.

A positive family history is important in clarifying the diagnosis. Were there siblings with neonatal jaundice (ABO or Rh isoimmunization or nonimmune hemolytic anemia)? Is there a family history of jaundice, anemia, early cholecystectomy, or splenectomy (hemolytic anemias)? What is the ethnic extraction (children with Niemann-Pick disease, Gaucher's disease, and Tay-Sachs disease are often Jewish; those with Fabry's disease are often Scandinavian; and those with thalassemia are often Greek or Italian)? What is the race (sickle syndromes occur commonly in blacks and those of Mediterranean descent)? Is there a family history of neurologic disease, retardation, or early unexplained death (lipidoses)? Is there a history of progressive liver disease and neurologic abnormalities (Wilson's disease)? Is there a family history of cystic fibrosis or autoimmune or collagen vascular disease (systemic lupus erythematosus, juvenile rheumatoid arthritis)? Is the child at risk for human immunodeficiency virus infection (although this infection is usually associated with hepatosplenomegaly)?

The past medical history is equally important. Has the child had repeated bouts of otitis media or seborrheic rashes (histiocytosis X)? Is there a history of heart disease (pericarditis, congestive heart failure) or mitral valve prolapse (subacute bacterial endocarditis)? Has the child had hepatitis or previously unexplained jaundice (portal hypertension)? Growth and development must be carefully assessed in ruling out chronic disease in general and the metabolic disease associated with mental retardation in particular. Has there been recent blunt abdominal trauma (subcapsular hemorrhage)?

A careful review of systems is essential. Has there been fever, fatigue, sore throat, or rash (cytomegalovirus or Epstein-Barr virus infection)? Has there been sudden jaundice, pallor, or dark urine (autoimmune hemolytic anemia)? Have there been systemic symptoms compatible with juvenile rheumatoid arthritis? Has there been fever, pallor, fatigue, or bone pain of a gradual onset (leukemia, lymphoma)? Unexplained abdominal or bone pains in black children may indicate Hb SC or Hb S β-thalassemia. Blood in the stool may indicate portal hypertension with varices or hemorrhoids. A history of repeated lower respiratory tract illnesses, diarrhea, and failure to thrive indicates cystic fibrosis as a possible cause. Was the spleen palpable in infancy in an otherwise asymptomatic child (cyst, cystic hygroma, or hemangioma)? Is neonatal or early childhood splenomegaly accompanied by jaundice, hypoglycemia, developmental delay, and cataracts (galactosemia)? Has the child had seizures as may be seen with congenital infection or with hypoglycemia due to fructose intolerance or storage disease?

Physical Examination

A careful examination is as important as the history. Most importantly, does the child appear acutely or chronically ill, or is the splenomegaly an incidental finding in an otherwise normal child? Is this spleen the soft, 1-cm spleen that may be normally palpated in a healthy child or a child recovering from recent viral infection(s)? Is the spleen tender to palpation? A tender and acutely enlarged spleen may indicate subcapsular hematoma or rupture as well as Epstein-Barr virus infection, other infection, or leukemia. Vital signs and growth parameters should be graphed, and any evidence of failure to thrive should be carefully noted.

Head examination may uncover puffy eyelids and pharyngitis seen in Epstein-Barr virus infection or chronic otitis

media as seen in histiocytosis. An eye examination may reveal the conjunctival comma vessels or proliferative retinopathy seen with sickle hemoglobinopathy, the scleral icterus of liver disease or hemolytic anemia, the cataracts of galactosemia, the cherry-red macula of Tay-Sachs disease, or the chorioretinitis seen in congenital infection or visceral larva migrans. Gum hypertrophy may indicate sarcoidosis or monocytic leukemia. The neck must be palpated to rule out masses or lymphadenopathy.

Cardiovascular examination should be concerned with jugular venous distention, heart sounds, murmurs, gallop rhythms, and clicks. Chest observation and percussion may reveal hyperexpansion compatible with the air trapping seen in cystic fibrosis. Auscultation may reveal the fine moist rales of heart failure, the more coarse rales of a pulmonary infiltrate, or the normal breath sounds heard in a child with chronic interstitial disease (e.g., histiocytosis).

The abdomen should be palpated and percussed for masses, hepatomegaly, and ascites. Hepatosplenomegaly may indicate infection, malignancy, congestive condition, storage disease, or heart failure. An anal examination should assess the presence of hemorrhoids. A thorough neurologic examination is vital, especially in diagnosing the metabolic disorders.

Generalized lymphadenopathy should be recorded. It is commonly seen in mononucleosis, histiocytosis, lymphoma, leukemia, juvenile rheumatoid arthritis, pseudolymphoma, and sarcoidosis. Bone and joint tenderness, as well as objective signs of arthritis, should be sought, and when these features are present, juvenile rheumatoid arthritis and leukemia should be considered.

The skin may provide a wealth of information. Pallor with or without jaundice may indicate a hemolytic anemia. Jaundice, telangiectasia, and spider angiomas indicate an underlying liver disease. Petechiae and ecchymoses may point to thrombocytopenia associated with infection or malignancy. Venous distention on the abdomen indicates portal vein obstruction. Seborrheic rashes are seen in histiocytosis. The "blueberry muffin" rash in the newborn invariably indicates congenital infection. Acute monocytic leukemia may be associated with subcutaneous nodules. Skin hemangiomas may be evidence of an associated splenic hemangioma. Signs of nonaccidental trauma should raise concern about a splenic blood collection or cyst. Clubbing of the nails may be seen in cystic fibrosis; splinter hemorrhages may occur in subacute bacterial endocarditis. Chronic and evanescent rashes of many descriptions are seen concomitantly with splenomegaly, and, although their presence may not be diagnostic, their absence is useful negative information.

Laboratory Tests

The aforementioned history and physical examination should both shorten the differential list and decrease the number of laboratory tests necessary to make the diagnosis. Ordering all possible laboratory tests is invariably expensive, painful, and unnecessary. A complete blood cell count, platelet count, reticulocyte count, sedimentation rate, carefully observed peripheral smear, Monospot or Epstein-Barr viral capsid IgM test, aspartate aminotransferase (SGOT) determination, bilirubin test, and chest roentgenogram are appropriate screening tests in a situation in which the history and physical examination do not alone clarify the diagnosis.

The results of the preliminary screening tests may indicate the need for further, more specific testing. Cytomegalovirus IgM antibody test, urine culture for cytomegalovirus, TORCH titers, PPD skin test, fungal serologic studies, blood cultures, stool culture and hematest, urinalysis for reducing substances, full liver chemistries, ceruloplasmin, antinuclear antibody test, Coombs' test, sickle cell preparation and hemoglobin electrophoresis, skull and long bone x-rays, and sweat chloride test may be indicated. The screening tests and the more specific laboratory studies combined with a thoughtful history and physical examination will make the diagnosis or rule out most of the possibilities.

MANAGEMENT

The clinical appearance of the patient rather than the degree of splenomegaly should dictate patient management. Mild splenomegaly in the absence of other symptoms or positive physical findings is usually related to a transient viral illness. Viral-induced splenomegaly may last for 6 to 8 weeks, but the spleen does not usually increase in size during this time. The asymptomatic child should be reexamined every 2 weeks until resolution of the splenomegaly. Any increase in spleen size or the development of any related symptoms should prompt the physician to repeat the screening laboratory tests immediately. In the presence of moderate or massive splenomegaly, the child should refrain from contact sports, and both the child and parent should be warned about the rare complication of splenic rupture.

The child with massive splenomegaly, despite an otherwise normal history and physical examination, should have a more thorough work-up. Any child with hypersplenism (splenic trapping and destruction of one or more cellular blood elements by the enlarged spleen) also requires immediate referral. It is clear from the list of etiologies that few of the diagnoses are themselves emergent problems. However, the child with sickle hemoglobinopathy and sequestration crisis, autoimmune hemolytic anemia, malignancy, sepsis, subacute bacterial endocarditis, Rocky Mountain spotted fever, serum sickness, congestive failure, or acute trauma requires immediate referral or treatment.

The otherwise normal child followed for 8 weeks without resolution of mild or moderate splenomegaly also requires further evaluation. Because of the usually chronic nature of the underlying disorder, these patients rarely require hospitalization. Their evaluations are most appropriately done by the pediatric hematologist, who is experienced in pursuing the work-up of those few patients with diagnostic enigmas whom the generalists refer. With the aid of the specialists in metabolic and gastrointestinal disorders, the hematologist may use skin, liver, rectal, or bone marrow biopsy, upper gastrointestinal tract films, splenic ultrasound examination, conventional or SPECT radionucleotide liver-spleen scan, and urine collections to rule out metabolic disease to define this small number of patients with chronic and pathologic splenomegaly.

ANNOTATED BIBLIOGRAPHY

Boles ET, Baxter C, Newton W: Evaluation of splenomegaly in childhood. Clin Pediatr 2:161, 1963. (Retrospective 12-year analysis in surgical patients with splenectomy, portal hypertension, and abdominal neoplasms.)

Eichner ER, Witfield CL: Splenomegaly: An algorithmic approach to diagnosis. JAMA 246:2858, 1981. (Thorough algorithm for causation of acute and chronic splenomegaly.)

McIntyre OR, Ebaugh FG: Palpable spleens in college freshman. Ann Intern Med 66:301, 1967. (Survey of the prevalence of splenomegaly in college students.)

McNicholl B: Palpability of the liver and spleen in infants and children. Arch Dis Child 32:438, 1957. (Prevalence of splenomegaly in the general pediatric population.)

Odom L, Tubergen D: Splenomegaly in children. Postgrad Med 65:191, 1979. (Concise, well-done review of the general problem.)

Stockman JA: Splenomegaly: Diagnostic overview. In Pochedly C, Sills RH, Schwartz AD (eds): Disorders of the Spleen: Pathophysiology and Management, pp 217–238. New York, Marcel Dekker, 1989. (Presents current diagnostic approach, including a discussion of diagnostic imaging.)

18

MUSCULOSKELETAL AND TRAUMATIC PROBLEMS

129

Developmental Dysplasia of the Hip (Congenital Dislocation of the Hip)

Lorin M. Brown

Developmental dysplasia of the hip (DDH) has replaced the term *congenital dislocation of the hip* (CDH) in an attempt to connote its varied pathologic conditions. It is divided into four major entities: (1) complete congenital dislocation of the hip, in which the femoral head is totally removed usually superiorly and posteriorly from the acetabulum (Fig. 129-1); (2) subluxation in which the femoral head is partially dislocated; (3) unstable in which there is a dislocatable or subluxable hip (i.e., the hip can be pushed usually superiorly and posteriorly out from under its acetabular coverage); and (4) other dysplasias of the hip joint, such as acetabular dysplasia. With this deformity, the acetabulum is flattened and elevated laterally in its coverage of the femoral head but the femoral head may or may not still sit well in the anatomic socket. At birth these cases may not be detected and the physical examination may be normal. Therefore, the hips must be repeatedly checked by the pediatrician during the first 2 years of life for late presentation of abnormal physical findings.

The physical signs of DDH do not have to be present at birth, or if they are present at birth they may later disappear. If not detected immediately at around the time of birth, most cases of DDH can be identified by 6 months of age. In late-onset DDH, the first detectable sign of dislocation appears many months after birth. Some cases of DDH, and especially acetabular dysplasia, cannot be physically detected until the second year of life or even later. It is important that the correct diagnosis be made as early as possible to allow for early treatment and thus a better end result.

PATHOPHYSIOLOGY

The reported incidence of dislocated hips varies between 1 to 11/1000 live births for dislocated hips and between 8 to 12/1000 live births for unstable dislocatable hips at birth. After 1 week of life, the incidence of DDH is reduced to 1/1000 because most unstable and some dislocated hips stabilize spontaneously during the first few days or week of life. Females are affected four times as often as males, and the left hip is affected 10 times as often as the right hip.

The cause of DDH is multifactorial and is not fully understood. Heredity is an important component. As many as one third of siblings will have an unstable hip if one parent and one other child have had an unstable hip. Another major etiologic factor is intrauterine posture. A term baby born in a breech position has a 14-fold increased likelihood of having a complete DDH. Simple capsular laxity is also believed to play a major etiologic role.

CLINICAL PRESENTATION

The infant who has a full DDH (i.e., with a dislocated hip) will present with either an adduction contracture of the hip or, more commonly, no overt physical findings. Developmental dislocation of the hip has no associated pain. There may be a calcaneovarus, equinovarus, or a calcaneovalgus posture of the feet. If the child is of walking age, a Trendelenburg limp will be present with a complete DDH. Later in life, associated degenerative arthritis may cause an antalgic gait.

DIFFERENTIAL DIAGNOSIS

The most important diagnosis to differentiate from DDH in the newborn is septic arthritis of the hip. Pus distends the

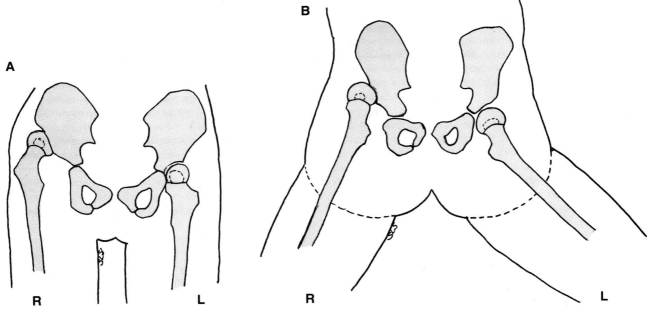

Figure 129-1. (**A**) Drawing of anteroposterior projection of right dislocated hip. (**B**) Drawing of the patient in froglike position showing right dislocated hip.

capsule, resulting in a subluxation or dislocation of the femoral head. The clinical findings are similar to those found with DDH except that pain will usually also be present and the infant will cry with motion of the hip (e.g., during diaper changes). Other diseases or congenital anomalies such as a congenital absence of the proximal femur will increase mobility of the hip joint on examination. A discoid meniscus, generalized joint laxity about the knee, or the snapping of the tensor fascia lata over the greater trochanter may also imitate the feel or sound of a dislocating hip. Later in life, a progressive DDH can occur with paralytic diseases such as cerebral palsy or spina bifida. In these diseases, the imbalance of the muscles about the hip will cause the hip to be progressively deformed and pulled out of the joint.

CLINICAL EXAMINATION

From birth until about the age of 3 months is the most opportune period in which to find the two classic signs of DDH: the *Ortolani sign* and the *Barlow sign*. The Ortolani (Fig. 129-2A) maneuver is performed with the hips held in 90 degrees of flexion. Each hip is tested independently while the opposite side of the pelvis is stabilized. The hip is first gently abducted while at the same time gentle pressure is placed on the greater trochanter to push the femoral head forward into the acetabulum (i.e., relocated), but when released, the femoral head again moves out of the acetabulum. If a sound is audible, which is often the case, it is actually that of a "thump" rather than the commonly de-

scribed "click." The Barlow maneuver (Fig. 129-2B) is positive when the hips are held in 90 degrees of flexion and pressure is applied over the lesser trochanter while adducting the hip, forcing the femoral head out of the acetabulum. When the pressure is released, the dislocatable hip usually returns to its acetabular position. In both supine and prone positions, the child with a complete dislocated hip may have asymmetric skin creases of the thighs. This finding may also be seen in normal children and is thus not pathognomonic of DDH. With unilateral DDH, the *Galeazzi sign* may be observed. With the child lying supine, the hips are flexed to 90 degrees and the knees are almost completely flexed. If

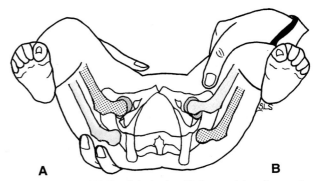

Figure 129-2. (**A**) Ortolini sign—with force of two fingers the dislocated hip is pushed into the acetabulum to the reduced position (*dotted femur*). (**B**) Barlow sign—with force of thumb the lax hip is dislocated out of the acetabulum to the dislocated position (*dotted femur*).

positive, the affected side will show an unequal shortened height between the knee joints because of shortening on the dislocated side. The femoral head is dislocated from the acetabulum (usually posteriorly) and will cause the leg on the dislocated side to appear shortened. This is termed a *positive Galeazzi test*. It is important to know that the pelvis must be held square to the table or this test is unreliable. After the age of 3 months, as the capsular tissue and ligaments about the hip tighten, there is limitation of motion about the hip. The fully mobile flexible infant becomes more like the adult with a decrease in range of motion of the joints. In the child with a dislocated hip, the adductor muscles become tightened and there is marked limitation of abduction of the dislocated hip. It is again stressed that absence of this sign in the young infant does not eliminate a diagnosis of dislocated hip, because without tightening of these structures there is no decrease in the limitation of motion. Moreover, as the hip becomes tighter and more limited in motion, the initial signs of Ortolani and Barlow disappear because the hip is held rigidly in its dislocated or subluxated position. Another sign is that of *telescoping*. In DDH, the femoral head and shaft can be pushed to and fro with the hip held in 90 degrees of flexion. This motion is due to the laxity of the hip capsule.

Another important aspect of the physical examination is that of the tightness of the hamstrings. In the child with DDH, the hamstrings are lax and allow a full extension of the knee when the hip and the leg are held in flexion and abduction in external rotation. Thus, if the knee can be completely extended, it is strongly suggestive that the hip is dislocated from the acetabulum (Fig. 129-3). If, however, the femoral head is in the anatomic acetabulum, the hamstrings should be firm with extension of the knees. Even in the congenitally lax-jointed child, there should still be some "check" to full extension of the knee by the hamstrings.

In the child over 18 months of age who is walking, *limping* is another sign of pathology. This is termed a *Trendelenburg gait*. Because the mechanical advantage of the hip joint is lost by the superior displacement of the pivot (femoral head) from the fulcrum (acetabulum), the abductor muscles of the hip joint become shortened, and therefore lax and weakened. This causes the pelvis to drop on the side opposite of the dislocation. Thus, as the child stands on the dislocated hip, the pelvis tilts downward on the opposite side because of the laxity and weakness of the abductor muscles on the dislocated side. The severity of the limp is compounded by the shortened leg. When both hips are dislocated, there is a bilateral Trendelenburg sign present without a leg length discrepancy. This results in a duck-type *waddling gait*. Congenital subluxation may also cause a Trendelenburg gait when the child is tired and the abductors are fatigued.

WORK-UP

The work-up for congenital dislocation or subluxation of the hip is relatively simple. Except in the immediate newborn period when a roentgenogram may be deferred if the physical findings are minor (e.g., a click only), an anteroposterior pelvis roentgenogram should be used whenever there is any reason to question the physical diagnosis. This view is usually adequate to identify pathology. The older the child, the more reliable will be this examination. The anteroposterior roentgenogram should be taken with the hips in neutral position to demonstrate whether the femoral head lies within the acetabulum, is partially dislocated, or is completely dislocated. The acetabular index is a measure of the covering of the acetabular roof. With dysplasia, this index will increase. Less than 28° is considered normal. With varying amounts of dysplasia, the angle progresses toward 45°. Other lines may be technically drawn to prove the positioning of the femoral head, but the radiographic positioning can usually be seen when the anatomy is understood without the need for drawing quadrants. Another useful sign is the *teardrop sign:* this is the distance from the medial metaphyseal side of the femoral neck to the lateral side of the medial wall of the acetabulum. This should be symmetric between the two hips provided both hips are normal. Asymmetry indicates subluxation or complete dislocation of one hip. The frog lateral view of the hips is useful to determine if a subluxed or dislocated hip will reduce into the acetabulum in the abducted position. Static nonstressed and dynamic ultrasonography has become a useful tool to limit

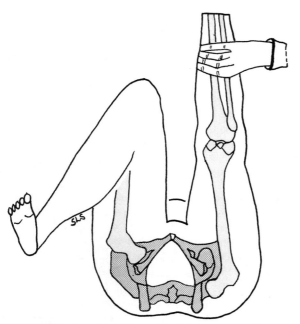

Figure 129-3. Lax hamstrings with full extension of the leg, suggesting a dislocated hip.

the number of roentgenographs in identifying and following DDH. Standard x-rays may be unreliable in the newborn period because of the limited ossification. Ultrasound can visualize all pelvic structures, and may even show pathology when there are no physical findings of DDH. Thus, the role of ultrasound in screening newborns at high risk for DDH is promising, but needs to be better defined. When performed by a skilled radiologist, ultrasound examination will show reduction, interposition, and acetabular coverage of the femoral head. Later, with treatment, magnetic resonance imaging or arthrography may be necessary to decide if there is any interposed tissue in the acetabulum. Computed tomography is another useful test if the diagnosis is questionable. Standard tomograms are occasionally useful to delineate the pathology; however, the simpler the test, the less the amount of radiation exposure the child receives. The more sophisticated tests should be reserved for the puzzling situations.

TREATMENT

Initially, treatment in the newborn nursery may consist of double or triple diapers to abduct the hips for a few days until the child can be reevaluated or examined by an orthopedist. This allows for a gentle initial stretch of the hips and adductor muscles and lessens the chances of avascular necrosis. The newborn is flaccid, and not much force is needed. However, once the infant has gained strength and can adduct his hips, the treatment by diapers is of no benefit. Acetabular dysplasia is treated by the orthopedic surgeon usually for an index over 28° if there is asymmetry between the hips. Some surgeons prefer to wait for an index of over 30° or possibly 35° if both hips are the same, but most surgeons will treat at a lower index if only one hip is involved. It is relatively easy to treat dysplasia in newborns, and waiting for a spontaneous resolution may not be wise because later the treatment becomes more difficult and the outcome may not be as favorable. These children, as well as those with dislocated hips, may be placed in an abduction Frejke pillow or a Pavlik harness. These are both safe means of treatment, whereas the metal types of abduction splints lead to a much higher incidence of avascular necrosis of the hip. Avascular necrosis, however, may develop no matter how careful or gentle the treatment. In acetabular dysplasia and DDH, the abduction device is used to maintain a safe concentric reduction of the femoral head until the capsular tissue has contracted to maintain the hip joint and a full acetabular coverage over the femoral head has developed.

If little or no acetabular dysplasia is present, minimal treatment is required for a simple *dislocatable* hip. Usually 2 months of bracing is sufficient to maintain a perfect reduction of the dislocatable femoral head. Developmental dysplasia of the hip found at birth will require between 6 and 12 months of bracing. Almost the same amount of time is required for acetabular dysplasia to resolve, but, some-times, a period greater than 1 year is necessary. When the dislocation is found beyond the newborn period, the child will require more time in a brace. A rule of thumb—the length of time of bracing is the age in months of the infant plus 9 to 12 months. After about 18 months of age, the child is usually too old for closed conservative treatment with bracing. Studies have shown that this age limit can be extended to 24 to 36 months of age, but the time required in the brace or harness for resolution of the problem is significantly increased.

Children older than the age of 2½ to 3 months discovered to have a dislocation or severe subluxation of the hip require traction to stretch the ligaments and neurovascular structures first to allow for a safe reduction of the femoral head into the acetabulum without increasing the risk of avascular necrosis. This traction may take from 1 week to months depending on the situation. The femoral head should be stretched down to below the triradiate cartilage center line to allow for an easy reduction of the femoral head into the acetabulum without undue stretch on the femoral vessels. The child is then taken to the operating room and placed under general anesthesia for an adductor tenotomy, followed by a closed reduction and the application of a spica cast. In the spica cast, it is essential that the child be placed in the safe "human position" to maintain the femoral head in the acetabulum and not overstretch the hips into abduction. This avoids new stress and compression of the vascular structures going to the femoral head. The human position, unlike that of the froglike position in which the legs are each forced into abduction of 90 degrees, limits the range of abduction to gravity force only.

The usual treatment for the child older than the age of 1½ to 2 years is an open reduction with an innominate or femoral osteotomy to replace the femoral head into the acetabulum. It is sometimes possible to obtain a closed reduction of the hip and later proceed with only an innominate or femoral osteotomy. It is desirable if a concentric reduction is obtained because the less surgery that is done about the femoral head the better the child's chances of avoiding an avascular necrosis of the hip. In the older child, the use of an Atlanta abduction brace may be necessary to maintain abduction and allow gait.

In a child with septic arthritis that caused the dislocated hip, the pus should be drained from the joint. Aspiration of the hip joint is not adequate and open drainage is required followed by intravenous therapy with antibiotics. Dislocations due to neuromuscular diseases such as cerebral palsy or myelomeningocele will require tendon lengthenings as indicated or even tendon transplantations to help rebalance the muscles about the hip and to try to maintain reduction of the hip if possible with osteotomies.

All children treated for DDH must receive regular and careful follow-up because not only may an apparently "cured" hip redislocate or subluxate but also the contralateral "normal" hip may, in the future, manifest joint abnormalities. Moreover, even the successfully treated hip may be prone to develop osteoarthritis.

ANNOTATED BIBLIOGRAPHY

Asher MA: Screening for congenital dislocation of the hip, scoliosis and other abnormalities affecting the musculoskeletal system. Pediatr Clin North Am 33(6), 1986. (Clinical discussion of acetabular dysplasia and its role in hip disease.)

Brown LM, Salter R: Examination of the lower extremities in the child: Part II. In Post M (ed): Physical Examination of the Musculoskeletal System, chap 10. Chicago, Year Book Medical Publishers, 1986. (Detailed and well-illustrated text.)

Brown LM, Sharrard WJW: Examination of the lower extremities in the child: Part I. In Post M (ed): Physical Examination of the Musculoskeletal System, chap 9. Chicago, Year Book Medical Publishers, 1986. (Detailed and well-illustrated text.)

Dunne KB, Clarren SK: The origin of prenatal and postnatal deformities. Pediatr Clin North Am 33(6), 1986 (Excellent illustrations of the Ortolani and Barlow test.)

Hensinger RN: Neonatal Orthopaedics, chap 10. New York, Grune & Stratton, 1981. (Specific and well written.)

Salter R: Textbook of Disorders and Injuries of the Musculoskeletal System, 2nd ed. Baltimore, Williams & Wilkins, 1983. (Excellent overview text of pediatric orthopaedics.)

Sharrard WJN: Pediatric Orthopedics and Fractures, 2nd ed. Oxford, Blackwell Scientific Publication, 1979. (Complete and well-documented.)

130

Toeing-in and Torsional Deformities

Edward Sills

Torsional deformity including, most commonly, in-toeing, must be understood in the context of the natural history, the site of involvement, the age of the child at the time of discovery, and the degree of disability.

During postnatal life, both the femur and tibia normally undergo a process of external rotation. If the normal processes of external rotation are interfered with by genetic or by environmental factors, the internal rotational postures will persist and will thus become one of the various deformities discussed in this chapter.

DIFFERENTIAL DIAGNOSIS

Torsional deformity of the lower extremity can occur because of an abnormality at any site between the foot and the hip. Some abnormalities are uncomplicated, occurring at a single level, whereas others are more complex. Multiple deformities may compensate each other as internal femoral

torsion and external tibial torsion, whereas others may be additive. An example of the latter occurs when mild femoral anteversion, internal tibial torsion, and metatarsus adductus combine to produce severe in-toeing. The major challenge to the examiner is to locate the site or sites of abnormality and to assess the degree of torsional deformity at the involved level.

PHYSICAL EXAMINATION

Most torsional deformities are present at rest. A dynamic deformity due to a muscular or neuromuscular disorder occasionally appears and is evident only with muscle activity. This discussion will be limited to those that are apparent at rest.

When examining the child, the physician should specifically assess the angle of gait, the excursion of hip rotation, the thigh−foot angle, and the shape of the foot.

The *angle of gait* is best defined as the angle between the line of progression (i.e., the direction in which the child is walking) and the axis of the foot. Most children and adults walk with their feet somewhat externally rotated. When there is any persistent internal gait or an external gait angle in excess of 30°, an abnormality exists. Most commonly, the problem is that of *in-toeing*. In-toeing tends to be more apparent in a tired child in whom fatigued mechanisms of compensation allow the underlying malrotation to become apparent.

Hip rotation is easiest to measure with the patient prone, the knees flexed to 90°, and the muscles relaxed. The legs are allowed to fall into full internal rotation after which the physician can measure the maximal internal rotation of the hip, first on one side and then on the other. Internal rotation is the angle between the vertical and the axis of the tibia when the hip is maximally internally rotated. External rotation is assessed in a similar manner. In the newborn, because of both the lateral orientation of the acetabula and the external hip rotation contracture induced by intrauterine positioning, external rotation and femoral neck anteversion are at their peak. The full-term newborn has an external rotation of close to 90°. This diminishes considerably as the more adult anterolateral positioning of the acetabula occurs. By childhood, external rotation gradually decreases to the extent that internal and external rotation are virtually comparable. Internal rotation is normally less than 60°. Femoral neck anteversion increases as the degree of internal rotation increases above normal. Once internal rotation exceeds 80°, there exists a severe femoral neck anteversion.

Tibial torsion is best measured by noting the angle between the axis of the foot (a line from the second toe to the midpoint of the heel) and the axis of the thigh when the prone patient is relaxed with the knee and ankle each at 90°. Medial or internal torsion of more than 10° in the infant indicates internal tibial torsion. Any medial rotation after 2 years of age indicates internal tibial torsion because the normal thigh—foot angle is 10 to 20° externally rotated. External rotation beyond 30° connotes external tibial torsion.

The bottom of the *foot* is examined with the child prone. Any convexity of the lateral border of the foot is indicative of *metatarsus adductus (varus)*.

METATARSUS ADDUCTUS

The most frequently diagnosed cause of in-toeing in infancy is metatarsus adductus (varus) or toeing-in of the forefoot. Metatarsus adductus (varus) is often bilateral and is usually due to abnormal intrauterine positioning. In the more common, supple form, the mild flexible deformity resolves spontaneously and requires no treatment other than passive stretching. If the forefoot is rigid and cannot be easily corrected with gentle manipulation of the forefoot with each diaper change, orthopedic assistance is usually required by 3 to 4 months of age. This persistent rigidity is often associated with internal tibial torsion and foot eversion. Rapid correction, usually in less than 1 month, can be effected by use of corrective long-leg casts. This can usually be accomplished either with a single application of a cast or with two serially abducted casts. Some orthopedists believe that the correction is best maintained with the use of outflared or reversed-last shoes after the casts are removed. If, following correction of the varus forefoot, there is a persistent internal tibial torsion, it can be treated with Denis Browne night splints. This latter treatment should not be applied to uncorrected metatarsus varus because the valgus part of the splint is exerted on the hindfoot as well as on the forefoot. If metatarsus varus persists and is not recognized until after 2 years of age, the deformity may be sufficiently "fixed" as to make attempts to correct the forefoot deformity force the heel into a slewfoot heel valgus. In such circumstances it may be appropriate to consider correctional intermetatarsal soft tissue releases. In the rare situation of a delay of diagnosis until school age, osteotomies may be required to correct the metatarsus varus. There is no indication that simple tendon release in the pretoddler is appropriate.

INTERNAL TIBIAL TORSION

Internal tibial torsion without metatarsus adductus (varus) is the most frequently diagnosed basis of in-toeing in the child who has begun to walk. It should be observed over time because most children self-correct over time. If the deformity is greater than 40° and it persists after the child has fully ambulated for about 6 months, the commonly accepted practice is to initiate splinting. This practice is sometimes deferred because of the danger that is presented by the action of the splints, which tends to force the feet into abduction and which can cause genu valgum and can also accentuate femoral neck anteversion. The child's usual everyday shoes are attached to a small bar at bedtime, with the side

or sides to be corrected set at an external rotation of 30°. Treatment is discontinued once the thigh—foot angle is 10° externally rotated. This usually occurs within a 9- to 15-month period. If genu valgum (knock-knee) and foot pronation are present, active night bar treatment is best deferred because this treatment tends to worsen the genu valgum and foot pronation. There is no indication that an initiation of night bar treatment beyond 3 years of age is beneficial. There have been no published studies to indicate that corrective shoes, wedges, or twister cables have any benefit in this disorder. A knowledge of biomechanical principles convinces me that a skeptical attitude toward the use of these devices in this disorder is warranted.

INTERNAL FEMORAL TORSION AND FEMORAL NECK ANTEVERSION

Internal femoral torsion and excessive femoral neck anteversion is the cause of in-toeing gait most often diagnosed after 3 years of age. Whereas the normal child has comparable internal and external hip rotation by this age, a child with this disorder has greater than 30° more internal than external hip rotation. It is a disorder that is usually bilateral and is seen most frequently in girls. After the age of 6 or 7 years, the deformity is compensated for by external tibial torsion. There is absolutely no justification for the use of any devices, splints, special shoes, wedges, twister cables, or casts to treat this "disorder." Orthopedic and pediatric studies have shown that none of these approaches is associated with outcomes better than the outcome of those left untreated. Although some youngsters with this condition experience quadriceps muscle cramps in the first decade and knee pain in adolescence, there are no data to support the contention that this condition leads to degenerative arthritis or to a functional disability. The exceedingly rare child, who is dysfunctional because of more than 90° internal hip rotation and severe anteversion, can undergo correction only with a major surgical derotational femoral osteotomy, a procedure that is rarely recommended.

The commonly offered advice to "sit like an Indian" or to "sit in a tailor position" is useful, not because of a direct therapeutic benefit but merely because it discourages the habit of sitting in a "W" or "reverse tailor" position, which tends to maintain the soft tissue contracture that holds the hip in internal rotation. This tends to increase fatigue in the responsible quadriceps muscles, which may, in turn, produce minor discomfort.

INDICATIONS FOR REFERRAL

Since most infants and young children with torsional deformity require no active treatment because their in-toeing will resolve spontaneously, referral should be judiciously infrequent. There are theoretical concerns, in fact, that unnecessary treatment may induce "overcorrection" as the self-correction is taking place. The rare youngster with persistent, rigid, nonflexible metatarsus adductus (varus) may benefit from a short course of casting, and the rare school-aged child with undiagnosed metatarsus adductus may require surgery. The child between 18 and 36 months of age with progressing internal tibial torsion is benefited by a night splint or bar, although overcorrection may accentuate femoral neck anteversion. The child who has internal femoral torsion with femoral anteversion does not benefit from the use of various devices. In view of the meager evidence that, with the few exceptions noted earlier, any intervention provides outcomes superior to those achieved spontaneously, there should be a general reluctance to subject children to the fashionable but unproven costly and inappropriate therapy with nonsurgical devices. The anxieties of parents and grandparents are better addressed with careful education than with unneeded appliance prescriptions.

ANNOTATED BIBLIOGRAPHY

Fabry G, MacEwen G, Shands A: Torsion of the femur: A follow-up study in normal and abnormal conditions. J Bone Joint Surg [Am] 55:1726, 1973. (Comprehensive discussion with a broad perspective of the major authorities.)

Salenius P, Vankka E: Development of the tibiofemoral angle in children. J Bone Joint Surg [Am] 57:259, 1975. (Elucidating guide to comprehending a dynamic process.)

Staheli L: Torsional deformities in children. J Cont Ed Pediatr 20:11, 1978. (Excellent perspective and good orientation to basic mechanisms with effective use of illustrative photographs.)

131

Bow Legs and Knock Knees

Edward Sills

In the normal course of development, infants have some degree of genu varus or bow leg until about 1 to 1½ years of age, at which time mild overcorrection spontaneously results in minimal genu valgus or knock knees. The tibiofemoral angle, as measured on a roentgenogram, is usually in excess of 15° of varus at birth; it approaches 0° in the middle of the second year; and it proceeds to as much as 10° of valgus by the third birthday. It gradually approaches the "normal" 5° of valgus by school age and remains relatively unchanged thereafter. Extreme bilateral or *any* unilateral genu varus is rare. Marked valgus is less rare and is often associated with an overweight child. In the child who clinically appears to exceed the limits of physiologic bowing (varus) or knock knee (valgus), roentgenograms should be obtained to ascertain whether there is an underlying condition that requires treatment to prevent a permanent deformity. The normal developmental pattern of early bow leg, transition to knock knee, and ultimate balanced straightening should be considered before subjecting a youngster with a moderate deformity to unnecessary investigation and treatment.

BOW LEG

The two most important causes of pronounced bow leg deformity are tibia vara (Blount's disease) and rickets.

Blount's Disease

Blount's disease, also termed *osteochondrosis deformans tibiae,* occurs in two forms: the infantile, bilateral progressive form and the milder juvenile (or adolescent) type, which is most often unilateral and usually appears late in the first decade. The infantile form is much more frequently encountered than the juvenile (adolescent) form. Blount's disease should be ruled out in any child older than 2 years of age with a persistent, unilateral or bilateral genu varus and a radiographically confirmed tibiofemoral angle in excess of 15° and in a child of *any* age with a radiographically confirmed tibiofemoral angle in excess of 25° of varus.

Infantile Blount's disease, often associated with substantial internal tibial torsion, involves a disturbance of growth in the epiphyseal and metaphyseal regions of the posteromedial aspect of the proximal end of the tibia. The precise etiology remains uncertain. One hypothesis, albeit controversial, is that the dysplastic ossification in this region results from abnormal forces transmitted over the medial tibial femoral compartment in early walkers. On the roentgenogram, the proximal tibia reveals varying 0° of metaphyseal fragmentation and epiphyseal depression, with the tibia bent abruptly medial and caudal at the proximal metaphysis. Over time, a hooked spur is formed, which radiographically indicates an advanced stage of Blount's disease.

Clinically, the major manifestation is a waddling gait. Knee, ankle, or foot pain occasionally results from excessive stress caused by the deformity. Medial swelling of the proximal tibia may be palpable. There is often significant internal tibial rotation, genu recurvatum, and pes planus with foot pronation.

The causes of acquired tibia vara include proximal tibial osteomyelitis, proximal tibial epiphyseal fracture, and proximal tibial enchondroma.

Treatment. If the angle has not begun to diminish by 18 months, or if, by 24 months, it has not fallen below 15° of varus, most authorities recommend treatment. If the deformity is less than 25° of varus, supportive shoes with a longitudinal arch and outer sole wedges are usually recommended. In those extraordinarily infrequent instances when the tibiofemoral angle exceeds 25° of varus, long-leg braces with genu varus pads to provide lateral force exertion are indicated to prevent a permanent deformity or dysfunction. Beyond 4 years of age, tibiofemoral angles in excess of

25° varus require an osteotomy to completely correct the deformity.

The juvenile (adolescent) type of tibia vara is associated invariably with a shortened extremity and an attendant limp. It is believed to be caused by trauma to the medial ossification center of the proximal tibia. The treatment is surgical; the lateral proximal tibia and the proximal fibula require epiphysiodesis, as do the proximal tibia and fibula of the opposite (i.e., uninvolved) leg to prevent leg length inequality sufficient to cause scoliosis.

Rickets

Rickets may cause severe and extreme bow leg deformity. It is a condition in which the deficiency of calcium or phosphate causes inadequate mineralization of the organic matrix of bone and cartilage. The two main causes of rickets are a lack of vitamin D (type I) and abnormal functioning of the renal tubules (type II). Vitamin D deficiency, due either to inadequate intake (e.g., from vegan or fad diets deficient in vitamin D) or inadequate absorption (e.g., from steatorrhea), is manifested by a combination of diminished intestinal absorption of calcium and phosphate and a decreased tubular reabsorption of phosphate with resultant hypocalcemia and hypophosphatemia. Type II rickets is caused by a deficiency of phosphate resulting from poor or absent renal tubular reabsorption of phosphate. Type III rickets is an end organ resistance to 1,25-dihydroxy vitamin D_3 and is associated with a low serum calcium.

On the roentgenogram the metaphyseal ends of long bones are poorly ossified and frayed. The epiphyseal plate is usually widened and cupped, and the cortices are thinned. The epiphyseal widening is associated with a bending of the softened shafts of the long bones. In addition, the femur and tibia often develop an anterior convexity.

Treatment. Rickets is treated by adequate (as defined by the underlying metabolic disorder) amounts of vitamin D or its essential metabolite, 1,25-dihydroxy vitamin D. Healing begins to occur promptly, and the acute healing is completed in weeks. Once the metabolic abnormality has been corrected, a more reasoned decision regarding splinting, bracing, and osteotomy can be made. The basis for these decisions generally follows those guidelines previously described for the treatment of Blount's disease. However, one must be especially careful to minimize immobilization so as to reduce the risk of recurrent osteoporosis.

KNOCK KNEES

Knock knees are measured by radiographically determining the angle between the lateral aspects of the femur and tibia. The clinical method is to measure the distance between the medial malleoli when the knees are fully extended, the medial femoral condyles are pressed together, and the patellae are facing upward.

The acute appearance of valgus deformity, especially if it is unilateral, should arouse suspicion of trauma, infection, or tumor. Stimulation of the proximal tibial epiphysis by the host's response to any of the above, for example, may lead to valgus, because of the tethering effect of an intact fibula.

If an epiphyseal fracture and rickets have been excluded as causes of knock knee, it is reasonable to defer diagnostic and therapeutic maneuvers in children younger than 7 years of age. If the feet are pronated in association with "physiologic" valgus, toeing-in can be promoted by using a longitudinal arch support; this arch support should be used if the pronation causes pain. If the child with genu valgus already toes in, or if there is no foot pronation, arch support is not indicated. There is no evidence that splints, twisters, casts, or braces play any useful role in managing the child with genu valgus who is younger than 7 or 8 years of age.

If, in the older child, there is an intermalleolar distance of 4 inches or more, or if valgus, as measured by the tibiofemoral angle exceeds 15°, operative intervention is indicated. The usual procedure is stapling or epiphysiodesis of the deformed bone (most commonly it is the medial distal femur), preferably when the epiphyses are still open so as to allow sufficient longitudinal growth to correct the deformity. Proximal tibia and fibula osteotomies are generally performed when valgus deformity is below the knee.

INDICATIONS FOR REFERRAL

The tibiofemoral angle normally progresses from genu varus in the newborn to genu valgus in the toddler. Extreme excesses in this development beyond the normal or "physiologic" expectation should raise the question of rickets or Blount's disease in the child with excessive bow leg. Trauma, tumor, infection, or, rarely, rickets must be ruled out in the child with bilaterally excessive knock knee beyond 7 years of age or at any age if unilateral.

With the exception of some rare instances of genu varus, orthosis, splints, twisters, and the like are generally considered to be inappropriate for these conditions. They certainly do not play a role in the management of knock knee. Correction of the underlying cause, if one is identified, is the first priority. In most instances of bow leg and in all cases of knock knee in which appliances and elaborate regimens are of little use, the primary physician has limited options: He or she may carefully monitor the child or may refer the child to an orthopedist for either additional reassurance or for guidance in management. A referral for orthopedic expertise is mandatory when, in the unusual extreme situation, staging of a surgical osteotomy or epiphysiodesis is considered.

ANNOTATED BIBLIOGRAPHY

Blount WP: Tibia vara. J Bone Joint Surg 19:1, 1937. (Sentinel report of an impressive study of this important disorder.)

Harrison HE, Harrison HC: Disorders of Calcium and Phosphate Metabolism in Childhood and Adolescence. Philadelphia, WB Saunders, 1979. (Lucid and thorough. There are more recent articles, but no better discussions.)

Howorth MD: Knock knees. Clin Orthop 77:233, 1971. (Useful clinical diagnostic and treatment perspective.)

Salenius P, Vankka E: Development of the tibiofemoral angle in children. J Bone Joint Surg 57A:259, 1975. (Elucidating, useful, superb graphs that enhance understanding most effectively.)

Sherman M: Physiologic bowing of the legs. South Med J 53:830, 1970. (Review that allows one to broaden a perspective on normal variation and abnormal extremes.)

132

The Limping Child

Helen M. Emery and Michael L. Miller

Limping may be the presentation of many problems, varying from a spinal cord tumor to a splinter in the foot. Determining why a child has a limp and instituting appropriate treatment can be a significant challenge to the physician.

WORK-UP

An analysis of the cause of the limp begins with a careful history. It is essential to determine if the limp is acute or chronic. When did the limp begin? How long has it been going on? Did it begin gradually or acutely? Preceding events (e.g., a fall) should be evaluated, but one should remember that trauma may be temporally associated with onset but not the real cause of the limp. Does the limp vary with the time of day or with certain activities? Is the limp painful, and, if so, where? Are there any relieving factors? Limping after strenuous activity suggests a musculoskeletal etiology such as a soft tissue strain or stress fracture. Constant pain, especially if it is increasing, suggests a tumor. Pain increasing with joint motion suggests a joint problem. Are there any systemic signs or symptoms such as fever, weight loss, rashes, or arthralgias?

Careful observations of the limp and gait pattern are usually most revealing about its cause. When watching the child walk, note signs of weakness, stiffness, or pain. Does the child bear weight on the leg yet refuse to walk, or does the child insist on being carried? An antalgic gait (a shortened stance [i.e., weight bearing] phase of walking) indicates pain, whereas a shortened or abnormal swing phase often suggests hip joint pathology. A waddling gait suggests that there is a weakness of the abductors, which is not uncommon in arthritis or other conditions that have caused children to be immobile. This is also characteristic of the gait seen in the child with uncorrected developmental dysplasia of the hip (see also Chap. 129). A flat-footed gait may result from the ankle being held in a fixed position, as a result of ankle arthritis.

A fixed back suggests a spinal or abdominal pathology such as diskitis or tumor in the spine. It should be remembered that pain from renal, abdominal, or spinal origin may be referred to the lower extremity or to the hip; from one site of the lower extremity to another (e.g., hip disease may present as knee pain), or to sites other than the lower extremity (e.g., hip pathology may be referred to the groin). If the whole leg is being dragged, a neurologic cause for the gait pattern is more likely, although this can occur occasionally with unilateral weakness caused by muscle pathology. The hip held in flexion suggests intra-articular pathology within that joint. *Hip-hiking* (i.e., elevation of the hip in the swing phase of gait) is seen in a child who keeps the knee in extension while walking, either because of pain on flexion or because of instability that is improved by locking the knee. If the knee is in flexion, the ankle is commonly plantar flexed and the child walks on his or her toes to equalize leg lengths.

The next stage in the examination is to ask the child to climb onto the examination table. Commonly, children favor the affected leg, especially if it is painful; they will usually use their good leg first to climb up onto the examination table.

When the child is on the examination table, the examination is begun with the child in a supine position. One should observe the position in which the child holds his or her body at rest. A spine that is held rigidly suggests a pathologic process, and usually the child avoids rolling or wiggling. Also one should watch for the "position of comfort" in a hip. The position of flexion and external rotation with a little abduction is common for intra-articular hip pathology. A knee held in approximately 45° of flexion is in the position of comfort for that joint. The distance on each side is measured from the anterior-superior iliac spine to the medial malleolus to eliminate leg-length discrepancy (a difference of greater than 2 cm may be considered significant).

Next the spine is examined for scoliosis. Close observation is necessary for evidence of atrophy or change in the skin and temperature over the affected area. Next, a neurologic examination is performed, including tests of reflexes, tone, and sensation. Proprioception is also easily tested in most children, often by using games like the "piggy game." The child can actively demonstrate the range of motion of the extremities, including sit-ups for the spine, while the examiner observes for pain, inability to perform a full range of motion, or weakness. Then, the entire extremity should be put through passive range of movement. After this, all joints are examined for stability and manual muscle strength testing is done, particularly to distinguish the subtle asymmetries. The presence of joint swelling or limited range of motion with pain reflects arthritis (see Chap. 133). Lastly, the examiner should note the family's reaction to pain or limitation, because it may provide clues to their degree of concern and also to any inappropriate manipulative behaviors.

DIFFERENTIAL DIAGNOSIS

The more common causes of a limp can be approached on an anatomic basis. The age of the child and chronicity of the limp are helpful in narrowing the range of diagnostic possibilities. Toxic synovitis and Legg-Calvé-Perthes disease must always be suspected in children between 4 and 8 years of age, and slipped capital femoral epiphysis should be considered in adolescents who limp. In most instances, trauma is the cause of an acute limp. The injury may be to bone (e.g., fracture), soft tissue (e.g., foreign body, abrasion, strain, or inflammation of a ligament or tendon) or to a joint (e.g., meniscal injury, sprain). Causes other than trauma (e.g., neuromuscular and leg length asymmetry) are more likely if the limp is chronic.

Spine

Diskitis, usually from a hematogenously spread staphylococcal infection, is one of the more common causes of back problems in a child, although it is not uncommon for the child to refer the pain to the abdomen or to the hip. One should look for rigidity of the spine and resistance to forward flexion or lateral movement. The paravertebral muscles are often also in spasm. Point tenderness can often be identified in one of the disk spaces. Spinal osteomyelitis can occur in this region, but it is less common. Spinal tumors are rare in children; they are often painful. Spinal cord tumors or cord compression can also present as a limp, as can tumors involving the nerve roots; and these are usually detected by an alteration in sensation, motor function, or atrophy. (Lower cord lesions will sometimes spare the extremities but cause bowel and bladder symptoms.) Intraabdominal pathology can also be referred to the back, and iliopsoas injuries or infections can be referred to the hip, causing children to walk with hip flexion.

Hip

Several important causes of a limp are caused by hip problems. These include soft tissue problems such as injuries to tendon insertions and ligaments; these are usually clearly activity related, and they improve with rest. As discussed in Chapter 129, in the ambulating child limping is the sign most often present in dislocated or dysplastic hips.

Pauciarticular juvenile rheumatoid arthritis presenting as a monoarticular arthritis in the hip is rare. Therefore, other conditions need to be differentiated. In the young child, the condition of *toxic synovitis* (transient synovitis), which usually presents with no or low-grade fever and sudden onset of hip pain, is a common, if not the most common, condition causing limp in children. The hip must often be tapped to exclude a septic process. Roentgenograms of the pelvis are normal, but a technetium bone scan shows a diffuse mild uptake over the hip joint. The white blood cell count, differential, and sedimentation rate are most often

normal, although the latter may be slightly elevated. The disorder is self-limited, and with bed rest, pain is often much improved within 48 to 72 hours, although it may last for 7 to 10 days. It is unusual for the synovitis to recur. A bacterially infected hip is usually much more painful and guarded, and the child is more toxic. Nonetheless, in some children with moderate sedimentation rate elevation and hip pain on range of motion, arthrocentesis is the only means of excluding bacterial arthritis.

The young child, especially in the age range of 4 to 8 years, is most vulnerable to idiopathic aseptic necrosis of the femoral head, *Legg-Calvé-Perthes* disease, which usually presents as limp and sometimes knee pain. The bone scan is helpful early, while roentgenograms later will show patchy sclerosis and collapse in the femoral head. The temperature, complete blood cell count, and sedimentation rate are all normal. In unusual cases, classic roentgenographic findings may take as long as 1 year to develop in *Legg-Calvé-Perthes* disease. Therefore, the diagnosis should be reconsidered in any child with persisting hip disease who does not respond to treatment for other conditions, even with previously normal roentgenograms.

In the older child, stereotypically the obese adolescent, *slipped capital femoral epiphysis* presents as a progressive limp and often knee pain. This condition is a surgical emergency and requires immediate non-weight-bearing status to prevent further slipping, sometimes traction to relieve spasm, and surgical pinning to stabilize the femoral head. It is most easily diagnosed by a roentgenogram that clearly shows the alteration of the alignment of the capital femoral epiphysis. There is also a less common condition, *chondrolysis of the hip,* that may follow pinning of a slipped epiphysis. This may occur spontaneously and may mimic an acute arthritic process in the hip. The roentgenogram shows joint space narrowing.

The femur is one of the more common sites for primary bone tumors, which may present with either hip or leg pain. These include primary osteogenic sarcoma, Ewing's tumor, and occasionally secondary tumors from neuroblastoma. Fortunately, these are much less common and usually are easily detectable by roentgenogram. Systemic malignancies including leukemias and lymphomas may present as limping. Benign tumors such as osteoid osteomas are usually apparent on a roentgenogram and demonstrate increased uptake on bone scan.

Knee

The knee is another common site for the origin of a limp. Several mechanical derangements of the knee related to trauma may present as limp, localized tenderness, and effusions. Meniscal injuries seldom occur before adolescence, however, and other causes must be sought in a younger child. *Osteochondritis dissecans,* which is usually detectable by roentgenograms especially with special sunset views, is more common in teenage boys and may cause knee locking because of loose bodies within the joint. *Chondromalacia patellae* is a common cause of knee complaints in older school-aged children, and the pattern of pain will usually be exacerbated by activities, especially those stressing quadriceps muscles. A positive patellar inhibition sign, which is pain inhibiting resisted contraction of the patella, and tenderness over the medial joint line accompanied by crepitus of the patellofemoral joint are characteristic of this condition. As with other joints, septic processes also need to be excluded. In *Osgood-Schlatter disease,* a limp often occurs after strenuous exercise. On physical examination, the tibial tuberosity will be painful and is usually swollen. *Plant thorn synovitis* represents a foreign body reaction. It is suspected based on history; the suggestion of a foreign body on a roentgenogram may require arthroscopy to exclude the diagnosis.

Leg

The tibia is vulnerable to *stress fractures,* particularly in young athletes. These are recognized by the pattern of pain after repetitive trauma, especially in athletes, and sometimes periostitis is visible on the roentgenogram. However, these features are often subtle, and a bone scan is more sensitive at demonstrating stress fractures.

Ankle

The ankle is very vulnerable to mechanical strains and sprains, particularly the medial and lateral ligaments. Often there is a clear-cut history of injury or recurrent injuries initiating the episode of limping. Common findings are point tenderness and a characteristic toe-walking gait to protect the ankle from weight bearing. Achilles tendonitis is also common in active youngsters and is often a cause of limp. The child feels more comfortable with the calf muscles flexed, placing less weight over the ankle, and avoiding stretching the tendon area. This is also a site for inflammation of tendons attaching to bones (enthesitis), which is a part of some arthritis syndromes. Heel pain is characteristic of ankylosing spondylitis and its variants, and may be accompanied by evidence of spurs on the calcaneus on the roentgenogram. The tarsus is another common site for aseptic necrosis, presenting as pain and limp, and this can usually be detected by bone scan early and later by roentgenography. Another major cause of problems in this area is a coalition between tarsal bones, either bony or fibrous. These cause an inflexible, painful flat foot and may require surgical intervention. The common familial flexible flat foot does not cause a limp.

Foot

Metatarsal phalangeal joints are commonly affected in arthritis. Involvement is often symmetric, and other objective signs of inflammation are usually present. Penetrating foot injuries, classically a child stepping onto a sharp object such as rusty nail that penetrates shoes and socks, often cause insidious problems in soft tissue, bone, and sometimes joints. Classically, *Pseudomonas* is one of the causative agents, but also tetanus and other unusual organisms can cause infection. By the time these infections are diagnosed, extensive bone or other tissue necrosis has often occurred, requiring surgical debridement for bacteriologic diagnosis and treatment.

LABORATORY TESTS

In a child with acute onset of a limp not readily explained by injury, investigation should focus on the most likely cause of the pain as determined by the history and physical examination. In general, roentgenograms are valuable for looking for fractures or tumors. Bone scans are much more sensitive for detecting areas of altered blood flow, such as aseptic necrosis of bone in the ankle or the femoral head or inflammation from infection, tumor, or arthritis. An erythrocyte sedimentation rate is useful; if the result is elevated, an inflammatory cause is suggested. However, it is not unusual for many tumors or even some arthritic processes to be associated with a normal sedimentation rate. If an intra-articular process is considered, the joint should be aspirated to both diagnose the cause and to relieve the risk of damage from pus under pressure inside an inflamed or infected joint. Further work-up beyond these tests is usually unnecessary.

TREATMENT AND REFERRAL

Most limps are likely to be on a mechanical basis. For the management of such problems, the reader is referred to Chapters 138, 140, and 141. However, a limp can indicate a more serious underlying cause that requires specific treatment. In evaluating a limp, the orthopedic surgeon is often one of the best resources, both because of experience with analyzing the gait for cause of a limp and also for understanding many of the mechanisms underlying it. A neurologist should be consulted for the infrequent neurologic causes of a limp (e.g., spinal tumors and peripheral neuropathies).

ANNOTATED BIBLIOGRAPHY

Hensinger RN: Limp. Pediatr Clin North Am 33:1355–1364, 1986. (Good clinical review.)

Jacobs BW: Synovitis of the hip in children and its significance. Pediatrics 47:558–566, 1971. (Thorough and still timely review.)

Perrin JCS, Badell A, Binder H et al: Pediatric Rehabilitation, Vol 6, Musculoskeletal and Soft Tissue Disorders. Arch Phys Med Rehabil 70:S183–189, 1989. (Includes symptom-based differential diagnosis of orthopedic causes of knee pain.)

Phillips WA: The child with a limp. Orthop Clin North Am 18:489–501, 1987. (Good review of orthopedic conditions.)

Renshaw TS: Pediatric Orthopedics, Major Problems in Clinical Pediatrics, vol 28, chap 4. Philadelphia, WB Saunders, 1986. (Good, practical discussions, especially of Legg-Calvé-Perthes disease; lists many references.)

Thompson G, Salter RB: Legg-Calvé-Perthes Disease. CIBA Clinical Symposia, vol 38, No. 1, 1986. (Lucidly presented comprehensive review.)

Tunnessen WW: Signs and Symptoms in Pediatrics, 2nd ed, chap 90. Philadelphia, JB Lippincott, 1988. (Excellent differential diagnosis of limp with "pearls" to direct the work-up.)

Wilkinson RH, Weissman BN: Arthritis in Children. Radiol Clin North Am 26:1247–1265, 1988. (Succinct radiologic review.)

133

Juvenile Rheumatoid Arthritis

Helen M. Emery and
Michael L. Miller

Arthritis is defined as an inflammation of one or more joints, suggested by objective findings of swelling, warmth, pain, and sometimes erythema. The definition of *juvenile rheumatoid arthritis* (JRA) accepted by the American Rheumatism Association is (1) objective signs of inflammation of one or more joints; (2) inflammation lasting at least 6 weeks; (3) onset before the 17th birthday; and (4) exclusion of other underlying causes of joint problems, such as infection or malignancy. An estimated 200,000 children in the United States (approximately 0.1% of the population) have JRA during childhood, making it the most common childhood rheumatic disease.

PATHOPHYSIOLOGY

The etiology of this condition remains unknown. Some studies have suggested that common childhood infections (e.g., viruses), in an immunologically predisposed host, will allow a persistent synovial inflammatory reaction to be initiated and perpetuated, secondarily causing damage to cartilage, bone, and surrounding structures. The association of various clinical patterns of JRA with specific HLA subtypes, identified by a polymerase chain reaction–based methodology, supports this hypothesis. However, much more information is needed to establish the causes and mechanisms.

CLINICAL PATTERNS

JRA is classified by the pattern of onset in the first 6 months into three major types: (1) systemic onset, (2) pauciarticular onset (fewer than five joints affected in the absence of classic systemic findings), and (3) polyarticular onset (five or more involved joints, again with the absence of classic systemic signs). A child will generally stay in one classification through the course of disease.

Systemic Disease

Systemic disease is characterized by fever of a particular pattern, arthritis, and characteristic extra-articular manifestations. It occurs equally in both sexes and has no age predilection.

Fever, by definition, lasts at least 2 weeks and may continue for months with one or two daily spikes to greater than 103°F (39.4°C) with a return to normal or subnormal temperatures between peaks. Commonly, the fever occurs in the afternoon or evening and is debilitating. Any other fever pattern is inconsistent with systemic onset disease.

An evanescent rash consisting of macules of almost fingernail size with central clearing often occurs over the trunk and extremities with the fever (or sometimes if the skin is warmed or traumatized.) This rash may be pruritic and often disappears completely when the fever subsides. Observation of this rash is helpful in confirming the diagnosis.

Almost one third of children with this variety of JRA will experience pericarditis or pleuritis. Clinical clues include tachycardia or tachypnea out of proportion to fever, splinted or shallow respiration in an effort to reduce pain from chest expansion, refusing to lie down (so pericardial or pleural fluid drains to diaphragmatic region), and abdominal pain (referred from the chest). About 5% of children with pericarditis develop myocarditis.

Enlargement of the liver, spleen, and lymph nodes is common, and anicteric hepatitis can also occur. This group also seems to be at special risk for salicylate hepatotoxicity.

Although arthritis must be observed to confirm this diagnosis, it can vary from limited and mild to extensive and severe, but it may be a less prominent feature of the illness than the extra-articular manifestations.

Laboratory Tests. Anemia can be quite profound in this group, and elevations of white blood cell count, platelets, and sedimentation rates can be striking. Tests for rheumatoid factor and antinuclear antibodies are always negative, and there is no test that confirms the diagnosis.

Pauciarticular Juvenile Rheumatoid Arthritis

Pauciarticular JRA can be classified into two subgroups according to the age and pattern of joint involvement.

One group affects predominantly young girls (average age at onset, 2 years; female-to-male ratio of 4:1) and usually affects large joints (e.g., knees, ankles, wrists, elbows, and neck and almost never hips). Frequent clues are morning stiffness, delayed motor milestones, or asymmetric accelerated growth around long bone epiphyses from increased vascularity. This group is at particular risk for developing asymptomatic chronic iridocyclitis, which can be diagnosed only by a slit lamp examination in its early, most treatable stages. The worst morbidity from this form of JRA is from eye complications (e.g., band keratopathy, cataracts, glaucoma, and visual loss) rather than joint disease.

Laboratory tests again do not confirm this diagnosis, because only nonspecific abnormalities (e.g., mild sedimentation rate elevations) occur and rheumatoid factor is absent. The test for antinuclear antibodies, however, does help identify the group at highest risk for eye complications (80% to 90% will have positive tests).

The second group with pauciarticular disease will have onset generally after the age of 8 years. This group is predominantly male and frequently has a family history for ankylosing spondylitis or other diseases now known to be related to the HLA-B27 tissue type in close relatives. The joints involved are often those of the lower extremity (e.g., tarsus, ankles, knees, and hips), and this disease may be a precursor to more classic ankylosing spondylitis that may take years to declare the classic findings (evidence of sacroiliitis on the roentgenogram and decreased lumbosacral mobility). These children are more at risk for the complications of ankylosing spondylitis (e.g., acute iridocyclitis and aortitis) than are children in the younger-onset group. Again, laboratory findings are nonspecific; these children do not have rheumatoid factor or antinuclear antibodies but more frequently carry the HLA-B27 tissue type. (It is not recommended to test for this gene because its presence or absence will not affect patient management.)

Polyarticular Juvenile Rheumatoid Arthritis

Children with polyarticular JRA usually present with multiple symmetric joint involvement, especially involving hands and feet. Some children will have a low-grade fever, malaise, and weight loss but not the characteristic systemic findings. Two distinct groups can be defined according to the presence or absence of rheumatoid factor. Those who have rheumatoid factor behave like those with young onset of adult rheumatoid arthritis. They are often teenagers at the time of presentation but may occasionally be very young. The disease is usually characterized by an aggressive, destructive course with all the potential complications of an adult-type disease: nodules, vasculitis, and lung complications not seen in the other childhood types. Fortunately, this kind accounts for only about 10% of all children with JRA. The children with polyarticular disease without rheumatoid factor generally are younger at age at onset. They often have a milder disease, and they are not at risk for the same extraarticular complications. Some of these children will prove positive for antinuclear antibodies.

DIFFERENTIAL DIAGNOSIS

Infections

Most acute infections are hematogenously carried into the musculoskeletal system (e.g., bones, joints, or immediately surrounding soft tissues). However, previous infections may cause a reactive arthritis, and sometimes an arthritis may be the product of a more generalized illness.

Acute Bacterial Infections

The age of the child suggests which organisms are most likely to occur. In newborns until 3 months, staphylococcus, group B streptococcus, and gram-negative organisms (including *Neisseria gonorrhoeae* if the child was exposed during the birth process) are most likely. General signs of a septic infant (e.g., temperature instability, poor feeding, jaundice) are usual, together with signs such as pseudoparalysis or pain when the infant is handled. Infections in bones and joints at this age often lead to severe growth abnormalities. Older children exhibit more acute signs, including high fever, toxicity, and localized complaints of pain that begin abruptly and progress rapidly. A septic joint will usually be painful, and the joint is held in a position of comfort (where maximum joint space can accommodate the pus and inflamed synovium). The child will resist using that joint with severe muscle spasm and guarding. This is in contrast to a child with osteomyelitis, who may have a sympathetic effusion in the adjacent joint but who usually shows most tenderness over the metaphysis rather than the joint itself and who also tolerates some active or passive range of motion.

The most useful tests confirm evidence of inflammation and identify the causative bacteria. For septic arthritis, aspiration of the joint is both diagnostic (white blood cell count is usually over 50,000 cells/mm^3; protein level is elevated; glucose concentration is low; and bacteria can be seen and cultured) and therapeutic. Relieving pressure from pus on cartilage to avoid further damage is especially critical in the hip. Especially in osteomyelitis, the bone scan can be helpful but may take a day or so to become positive. Aside from soft tissue changes, roentgenographic changes may be absent for up to 2 weeks and, if seen, reflect bone and joint damage that could have been avoided by early initiation of treatment. Situations that cause confusion include pretreatment with antibiotics, which masks acuity of joint findings; a compromised host (e.g., a child on corticosteroids or immunosuppressive therapy); and penetrating bone and joint injuries, which are often more insidious and involve unusual and often mixed organisms and require surgical debridement.

Postinfectious arthritis is often precipitated by viral (e.g., rubella, echoviruses) or bacterial (e.g., *Salmonella, Yersinia*) infections. These are usually self-limiting (less than 6 weeks). However, severe chronic arthritis can develop. Lyme disease, resulting from infection with the spirochete *Borrelia burgdorferi*, should be considered in all children presenting with arthritis who live in endemic areas or who have been exposed to tick bites. Serologic testing should be obtained, even when erythema chronicum migrans or other organ manifestations (e.g., cardiac or neurologic) are absent.

For a detailed discussion on lyme disease, see Chap. 206. Arthritis may occur as a prodrome to other immune complex processes (e.g., serum sickness and hepatitis).

Malignancies

About 50% of children with malignancies have musculoskeletal pain at the time of diagnosis, which may simulate arthritis. These include both localized forms (e.g., osteogenic sarcoma), metastatic processes (e.g., from neuroblastoma), or systemic forms (e.g., leukemia or lymphoma). Useful clues are pain at night or at rest, pain out of proportion to physical findings, and systemic illness (e.g., fevers, weight loss). Roentgenograms, bone scans, and bone marrow aspiration are most useful in diagnosing these tumors and may be positive before blood parameters are altered. Many childhood malignancies are curable if early treatment is initiated; thus, it is critical to diagnose a disease in this group.

Mechanical Noninflammatory Disorders

Benign limb pain of childhood (growing pains) is an inclusive term, but is a diagnosis of exclusion. Young children (often 2 to 5 years of age) wake up at night with apparent deep calf or thigh pain, often after an active day. This pain is relieved by heat, rubbing, and simple analgesics. It is nonprogressive (although the rewards of midnight crying may escalate this behavior), and the child is otherwise totally well. Reassurance is the best treatment.

Benign hypermobile joint syndrome is usually hereditary. These children will complain of pain after activity and can be identified by physical findings of diffuse ligamentous laxity including hyperextension to more than 90 degrees at metacarpophalangeal joints, more than 15 degrees at the elbows, recurvatum of the knees, and hypermobility of the spine. This may be a benign variant of *Ehlers-Danlos syndrome*. Such children are often encouraged in gymnastics and dance to exaggerate these tendencies and consequently increase their complaints.

Aseptic necrosis of bone most commonly occurs at the hip (*Legg-Calvé-Perthes* disease) but can occur at other sites. Pain is often insidious in onset, or a limp or referred pain is noted. Roentgenograms and bone scan are the best diagnostic tools. The treatment varies with the site and severity of pain (see Chap. 132).

Trauma

Injury is the most frequent explanation of musculoskeletal pain in children but may also be misleading, because parents may attribute the onset of symptoms to an unrelated incident. In contrast, an injury from subtle child abuse may lead to an evaluation for other causes of pain. Sports injuries (e.g., little leaguer's elbow, runner's knee) must also be considered in a child with persistent pain (see Chap. 137).

Metabolic Disorders

Although these are rare in children, hematologic disorders (e.g., hemophilia, sickle cell disease), immunodeficiency (IgA and IgG deficiency), gout (from inborn errors of purine metabolism pathways), and true connective tissue diseases all present as musculoskeletal pain and sometimes frank arthritis.

Systemic Inflammatory Disorders

Inflammatory bowel disease (ulcerative colitis and Crohn's disease) may present as musculoskeletal pain or true arthritis before the classic gastrointestinal findings are present. Clues include a failure of linear growth, weight loss, and decreased appetite. Anemia, occult blood loss, and low serum albumin levels may suggest that an evaluation of the intestinal tract (by endoscopy or contrast radiography) is needed (see also Chap. 107).

Rheumatic Diseases

Any rheumatic disease may present as either arthritis or other musculoskeletal complaints.

Rheumatic fever usually has an acute migratory (i.e., lasting only a few days in any one joint) polyarthritis pattern involving primarily knees, ankles, elbows, and wrists. However, the arthritis can sometimes be "additive," in that arthritis may persist in initially involved joints as it affects new ones. In addition to other criteria (e.g., carditis, erythema marginatum, subcutaneous nodules, or chorea), there must be either culture or antibody evidence of a preceding streptococcal infection. Arthralgia is a minor criterion, and all musculoskeletal symptoms disappear rapidly with treatment with salicylates or corticosteroids and are self-limited even if untreated.

Systemic lupus erythematosus has arthritis as a presenting complaint in most cases but is usually accompanied by evidence of other systemic disease (e.g., most often Raynaud's phenomenon, nephritis, and hematologic disorders) and almost always has a strongly positive test for antinuclear antibodies and low complement levels secondary to immune complex formation.

Dermatomyositis presents as weakness, muscle tenderness, and a classical heliotrope rash over eyelids and hands and sometimes on the trunk. The childhood variant is commonly associated with systemic vasculitis, although not with underlying malignancies. Elevated muscle enzyme levels usually confirm the clinical picture, although electromyography and muscle biopsy may sometimes be needed.

In the absence of a classic rash, however, polymyositis may be difficult to differentiate from muscular dystrophy or other myopathic processes, and a biopsy, nerve conduction times, and electromyograms may be required. Children may present with a chronic synovitis indistinguishable from JRA, particularly when rheumatoid factor and antinuclear antibody tests are positive (as is the case in at least 10% of dermatomyositis patients). The presence of muscle weakness out of proportion to synovitis in any child should raise the suspicion of dermatomyositis or polymyositis. Results of the appropriate enzyme studies will indicate whether further tests are necessary.

Vasculitic syndromes (e.g., Henoch-Schönlein purpura, Kawasaki disease, and polyarteritis nodosa, which are the most common in children) usually have inflammatory musculoskeletal components and can usually be recognized by the associated physical findings, but laboratory tests may be nonspecific.

WORK-UP

History and Physical Examination

The general approach to the evaluation of a child with arthritis is similar, regardless of the etiology of the swollen joint(s). There must be a careful assessment of the pattern of pain, noting particularly the location, radiation, fluctuations of symptoms either with activity or time, and duration. The progression and preceding events are the best guide to the underlying process. Furthermore, an evaluation of non-specific findings, such as fever, malaise, or weight loss, and a complete review for evidence of involvement of other organ systems is essential.

The history is supplemented by a careful physical examination. A clinician who does not perform a complete musculoskeletal examination may miss subtle physical findings. The general principles of inspection, palpation, and moving the affected part both actively and passively, while carefully observing for evidence of pain in the child's nonverbal as well as verbal reactions, are the mainstay of the physical examination. Remember that pain is often referred distally in children (e.g., a knee complaint commonly originates in the hip).

MANAGEMENT

Medications

The usual first line of treatment is salicylates in therapeutic doses (80 to 90 mg/kg/d in four divided doses for children younger than 20 kg; 60 to 80 mg/kg/d for older children) to achieve a level of 20 to 30 mg/dL. Recently, some pediatric rheumatology centers have started to recommend nonsteroidal anti-inflammatory medications (e.g., ibuprofen, 30–40 mg/kg/d in three doses) instead. Parents need to know about the complications of salicylates (e.g., easy bruising, stomach upset) and the signs of toxicity (e.g., hyperventilation, decreased hearing, drowsiness or irritability, and progressive vomiting). If there is a question of toxicity, the parents should be asked to stop the aspirin and a salicylate level should be determined. If the child does not tolerate aspirin, a nonacetylated salicylate (e.g., choline salicylate or magnesium choline salicylate) or a nonsteroidal anti-inflammatory agent (e.g., sodium tolmetin in a dose of 20

to 30 mg/kg/d) can be substituted. All of these medications will take at least several weeks to suppress inflammation. Thus, a trial of 3 to 6 months will usually be done before deciding to add a disease modifying antirheumatologic drug (DMARD).

The choice of a DMARD (e.g., oral or intramuscular gold salts, D-penicillamine, hydroxychloroquine) is not always simple and should be decided only after a full discussion of side effects and anticipated outcome with the child and family. For children who have an unresponsive, destructive disease, low doses of methotrexate have been used but are regarded as experimental. In general, DMARDs are reserved for children with aggressive polyarticular JRA. Some children with aggressive pauciarticular disease affecting a large joint such as the knee may also benefit from therapy with a DMARD. Gold salts have been reported to cause a coagulopathy in some children with systemic JRA and should be avoided in this subtype.

Oral corticosteroids have a limited role in the management of childhood arthritis and are used mainly for severe systemic manifestations (e.g., pericarditis, pleuritis, and severe anemia). The side effects of sustained corticosteroids (e.g., osteoporosis, increased susceptibility to infections, growth failure, risks of diabetes, and hypertension) are not warranted in light of the fact that corticosteroids, while making the patient feel better, do not prevent (and may even hasten) joint destruction. Furthermore, their effectiveness may decrease over time. Topical corticosteroids (combined with mydriatics) are valuable in controlling eye disease, and occasional intra-articular corticosteroids are used, usually in conjunction with initiation of DMARDs and an intensive therapy program.

Physical and Occupational Therapy

The goals of management are to reduce inflammation and to maintain function in joints. All children with JRA and their parents should learn the normal range of movement and be alert to even a subtle loss of range. If this occurs, a therapist can show parents how to work with the child to maintain full joint range and prevent losses (e.g., laying prone during television time for hip disease.) For children with morning stiffness, a hot bath in the morning followed by range of motion exercises will enable them to be more functional. Resting splints (e.g., for wrists or knees) will allow the joints to remain in a functional position and prevent the formation of flexion contractures.

For children with more extensive disease, especially lower extremity contractures, a more aggressive program of range of motion exercises and strengthening, gait training, functional skill development, and outpatient or sometimes even inpatient treatment by an experienced therapist is necessary.

Management of behavior is as important as management of the disease. Both child and parent should be fully informed about what to expect in terms of taking medications and undertaking a therapy program. Parents should be encouraged to avoid overprotecting their child while under the misapprehension that inactivity will spare their child pain. In fact, moving the joint helps the child loosen up, and muscle strength will provide stability around inflamed joints. The child should be educated to respect his or her joints but should not be restricted except in unusual circumstances (e.g., somersaults are not encouraged in children with neck involvement). Encouraging self-esteem and appropriate assertiveness will facilitate independence and the achievement of developmental goals. Simple behavior modification techniques (e.g., encouraging a child through a painful exercise instead of focusing on crying, sticker charts, and rewards to facilitate compliance with splints and medicines) are invaluable.

Ambulation is critical in a child with JRA. Once osteoporosis, weakness, and contractures are established, they are difficult to reverse. Wheelchairs should be avoided at all costs: besides the invalid image they convey, the flexion positions of hips and knees, and the weakness from inactivity undermine the therapeutic goals. The alternative is a tricycle or walker, which encourages weight bearing and use of available range and strength.

PROGNOSIS

There is great variability in outcomes for children with JRA. In general, the younger-onset pauciarticular group almost never have a permanent disability from their arthritis (although they may from eye disease). However, between one third to one half of children with polyarticular rheumatoid factor–positive disease or the systemic-onset variety will have residual deformities and functional limitations. It is hoped that these figures will improve as better treatment becomes more widely available.

INDICATIONS FOR REFERRAL

All parents should be encouraged to contact their local chapter of the Arthritis Foundation–American Juvenile Arthritis Organization to obtain information on JRA, such as medication pamphlets and brochures informing schools about arthritis. Many also have parent support groups and facilitate networking between children and parents.

The following specialties are often involved in the comprehensive management of children with arthritis:

- Pediatric rheumatologist: When the diagnosis is uncertain, DMARDs are being considered, or the child is developing flexion contractures or functional limitations, a referral is indicated for assistance in decision-making.
- Orthopedist: The role of surgery for children with JRA is limited. A fixed flexion contracture unresponsive to aggressive therapy may benefit from soft tissue release; an end-stage joint may be replaced in a child who has completed skeletal growth with marked relief of pain and improvement in function. However, only a very experienced

arthritis surgeons working with a pediatric rheumatologist, therapists, and a motivated patient should undertake these procedures.
- Ophthalmologist: All children with JRA should be screened annually. The highest risk group (young-onset pauciarticular JRA) should be seen at 3- to 4-month intervals for a slit lamp examination to exclude uveitis.
- Social worker/psychologist: Financial demands of the child's illness can be a major burden to any family with a chronically ill child. Most states cover JRA under their Crippled Children's Program. A social worker can assist in determining if the family is eligible and can facilitate the referral. These professionals can also help the entire family adjust to the chronic illness and help establish behavior programs when needed.
- Physical and occupational therapists: Therapists should evaluate the child initially and help teach families normal range and simple exercises. Specific directions for splinting, joint protection techniques, and more aggressive range and strengthening programs should be developed with the physician as required.

ANNOTATED BIBLIOGRAPHY

Cassidy JT, Petty RE: Textbook of Pediatric Rheumatology, 2nd ed. New York, John Wiley & Sons, 1990. (Most comprehensive text on the subject.)

Maksymowych WP, Van Kerckhove C, Glass DN: Juvenile rheumatoid arthritis, human leukocyte antigen, and other immunoglobulin supergene family polymorphisms. Am J Med 85(6A):26–28, 1988. (Overview of role HLA antigens probably play in juvenile rheumatoid arthritis.)

Miller ML (ed): Pediatric rheumatology. Pediatr Clin North Am 33(5), 1986. (Highlights physical and occupational therapy, psychosocial aspects, and community and school programs for children with rheumatic diseases and also contains current and comprehensive reviews of the major childhood arthritides and Kawasaki syndrome.)

Schaller JG: Arthritis in children, Pediatr Clinic North Am 33(6): 1565–1580, 1986. (Brief, yet good overview.)

134
Torticollis
Murray A. Braun

Torticollis is characterized by a contracted state of the cervical muscles causing rotation of the head and neck and an unnatural head tilt.

PATHOGENESIS

Because of its diverse etiology, several loci of pathology may be involved in causing torticollis. These include the upper cervical spinal cord, which gives rise to cranial nerve XI and supplies the sternocleidomastoid and trapezius muscles; the bony spine and spinal canal; the base of the skull (where cranial nerve XI enters the foramen magnum and exits through the jugular foramen), the posterior fossa, and the brain stem; the soft tissues, including the skin (*pterygium colli*) of the neck; the sternocleidomastoid muscle; and the basal ganglia.

Congenital muscular torticollis may be due to an unusual fetal posture or mechanical constraint in utero in late gestation. Factors associated with this disorder are deformities (e.g., metatarsus adductus, hip dislocation, and flattened auricles); infants with greater than average birth weight who are born to primigravidas; birth trauma; breech presentation; and forceps delivery. Torticollis may be coincident with *plagiocephaly* (a rhomboid-shaped head), itself due either to mechanical constraint in utero or premature closure of the cranial sutures. Hereditary factors, muscular ischemia secondary to venous occlusion in utero, myositis, and anterior horn cell dysfunction are also hypothesized to play a role in the genesis of congenital muscular torticollis.

CLINICAL PRESENTATION AND DIFFERENTIAL DIAGNOSIS

Congenital Torticollis

Congenital torticollis is generally due to bony anomalies, a skin abnormality (skin web), central nervous system disorders, or, most commonly, a focal or localized neuromuscular abnormality. Congenital torticollis, when presenting as a hard, fusiform, olive-like mass ("tumor") of the sternocleidomastoid muscle, is usually the result of localized sternocleidomastoid muscle fibrosis. The tumor appears in the first weeks of life but may not be evident for months. Initially, the tumor tends to increase in size and usually disappears in 5 to 8 months, although it may persist for years.

The tumor seen in congenital muscular torticollis must be distinguished from other neck masses presenting in infancy. *Fibrodysplasia ossificans progressiva,* resulting in an enlargement of the sternocleidomastoid or other neck muscles, may be present (see also Chap. 84).

Pseudotorticollis may be secondary to abducens or other oculomotor palsies and occurs in *spasmus nutans* and *congenital nystagmus.* In the latter, the torticollis is compensatory to achieve binocularity with fusion.

Acquired Torticollis

Acquired torticollis either is short-lived and reversible or is progressive. It is commonly due to an inflammatory process, with lymph node involvement either overlying the muscle, causing it to contract, or at some distant site, with its direct role in causing spasm of the sternocleidomastoid muscle less clear. Upper respiratory tract infection, tonsillitis, sinusitis, mastoiditis, cervical adenitis, retropharyngeal abscess, and cellulitis are most commonly the cause of cervical node enlargement.

Direct trauma to the sternocleidomastoid muscle, with resultant hematoma, can cause muscular spasms. Traumatic torticollis may also result from either atlantoaxial subluxation or basal ganglia injury. Even in inflammatory torticollis without trauma, subluxation of the atlantoaxial joint may occur. This is believed to result from hyperemia and pathologic relaxation of the transverse ligament of the atlantoaxial joint.

An idiosyncratic response to *phenothiazines* or *metoclopramide* may cause a highly reversible torticollis.

Other causes of benign, reversible torticollis in infancy include *paroxysmal torticollis of infancy* and *Sandifer's syndrome.* Paroxysmal torticollis of infancy is an infrequent disorder that may be associated with vestibular dysfunction. It and benign paroxysmal vertigo of childhood may be related to migraine (so-called *migraine equivalent*), especially in the setting of other migrainous symptoms and positive family history. Paroxysmal torticollis of infancy has its onset between 2 and 8 months of age. When torticollis occurs, the child is distressed and pale. Older children may describe vertigo. Ataxia and rolling or deviation of the eyes may be present.

Sandifer's syndrome is caused by *gastroesophageal reflux* with or without hiatal hernia and leads to bizarre dystonic features including torticollis. Vomiting and feeding difficulties early in infancy are then followed by posturing of the neck during feeding in later infancy and early childhood; these features subside with fasting. Shortening of the sternocleidomastoid muscle is not observed in these patients.

When *progressive,* torticollis may result from a variety of etiologies. In children, progressive torticollis is most commonly caused by an *infratentorial tumor.* Other structural lesions include a *colloid cyst of the third ventricle* and *syringomyelia,* which may occur in the cervical spinal cord with or without a spinal tumor. Syringomyelia may be associated with a *Klippel-Feil syndrome* (short or webbed neck, fused vertebral bodies). A *sarcoma* may invade the basilar skull with consequent entrapment of cranial nerve XI. Muscular disease is not a major cause of torticollis, but it may be associated with *myositis* of the sternocleidomastoid muscle. The basal ganglia may be affected by abnormal copper metabolism and deposition, leading to hepatolenticular degeneration (*Wilson's disease*) or may be involved in the pathogenesis of *dystonia musculorum deformans,* in which torticollis is often a prominent finding.

In adults, but sometimes in adolescence, *spasmodic torticollis* occurs and tends to be of extrapyramidal origin. This form of focal dystonia may either be idiopathic or familial.

Hysteria or a *conversion reaction* may also be associated with torticollis.

TORTICOLLIS 511

WORK-UP

History

Prenatal, perinatal and postnatal characteristics, as noted above, must be sought in the evaluation of the infant with congenital torticollis.

Hereditary factors may provide a clue to progressive and degenerative disorders causing torticollis. For example, a disproportionate number of Ashkenazi Jewish families have been reported to be afflicted with focal dystonia.

A history of recent illness should be sought. In acute torticollis, an infection such as tonsillitis or cervical adenitis may occur concurrently. Recent drug exposure should also be explored.

Torticollis in the child with Sandifer's syndrome may improve with fasting and when gastroesophageal reflux is reduced.

Paroxysmal disorders (migraine equivalent) will be diagnosed with careful assessment for family history of migraine and of reported symptoms, such as intermittent facial pallor, ataxia (unsteadiness), vertigo (dizziness), and nystagmus (abnormal eye movements).

Physical Examination

In congenital torticollis, appreciation of shortening of the sternocleidomastoid muscle may be difficult in the young infant who ordinarily has a short neck. A mass within the midsection of the cervical muscle may be palpated in early infancy, and facial asymmetries may only become evident after many weeks postnatally. The shape of the skull should be assessed. Careful ocular motility and ophthalmologic evaluation is indicated when plagiocephaly, spasmus nutans, or congenital nystagmus is present. Cervical scoliosis will be noted only in later infancy, but some syndromes such as the Klippel-Feil syndrome may be noted in infancy. Other deformities associated with congenital torticollis in the newborn should be noted.

The head and neck should be examined carefully for infection and lymphadenopathy since acute infection of the pharynx and cervical lymph node involvement are the most common causes of childhood torticollis. If such causes are not obvious, a careful neurologic examination including fundoscopic is mandatory.

Progressive and degenerative diseases will have associated findings such as liver disease, altered sensation, and movement disorder (e.g., tremor).

Laboratory Tests

Plain roentgenography in the infant with *congenital* torticollis, with or without a palpable neck mass, will usually be necessary to demonstrate cervical bony anomalies. Magnetic resonance imaging (MRI) may be needed to interpret complicated cervical anomalies or to reveal an anomaly not apparent on plain films. MRI or an enhanced computed tomographic scan of the neck will distinguish fibrodysplasia ossificans progressiva from congenital muscular torticollis in early disease. Computed tomography and MRI of the neck are most sensitive for evaluating the atlantoaxial joint. Rarely will open-muscle or fine-needle biopsy be needed to differentiate a benign muscle tumor of congenital muscular torticollis from a malignancy or other mass.

The child suspected of having Sandifer's syndrome should have a barium swallow and esophageal *p*H probe investigation to rule out gastroesophageal reflux (see Chap. 102).

Calcification of the intervertebral disk is readily diagnosed by routine spine roentgenograms. Vertebral osteomyelitis and diskitis may require a combination of imaging modalities, including radionuclide scans and MRI.

A complete blood cell count and erythrocyte sedimentation rate may point to an infectious process. Sinus and mastoid bone films may disclose localized infection, which is also readily visualized by MRI.

Results of electroencephalography and caloric tests in paroxysmal torticollis of infancy are usually normal, but results of auditory testing may be abnormal.

Investigation of *progressive* torticollis requires more extensive testing. Work-up usually includes MRI and radiographic imaging of the head and neck; slit lamp examination for Kayser-Fleischer corneal ring, measurement of serum hepatic enzyme levels, copper and ceruloplasmin determinations, 24-hour urinary copper excretion to rule out Wilson's disease; and serum creatine phosphokinase determination to rule out myopathies. Other tests will be determined by the results of the physical examination and in consultation with a specialist.

TREATMENT

The hallmark of treatment of congenital muscular torticollis is passive stretching. This is performed by lateral flexion of the head to the side opposite the torticollis and rotation of the chin to the affected side. The infant's rooting reflex will also cause the head to rotate. Massage of the contracted sternocleidomastoid muscle, relocation of the crib, and use of a halter or strapping (quite uncomfortable) are also advocated. The majority of conservatively treated cases with congenital muscular torticollis will resolve by 1 year of age; if these cases are not resolved by then, they are unlikely to do so without surgery (tenotomy and resection). When applied at 5 to 6 months of age, a fitted plastic helmet that puts pressure against the growing skull may remediate persistent torticollis-associated plagiocephaly.

Treatment of acquired inflammatory torticollis consists of treating the underlying infection with systemic oral antibiotics. Uncommon infectious etiologies such as vertebral osteomyelitis, diskitis, and mastoiditis initially require intravenous antibiotics. A soft cervical collar may provide symptomatic relief of discomfort.

Patients whose torticollis is secondary to muscle spasm, to strain, and to calcification of the intervertebral disk will respond to local heat, analgesics, and antispasmodics within 5 to 7 days.

Torticollis from ingestion of and idiosyncratic response to phenothiazines and metoclopramide is treated with intravenous diphenhydramine and diazepam, respectively.

Benzodiazepines and anticholinergics are occasionally effective in treating patients with spasmodic torticollis. Other adjunctive treatment modalities include physical therapy, electromyography—biofeedback, and neurosurgical lesions of the spinal roots and thalami. Local anesthesia and, recently, injection of botulinum toxin has shown promise in the treatment of spasmodic torticollis in adults.

INDICATIONS FOR REFERRAL OR HOSPITALIZATION

Patients with mastoiditis and retropharyngeal abscess should be referred to an otolaryngologist. Other torticollis-associated upper respiratory tract infections need only medical treatment. Severe infections require that the patient be hospitalized and treated with intravenous antibiotics.

The choice of an orthopedic or neurologic surgeon in cases of atlantoaxial subluxation will depend on the availability and expertise of the surgeon. Traction is successful in patients with atlantoaxial subluxation but may have to be used for months.

Evidence of focal neurologic signs, other than the contracted sternocleidomastoid muscle, or raised intracranial pressure should prompt immediate referral to a neurologist.

Any progressive disorder either heralded or accompanied by torticollis should also be referred to a neurologist. Often hospitalization will be necessary to coordinate a multidisciplinary approach to diagnosis and management.

ANNOTATED BIBLIOGRAPHY

Bray PT, Herbst JJ, Johnson DG et al: Childhood gastroesophageal reflux (neurologic and psychiatric syndromes mimicked). JAMA 237:1342, 1977. (Reports that late diagnosis is often the rule in Sandifer's syndrome.)

Clarren SK: Plagiocephaly and torticollis: Etiology, natural history, and helmet treatment. J Pediatr 98:92, 1981. (Stresses diligent early therapy for both entities.)

Menkes JH: Textbook of Child Neurology, 3rd ed. Philadelphia, Lea & Febiger, 1985. (Overview of several forms of idiopathic torticollis.)

Parker W: Migraine and the vestibular system in childhood and adolescence. Am J Otol 10:364, 1989. (In-depth review of paroxysmal torticollis of infancy.)

Swaiman KF (ed): Pediatric Neurology: Principles and Practice. St. Louis, CV Mosby, 1989. (Includes exhaustive differential diagnosis.)

Volpe JJ: Neurology of the Newborn, 2nd ed. Philadelphia, WB Saunders, 1987. (Discussion of congenital torticollis as a restricted neuromuscular disorder.)

135
Pectus Deformities of the Chest Wall

Daniel P. Ryan

Deformities of the chest wall are often seen in children throughout the course of routine care. The presence of a deformity should alert the physician to look for associated problems, but the indications for surgical referral and correction are not well-defined. In recent years there has been increasing controversy concerning the physiologic versus the cosmetic benefits of surgical correction.

PATHOPHYSIOLOGY

The degree of the pectus deformity and the physiologic impairment are difficult to quantify. There is general agreement that nearly all children with pectus deformity have no symptoms related to the abnormal chest wall. Mild degrees of impaired cardiorespiratory function may be evident with exercise but not at rest. Improvement of physiologic parameters during exercise have been reported after repair of the deformity, but these studies usually failed to document the degree of the sternal depression present before and after the surgery. Other studies have failed to show any physiologic benefit to the patient by correcting the chest wall deformity, but, again, the degree of deformity in these patients is rarely quantified.

A proposed mechanism for improved maximal cardiac output and exercise tolerance is that the left and right atria are compromised by the displaced position of the heart into the left side of the chest. One can imagine that with increasing degrees of sternal depression, the area for expansion of the atria would become more and more limited. At rest the cardiac output is not likely to be affected; however, during exercise there may be space restrictions to atrial filing and therefore a limitation to maximal cardiac output. Improvement in the aeration of the lower lobes of the lungs is probably less of a factor in improved cardiac output and exercise tolerance but may be contributory, especially if some degree of ventilation–perfusion mismatch is present because of less-than-maximal excursion of the chest wall during maximal ventilation.

CLINICAL PRESENTATION

Deformities of the ribs and sternum that fall into the categories of *pectus carinatum* (pigeon breast) or *pectus excavatum* (funnel chest) are often present at birth. Nearly 85% of patients have the deformity noticed in the first year of life. Some patients, however, describe a rather sudden change in the contour of the chest wall over a few weeks during a pubertal growth spurt. Usually the child is evaluated because of the parent's wishes or in adolescence or adulthood because of the patient's perception of the deformity and a wish for "normality."

The presence of a pectus deformity should alert the physician to a number of associated syndromes and latent problems. The most common and potentially most lethal associated problem is *Marfan's syndrome*. Patients with Marfan's disease should be evaluated for coexisting cardiac and aortic involvement and should be counseled concerning their condition. Avoiding stressful physical exertion such as weight-lifting and competitive sports is probably wise so as to decrease the chances of sudden death. If Marfan's syndrome is suspected, full cardiac evaluation should be done before any decisions are made regarding surgical procedures on the chest wall. Ligamentous and ocular disease are not always present, even when there is severe valvular heart disease, congestive heart failure, or aortic enlargement.

Cardiac problems have been associated with chest wall deformities without coincident Marfan's syndrome. Cardiac dysrhythmias such as atrial fibrillation and paroxysmal supraventricular tachycardia have been described in patients with pectus excavatum; the etiology is unclear. Clearly, however, there is an increased incidence of Wolff-Parkinson-White syndrome in patients with pectus excavatum (as high as 4%). In addition, many patients with pectus excavatum have echocardiographic evidence of mitral valve prolapse. Some of the patients with mitral valve prolapse will have their findings resolve after the chest wall deformity is corrected.

Scoliosis is present along with pectus deformities in about 20% of patients. From 14% to 18% of patients with combined pectus and scoliosis require therapeutic intervention for the scoliosis ranging from bracing of the thorax to surgical arthrodesis of the vertebrae.

Poland's syndrome is often easily distinguished from simple pectus excavatum. The constellation of anomalies in this syndrome include absence of the pectoralis major and pectoralis minor muscles, hand anomalies, absence of ribs, chest wall depression, athelia and/or amastia, absence of axillary hair, and limited subcutaneous fat on the chest. Any patient may have any number of the anomalies, and the defects range from relatively mild to very severe.

The chest wall problem that leads to most symptoms and most severe deformity is the absence of ribs. Even small areas of absent ribs in infants can result in the "flail chest" physiology of increased respiratory work, lung herniation, atelectasis, or recurrent pneumonia. In addition, the contralateral chest wall often has a carinate deformity and the sternum is usually very rotated. Such patients are best treated with repairing the rotational defect of the sternum, by resecting the deformed costal cartilages, and by stabilizing the chest wall defect due to the absent ribs by using autologous rib from the opposite side.

WORK-UP

All children with moderate to severe chest wall deformities should be evaluated for the associated problems listed earlier. Unless surgical intervention is contemplated, there is no indication to do any specific evaluation of the pectus deformity itself. Documentation of the degree of sternal deformity is best done with simple posteroanterior and lateral chest roentgenograms. Although computed tomographic scans have also been used to document the amount of deformity, the extra cost is not justified. Evaluation with pulmonary function testing or other sophisticated exercise testing is also not necessary, unless a patient has specific symptoms.

INDICATIONS FOR REFERRAL

Because of the controversy surrounding the surgical repair of a pectus deformity, any patient who wishes to contemplate surgery should be evaluated by a pediatric surgeon who is trained to perform the repair. In some areas of the country, qualified adult thoracic surgeons may be appropriate for older children. Plastic and reconstructive surgeons have described various methods to fill the depression in the chest, but none of these techniques improve the bony deformity that may be contributing to physiologic impairment.

In some patients with coexisting pectus excavatum and heart disease, closing the chest following corrective cardiac surgery may necessitate elevation of the sternum to prevent pressure on the right ventricle and pulmonary outflow tract or on surgically constructed conduits. Yet, simultaneous repair of the chest wall deformity and cardiac surgery is possible if adequate preparation in made. The chest wall preferably should be repaired before any cardiac surgery to prevent difficulties with bleeding into the mediastinum from costal cartilage resection done at the time of cardiac surgery. The accepted techniques for pectus repair usually do not interfere with the performance of a median sternotomy after healing takes place. The approach for each patient should be coordinated between the cardiologist, cardiac surgeon, and pediatric surgeon for optimal results.

Patients with significant scoliosis should also be evaluated by an orthopedic surgeon before repair of the chest wall. The best results can be obtained by a combined approach to the spine and chest wall. Often in these cases, the spine is of paramount importance and repair of the curvature will also improve the appearance and function of the chest wall.

Children with absent ribs and Poland's syndrome should be referred early for evaluation before the development of associated pulmonary problems. Stabilization of the chest wall using autologous rib grafts in the area of absent ribs offers the best choice for a good result. The rib is harvested from a normal area on the opposite side, leaving the periosteum intact to allow for regeneration. The rib graft may be split longitudinally to allow for correction of the deformity with the least tissue removed from the normal area. Repair of the chest wall deformity is usually done prior to any breast reconstruction, although techniques using the ipsilateral latissimus dorsi muscle as a flap along with rib grafts may accomplish breast reconstruction as a single operation. In boys with absent ribs, use of the latissimus dorsi muscle should probably be avoided because it provides much of the shoulder stability in these patients with absent pectoralis muscles.

Many techniques of repair of the chest wall deformity in pectus excavatum and carinatum have been described, and good results are reported with all techniques. Most techniques used today involve resecting the deformed lower costal cartilages in a subperichondrial plane to free the sternum. The sternum is then elevated to a normal or even to an "overcorrected" position, usually with the assistance of an anterior osteotomy below the level of the manubrium and with resection of the xyphoid process. Rotational deformities are corrected by performing the osteotomy at an oblique angle to correct both the depression and rotation simultaneously.

The sternum is then secured in place using the pectoral muscles and fascia or internal stents of either metal or autologous bone graft from a flat rib. The necessity of internal fixation is a matter of debate. The presence of metal struts usually necessitates a second procedure to remove them a number of months after the original procedure; however, the removal is usually done in an outpatient setting, occasionally with the patient under local anesthesia.

The recovery period varies with the age of the patient. Children in the 4- to 7-year age group are usually in the hospital for 3 or 4 days following the operation. Teenagers often require 5 to 7 days before they are comfortable enough to go home. With the use of continuous epidural analgesia postoperatively, much of the discomfort can be prevented. The complication rate from the surgery, including problems ranging from pneumothorax, wound seroma, hematoma, or infection is less than 2%. The risk of recurrence following surgical repair is also very low.

ANNOTATED BIBLIOGRAPHY

Hawkins JA, Ehrenhaft JL, Doty DB: Repair of pectus excavatum by sternal eversion. Ann Thorac Surg 38:368–373, 1984. (Description of a procedure to repair the deformity and how it can be done in conjunction with cardiac surgery.)

Haller JA, Colombani PM, Miller D, Manson P: Early reconstruction of Poland's syndrome using autologous rib grafts combined with a latissimus muscle flap. J Pediatr Surg 19:423–429, 1984. (Good description of the problems unique to Poland's syndrome and their surgical treatment.)

Ravitch MM: The chest wall. In Welch KJ, Randolph JG, O'Neill JA Jr, Rowe MI (eds): Pediatric Surgery, 4th ed, vol 1, pp 563–589. Chicago, Year Book Medical Publishers, 1986. (Classic description of the problem and the original corrective procedure by its originator.)

Shamberger RC, Welch KJ: Cardiopulmonary function in pectus excavatum. Surg Gynecol Obstet 166:383–391, 1988. (Exhaustive review of the literature concerning the functional changes with pectus excavatum.)

Shamberger RC, Welch KJ: Surgical repair of pectus excavatum. J Pediatr Surg 23:615–622, 1988. (This largest single experience with pectus excavatum repair reviews over 1000 surgical cases.)

136
Scoliosis

Anthony E. Webber

There has been a recent explosion of awareness and interest in scoliosis that has penetrated both the lay and medical worlds. Since the founding of the Scoliosis Research Society in 1966, the level of care for scoliosis has improved considerably. This includes detection in school screening programs to improved surgical techniques and instrumentation systems. It is in this milieu that the pediatrician should have the examining skills necessary to manage the vastly increased numbers of adolescents discovered by the school screening programs and also to be aware of those children with more severe curves that may require bracing and possibly surgery. Although the majority of minor curves detected by school screening will not progress to the severity requiring intervention by the orthopedic surgeon, it is the role of the pediatrician to be aware of the potential for progression of minor curves and to refer patients to the orthopedist when appropriate.

DEFINITION AND CLASSIFICATION

Scoliosis is defined as a lateral curvature of the spine. This may involve the spine from the cervical through to the lumbar spine. The presence of scoliosis is not a normal finding, but it is usually unrecognized by the child and his family.

Kyphosis is a curve that is concave anteriorly when viewed from the lateral projection, giving a hunchback appearance. It is normally present in the thoracic spine.

Lordosis is a curve that is convex anteriorly when viewed from the lateral projection, giving a swayback appearance. It is normally present in both the cervical and lumbar spine.

Although the causes of scoliosis are many (Table 136-1), the vast majority of scoliosis noted in both the pediatrician's office and in a referral scoliosis clinic is termed *adolescent idiopathic scoliosis.*

The diagnosis of idiopathic scoliosis should only be made after excluding nonstructural scoliosis, neurologic causes of scoliosis by a careful history and physical examination, and congenital scoliosis with a roentgenogram.

The patterns of curvatures are defined by the position of the curve within the spine and also by the direction of the convexity of the curve. In idiopathic scoliosis, the more common curve patterns are right thoracic and left lumbar double major curves; right thoracic and right thoracolumbar curves; and left lumbar curves.

The clinical detection of these curves results from rotation of the spine that occurs in conjunction with the lateral curvature. The rib and lumbar humps that manifest in the forward bend test for scoliosis are due to the rotational component of the laterally curving spine.

ETIOLOGY

The etiology of idiopathic scoliosis remains unknown, but certain factors are known to play a role. Genetic factors are important; daughters of mothers who have had scoliosis have a greater risk for developing scoliosis. The mode of inheritance is uncertain, and both dominant and multifactorial modes of transmission have been suggested.

In minor curves of less than 10° the male-to-female ratio is 1:1. However, as the curve magnitude increases, the ratio of female to male increases significantly, indicating that sex has a significant role in the pathogenesis of scoliosis. In curves greater than 20°, the female-to-male ratio is 5:1.

CLINICAL PRESENTATION

The pediatrician will encounter scoliosis in many scenarios, but most frequently it will be the result of referral from a school screening program or an incidental finding in a routine physical examination. The office visit should include a family history and possible neurologic causes of scoliosis. The history should elicit information regarding sexual development, since the onset of menses indicates limited growth potential and thus less potential for progression of the curve. If pain is the presenting symptom in a child with scoliosis, idiopathic scoliosis is unlikely to be the diagnosis.

The physical examination involves a careful neurologic examination, evaluation of the skin for café-au-lait spots, and evaluation of secondary sex characteristics (Tanner staging). Local evaluation of the back for hairy patches, dimples, and lipoma may indicate the presence of a congenital scoliosis. Assessment of leg lengths is relevant in that inequality may result in a nonstructural scoliosis that disappears with sitting or with the pelvis balanced by appropriate blocks beneath the short leg.

The specific examination for scoliosis includes evaluation of shoulder height, rib, and waist and breast asymmetry. The *forward bend test* is most helpful for assessing the presence of and the severity of scoliosis (Fig. 136-1). As the patient bends forward, the rotation of the vertebra associated with the scoliosis results in the presence of a rib and/ or a lumbar hump. It is this forward bend test on which school screening programs rely. The size of the hump can be measured in centimeters or by the use of a scoliometer

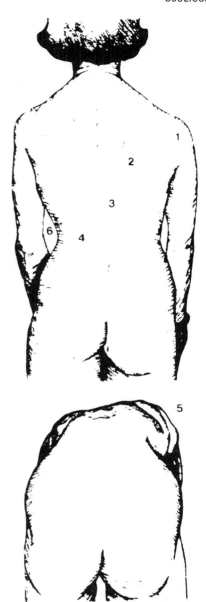

Figure 136-1. The forward bend test. Signs of scoliosis on a screening examination include (**1**) depression (or elevation) of shoulder; (**2**) asymmetry of scapulae; (**3**) visible curvature of spine; (**4**) sacral tilt (or asymmetry of hips); (**5**) rib hump (lumbar or thoracic); (**6**) asymmetry in distance between arms and body. In addition, failure of occiput to line up directly over buttocks' crease may be noted. (Berwick DM: Scoliosis screening. Pediatr Rev 5:238–247, 1984)

that quantifies the slope of the spine at the highest point of the hump. The scoliometer is a useful technique of serial examination in the child with scoliosis. A scoliometer reading of 6 degrees or less indicates that a curve is minor and does not require active intervention.

(Text continues on p. 517)

Table 136-1. Classification of Structural Scoliosis

I. Idiopathic Scoliosis—This group, which makes up about 65% of all patients seen, is subdivided according to the age at which the scoliosis is first noticed. There can be a considerable lapse between the time when scoliosis first develops and when it is first noticed. Each subdivision has certain definite characteristics that distinguish it from the others.
   A. *Infantile Scoliosis*—spinal curvature develops during first 3 years of life
      1. Progressive
      2. Resolving
   B. *Juvenile Scoliosis*—spinal curvature develops between skeletal ages of 4 and 12 years in girls and 4 and 14 years in boys
   C. *Adolescent Scoliosis*—spinal curvature develops after skeletal age of 12 years in girls and of 14 years in boys
II. Congenital Skeletal Abnormalities—This group makes up about 15% of patients seen with scoliosis, and the deformity is caused by anomalous bony development.
   A. *Vertebral Anomalies*
      1. Open vertebral canal
         a. With neurologic deficit
            (1) Myelomeningocele
         b. Without neurologic deficit
            (1) Spina bifida occulta
            (2) Myelomeningocele
      2. Closed vertebral canal
         a. With neurologic defect
            (1) Diastematomyelia
            (2) Other forms of spinal dysrhaphia
         b. Without neurologic defect
            (1) Failure of formation of vertebral elements
               (a) Wedged vertebra
               (b) Hemivertebra
            (2) Failure of segmentation of vertebral elements
               (a) Partial—vertebral bar
               (b) Complete—vertebral coalition
   B. *Extravertebral Anomalies*
      1. Rib coalition
III. Neuromuscular Abnormalities—This group makes up about 10% of patients seen with scoliosis.
   A. *Neuropathic*
      1. Upper motor neuron lesion
         a. Cerebral palsy
         b. Spinocerebellar degeneration
            (1) Charcot-Marie-Tooth disease
            (2) Friedreich's ataxia
            (3) Roussy-Lévy syndrome
         c. Syringomyelia
         d. Spinal cord tumors
         e. Spinal cord injury
      2. Lower motor neuron lesion
         a. Poliomyelitis
         b. Other types of viral myelitis
      3. Progressive spinal muscular atrophy
         a. Infantile (Werdnig-Hoffmann syndrome)
         b. Juvenile (Kugelberg-Welander syndrome)
      4. Nonprogressive juvenile spinal atrophy
      5. Dysautonomia (Riley-Day syndrome)
   B. *Myopathic*
      1. Muscular dystrophy
         a. Pseudohypertrophic muscular dystrophy
         b. Limb-girdle muscular dystrophy
         c. Facioscapulohumeral muscular dystrophy
      2. Myotonia atrophica (Steinert's disease)
      3. Myotonia congenita (Thomsen's disease)
      4. Arthrogryposis
      5. Hypotonia
IV. Scoliosis Associated With Neurofibromatosis—This group makes up about 5% of patients seen with scoliosis.
V. Mesenchymal Disorders
   A. *Congenital*
      1. Marfan's syndrome
      2. Ehlers-Danlos syndrome
   B. *Acquired,* i.e., rheumatoid arthritis
VI. Trauma
   A. *Fractures of the vertebral body*
   B. *Surgical insult*
      1. Damage to vertebral growth plates
      2. Laminectomy
      3. Extraspinal—thoracoplasty
   C. *Irradiation*
VII. Extraspinal Contractures
   A. *Postempyema*
   B. *Burns*
VIII. Osteochondrodystrophies
   A. *Diastrophic dwarfism*
   B. *Mucopolysaccharidoses* (Morquio's disease, and others)
   C. *Spondyloepiphyseal dysplasia*
   D. *Multiple epiphyseal dysplasia*
   E. *Other*
IX. Infection of Bone
   A. *Acute*
   B. *Chronic*
      1. Tuberculosis
X. Metabolic Disorders
   A. *Osteomalacia*
      1. Rickets
   B. *Osteoporosis*
   C. *Osteogenesis imperfecta*
   D. *Homocystinuria*
XI. Thoracogenic Disorders
   A. *Post thoracotomy*
XII. Related to Lumbosacral Joint
   A. *Related to spondylosis and spondylolisthesis*
   B. *Congenital anomalies of the sacrum and sacroiliac joint*
XIII. Tumors
   A. *Vertebral column*
      1. Osteoid-osteoma
      2. Hemangioma
   B. *Spinal cord*
      1. Astrocytoma
      2. Teratoma
      3. Intermedullary cysts
      4. Lipoma
      5. Ependymoma

Reprinted with permission from Riseborough EJ, Herndon JH: Scoliosis and Other Deformities of the Axial Skeleton, p. 22. Boston, Little, Brown & Co., 1975

The flexibility of the curve can be determined by asking the patient to rotate to the right and the left while in the forward bending position. A curve that is more rigid is suggestive of a congenital scoliosis or may indicate a curve that will be less responsive to bracing or surgery.

The use of spinal roentgenograms should be limited to those children in whom the clinical findings are suggestive of a scoliosis of at least 10 degrees. A single anteroposterior view of the spine will, in most cases, be sufficient to assess the nature and severity of the curvature. Multiple and repeated roentgenograms of the spine should be avoided, and lateral projections should be ordered only if the normal kyphotic and lordotic curves are not present. The Cobb method of assessing severity of curves (angles drawn on the spine roentgenogram) is routinely used to quantify the degree of curvature of the scoliosis.

Moiré or fringe topography can be used to monitor a patient with a known scoliosis. By serially evaluating the pattern of interference fringes that are cast on the back when light is shone through a screen of closely spaced wires, progression of a scoliosis can be reliably and safely detected.

MANAGEMENT

The management of scoliosis aims to prevent the deterioration of curves through the growing years. It is the large curves of greater than 50 to 60 degrees that will result in cosmetic deformity, pulmonary problems, and possibly pain, and therefore must be avoided.

Unfortunately, it is not possible to reliably predict the course of the majority of adolescents with mild scoliosis. Thus, even if scoliosis is mild, serial evaluation is necessary to assess for progression of the curve. Depending on the rate of growth of the patient, this evaluation should be performed every 4 to 6 months. It is especially important to closely follow children who are undergoing rapid growth, since they are at greatest risk for progression of their scoliosis.

In the child with a mild curve (i.e., less than 20° to 25°), no active intervention is required because it has little or no functional or cosmetic significance. Exercises, physical therapy, and chiropractic manipulation have no role in the treatment of minor curves, since they have not been shown to alter the natural history of the disease. The patient should be allowed to participate in physical education and sporting activities and should be encouraged to have a normal lifestyle. It is common for the teenager to be concerned about his or her curve. He or she should be counseled appropriately and reassured that most curves do not progress.

In the child with a progressive curve that is greater than 20° or 25° degrees, and if the child has growth potential, brace treatment will usually be indicated. The low-profile Boston brace and high-profile Milwaukee brace are two of the more commonly used braces for progressive scoliosis. When appropriately used, bracing has an excellent chance to prevent deterioration and progression of curves. These braces are generally worn for 18 to 24 hours per day until the end of skeletal growth. An exercise program is combined with bracing to maintain adequate flexibility and strength of spinal muscles. It is important to counsel families that bracing will not result in correction of the curve and a straight spine, but will prevent progression of the curve in up to 85% to 90% of children who, if left untreated, would require surgical intervention.

Some clinicians have advocated the use of electrical stimulation of the paraspinal musculature instead of bracing for progressive curves. This technique is not used widely, since results have been less reliable and less predictable than bracing.

The psychological and social stresses on the adolescent who wears a brace for up to 24 hours a day are often immense. Compliance may be poor, and families and patients should be given needed support.

In the child who fails a brace program because of noncompliance, or who has a progressive curve despite adequate bracing, fusion and instrumentation of the spine is indicated. With the advent of better surgical techniques and instrumentation systems (e.g., Luque, Cotrel-Dubousset), the postoperative period has been easier for the patient. A plastic brace and at times no bracing at all has replaced the 3- to 6-month period of body jacket casting. Success rates are very high in preventing progression of scoliosis, although late long-term effects of spinal fusion of lumbar vertebrae may be an increasing problem.

INDICATIONS FOR REFERRAL

Children with scoliosis should be referred to an orthopedist when the objective examination indicates that the scoliosis is progressing (i.e., a change of at least 5°) or when the curvature on initial examination is greater than 15° in a growing child. Those children whose scoliosis is secondary to one of the conditions listed in Table 136-1 are usually already followed by an appropriate subspecialist (e.g., orthopedist, neurologist); if they are not, consideration should be made for subspecialty consultation.

ANNOTATED BIBLIOGRAPHY

Berwick DM: Scoliosis screening. Pediatr Rev 5:238–247, 1984. (Critical review of principles of screening for scoliosis, emphasizing that few of those children with positive screening tests have problems requiring intervention and that screening, if done at all, should be concentrated in age groups with rapid growth.)

Bjure J, Nachemson A: Non-treated scoliosis. Clin Orthop Rel Res 83:44–52, 1973. (Review and report on long-term consequences of severe scoliosis, emphasizing that surgical correction is indicated only in a small proportion of cases.)

Lonstein JE, Bjorklund S, Wanninger MH, Nelson RP: Voluntary school screening for scoliosis in Minnesota. J Bone Joint Surg [Am] 64:481–488, 1982. (Description by pioneering American group of the organization and results of a state-wide screening program that showed that of the 3.4% with positive tests, about one third had scoliosis on follow-up evaluation.)

Rogala EJ, Drummond DS, Gurr J: Scoliosis: Incidence and natural history. J Bone Joint Surg [Am] 60:173–176, 1978. (Prospective epidemiologic study of idiopathic scoliosis in 1122 school children, with a 2-year follow-up of 603 in which progression of curvature was observed in 6.8% of cases and spontaneous improvement occurred in 3%.)

Torrell G, Norwell A, Nachemson A: The changing pattern of scoliosis treatment due to effective screening. J Bone Joint Surg 63 [Am]: 337–341, 1982. (Presents data suggesting that screening in Sweden may have reduced the proportion of cases ultimately requiring surgery.)

137

Soft Tissue Injuries

Charles F. Sanzone

Soft tissue injuries include *sprains* (involving ligaments), *strains* (involving muscles and tendons), and *contusions* (bruises). These terms are often used incorrectly or inexactly. Moreover, it may be difficult to differentiate these injuries from each other. The most common soft tissue injuries to children are minor contusions and are often sports related. Sprains and strains are far less common than fractures in growing children.

This chapter covers principles in the management of soft tissue injuries, which are similar for sprains, strains and contusions. Fractures are discussed in Chapter 138, and skin lacerations and abrasions are discussed in Chapter 143. Injuries involving upper extremities, knees, and feet are discussed in separate chapters (see Chaps. 139 through 141. *Overuse injuries* in children are sports related but are presented here instead of in the chapter on sports medicine because principles for their treatment are similar to those of other soft tissue injuries.

PATHOPHYSIOLOGY

Ligaments are richly supplied with nerve endings as part of the proprioceptive apparatus. Physical disruption of a ligament (sprain) and direct contusion are the only mechanisms causing pain in a ligament. In children whose growth plates (physes) are still open, severe sprains are rare injuries because the ligaments are usually stronger than the cartilaginous physes, when both are subjected to tension. Muscles and tendons can be ruptured (strains, single macrotrauma episodes), injured by repetitive small stresses (microtrauma and overuse syndromes), or fatigued (accumulation of metabolites). The origins and insertions of muscles and tendons are usually mediated by cartilaginous structures similar to growth plates (apophyses). Where apophyses exist, avulsion fractures are far more common than ruptures to either tendon or the muscle. Sudden forces may also result in avulsions of muscles, tendons, or ligaments from their insertions. Injuries to nerves are not considered in this chapter.

Injuries occur from trauma, which may or may not be sports related. Regardless of etiology, bleeding and edema result. In general, the more severe the injury, the greater the extent of bleeding and damage to the underlying tissue. Bleeding leads to edema, which in turn results in loss of motion and pain. Most injuries are mild and do not cause loss of function. Loss of stability implies a serious sprain or strain because the ligament, tendon, or muscle is disrupted, either partially or completely.

Overuse injuries are caused by repetitive microtrauma to any area in the musculoskeletal system and may result in sprains, strains, tendinitis, bursitis, apophysitis, and stress fractures. Since children are training more intensely and competing earlier, overuse injuries are presenting more frequently in the pediatric population. As outlined in the American Academy of Pediatrics' sports medicine handbook, causes include a change in the child's training (e.g., increase in rigor or the addition of a new technique such as weight training); incorrect biomechanics (e.g., poor technique); improper environment (e.g., running on concrete); anatomic malalignment (e.g., leg length discrepancy, flat feet, pronation); improper equipment (e.g., worn out athletic shoes); growing cartilage (which is sensitive to stress); and associated diseases (e.g., arthritis). The most common overuse syndromes in children are *apophysitis of the posterior calcaneus (Sever's disease), plantar fasciitis, achilles tendonitis, Osgood-Schlatter disease, shin splints, chondromalacia patellae, shoulder impingement syndromes* (e.g., "swimmers' shoulder"), and *epiphysitis of the medial epicondyle* (e.g., "pitcher's elbow").

CLINICAL PRESENTATION

Sprains

Sprains are divided into grade 1 (mild), grade 2 (moderate), and grade 3 (severe) injuries. Grade 1 is most common and results in microscopic tearing of the ligament without elongation. Swelling is minimal; function and stability are preserved. Grade 2 sprains result in a partial loss of function caused by a larger, although incomplete tear causing detectable laxity. In grade 3 strains, a complete tear causes marked laxity and loss of stability. Swelling is usually present, as are pain and tenderness.

Strains

Strains are also graded, but this categorization is probably less clinically useful than for sprains. The most common strain is mild grade 1 and usually results from overstretching of the muscle. There may be muscle spasm, and pain occurs when the muscle is used, but there is no loss of strength. An immediate onset and rapidly appearing hematoma suggest a more severe strain. A grade 2 strain has a partial disruption causing some loss of function. With a grade 3 strain, there is a complete tear in the muscle or tendon that can often be palpated as a gap, and the function is lost. As with sprains, the child complains of pain and tenderness. Swelling, often recognized a hematoma, is seen in grade 2 and 3 strains but may be appreciated as only slight bogginess with a grade 1 strain.

Contusions

Contusions are bruises without disruption to the overlying skin. With mild contusions edema may not be present. They usually heal uneventfully, but an injury to the quadriceps ("Charley horse") warrants concern since *myositis ossificans* may result from an otherwise unremarkable bruise.

DIFFERENTIAL DIAGNOSIS

The cause of the complaint or injury is usually apparent either by the history or by the examination, and seldom does a differential diagnosis need to be generated. However, confusion may arise, and infection, inflammation (e.g., from a collagen vascular disorder), tumor, vascular disorder (e.g., hemangioma, arteriovenous malformation, lymphangioma, bleeding diathesis), neuropathy, or connective tissue disease (e.g., Ehler-Danlos syndrome) may need to be considered. Child abuse must be suspected when lesions are multiple or atypical or when circumstances of the injury are unusual.

Although a soft tissue injury may be the most obvious or indeed the only apparent lesion, the possibility of a more serious occult lesion (e.g., splenic rupture in the presence of a contusion to the abdomen) must always be ruled out.

WORK-UP
History

The circumstances, time of onset of the injury, and, most importantly, a description of the mechanism of the injury should be determined. This will often provide a clue to the diagnosis. For example, the type of injury from a fall while jumping (low impact) will likely be different than a fall caused by a moving object such as a car. High-impact injuries are more likely to produce fractures, dislocations, or ligament injuries in addition to soft tissue injuries. However, low-impact injuries may also produce serious soft tissue injuries. Was pain immediate or did it occur several hours later? Grade 1 sprains or strains may have a delayed onset. In general, the more serious the injury, the sooner will the symptoms occur. Did swelling occur immediately?

Swelling due to hemorrhage is usually of prompt onset (minutes to a few hours), whereas edema and effusion often take 6 to 12 hours to appear. This is an important point in distinguishing traumatic effusions from acute hemarthroses. Was ice applied immediately after the injury? This could alter the physical findings and have the injury appear less serious. The reporting of a "pop" or "snap" usually indicates a serious injury, often a complete tear. Is there reluctance to use the injured joint, limitation of motion, instability, or "giving way"? Details of preexisting diseases should be obtained.

Physical Examination

A detailed examination of the affected part must be performed, but this may not always detect the severity of the injury. Grade 1 sprains are diagnosed on the basis of direct tenderness over a ligament, indirect tenderness in the ligament on stress, and stability to stress. Grade 2 sprains have some instability, and grade 3 sprains have complete instability. With grade 1 strains there is tenderness over the muscle without a hematoma, and grade 3 strains have palpable defects in the muscle with loss of function.

The observer should first inspect the injury. The alignment of the extremity should be noted. A deformed limb should be splinted, have its circulation monitored closely, and be regarded as an emergency. Swelling usually indicates the specific area to be evaluated. It is important to reserve maneuvers that may be painful until the end of the examination to maintain the patient's cooperation.

Palpation for *direct bony tenderness* is important. In the traumatic setting, direct bony tenderness indicates the presence of a fracture until proven otherwise. Similarly, in the vicinity of a joint, direct bony tenderness indicates a fracture, avulsion, or growth plate injury, rather than a sprain. In the inflammatory setting, direct bony tenderness indicates osteomyelitis until proven otherwise. Both the medial and lateral sides of the joint should be palpated. If the anatomy of the individual ligaments is known, each ligament and each component of the ligament should be palpated. Once direct tenderness has been evaluated, the examiner should test for *indirect tenderness,* confirming a disruption of the soft tissue in question and assessing its stability. Indirect tenderness is elicited by applying a stress without touching the structure. For example, to stress the medial collateral ligament of the elbow, one hand is placed on the lateral aspect of the joint while the other hand grasps the forearm near the wrist. Pushing the hands toward each other exerts a valgus force at the elbow, placing the medial collateal ligament on stretch. The entire range of motion of the injured extremity must be evaluated as well as that of the uninjured extremity. Finally, the integrity of the skin, circulation, and neurologic function must be accurately documented.

Because *instability* differentiates serious injuries from

minor ones, it is most important to determine if there is instability of the joint or loss of function. The extent of the swelling and ecchymosis should be noted, but even with severe injuries, these findings may be minimal if ice and compression were applied immediately after the injury.

Gentle palpation early, before the onset of generalized edema, can often delineate the site of injury. Massive edema obliterates the point of maximal tenderness.

Erythema is a late sign of most musculoskeletal inflammatory conditions, with the exceptions of superficial bursitides such as those of the prepatellar and olecranon bursae.

Laboratory Tests

Grade 1 sprains or strains usually do not require roentgenographic examination. If, however, symptoms increase or do not resolve after 48 to 72 hours of treatment, a roentgenogram should be obtained. Roentgenograms should usually be obtained for grade 2 and always grade 3 sprains and any strain near bony attachments. The presence of a fracture, dislocation, or major ligamentous damage will usually be visible on both anteroposterior and lateral roentgenograms of the injured part. Failure to demonstrate a fracture roentgenographically is *not* proof that a fracture does not exist. Subtle signs of fracture include all those indicative of deep soft tissue swelling, such as displacement or effacement of fat pads and soft tissue planes. If the roentgenographic interpretation is uncertain, it is useful to obtain roentgenograms of the opposite, uninjured body part. Stress views may result in additional injury and are best ordered by an orthopedist.

Magnetic resonance imaging may be useful when the extent or exact location of the injury needs to be clarified. Arthrocentesis of large post-traumatic effusions and all nontraumatic effusions may be diagnostic as well as therapeutic.

In the nontraumatic setting, however, deep soft tissue swelling indicates infection or neoplasm. If either is suspected, it is often useful to obtain a hemogram with a white blood cell count and differential, erythrocyte sedimentation rate (to help rule out osteomyelitis, septic arthritis, and systemic inflammatory disease), and hemoglobin electrophoresis (to rule out sickle cell crisis).

Treatment

RICE is the acronym for the treatment of all soft tissue injuries.

- *R* (for rest): The injured area should be rested for the first 24 to 72 hours, until the pain resolves. This is to minimize further bleeding into the injured tissue. If pain is still present after 72 hours, the child should be reevaluated because other diagnoses such as fractures may be present. Slings, crutches, or newer devices such as inflatable

splints for sprained ankles may encourage rest or permit protective function.
- *I* (for ice): Cryotherapy has been demonstrated to be effective, particularly when applied immediately or at least within the first 6 hours. Indeed, all soft tissue injuries should be "iced." Ice decreases pain by reducing nerve impulses, limits hemorrhage by vasoconstriction, and prevents further tissue damage by decreasing catabolism.

Ice chips are most effective and should be applied for 20 minutes every 4 hours while the child is awake until the bleeding stops and the swelling is reduced. The ice pack should be applied over a layer of wet elastic wrap, with the rest of the bandage then applied over the ice pack to hold it in place. This technique prevents frostbite and achieves compression. Frozen gel or packages of small frozen vegetables (e.g., corn) are effective alternatives to ice packs, are reusable, and can be contoured to the injury. The "instant ice" bags produce cold by an endothermic reaction but are not as effective as ice packs because they do not become as cold, and the cold lasts only 10 minutes. Heat should not be used acutely for soft tissue injuries.
- *C* (for compression): Elastic bandages are crucial for decreasing bleeding and swelling. The injured part should be bandaged continuously for several days until all edema is resolved. Good technique in applying the elastic wrap is important. When there is a depression (e.g., ankle injury), padding must be used under the bandage and the wrap then applied from bony prominence to bony prominence. The bandage should not be applied too tightly for fear of vascular compromise.
- *E* (for elevation): Elevation above the level of the heart reduces hydrostatic pressure, which in turn reduces edema.

In addition to the above therapies, analgesics are often symptomatically helpful. Nonsteroidal anti-inflammatory drugs may be preferable to acetaminophen because of their combined analgesic and anti-inflammatory properties. Aspirin should be avoided because it has greater anticoagulant effects than the nonsteroidal anti-inflammatory agents.

For grade 1 sprains, range of motion exercises are instituted within the week when swelling has stabilized, but weight bearing is delayed until the pain has disappeared. Participation in sports should be deferred until pain has subsided and full range of motion has been achieved. The devoted athlete may be allowed to participate, provided that he or she understands the possibility of worsening his injury and that some protection in the form of a brace (not an elastic sock) or taping is provided.

Contusions are treated in the same manner as sprains and strains. If myositis ossificans develops, the child should be restricted from activity until movement may be performed painlessly.

A detailed discussion of overuse injuries is beyond the scope of this chapter, but therapeutic principles are similar to other soft tissue injuries. Namely, the examiner should have an understanding of the anatomy, or if uncomfortable with managing these injuries, he or she should refer the patient to a more experienced clinician. The injured part should be rested, and ice should be applied. Anti-inflammatory medication may also be part of therapy. Most injuries get better when activity is discontinued, but healing may take up to 12 weeks. The major therapeutic difference between soft tissue and overuse injuries is the central role of compression in the former and correction of the underlying cause such as improper training in the later.

INDICATIONS FOR REFERRAL

The injured, dedicated athlete in organized sports would likely benefit by referral to an orthopedist. Grade 2 sprains require some judgment with regard to referral. In complex or inherently unstable joints such as the knee, the patient should be referred to an orthopedic clinician. All grade 3 sprains and strains should also be referred to an orthopedic surgeon. Many will require surgical repair. Joint effusion should also be referred.

A discussion of rehabilitation is beyond the scope of this chapter and usually beyond the expertise of the primary care clinician. Its goals are to reestablish muscle strength and endurance, and it should never be undertaken when pain is present. Referral to a physiotherapist, trainer, or orthopedist is best to determine when to institute an optimal rehabilitation program. In addition to isometric, isotonic, or isokinetic exercises (singly or in combination), other modalities such as ultrasound examination and galvanic stimulation may be useful.

ANNOTATED BIBLIOGRAPHY

American Academy of Pediatrics: Sports Medicine: Health Care for Young Athletes, 2nd ed. Elk Grove Village, IL, American Academy of Pediatrics, 1991. (Good reference with excellent chapters on overuse syndromes and initial management of minor soft tissue trauma.)

American Academy of Orthopedic Surgeons: Injury and Repair of the Musculoskeletal Soft Tissues. Park Ridge, IL, American Academy of Orthopedic Surgeons, 1988. (Focuses on the structural aspects of soft tissue injury.)

Garrick JG, Webb DR: Sports Injuries: Diagnosis and Management, Philadelphia, WB Saunders, 1990. (Another good overall reference, particularly the chapter on soft tissue injuries.)

Iverson LD, Clawson DK: Manual of Acute Orthopaedic Therapeutics, 3rd ed. Boston, Little, Brown & Co, 1987. (Excellent and concise, with many "how-to" hints not found in other publications.)

Rang M: Children's Fractures, 2nd ed. Philadelphia, JB Lippincott, 1983. (Unique, folksy and amusing presentation of the basics of pediatric orthopedic trauma, making each chapter memorable; a good starting point for those interested in pediatric orthopedics.)

Rockwood CA, Wilkins KE, King RE: Fractures in Children. Philadelphia, JB Lippincott, 1984. (Excellent, encyclopedic, multicontributor textbook.)

138

Fractures: Guidelines for Initial Management

Lorin M. Brown

Fractures of the child's skeleton are unlike those in the adult because of the child's ongoing growth. The child will double in size between birth and 2 years of age and again between 2 and 10 years of age. During these times of accelerated growth, the body has both a forgiving and an unforgiving attitude toward the reshaping and future length of the remodeling skeleton. Distal to the long bones are growth plates that connect the epiphyseal ends to the shafts of the bones. The growth plates consist of soft cartilaginous cells structured in five different layers. During childhood and early adolescence, these plates are softer and much more easily injured than are the tough ligaments and capsular tissue that attach to the epiphyses to form the joints. Therefore, when an injury occurs at a joint in the growing child, it is more likely to be a growth plate fracture than a ligamentous sprain or tear.

TYPES OF FRACTURES

The five types of fractures involving the growth plates have been categorized in the Salter-Harris classification (Fig. 138-1).

There are fewer residual complications and much more forgiving remodeling of the bone with a Salter-Harris type I or II fracture. A Salter-Harris type I fracture is usually seen on the roentgenogram as a rarefaction in the epiphyseal line. When it is nondisplaced there is no displacement of the metaphysis on the epiphysis itself. Due to projection difficulties while taking roentgenograms, it may be that no difference in the epiphyseal width is seen. However, with swelling over the distal epiphysis and with point tenderness to palpation of the epiphyseal line, such as the distal fibular head, the clinical diagnosis of a Salter-Harris type I fracture may be made.

The closer to a joint or epiphyseal line that a fracture occurs, and the younger the child at the time of the fracture, the greater will be the chance for remodeling or restructuring of that bone. Conversely, the farther from a joint and the older the child, the less chance there is of the bone regrowing on its own into a more suitable posture. Type II fractures have a similar prognosis to type I fractures. Salter-Harris type III and IV fractures have a worse prognosis. If there is displacement, an open surgical reduction will usually be required to anatomically realign the joint and the growth plates. The Salter-Harris type V fracture has the

(Text continues on p. 523)

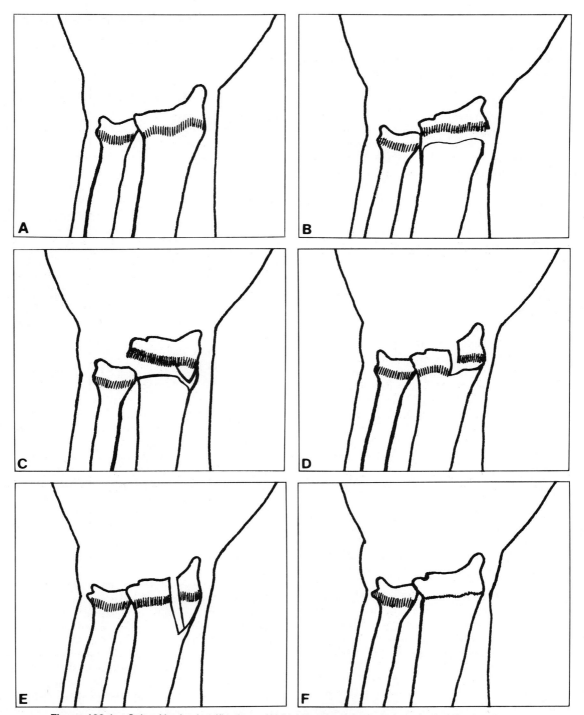

Figure 138-1. Salter-Harris classifications: (**A**) Uninjured epiphyseal plates in the distal radius and ulna. (**B**) Type 1 epiphyseal plate injury. The epiphyseal plate is disrupted, and the epiphysis is, to some degree, displaced from the metaphysis. (**C**) Type 2 epiphyseal plate injury. The epiphyseal plate is disrupted, and a piece of the metaphysis displaces with the plate and epiphysis. (**D**) Type 3 epiphyseal plate injury. The plate and epiphysis fracture as in a type I or II injury, but there is also an intra-articular break that separates both portions. (**E**) Type 4 epiphyseal plate injury. The epiphysis and epiphyseal plate break, taking along a portion of the metaphysis. (**F**) Type 5 compression epiphyseal plate injury. The epiphyseal plate is partially or totally destroyed by a compression fracture that pushes the epiphysis into the metaphysis.

worst prognosis. There is impaction and crushing of some or all of the growth plate, resulting in a bony bridge across the epiphyseal plate that will not allow further growth. If there is growth, it will occur in an angulated direction.

Other types of fractures that may be found are *simple* fractures through the metaphysis or diaphysis of the long bones. If they occur straight across they are called *transverse* fractures. If they are at an angle, they are termed *oblique* fractures. If a twisting motion resulted in the oblique fracture, it is referred to as a *spiral* fracture, where the fracture twists the bone from the torquing motion. When a transverse fracture occurs, the mechanism of injury is either a direct blow or a pathologic fracture. Pathologic fractures occur in various conditions ranging from a simple bone cyst to a malignancy. A fracture found in multiple pieces is termed *comminuted*. This would more likely occur with severe trauma or a crushing blow. If the bone is protruding from the skin, it is referred to as a *compound* fracture. These fractures must be surgically irrigated and reduced to prevent bone infection.

In addition to the type of fracture, the position of the fracture is important for the reduction, immobilization, and prognosis for fracture healing. The bone is angulated if it is in any way bent off its normal plane. The direction of the bend is used to describe that position. If, for example, the bone is bent at the distal radius toward the palm, it is described as volar or palmer angulation. The outcome of these types of fractures is based on the degree of final bony contact at the fracture site as well as on the alignment at the end of treatment.

Whether the fractured bone encompasses a dislocation is also important. When the bone is fractured and displaced from the joint, it is termed a *fracture-dislocation*. For example, if the olecranon at the elbow joint is fractured and displaced it would be called a fracture-dislocation of the elbow.

CLINICAL PRESENTATION

The child presents to the pediatrician because of having fallen or in some way injured a limb. There will usually be swelling and pain. Some children, however, are more stoic than others, and some fractures, such as torus-impaction types, are more stable and less painful. Joint effusion may result from intra-articular injury, including epiphyseal damage. The younger child will commonly splint the limb against his or her body. He or she will resist allowing the fractured limb from being touched and will cry when it is moved.

DIFFERENTIAL DIAGNOSIS

The differential diagnosis of fractures includes infection of the joints, sympathetic effusion from an osteomyelitis of bone juxtapositioned to the joint, synovitis, cellulitis, and soft tissue trauma (see also Chap. 137). Foreign bodies, especially in the feet and hands, must be ruled out. The older child is more likely to have a tendonitis or sprain. Portions of the ligaments around the joints can tear. A limp upper extremity in a child usually younger than 5 years of age is most likely secondary to a subluxed radial head at the elbow. It may also appear that the shoulder, elbow, or wrist is involved.

WORK-UP

History

The child or the parents of the younger child should be asked how the injury occurred and also the time of onset of when the swelling or pain was first noticed. The history of a fever, recent illness, and/or prior joint swelling should be obtained. Any unusual or suspicious circumstances should be carefully delineated (e.g., whether a new babysitter was with the child). Child abuse should also be ruled out in children with multiple fractures.

Physical Examination

A fracture from a fall may also be accompanied by head trauma or other related fractures; therefore, the entire body should be examined for injuries, including swelling. Especially in the young child, the skin should be checked for evidence of abuse or neglect, such as burns or multiple hematomas. Over approximately a 10-day period, a hematoma will resorb, turning from blue to green and finally to yellow. Thus, the age of the bruise can be approximated. Joint swelling surrounded by an area of warmth or erythema may indicate infection. In the absence of a history of trauma, infection is more likely than a fracture. Active or passive motion produces significant pain in either condition.

Laboratory Tests

The definitive test to diagnose a fracture is the roentgenogram. Swollen joints should be x-rayed, because a child will rarely have "just a sprain." One does not want to overlook a nondisplaced or a displaced epiphyseal fracture that may later result in a growth disturbance, residual deformity, and arthritic problems. Roentgenograms may include the joint above and below as well as the entire shaft of the bone involved. At least two views (i.e., anteroposterior and lateral) should be taken at 90° to each other. In addition, an oblique view may also be useful. One specific roentgenographic sign noted at the elbow is termed a posterior *fat pad sign*. This is seen on a true lateral roentgenogram of the distal humerus and presents as a blackened shadow behind the humeral condyles where a hemorrhage between the fat pad and the fractured joint has pushed the posterior fat away from the humerus. In the absence of a grossly visible displaced fracture, this represents a Salter-Harris type I epiphyseal fracture of the distal humerus or a nondisplaced supracondylar or radial epiphyseal fracture. This finding, combined with pain about the elbow, has such a high correlation with an actual fracture that it should be considered as pathognomonic for a fracture.

Selectively, tomogram films (laminograms), computed tomograms, or bone scans may be helpful in the diagnosis and treatment of the injured child. If roentgenograms fail to reveal a fracture, appropriate laboratory tests such as a complete blood cell count, sedimentation rate, antinuclear antibodies, and rheumatoid factor may be ordered to evaluate for arthritis, collagen vascular disease, or an underlying infection.

TREATMENT

Nondisplaced fractures of fingers are best treated by *buddy taping*. First, a stretchable type of adhesive tape may be used to fasten the fractured finger to the adjacent finger to stabilize it from rotation. They are then splintered in a position of function termed *intrinsic plus*. This holds the metacarpophalangeal joints at 90 degrees of flexion, 20 degrees at the proximal interphalangeal joint and 10 degrees at the distal interphalangeal joint. In this posture, the ligaments are stretched to their longest and therefore have the least chance of becoming shortened and causing a contracture. Splinting is maintained for approximately 3 weeks, at which time guarded active range of motion is allowed for the next 3 weeks. This, however, assumes adequate healing has been obtained on roentgenographic examination.

When the child has caught a finger or fingers in a door or desk top (which is a common occurrence), lacerations of the nail bed must be repaired. An avulsed nail is usually discarded and the repaired nail bed covered with lubricated gauze. If there is not a partial amputation, the main concern is that an epiphyseal fracture of any type has occurred. For this reason, roentgenograms are required to rule out the need for an open reduction or a closed reduction of the fractured joint epiphysis. Fractures of the *metacarpal* bones of a child are best treated by a short-arm cast. Depending on the age of the child, 3 to 5 weeks of immobilization is required, followed by an average additional 3 weeks of guarded active range of motion. Fractures of the carpals are rare in children because these bones consist largely of cartilage and have no distinct growth plates. In the adolescent, nondisplaced fractures of the carpal navicular bone are more common and should be treated by a short-arm cast extended to include the proximal phalanx of the thumb (see Chap. 139 for a discussion on hand injuries).

Displaced fractures of the distal *radius* are best treated by a closed reduction (straightening the bone without surgically opening the limb) if at all possible. Open reductions can lead to excessive callus formation and bridging across the interosseous space of the forearm, which would cause a loss of pronation and supination. Correct alignment and angulation must be attained to maintain a full range of motion and position. Fractures of the proximal ulna and radius, if displaced, are harder to align and may require an open reduction. Fractures of the distal humerus, if nondisplaced, should be treated initially by a posterior mold extending from the proximal humerus to the palm. Because of excessive swelling in this area, circumferential or compression bandaging, which could impair the circulation, should be avoided. For this reason, immediate circular casting is ill-advised unless a box configuration is used at the elbow joint or close observation and bulky padding is used. Similarly, to avoid compromising the circulation with tight casting, displaced fractures may require either surgical pinning or skeletal traction to attain and maintain correct alignment. A broken shaft of the proximal humerus is best treated by means of either a *hanging cast* (a long-arm circular cast that hangs from the neck forming a portable traction) or *sugar-tong splint* and swathe-type immobilization. A sugar-tong splint is similar in principle to the hanging cast. Its major advantage is that it is lighter and not circularly restrictive.

Clavicular fractures are commonly seen by the pediatrician in his office. Fractures of a greenstick type should not be manipulated but rather allowed to heal and remodel on their own unless there is a significant amount of angulation. The main treatment principle is to keep the shoulders pulled backward so as to keep the bones within their periosteal sleeve on stretch and not allow the bone edges to rub, thus causing pain and further bleeding. Rarely, there may be interposition of soft tissue that prevents healing of what is commonly believed to be a fracture that usually heals without complications. If there is a severely displaced fracture, there is a possibility that one of the bone edges may have pierced into the lung cavity, causing a partial or complete pneumothorax. The major blood vessels below the clavicle may also be torn, causing a hemothorax or subcutaneous emphysema. A child with a clavicular fracture should be immobilized for between 3 and 4 weeks by means of a figure-of-eight shoulder hyperextension device. This may be augmented with a sling if the child is more comfortable. It is generally more comfortable for the child to sleep flat on his back with a small raise between the scapulae allowing his shoulders to fall backward. In children with epiphyses open, it is rare to have an acromioclavicular dislocation. If there is pain in the distal clavicle, there is probably a Salter-Harris type I or II fracture of the distal clavicular epiphysis. A modified type splinting device similar to that for an acromioclavicular dislocation should be employed if there is significant displacement. Otherwise, the same treatment used for simple clavicular fractures should suffice. Pain with apparent dislocation of the medial end of the clavicle of a growing child is rarely caused by a dislocation of the clavicle; a Salter-Harris type I fracture of the clavicle from the medial clavicular epiphysis is more likely. This fracture should be reduced onto the epiphysis as with any epiphyseal fracture and may require an open reduction to align it and a shoulder spica cast to maintain it.

Complications from fractures of the *tibial* shaft can be insidious. A fractured tibia may bleed slowly and may develop into a *compartment syndrome*. This occurs because the tibial bleed is enclosed within the fascia of the lower leg muscles that envelop the tibia. There is no continuation of these compartments, especially in the anterior leg, and a significant hemorrhage can lead to compression of the neurovascular structures of the lower extremity. Ischemic contractures with death of the muscles that move the foot and ankle may then result. Immediate circular casting for displaced tibial fractures is contraindicated without close observation in a hospital. Fractures of the *femoral* shaft usually require traction followed by a body spica cast; although it is a large bone it is not difficult to fracture. In children younger than 2 years of age the most common cause of femoral fracture is child abuse; however, this type of fracture is not pathognomonic for abuse. *Hip* fractures require traction if they are nondisplaced. It also may require very little trauma to dislocate the hip of a very young child. More commonly, hip fractures are displaced and will require immediate open reduction with internal fixation. Fractures of the knee, foot, and ankle are covered in Chapters 140 and 141.

Children may present with low back pain, especially those who participate in athletics such as football, track, and gymnastics. This may be the result of a fracture of the pars interarticularis of the posterior ring of the lumbar vertebrae. Oblique roentgenograms aid in making this specific diagnosis. A bone scan should be obtained if a fracture is found in the absence of spondylolysthesis (forward slippage of the proximal spinal column on the distal). If radioactive isotope uptake is increased in these posterior structures without further evidence of an underlying neoplasm, a relatively fresh fracture is most likely. Immobilizing the child in a body cast from the abdomen to the ipsilateral knee for 12 weeks or in a custom-made, lumbar-flattened, low-fit thoracolumbosacral orthosis may result in union of the pars interarticularis. Failing union, the child is treated symptomatically by means of the custom-made orthosis for sports or as symptomatically needed to prevent further slippage. Periodically the spine is checked for spondylolysthesis with a lateral roentgenogram. Should there be significant movement of the vertebral bodies or intolerable back pain, operative fusion of the specific vertebral level is indicated.

INDICATIONS FOR REFERRAL

The physician should refer the child with a fracture or injury based on his training and skill in the treatment of fractures. If he does not feel confident in dealing with the undisplaced, angulated, or intra-articular fracture, it would be best to refer the child. All fractures should be seen as soon as possible. Excessive swelling, especially at the elbow, forearm, or shin need immediate attention. Compound fractures need immediate dressings and prophylactic antibiotics to protect against osteomyelitis. Specifically, antibiotics of the penicillin-resistant staphylococcal spectrum are needed for 5 days to treat a contaminated wound. Sterile debridement, closure, and reduction are also needed.

Torus or mild greenstick fractures can be splinted and then put in a cast within a few days. Hand and finger fractures should not be treated casually. There may be a subtle angulation at the epiphysis, displacing the finger into adduction or abduction. The fingers will then heal that way if the fracture is not reduced. Some nondisplaced fractures, especially of the hip and elbow, may become displaced if not immobilized. Correct immobilization should hold the fractured area as well as the joints above and below it. If the fracture is in a joint, the entire bone shafts on either side of that joint need to be immobilized. Any material may be used as a splint (e.g., magazines, pillows or boards). A shoulder or clavicle can be held with a sling. A femur that is injured is immobilized by strapping the two legs together or applying straight constant traction to the affected leg.

Ideally, strips of plaster or fiberglass casting material for splinting peripheral extremities should be kept in the office setting. After an underpadding of cotton is rolled over the affected extremity several layers thick, a plaster or fiberglass splint is applied to the length desired. No compression dressing should be used. This will decrease the chances of creating a Volkman ischemic contracture or other circulatory problem. If there is a loss of pulse or swelling compatible with a developing compartment syndrome, an orthopedic surgeon should be consulted immediately. A *compartment syndrome* consists of increasing pain, decrease in sensation, and decrease in capillary filling and/or pulse. Any of these symptoms should be regarded as a danger signal, and further compartment pressure testing or immediate surgery is necessary.

If a significant neck or spine injury is diagnosed or suspected, one should place the child on a hard full body board splint, with the child strapped and packed into position until the injured area is x-rayed and appropriately treated.

ANNOTATED BIBLIOGRAPHY

Rang M: Children's Fractures, 2nd ed. Philadelphia, JB Lippincott, 1983. (Simple, complete volume on fractures in children.)

Rockwood C Jr, Wilkins KE, King RE: Fractures in Children, 3rd ed. Philadelphia, JB Lippincott, 1991. (Excellent authoritative book on fractures in children.)

Salter RB: Textbook of Disorders and Injuries of the Musculoskeletal System, chaps 15–17. Baltimore, Williams & Wilkins, 1970. (Authoritative and concise.)

Sharrard WJW: Paediatric Orthopedics and Fractures, 2nd ed, vol 2, p 1484. Oxford, Blackwell Scientific Publications, 1979. (Complete and extremely well-documented.)

139

Injuries to the Upper Extremity

Charles F. Sanzone

While the lower extremity is primarily adapted to the single function of locomotion, the upper extremity functions both as an effector organ and secondarily as a sensory organ. The extremity begins at the shoulder girdle, the most mobile joint of the body. It is attached to the axial skeleton at one point only, the sternoclavicular joint. It ends at the hand, a uniquely human organ endowed with extraordinary suppleness and strength as well as exquisite sensitivity. This unique combination of functions makes the hand a major channel for interaction with the environment and one of the most frequently injured body parts.

With the exception of injuries to the hand, indirect trauma, such as falls onto the outstretched hand, accounts for most injuries to the upper extremity. The hand itself is more liable to direct trauma, especially in the inquisitive toddler and the newly assertive adolescent.

A general discussion of the types of fractures and their initial management is found in Chapter 138.

WORK-UP

History

The history of most injuries is straightforward. The magnitude and direction of the trauma should be noted. The presence or absence of complaints referring to changes in neurovascular function should also be recorded. When lacerations or abrasions are involved, the status of tetanus immunization must also be determined.

The way in which the trauma occurred is important to determine because specific mechanisms of injury are regularly associated with specific patterns of injury. A *fall onto the outstretched hand,* for example, causes fractures of the carpal scaphoid and distal radius, midshaft fractures of the radius and ulna, supracondylar and condylar fractures of the humerus, or fractures of the clavicle. A *fall onto the point of the shoulder* causes acromioclavicular separations, disruption of the physis at the proximal end of the clavicle, or traction injuries to the brachial plexus.

Crush injuries, especially those involving rollers such as are found in grocery store conveyor belts and in escalators, can cause edema out of proportion to the apparent severity of the injury. Even when the force of the injury is insufficient to cause fractures or major skin trauma, the deep pressure wave caused by the roller can disrupt the muscles of the hand and forearm, which are housed in tight, inelastic compartments. Hemorrhage and/or edema from the muscle injury can then cause an increase in the pressure within the compartment, resulting in ischemia and a full-blown *compartment syndrome.*

Bites, animal or human, combine the dangers of penetration with the introduction of bacterial flora and sometimes crushed, devitalized tissue. Any abrasion or laceration incurred during a fight is potentially dangerous and should be treated promptly, adhering to the principles of proper wound management (see Chaps. 143 and 144).

Injection injuries, caused by grease guns, paint guns, or other high-pressure aerosol devices are particularly dangerous because foreign substances can be forced great distances along tissue planes or tendon sheaths. Adequate debridement of such injuries cannot be achieved in the emergency department or office. These patients should be referred to a hand surgeon.

Physical Examination

Inspection of the upper extremity begins with casual observation of the patient. If the limb is not in a sling, most children will support the injured limb with the uninjured one. The patient should disrobe from the waist up. For comfort, the shirt should be removed from the uninjured limb first. When modesty is an issue, an examining gown slung over the uninjured shoulder sarong fashion allows complete visualization of the limb from the sternoclavicular joint to the fingertips. Swelling, erythema, and ecchymosis should be sought. The normal contours should also be assessed. Absence of, or increase in, the prominence of the proximal clavicle may indicate separation of the proximal clavicular physis or dislocation of the sternoclavicular joint. An increase in the prominence of the distal clavicle is a sign of distal clavicle fracture or acromioclavicular separation. Loss of the contour of the shoulder laterally indicates the possibility of glenohumeral dislocation. Prominence of the elbow laterally may indicate a supracondylar fracture of the distal humerus or lateral dislocation of the radial head. An unusual bow of the forearm may indicate the presence of fractures of both bones. The "dinner fork" deformity of the wrist is indicative of a distal radius fracture.

Inspection of the hand is straightforward, but describing the results can be difficult. One's findings should be recorded on a simple drawing in the record and include landmarks such as flexion creases, palm creases, and knuckle pads. Drawing permits accurate portrayal of even complex findings with minimal effort and expenditure of time. Since the skin of the volar surface of the hand is held in place by dense connective tissue septa, most edema will present dorsally, regardless of the side of the causative lesion. Several patterns of swelling may be noted. *Uniform swelling* of a digit is characteristic of suppurative tenosynovitis, whereas *fusiform swelling* occurs with synovitis of the interphalangeal joints, as in rheumatoid arthritis. The flexor tendon sheaths of the thumb and little finger are so close to each other at the base of the palm that infection can easily spread from one to the other, causing the characteristic *horseshoe abscess.*

All of the bones of the upper extremity, except the proximal thirds of the humerus and radius and the body of the scapula, are palpable along their subcutaneous borders. Palpation for *direct bony tenderness* is most important. In the setting of trauma, it is diagnostic of fracture. The same tenderness in the vicinity of a joint indicates a sprain or physeal fracture. If the anatomy of the individual ligaments is known, each ligament and each component of the ligament should be palpated. Once direct tenderness has been evaluated, the examiner should test for *indirect tenderness* to confirm a disruption of the ligament in question and to assess its stability. Indirect tenderness is elicited by applying a stress without touching the structure; for example, to stress the medial collateral ligament of the elbow, one hand is placed at the lateral aspect of the joint while the other hand grasps the forearm near the wrist. Pushing the hands toward each other exerts a valgus force at the elbow, placing the medial collateral ligament on stretch. If there is a strong suspicion of instability, this should be done in the radiology suite with radiographic documentation.

No examination of a traumatized extremity is adequate unless the integrity of the skin, circulation, and neurologic function has been documented. Open fractures, traumatic arthrotomies, neurovascular disruptions, and compartment syndromes (i.e., all limb-threatening emergencies) are thus ruled out.

Laboratory Tests

Judicious use of the laboratory is recommended to assess infections and systemic diseases that may manifest in the hand and upper extremity. Roentgenography, however, is essential. To be adequate, the examination must contain at least two views separated by 90° (i.e., anteroposterior and lateral), include the entire bone in question, and include the joints distal and proximal. The shoulder girdle, however, may require more extensive radiologic evaluation. Documentation of sternoclavicular separations often requires computed tomography, as do fractures of the scapula. Acromioclavicular separations require stress views—anteroposterior views of both shoulders with and without 10-pound weights attached to the wrists. While the upper humerus can be evaluated adequately by two anteroposterior views in internal and external rotation, the glenohumeral joint requires anteroposterior and axillary lateral views.

Plain roentgenograms of the hand are difficult to read because of the multiple structures and their superimposition on each other. Several strategies can simplify the evaluation of hand roentgenograms. First, an anteroposterior and lateral view of only the part in question is ordered (e.g., index finger or carpus). Second, the parts of *least* interest are evaluated first, lessening the chance of forgetting to evaluate everything on the roentgenogram by overconcentration on the area in question. Third, each structure on the film is evaluated in turn (i.e., soft tissues first, then the bones, then the joint spaces). The more sophisticated radiographic techniques are generally of little use, but in specific instances they are invaluable. Scintigraphy is useful in detecting occult fractures of the carpal scaphoid and in delineating some tumors. Magnified views can demonstrate subtle fractures of the carpus. Arthrography can demonstrate injuries to the intercarpal joints and tears of the triangular fibrocartilage on the ulnar side of the wrist. Computed tomography is the best means of evaluation the distal radioulnar joint. It should be remembered that a "negative" roentgenogram does not always exclude a fracture. Deep soft tissue swelling, as evidenced by displacement of superficial or deep fat pads, should raise the examiner's suspicions.

TREATMENT

The Shoulder Girdle

The shoulder girdle can be conceptualized as a complex of three bones—the clavicle, the scapula, and the upper humerus—and four joints—the sternoclavicular, acromioclavicular, scapulothoracic, and glenohumeral.

The growth plate of the proximal clavicle is the last to close (at about 21 years of age). Therefore, dislocations of the scapulothoracic joint, while very rare in the general population, never occur in the pediatric population. Fracture separations of the growth plate, however, do occur. Neurovascular compromise occurs almost exclusively in posterior dislocations. The anatomy of the lesion should be clearly demonstrated by computed tomography in such cases. Uncomplicated fractures require only symptomatic care (sling and analgesics) as long as there is no neurovascular compromise. Injuries associated with neurovascular compromise should be referred for immediate reduction.

In children younger than 10, fractures of the shaft of the *clavicle* seldom require reduction. Only severely angulated fractures should be referred as emergencies. A simple sling, a "figure of eight" splint, or both are all that is required as needed for comfort. In teenagers, moderately to severely angulated fractures should be reduced with the use of regional anesthesia and maintained in a figure-of-eight splint.

Injuries to the *acromioclavicular joint* usually result from a blow or a fall directly on the point of the shoulder. Prior to the teen years, the same injury usually produces fractures of the distal clavicle. The unique feature of these injuries is that no matter how displaced the fragments become the coracoclavicular ligaments remain attached to the periosteum, ensuring that any malposition will be corrected by remodeling over a period of 3 months to a year. Only comfort measures and support are required.

Sprains are graded (I–IV) by a standard stress roentgenogram. The stress film will show no displacement in grade I sprains (partial tears of the capsule). Displacement of the distal clavicle relative to the acromion but leaving the joint surfaces in contact defines a grade II sprain (complete rupture of the capsule and elongation of the coracoclavicular ligaments). A complete dislocation of the acromioclavicular joint is a grade III sprain (complete disruption of the coracoclavicular ligaments). Grade IV sprains represent the extremes of displacement of grade III injuries.

There is no controversy about the treatment of grade I sprains. Relief of stress by means of a sling and appropriate local measures, such as cold packs, produce uniformly good results in 2 to 3 weeks. Sports are forbidden during this time.

The prominence of the distal clavicle is easily visible in grade II and III sprains of the acromioclavicular joint. Pain and tenderness are localized to the acromioclavicular joint. Excessive motion of the joint is demonstrated by depressing the distal clavicle while pushing the humerus up, reducing the joint (piano key sign). Indirect stress, applied by pulling on the arm, causes pain.

Grade II and III sprains may be treated operatively or nonoperatively. An ordinary sling is not adequate treatment for the more severe sprains. Some means of maintaining the joint reduced while supporting the upper extremity is required. This can be accomplished by means of a sling combined with strapping encircling the upper extremity from the elbow to a point just proximal to the coracoid process. Prefabricated splints (Kenny-Howard sling) are available. For such treatment to succeed, the reduction must be maintained *constantly* for 4 to 6 weeks. The immobilization may lead to skin irritation and necrosis beneath the straps, maceration of the axilla, and hidradenitis suppurativa. Patients have difficulty cooperating with such a regimen. Operative management of the injury consists of exploration of the acromioclavicular joint and repair of the coracoclavicular ligament. Whichever surgical technique is selected, the complications of surgery include scaring, infection, and failure to achieve or maintain reduction. The usual management is immobilization for grade II injuries and surgery for grade III injuries.

Injuries to the capsular ligaments of the *glenohumeral joint* are not diagnosable by ordinary clinical or radiographic means. Injuries to these ligaments lead to recurrent anterior subluxation and dislocation of the shoulder. Acute dislocations are treated by prompt reduction using adequate analgesia, followed by a minimum of 4 weeks of immobilization in a sling and swathe. Chronic dislocations exist after three recurrent dislocations have occurred. Some younger adolescents are able to dislocate the joint voluntarily. Treatment for this disorder is behavioral.

The *rotator cuff* is an extrinsic component of the glenohumeral joint, composed of the tendons of the supraspinatus and infraspinatus, teres minor, and subscapularis muscles. These muscles, acting in concert, initiate abduction of the shoulder. In young patients the rotator cuff may be torn by

violent forces acting about the shoulder in abduction and external rotation. The diagnosis is based on the inability to initiate abduction of the involved shoulder and the inability to adduct the shoulder smoothly from full abduction (drop arm sign). The treatment is symptomatic, with early rehabilitation. If weakness persists beyond 6 weeks, the patient should be referred for consideration of operative repair.

The Elbow

Supracondylar fractures of the humerus are potentially serious injuries that require immediate evaluation and treatment. The fracture usually results from a sudden and forceful hyperextension of the elbow. Acute pain and swelling rapidly develop. If the fracture is displaced, a sharp edge of bone frequently tears the adjacent brachial artery or vein. Either this bleeding or the swelling can cause a compartment syndrome which, if untreated, may result in Volkmann's ischemic contracture. Even if the fracture is nondisplaced, vascular and neural function must be followed closely, and some authorities recommend hospitalization to ensure that good perfusion is maintained. Displaced fractures require emergency treatment, usually open reduction, and internal fixation of the fracture, followed by hospitalization to monitor circulation and function.

The elbow joint is intrinsically stable because of the congruency of the ulnohumeral joint. The medial and lateral collateral ligament complexes are very strong, and injuries to them are usually associated with dislocation or subluxation of the joint. Such injuries should be referred to the care of an orthopedic surgeon.

Avulsions of the medial and lateral epicondyles are not rare. The wrist and finger flexors originate from the medial epicondyle, as does the medial collateral ligament. The extensors originate from the lateral epicondyle. Strong varus or valgus stresses acting in conjunction with contraction of these muscle masses can produce acute avulsions. Repetitious exertion of forces of lesser magnitude over a period of time can result in apophysitis (medial = *pitcher's elbow;* lateral = *tennis elbow*). *Avulsions* should be referred to an orthopedic surgeon for consideration of operative intervention, but apophysitides can be managed with rest followed by strengthening exercises.

Ice is recommended initially to control inflammation and swelling (20 minutes four to six times a day for 3 days). If the apophysitis is mild, icing after the activity may be all that is necessary to relieve symptoms.

A correction of technique can also be curative for a pitcher or tennis player with apophysitis.

One elbow injury occurs with such frequency that it merits special mention: the *pulled elbow* or *nursemaid's elbow*. The injury is caused by a sudden traction on the forearm. This force causes a widening of the lateral joint space with interposition of the annular ligament of the radius between the joint surfaces, blocking spontaneous reduction.

The child is irritable and often has a pseudoparalysis of the involved extremity. A roentgenogram has limited value in establishing the diagnosis, but the prompt return of function with a reduction of the radial head is diagnostic, as is the click that is usually felt on reduction. The reduction maneuver consists of gentle traction on the wrist followed by full, forced supination. No immobilization is required for first subluxations. For repeat injuries, however, a posterior splint is applied for several days.

Wrist

The ligament complexes about the wrist are composed of ligaments that are both short and stout. Consequently, wrist sprains, which are often diagnosed, rarely occur. Older children may develop instability of the wrist due to a disruption of the intercarpal ligaments. An accurate diagnosis of these injuries requires a stress series of roentgenograms, consisting of true lateral and anteroposterior views in neutral, radial, and ulnar deviations as well as an anteroposterior view with the fist clenched. In the lateral projection, the radius, lunate, and capitate should be coaxial. In the anteroposterior view, any increase in the scapholunate distance is abnormal. Patients suspected of having ligamentous disruptions about the wrist should be referred to a hand surgeon.

The Hand

Fractures. The most common finger injury is the crush of the fingertip, usually by a door. A conminuted fracture of the nonarticulating portion of the distal phalanx often results. The fingernail acts as a natural splint for this fracture; thus, it should be preserved. A protective splint is usually all that is necessary until the tenderness has subsided. The resulting subungual hematoma is a source of pain. Burning through the nail with a red-hot paper clip provides prompt relief. If the nail has been avulsed, it should be replaced under the eponychium to serve as a splint and to prevent adhesions of the eponychium to the nail bed, which result in troublesome nail deformities. Lacerations of the nail bed should be repaired with 5-0 absorbable sutures prior to replacing the nail. A blow to the tip of the finger in a longitudinal direction will result in the avulsion of the terminal tendon of the extensor apparatus. The same mechanism in a child with open physes will result in a fracture separation. If the fragment is less than 50% of the joint surface, and the joint remains reduced, this "mallet" (also called "baseball") finger is treated with continuous splinting in extension for 6 weeks. If the joint is dislocated or subluxed, and the fragment represents a sizable proportion of the joint surface, a referral for operative management is indicated.

The distal articular surfaces of the proximal and middle phalanges are composed of radial and ulnar condyles. Condylar and bicondylar fractures are common athletic injuries. Nondisplaced fractures can be treated with immobilization for 10 days to 2 weeks, followed by buddy taping for 2 more weeks. Fractures of the phalangeal neck usually result from forceful hyperextension of the interphalangeal or metacarpophalangeal joint most often by a closing door. Closed manipulation and splinting are adequate treatment in moderately and minimally displaced fractures. Severely displaced fractures and irreducible fractures should be referred for open treatment. Transverse fractures of the shaft of the phalanges may be reduced and splinted. When the fracture is through the middle phalanx proximal to the insertion of the flexor superficialis tendon, the finger is splinted in extension; when it is distal to the flexor insertion, the finger is splinted in flexion. Oblique and spiral fractures of the shaft, however, should be referred for consideration of operative reduction and fixation. The proximal end of the phalanx is its epiphyseal end. Salter-Harris type III injuries of this physis should be referred, but Salter-Harris type II injuries may be reduced and splinted. Radial and ulnar angulation of proximal phalanx fractures are best corrected by placing a pencil or pen in the web space to act as a fulcrum. Fractures of the finger metacarpals are unusual in children with open physes. They are common in adolescents, however. The most common mechanism of injury is longitudinal compression, as in punching. It is, therefore, essential to inspect the knuckle to rule out penetration of the joint by a tooth in any patient presenting with a metacarpal fracture. If there is penetration of the joint, the child should be referred to a hand specialist. Dorsal angulation of up to 50 degrees may be accepted in fractures of the metacarpal neck; these are treated by closed reduction and immobilization in a gutter splint for 4 weeks. The thumb metacarpal may be fractured through the metaphysis or the physis. Metaphyseal or Salter-Harris type II injuries are treated with closed reduction and casting in a below-elbow cast extending to the base of the thumb nail. Salter-Harris type III injuries, however, require accurate open reduction to avoid joint incongruity and progressive deformity. Fractures involving the proximal articular surface of the thumb metacarpal (Bennett's fractures) are rare in children with open physes. In older children, they should be referred. Fractures of the carpal bones prior to adolescence are also rare because the relative weakness of the distal radial physis has a protective effect on the strongly supported carpus. With fusion of the distal radial physis, this protection is lost and carpal injuries become more common.

Dislocations. Open physes protect against dislocations. In the older adolescent, however, dislocations occur. Interphalangeal joint dislocations are easily reduced by exaggerating the deformity, by applying longitudinal traction, and by applying thumb pressure or flexing. Dorsal dislocations are most common, followed by radial and ulnar dislocations. The metacarpals dislocate dorsally, usually in association with other severe, high-energy hand injuries. Open reduction and pinning are usually required to maintain the reduction. Dislocations of the wrist are serious injuries with a high incidence of associated neurovascular injuries. Immediate neurovascular assessment, splinting, and referral are mandatory.

Sprains. As in dislocations, open growth plates protect against sprains in the young child. Older children may suffer disruptions of the intrinsic ligaments of the hand. The collateral ligaments of the interphalangeal and metacarpophalangeal joints are vulnerable. Instability is assessed with the interphalangeal joints in extension, but the metacarpophalangeal joints should be stressed in 90 degrees of flexion. Treatment of even third-degree sprains is nonoperative, with splinting and buddy taping. The metacarpophalangeal joint of the thumb is an exception. Operative repair is indicated if stress roentgenograms demonstrate a complete disruption of the ulnar collateral ligament. If any of the intercarpal ligaments are ruptured, the scapholunate interosseous ligament is usually involved. A disruption of this ligament results in a widening of the scapholunate joint space on a regular or stress (clenched fist) roentgenogram. The wrist collapses into either dorsal or volar instability patterns. The treatment is surgical (see also Chap. 137).

Amputations. In young children, complete or partial amputation of almost any body part is an indication for replantation of that part. The criteria for the selection of adolescents and young adults for replantation or revascularization, however, are more stringent. Replantation of the thumb, multiple digits, partial amputation of the hand through the palm or wrist, or a clean relatively transverse amputation above the wrist is indicated. Replantation of single digit amputations may be indicated if the level of amputation is above the flexor superficialis insertion (distal to the proximal third of the middle phalanx). The attending physician should make direct contact with the surgeon who will be accepting the patient. Detailed instructions for preparation of the amputated part should be obtained. This usually involves placing the amputated part in a plastic bag filled with saline and placing the bag on ice. There should be no unnecessary delay in transportation to the microvascular surgeon because maximum allowable cold ischemia time not under the surgeon's direct supervision is about 6 hours. Fingertip amputations do not require such highly specialized intervention. Their treatment centers on three concerns: (1) preservation of sensation, (2) preservation of the cushioning function of the pulp, and (3) preservation of the nail. There is little controversy that in transverse injuries with no bone exposed healing by secondary intention provides the best results in terms of sensation and function. In amputations whose obliquity is from dorsal to volar, the main problem is a loss of digital pulp. Such complicated strategies as advancement flaps and pedicle flaps may be justified. Injuries to the nail bed should be referred to a hand surgeon. Ring avulsion injuries, in which an encircling band caught on something and degloves a digit, are treated by resection of the digit and its metacarpal.

ANNOTATED BIBLIOGRAPHY

Cox JS: The fate of the acromioclavicular joint in athletic injuries. Am J Sports Med 9:50–53, 1982.

Green DP (ed): Operative Hand Surgery, 2nd ed. New York, Churchill Livingstone, 1988. (Very complete, three-volume multiauthor text.)

Iverson LD, Clawson DK: Manual of Acute Orthopaedic Therapeutics. Boston, Little, Brown, & Co, 1977. (Excellent and concise, with much practical instructions not found in other publications.)

Ogden JA: Skeletal Injury in the Child. Philadelphia, Lea & Febiger, 1982. (Scholarly tome filled with unique photographs of anatomic specimens and histologic preparations butits exhaustive analysis of most injuries makes it too cumbersome for quick reference.)

Rang M: Children's Fractures, 2nd ed. Philadelphia, JB Lippincott, 1983. (Unique, folksy and amusing yet thorough presentation of the basics of pediatric orthopedic trauma, making each chapter unforgettable; a good starting point for those interested in pediatric orthopaedics as well as a good quick reference.)

Rockwood CA, Wilkins KE, King RE: Fractures in Children. Philadelphia, JB Lippincott, 1984. (Excellent, encyclopedic, multicontributor textbook with excellent entries on all subjects, exhaustive listing of alternative treatments, and a statement of the author's preferred treatment for each disorder.)

Tachdjian MO: Pediatric Orthopaedics, 2nd ed. Philadelphia, WB Saunders, 1990. (Greatly expanded from previous edition with four very up-to-date encyclopedic volumes.)

140
The Injured Knee

Lorin M. Brown

The child's knee is as much at risk from sports and accidents as is the adult knee. Damage to the epiphyseal plates of the distal femur, the proximal tibia, and the proximal fibula may also complicate the kind of problems that can occur with the knee. The epiphyseal plates, in addition to the tibial spine, which is located on top of the tibial epiphysis, are easier to fracture in the growing child than it is to tear the adjacent ligaments. Epiphyseal fractures should not be overlooked since these could result in a growth disturbance later on. Therefore, until the end of adolescence, a traumatically swollen knee is more likely to be the result of a fracture than a ligamentous tear. Later in life, the menisci, cruciate ligaments, collateral ligament, and the capsule are the first areas injured. It must be remembered, however, that any type of injury may occur at any age. The child's radiologic evaluation is more complicated because large portions of the joint structures in the younger child are cartilaginous and thus invisible. In addition, the normal laxity in the growing child's knee can confuse the picture when evaluating for ligamentous damage, especially to the anterior cruciate ligament.

PATHOPHYSIOLOGY

Injuries about the knee can occur in any type of sport or activity that the child is undertaking. Falling onto flexed knees, jumping or falling from monkey bars or other gymnastic equipment, and falling off of a bicycle are a few of the ways in which a child can injure his or her knee. A simple fall or a medial to lateral blow to the involved patella is sufficient to cause a patellar displacement. There is usually an increased valgus angle to the knee and leg as well as joint laxity that predispose to patellar instability. Sports activities cause adult-type injuries in the older child. "Clipping" and "tackling" injuries cause epiphyseal separations or disruptions of the collateral and cruciate ligaments of the knee. The child will have a tibial avulsion fracture instead of a cruciate ligament tear. Rotatory injuries will cause tearing or shearing of the menisci of the knee. The injuries become more related to the soft tissues and internal structures of the knee as the child's ligaments become thinned and the epiphyses fuse. A congenital deformity may present as early as 2 to 3 years of age when a congenital discoid meniscus may become symptomatic.

Osteomyelitis tends to occur about the knee due to the increased matrix of capillary vessels in the metaphysis of the distal femur and proximal tibia. These form static spaces in which the bacteria grow. When the pressure becomes great enough, it may then decompress through the bone into the knee joint and be first identified as a septic joint. A hematoma from trauma may breed bacteria and proliferate in the same fashion. The bursae about the knee (especially the prepatellar and infrapatellar bursae) are highly susceptible to falls and may become lacerated or otherwise inflamed from falling, sharp objects, or repeated trauma. *Osgood-Schlatter disease* is either a stress fracture or apophysitis of the tibial tubercle caused by repeated trauma and stress to the apophysis. The degree of pain varies with the psychological and physiological make-up of each child. The epiphyseal area becomes tender to palpation and motion because it is the site of the attachment of the patellar ligament, which is the ultimate insertion of the quadriceps mechanism. With the knee in full extension, this area is highly vulnerable to injury and stress.

Fractures of the epiphysis are described in Chapter 138. Any of the five types of fractures of the Salter-Harris classification may occur about the epiphyses of the knee. Salter-Harris type I and II fractures are most prevalent. These types occur in an identical biomechanical fashion as they do in adult knee injuries where they result in ligamentous, meniscal, and/or cruciate ligament tears. A blow from the lateral side of the knee will open the epiphysis on the medial side. Depending on the angle and velocity, a force can result either in a Salter-Harris I fracture (that cannot be discerned as a fracture unless a stress roentgenogram is performed) or with a portion of the metaphysis being torn off with the epiphysis, resulting in a Salter-Harris type II injury. A forward blow directly to the knee of a child may dislocate the epiphyseal plate of the knee posteriorly or anteriorly or fracture the tibial spine off of the articular plateau of the proximal tibia. The analogous injury in the skeletally mature patient is a dislocated knee or a tear of one or both cruciate ligaments. Other rotatory injuries that tear the meniscal tissue in the adult may instead produce various Salter-Harris type III and type IV injuries, taking off portions of the epiphyses or tearing the meniscal tissue. Past puberty, the epiphyseal plates become partially bridged and injuries will most likely result in ligamentous tears and meniscal damage as seen in the adult. The worst case of all occurs with a combination injury that not only tears the soft tissue but also damages both the growth center and the articular surface of the growing joint.

CLINICAL PRESENTATION

The injured child presents with a swollen or erythematous warm knee. The history is critical since the appearance may be the same whether it is septic or traumatic. The knee will be painful and the range of motion will be limited, regardless of the etiology.

CLINICAL EXAMINATION

With a history of trauma, the child should first be examined by roentgenography. This is important in that a nondisplaced tibial spine fracture or epiphyseal plate injury may become displaced by the initial physical examination of the knee. It is more important in the child than in the adult, because of the likelihood that the injury resulted in a fracture rather than only a ligamentous or meniscal tear. After a fracture has been ruled out, the knee should be examined to ensure that there is no ligamentous tear, or Salter-Harris type I injury that was not seen on the initial roentgenograms. The knee should be stressed with the leg in extension into both varus and valgus positions. This is accomplished by placing one palm against the distal femur and by using this palm as a fulcrum while pushing the tibia laterally, thus placing a valgus stress on the knee. This will open the medial side of the knee if there is an epiphyseal fracture or a tear of the medial collateral ligament. With the knee in extension, the posterior capsule must be torn for instability to occur. If the same examination is performed with the knee in 30 degrees of flexion, instability will more likely be related to only ligamentous or epiphyseal damage than to capsular injury. The reverse maneuver is then applied, pulling the leg into varus. This will indicate whether there is a tear of the lateral collateral ligament. The fibular head may be fractured, causing laxity in the lateral collateral ligament because this is what the ligament attaches to. The knee is then flexed to 90 degrees and, with pressure applied to the posterior proximal tibia, the flexed knee should be pulled forward. With the foot held stable, usually by the examiner sitting on the patient's forefoot, an increased forward laxity of the injured knee compared with the opposite knee may be found with an anterior cruciate ligament tear. This is known as the *Drawer sign*. Posterior stress laxity of the tibia relative to the well knee may indicate a posterior cruciate tear. The same maneuver can be performed with the knee at 30 degrees of flexion. In this position, it is known as the *Lachman test*. The knee that presents as "locked" in the child may not be a meniscal injury, as it is usually in the adult, because a child will "freeze" his knee more readily when it hurts than the adult. The examiner must be sure that the child is not just holding his or her knee stiff from a contusion. A *McMurray sign* can be elicited with a significantly torn meniscus and with a discoid meniscus. For this maneuver, the child lies flat on his or her back with the hip and knee flexed and then, while internally or externally rotating it, the knee is pulled into extension. The knee will have a rubbery snap or popping sound and will be shifted in position if the meniscus is torn. If the tear is not complete, this will also elicit pain as the femoral condyles are rotated and pushed onto the meniscus, pulling the attached capsule with the meniscal fragment.

If the history suggests that the patella is the source of pain, the examination proceeds as follows. The leg is held in extension and manual force is exerted against the medial side of the patella, pushing it in a lateral direction. If the child screams or grabs for the knee and tries to prevent this maneuver, it is termed a *positive apprehension test*. The child, having recently had the patella dislocate laterally (as is almost always the case), will be on guard against a recurrence and will try to prevent the examiner from reproducing the pain. In addition, if the patella was completely dislocated, the anteromedial structures of the knee joint will be torn, swollen, and painful when palpated. If there is not a gross effusion, there may still be a mild effusion that can be detected by the *ballottement test*. The suprapatellar pouch (area proximal to the patella) is compressed, pushing any blood or effusion in this area down into the knee joint. The patella may then be pressed in an anterior to posterior manner and will ballotte front to back when compressed and released.

DIFFERENTIAL DIAGNOSIS

The differential diagnosis in a young child is most often between infection and trauma. The infection is usually from a juxta-articular osteomyelitis, an intra-articular sepsis, or an infection of a bursa. Cellulitis overlying the knee is usually readily diagnosed, although the location of infection may not always be apparent, especially if it is deep. Other causes of effusion include arthritis and, far less commonly, malignancy. Polyarthritis can result from any cause of arthritis (e.g. JRA, rheumatic fever) or may be a transient synovial reaction to a systemic illness (e.g., bacteremia and virtually any viral illness). Osgood-Schlatter condition is an inflammation or stress fracture of the tibial tubercle, and it occasionally combines with a tendonitis of the patellar ligament to produce a painful prominence under the anterior knee.

Congenital dislocations of the patella versus a traumatically dislocated patella is usually easily differentiated. A congenitally dislocated patella is usually dislocated laterally. Flexion of the knee reveals the femoral condylar sulcus without a patella present. A traumatically dislocated patella is almost always associated with severe pain and immediate swelling following a traumatic episode.

WORK-UP

If trauma is not the obvious cause, a complete blood cell count, erythrocyte sedimentation rate, rheumatoid factor, ASO titers, and antinuclear antibody test should be ordered to rule out a septic disease, juvenile rheumatoid arthritis, other arthritis, or rheumatic fever. Later, a slit lamp eye examination may be necessary for juvenile rheumatoid arthritis evaluation. Juvenile rheumatoid arthritis and a septic knee can be difficult and occasionally impossible to differentiate. It is commonly necessary in the infant and child to perform a technetium or gallium scan to rule out infection or fracture. An infant's knee may have been injured by child abuse, and trying to differentiate this from a septic knee with only plain roentgenograms may not be possible. One should not hesitate to repeat any tests if the clinical presentation or diagnosis remains unclear. Aspiration of the fluid from the knee joint may also be performed. A bloody effusion is usually pathognomonic for trauma, a synovial effusion more indicative of arthritis, and "puslike" fluid could be either from a septic knee or juvenile rheumatoid arthritis. An arthrogram, in which dye is injected into the knee joint to visualize the shape and contour of the menisci that are invisible on routine roentgenograms, may be performed if the problem does not subside with conservative treatment and if the symptoms are highly suggestive of a traumatic meniscal tear or congenital malformed discoid meniscus. Magnetic resonance imaging provides a good picture of the internal structures of the knee, and has largely replaced arthrograms as a diagnostic tool.

Arthroscopy may be the final and ultimate examination of the knee. It is possible to examine the knee with either a smaller pediatric arthroscope or the adult-sized arthroscope. This procedure is not without complications, and more damage can occur from the unskilled arthroscopist or large arthroscopic instruments than the disease process itself. The knee in the young child has not had the stresses of the adult knee, and the joint space itself is small. Arthrotomy, usually of a small incision size, may be necessary to remove pieces of meniscus or large bony fragments that cannot otherwise be easily removed or replaced in the child or adolescent's knee. Specialized procedures such as these, especially on a young child, are best performed by an experienced arthroscopist.

TREATMENT

Fractures that displace the epiphyseal plates of the distal femur or proximal tibia and that extend intra-articularly must be reduced and possibly internally fixated surgically. A displaced fracture of the tibial spine may also need to be wired or pegged with an absorbable peg into position. Some fractures of the distal femur or proximal tibia may need to be gently manipulated back into an anatomic position. General anesthesia may be required in some instances. Disruption of the tibial tubercle may likewise need a surgical reduction to reattach the tubercle. Care must be taken to avoid closure of the epiphysis or apophysis, which could cause the proximal tibia to grow into recurvatum. Furthermore, if a fracture of the cartilaginous surface of the patella causes the patellar ligament to pull off the inferior surface of the patella (sleeve fracture), a complete disruption in the extensor mechanism of the leg results.

Minor fractures, such as Salter-Harris type I, may be treated by long-leg or cylinder casting, whereas type II fractures of the distal femoral epiphysis usually require a body spica cast to prevent the hamstring muscles and quadriceps mechanism from redisplacing the epiphysis. Ligaments may be damaged in a child and will usually heal rapidly by casting in the appropriate position. With medial collateral ligament tears early range of motion exercises are advisable. After several weeks in a cast, the leg is allowed flexion and extension range of motion in a specific brace that allows only this motion. An open repair of the collateral ligaments is rarely indicated. The reconstruction of a completely torn cruciate ligament is indicated if the child is having instability with walking or running and the epiphyses are closed. A specialized brace may be used for sports in the future. If the leg is stable and there is normal walking and running, cruciate surgical repair is purely elective. Peripheral meniscal tears will most likely heal in a child. In the young child, it is highly unlikely for a meniscus to be detached, and damage may well be the result of a congenitally malformed and biomechanically weakened discoid meniscus that will require surgical removal. Osteochondral fragments may be drilled arthroscopically to try to hasten fusion of the fragment. Osteochondral fragments, which are found to be totally detached, are best treated by removal if there is no living osseous condylar portion. If the surface areas are bulging or depressed and a roentgenogram shows a persistent osteochondral fragment that is clinically significant, arthroscopic drilling through the cartilage into the bony bed may possibly allow for ingrowth of bone matrix and a faster healing of the fractured or avascular fragment. Surgery, however, should be reserved for the patient with the aforementioned findings who has also effusion and pain or delayed healing. The extent of articular damage can be seen directly. In addition, a septic or arthritic knee can be evaluated and fully cleansed with minimal incisions through arthroscopic surgery.

ANNOTATED BIBLIOGRAPHY

Post M (ed): Physical examination of the musculoskeletal system. In Brown LM, Sharrard WJW (eds): Examination of the Lower Extremities in the Child. Chicago, Year Book Medical Publishers, 1987. (Complete description of the physical examination.)

Rang M: Children's Fractures, 2nd ed, chap 18. Philadelphia, JB Lippincott, 1983. (Excellent general reference.)

Rockwood C, Rockwood K: Fractures in Children, chap 11. Philadelphia, JB Lippincott, 1984. (Excellent general reference.)

Sharrard WJW: Paediatric Orthopedics and Fractures, 2nd ed. Oxord, Blackwell Scientific Publications, 1970. (Excellent general reference.)

141

The Injured Foot

Lorin M. Brown

The child's foot is vulnerable to injury from birth. It is the basis for support of the body, and it is exposed to tremendous stress incurred by walking and running. There are multiple type of fractures ranging from stress fractures to compound comminuted fractures that can be acute as well as chronic problems and may last a lifetime. Thus, foot injures should not be taken lightly and should be carefully evaluated.

PATHOPHYSIOLOGY AND CLINICAL PRESENTATION

Cuts on the foot often occur from a child stepping on glass, a pin, or a nail. A wound may be self-inflicted by a child tearing at his or her toe nails or by cutting the nail back in such a way that an *ingrown nail* develops. With infection, an erythematous swollen area may be seen either around the cuticle bed of the nail or on the foot. Cellulitis can rapidly develop and spread either in the streaking manner of a lymphangitis following the lymph channels proximally up the leg, or the infection can form a large abscess. Both can be life threatening. Certain children, such as those with an immunodeficiency and juvenile diabetes must be carefully observed, because they are at greater risk for rapidly developing and chronically sustaining infections of the feet.

The foot is exposed to trauma by the child stubbing his or her toe. The likelihood of injury becomes great when the child is able to go outdoors. A foreign body must always be considered as the cause of a chronic soft tissue infection. Fractures of the toes are significant when they involve an articular surface or an epiphyseal plate, especially of the great toe. As 50% of push-off occurs at the phalangeal-metatarsal joint of the great toe, an intra-articular fracture of this joint surface must be fully treated. Fractures of the shafts of the other bones can occur as well as dislocations of all joints of the phalanges of all toes. With the increasing popularity of athletic competition, *stress fractures* seen formally only in older adolescents are now also commonly found in the younger athlete. These fractures, although they may initially be invisible on a normal roentgenogram, may eventually prove to be nondisplaced fractures requiring treatment.

More violent trauma can result in complete dislocations of the hind and midfoot and occasionally may become surgical emergencies. The heel may become inflamed from constant trauma and may develop a tendonitis at the Achilles insertion. Tendonitis may also be present over the peroneal tendons laterally, the posterior tibial tendon medially, the extensor tendons dorsally, or the flexor tendons medially and plantarly. Another cause of heel pain is an apophysitis of the calcaneus (Sever's disease).

DIFFERENTIAL DIAGNOSIS

Infections of the foot must be differentiated from underlying fractures. It should be remembered that in children with paralytic conditions such as spina bifida, what appears to be a warm erythematous infection is most likely the response pattern to a fracture.

Dislocations of the toes must be differentiated from displaced or angulated fractures. A simple toe fracture that can be treated with a minimum amount of effort leaves a less than optimal result if a dislocation of one of the phalangeal joints is overlooked. A strand of hair may become wrapped around an infant's toe and eventually amputate it if the hair is not found and removed. Midfoot pain may be secondary to either a fascial or tendon sprain, or it may be the result of a midfoot or hindfoot bone fracture. It is essential to differentiate a septic joint from an arthritic one. A red, swollen joint is much more likely to be infected, but an underlying arthritis such as juvenile rheumatoid arthritis must be considered. Gout is possible, although quite uncommon in the child. Pain in the foot may also be the result of an avascular necrosis. These include *osteochondritis dissecans*, which may be present about the talus, and *Kohler's disease,* which involves the tarsal navicular. *Sever's disease* is sometimes considered an avascular necrosis of the posterior calcaneal apophysis. Finally, *Freiberg's avascular necrosis* involves a flattening and arthritic degeneration of one of the phalangeal metatarsal joints. These have multiple etiologies, and they may be the result of trauma. Congenitally formed bars between various midfoot and hindfoot bones should also be considered in the differential diagnosis of foot pain with relatively little trauma. The roentgenographic appearance depends on whether there is partial or complete ossification.

WORK-UP

The child's foot must be carefully examined. The areas of pain or tenderness are palpated. Usually with a cellulitis,

the red demarcated area will be painful over the erythematous tissue and nonpainful peripheral to this area. However, with an underlying fracture, the erythematous area may be just the surface manifestation of the fracture. Hemorrhage and pain may also be present over the nonerythematous areas, since the underlying bone is in continuity with the fracture. Palpation of the tendons about the foot is essential in differentiating tendonitis from ligamentous or bony involvement.

To help differentiate infection and arthritis, it is essential to obtain a complete blood cell count, sedimentation rate, C-reactive protein, rheumatoid factor, antistreptolysin-O, and antinuclear antibody titers.

Fractures must be ruled out by regular anteroposterior and lateral as well as probably oblique roentgenograms of the foot. Special views such as axial views of the calcaneus may be necessary. Is one fails to reveal a fracture or an infection by means of conventional roentgenography, a technetium three-phase bone scan or a gallium scan may be needed but may be of limited value when imaging the small phalanges of the toes. These will show stress fractures and even show generalized stress areas in the limbs without a fracture present. They will also demonstrate an infection. Conventional tomograms or computed tomograms may be necessary to evaluate three-dimensional fractures of the bone, such as the navicular or talus, and in conditions causing pain, such as congenital fusions found between various hindfoot and midfoot bones. If infection is suspected, aspiration of the area may be helpful in obtaining an organism. Often, however, nothing grows on the culture media. Arthroscopy of the ankle joint is of limited value in the smaller child and adolescent.

TREATMENT

Fractures of the child's foot are usually treated by means of a short-leg cast. In the more distally based fractures of the metatarsal necks and toes, it is necessary to extend the platform forward of a short-leg cast to support these structures. After manipulation to the desired alignment, fractures of the individual toes may be maintained by buddy taping with stretchable tape to prevent strangulation necrosis of the distal portion of the soft tissues. Since the toes may swell from walking, a circumferentially applied bandage that is not made of a stretchable type of material or a spiral-type application can result in an iatrogenic amputation of the toe.

It is essential to reduce any dislocated joint to prevent an osteoarthritic deformity later. An open reduction is rarely needed unless there is a major dislocation in the position of a bone or it is an open wound. Metatarsals and phalanges, as long as they are in adequate alignment, should heal well without complications or sequelae. A fracture of the navicular in the longitudinal plane may require a long time for healing because it is relatively avascular and may become a nonunion. Fractures of the talus are rare in children but are dangerous and should be referred immediately for emergency treatment. Open reduction may be required to maintain blood supply to the involved fractured area.

Large areas of cellulitis, spreading lymphangitis, deep puncture wounds, or a systemically ill child require therapy with intravenous antibiotics until the infection is controlled. Then if parental care is reliable, oral antibiotics may be given. It is usually not necessary to decompress an early osteomyelitis with surgery, but it may occasionally be needed. A large abscess will not resolve without drainage. Although small fragments of foreign material may become encased in the foot and may never cause a problem, certain objects (most often, pins) caught perpendicular to the planes of motion will continue to fester and will not resolve even when treated with antibiotics. These objects should be removed. Chronic infections of the toes caused by ingrown toe nails will likewise require systemic antibiotics and may not heal until the nail has been at least partially surgically removed.

A referral will usually be required for most nontrivial injuries.

ANNOTATED BIBLIOGRAPHY

Brown LM, Sharrard WJW: Examination of the lower extremities in the child, p 186. In Post, M (ed): Physical Examination of the Musculoskeletal System, chap 9. Chicago, Year Book Medical Publishers, 1987. (Complete description of the physical examination.)

Morrissy RT (ed): Lovell and Winter's Pediatric Orthopedics, 3rd ed, chaps 27–31, pp 963–1024. Philadelphia, JB Lippincott, 1990.

Rang M: Children's Fractures, 2nd ed, chap 21. Philadelphia, JB Lippincott, 1983.

Rockwood C, Rockwood K: Fractures in Children, chap 13. Philadelphia, JB Lippincott, 1984.

Salter RB: Textbook of Disorders and Injuries of the Musculoskeletal System. Baltimore, Williams & Wilkins, 1970.

Sharrard WJW: Paediatric Orthopedics and Fractures, 2nd ed., chap 8. Oxford, Blackwell Scientific Publications, 1979. (This reference and the previous three references are all excellent general, yet comprehensive references.)

142

Burns: The Outpatient Management

Laurie A. Latchaw

It is estimated that 440,000 children are burned each year. Cutaneous burns result when excessive heat energy is transferred into the skin, causing cellular protein coagulation and destruction of enzyme systems. This, in turn, allows cellular fluid to leak out and bacteria to invade.

PATHOPHYSIOLOGY AND CLINICAL PRESENTATION

The depth and extent of the burn must be carefully assessed since this determines optimal medical management.

First-degree burns involve only the epidermis and are characterized by erythema, moderate pain, and edema. They heal in 5 to 10 days without the risk of scarring or infection. Sunburns and most hot water scald burns are first-degree injuries.

Second-degree burns involve the dermis and are characterized by blisters, severe pain, and edema. Second-degree burns may be superficial or deep. Superficial second-degree burns are bright red under the blister and heal in 10 to 14 days with temporary depigmentation. They may become infected if not cared for properly. Deep second-degree burns, however, are white beneath the blisters, may take up to 1 month to heal, and may have severe scarring. Infection may convert a deep second-degree burn to a third-degree burn. Grease burns are usually second-degree injuries. However, in small children with relatively thin skins, even hot water scald burns can be second-degree burns.

Third-degree burns involve the entire skin down to the subcutaneous tissue. They are white or charred in appearance and painless. Healing occurs from the burn edges at the rate of 1/8 inch per week. Severe scarring and contracture will occur unless skin grafts are applied. Susceptibility to both wound and systemic infection is high. Most flame injuries in older children are full-thickness burns.

In determining depth of injury, it is always safer to err toward the more serious diagnosis initially to avoid inappropriate outpatient therapy in a child who would be better treated by hospitalization. Differentiating a deep second-degree from a third-degree burn may be impossible.

The extent of the burn should be determined by plotting all second- and third-degree areas on a Lund and Bowder chart. This chart allows for the inversely changing proportionate size of a child's head and extremities with age.

WORK-UP

The work-up for any burned child should include a documentation of the heat source, the duration of the heat exposure, and how the burn was acquired. Tetanus immunization must be documented as well as a history of congenital heart disease, implanted prosthetic material, or a recent streptococcal infection. If the appearance or location of the burn is inconsistent with the history, child abuse must be suspected. Minor burns do not warrant baseline laboratory tests, but with extensive or deep burns, the clinician should obtain a complete blood cell count with differential white blood cell count, electrolytes, glucose, and blood urea nitrogen. "Strep screen" throat cultures are recommended in all patients with third-degree burns as well as those with second-degree burns of the hand. Patients who have extensive burns also require arterial blood gas analysis and determination of serum and urine osmolalities and carbon monoxide levels if an inhalation injury is suspected.

TREATMENT

Minor burns cover less than 10% of the total body surface area. Over 90% of burned children have minor injuries that can safely be managed in an ambulatory setting.

Burn treatment begins with removing the heat source and cooling the injury. This is accomplished by placing the burned area under a briskly flowing cold water faucet. Even chemicals can be safely "flushed off" with large-volume, high-pressure tap water because the chemical is diluted and is removed instantaneously.

Thirty minutes before outpatient burn cleansing and debriding, the child should be sedated with either codeine, 1 mg/kg orally, or chloral hydrate, 50 mg/kg orally. The burned area is cleansed gently with a sterile saline or a diluted povidone-iodine solution.

Blebs and blisters that are intact may be left as a physiologic dressing. Aspiration of the blisters to remove the fluid potentially contaminates the burn and is not recommended. Blebs and blisters that are broken or leaking should be debrided completely to ensure that bacteria are not trapped under the burned skin. Debridement can usually by done by simply wiping away the dead skin with a gauze sponge. Sharp debridement with sterile scissors is occasionally necessary. A thin coat of silver sulfadiazine is applied as a topical antibiotic. Silver sulfadiazine 1% cream is the preferred topical agent in children with burns because of its soothing quality, anti-*Pseudomonas* activity, and lack of significant side effects.

Minor burn dressings should provide protection, comfort, and, if possible, joint mobility. The standard dressing after application of 1% silver sulfadiazine is a soft, bulky gauze wrap. A hand dressing that separates each web space with gauze prior to wrapping the hand with the fingers extended is imperative for proper hand healing and function.

The burns may alternatively be covered with a transparent adhesive dressing (e.g., OpSite, Tegoderm, or Bioclusive), leaving at least a 3-cm sealed margin. Little "gloves" may be fashioned by placing the hand palm down on a sheet of transparent adhesive dressing and then covering it with another sheet. Generous 2- to 3-cm sealed margins should be left around each finger. The top is taped to the wrist. This dressing may take practice to apply but affords comfortable yet flexible hand coverage.

A third dressing choice is a biosynthetic compound (Biobrane) that is applied directly to the cleansed or debrided burn and then wrapped with elastic gauze. The dressing is checked every day, and any fluid or air pockets that have accumulated are aspirated dry. Adherence between the wound and the Biobrane should occur in 1 to 2 days. It is then left intact until the burn has reepithelialized. Biobrane gloves of various sizes are available for hand burns. This dressing provides comfort and flexibility and, once adhered, eliminates painful dressing changes.

Tetanus prophylaxis is given if immunizations are not current. No systemic antibiotics are prescribed unless the child has a valvular heart disease or a concomitant streptococcal infection.

The parents are instructed to increase the child's enteral fluid intake by 1% per burned body surface area but to avoid excessive free water intake. They should return in 1 to 2 days for a dressing check or immediately if the dressing falls off or if the child's temperature exceeds 102.2°F (39°C).

The initial gauze dressing should be changed in 2 days by a clinician. The burn must be completely cleansed of all fibrinous debris, serous exudate, and silver sulfadiazine because this combination simulates purulence. The burn, once cleaned, must be inspected for signs of infection. Patients with infected burns require hospitalization for systemic therapy with antibiotics and frequent dressing changes. Clean burns are redressed after an application of silver sulfadiazine. Parents may be instructed to do the subsequent dressing changes at home, but the physician should inspect the burn wounds once a week to ensure proper healing.

Very small burns to the face may be treated open. An antibiotic ointment is applied after cleansing and debriding. Frequent reapplication of the ointment is usually necessary, and the child may require "mittens" to keep the area from being touched.

INDICATIONS FOR REFERRAL OR ADMISSION

Critically burned patients have injuries involving more than 30% of their body surface area or have inhalation or electrical injuries. These children should be transferred to a regional burn center.

A major burn injury encompasses more than 10% of the total body surface area or is composed of more than 2% third-degree injury. These children require hospitalization for their burn care and fluid resuscitation. Other criteria for hospitalization include burns in children younger than 2 years of age because of increased fluid needs; burns to the face and perineum, which are often difficult to keep clean; and burns to the hands or feet, which may benefit from early tangential excision and grafting. Hand and/or foot burns that are superficial and less than one fourth of the hand surface area do not require admission to the hospital.

It may be desirable to admit a child with minor burns whose family or social environment precludes proper outpatient care and follow-up.

ANNOTATED BIBLIOGRAPHY

Ahlgren L: Burns. In Gellis SS, Kagan BM (eds): Current Pediatric Therapy, 12th ed, pp 685–687. Philadelphia, WB Saunders, 1986. (Current review of pediatric burn care.)

Kiher RG, Carvagal HF, Milcah RP et al: A controlled study of the effects of silver sulfadiazine on white blood cell counts on burned children. J Trauma 17:835–836, 1977. (Study confirming silver sulfadiazine as best topical burn agent for children.)

Larkin JM, Moylar JA: The role of prophylactic antibiotics in burn care. Am Surg 42:247, 1976. (Original article throwing doubt on the prophylactic use of penicillin for burns.)

143

Lacerations and Abrasions

Daniel P. Doody

Skin injuries are often encountered by the pediatrician. In this chapter the principles of wound management to achieve optimal closure with restoration of function at the site of injury are reviewed.

LACERATIONS

Pathophysiology

Lacerations are a break in dermal and epidermal integrity most often caused by penetrating injuries. This energy is transmitted primarily to the skin and is associated with less damage to neighboring tissue. Compressive injuries from blunt trauma generate higher kinetic energies that are dispersed in the surrounding tissue and cause bruising and local tissue ischemia. These complex wounds tend to be more prone to bacterial infection.

The concentration of normal skin flora varies in different anatomic areas, with the axilla, perineum, and anorectal areas having especially high density. An important additional area that has been identified with high concentrations include the areas of the nail beds on the hands and feet. At these points, bacterial concentrations can be as great at $10^6/cm^2$. Extremities and truncal areas have an average of 1000-fold less bacterial count per unit area. Therefore, wounds in proximity to areas where bacterial concentration is higher are more prone to infection. In the oral cavity, bacterial concentration in the gingiva and crevasses have an extraordinarily high bacterial load, and this is the primary reason for the high infection rate of wounds resulting from human or animal bites (see Chap. 144).

Other factors that play a role in determining if a wound will become infected include vascularity and anatomy of the area, time elapsed in caring for the wound, and the implantation of particulate matter from the soil or ground. Surprisingly, elements of the soil have infection promoting factors, acting as inhibitors at the cellular and humoral level. These factors, often found in swampy areas and in areas with high clay concentration, act to decrease the phagocytic capabilities of leukocytes while interfering with the normal activity of neutrophils. Therefore, injuries and lacerations that occur in swampy areas or at excavation sites containing clay subsoil are at increased risk of becoming infected. Puncture wounds through tennis shoes have a high incidence of *Pseudomonas* infection, and this inoculum should be treated with oral antibiotics to prevent soft tissue infection in the sole.

CLINICAL PRESENTATION

When a child presents with a laceration, one must remember that other potentially life-threatening injuries may coexist. An immediate survey should identify these problems. If massive bleeding is present, blind attempts to control bleeding with clamps should be avoided. Rather, direct pressure is the most efficient and safest means of stopping hemorrhage. The clinician should expose the wound and apply direct pressure using a sterile gauze over the site. If this maneuver fails to control bleeding, the extremity can be elevated for a brief period of time. A sphygmomanometer may be placed proximal to the laceration to an inflated pressure that is greater than systolic pressure. This type of pressure will greatly reduce bleeding and can be maintained for 30 to 60 minutes without ischemic damage to the distal nerves and vessels.

Once the initial stabilization is achieved, careful examination of the laceration is performed using sterile technique. It is important during this time that a mask and sterile gloves be used by the examiner. Not all traumatic injuries are heavily contaminated. The health professionals dealing with a lacerations should use universal precautions to protect themselves and to reduce the likelihood of introducing bacteria into the exposed integument and subcutaneous tissue.

Once the injured site is examined, one should determine if any neurovascular compromise distal to the injury site is present. This is particularly important prior to infiltrating the area with an anesthetic agent that may effect a motor as well as a neurosensory block. The practitioner should carefully palpate the underlying bone at the site of the injury to identify an open fracture that requires urgent surgical evaluation for debridement and closure. The complication of osteomyelitis is greatly increased as the time from injury to closure is increased over 6 hours. Appropriate roentgenographic studies should be expediently obtained to determine if a fracture is present.

TREATMENT

The treatment of simple lacerations is designed to promote optimal healing of the wound with the lowest chance of developing a wound infection. An important concept in this care is appropriate administration of a local anesthetic agent to allow adequate debridement of devitalized tissue, careful examination of the wound for particulate matter and appropriate cleansing, and finally closure of the injury without tension.

Anesthesia

Anesthetics may be injected or applied topically. The injection technique, using an amide-type local anesthetic agent such as lidocaine or bupivacaine, is most common. Lidocaine in a 1% concentration has a rapid onset (usually within 2 to 3 minutes) but a short half-life, providing the clinician with approximately 60 minutes of complete anesthesia. On the other hand, bupivacaine at a concentration of 0.25% to 0.5% has a delayed onset with as long as 10 minutes being required before full anesthesia is achieved. The duration of action is 4 to 6 hours and is significantly longer than lidocaine.

The addition of epinephrine at a concentration of 1:200,000 decreases absorption of the anesthetic agent at the wound site and potentiates the local effect of the anesthetic agent; however, it delays the onset of action. Experimentally, the vasoconstriction from epinephrine may promote bacterial invasion and increase the incidence of wound infection. This potentially detrimental effect of epinephrine should be considered if the wound is particularly complex or dirty and the risk of wound infection is great.

The technique of wound infiltration is equally important. Rapid intradermal injection of any fluid is painful. Injection into the subcutaneous tissue through the edges of the wound is less painful for the patient. The use of the smallest available needle (27 or 30 gauge) also decreases the amount of pain, primarily by allowing a slower and more controlled delivery of the anesthetic.

Until the introduction of TEC (a solution of 0.5% tetracaine, 1:2,000 epinephrine, and 11.8% cocaine), topical anesthesia was ineffective in providing adequate analgesia to allow appropriate closure. The introduction of TEC in 1980 has enabled the use of topical solutions as a means of providing anesthesia without injection. The solution is dripped into the wound, and an additional 1 to 2 mL soaked in a small gauze pad is placed over the wound and left in contact for 10 to 15 minutes. This topical agent has equivalent efficacy of anesthesia as the infiltration technique using lidocaine. Complications are infrequent, although a fatality has been reported with this solution when an inappropriately large volume was placed near the nasal mucous membranes, resulting in excessive drug absorption. To avoid excessive absorption, TEC should not be applied to mucosal surfaces and should not be reapplied if initial analgesia is unsuccessful. While some centers are currently not using this topical agent, many others are reporting great success with its use.

Preparation

The preparation of the surgical site depends on removal of particulate matter as well as infective organisms. Debridement of devitalized tissue is the final step in optimizing the wound for closure. The use of a high-pressure irrigating solution of saline effectively removes particulate matter. To facilitate the irrigation, a 35-mL syringe and a 19-gauge needle should be used. This promotes a jetlike action of the irrigant to adequately wash the wound.

Obviously devitalized tissues need to be removed. Tissue of questionable viability should be preserved. Many times, if this tissue can be closed without tension, it will survive. In certain areas, such as the face, the practice of minimal debridement should be followed. Use of an antibacterial agent to clean the wound is important. Unfortunately, povidone-iodine solutions are known to be cytotoxic. As a result, they may lessen the ability of the neutrophils to clear the bacterial inoculum. Similarly, chlorhexidine solutions damage white blood cells. Although these theoretical problems exist, both solutions can be diluted and have been used successfully for many years.

Once the wound is appropriately cleansed, closure is achieved using standard methods. Skin closure is best achieved with the use of a monofilament suture material such as nylon. Prolene has also been used in these cases; however, the expense engendered by the use of this suture material is rarely justified. In the smaller child, fine plain gut sutures can be used to achieve excellent approximation without the subsequent difficulty encountered with suture removal. The plain gut suture made from collagen derived from sheep or bovine intestine is an absorbable suture that lasts 7 to 14 days. It rarely causes suture reaction, unlike longer lasting absorbable suture materials such as chromic, polyglycolic acid (Dexon), polyglactin (Vicryl), and polydioxanone (PDS). These sutures, lasting from 3 to 6 weeks, are associated with suture reaction in 15% to 20% of cases. As a result, they are inappropriate to use on the skin in a traumatic setting.

Since many lacerations are under tension when they are closed, the use of subcuticular sutures is usually not indicated. These sutures need to be placed in a tension-free incision to obtain the best cosmetic results. Moreover, the subcuticular closure creates a closed environment that may promote bacterial proliferation in these potentially contaminated wounds. With debridement of devitalized tissue, these lacerations should have the edges approximated by simple interrupted sutures without tension to provide the best outcome.

The optimal time for removal of sutures depends on the site of injury, the complexity of the injury, and the presence of tension at closure. Removal of the suture material on the head and neck is performed after 4 to 5 days. Skin closure can be continued by the use of a tape closure (Steri-strips). On extremities, sutures should be removed after 7 to 8 days to prevent the suture tracks that occur with epithelialization around the suture material. Sutures on the feet and over the joints should be left in place for 2 weeks.

Use of tape as a form of skin closure can be applied for superficial lacerations that lie in good approximation. Ten to 15% of lacerations seen in the emergency department fall into this category. Tape closure is inappropriate if dermal fat is exposed. Tape closures have a lower incidence of infection than any form of suture closure. Moreover, in clinical series, the use of tape without any underlying sutures except for fascial sutures has been associated with excellent cosmetic outcome. In other series, the tape does not evert the skin edge and the eventual outcome leaves the patient with a depressed scar that is not as satisfying as those that are achieved with suture closure.

Postsuture Care

Once closure is achieved, epithelialization across the laceration occurs rapidly. Experimentally, the skin is sealed within 72 hours and it is recommended that the wound be covered for that period of time. In simple lacerations, gauze placed over the suture line and then covered with any type of occlusive dressing is appropriate. More complex lacerations or injuries extending over joints should be immobilized for 5 to 7 days by a bulky dressing or the use of a splint. While antibiotics are rarely needed for clean lacerations, the use of broad-spectrum oral antibiotic prophylaxis is indicated if the wound is "dirty."

Tetanus Immunization

Clinical features of the wound as well as history of previous tetanus immunizations will determine whether a booster of a tetanus toxoid or the more protective tetanus immune globulin (TIG) needs to be given. Features of the wound including length of time from injury to treatment, complexity of the wound, type of particulate matter that is present, evidence of significantly devitalized tissue, or the presence of a contaminant affect the risk for tetanus. In those instances, the clinician should give tetanus toxoid as a booster if none has been given in the past 5 years. It is currently recommended that the child receive TIG in addition to the tetanus toxoid if there is a tetanus-prone wound in a child with an uncertain tetanus toxoid immunization history or if the child has received fewer than four immunizations. The only specific contraindication to the use of tetanus toxoid is a previous severe hypersensitivity reaction. Local reactions are common and should not be considered an allergy.

ANIMAL AND HUMAN BITES

Animal and human bite wounds are complex lacerations that frequently need surgical evaluation for best outcome. Often the bite injury causes significant underlying tissue damage because of the crushing nature of the injury. Moreover, wound contamination secondary to the bite injury is common because of the high bacterial inoculum that is present in the oral cavity. Any resulting infection caused by the aerobic and anaerobic mouth flora can be severe and life threatening.

If the wound is clean and the time from injury to treatment is short, oral antibiotics in the form of amoxicillin-clavulanate (Augmentin) is effective for both animal and human bites. If there is any evidence of systemic infection, if the patient presents late after the injury, or if the method of injury is severe, parenteral antibiotics are indicated. Penicillin G plus a β-lactamase–resistant penicillin are effective when given in combination. Cefoxitin or ticarcillin-clavulanate (Timentin) are effective as single-drug therapies for most infections from bites. Surgical debridement remains the mainstay of treatment in severe infections from bites. In those instances, parenteral administration of antibiotics for up to 4 weeks may be necessary. As in dirty wounds, tetanus status needs to be determined and appropriately treated. (The reader is referred to Chapter 144 for a more complete discussion of animal and human bites.)

Abrasions

Abrasions are one of the most painful injuries because the denuding injury exposes dermal pain fibers. The loss of the epidermal elements opens a tender and weeping dermis that may be prone to infection. Although many of these wounds will heal without the need for treatment, the biology of wound healing suggests that a moist occlusive dressing will promote neoepithelialization and a more rapid closure of the wound. All abrasions benefit from moist occlusive dressings, but those greater than 8 cm² should have a biosynthetic dressing applied. Dry dressings promote scab formation by drying of the proteinaceous exudate. Within 18 to 20 hours, the underlying dermal layers will similarly dry. This hinders growth of the epidermal elements from the skin appendages. By providing a moist rather than dry environment, epidermal growth and coverage of the dermal matrix is promoted.

Use of the biosynthetic dressings (OpSite and Tegaderm) have been shown to facilitate healing of skin donor sites in the treatment of burn wounds. Since the donor site is similar to the injury seen in abrasions, it is assumed (although not proven) that similar treatment of abrasions would be beneficial. The water vapor–permeable dressings have a slightly increased incidence of wound infections as compared with fine mesh gauze but provide the definite advantages of promoting rapid epithelialization (time to healing—67% of dry gauze) while achieving an almost pain-free environment. For most children, these advantages outweigh the slightly increased incidence of wound infections. With a clean abrasion, the healing benefits of these biosynthetic membrane barriers may be used to best advantage. Use of petroleum jelly–impregnated gauze often dries on the abrasion site and removal is often painful. This problem does not occur with the use of the polyurethane adhesive membranes.

When particulate matter is imbedded into the dermal matrix, a traumatic tattoo may result. Early removal of the foreign material is important to achieve optimal cosmetic result. If it cannot be achieved easily in the office, general anesthesia for surgical scrubbing and occasionally dermabrasion is necessary to prevent this long-term complication. Delayed treatment generally results in a less satisfactory result.

INDICATIONS FOR REFERRAL

Simple dermal injuries in the form of abrasions and lacerations can often be handled in the practitioner's office by the use of simple surgical techniques. Complex lacerations that may require significant debridement should be referred for surgical evaluation and expertise. Lacerations with concomitant neurovascular or musculoskeletal injuries should be referred emergently for surgical treatment. Although some clean bites can be irrigated, left open, and treated with outpatient oral antibiotics if indicated, more complex bite wounds with a complicating infection or in a dangerous site (i.e., face, joints, and hands) should be referred for possible parenteral antibiotic therapy and surgical debridement. Abrasions with tattooing should be seen in an emergency department if the particulate debris cannot be removed completely in the office. Finally, it is important to consider the psychological advantages to the child and parents if extensive debridement is necessary, and, in those instances, referral for surgical care under general anesthesia may be preferable.

ANNOTATED BIBLIOGRAPHY

Barnett A, Berkowitz RL, Mills R, Vistnes LM: Comparison of synthetic adhesive moisture vapor permeable and fine mesh gauze dressings for split-thickness skin graft donor sites. Am J Surg 145:379, 1983. (Comparative trial establishing superiority of occlusive adhesive barriers over conventional fine mesh gauze.)

Bonadio WA, Wagner V: Efficacy of TAC topical anesthetic for repair of pediatric lacerations. Am J Dis Child 142:203, 1988. (Topical anesthetic application in pediatric population demonstrating equal efficacy to local infiltration anesthetic technique.)

Brook I: Human and animal bite infections. J Fam Pract 28:713, 1989. (Collective review of pathogens found in bite wounds with specific antibiotic rationale.)

Edlich RF, Rodeheaver GT, Morgan RF et al: Principles of emergency wound management. Ann Emerg Med 17:1284, 1988. (Excellent review of the pathophysiology of wound management and principles of repair.)

Rappaport NH: Laceration repair. Am Fam Physician 30:115, 1984. (Review article that addresses the specifics of surgical wound care.)

144

Animal and Human Bites

Robert A. Dershewitz and
Sonia Lewin

Animal bites occur commonly, with children being victims approximately 75% of the time. Although most bites are relatively minor, some result in serious infection, loss of function, disfigurement, or psychological trauma. Over 1 million dog bites occur each year; the ratio of dog to cat bites is 10:1. Approximately 10 children per year are killed by dog attacks, usually by family or neighbors' dogs. Con-

trary to common belief, only 10% of bites are inflicted by stray dogs. Boys are twice as likely to be bitten by dogs than are girls, whereas girls are twice as likely to be bitten by cats. Human bites are not as common as other bites but are potentially more serious.

Although principles for treating animal and human bites are similar, the optimal management of a bite must be individualized. The type, location, time, and circumstances of the bite, and the kind of animal and its condition are important considerations. Even when this information is known, "hard" data are scarce, resulting in varying recommendations for treatment.

PATHOPHYSIOLOGY

Infection of the surrounding soft tissues is the most common complication of a mammalian bite. Cellulitis and abscesses are the two most common infections. Lymphangitis and lymphadenitis also occur frequently as does cat-scratch disease (see Chap. 207). Rabies, although rare, is the ever-present dreaded outcome of an animal bite. Infection of tendons, periosteum, and joint spaces are also serious potential complications.

Pasteurella multocida is present as normal mouth flora in 10% to 60% of dogs and 50% to 70% of cats and is the causative agent in 20% to 50% of infections from dog bites and 80% from cats. It is a virulent pathogen, usually producing clinical signs of infection within 24 hours after the bite. Dog bites may also become infected with *Staphylococcus aureus* and *S. epidermidis,* α-hemolytic and other streptococci, and *Enterobacter* species. The human mouth has more organisms than other animals. Infections from human bites are most often caused by mixed flora, including *Streptococcus viridans, Staphylococcus aureus, Eikenella corrodens,* and other gram-negative rods and anaerobes such as bacteroides and *Fusobacterium* species.

Streptobacillus moniliformis, found in mouth flora of rats and mice, can cause bite infections and may lead (rarely) to rat-bite fever.

Although one cannot predict which bite will become infected, certain factors predispose to infection. Cat bites become infected more frequently than dog bites (20% to 50% vs. 5% to 10%) because they usually produce punctures that inoculate bacteria deep into the wound, close quickly, and are difficult to clean and debride. Because cats often lick their paws, infection due to *P. multocida* may occur from deep cat scratches as well as from bites. Dog bites create lacerations that can usually be well irrigated and debrided. Large dogs may produce considerable crush injuries. Even if adequately debrided, these wounds are prone to infection, as are bites to relatively avascular areas. The rate of infection is highest for bites to the hand and lowest for bites to the face. In infants, however, the risk of skull penetration and subsequent deep-seeded infections following bites to the scalp or face must be considered, and skull roentgenograms should be obtained when indicated. Human bites (especially to the hand) have a high rate of infection, but those inflicted by young children become infected less frequently. The time in seeking medical attention after the bite is another very important risk factor for infection. In one study, 59% of all patients with infected animal bites had delays of more than 24 hours in obtaining medical care.

Any bite on the hand, but especially by a human, is potentially devastating. The metacarpophalangeal joints on the dorsum of the hand are most often bitten when a clenched fist hits an opponent's tooth, producing either a puncture wound or crush injury. If a tendon or joint is penetrated, a rapid and fulminant closed-space infection (tenosynovitis) may develop.

MANAGEMENT

Although management recommendations for animal bites are controversial, there is consensus on the importance of good wound care. Initial surveillance cultures of bites are not recommended because of poor correlation with subsequent cultures of infected wounds.

Wound Care

In Callaham's study (see bibliography), 12% of irrigated wounds became infected compared with 69% of those not irrigated. Soaking the wound is not effective; scrubbing the surrounding area is indicated. Copious irrigation under pressure (e.g., using a 19-gauge needle and 35-mL syringe or Water Pik) is the critical step to reduce the total bacterial load of the wound. A saline solution is adequate, although some authors recommend adding an antiseptic to the solution such as 1% povidone-iodine diluted to one tenth of its original strength. Depending on the size and location of the bite, at least 150 to 1000 mL of saline should be used to irrigate the wound, and the stream should be aimed in all directions so as to debride all surfaces. Although controversial because puncture wounds close quickly and tissue damage may result from pressure irrigation, puncture bites should also be irrigated by hydraulic pressure.

All wounds, unless small and superficial, should be debrided to further reduce the risk of infection. Foreign bodies, such as strands of clothing, must be meticulously removed. Jagged edges should be trimmed judiciously for a better cosmetic result. Debridement also provides additional exposure of the wound, so irrigation should be repeated after thoroughly debriding the area (see also Chap. 143).

Primary Versus Secondary Healing

Puncture wounds and other bites likely to become infected (i.e., in relatively avascular areas, in immunocompromised hosts, older than 12 hours, with extensive tissue injury, and deep human bites) should not be sutured. In questionable situations, it is preferable to leave the wound open. If thoroughly irrigated, dog bites to the face that are sutured seldom become infected. (Even without prophylactic antibiotics, Guy and Zook [see bibliography] reported an infection rate of only 1.4%). Although increasing numbers of physicians in emergency departments suture bites on the hand, current recommendations state that bites on hands (especially by humans) should *not* be sutured. The rationale is that it is wiser to forego the better cosmetic result of primary repair than to risk infection with its resultant morbidity and potential hospitalization. Parents should be advised that the scar will "look better" over time and that it can be subsequently revised if cosmesis is a concern. An alternative to suturing is the use of paper tape for "loose" primary closure to minimize both the scar and the risk of infection.

Prophylactic Antibiotics

Although the efficacy of prophylactic antibiotics has not been established, some authors advocate a 5-day course for all bites. A more rational approach is to individualize their use. Prophylactic antibiotics should not be given for superficial bites in well-vascularized areas that are treated immediately with appropriate wound care because they are at low risk of becoming infected. Prophylactic antibiotics, however, are recommended for hand and deep face bites (where infection may be devastating), for cat bites, and for other bites likely to become infected (see listing in previous section on primary versus secondary healing).

No single antibiotic will effectively cover all potential pathogens. The most appropriate choices are penicillin or amoxicillin/clavulanate (Augmentin) for 5 days. Penicillin is the most active agent against *P. multocida*, and it also covers streptococci and many anaerobes. It is probably the drug of choice for cat and dog bites, but if *S. aureus* is also suspected, a penicillinase-resistant penicillin or cephalosporin must be added. Augmentin gives good coverage of *S. aureus*, streptococci, *Eikenella corrodens*, *P. multocida*, and anaerobic bacteria including β-lactamase producers. It is probably the drug of choice for human bites because up to 45% of *Bacteroides* strains in human oral flora produce β-lactamase. Clindamycin, first-generation cephalosporins, and penicillinase-resistant penicillins have very poor activity in vitro against *P. multocida* and *Eikenella corrodens*, but they have been used effectively in vivo to prevent bite wound infections. Cefuroxime axetil, a second-generation cephalosporin, cefixime, a third-generation cephalosporin, and the fluoroquinolones are effective against *P. multocida* and other organisms commonly isolated from bite wounds.

If the patient is allergic to penicillin, erythromycin or, in the older child, tetracycline may be used. About 50% of *P. multocida* strains and many anaerobes and *S. aureus* are resistant to erythromycin.

Concern About Rabies

In the United States, rats, mice, prairie dogs, hamsters, gerbils, chipmunks, squirrels, rabbits, and hares are virtually rabies free. If the biting animal is potentially rabid, the physician should decide if postexposure rabies prophylaxis is indicated. The rabies virus may also be transmitted by licking mucous membranes, fresh wounds, or abrasions. An ill animal, one that behaves strangely, or one that bites without provocation is more likely to be rabid. If the bite was provoked and the animal can be observed, it should be watched or quarantined for 10 days. If the animal remains healthy, no prophylaxis is required; if it behaves strangely or become sick, it must be sacrificed and its brain tested for rabies. Empiric rabies prophylaxis should be administered after bites from bats and wild carnivores such as skunks, raccoons, foxes, coyotes, and bobcats because of their greater chance of being rabid. If the animal is caught, it should be killed without damaging the head. If the head cannot be delivered immediately to the health department, it should be stored in a refrigerator (not a freezer). Contact the state or local health department for help in management. If a biting dog or cat escapes, rabies prophylaxis may not be necessary if there have been no reported rabid dogs or cats in that geographic area.

It is safe to delay postexposure prophylaxis up to 1 week. A negative fluorescent rabies antibody test on an acceptable brain specimen obviates the need for prophylaxis. If the specimen is positive for rabies or if there is a possibility that the animal may be rabid, both rabies immune globulin (RIG) and human diploid cell vaccine (HDCV) must be given. Up to half a single dose of RIG (20 IU/kg) is infiltrated into the area of the wound and the rest is given intramuscularly, at a separate site from HDCV. A total of five intramuscular doses of HDCV, each 1 ml, are given on days 0, 3, 7, 14, and 28.

Tetanus Prophylaxis

Although the risk of tetanus is not great, the immunization status of the child should be determined. If the patient is not completely immunized (i.e., is not up to date with the primary vaccination series or has not had a booster dose within 5 years for a contaminated wound or 10 years for a superficial bite) 0.5 mL tetanus toxoid, TD or Td is given intramuscularly. If the child is younger than 6 years old and needs pertussis immunization, give DPT if it is not contraindicated for other reasons. Only Td should be given to children 8 years of age and older. An incompletely immunized patient with a tetanus-prone injury (e.g., deep or contaminated) should also receive human tetanus immunoglobulin (TIG) 250 to 500 units intramuscularly at a separate site.

INDICATIONS FOR REFERRAL AND ADMISSION

Despite appropriate, timely wound care and the use of prophylactic antibiotics in patients presenting early with uninfected bites, 8% to 16% of bite wounds will become infected. Hospitalization is indicated if the infection is rapidly progressing, does not respond to oral antibiotics, is deep (e.g., involves a tendon or joint space), or is on the hand or face. Most infections are uncomplicated and can be readily managed by the primary care physician. The initial choice of antibiotic(s) pending culture results should be based on a Gram stain. A penicillinase-resistant penicillin is used if gram-positive cocci are seen in clusters. Combination therapy is warranted if the Gram stain is not useful. A reasonable initial choice is amoxicillin/clavulanate or penicillin and a penicillinase-resistant penicillin. The involved extremity should be elevated and immobilized. If a sutured bite becomes infected, the sutures are removed and any pus is drained. Any retained foreign bodies should be sought and removed. Consultation with an infectious disease specialist or a surgeon may be helpful, especially for wound drainage.

Human bites on the hand and any bite over a joint require a special protocol. The depth and extent of the injury must be determined since even a relatively minor closed-fist injury may penetrate the tendon and joint capsule, requiring operative debridement and repair. The patient should be referred to an experienced surgeon because special expertise for assessing this type of wound is required.

PATIENT AND PARENTAL EDUCATION

Patients or parents are instructed to observe for signs of wound infection and to return immediately if they are noted. Children should be taught how to, and when not to, approach animals because adherence to basic safety rules will prevent many animal bites.

ANNOTATED BIBLIOGRAPHY

Brook I: Microbiology of human and animal bite wounds in children. Pediatr Infect Dis J 6:29–32, 1987. (Study demonstrating the polymicrobial aerobic-anaerobic nature of most human and animal bite wounds.)

Brook I: Human and animal bite infections. J Fam Pract 28:713–718, 1989. (Thorough review of the topic that stresses the need for scrupulous wound care and provides a well-referenced discussion on the use of antibiotics.)

Callaham ML: Controversies in antibiotic choices for bite wounds. Ann Emerg Med 17:1321–1330, 1988. (Provocative review that shows that human bites [except closed-fist injuries] do not have a higher rate of infection than other animal bites and questions the advantage of amoxicillin/clavulanate over less expensive antibiotics with fewer side effects.)

Centers for Disease Control: Rabies. MMWR 33:26S–28S, 1984. (Complete guide on rabies prophylaxis.)

Galloway RE: Mammalian bites. J Emerg Med 6:325–331, 1988. (Excellent overview that outlines the risk factors for infection and gives a detailed plan for proper wound cleansing.)

Guy RJ, Zook EG: Successful treatment of acute head and neck dog bite wounds without antibiotics. Ann Plast Surg 17:45–48, 1986. (Prospective study of wounds treated within 6 hours with vigorous irrigation, debridement, and repeat irrigation; infection rates were equally low with or without antibiotics.)

Lewis RC: Infections of the hand. Emerg Clin North Am 3:271–274, 1985. (Comprehensive discussion on management of [mainly human] hand bites.)

Mann JM: Systematic decision-making in rabies prophylaxis. Pediatr Infect Dis 2:162–167, 1983. (Logical and practical guide in deciding which bites require rabies prophylaxis.)

Mofenson HC, Greensher J: Accident prevention. In Hoekelman RA (ed): Primary Pediatric Care, pp 237–239. St. Louis, CV Mosby, 1987. (Sound recommendations on teaching children about animals with safety rules for meeting a strange dog.)

Trott A: Bite wounds. In Trott A (ed): Wounds and Lacerations: Emergency Care and Closure, pp 227–246. St. Louis, CV Mosby, 1991. (Current and comprehensive discussion on mammalian bites with well-referenced guidelines for wound management and the use of antibiotics.)

145

Trauma to the Oral Cavity

Joan M. O'Connor

Trauma to the oral cavity is common. The types and extents of injuries are diverse, and the emergency situation is usually stressful for both the parents and the child. The pain accompanying soft tissue lacerations makes the examination uncomfortable, and the physical and psychological impact this injury will have on "the smile" produces anxiety. The most common site of injury is the maxillary central incisor. Most injuries to the primary teeth occur at between 18 and 30 months of age, a time when the child gains independence and mobility but still lacks stability and coordination. Children who are 9 to 10 years old are in the most common group to have traumatic injury to the permanent dentition. Boys sustain fractures to the permanent anterior teeth twice as often as girls.

PATHOPHYSIOLOGY AND CLINICAL PRESENTATION

The alveolar bone supporting the primary incisors is immature and pliable. Displacement, particularly *intrusion*, rather than fracture, is the more common injury in this dentition, whereas the denser bone of the older child seems to stabilize the permanent tooth, rendering it more susceptible to a fracture. The intrusion is characterized by a partial or complete disappearance into the alveolar bone. If there is swelling of the surrounding soft tissue, the damage appears worse than it actually is. In the intrusion type of displacement of the primary dentition, a risk of damage exists to the underlying permanent tooth; the extent of damage depends on the state of development of the tooth and the degree of displacement that occurs. In the permanent dentition, *extrusion* is a much more common type of displacement than intrusion. Extrusion is rare in the primary teeth except when the root is fractured. A partial displacement of a tooth, especially laterally, has a better prognosis when root development is not complete. The open apex allows for hyperemia of pulpal vessels that are often strangulated in a completely formed root with a small apex. In general, a tooth traumatized but not fractured usually receives a greater shock than one that is chipped, probably because the energy of the blow is dissipated in fracturing the tooth rather than absorbing the energy internally.

When a total displacement (*avulsion*) occurs, the prognosis of the affected tooth or teeth is uncertain: some reestablish normal attachment, some become ankylosed (fused to bone), and others fail completely. The primary reasons for failure are external resorption of the root and periapical abscess.

Discoloration of a tooth following trauma is usually the result of some seepage from the pulpal vessels into the dentinal tubules. A loss of vitality of the pulp is variable. If there is no resulting pulpal damage, the discoloration tends to lighten in time.

Minor crown fractures are not common in the primary dentition, probably because the stubby shape of the tooth, the thin layer of enamel, and the relatively large pulp cause fractures to involve the pulp. Coronal fractures of enamel and dentin without pulpal exposure constitute 60% to 70% of all fractures involving permanent teeth.

Root fractures should be suspected in teeth that are mobile but seem to pivot short of the apex. Successful healing may occur if fragments are in close apposition, if infection is absent, and if the fracture has occurred more closely to the root apex than the crown of the tooth.

Injury to the developing permanent tooth can occur as a sequela to primary dentition trauma, either through direct impact of the primary tooth against the permanent tooth or as a result of an infection of the primary tooth, which affects the enamel of the permanent tooth. Enamel hypoplasia (staining or rippling of the enamel), dilaceration of the root (malalignment of the long axis of the tooth occurring at the point of development that the tooth was at when the insult occurred), and cessation of root formation are common effects on the permanent tooth following trauma to the primary tooth.

Oral burns, almost exclusively the result of electrical burns, are more commonly seen in emergency departments than in the pediatrician's office. Such burns can cause severe constriction, scarring, and deformation of the lip.

DIFFERENTIAL DIAGNOSIS

Child abuse should be suspected if there are signs of old wounds or if the history is inconsistent with the trauma.

WORK-UP

History

The history is significant for the following:

- *Age:* Age will give an indication of the extent of tooth eruption and root formation/resorption. The loss of maxillary central incisors may be as simple as a bump near the time of exfoliation or a complete avulsion of teeth with fully formed roots. A severe blow to a young tooth in which root formation is incomplete has a wide apical passageway for emerging vessels. This results in a much more favorable prognosis than the tooth with advanced apical development allowing only a narrow passage for vessels. The situation in a child with a fractured tooth may look much worse than it actually is if the tooth had only partially erupted prior to the incident.
- *Time of injury:* Successful treatment to an injured pulp or reimplantation of avulsed teeth is inversely proportional to the time that has elapsed. Injuries to the teeth frequently involve legal or insurance claims; thus, time notation in the record is also important.
- *Patient complaints:* These complaints are often invaluable in determining the extent of damage. Sensitivity to biting in a position of normal occlusion may indicate a displacement or an extrusion not initially detected. A reaction to thermal change indicates hyperemia of a vital dental pulp and treatment is necessary.

Physical Examination

Soft Tissue Trauma. The lip and tongue should be examined thoroughly for internal/external (through-and-through) lacerations. The wound should also be examined for tooth fragments and particles of glass, rock, asphalt, or other puncturing objects imbedded deeply.

Hard Tissue Trauma. A direct blow to the chin may result in condylar head fractures. Particular attention should be paid to tenderness in this area or a limited range of motion on opening or closing of the jaw. The dentition should be examined closely for missing or fractured teeth, and attempts should be made to account for the missing pieces by a close examination of the soft tissue. Fractured teeth should be examined to determine the extent of damage (e.g., exposure of dentin, pulp, and the presence of root fragments).

Any suspected fracture of the jaw should be x-rayed with either a panoramic or lateral jaw film. A fracture of the root can be verified by occlusal films taken by the child's dentist.

MANAGEMENT

Soft Tissue Lacerations

When treating soft tissue lacerations, local anesthetic infiltration with a 2% lidocaine solution will ease debridement with hydrogen peroxide and saline. Suturing, if necessary, can then be completed. Prophylactic antibiotic coverage should be considered if the wound is "dirty," if it is punctured by a foreign object, or if there is skin to oral mucosal communication.

Gingival lacerations usually first appear much worse than they actually are. Displaced tissue can usually be repositioned easily after a thorough cleaning with hydrogen peroxide. If the gingiva can be repositioned (as is the case in most patients) so that it is well apposed to the surrounding tissue, healing will generally occur without any complications, since the area is so vascular. If the tissue appears greatly displaced, single sutures of resorbable gut, placed between the teeth from the labial to the palatal surface to restore the normal contour of the tissue, will ensure proper and rapid healing. Warm saline rinses and gentle swabbing with a cotton gauze are advisable for cleaning the area until healed, because the area will be too uncomfortable to clean with a toothbrush.

Hard Tissue Trauma

When intrusion-type displacements are sustained, the damage, if any, occurs at the time of impact. No further damage will occur if the affected tooth is observed closely. Reeruption can be expected within 3 to 4 weeks. The parents must be cautioned that a severely intruded tooth frequently becomes nonvital with ensuing pulpal necrosis. When the affected tooth is a primary tooth, periapical necrosis could affect the developing permanent successor. Any tenderness on eating that develops over that tooth should be reported to the dentist and a roentgenogram to view the periapical area should be taken within several weeks to detect abscess formation. A tooth that fails to re-erupt should be considered for extraction, particularly in the primary dentition, to prevent interference with the normal path of eruption of the permanent tooth.

When extrusion of a primary tooth with a root fracture occurs, extraction is usually recommended. Extrusions of the permanent teeth should be referred to the dentist to rule out a fracture of the root. A root fracture that is closely apposed and does not occur in the cervical third has a good chance for successful healing if properly stabilized and if occlusal interferences are removed. Lateral displacements can often be repositioned by the parent or physician with light finger pressure. The area is often tender because of soft tissue injury; therefore, the patient will not use this area very much, allowing the tooth to stabilize without any splinting. If the displacement is extreme but with minimal damage to the alveolus, it may be necessary for the dentist to apply a small acrylic splint.

Avulsion of a primary tooth is usually not replanted because of the high incidence of root resorption following such a procedure. The sequelae of possible pulpal necrosis and attendant cost considerations must be weighed against the length of time the tooth would be expected to be a functioning component of the arch.

If a primary tooth is lost either to avulsion or extraction, the need for space maintenance must be considered. In general, if the primary cuspids have erupted (at about age 8 months), there is little space loss in the anterior region when a tooth is lost prematurely.

Avulsed permanent teeth should be replanted in their sockets as soon as possible. If replantation occurs within the first few minutes after avulsion, root canal therapy may not be required because there is a possibility of revascularization of the blood supply to the pulp and reattachment of the periodontal membranes. Studies have shown that when a tooth is out of its socket less than 30 minutes, replantation is successful in 90% of cases. When the time lapsed is 30 to 90 minutes, the success rate drops to 43%, and after 90 minutes, the success rate is only 7%.

If a telephone call is received from the parent, school nurse, or team coach prior to arriving at the office, the person should attempt to reimplant the permanent tooth back in its socket. If this reimplantation is unsuccessful, the avulsed tooth should be transported in milk or saliva. The tooth can also be carried in the mucosal fold of the lower lip if the patient is cautious not to swallow it.

Before replanting, the tooth should be gently washed with saline. Harsh scrubbing that may fragment the periodontal ligament must be avoided. Once the tooth has been replanted, splinting by way of orthodontic brackets or an acrylic splint is recommended. If considerable time has elapsed, the pulp may be nonvital. A referral to the patient's dentist may be advisable for root canal treatment of the tooth prior to insertion and, if necessary, a curettage of the socket should be done to reinsert the tooth.

A tooth that is discolored by a traumatic blow should be monitored by the dentist on routine visits to ensure that no pathology of the pulp is present.

When a fracture of a tooth involving only enamel occurs, the preferred treatment (if sought at all) is minimal, requiring only a smoothing of the edges that are rough and that irritate the lips or tongue. If the pulp cannot be seen but the tooth is sensitive to cold or air, a covering of calcium hydroxide and acrylic should be applied to provide relief and protect the pulp. An application of topical fluoride to the exposed dentin will also decrease sensitivity. When the pulpal tissue is exposed, removal of vital pulp tissue (pulpotomy), extraction of the entire pulpal chamber with replacement by a zinc oxide, eugenol, and formocresol material (pulpectomy), or an extraction should be performed by the dentist after consideration of factors such as time elapsed, root development, root resorption, and the proximity to the permanent tooth. If pulpal therapy is provided, the fractured crown can then be restored by means of composite (acrylic) crowns.

INDICATIONS FOR REFERRAL

A referral for extensive lacerations of the soft tissue should be made to an emergency department or plastic surgeon or to an emergency department for electrical burns. In the case of electrical burns, an appliance with commissure posts is often made by a dentist in cooperation with the plastic surgeon to reduce the constriction and scarring that occur during healing. The appliance is worn for about 1 year and may eliminate the need for surgery, or at least reduce the number of operative procedures.

A referral to a dentist should be made for any suspected fractures of the roots of teeth, for exposures of the dental pulp, and when splinting is preferred.

PATIENT EDUCATION

A reduction of the incidence of oral trauma involves education of the supervising adult and the use of preventative measures and appliances.

The environment should be studied to reduce the common situations that lead to facial trauma. The young child should be restrained in an acceptable car seat while riding in a motor vehicle. The child should be taught safety precautions for the bathtub, stairways, and so forth. Electrical cords should be inaccessible to the child.

Children who have a severe protrusion of the maxillary teeth should be treated as early as possible because these teeth are more prone to injury.

Children should be outfitted with mouthguards before participation in athletics. These devices should be either custom fitted, those made to fit over orthodontic appliances, or the type available in sporting goods stores that are readily molded in warm water.

ANNOTATED BIBLIOGRAPHY

Andreasen JO, Andreasen FM: Essentials of Traumatic Injuries to the Teeth. St. Louis, CV Mosby, 1990. (Comprehensive treatment of all aspects of dental trauma.)

Andreasen JO, Hjoring-Hansen E: Replantation of teeth: I. Radiographic and clinical study of 110 human teeth replanted after accidental loss. Acta Odontol Scand 24:263–286, 1964. (Discussion of the effects of trauma by one of the foremost authorities on the subject.)

Ellis RG, Davey KW: The Classification and Treatment of Injuries to the Teeth of Children. Chicago, Year Book Medical Publishers, 1970. (Excellent classification according to the extent of injury with corresponding particularly detailed treatment for each classification that is probably more helpful to the dentist than the pediatrician.)

Hill C: Oral trauma to the preschool child. Dent Clin North Am 28:177–186, 1984. (Concise and practical for trauma of the primary dentition.)

McDonald RE, Avery DR: Management of traumatic injuries to the teeth and supporting tissues. In McDonald RE, Avery DR (eds): Dentistry for the Child and Adolescent, 5th ed, pp 512–572. St. Louis, CV Mosby, 1987. (Thorough general text of pediatric dentistry.)

Ripa L, Finn SB: The care of injuries to the anterior teeth of children. In Finn SB (ed): Clinical Pedodontics, 4th ed, pp 224–270 Philadelphia, WB Saunders, 1973. (Comprehensive, well-illustrated discussion of trauma, particularly of treatment.)

19

NEUROLOGIC PROBLEMS

Elizabeth C. Dooling, Section Editor

146

The Floppy Infant

Kalpathy S. Krishnamoorthy

Floppiness (*hypotonia*) is a common clinical manifestation of an underlying neurologic disorder in infancy. To some degree, hypotonia is subjectively based on the experience of the examiner. It is strongly suspected, however, when there is a diminished resistance of the joints to passive movement, when there is an increased range of joint motion, or when the infant assumes abnormal postures. Gross motor delay is one of the hallmarks of this condition. The parents are often the first to suspect this abnormality.

PATHOPHYSIOLOGY

The control and maintenance of muscle tone is complex. Several aspects of this function are not well understood. Hypotonia may be due to a specific neuromuscular disorder or an associated finding of a wide variety of apparently unrelated metabolic conditions, as in malnutrition or in renal tubular acidosis. The muscle tone is maintained by suprasegmental pathways (upper motor neuron system) and their influences through the lower motor neuron system. The suprasegmental influences originate in the central nervous system through the corticospinal-corticobulbar pathways, basal ganglia, cerebellum, and some descending spinal tracts. These upper motor neuron connections exert a strong influence on the muscle tone through the motor unit. The latter, also known as the *lower motor neuron system,* includes the anterior horn cell, its axons along the peripheral nerve, the neuromuscular junction, and the innervated muscle fiber. Hypotonia may thus occur due to disorders in the integrity of the upper or the lower motor neuron system.

CLINICAL PRESENTATION

The clinical picture will depend on the age of the patient, the location of the lesion, and specific features of an underlying disorder. To some extent there are certain common features that apply to most floppy infants. In the neonatal period the diagnosis of a floppy infant is suggested by the following: poor sucking, swallowing, and coordination; a weak cry; a lack of spontaneous motor activity; an abnormal posture; and respiratory distress. As they get older, floppy infants characteristically manifest a lack of normal gross motor development. They may also show feeding difficulties, recurrent aspiration pneumonia, or obvious skeletal anomalies. They usually show a delay in sitting, walking, running, and other common gross motor functions. In other instances, they may also show subnormal cognitive speech and language skills. Their neurodevelopmental skills may either remain static or deteriorate, depending on the underlying condition. Certain distinct clinical features may aid in the diagnosis (e.g., fasciculations of the tongue in Werdnig-Hoffmann disease or facial diplegia in myotonic dystrophy). Other specific abnormalities are described under the clinical examination.

DIFFERENTIAL DIAGNOSIS

The differential diagnosis is best organized around the anatomic localization of the lesion, with evaluation usually proceeding in a cephalocaudal direction (Fig. 146-1). The motor development and examination of floppy infants is uniformly abnormal. This finding, with a combination of other clinical and laboratory features, will usually aid in making a specific diagnosis. Several conditions that produce transient hypotonia such as sepsis or drug intoxications are not included in this discussion.

In some cases the examiners cannot find hard evidence for a neuromuscular disorder. Close follow-up is necessary in such instances. The term *benign congenital hypotonia* is no longer considered a tenable diagnosis.

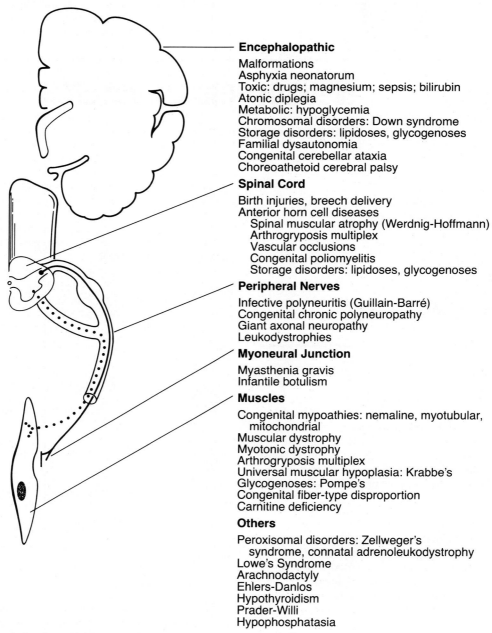

Encephalopathic

Malformations
Asphyxia neonatorum
Toxic: drugs; magnesium; sepsis; bilirubin
Atonic diplegia
Metabolic: hypoglycemia
Chromosomal disorders: Down syndrome
Storage disorders: lipidoses, glycogenoses
Familial dysautonomia
Congenital cerebellar ataxia
Choreoathetoid cerebral palsy

Spinal Cord

Birth injuries, breech delivery
Anterior horn cell diseases
    Spinal muscular atrophy (Werdnig-Hoffmann)
    Arthrogryposis multiplex
    Vascular occlusions
    Congenital poliomyelitis
    Storage disorders: lipidoses, glycogenoses

Peripheral Nerves

Infective polyneuritis (Guillain-Barré)
Congenital chronic polyneuropathy
Giant axonal neuropathy
Leukodystrophies

Myoneural Junction

Myasthenia gravis
Infantile botulism

Muscles

Congenital mypoathies: nemaline, myotubular,
    mitochondrial
Muscular dystrophy
Myotonic dystrophy
Arthrogryposis multiplex
Universal muscular hypoplasia: Krabbe's
Glycogenoses: Pompe's
Congenital fiber-type disproportion
Carnitine deficiency

Others

Peroxisomal disorders: Zellweger's
    syndrome, connatal adrenoleukodystrophy
Lowe's Syndrome
Arachnodactyly
Ehlers-Danlos
Hypothyroidism
Prader-Willi
Hypophosphatasia

Figure 146-1.   Differential diagnosis of a floppy infant.

Some of the common causes of floppy newborns include asphyxia, Werdnig-Hoffmann disease, cerebral anomalies, metabolic disorders, myotonic dystrophy, congenital fiber-type disproportion, and congenital myopathies. In later infancy the following are some of the important considerations: atonic cerebral palsy, degenerative disorders (lipidoses), Werdnig-Hoffmann disease, congenital structural myopathies, myotonic dystrophy, Duchenne pseudohypertrophic muscular dystrophy, infantile botulism, Pompe's disease, and metabolic mitochondrial myopathies. Certain nonneurologic disorders may also present as hypotonia (e.g., arachnodactyly, Ehlers-Danlos syndrome, renal tubular acidosis, Lowe's syndrome, and Prader-Willi syndrome).

WORK-UP

History

The clinician must focus on important additional clues to arrive at a tentative diagnosis. The parents' chief concerns need to be carefully assessed to know the severity of the situation, especially the sequence of milestones and the extent of motor delay. The physician should determine if the condition is transient or progressive; if it is a familial-genetic or a sporadic case; if the child is globally delayed or merely slow in the motor skills; and if there are systemic disorders (e.g., renal, cardiac).

The physician should ask the mother about her pregnancy, labor, delivery, and the neonatal period of the child. Evidence of fetal distress, difficult delivery, and low Apgar scores may all be clues for asphyxia. In the newborn, however, a primary neuromuscular disease may coexist with an asphyxial injury as in myotonic dystrophy. In the latter, the mother should always be examined carefully for evidence of myotonic dystrophy since 90% of the infants with myotonic dystrophy are born to an affected mother. These women may have a characteristic myopathic facies, a typical history of increasing muscular weakness during pregnancy, and uterine dystocia during delivery. Percussion myotonia is a characteristic finding in these women. The physician should also ask if there was diminished fetal activity, which is typical of Werdnig-Hoffmann disease and Prader-Willi syndrome.

During the first days or weeks of life, characteristics of a floppy infant may be recognized that may later evolve into a distinct entity. Examples of such conditions include cerebral malformations, Werdnig-Hoffmann disease, congenital myopathies, or myotonic dystrophy. These infants typically have feeding difficulties, lethargy, poor activity, and respiratory difficulties; later on, they exhibit characteristic findings.

A detailed survey of all of the milestones should be performed by the clinician. Very-low-birth-weight premature infants are usually slower in acquisition of gross motor milestones until their second birthday. Additional information should be sought regarding a family history of neuromuscular disorders, hypoglycemia, seizures, enlarged liver (glycogen storage disorders), preceding viral illness (polyneuropathy), ingestion of honey and constipation (infantile botulism), hyperextensibility of the joints (Ehlers-Danlos syndrome), voracious appetite, and an abnormal increase in weight gain (Prader-Willi syndrome). Rapid deterioration of neurologic functions favors a neurodegenerative disorder or metabolic myopathy.

Physical Examination

The physical examination offers the most valuable information in the evaluation of floppy infants. The evaluation should include a general examination and a complete neurologic evaluation, the latter encompassing a detailed developmental hearing and visual assessment.

By this approach, a distinction can be made between an upper motor neuron disorder versus a lower motor neuron lesion. An upper motor neuron lesion is generally characterized by a lack of muscle weakness, normal muscle bulk, preserved tendon reflexes, and, in some cases, evidence for cerebral dysfunction. In lower motor neuron lesions, however, there may be fasciculations, muscle atrophy, muscle weakness, and diminished or absent tendon reflexes. These children are generally appropriate in their cerebral functions such as cognitive skills and speech and language functions. It is worth emphasizing that this is only a general rule and that there are exceptions. For instance, infants with muscular dystrophy or myotonic dystrophy may show evidence for cerebral dysfunction. The physician needs to estimate the patient's overall intelligence and psychomotor development. Specific features of various conditions should then be looked for systematically.

The general examination should include the head circumference, palpation of the abdomen for hepatosplenomegaly, and auscultation of the heart for cardiac murmur. This examination may disclose somatic anomalies, clues for neurometabolic disorders (e.g., glycogenoses), or evidence for specific syndromes (e.g., Down syndrome). A meticulous examination of the face may offer clues to myotonic dystrophy and myopathies. These abnormalities include facial diplegia, a tented upper lip, a fishlike mouth, and a myopathic face.

During the neurologic examination the physician should especially look for the following abnormalities: ophthalmoplegia and ptosis (metabolic myopathies and infantile botulism); fasciculations of the tongue (Werdnig-Hoffmann disease); macroglossia (glycogenosis or hypothyroidism); microcephaly or macrocephaly (cerebral dysgenesis, lipidoses); arthrogryposis (myotonic dystrophy); scoliosis (congenital myopathy); and ptosis (congenital myopathic disorders, myasthenia gravis). The muscles should be carefully inspected. In congenital fiber-type disproportion and in Werdnig-Hoffmann disease, atrophy is a common finding, whereas pseudohypertrophy of calf muscles may be noted in Duchenne pseudohypertrophic muscular dystrophy.

The examiner should also note that the deep tendon reflexes are normal or increased in cerebral conditions, normal or diminished in muscle disorders, and always diminished or absent in anterior horn cell disorders and polyneuropathy. The clinician should also elicit Gowers' sign, which is usually diagnostic of Duchenne pseudohypertrophic muscular dystrophy or in neurogenic myopathies such as spinal muscular atrophy.

A thorough clinical examination will also offer clues to other conditions that produce hypotonia such as in Down syndrome, Prader-Willi syndrome, Lowe's syndrome, arachnodactyly, Ehlers-Danlos syndrome, renal tubular acidosis,

Riley-Day syndrome, Leigh disease, giant axonal neuropathy, and leukodystrophies.

There are some children who show minor anomalies, moderate hypotonia, and gross motor delay in whom it may be difficult to arrive at a specific diagnosis. Some of these children may go on to exhibit gross and fine motor immaturities, speech and language dysfunction, and learning disabilities.

Laboratory Tests

If the patient's history and physical findings suggest a cerebral cause, investigations such as a computed tomographic brain scan, magnetic resonance imaging, electroencephalogram, and chromosomal analysis may be useful. Magnetic resonance imaging alters the advantage of showing structural anomalies and disorders of myelination, both of which may be seen in infants with cerebral hypotonia. If a systemic metabolic cause is suspected, appropriate studies should be ordered, such as thyroid screening, amino and organic acid screening, and determination of lactate, pyruvate, carnitine, serum electrolytes, and arterial ammonia levels.

If the clinical examination suggests a lower motor neuron disorder, the following studies may be useful.

Cerebrospinal Fluid. A lumbar puncture is indicated in postinfectious polyneuropathy. The cerebrospinal fluid protein level is usually elevated, and there is no significant leukocytosis.

Serum Muscle Enzymes. The most frequently elevated muscle enzymes in muscle diseases are creatine phosphokinase (CPK), aldolase, and aspartate aminotransferase (SGOT). The CPK value is not elevated in all muscle disorders; thus, normal values are likely in myotonic dystrophy and in most congenital myopathies. CPK is typically high in Duchenne pseudohypertrophic muscular dystrophy. Determination of enzyme levels is not useful in other lower motor neuron disorders. Determination of aldolase is comparable to that of CPK in its usefulness.

Nerve Conduction Velocity. An estimation of nerve conduction velocity (NCV) is a valuable test to investigate the disorders of peripheral nerves. The ulnar and peroneal nerves are commonly studied. The NCV is abnormal in both acquired and congenital polyneuropathies associated with demyelination or failure of myelination. The NCV is normal in disorders of muscles and in the early stages of disorders of anterior horn cells.

Electromyography. The use of electromyography (EMG) provides valuable information about the electrical activity of muscle at every level of the motor unit. The test thus helps to localize the lesion at the anterior horn cells, peripheral nerves, axons, and the muscle fibers. Typically, EMG is useful in Werdnig-Hoffmann disease, polyneuropathy, myopathies, muscular dystrophy (especially Duchenne), and myotonic dystrophy. The typical EMG finding in myotonic dystrophy ("dive bomber" sound) is not commonly noted in infancy, although this is typical in the adult with myotonic dystrophy. However, an EMG study may not always result in a conclusive diagnosis.

Muscle Biopsy. An examination of a biopsied muscle is the most definitive test in the evaluation of the floppy infant with a suspected lower motor neuron disorder. Besides the usefulness in establishing the diagnosis, this test helps in the determination of prognosis and in genetic counseling. Since there are difficulties in the interpretation of neonatal muscle biopsies, we recommend that a biopsy be performed *after* the age of 2 months unless there is an emergent situation. Muscle biopsies are used to study the histology, histochemistry, and electron microscopy. The muscle biopsy is typically useful in the diagnosis of Werdnig-Hoffmann disease, congenital structural and metabolic mitochondrial myopathies, muscular dystrophy, fiber-type disproportion, and polyneuropathy. It is obviously not useful in the upper motor neuron disorders.

Miscellaneous Tests. When myasthenia gravis is suspected, edrophonium (Tensilon) or neostigmine (Prostigmin) tests should be performed. Urine and white blood cell lysosomal enzyme assays are useful in suspected cases of Pompe's disease and lipid storage disorders. Blood and cerebrospinal fluid lactate and pyruvate levels are important in the evaluation of mitochondrial encephalomyopathies. Both EMG and stool culture for Clostridia are diagnostic in infantile botulism. Appropriate blood studies will be indicated in infants with suspected peroxisomal disorders. Technologic advances in high-resolution banding have been very useful in the detection of chromosomal deletions including Prader-Willi syndrome. Skin biopsy for fibroblast cultures to determine the lysosomal enzymes is useful in the diagnosis of lysosomal storage disorders (e.g., ceroid lipofuscinosis).

MANAGEMENT

It is essential that the physician determines if the condition is static or progressive. This will enable the physician to discuss with the parents the diagnosis, their concerns, and the prognosis. Parental support is essential because there will usually not be a specific treatment available. The help of allied professionals such as social workers and nurse practitioners will be particularly useful for the parents to vent their feelings, anxiety, and depression. These professionals should be readily accessible for the parents to provide ongoing support and counseling, especially in the early stages.

Unfortunately, many conditions are not amenable to drug treatment. The use of biotin, vitamin E, zinc, and drugs such as quinidine and phenytoin has not been promising.

The children should be enrolled in a comprehensive rehabilitation program that will include physical, occupational, and speech therapists. Enrollment in the early stages often enables these children to enhance their maximal developmental potential. Furthermore, it helps the parents deal with the situation and also provides appropriate long-term planning for special educational needs in many of these children. The role of other professionals such as physical therapists, occupational therapists, and orthopedists cannot be underestimated in the care of these youngsters, especially on a long-term basis. Those patients with specific neuromuscular muscle diseases may be referred to the local chapter of the Muscular Dystrophy Foundation, which provides parental support groups, financial assistance, and other forms of aid for the long-term care of these children. Finally, genetic counseling is indicated when a genetically transmitted disorder (e.g., myotonic dystrophy, Duchenne pseudohypertrophic muscular dystrophy) is diagnosed. Continuing and rapid advances in molecular genetics using DNA analyses make it possible to investigate presymptomatic cases, detect carriers, and make a prenatal diagnosis in certain specific disorders (e.g. myotonic dystrophy, Duchenne pseudohypertrophic muscular dystrophy, Werdnig-Hoffmann disease). These studies will become increasingly important in genetic counseling.

INDICATIONS FOR REFERRAL AND ADMISSION

Any infant whose condition is severe or rapidly progressive should be referred for a neurologic evaluation. If the condition is not rapidly progressive, then there is a need for at least a one-time neurologic consultation to help determine the etiology. In most instances, the work-up can be performed on an outpatient basis (e.g., muscle enzymes, nerve conduction studies, EMG, and computed tomography). However, if a muscle biopsy is necessary or if the patient's health is declining rapidly, a brief hospitalization may be necessary to complete the work-up.

ANNOTATED BIBLIOGRAPHY

DiMauro S, Bonilla E, Zeviani M et al: Mitochondrial myopathies. Ann Neurol 17:521–538, 1985. (Current review of mitochondrial myopathies; excellent reference source.)

Dubowitz V: The Floppy Infant. London, Spastics International Medical Publications and Heinemann Medical Books, 1975. (Excellent monograph on floppy infants.)

Gamstrop I: Nondystrophic myopathies with onset in infancy and childhood. Acta Pediatr Scand 71:801–886, 1982. (Description of myopathic disorders.)

Gamstrop I, Sarnat HB: Progressive Spinal Muscular Atrophies. New York, Raven Press, 1984. (Textbook discussing the entire spectrum of spinal muscular atrophy.)

Hanson PA: Myotonic dystrophy and infancy and childhood. Pediatr Ann 13:123–127, 1984. (Good review of this condition.)

Parker RJ, Brown MJ, Berman PM: The diagnostic value of EMG in infantile hypotonia. Am J Dis Child 136:1057–1059, 1982. (Discusses the value of electromyography.)

Swaiman KF: Pediatric Neurology: Principles and Practice, vol II. St. Louis, CV Mosby, 1989. (Excellent reference on neuromuscular diseases in infancy.)

Zellweger H: The floppy infant: A practical approach. Helv Paediatr Acta 38:301–306, 1983. (Current review on the clinical approach to this problem.)

147
Muscle Weakness

Charles N. Swisher

Since weakness is a common sign of systemic disease, a careful evaluation of other systems should be undertaken before the focus narrows to the neuromuscular examination. Weakness can be either local or generalized and, depending on the location of the lesion, hypotonia rather than weakness may result. One should distinguish between muscle weakness, hypotonia, and myotonia. Muscle weakness refers to a reduction of motor power. Hypotonia refers to a reduction of muscle tone and is discussed extensively in Chapter 146. Myotonia refers to the infrequent occurrence of a pattern of sustained muscle contraction with slow relaxation that clinically presents as "stiffness" relieved by exercise. The primary emphasis of this chapter is on neuromuscular diagnosis based on the concept of the *motor unit,* which consists of the anterior horn cell, motor root, peripheral nerve, neuromuscular junction, and muscle fiber itself.

PATHOPHYSIOLOGY

The etiology of weakness from systemic causes other than the neuromuscular system can be any combination of infectious, metabolic, and immunologic components that results in a general pattern of debility. Several hereditary, infectious, toxic, immunologic, and metabolic conditions can act on individual components of the motor unit, resulting in characteristic clinical and electrophysiologic (and in some cases biochemical) findings. For example, the anterior horn cell can be affected either by a hereditary predisposition to cell loss such as Werdnig-Hoffmann disease or acquired infections such as poliomyelitis or coxsackievirus. The motor root can be affected by a postinfectious immunologic process such as Guillain-Barré disease.

The lower motor neuron may be involved alone in traumatic injury and toxic neuropathy and is consistently involved in some of the progressive degenerations of the central nervous system. In the demyelinating leukodystrophies such as metachromatic leukodystrophy and Krabbe's disease, there is involvement of the peripheral nerve and slowing of the nerve conduction velocity.

CLINICAL PRESENTATION AND DIFFERENTIAL DIAGNOSIS

The clinical presentations of muscle weakness are discussed together with a differential diagnosis.

Anterior horn cell disease may be produced by various conditions. Spinal muscular atrophy refers to hereditary muscle atrophy and weakness associated with degeneration of the anterior horn cells of the spinal cord. Involvement varies from severe to mild. Various forms of anterior horn cell involvement also have a different chronologic presentation. The most severe form (*Werdnig-Hoffmann disease*) has an early onset, either in utero (reduced or absent fetal movements) or within the first 2 to 3 months of life. Owing to respiratory failure, survival is rare after 1 year of age. The intermediate form usually presents after the first 6 months of life, and respiratory difficulty is later and milder, with survival to adolescence or adulthood. The mild form, *Kugelberg-Welander disease,* presents with a mild weakness after the child has begun to walk. The weakness is located primarily in the pelvic girdle, resulting in difficulty climbing stairs and limited exercise tolerance.

Lesions affecting the motor root that produce muscle weakness are predominantly acquired. The most frequent example is *Guillain-Barré disease,* in which a previously healthy child presents with an ascending pattern of progressive weakness and areflexia. The condition that usually appears a few days after a minor infection may have an associated mild sensory disturbance, such as back pain, dysesthesias, and diminished sensation.

Although focal muscle weakness can result from traumatic motor root and peripheral nerve injury such as in *Erb-Duchenne palsy* after a brachial plexus injury, some peripheral nerve lesions in childhood have a hereditary basis such as *Charcot-Marie-Tooth disease* and *Déjérine-Sottas disease.*

Disorders of the neuromuscular junction producing weakness are immunologic or toxic. Immunologic disorders include the various *myasthenic syndromes,* including infants of myasthenic mothers and congenital and childhood-onset myasthenia. Infants of myasthenic mothers occasionally have a transient pattern of hypotonia and weakness resulting from transplacental passage of maternal antibodies that is responsive to neostigmine (Prostigmin) or pyridostigmine (Mestinon) and resolves in a few days. The congenital and childhood-onset forms are of long standing and require ongoing treatment with neostigmine or pyridostigmine. The classic toxin affecting the neuromuscular junction is *botulism,* which is associated with both palatal paralysis and nasal speech, as well as diffuse weakness and hypotonia in the older child and descending weakness, constipation, and sometimes dysautonomia in *infantile botulism.*

Primary muscle disease may be congenital or acquired. Congenital muscle disease may be either a myopathy, with abnormal muscle fibers, or a muscular dystrophy, with progressive degeneration of skeletal muscle fibers. *Congenital muscular dystrophy,* in contrast to later developing forms, is most active in early postnatal life but tends to stabilize rather than progressively deteriorate as the patient ages. One cannot clinically distinguish between the various congenital myopathies because they tend to present in a similar pattern of early hypotonia and weakness. Such weakness may be predominantly of a limb girdle pattern or may be more generalized. Electrophysiologic studies are helpful, but an appropriate diagnosis requires a muscle biopsy with histochemical studies.

The most common form of dystrophy is the *Duchenne type,* which involves the pelvic girdle; this type is severe and progressive with death late in the second or early third decade of life. The onset of weakness is noted usually between the ages of 2 and 4, and it may be associated with a learning disability or mild retardation. Characteristically, there is a pseudohypertrophy of the calves, with dystrophic calf muscle replaced with fat tissue. A later-onset dystrophy, similar in clinical appearance to Duchenne but milder in degree, is *Becker's dystrophy.* Children with Becker's dystrophy remain ambulatory after 16 years of age, in contrast to children with Duchenne dystrophy who are nonambulatory at that age. Both Duchenne and Becker's dystrophies are inherited in an X-linked recessive manner but differ on the basis of muscle dystrophin. Carrier females may be detected by serum creatine phosphokinase evaluations, although the CPK level tends to drop with age. An autosomal dominant form of dystrophy is *myotonic dystrophy,* which is characterized by a slow progression, distal weakness and wasting, a variable degree of weakness, low IQ scores, joint contractures, and respiratory difficulties in infancy. An examination of other family members is helpful because the disease is frequently more striking in the adult than the child. Rarer muscular dystrophies are *limb girdle dystrophy,* which is often inherited in an autosomal recessive manner, and *facioscapulohumeral dystrophy,* which is inherited in an autosomal dominant fashion. Both conditions are relatively mild with a slow progression and presentation in adolescence or adult life.

One confusing and difficult area in the pathophysiology of weakness is the group of *periodic paralyses,* which are characterized by attacks of weakness and hypotonia, with a pattern of remission and relapse. A family history is important because these conditions are largely inherited in an autosomal dominant form. Hyperkalemic and hypokalemic forms exist as well as a normokalemic variety.

Muscle weakness can be associated with various endocrine and metabolic disorders. These disorders are important to identify because specific treatments are often available. *Hyperthyroidism* can lead to a constant or a periodic pattern of muscle weakness, or myasthenia. *Hypothyroidism* can be associated with a slowness of movement as well as easy fatigability, which is frequently associated with mental depression. *Cushing's syndrome* is associated with a weakness of the lower limbs. More commonly, muscle weakness can occur as a result of corticosteroid therapy, and this factor may complicate the diagnosis in the case of corticosteroid-treated dermatomyositis, in which the primary weakness is prominent. *Malnutrition* may result not only in weakness but also in associated hypotonia and hyporeflexia. Other rare causes of muscle weakness include the glycogenoses and carnitine deficiency. Carnitine deficiency is characterized by congestive heart failure, weakness, and hypotonia.

Inflammation can lead to muscle weakness either as a connective tissue disorder, such as dermatomyositis, or as a myositis due to bacterial, viral, or parasitic involvement. Viral infection (particularly coxsackievirus infection) has been implicated in polymyositis. In sarcoidosis there is frequently an involvement of muscle with either localized or general weakness. Rarely, trichinosis may produce weakness and pain and should be suspected in children with eosinophilia and a history of eating undercooked pork.

WORK-UP

History

The history is important in the evaluation of a child with muscle weakness. The physician should inquire if the weakness is proximal or distal, localized or generalized, lifelong or recent, continuous or episodic, or related to activity patterns. A family history is of particular interest in a child with apparent congenital weakness or a pattern of weakness of insidious onset. Was there exposure to infectious agents or toxins? A past history of systemic illness, malnutrition, a change in foods for an infant, and constipation or other contributing causes to weakness should be noted. The physician should also inquire about other or related symptoms of muscle disorder in childhood such as a delay in motor milestones, an abnormal gait, a tendency to fall, hypotonia, or muscle cramps. An inability to run or jump in a young child after the age of 3 may indicate a significant muscle weakness.

Physical Examination

The physical examination is best assessed both informally and formally. In a play setting, the child can frequently be observed to demonstrate details of gait and posture that may be inhibited in the examining room. Play activity such as handling and reaching for small toys can illustrate the presence or absence of weakness and may help to localize the pattern. The physician should test for gross motor milestones of the child. Jumping should be accomplished by 3 years of age and hopping on one foot by 4 or 5 years of age. *Gowers' sign*, in which the child compensates for weak pelvic girdle muscles with relatively stronger distal upper extremity muscles by "climbing up himself" with the hands

while attempting to move from prone to standing, is characteristic of proximal muscle disease.

Additional observations to make during the physical examination are the presence of muscle enlargement or wasting, the presence and degree of deep tendon reflexes, and a tightening of the heel cords, which may be noted in muscular dystrophies, as contrasted to the "dropfoot" of the child with a peripheral neuropathy. Associated problems such as scoliosis and respiratory difficulties with a characteristic "bell-shaped" chest should also be noted. Joint contractures can occur in children who have not been ambulatory for a long time. Erythematous skin lesions involving the extensor surfaces of joints, particularly those of the fingers, are frequently seen in dermatomyositis and should be noted.

Laboratory Tests

Initial laboratory studies should complement the history and physical examination to eliminate systemic causes of weakness such as dehydration, infection, or malnutrition. These tests might include blood and urine electrolyte studies, thyroid studies, blood glucose and ammonia determinations, and blood and urine cultures. The cerebrospinal fluid may show the typical albuminocytologic dissociation (i.e., few cells and elevated protein) in patients with Guillain-Barré syndrome. In rare cases, specific biochemical studies may be definitive in degenerative disorders with weakness and a known biochemical abnormality such as the deficient urinary aryl sulfatase in metachromatic leukodystrophy; deficient leukocyte enzymes in the glycogenoses; and elevated lactate and pyruvate levels in blood and cerebrospinal fluid in mitochondrial myopathies. Neuromuscular disorders should be pursued once various systemic causes have been eliminated. The three primary investigations in this area are serum enzyme determination, electrophysiologic studies, and a muscle biopsy. The serum enzyme (aspartate aminotransferase, creatine phosphokinase, and aldolase) levels are elevated when muscular dystrophy is present and may, in the case of Duchenne pseudohypertrophic muscular dystrophy, precede the observation of weakness by many months. However, children who have had recent bruises, intramuscular medication, or vigorous exercise may also have elevated creatine phosphokinase values. Isolated elevated creatine phosphokinase levels may alert the physician to potential malignant hyperthermia. Recent developments in the basic sciences have made possible more precise diagnosis of the muscular dystrophies. The abnormal dystrophin gene that results in Duchenne or Becker's dystrophy has been isolated, and a quantitative study of the dystrophin gene in muscle biopsies of suspected affected patients is available. After this initial muscle biopsy is performed, linkage analysis and DNA testing can be done on peripheral leukocytes of suspected carriers.

Electrophysiologic studies to determine the cause of muscle weakness include electromyography (EMG) and nerve conduction studies. EMG studies are best performed in subjects who voluntarily contract their muscles; these studies may be equivocal in young children. Stool samples should be collected for assay of botulinum toxin in infants before proceeding to a muscle biopsy. Nerve conduction studies are valuable in differentiating between neuropathic and myopathic weaknesses.

A muscle biopsy can be valuable in determining the etiology of muscle weakness, but it must be carefully planned in regard to biopsy technique and tissue study. A segment of muscle is removed parallel to the muscle fibers and is frozen for a histologic study while separate samples are fixed for electron microscopy. Dystrophin is analyzed when Duchenne and Becker's dystrophies are considered. In 99% of the cases, boys with Duchenne dystrophy have no dystrophin while children with Becker's dystrophy have abnormal dystrophin. Several stains are done routinely on every muscle biopsy and, when taken together, can provide information not only of morphologic features but also of individual fiber types and specialized structural and biochemical features.

MANAGEMENT

The treatment of muscle weakness resulting from systemic illness is the treatment of the underlying disease or deficiency. Dehydrated and malnourished children who are unable to lift their heads or raise to a sitting position can make rapid and dramatic improvement with treatment. Infants with botulism require antibiotics and supportive care, including ventilatory monitoring and assistance. Use of intravenous gamma globulin has shown promising results in children with Guillain-Barré syndrome and is an effective alternative to plasmapheresis. Children with myasthenia placed on neostigmine or children with dermatomyositis placed on corticosteroids can demonstrate gratifying recovery.

L-Carnitine is a natural substance that transports fatty acids into mitochondria and is now available for oral treatment of systemic carnitine deficiency. Although primary carnitine deficiency is rare, secondary deficiency occurs in nutritional states. (L-Carnitine administration may also reverse occasional side effects of valproate administration such as drowsiness.) Plasma and urine carnitine levels can be obtained to evaluate the child with unexplained hypotonia or weakness.

The treatment of many children with myopathies, neuropathies, and muscular dystrophies in ambulatory pediatric practice requires an organized team approach, with the pediatrician often serving as the advocate for the child. An accurate assessment of the current degree of motor weakness and functional disability allows efforts to be made by an interdisciplinary team of physiatrists, physical therapists, orthotists, educators, and social workers to plan for the most appropriate home and school environment for the child. For the ambulatory child, polypropylene braces and home equipment such as bathtub chairs and special handholds installed at critical areas (e.g., stairs) around the house are invaluable. A school bus taking the child to classes and a school located on one level with reasonably short distances between classes is important. Ongoing physical therapy is mandatory, serving a dual purpose of monitoring home exercises and assessing the current level of motor function. For the nonambulatory child, appropriate wheelchairs need to be provided and further transportation issues need to be resolved. Occupational therapy is an additional modality to help maximize independence in activities of daily living.

Just as a systemic disease can cause muscle weakness, a chronic muscle disease can cause problems in other systems. These problems need to be addressed directly as part of a therapeutic plan. Respiratory deficits are a major problem in a variety of chronic muscle disorders and result in pneumonia, which is the cause of death in most children with Duchenne muscular dystrophy and Werdnig-Hoffmann disease. Intercostal and diaphragmatic muscle weaknesses are also problems in many other forms of myopathy and need to be managed with prompt treatment of upper respiratory tract infections, good respiratory toilet with suctioning, provision of adequate humidity, and postural drainage when appropriate. A difficult medical-ethical problem relates to the use of a respirator in children with chronic respiratory insufficiency resulting from motor neuron or primary muscle disease. It is best in these cases to talk with parents about the possible use or nonuse of artificial ventilation prior to the development of a crisis.

Orthopedic problems commonly accompany chronic muscle weakness and result in progressive scoliosis, heel cord shortening, and other joint contractures. Early and periodic consultation with a pediatric orthopedic surgeon can add years of ambulation to a child with muscular dystrophy and may preserve a similar function for prolonged periods of time for other children with neuromuscular disability.

Although the management of many congenital myopathies and dystrophies is similar, an accurate diagnosis of a neuromuscular condition is an essential prerequisite to genetic counseling. The aid of clinical geneticists should be sought whenever one is dealing with chronic familial conditions of variable or uncertain outcome, because casual or incomplete genetic counseling may lead to planned pregnancies resulting in lifelong unanticipated disability.

INDICATIONS FOR REFERRAL OR ADMISSION

There has been a proliferation of sophisticated electrophysiologic devices in outpatient settings and community hospitals. Since neuromuscular disease in childhood is complex, it is imperative that muscle biopsies on children be performed by laboratories skilled in this procedure and using the complex histochemical and electron microscopy available for their interpretation. EMG studies should likewise be performed by those persons who have considerable experience in the EMG evaluation of children.

Hospitalization for children who have an acute onset of weakness is mandatory in a facility where close attention can be paid to respiratory status and appropriate action taken in case of respiratory decompensation, often seen in Guillain-Barré disease or infantile botulism. Acute respiratory decompensation is also common in children with pre-existing muscle disease who initially have a mild upper respiratory tract infection. Therefore, children with a known myopathy should be hospitalized for observation whenever such an infection produces a deterioration in respiratory function. Hospitalization is indicated for those children with weakness of unknown etiology, which may be related to dermatomyositis or a metabolic or degenerative condition requiring further investigation and initial inpatient management. Hospitalization is also indicated for surgical procedures used in the management of chronic myopathic or neuropathic conditions such as heel-cord lengthening.

ANNOTATED BIBLIOGRAPHY

Breningstall GN: Carnitine deficiency syndromes. Pediatr Neurol 6:75–81, 1990. (Lucid review on a difficult topic.)

Brooke MH: A Clinician's View of Neuromuscular Diseases. Baltimore, Williams & Wilkins, 1986. (Comprehensive review of muscle disorders of children with excellent illustrations.)

Downey JA, Low N (eds): The Child with Disabling Illness. Philadelphia, WB Saunders, 1974. (Practical management suggestions and discussion of pathophysiology, especially Chapter 11 on diseases of muscle.)

Dubowitz V: The Floppy Infant, 2nd ed. Philadelphia, JB Lippincott, 1980. (Primarily a discussion of hypotonia, with many good observations on the evaluation of weakness.)

Dubowitz V: Muscle Disorders in Childhood. Philadelphia, WB Saunders, 1978. (Classic reference on muscle disorders affecting motor function.)

Edward RH, Wiles CM, Mills KR: Quantitation of muscle contraction and strength. In Dyck PJ, et al (eds): Peripheral Neuropathy, chap 48. Philadelphia, WB Saunders, 1984. (Exhaustive survey of neuropathic weakness and its clinical syndromes; see especially the chapter on quantitation of muscle contraction and strength.)

Hoffman EP et al: Dystrophin in human muscle biopsy specimens. N Engl J Med 318:1363–1368, 1988. (Classic article on recent diagnostic techniques.)

Menkes JH: Textbook of Neurology, 4th ed, chap 13. Philadelphia, Lea & Febiger, 1990. (Clinically oriented with extensive bibliography of recent literature on diseases of the motor unit.)

Schreiner MS, Freld E, Ruddy R: Infant botulism: A review of 12 years' experience at the Children's Hospital of Philadelphia. Pediatrics 87:159–165, 1991. (Excellent clinical summary with epidemiologic background.)

Shahar E, Murphy EG, Roifman CM: Benefit of intravenously administered immune serum globulin in patients with Guillain-Barré syndrome. J Pediatr 116:141–144, 1990. (Discusses benefits of IV γ-globulin versus plasmapheresis in the treatment of three pediatric patients with GBS.)

Vinken PJ, Bruyn GW (eds): Handbook of Clinical Neurology, Vols 40 and 41, Diseases of Muscle. New York, Elsevier, 1979. (Exhaustive survey of clinical presentation and pathophysiology of muscle disease.)

148
Microcephaly
Elizabeth C. Dooling

Microcephaly, or small head size, refers to a head circumference that is smaller than 2 standard deviations below the 50th percentile for the child's age. It may be classified as primary or secondary microcephaly. *Primary microcephaly,* sometimes called *microcephaly vera* or *microcrania,* may be inherited on an autosomal dominant or recessive basis, or it may occur sporadically. *Secondary microcephaly* results from trauma, vascular insults, or infections to the brain that occur later in gestation to an already well-formed brain.

PATHOPHYSIOLOGY

The brain begins as a vesicular structure with large germinal centers that are composed of neuroblasts that migrate to the cortex by means of "guiding" radial fibers in two waves of migration: (1) between 6 and 12 weeks and (2) between 16 and 24 weeks. By the end of the second trimester the normal cortical laminar pattern has been completed and primary fissuration of the brain has occurred. The developing brain is sensitive to various neurocytotoxic agents, including radiation, alkylating agents, alcohol, tobacco, aminoacidurias (e.g., phenylketonuria), and certain viruses. Infants of mothers with diabetes and uremia may have microcephaly. A large cerebral growth spurt normally occurs after the 26th week of gestation. Secondary fissures and gyri can be recognized. The germinal matrix regresses and astrocytes, both reactive and myelinative, appear.

Primary microcephaly will result if there is a primary failure or interruption of neuronal migration. Other organs, such as the eye, that are growing and developing concurrently may be abnormal. Multiple craniofacial and somatic anomalies are also present in children with chromosomal disorders. Children who have familial microcephaly may not have associated dysmorphic features. When the infant is subjected to an intrauterine infection (viral or bacterial), ischemia, hemorrhage, or hypoxia in the late third trimester or is asphyxiated at or shortly after birth, secondary microcephaly may develop.

Clinical Presentation

The infant with primary microcephaly has an obviously small head size at birth. The head circumference is less than or equal to 31 cm in a full-term infant, while weight and length may be appropriate for the gestational age. The palpebral fissures are also short. There is a flattening of the posterior aspect of the head with underdevelopment of the normal parieto-occipital fullness. The forehead is broad and sloping. The eyes are prominent and may look froglike. The facial features may be coarse. The ears are often posteriorly rotated. Other somatic anomalies may be readily recognized. The older child is usually also distinctive in appearance because of the small head size in proportion to a more normally developed body, although the overall stature may be small, giving him or her a dwarflike appearance. The child is often hyperactive and easily distractible, and he or she may have a seizure disorder.

The infant with secondary microcephaly has a normal head circumference at birth as well as an appropriate body weight and length and normal length of palpebral fissures. As the child grows older, the slow rate of head growth becomes apparent. As the child's head circumference deviates farther from the normal curve for age, the head size sometimes conforms to the child's own percentile, over years. At other times it plateaus after 12 to 18 months of age. Developmental delay occurs and may be associated with spastic paraparesis, hemiparesis, or quadriparesis as well as sensory deficits, including blindness and deafness.

DIFFERENTIAL DIAGNOSIS

Primary microcephaly can usually be differentiated from secondary microcephaly on the basis of the prenatal and birth histories and the head circumference of the infant at birth. (See the display on causes of microcephaly.)

WORK-UP

History

The gestational history must be carefully reviewed to assess the occurrence of any teratogenic exposure (e.g., alcohol, drug, and tobacco abuse, anticonvulsants, and retinoic acid), exposure to radiation, and infections in the first and second trimesters. Prenatal records should be reviewed in the event that the mother is unable to recall minor points that may be contributory. The family history should also be reviewed in depth to ascertain the range of head sizes, and, more importantly, the incidence of other affected children. The birth records should be reviewed critically to determine whether a hemorrhage, a period of hypoxic ischemia, or sepsis occurred.

Physical Examination

The head circumference should be carefully measured with a metal or nonstretching cloth tape. The size of the anterior

Some Causes of Microcephaly

PRIMARY

Familial
  "Benign" associated with normal physiognomy and intelligence
  Associated with inferior intelligence ± seizures ± hyperactivity
Inductive-migrational disorders
  Agyria
  Pachygyria
  Microgyria
  Polymicrogyria
  Lissencephaly
  Agenesis of the corpus callosum
  Schizencephaly
  Chromosomal disorders (trisomies, rings, deletions, Prader-Willi syndrome, lissencephaly)
  Nonchromosomal disorders (Smith-Lemli-Opitz, Cornelia de Lange, Hallermann-Streiff, and Rubinstein-Taybi syndromes)
Toxic-metabolic
  Radiation
  Alkylating agents
  Alcohol
  Illicit drugs
  Tobacco
Infectious
  Rubella
  Mumps
  Cytomegalovirus
  Toxoplasmosis
  Syphilis
  Herpes simplex, types 1 and 2
  Listeriosis
  Human immunodeficiency virus

SECONDARY

Vascular (asphyxia, placental separation, or septic shock) resulting in:
  Porencephaly
  Hydranencephaly
  Cystic encephalomalacia
  Laminar necrosis
Metabolic (maternal uremia or diabetes)

fontanelle and eyes should be noted. The sutures should be palpated to assess their overlapping. The infant should be examined for major and minor anomalies that would suggest a chromosomal disorder or classified syndrome. Localized, discrete, or generalized vesicular eruptions, generalized petechiae, hepatosplenomegaly, jaundice, and other evidence of active viral infection should be evaluated.

Laboratory Tests

Vesicular lesions, cerebrospinal fluid, urine, stool, and throat washings should be cultured for virus in nonasphyxiated infants. TORCH titers should be drawn on the mother and infant. IgM titers of the infant should also be obtained. Human immunodeficiency virus testing may be appropriate in certain cases. Chromosomes should be checked if there are associated somatic anomalies. Roentgenograms of the skull may show early fusion of the sutures caused by a failure of growth of the underlying cerebral tissue. Computed tomographic scans are sensitive in detecting small areas of periventricular or intraparenchymal calcification as sequelae of an intrauterine infection. Magnetic resonance imaging shows heterotopias and other evidence of cerebral dysgenesis.

MANAGEMENT AND REFERRAL

If the family history is clearly supportive of a familial etiology, an otherwise entirely healthy child is likely to develop and perform like other family members. Reassurance may be sufficient in such cases. If, however, the infant has microcephaly of a sporadic type, deficient intelligence may be present. Martin and Sells have found that approximately 7.5% of children with the sporadic type of microcephaly have normal intelligence. Sporadic cases of microcephaly should be referred to a geneticist after the basic evaluations have been completed. (For the management of microcephaly from craniosynostosis, see Chap. 149.)

ANNOTATED BIBLIOGRAPHY

Caffey J: Pediatric X-ray Diagnosis. Chicago, Year Book Medical Publishers, 1961. (Good basic introduction to normal and abnormal growth of the skull.)

Menkes JH: Textbook of Child Neurology, 4th ed, pp 188–208. Philadelphia, Lea & Febiger, 1990. (Well-referenced chapter on chromosomal disorders.)

Swaiman KF: Pediatric Neurology, pp 343–345. St. Louis, CV Mosby, 1989. (Excellent textbook presenting a comprehensive tabulation of common and uncommon causes of abnormal head growth.)

149

Craniosynostosis

Brooke Swearingen and Paul H. Chapman

Abnormalities of skull shape are medically, socially, and cosmetically important. In modern pediatric practice, consideration of the diagnosis often arises from parental concern over the cosmetic deformity. The relationship among multiple sutural fusion, intracranial hypertension, and developmental delay is important although often misunderstood.

The classification of the craniosynostoses (premature closure of the suture[s]) can be based on the skull shape or on the suture fused (Fig. 149-1). *Scaphocephaly or dolichocephaly* refers to a narrow, elongated skull that is associated with fusion of the sagittal suture. *Trigonocephaly* is a nar-

row forehead with hypotelorism and a median supraglabellar ridge occurring with fusion of the metopic suture. Fusion of the coronal sutures bilaterally results in *brachycephaly,* which refers to a broad skull with a high forehead. The term *oxycephaly* has been used to describe the high conically shaped head resulting from coronal with sagittal or lambdoidal synostosis. *Plagiocephaly* refers to an asymmetric skull with a sloped occiput or forehead resulting from unilateral lambdoid or coronal fusion. The cloverleaf skull (or *Kleeblattschade*) may arise from multiple fusions involving the coronal, sagittal, and lambdoid sutures. Complex genetic syndromes (e.g., Crouzon's or Apert's syndromes) may involve multiple premature synostoses and also other facial and skeletal abnormalities.

PATHOPHYSIOLOGY

The factors involved in skull morphogenesis are poorly understood and involve an interaction between the brain, dura, skull base, and the developing calvaria. Sutures form over dural reflections connecting the basicranium and calvaria, which in turn reflect the underlying form of the brain. The sagittal and metopic sutures overlie the falx cerebri; the coronal suture overlies the dural reflection originating at the sphenoid wing; and the lambdoid suture overlies the transverse sinus and the tentorium cerebelli. Ossification centers form in central zones delineated by these reflective bands between 12 and 16 weeks' gestation. Bone forming activity normally halts at the reflective bands, where a suture then forms. Any underlying abnormality of the brain that has altered the normal pattern of dural reflection should also alter the pattern of suture formation. This has been found to occur in some cases of holoprosencephaly, craniopagus, and dicephaly. Premature fusion of sutures arises, according to one theory, when changes in the skull base alter the pattern of dural reflection. Others have emphasized the influence of local factors, with changes in the skull base as a secondary phenomenon. Sutures can be experimentally fused by transplanting the periosteum or by applying cyanoacrylate. Reports in the literature suggest that intrauterine head constraint may be contributory in isolated cases. It is interesting to note, however, that artificial skull binding, as practiced by some primitive tribes, produces skull shape abnormalities without premature synostosis.

Finally, the craniosynostoses may occur as a result of a generalized metabolic abnormality, such as rickets and hyperthyroidism.

CLINICAL PRESENTATION

Since craniosynostosis occurs during infancy, the abnormality is most often evident on inspection by the parent or pediatrician. Single fusions are usually asymptomatic. Complex multiple fusions have been associated with headaches, visual loss, and retardation. The incidence of headache varies with the age of the child and the number of

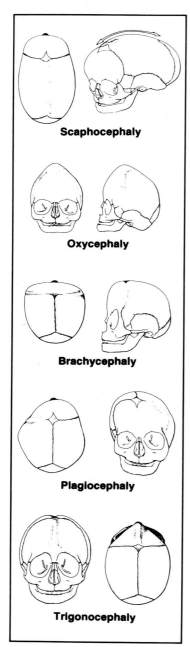

Scaphocephaly

Oxycephaly

Brachycephaly

Plagiocephaly

Trigonocephaly

Figure 149-1. The classification of the craniosynostoses based on skull shape. (Courtesy of the BNI Quarterly II[1]:30, 1986)

sutures fused; it is most common in the older child with multiple synostoses. A loss of vision, although rare, requires further evaluation. The incidence of papilledema is 20% to 40% in those children with multiple fusions. The case for craniosynostosis as a cause of retardation is difficult to prove, but a higher incidence of retardation is apparent in those children who have multiple synostoses. This is more

commonly seen with the complex deformities and only rarely with a single fusion.

DIFFERENTIAL DIAGNOSIS

The differential diagnosis of an abnormal skull shape is not extensive, and the appearance of the simple synostoses is characteristic. Multiple fusions associated with a facial abnormality should prompt a consideration of the craniofacial syndromes (e.g., Crouzon's syndrome, Apert's syndrome) along with their other systemic abnormalities. When primary microcephaly produces synostosis, computed tomography may reveal an underlying loss of brain substance. Positional molding, either prenatally or postnatally, may appear identical to the true premature fusion. This is particularly true for the unilateral occipital flattening that is reminiscent of lambdoidal synostosis. These infants have sutures present radiographically, but they clearly have an abnormal head shape. The abnormality can usually be corrected simply by preventing the infant from sleeping on the defect.

WORK-UP

The diagnosis is made on the basis of a physical and radiographic examination. Historical details (e.g., the presence of a familial syndrome) may occasionally be important, but recognition of the characteristic appearance is essential. Palpation of the sutures in the infant may be useful, and synostosis is unlikely if the plates are clearly mobile. The entire length of the suture must be felt, because a short bony segment can prevent growth. A palpable bony ridge is often appreciated along the fused sagittal or metopic sutures. The fontanelle may provide an indication of elevated intracranial pressure. Papilledema, although usually seen only in cases of multiple fusions, is an important finding.

The most useful radiographic study is the plain skull roentgenogram. The sutures should be well demonstrated; this may require oblique views. The region of bony fusion will appear as a loss of normal suture lucency with perhaps an increased density. In cases of multiple fusions, the orbit and sphenoid wing may have a characteristic appearance. Computed tomography can be useful in cases of multiple fusion or when hydrocephalus is suspected, but it adds little to the evaluation of the simple fusions.

TREATMENT

The primary indication for surgery for a single synostosis is the desire for plastic reconstruction: the risk of developing intracranial hypertension or retardation in these children is minimal. The risk of intracranial hypertension is greater in cases of multiple suture fusion. The timing of surgery is important; better results are obtained when the surgery is performed at an early age because skull remolding takes advantage of a rapidly growing brain in infancy. A single synostosis is generally best corrected within the first few months of life. When there is a question of head molding rather than true synostosis (e.g., unilateral occipital flattening) the physician may wish to temporize while positioning measures are tried. Such decisions should generally be made in consultation with a pediatric neurosurgeon. The child's appearance may worsen as he or she grows, necessitating more complex procedures. Operating on a newborn is not necessary; deferring the procedure until the infant is 6 weeks of age allows for a larger blood volume and less anesthetic risk.

The surgical procedure currently performed involves an excision of the fused suture (strip craniectomy) sometimes with morcellation of the abnormally shaped bone. The correction of more complex fusions may involve the manipulation of a larger bone fragment such as supraorbital ridges. Surgical complications include the risk of excessive bleeding, a dural tear with resulting cerebrospinal fluid leak and a "growing skull defect," and the ongoing risks of infection and anesthesia. Postoperatively, the child needs to be observed closely for 1 to 2 days for a continued drop in hematocrit. Significant scalp and facial edema are common for 3 to 5 days.

INDICATIONS FOR REFERRAL

The craniosynostoses are often diagnosed by the pediatrician during the newborn or early infancy well-baby examinations. The parents should be informed that the deformity in simple fusions is primarily cosmetic and that the risk of intracranial hypertension is small. Reconstructive surgery can be performed at the appropriate time if the appearance is objectionable. Early neurosurgical referral is appropriate in any suspected case.

ANNOTATED BIBLIOGRAPHY

Davis CH, Alexander E, Kelly D: Treatment of craniosynostosis. J Neurosurg 30:630–636, 1969. (Description of surgical procedures for sagittal, coronal, and multiple synostosis.)

Mohr G, Hoffman H, Munro I et al: Surgical management of unilateral and bilateral coronal craniosynostosis: 21 years of experience. Neurosurgery 2:83–92, 1978. (Series of 116 patients presented from the Hospital for Sick Children, Toronto.)

Moss ML: Functional anatomy of cranial synostosis. Child Brain 1:22–33, 1975. (Describes a theory of the pathophysiology of craniosynostosis relating sutural fusion to changes in the skull base.)

Renier D, Saint-Rose C, Marchac D, Hirsch J: Intracranial pressure in craniostenosis. J Neurosurg 57:370–377, 1982. (Report of use of epidural sensor to monitor intracranial pressure in 92 cases of craniosynostosis: the intracranial pressure was found to be normal in one third, borderline in one third, and abnormal in one third, with elevations primarily in those cases of multiple fusions; a correlation was found between intracranial pressure and mental ability.)

Shillito J, Matson DD: Craniosynostosis: A review of 519 surgical patients. Pediatrics 41:829–853, 1968. (Review of the Boston Children's Hospital experience stressing the importance of early surgery.)

Whittle I, Johnston I, Besser M: Intracranial pressure changes in craniostenosis. Surg Neurol 21:367–372, 1984. (Proposal that continuous intracranial pressure monitoring be used as an adjunct to decide the indications for surgical therapy; of the 20 patients, 7 (35%) had associated hydrocephalus and 15 had multiple sutural fusions or complex deformities.)

150

Macrocephaly

Elizabeth C. Dooling

Macrocephaly, or large head size, refers to a head circumference that is greater than 2 standard deviations above the 50th percentile for the child's age. It may be classified as primary or secondary macrocephaly. *Primary macrocephaly,* sometimes called *macrocrania,* is often inherited on an autosomal dominant basis, and, less frequently, occurs sporadically. *Secondary macrocephaly* may arise from conditions that cause overgrowth of the cerebral tissues, such as space-occupying lesions, or obstruction of the cerebrospinal fluid (CSF) circulation.

PATHOPHYSIOLOGY

Most of the growth and differentiation of the skull occurs during the first and second years of life. Thus, most of the features of the adult skull are present by a child's second birthday. Growth of the skull is slowest from the second year to puberty, after which the velocity of growth increases for 1 or 2 years. The skull usually attains its definitive size by age 20.

The fontanelles and sutures become smaller and narrower by the ingrowth of bone into the remnants of the fetal membranous and cartilaginous skull. This process varies from child to child and even on both sides of the skull; thus, the skull is usually asymmetric and the left side is often larger in the frontal region than the right. The anterior fontanelle is usually reduced to fingertip size during the first half of the second year. The posterior fontanelle may be palpable at birth but usually disappears by 2 months of age. The frontal suture begins to close in the second year but persists throughout life in approximately 10% of persons.

The CSF is produced in the choroid plexuses that arise from the lateral ventricles in frondlike projections from the walls of the posterior horns and the third and fourth ventricles. If the flow of the CSF is obstructed, the volume of

CSF (which is produced at a regular rate of approximately 20 mL/h) will not circulate normally. To accommodate the increased volume, the lateral ventricles usually expand with concomitant compaction of the adjacent central white matter of the cerebral hemispheres. When the anterior fontanelle is open, it may bulge as an indicator of expanding ventricular size. The sutures may separate more widely than they normally do, and clinical signs of increased intracranial pressure may develop. Rapid head growth occurs and can be detected by careful serial measurements of the head circumference.

CLINICAL PRESENTATION

The clinical presentation of the child with macrocephaly varies according to the underlying cause of the large head size. An infant may have no dysmorphic features at birth but may have an obviously large head in proportion to weight and length. He or she may present with multiple congenital anomalies, including dysraphism with a myelomeningocele or faciopalatal clefts. An otherwise healthy infant may have too large a head to fit a baby bonnet comfortably, or it may be difficult to pull a shirt over the infant's head. The head circumference should be measured regularly during routine examinations and preferably by the same person with a metal or plastic-coated cloth tape to ensure precision of measurement. When an infant's head circumference falls above the 98th percentile for age, it is necessary to measure the head circumference of both parents to determine whether they conform to similar percentiles. The child's height and weight should be plotted on growth charts to assess the proportionality of the head and body growth. The infant should be checked at intervals of 2 to 4 weeks or even weekly if necessary to determine how quickly the head is growing. The head may grow more rapidly than the body, so that a discrepancy between weight, length, and head circumference becomes apparent. When the head enlarges because of an underlying increase in the total volume of the cranial cavity (e.g., from a structural malformation, blood, neoplasm, infection, or increase in volume of CSF because of obstructed CSF pathways), the child will present with signs of increased intracranial pressure (ICP). The earliest signs in a young child or infant younger than 6 months of age will be a bulging or tenseness of the anterior fontanelle followed by, or associated with, a change in eating or sleeping habits. The infant may be irritable and will not be comforted by feeding or rocking. Feedings may be vomited in a projectile manner, and the infant may be disinclined to nurse or suck. The infant may sleep for longer periods and may need to be awakened for feedings. There may be decreased visual responses and poor ocular fixation.

Altered feeding and sleeping habits may be more easily recognized in the older infant. If the fontanelle is open, it may be tense. The cranial sutures may be palpably spread. The toddler may fall more frequently or may be content to sit and show less interest in normal activities. Associated with discernible broadening of the forehead with frontal bossing, a sunsetting appearance of the eyes may develop because of pressure on midbrain structures that govern upward gaze.

The older child may complain of having a headache, or may hold the front or sides of the head. He or she may vomit most frequently on awakening in the morning or after naps. A gait disturbance may become apparent. The ability to perform gross motor skills such as riding a bicycle or skating may be impaired. The child may show a disinterest in playing or may tire easily. Complaints of diplopia or blurred vision may not be made until late in the development of increased ICP. However, strabismus or changes in the child's visual acuity, as evidenced by holding books closer, sitting closer to the television, or deterioration in school work, may suggest a decline in visuomotor function due to intracranial hypertension.

DIFFERENTIAL DIAGNOSIS

The differential diagnosis of macrocephaly is presented in the display on Differential Diagnosis of Macrocephaly in order of frequency of occurrence.

WORK-UP

History

The family history is important in the otherwise healthy child with a large head. A review of earlier medical records, including maternal infections during pregnancy and head circumference at birth, helps to determine what the rate of head growth has been and if there has been a recent deviation from the child's curve. A history of change in eating or sleeping habits, in personality, or in school performance must be sought. The physician should ask about the occurrence of birthmarks in close family members to ascertain the incidence of neurofibromatosis or tuberous sclerosis, which are disorders that may be associated with a large head size or macrocephaly.

Physical Examination

A careful measurement of the head circumference in its greatest diameter is essential. The size and tension of the anterior fontanelle should be assessed. The craniofacial ratio should be approximated. (The face is about one-third of the size of the cranial vault in the infant. In adults, the face-cranium ratio is approximately 1:2.) A survey of the skin in bright sunlight and then with Wood's light should be made to look for hypopigmented or café-au-lait spots. An examination of the back for evidence of a dermal sinus may indicate underlying spinal dysraphism. Other dysmorphic features should be noted. An enlargement of the liver and

Differential Diagnosis of Macrocephaly

I. Congenital
  A. *Familial*
  B. *Sporadic*
II. Acquired
  A. *0–6 Months*
    1. Post-hemorrhagic—higher in premature infants
    2. Postinfectious
       a. Intrauterine
       b. Postnatal
    3. Post-traumatic
    4. Malformative (e.g., hydranencephaly, aqueductal stenosis)
       a. Familial X-linked
       b. Sporadic
       c. Arnold-Chiari types I or II
    5. Neoplasm
       a. Primary—choroid plexus papilloma, teratoma
       b. Metastatic—Wilms' tumor, neuroblastoma
    6. Metabolic
    7. Storage or neurodegenerative
  B. *6–12 Months*
    1. Aqueductal stenosis
    2. Post-traumatic
    3. Postinfectious
    4. Metabolic
    5. Neurocutaneous syndrome
    6. Neoplasm—choroid plexus papilloma, ependymoma, desmoplastic astrocytoma of infancy, primitive neuroectodermal tumor, medulloblastoma
    7. Neurodegenerative
  C. *1–6 Years*
    1. Post-traumatic
    2. Postinfectious—abscess, arteritis
    3. Aqueductal stenosis
    4. Neoplasm
       a. Posterior fossa—medulloblastoma, astrocytoma, ependymoma
       b. Brain stem—astrocytoma, ependymoma
       c. Cerebral hemispheres—primitive neuroectodermal tumor, astrocytoma, choroid plexus papilloma, germinoma
    5. Metabolic
    6. Neurodegenerative

spleen, chorioretinitis, and other findings consistent with an intrauterine infection should also be noted. Bruits or venous distention over the cranium may reflect a vascular anomaly such as the vein of Galen malformation.

Laboratory Tests

The child with primary or familial macrocephaly can be monitored at regular intervals by his or her primary physician. Skull roentgenograms and computed tomographic (CT) scans are not necessary when a positive family history has been obtained or if the child is *asymptomatic* (i.e., if there is no developmental delay and signs of ICP are absent). When the fontanelle is still open, cranial ultrasound examination is useful in determining ventricular size without ex-

posure to x-rays. If the child is *symptomatic,* the physician should assume that secondary macrocephaly is present and appropriate studies should be made.

The child with secondary macrocephaly requires investigation. TORCH titers should be drawn from the child and the mother. A premature infant known to have had an intracranial hemorrhage may be followed with serial cranial ultrasound examinations for an assessment of ventriculomegaly. A midline shift of the intracranial structures and some congenital malformations such as agenesis of the corpus callosum or holoprosencephaly may be apparent on cranial ultrasound examination. The delineation of processes in the subdural or subarachnoid spaces, however, cannot be made with ultrasound examination. Intracranial calcifications indicating an intrauterine infection or tuberous sclerosis are readily seen on CT scans. If a history of preceding infection, trauma, or seizures is obtained, a CT scan will provide information about processes such as subdural collections that necessitate prompt treatment. Plain skull roentgenograms are helpful in assessing the chronic changes of increased ICP but rarely are ordered because a CT scan is more useful in localizing a focal abnormality, assessing hydrocephalus, and guiding surgical intervention when indicated. A plain CT scan allows the assessment of the extent and width of the cerebral mantle, ventricular size, and intracranial hemorrhage and will also show shifts of intracranial structures from the midline. A contrast-enhanced CT scan permits an assessment of the neovascularity of mass lesions and vascular malformations. Magnetic resonance imaging (MRI) may show a process that cannot be visualized within the sensitivity of the CT scan. The MRI scan is superior for imaging the posterior fossa and brain stem disorders and should be obtained in the cases in which a strong suspicion of disease exists but a disorder is not visualized by a CT scan. Also, baseline MRI studies allow serial studies to be obtained and compared without repeated x-ray exposure to the child.

INDICATIONS FOR REFERRAL

The child with uncomplicated macrocephaly needs no further evaluation in contrast to a child who has been found to have intracranial hypertension due to a space-occupying lesion, CSF flow obstruction, or a storage disorder. The latter child should be referred to a neurosurgeon and a pediatric neurologist.

ANNOTATED BIBLIOGRAPHY

Caffey J: Pediatric X-Ray Diagnosis. Chicago, Year Book Medical Publishers, 1961. (Good basic introduction to normal and abnormal growth of the skull.)

Menkes JH, Till K, Gabriel RS: Malformations of the central nervous system. In Menkes JH (ed): Textbook of Child Neurology, 4th ed, pp 209–283. Philadelphia, Lea & Febiger, 1990. (Extremely well-referenced chapter that covers many aspects of developmental disorders that produce macrocephaly and hydrocephalus.)

Swaiman KF: Pediatric Neurology, pp 335–342. St. Louis, CV Mosby, 1989. (Excellent textbook presenting a comprehensive tabulation of common and uncommon causes of abnormal head growth.)

151

Headache

Verne S. Caviness, Jr. and
A. Alyssa LeBel

A headache is a symptom experienced by virtually everyone at some time in his or her life. Recurrent headaches may cause sufficient disability in 20% of the population to warrant medical consultation, and rank with obesity as a principal cause of chronic morbidity among children. Most headache disorders, including the most severely disabling, are the expression of a "benign," physiologic state. A headache infrequently may be a symptom of a host of systemic and intracranial disorders. The alert physician tries to distinguish between the benign and symptomatic headache disorders on the basis of a history and physical examination supplemented by appropriate diagnostic tests.

CLINICAL PRESENTATION

The most prevalent of the headache disorders are the benign forms. The majority encountered in the clinical practice of pediatrics may be subdivided into the following three syndromes.

Migraine

The migraine syndrome includes a remarkable spectrum of symptoms and signs. The migraine headache is typically throbbing in quality and predominantly hemicranial in distribution. Other complaints are common. These include sensations described as aching, stabbing, squeezing, burning, tingling, or crawling. Typically, the discomfort is more intense on one side initially, but does not affect the same side each time. Discomfort is generally most intense in the frontal, temporal, and orbital regions but may occur in the occipital and cervical regions.

A migraine attack is paroxysmal, reaching maximum intensity in 1 or at most a few hours. It may last no more than 1 hour, but more often it continues through much of a day and may be terminated by sleep. Less commonly, severe episodes of migraine may continue with declining severity over 2 or more days. The headache may be preceded by a premonitory sense of fatigue, dread, anxiety, or even excitement and is usually accompanied by light and sound intolerance or nausea and vomiting. Focal neurologic symptoms may be dramatic and when encountered for the first time are justifiably alarming for both the patient and the physician. The most common of these symptoms are visual and may include scintillations, scotomas, or field defects that may be unilateral or bilateral. There may be complete blindness, characteristically a sensation of "blackness." There may be "heaviness," weakness, or clumsiness of one or both extremities on a side and tingling or numbness involving variably the face, arm, and leg on one side of the body. Ophthalmoplegia, vertigo, confusional states, dysarthria or dysphasia, or ataxia may also be present. Transient hemiparesis, sometimes shifting from side to side, may occur with, or at other times independently of, the headache. Typically, these focal neurologic symptoms and signs last for a short time and recovery is complete. Rarely a deficit persists. By convention, a migraine accompanied by any of these focal neurologic manifestations is designated as *classic* migraine and without these manifestations it is designated as a *common* migraine.

The focal neurologic signs and symptoms associated with a migraine are particularly prevalent in children. *Ophthalmoplegic* migraine is essentially a disorder of childhood and invariably has its first expression before the age of 12. The pattern of a migraine is additionally distinctive in children in that it may coexist with, and appears to be related to, the so-called *periodic syndrome:* recurrent abdominal pain, nausea and vomiting, benign vertigo or motion sickness, and high fevers. Somnambulism and syncope are also relatively prevalent among children with a migraine.

Tension Headache

The tension headache is a dull aching discomfort that is distributed typically in a bandlike fashion around the head. A cervical ache and stiffness are common. The symptoms may wax and wane over many hours on a particular day or over many days. Not uncommonly a headache may persist without relief for weeks, months, or even years. Typically, a tension headache more than a migraine is more "purely" a headache disorder, although it is often associated with light and sound intolerance and a queasiness in the abdomen.

Cluster Headache

Pain is extreme and is described as a burning, searing, or stabbing sensation. It is concentrated in the eye or orbit and is typically associated with lacrimation, ocular injection, and rhinorrhea, which are most conspicuous on the affected side. In less than 10% of episodes, ptosis and miosis are present on the same side. Pain is typically abrupt in onset and lasts from minutes to 1 or 1½ hours. In the pediatric population and in about 90% of affected adults, the attacks are clustered, occurring one or many times per day over a period of weeks to 2 or 3 months. It is the least common type of headache in children.

PATHOPHYSIOLOGY

Pathophysiologic mechanisms of the headache syndromes are not well understood. Current opinion holds that the full syndrome, including both pain as well as other broadly ranging symptoms, originates centrally, possibly initiated as a physiologic disturbance within the hypothalamus. This disturbance is variably modulated by genetic predisposition, circadian rhythms, endocrine changes, emotional stress, or excessive afferent stimuli. The headache pain component is believed to arise at least in part from neurogenically induced "inflammation" in the dura, a mechanism induced in blood vessels by way of sensory nerves. Multiple peptide transmitters, such as monoaminergic substances, substance P, calcitonin-gene-related peptide, neurokinins A and B, neuropeptide K, and vasoactive intestinal polypeptide are believed from experimental studies to mediate these vascular changes. The complexity of interaction of multiple neural systems in these phenomena, including the actions of multiple transmitters, may explain why such a wide range of pharmacologic substances is variably effective in relieving headache.

Migraine and tension headaches appear to be closely related pathophysiologic states in that they typically occur together in the same person. Also, the threshold for expression of both headaches is modulated by the same genetic, hormonal, and exogenous factors. The familial prevalence has been estimated at 50% to 90% for both syndromes. The strong prevalence of migraine and tension headaches among women, the tendency to initial expression at menarche, or a strong crescendo expression in early pregnancy, at menopause, or while on birth control pills underlines the role of estrogen fluxes as a potent modulator of headache threshold. Other exogenous factors that variably lower the threshold for expression of these headache disorders include alcohol, particularly red wine, nitrates and monosodium glutamate (e.g., hot dogs, Chinese food), chocolate, and milk products (at times an expression of lactose intolerance). Psychological stress is another critical determinant. Typically, depressive symptoms such as fatigue, nonrestful sleep, or a "down feeling" accompany or even precede a crescendo of headache. It should be emphasized that a major psychiatric disturbance, including disabling neurosis or psychosis, is no more prevalent among persons disabled by a headache than in the general population.

The pathophysiology of a cluster headache appears to differ from that of the other two benign headache syndromes in that it is almost unique to men (90%) and has no familial predilection. However, it shares some of the exogenous modulating factors, alcohol, in particular.

DIFFERENTIAL DIAGNOSIS

Although most headache disorders are benign, a headache may be a presenting manifestation of a wide variety of neurologic and systemic disorders, some of which are treatable and others lethal if not treated. A severe headache of acute onset in a child not subject to recurrent headache poses a different set of diagnostic possibilities than recurrent headache disorders. An acute, severe headache associated with nausea, vomiting, prostration, and, not infrequently, fever in the absence of a history of similar episodes should lead one to suspect subarachnoid hemorrhage, meningitis, or parameningeal infection, such as epidural abscess or other causes of increased intracranial pressure. When gradual evolution over hours has occurred and there is meningismus with or without other evidence of systemic infection and when papilledema is not present, an immediate lumbar puncture is indicated to exclude meningitis. When an abrupt onset is associated with meningismus and, possibly, focal neurologic signs, the initial preferred diagnostic procedure is a computed tomographic (CT) scan. This should be done primarily without contrast medium infusion so that blood will be recognizable. A follow-up image may be done with contrast medium infusion if a tumor or an abscess is suspected. A lumbar puncture may be done subsequently if the CT scan is normal and should be done especially if the question of subarachnoid hemorrhage has not been satisfactorily answered (see also Chap. 153).

WORK-UP

History

The differential diagnosis of benign versus symptomatic recurrent headache does not hinge on the character and distribution of the individual headache itself. It depends, rather, on an integrated analysis emphasizing an attack pattern, family history, context of appearance, and a general medical and physical examination. Critical historical points are the attack pattern and the localization of headache. Where severe headaches, separated by headache-free intervals, have recurred over 6 months or longer, the probability of an intracranial mass is low. The benign forms of headache vary in localization, often shifting sides and spreading across the midline. A highly localized, more or less persistent headache, lasting for a few days to a few weeks, is significant, particularly if the pain awakens the child from sleep or is present on awakening in the morning. Pain occurring in sharply focal fashion over the eye, when associated with signs of third nerve paresis, must be assumed to be a manifestation of a posterior communicating or internal carotid artery aneurysm until proved otherwise by arteriography. Pain located in the cervical-medullary junction and associated with resistance to neck flexion raises the possibility of posterior fossa tumor or malformation. A sinus abscess will be associated with local point tenderness often with local erythema and heat. A symptomatic temporomandibular joint will be painful when compressed or associated with decreased movement or pain on movement of the jaw.

Physical Examination

The completely normal general medical and neurologic examination may be taken as strongly reassuring. Disorders caused by increased intracranial pressure, including mass lesions, hydrocephalus, and pseudotumor cerebri, will be associated with abnormal physical findings before a disabling headache leads to neurologic consultation. Lateralizing hemispheric signs, papilledema, disturbances of gaze or individual cranial nerve function, ataxia, and disturbances of gait and reflex are highly sensitive indicators. Elevated blood pressure should alert one to the unlikely possibility of pheochromocytoma. The cutaneous lesions of the phakomatoses, visceromegaly, large lymph nodes, or purpuric lesion, are tell-tale signs of generalized disorders that might be correlated with an intracranial mass, arterial disease or inflammatory processes. Arteriovenous malformation may be suspected from the presence of cutaneous angiomas.

Laboratory Tests

Routine blood and urine studies are recommended for all patients seen in consultation for a disabling recurrent headache, even when the history and physical examination are reassuring. The specific tests include a complete blood cell count, sedimentation rate and determination of calcium and blood glucose levels. Such values, when normal, are an essential baseline starting point for several medications that might be used in the treatment of a headache.

Other diagnostic tests should be tailored to the historical and physical indications. A CT scan or magnetic resonance imaging (MRI) scan will be indicated in subacutely expressed headache disorders, particularly if pain is highly localized. CT and MRI scans are always indicated in subacute and chronically established headache disorders in which a neurologic examination is abnormal, papilledema is present, or the history suggests the child is having seizures. It is only when the question of seizures is raised that an electroencephalogram is likely to be helpful diagnostically. Plain roentgenograms of the skull and sinuses, particularly if CT and MRI scans are unavailable, or of the temporomandibular joint may be required to clarify symptoms relating to these respective localizations.

TREATMENT

When a headache is symptomatic of an underlying cranial, intracranial, or systemic disease, quite different approaches,

appropriate to the underlying disease, will be required. These are beyond the scope of the present discussion. The approach to therapy for benign headaches reflects the fact that young adults, aged 18 to 20, often regard the pediatrician as their primary physician and that it is among this population that many of the most disabling headache disorders are encountered.

The pediatrician should undertake three critical basic components of headache management: (1) identification and elimination of specific provocative factors, (2) reassurance, and (3) pharmacologic intervention. It will also be the responsibility of the pediatrician to initiate a neurologic or psychiatric referral if warranted.

Elimination of Exogenous Substances

Frequently, exogenous substances ingested by the patient play a role in bringing on the headache. Some of these items include alcohol, cheeses, and foods containing monosodium glutamate. Avoidance of such offending substances may be a partial, although rarely a complete, solution. Birth control pills require particular emphasis. Used increasingly over the past 2 decades by adolescent girls, the pill has been a consistent offender and, possibly, may place a young woman who has headaches at increased risk for stroke, especially if she smokes. The physician must inquire about the use of birth control pills, which will require great tact if the parents are unaware. When a headache crescendo is found to occur in association with use of birth control pills, the physician must make the strongest possible argument that these pills be discontinued. Furthermore, it is completely unjustified for the physician to provide the patient with potentially toxic medications for headache provoked by birth control pills. The use of birth control pills in the management of severely symptomatic endometriosis, which coexists with a disabling headache, is an exceptional circumstance. Here, a compromise approach such as a reduction of the estrogen dose or intermittent estrogen therapy may be worked out with the patient's gynecologist.

Reassurance

The importance of reassurance cannot be underestimated. Quite reasonably, the patient and the parents may seek consultation because they are anxious about its cause. They may be concerned specifically about the possibility of a brain tumor. It is critical that they be convinced that the physician has also considered and excluded this as well as other feared diagnoses. It is best to discuss this concern openly. For example, the patient or family will realize that a normal examination and a recurrent headache history continuing over 1 year or more make the existence of a tumor highly improbable. At least as far as the diagnosis is concerned, many patients will be reassured when it is brought to their attention that other members of their families have suffered similar headache disorders or by the observation that the headache is consistently provoked by an ingested substance. When diagnostic uncertainty or the family's anxiety justifies a CT or MRI scan, the family must be helped to understand that a normal study *does* resolve the issue and is not a failure to find the underlying sinister cause.

Pharmacologic Intervention

Rather than behavioral therapies such as biofeedback, pharmacologic intervention is the choice of most patients and physicians. (When *biofeedback* is available in a community and its requirements of time and personal discipline are appropriate to patient and family, this mode of therapy should also be given consideration. It is as effective as medications in some patients, and it is safe.) Mild analgesics such as aspirin or acetaminophen provide satisfactory relief for most patients who have an occasional migraine or tension headache of mild to moderate severity. Headaches unresponsive to these medications require a dual strategy involving prophylactic suppression of headaches as well as treatment of the individual headaches as they occur. Cluster headache, only rarely encountered by the pediatrician, generally requires relatively extreme pharmacologic measures.

Whatever medication is chosen, several practical points are useful to keep in mind. Any drug chosen may have alarming side effects and potential toxicities. In particular, the physician should be cautions about the use of potentially teratogenic preparations for headaches occurring in the course of an undisclosed pregnancy. The patient or family should be offered reasonable expectations of the effectiveness, the potential side effects, and overall time required for medical treatment. Unexpected side effects of drugs, disappointment in the face of unrealistic expectations for relief, and an "open ended" medication schedule without a "game plan" are all potentially defeating sources of anxiety. Thus, the patient should be cautioned about the possibility of side effects, with emphasis on the possibility that unexpected side effects may occur, and should be cautioned that a particular preparation may not be effective.

The patient or family should understand that the development of an optimal program may require a trial of one or more preparations and that with even the most effective medication, a series of trials and errors may be required to get the optimum dose. Although several days or weeks may be required to achieve an effective dose, it is well to begin each medication at a low, tolerated dose and increase the dose only as tolerated. (Patients who are frightened by the side effects of a drug advanced too quickly may refuse to use that drug in the future, even though it might be the best choice.) The tolerated drug should be used aggressively, increasing the dose to a maximal safe dose or until the desired effect is achieved. Often a potentially effective drug is abandoned too early without a satisfactory trial at maximum dose. Ready access to the supervising physician is essential to the success of pharmacologic therapy; the patient should not become anxious if the initial course of therapy does not fulfill his or her expectations immediately.

A relatively large number of drugs, representing multiple, pharmacologic classes, have been variably effective in the prophylactic management of headaches. These include β-adrenergic receptor blockers, calcium channel antagonists, anticonvulsants, tricyclic antidepressants, phenothiazines, antihistamines, benzodiazepines, nonsteroidal anti-inflammatory preparations, lithium carbonate, methysergide, and corticosteroids. The efficacy of each of these classes, in terms of reduction of headache frequency, has been variously estimated at 50% to 75%. In interpreting this figure, the physician should remember that the placebo effect of pharmacologic prophylaxis in benign headache disorders has been estimated to be between 40% and 50%.

Various factors will influence drug choice, including the physician's prior experience with a particular preparation, the preference of the patient or the patient's family, the ease of administration, and the experienced side effects. Propranolol and verapamil are recommended because of their relative freedom from toxicity and side effects, in particular psychotropic and sedating effects. One must be alert to the appearance of bradycardia and orthostatic hypotension, generally signaled by lightheadedness. These drugs are occasionally a nuisance for the active child because of the necessity of administration several times per day. The antihistamine cyproheptadine and the tricyclic antidepressants may be effective choices for both migraine and tension headache disorders. The anticonvulsant phenytoin may be useful in migraine and may be given at relatively low risk, although the physician must be alert to the possibility of hematologic or hepatic toxicity. These drugs may be taken as a single dose at bed time. Among the tricyclic antidepressant preparations, desipramine is particularly reliable when, as is often the case, fatigue and sleep disturbance precede or are associated with a crescendo headache disorder. If desipramine is used, it is wise to pair it with small doses of a benzodiazepine such as diazepam (Valium) for the first week. A baseline electrocardiogram should be attained for evaluation of dysrhythmias exacerbated by the tricyclics. Otherwise, an alarming agitation may bias the child or family against continued use of the drug.

When prophylactic medications are used, they will generally be needed for only several months. When prophylactic treatment is required for 4 to 6 months or longer, a succession of different drugs may be required as the disorder "escapes" from an initially effective medication. For example, escape from propranolol and verapamil occurs particularly when treatment must be prolonged for several months. After 4 to 6 weeks of effective headache control, the patient should gradually taper and discontinue the drugs if headaches do not recur. When the relatively safe drug classes listed above fail in the prophylaxis of a recurrent headache, it is possible that one of the other classes of drugs will be effective. For two reasons the pediatrician might prefer referral at this juncture. First, the other drug classes are potentially more toxic. Second, when the safer drugs fail, it is often the case that the solution will not be a pharmacologic one.

Migraine Headache Treatment

Migraine, in particular, is typically associated with nausea, vomiting, and agitation. If over-the-counter preparations do not afford effective relief, other medications are necessary to alleviate these distressing symptoms as well as the pain itself. Preparations containing butalbital, acetaminophen, caffeine, ergotamine tartrate (Fiorinal, Esgic, Wigraine, Cafergot) are generally reliable choices that for most patients are well tolerated and acceptably free of risk. However, one must be alert to excessive use, signaling dependency on these preparations. Their regular use on as many as 3 to 4 days per week over several months means that an effective prophylactic program is needed. Ergotamine, when used excessively, has risks associated with arterial spasm; it may cause uterine cramps, and it is absolutely contraindicated in pregnancy.

Patients with severe migraine headaches unresponsive to substantial doses of a simple preparation may be encountered in medical clinics and emergency departments and may require narcotic injections for relief. Chlorpromazine is recommended not only by its efficacy but also by the fact that the patient or parent may give the drug at home, that it is nonaddictive, and that it is relatively well tolerated and safe when used only intermittently for episodic headache. The small risk of extrapyramidal side effects or of hepatic toxicity when chlorpromazine is given intermittently is preferable to the risks, side effects, and inconvenience of narcotic injections. Relatively large doses may be required, and failure to use sufficient amounts is a principal cause of an unsatisfactory response. For a teenager, depending on experience gained on several trials, 25 to several hundred milligrams may be required over 2 to 4 hours. This may be given with 2 to 4 Cafergot tablets. Suppositories are effective when severe nausea and vomiting initially preclude oral use of the drug. Metoclopramide and trimethobenzamide (Tigan) are other substances that may be similarly used.

Headache specialists may resort to more unusual treatment strategies for intractable migraine headaches under circumstances when the patient is under observation within a clinic or hospital. These measures include intravenous administration of dihydroergotamine in dosages ranging from 0.5 to 1.0 mg every 8 hours over a period of 3 to 5 days. In adolescents and young adults, a bolus of intravenous lidocaine may also be effective in terminating a prolonged migraine headache. Intravenous hydrocortisone is yet another option in the treatment of severe refractory migrainous headache.

Cluster Headache Treatment

This type of headache may be treated prophylactically with lithium carbonate, corticosteroids, methysergide (Sansert), or chlorpromazine, singly or in combination. Individual headaches may respond to rapidly absorbed inhalant or sublingual ergotamine preparations.

INDICATIONS FOR REFERRAL OR ADMISSION

Referral or admission to a hospital is indicated when it is established or probable that a headache is a symptom of significant intracranial or systemic disease. Indications for referral to a neurologist, specialty headache clinic, or psychiatrist may be less obvious when one is dealing with the benign headache syndromes. The following guidelines for referral are recommended: when the diagnosis remains in doubt despite clinical analysis, CT or MRI scan, and other laboratory tests, and when the response to therapy is unsatisfactory or unexpected. Drugs with which the pediatrician is sufficiently experienced, including those that he or she views as acceptably free of risks, may have failed to provide satisfactory relief. Alternatively, the use of such drugs may have been associated with bizarre side effects or the patient may have been intolerant to drugs that should have helped. Extreme drug intolerance and bizarre side effects are clues that there is a substantial underlying anxiety state or other psychological disorder and that a psychiatric consultation is indicated.

ANNOTATED BIBLIOGRAPHY

Barlow CF: Headaches and Migraine in Childhood. Philadelphia, JB Lippincott, 1984. (Excellent review; comprehensive and thoughtful.)

Fields HL, Barbaro NM, Heinricher MM: Brain stem neuronal circuitry underlying the antinociceptive action of opiates. Progr Brain Res 77:245, 1988. (Current state of research on pain-related neural circuitry.)

Headache Classification Committee of the International Headache Society: Classification and diagnostic criteria for headache disorders, cranial neuralgias and facial pain. Cephalalgia, suppl 7, 8: 1–96, 1988. (Current full classification system.)

Honig PJ, Charney EB: Children with brain tumor headaches. Am J Dis Child 136:121, 1982. (Discussion of abnormal physical signs that are generally present when a headache is associated with a brain tumor.)

Maciewicz RJ, Chung RY, Strassman A et al: Relief of vascular headache with intravenous lidocaine: Clinical observations and a proposed mechanism. Clin J Pain 4:11, 1988. (Preliminary experience with a new treatment for severe headache.)

Maratos J, Wilkinson M: Migraine in children: A medical and psychiatric study. Cephalalgia 2:179, 1982. (Perspective on the relationship of psychological stresses and headache in children.)

Raskin NH, Schwartz RK: Interval therapy of migraine: Long-term results. Headache 20:336, 1980. (Although concerned with adults, the study treats well the vagaries of headache response to various medications over time.)

Sillanpaa M: Changes in the prevalence of migraine and other headaches during the first seven school years. Headache 23:15, 1983. (Presents [along with the following article] the epidemiology of headache among children in a northern European country.)

Sillanpaa M: Prevalence of headache in prepuberty. Headache 23:10, 1983.

152

Head Trauma

Elizabeth C. Dooling

Approximately 200,000 children are hospitalized each year in the United States because of head trauma. Boys are injured two to three times as frequently as girls. Accidents are the most common cause of death in children between 1 and 14 years of age, and many fatalities result from head injuries. Head injuries may be classified as focal and diffuse. The morbidity associated with head trauma is high. Many children are left with permanent disabilities and require special educational programs and ongoing rehabilitative care.

PATHOPHYSIOLOGY

The skull is covered by a fibrous sheet known as the *epicranium aponeurotica or galea aponeurotica.* The galea is firmly adherent to the overlying skin of the scalp but is applied only loosely to the pericranium. Fusing on each side to the temporal fascia just above the zygomatic arches, these attachments limit the spread of subgaleal effusions. Under the skull itself is the dura, which is a thick and tough bilayered membrane composed of dense collagenous tissue. The dura has the consistency of plastic wrap in the infant and waxed paper in the older child. The outer layer of the dura is fused with periosteum. The inner layer or dura proper is separate from the outer layer at certain points and forms folds that project into the cavities formed between the cerebral hemispheres, between the occipital lobes and cerebellum, and in the midline of the posterior fossa. The arachnoid, an avascular structure, lies under the dura. The cerebrospinal fluid (CSF) circulates between the arachnoid and the pia, a weblike membrane in which the blood vessels ramify. The pia is thinner over the cortex and thicker over the brain stem; thus, the cerebral tissue is protected by the bony cranium and its overlying and underlying collagenous or membranous structures.

CLINICAL PRESENTATION

Head injuries may range from superficial lacerations of the skull to penetration of foreign bodies or skull fragments through the scalp, skull, and cerebral tissue to the ventricular system. There may be a total preservation of consciousness, transient "lightheadedness," a brief loss of consciousness, or a prolonged coma, usually in proportion to the severity of the injury. The child who is struck by an automobile may sustain injuries to other major organs and may thus be further compromised by hemorrhage or shock. Usually, an acute event causes the head injury. Less commonly, a subacute or chronic course may follow trauma.

A newborn who is subjected to a traumatic delivery may present with a simple scalp swelling under which there may or may not be a skull fracture or a skull fracture associated with an epidural hematoma of arterial or venous origin. Young children most often sustain head trauma related to accidents while playing, riding in cars, or during a seizure. Other children and adolescents will incur injuries at play, at work, or while driving a car. Scalp swelling may be classified as follows:

- *Subgaleal hematoma* resulting from bleeding beneath the galea aponeurotica. It is the most common cause of swelling from head trauma beyond the newborn period.
- *Caput succedaneum* resulting from scalp edema due to local pressure and trauma during labor. It is most easily differentiated from a cephalohematoma in that the swelling is diffuse and often crosses sutures.
- *Leptomeningeal cyst* referring to a fluid-filled space between the arachnoid and pia and to arachnoid herniation through a contiguous dural tear.
- *Cephalohematoma* or hemorrhage beneath the external periosteum of the skull, usually in the parietal region.

For these conditions, surgical intervention is necessary only in the case of the leptomeningeal cyst.

If the swollen area is transilluminated, there is a diffuse increase in infants with caput succedaneum, a focal increase in a child with a leptomeningeal cyst, a diffuse decrease in a child with subgaleal hematoma, and a focal decrease overlying a cephalohematoma.

Skull fractures may be suspected clinically by direct palpation of the skull or by crepitus on palpation of the skull. Skull fractures may be classified as follows:

- *Linear fractures:* About 75% of all skull fractures in children are linear. No specific treatment is usually necessary, but careful observation for 18 to 24 hours is necessary.
- *Depressed fractures:* The outer and inner tables of the calvarium are disrupted. Tangential roentgenograms of the skull may be necessary to identify the extent of the depression. When the depression is 5 to 10 mm in depth, surgical elevation is indicated.
- *Compound fractures:* Bone fragments protrude through

the scalp laceration. Surgical debridement with elevation and antibiotic prophylaxis are necessary.

- *Basal fractures:* These fractures are often not evident on plain roentgenograms but may be apparent on computed tomographic (CT) scans in the axial plane. When epistaxis, hemotympanum, or hemorrhage in the nasopharynx, mastoid, postauricular, or periorbital area occurs, a basal skull fracture is likely. Cranial nerve palsies and CSF leakage may be present.
- *Diastatic fractures:* These fractures result from separation of the cranial bones at one or more suture sites, especially the lambdoid, and occur usually in early childhood.
- *"Growing" fractures:* These develop within the first 6 months following linear or diastatic fractures. The parietal bone is most frequently affected. Children younger than 3 years old are most susceptible. The fracture is prevented from healing because of the coexisting arachnoid cyst that prevents apposition of the bony margins.

A *cerebral concussion* is characterized by a transient loss of consciousness of varying duration (seconds, minutes, or, less often, hours) and is more likely to occur when the head is not fixed at the time of blunt injury. A concussion is associated with temporary retrograde amnesia of events remotely preceding the injury and temporary posttraumatic or anterograde amnesia that may last for several hours after the accident. The *postconcussive* syndrome is characterized by headache, dizziness, irritability, nervousness, difficulty in concentrating, and, sometimes, changes in behavior or intellect. It is usually self-limited, with recovery in 4 to 8 weeks, but it occasionally evolves into a more chronic condition.

A *cerebral contusion* or *laceration* indicates bruising or tearing respectively of brain tissue. Such lesions can cause indirect trauma to tissue directly beneath the site of blunt or penetrating injury or directly or diagonally opposite to the area of impact. These lesions are called *coup* when contiguous tissue is affected or *contrecoup* when tissue contralateral to the traumatized area is involved. These injuries are important because of their relationship to the development of post-traumatic epilepsy.

Hematomas may be *epidural* or *subdural* in location. They may result from relatively mild preceding head trauma; they may not be able to be differentiated from each other. An epidural hematoma is rarer than a subdural hematoma; it is usually unilateral; it is associated with a skull fracture; and it most often occurs in children older than 2 years. A subdural hematoma usually occurs in children younger than 1 year of age; it has an underlying skull fracture; it is often bilateral; the source is venous in origin; and it is more likely than an epidural hematoma to be associated with seizures. A transient period of lucidity or near-normal behavior may follow a period of depressed consciousness immediately after the injury. In the third phase, a decreased or deepening level of consciousness may supervene in a child with an epidural hematoma. Recurrent seizures, anemia, and irritability occur more often in a child with a subdural hematoma. In either case, the hematoma is a space-occupying lesion within the fixed volume of the cranial cavity and thus produces increased intracranial pressure. Lethargy, vomiting, a full fontanelle even when upright, separation of the sutures, sixth and third nerve weakness, headache, papilledema, and Cushing's triad of elevated systolic blood pressure, decreased pulse, and slow respirations may be found in a child with raised intracranial pressure. Third nerve weakness and hemiparesis may develop when there is an incipient herniation of the uncus or temporal lobe.

Fractures of the occipital bone in proximity to the transverse sinus and vascular tentorium may be complicated by infratentorial epidural (venous) bleeding. Patients with posterior fossa hematomas present with altered consciousness, vomiting, meningismus, ataxia, and abnormal respirations. Rarely, children who have sustained mild head trauma with lacerations may have no sequelae directly related to the injury but may have apparent unmasking of coexisting problems, such as neoplasm.

Diffuse changes in the cerebral white matter have become recognized as important as focal hematomas in affecting the outcome of the head-injured patient. Formerly described as shearing of the white matter, diffuse axonal injury takes 18 to 24 hours to develop and may be identified in some cases by neuroimaging studies. In others, it is seen macroscopically at autopsy.

DIFFERENTIAL DIAGNOSIS

The child who has a head injury does not usually present as a diagnostic dilemma because of external evidence of trauma and, usually, the observations of witnesses to the accident. The possibility of child abuse in an infant or a toddler should always be considered, even with a witness who reports otherwise.

A differential diagnosis must be formulated for the child who is found unconscious. In addition to closed head trauma—with or without external evidence of injury—other causes of coma must be considered. Most common is ingestion of drugs and poisons. Other common causes include metabolic disorders such as diabetic ketoacidosis, fulminant central nervous system infection, acute encephalopathy, postictal state, and rupture of a congenital vascular malformation.

WORK-UP

History

It is imperative to obtain information from the person(s) present at the scene when the child was injured. The child's behavior antecedent to the accident should be noted (e.g., to exclude preceding seizure activity that may have predisposed to a fall from a bicycle). The child may be unaware of losing consciousness after an injury that produces a concussion but may be amnestic when questioned closely. A history of evolving depressed consciousness, vomiting, recurrent seizure activity, increasing weakness of arms or legs, sleepiness, or vision changes such as diplopia dictates exclusion of an expanding intracranial lesion.

Physical Examination

Vital signs must be taken and monitored. The level of consciousness must be assessed, and adequate ventilation and circulation must be maintained. A careful inspection of the scalp and body to assess abrasions, lacerations, and swellings is necessary. The nasopharynx and ears should be checked for evidence of fresh blood. The neck should be immobilized with a cervical collar before the patient is moved. The abdomen should be palpated for evidence of visceral bleeding.

Most importantly, signs of increased intracranial pressure should be systematically sought. Most commonly, these signs include a full fontanelle or separated sutures, changes in the child's level of responsiveness, and changes in the pattern and rate of respirations. The most common clues in the older child are headache and papilledema. The pupillary size, equality, and reaction to light must be recorded, as must ocular movements and retinal hemorrhages. A unilateral dilated and sluggish (or fixed) pupil may represent a compression of the third nerve by a herniating portion of the temporal lobe. In the unresponsive child, the eye movements may be assessed by moving the child's head passively (if there are no cervical fractures), or, if the eardrums are intact, by instilling ice water to stimulate oculovestibular reflexes. Asymmetric reflexes, absent motor function, and abnormal resting posture should be assessed because these findings may signal impending herniation. Even more ominous is decorticate posturing (characterized by flexion and adduction of the arms and extension of the legs) or decerebrate posturing (characterized by extension and internal rotation of the arms and extension of the legs).

Laboratory Tests

A hematocrit should be obtained because intracranial bleeding, especially in the newborn and young infant, may result in anemia. If there is obvious blood loss in large quantity, a sample should be sent to the blood bank for type and should be cross-matched in anticipation of a blood transfusion. If there is an associated neck or spine injury, the patient's head and neck should be immobilized with a cervical collar or sandbags before being moved to the radiology department. A child with minor head trauma who is fully alert and without neurologic signs usually does not need skull roentgenograms. Skull and cervical spine roentgenograms are rec-

ommended in a child with any of the following: significant scalp swelling, localizing neurologic signs, unconsciousness for more than 5 minutes, palpable findings suggestive of a depressed or compounded skull fracture (i.e., bony malalignment), signs suggestive of a basilar skull fracture, and a progressive worsening of the neurologic status. Roentgenograms of the facial bones and orbits should be obtained if facial trauma has also occurred. CT scans should be ordered in children who have had severe head trauma or who have serious neurologic signs. A plain CT scan will disclose intracranial bleeding such as epidural or subdural hematomas, intracerebral hematomas, and posterior fossa hemorrhages and will show areas of cerebral contusion. Mass effect and midline shifts will be readily apparent on CT scans. Fractures of the basal skull may be more easily identified on CT scans than on routine skull roentgenograms. CT scanning has largely eliminated the need for cerebral angiography and may supplant tomography of the base of the skull when hemotympanum, otorrhea, or rhinorrhea is present.

MANAGEMENT AND REFERRAL

If there is a fracture of a bone at its suture point, a careful follow-up including a head measurement is indicated to ensure that the fracture heals completely. If the child sustains a brief loss of consciousness (i.e., 1 to 10 minutes), close observation for the first 24 to 48 hours is necessary. If the parents are reliable and competent, this observation may be done at home after an initial medical evaluation. Hospitalization is advised if there is any doubt about the responsibility of the child's caretakers or if there is any abnormal neurologic sign or symptom. Parents should be instructed to monitor the child's level of consciousness—how readily the child can be aroused and how coherent the child is, respiratory pattern, pupil size and reactivity—at regular intervals of 1 to 2 hours. Delayed cerebral edema from cerebral contusion may occur within 8 to 12 hours after the injury. (Maximal cerebral edema usually occurs within 48 to 72 hours after the injury.) A child with a loss of consciousness for 10 to 30 minutes or more should be hospitalized for monitoring. A child with a seizure at the onset of the injury need not be treated with anticonvulsants if the seizure is brief and generalized (i.e., less than 10 minutes, but such a child should be hospitalized for observation). Any child with signs of increased intracranial pressure (e.g., third cranial nerve palsy, sixth nerve palsy, dilated and fixed pupils, anisocoria, Cushing's triad) requires immediate therapy to prevent brainstem herniation, with its resultant high morbidity and mortality. Similarly, the child with signs of herniation (e.g., decorticate posture) or impending herniation (e.g., unequal pupil) as well as the child who sustains multiple injuries or an open-head injury should be admitted to an intensive care unit for close monitoring. The placement of an intracranial pressure gauge bolt is often necessary, and additional treatment to keep the intracranial pressure below 20 mm Hg by using hyperventilation to reduce the PCO_2 to 25 mm Hg, mannitol or other osmotic diuretics, and fluid restriction can be implemented. Likewise, children with epidural, subdural, and intracranial hemorrhages should be admitted to an intensive care unit. Epidural hematomas are surgical emergencies. A "lucid" phase may be interspersed between periods of coma or depressed consciousness. With signs of increased intracranial pressure, subdural hematomas may need to be tapped or evacuated. Comprehensive management of the seriously injured child requires the facilities of a pediatric tertiary center and a multidisciplinary staff.

Post-traumatic epilepsy following head trauma occurs in approximately 1% of all children, but in about 5% of children hospitalized for head trauma. The more serious the injury, the greater will be the chance of the child developing a learning disability and intellectual impairment (e.g., memory and motor deficits and seizures). An increased incidence of neurologic sequelae occurs in those patients who are hospitalized for more than 24 hours. Approximately 75% of patients who are in a coma for more than 3 weeks are more likely to remain dependent in caring for themselves. Overall, children younger than 16 years of age recover more function. Memory deficits contribute greatly to dependency needs. Cognitive dysfunction and personality changes may be subtle and go unrecognized in the early convalescent stage.

Chronic seizure disorders are often associated with a poor long-term functional outcome. Three risk factors were identified by Jennett and Teasdale (see bibliography) for development of post-traumatic seizures: (1) the occurrence of seizures within the first week of head injury; (2) the presence of an intracranial hematoma; and (3) the presence of a depressed skull fracture. Seventy percent of head-injured patients who developed post-traumatic epilepsy had seizures within the first 6 months after head injury.

Families with head-injured children may seek information from the National Head Injury Foundation, 18A Vernon Street, Framingham, Massachusetts 01701.

ANNOTATED BIBLIOGRAPHY

Adams JH, Graham DI, Gennarelli TA, Maxwell WL: Diffuse axonal injury in non-missile head injury. J Neurol Neurosurg Psychiatry 54:481–483, 1991.

Berger MS, Pitts LH, Lovely M et al: Outcome from severe head injuries in children and adolescents. J Neurosurg 62:194–199, 1985. (Prospective study of mostly direct admissions to San Francisco General Hospital: outcome was assessed for more than or equal to 6 hours; the mortality rate was 33% and persistent elevation of intracranial pressure was usually associated with a poor prognosis.)

Bruce DA, Alavi A, Bilianuk D et al: Diffuse cerebral swelling following head injuries in children: The syndrome of malignant brain edema. J Neurosurg 54:170–178, 1981. (Report of diffuse brain swelling found on 29% of computed tomographic scans of 214 patients; the authors postulate that severe cerebrovascular changes [i.e., vasodilatation and initial hyperemia] are responsible for swelling, not disturbed autoregulation.)

Chadwick O, Rutter M, Shafter D, Shrout PE: A prospective study of children with head injuries: IV. Specific cognitive defects. J Clin Neuropsychol 3:101–20, 1981. (Serial studies of 25 children with head injuries causing amnesia for more than or equal to 1 week matched to 25 children with orthopedic injuries showed subtle impairment of visuomotor or visuospatial performance in a few cases.)

Eiben CF, Anderson TP, Lockman L et al: Functional outcome of closed head injury in children and young adults. Arch Phys Med Rehabil 65:168, 1984. (Retrospective review of the outcome of closed head injuries.)

Hahn YS, Chyung C, Barthel MJ et al: Head injuries in children under 36 months of age. Child Nerv Syst 4:34–40, 1988. (Excellent analysis of outcome of head-injured children admitted to Children's Memorial Hospital, Chicago, between 1981 and 1985 who were younger than 3 years of age. This group accounted for 43% of the admissions; 75% had a fall. Their patients with a Glasgow Coma Scale score of 5 or 6 had a variable outcome when they adapted the Glasgow Coma Scale to a Children's Coma Scale.)

Jennett B, Teasdale G: Management of Head Injuries. Philadelphia, FA Davis, 1981. (Excellent and comprehensive text addressing authors' experience with a head-injured [mainly adult] population, including prognosis and objectives of care.)

Kalinsky Z, Morrison DP, Meyer CA et al: Medical problems encountered during rehabilitation of patients with head injury. Arch Phys Med Rehabil 66:25, 1985. (Discussion of the range of problems presenting in head-injured patients and the roles of the specialists in coordinating health care.)

153

Meningitis

Mark S. Pasternack and Elizabeth C. Dooling

Meningitis, an inflammatory process involving the meninges of the brain and the fluid within the spaces enclosed by the pia-arachnoid, may result from bacterial, viral, fungal, parasitic, or protozoan infections. A high level of suspicion is crucial to diagnose meningitis promptly and to initiate proper therapy with the hope of minimizing morbidity and mortality.

This chapter is intended to present an overview of bacterial meningitis. Since a more detailed discussion is critical for its diagnosis and management (but beyond the scope of this chapter), the reader is encouraged to refer to a major textbook of pediatrics or infectious diseases for more specific "in-hospital" guidelines, especially with reference to characteristics of the cerebrospinal fluid (CSF) in the newborn with infection, to therapy, and to short-term complications.

PATHOPHYSIOLOGY

Bacterial meningitis generally develops as a consequence of transient or sustained bacteremia. Meningitis may arise after a brief prodrome of fever without an apparent focus of infection, or may complicate a focal suppurative process such as otitis media, sinusitis, or mastoiditis. Direct seeding of the CSF may occur following penetrating head injuries or neurosurgery or from congenital sinus tracts in the neuraxis. Hematogenous meningitis usually involves a single organism, whereas meningitis due to a contiguous focus or direct inoculation is occasionally polymicrobial.

The presence of bacteria in the CSF leads to hyperemia of the meningeal vessels and is followed closely by a migration of neutrophils into the subarachnoid space. The subarachnoid exudate increases rapidly and extends over the convexity to the base of the brain and into the sheaths of the cranial and spinal nerves and, for a short distance, into the perivascular spaces of the cortex. Initially, polymorphonuclear leukocytes, often containing phagocytized bacteria, predominate; lymphocytes and histiocytes or macrophages become more dominant after a few days. Plasma cells subsequently appear and increase in number. The presence of pus in the subarachnoid space incites an inflammatory response in the meninges and thus causes symptoms and signs similar to those caused by the presence of blood or neoplastic cells.

Experimental investigations have shown that the characteristically observed pleocytosis is a response to proinflammatory cytokines (e.g., tumor necrosis factor, interleukin-1) elicited by certain bacterial products (gram-positive cell wall proteoglycan, gram-negative lipopolysaccharide). The pleocytosis is not effective at eradicating infection (which is accomplished by the bactericidal antibiotics employed in therapy). Rather, it is responsible for the disruption of the blood–brain barrier and for the inflammatory sequelae that result in intracranial hypertension, hypoperfusion, and vascular injury.

Clinical Presentation

Neonatal meningitis is usually due to the dominant neonatal bacterial pathogens such as group B streptococci (*Streptococcus agalactiae*) and enteric gram-negative bacilli, although *Listeria monocytogenes* is an important pathogen, causing approximately 10% of cases. *Early-onset neonatal meningitis* occurs within the first week of life and is more frequently observed in "high-risk" infants (e.g., prematurity, prolonged prepartum rupture of membranes, invasive fetal monitoring). Early-onset infection is often fulminant, with the clinical picture dominated by hypotension and/or group B streptococcal pneumonia rather than the signs or symptoms of meningitis. *Late-onset meningitis* occurs after the first week of life and may develop at any time during the first 3 months of life. Many of these infections develop in otherwise normal infants with uncomplicated perinatal courses; in these patients the meningitic process dominates the clinical picture (see also chap. 196).

The signs and symptoms of meningitis in newborns are generally nonspecific and nonlocalizing. Fever is usually present, although in newborns a temperature of more than 102 °F (38.9 °C) is infrequent. Neurologic signs may be limited to poor feeding, hypotonia, and lethargy or, conversely, to increased motor tone and irritability. The fontanelle may be full, but it is not a consistent finding. Classic signs of meningismus, such as a stiff neck or positive Kernig's and Brudzinski's signs, are rare. Consequently, all newborns with fever require careful neurologic assessment and lumbar puncture as part of the initial evaluation.

In older infants and children during the first few years of life, bacterial meningitis is caused almost exclusively by the encapsulated pathogens *Hemophilus influenzae* type b, *Streptococcus pneumoniae,* and *Neisseria meningitidis.* In children 6 to 24 months of age with acute febrile illnesses with a temperature exceeding 103 °F (39.4 °C), there is a significant incidence of bacteremia due to *S. pneumoniae* and *H. influenzae,* and approximately 2% of these cases are complicated by the development of meningitis. In some children, primary foci of infection such as otitis media, pneumonia, cellulitis, or septic arthritis may be present, but frequently, no primary focus is identifiable. The typical presentation is a prodromal febrile illness of 1 or a few days' duration with progression to include high fever, vomiting, headache (in older children), and a stiff neck. Lethargy and obtundation usually develop and may progress to stupor or even coma. Grand-mal seizures may occur due to cortical inflammation and/or cortical venous thrombosis, but most often represent fever-associated seizures. A petechial exanthem usually indicates meningococcemia, but meningococcal infection may be associated with maculopapular eruptions or occur without cutaneous involvement. *H. influenzae* type b may occasionally produce significant thrombocytopenia and similar cutaneous changes and, conversely, petechial eruptions may occasionally be seen with enteroviral disease such as coxsackievirus infection.

Differential Diagnosis

In most instances, the diagnosis of bacterial meningitis is based on the clinical features and characteristic CSF findings. However, on occasion, certain viral meningoencephalitides such as mumps, lymphocytic choriomeningitis virus, or enterovirus will generate a granulocyte-predominant pleocytosis with hypoglycorrhachia, and, in selected instances, uncertainty in diagnosis will necessitate empiric antibiotic therapy for bacterial meningitis. In addition, parameningeal infections (e.g., subdural empyema, brain abscess, or bacterial cerebritis) may produce a granulocytic pleocytosis suggestive of bacterial meningitis. Noninfectious etiologies that may produce fever, headache, and meningismus include subarachnoid hemorrhage due to a ruptured vascular malformation or congenital aneurysm, collagen vascular disease, intracranial neoplasm, or toxic ingestions of barbiturates, phenylpropanolamine, or illicit drugs. Clinical features and imaging studies are important in distinguishing among these diverse possibilities.

Reye syndrome may follow a respiratory or gastrointestinal illness or varicella, and it may begin with a fever, vomiting, and an altered mental state. A child who has lead poisoning may be confused or show signs of increased intracranial pressure. Children who have metabolic disorders such as hypernatremia or hyponatremia, hypoglycemia, or hemolytic uremic syndrome may be acutely febrile and unresponsive. A patient who has pseudotumor cerebri may complain of a headache or stiff neck, and may vomit. Osteomyelitis of the spine may be associated with fever and meningismus.

WORK-UP

History

Diagnostic efforts should be focused and dovetailed with the institution of supportive measures. Rapid initiation of therapy minimizes the risk of metastatic infection or cardiovascular collapse, particularly with meningococcal or *H. influenzae* type b infection, and may reduce the risk of developing sensorineural hearing loss. The past medical history should be quickly reviewed to verify prior *H. influenzae* type b immunization, to ascertain the extent of prior middle ear and sinus disease, surgery, and head trauma. Recent use of oral antibiotics should be noted, since sterile CSF is sometimes due to such prior therapy, resulting in partially treated bacterial meningitis. The presence of possible allergies, particularly immediate hypersensitivity (urticaria, angioedema, or anaphylaxis) to β-lactam antibiotics should be reviewed.

It is important to check on recent exposure to patients with infectious illnesses among family members or day-care contacts (e.g., meningitis); preceding illness; travel to an area of endemic infections (e.g., Lyme disease); the presence of congenital defects including heart disease, spinal dysraphism, or fistulas; or indwelling foreign bodies such as heart patches or valves, catheters, or ventriculoperitoneal or ventriculoatrial shunts. It is also important to inquire about concurrent diseases such as immunodeficiency states including gammaglobulinopathies, chronic renal disease, leukemia, or other illnesses that require immunosuppressant therapy.

Physical Examination

The examination should document the initial hemodynamic and neurologic status of the child and provide possible information regarding etiology. Respiratory precautions should be employed throughout the initial evaluation. After obtaining vital signs, the skin should be examined for the presence of a petechial or maculopapular eruption or needle marks. The scalp must be inspected carefully to look for pustules or vesicles, insect bites, and ticks. Head and neck examination should include careful inspection of the tympanic membranes with pneumatic otoscopy and the presence of tenderness or inflammatory changes at the sinuses and mastoid processes. Neck stiffness should be assessed, including testing for both *Brudzinski's sign* (flexion of the neck causing involuntary flexion of the hips) and *Kernig's sign* (inability to extend the legs with the hips flexed). Auscultation of the chest should be performed to rule out pneumonitis (primary pneumonia or secondary aspiration pneumonia) and pathologic murmurs suggesting infective endocarditis. The extremities should be examined for possible metastatic infection such as septic arthritis or osteomyelitis. A neurologic examination should assess the level of consciousness, orientation, ability to follow commands, as well as motor strength and reflexes. The presence of possible cranial nerve paresis, particularly abducens (sixth cranial) nerve paralysis, should be assessed. Although papilledema is infrequent among patients with bacterial meningitis because of the rapidity of onset of their illness, funduscopic examination is important prior to performing a diagnostic lumbar puncture. The presence of focal neurologic deficits, together with papilledema, mandates immediate consultation with a neurologist or neurosurgeon and urgent cranial imaging studies *before* lumbar puncture.

TREATMENT

Appropriate antibiotic therapy should be initiated as soon as the diagnosis of bacterial meningitis is suspected (Table 153-1). If difficulty arises in performing the lumbar puncture, it is appropriate to administer antibiotic therapy promptly prior to a subsequent successful lumbar puncture, rather than to delay initial treatment for hours. Gram stain of the CSF will confirm the diagnosis of bacterial meningitis in the majority of instances, but empiric antibiotic therapy should be administered to all patients with compatible clinical illnesses and CSF findings while awaiting the results of CSF culture for 48 to 72 hours. Most patients with viral meningitis are less toxic in appearance than those with bacterial disease, have a typical lymphocyte-predominant CSF profile with normal glucose and normal or minimally elevated protein levels, and may be observed expectantly. However, in infants younger than 12 months of age, or in those children with low glucose or granulocyte-predominant pleocytosis in the CSF, it is appropriate to begin therapy for bacterial meningitis until final culture data are available.

Initial therapy is guided by the child's age and clinical findings as well as by the Gram stain and antigen detection results, based on the expected spectrum of pathogens. Newborns are generally treated with ampicillin and gentamicin, which provide synergistic bactericidal therapy against group B streptococci and *Listeria monocytogenes*. When the Gram

Table 153-1.   Antimicrobial Agents for Treatment of Meningitis

REGIMEN	NEWBORNS 0–7 Days of Age	NEWBORNS 8–28 Days of Age	INFANTS AND CHILDREN
	DAILY DOSE		
Penicillin G	100,000–150,000 U/kg/day ÷ q12h	150,000–200,000 U/kg/day ÷ q8 or q6h	250,000 U/kg/day ÷ q6 or q4h
Ampicillin	100–150 mg/kg/day ÷ q12h	150–200 mg/kg/day ÷ q8 or q6h	200–300 mg/kg/day ÷ q6h
Kanamycin	15–20 mg/kg/day ÷ q12h	20–30 mg/kg/day ÷ q8h	
Gentamicin*	5 mg/kg/day ÷ q12h	7.5 mg/kg/day ÷ q8h	
Tobramycin*	4 mg/kg/day ÷ q12h	6 mg/kg/day ÷ q8h	
Amikacin*	15–20 mg/kg/day ÷ q12h	20–30 mg/kg/day ÷ q8h	
Chloramphenicol*	25 mg/kg/day ÷ q12h	50 mg/kg/day ÷ q12h	75–100 mg/kg/day ÷ q6h
Cefotaxime	100 mg/kg/day ÷ q12h	150–200 mg/kg/day ÷ q8 or q6h	200 mg/kg/day ÷ q6h
Ticarcillin	150–225 mg/kg/day ÷ q12 or q8h	225–300 mg/kg/day ÷ q8 or q6h	
Methicillin	100–150 mg/kg/day ÷ q12 or q8h	150–200 mg/kg/day ÷ q8 or q6h	
Oxacillin	100–150 mg/kg/day ÷ q12 or q8h	150–200 mg/kg/day ÷ q8 or q6h	
Nafcillin	100–150 mg/kg/day ÷ q12 or q8h	150–200 mg/kg/day ÷ q8 or q6h	
Vancomycin	20 mg/kg/day ÷ q12h	30 mg/kg/day ÷ q8h	40 mg/kg/day ÷ q6h
Ceftriaxone			100 mg/kg/day ÷ q12h
Ceftazidime	60 mg/kg/day ÷ q12h	90 mg/kg/day ÷ q8h	125–150 mg/kg/day ÷ q8h

*Serum concentrations should be monitored and dosages adjusted accordingly.
(Adapted from Klein JO, Feigin RD, McCracken GH Jr: Report of the Task Force on Diagnosis and Management of Meningitis. Pediatrics [Suppl] 78[5]: 971, 1986)

stain of the CSF reveals enteric gram-negative bacilli, ampicillin and a third-generation cephalosporin such as cefotaxime may be considered. Although the latter agent is remarkably potent, has a broad spectrum of activity, and achieves excellent levels in the CSF, the outcome of infants with gram-negative bacillary meningitis treated with third-generation cephalosporins has not been shown to be superior to conventional treatment with aminoglycosides. However, cephalosporin therapy has the benefits of a favorable safety profile and does not require drug level monitoring. If the initial Gram stain is negative, either regimen is acceptable and may be revised once a pathogen is isolated and sensitivities are confirmed. Therapy in neonatal meningitis is usually maintained for 3 weeks because of a significant rate of relapse observed after briefer courses of therapy. Gentamicin is usually stopped after several days of synergistic therapy in streptococcal or listerial disease unless the group B streptococci demonstrate "tolerance" (i.e., a resistance to the bactericidal activity of penicillin).

Bacterial meningitis in older infants and children has traditionally been treated with ampicillin and chloramphenicol. However, the third-generation cephalosporins such as cefotaxime and ceftriaxone provide effective monotherapy with improved patient tolerance, and the long half-life of ceftriaxone has facilitated every-12-hour therapy for bacterial meningitis.

Meningococcal meningitis is usually treated for 7 days, *H. influenzae* disease for 7 to 10 days, and pneumococcal meningitis for 10 to 14 days. In part, the extended therapy for pneumococcal meningitis is based on the frequent presence of a parameningeal focus of infection such as sinusitis, which requires extended therapy.

A history of late morbilliform rash as an adverse effect of penicillin therapy does not preclude cephalosporin therapy, but a history of immediate hypersensitivity to β-lactams necessitates the use of chloramphenicol or (rarely) desensitization to a β-lactam agent. Recent clinical studies have shown that the administration of dexamethasone, 0.15 mg/kg/q6h, for the first 4 days of therapy beginning with the first dose of antibiotic therapy may reduce the risk of sensorineural hearing loss and is gaining increasing acceptance among clinicians.

Ancillary measures are important as well. Patients with bacterial meningitis are initially treated in the intensive care unit. Those patients with meningitis due to *H. influenzae* type b or *N. meningitidis* and those patients with purulent meningitis due to an as yet unknown pathogen are managed with respiratory precautions for the first 24 hours of therapy. The airway should be protected if the child is obtunded and the gag reflex depressed. In an attempt to control possible cerebral edema, fluids are restricted to two thirds of calculated needs for the first 48 hours, and the patient's neurologic status is monitored frequently. In infants, the head circumference should be measured daily to detect the development of hydrocephalus and/or subdural effusions. Increasing head circumference should be monitored by ultrasound examination or computed tomography. For the first 48 to 72 hours required fluids are administered parenterally to minimize the risk of aspiration. Since meningococcal and *H. influenzae* meningitis have a significant risk of secondary spread within households, rifampin prophylaxis should be administered to household contacts at the time of diagnosis. The index patient should receive prophylaxis at the completion of parenteral therapy. See Chap. 199 for a detailed discussion on prophylaxis.

INDICATIONS FOR REFERRAL

Although antibiotic failure leading to recrudescence or relapse is quite rare, persistent fever is common, especially with *H. influenzae* type b meningitis. In such cases, management must be individualized but possible drug fever, metastatic infection, intracranial complications including subdural effusion or even subdural empyema, extracranial secondary infections such as pneumonia, urinary infection, intravenous catheter-associated bacteremia, and noninfectious processes such as phlebitis must be considered. Repeat lumbar puncture, appropriate imaging studies, and change of antibiotic therapy to chloramphenicol instead of a β-lactam agent may be appropriate. Evaluation by an infectious disease consultant is often helpful, and the presence of extensive subdural collections in the presence of persistent fever or obtundation should be evaluated by a neurosurgical consultant. In occasional cases of meningitis, drainage of a sinus or otitic parameningeal focus of infection may be necessary, requiring consultation with an otolaryngologist.

PROGNOSIS

Up to 30% of newborns develop postinfectious hydrocephalus. There is a increased risk of neurologic deficits and seizure disorders especially in newborns, but also in older children. Children with bacterial meningitis are at risk for mental retardation and learning disabilities. Since as many as 20% of children develop an auditory nerve dysfunction, an auditory evaluation (brain stem evoked response or audiogram) should be obtained either prior to or shortly after hospital discharge. The prognosis of children who have viral (aseptic) meningitis is considerably more favorable, although seizures, learning, and behavioral disorders may occur afterward, especially when enteroviral meningitis develops in infants.

ANNOTATED BIBLIOGRAPHY

Converse GM, Gwaltney JM Jr, Strassburg DA, Hendley JO: Alteration of cerebrospinal fluid findings by partial treatment of bacterial meningitis. J Pediatr 83:220–225, 1973. (Most patients with acute bacterial meningitis who received antibiotics prior to lumbar puncture retained the typical cerebrospinal fluid features of bacterial meningitis, but occasional patients may have significant alterations in one or more cerebrospinal fluid parameters.)

Donat JF, Rhodes KH, Groover RV, et al: Etiology and outcome in 42 children with acute nonbacterial meningoencephalitis. Mayo Clin Proc 55:156–160, 1980. (Prospective study with follow-up to 1 year: 19 cases of California and 8 cases of enterovirus disease were identified by counterimmunoelectrophoresis and culture, and morbidity and mortality occurred in approximately one half of the cases.)

Haslam RHA: Role of computed tomography in the early management of bacterial meningitis. J Pediatr 119:157–159, 1991. (Review of appropriateness of CT scanning in patients with acute meningitis.)

Klein JO, Feigin RD, McCracken GH: Report of the Task Force on Diagnosis and Management of Meningitis. Pediatrics 78(Suppl): 959–982, 1986. (Good reference for the office-based pediatrician.)

Lebel MH, Freij BJ, Syrogiannopoulos GA et al: Dexamethasone therapy for bacterial meningitis: Results of two double-blind, placebo-controlled trials. N Engl J Med 319:964–971, 1988. (Two large prospective, double-blind, placebo-controlled trials demonstrated that dexamethasone therapy in childhood bacterial meningitis hastens normalization of cerebrospinal fluid abnormalities and reduces the incidence of sensorineural hearing loss.)

Lin T, Nelson JD, McCracken GH Jr: Fever during treatment for bacterial meningitis. Pediatr Infect Dis 3:319–322, 1984. (Fever often persists despite successful medical therapy of childhood meningitis, especially with *H. influenzae* type b. Drug fever, metastatic infection, and subdural effusions were generally associated with prolonged fever. Secondary fevers were associated with nosocomial infections or subdural effusions.)

Nadol JB: Hearing loss of sequelae of meningitis. Laryngoscope 88:739–755, 1978. (Retrospective study of 547 patients with meningitis: 235 bacterial, 304 viral; 21% had sensorineural hearing loss during acute and recuperative stages, and permanent hearing loss did not occur in children with aseptic meningitis.)

Odio CM, Faingezicht I, Paris M et al: The beneficial effects of early dexamethasone administration in infants and children with bacterial meningitis. N Engl J Med 324:1525–1531, 1991. (Dexamethasone therapy was associated with improvement in cerebrospinal fluid pressure, levels of inflammatory cytokines, clinical status, and improved neurologic and audiologic outcomes in children with bacterial meningitis.)

Pomeroy SL, Holmes SJ, Dodge PR, Feigin RD: Seizures and other neurologic sequelae of bacterial meningitis in children. N Engl J Med 323:1651–1657, 1990. (Review of risks for epilepsy in a prospective study of 185 infants and children with acute bacterial meningoencephalitis who were followed for a mean of 8.9 years.)

Schaad UB, Nelson JD, McCracken GH Jr: Recrudescence and relapse in bacterial meningitis of childhood. Pediatrics 67:188–195, 1981. (Antibiotic failures in childhood meningitis are rare [<1% of cases] and are limited to infants younger than 2 years of age. Cerebrospinal fluid findings and fever course were not predictive of failure. Routine test-of-cure lumbar punctures are not necessary.)

Taylor HG, Mills EL, Ciampi A et al: The sequelae of *Haemophilus influenzae* meningitis in school-age children. N Engl J Med 323:1657–1663, 1990. (Retrospective study of 97 of 519 children treated for *H. influenzae* meningitis at mean age of 17 months; relatively few children had persistent neurologic problems.)

154

Cerebral Palsy

Margaret L. Bauman

Cerebral palsy is a term used to define a group of nonprogressive neuromotor disorders of central nervous system (CNS) origin that become apparent during development and probably result from multiple causes. The incidence of these disorders is estimated to be 1.5 to 5.0 per 1000 live births, with a prevalence of approximately 400,000 living affected children in the United States. It is believed that cerebral palsy affects at least 1 of 500 school-aged children and is one of the major handicapping conditions of childhood.

PATHOGENESIS

In 1862, William J. Little first described what is now believed to be the spastic form of cerebral palsy and was convinced that its cause was birth related. Most modern hypotheses pertaining to cerebral palsy continue to place the major blame for these disorders on birth trauma and problems of delivery. In all likelihood, multiple factors contribute to their development.

Evidence from recent retrospective and prospective studies indicates that prenatal factors probably contribute to at least 50% of the cases of cerebral palsy. Evaluation of these children has revealed such risk factors as maternal mental retardation, third-trimester proteinuria, siblings with cerebral palsy, the administration of thyroid hormone or estrogen during pregnancy, congenital malformation of the CNS and/or other body organs, recognizable syndromes, third-trimester bleeding, and multiple dysmorphic features unassociated with a recognizable syndrome. Many of these children have been small for gestational age at the time of delivery, with all forms of cerebral palsy being represented in this group.

Evidence for a perinatal cause is found in approximately one third of the children with cerebral palsy. Risk factors in this group include perinatal asphyxia, cardiorespiratory arrest, and intraventricular hemorrhage. Many of these children include infants who were small for gestational age or who were premature (<2500 grams). Low birth weight appears to be one of the major risk factors and may contribute to as many as 30% to 40% of the children who are later diagnosed as having spastic diplegia. Full-term infants whose birth has been complicated but who are asymptomatic in the newborn period have shown no increased risk of developing cerebral palsy. A careful review of perinatal events suggests that only approximately 6% of birth-related factors could be considered preventable. These preventable events include asphyxia secondary to breech delivery and placenta previa.

Postnatal causes for cerebral palsy can be found in about 10% of the cases and generally include events occurring after the seventh day of life. Risk factors in this group include head trauma largely secondary to child abuse, meningitis, anoxia related to aborted sudden infant death syndrome (SIDS), and disorders leading to acute infantile hemiplegia. It is estimated that approximately one third of the children who later present with hemiplegia are in this etiologic category. Other possible risk factors for the development of later cerebral palsy include the presence of seizures within the first year of life and neonatal seizures in conjunction with a low Apgar score and abnormal neonatal signs.

Thus, it is probable that one or more of multiple processes may occur to produce a child with cerebral palsy and that our ability to reliably predict which children may be at particularly high risk in any individual circumstance is poor.

CLINICAL PRESENTATION

Much of the difficulty encountered in understanding the causes and outcome of cerebral palsy relates to inconsistencies in definition and terminology. A functionally oriented classification was prepared by Vining and colleagues in 1976 (see bibliography) and has been used subsequently by most authors, thus improving communication and discussion among researchers and clinicians. Topographic patterns of motor dysfunction have been found to be useful in designating the spastic forms of cerebral palsy and include the following:

- *Hemiplegia:* spasticity involving two limbs on the same side of the body
- *Double hemiplegia:* spasticity involving all four extremities with the upper limbs being predominantly affected
- *Quadriplegia:* spasticity involving all four extremities, with the lower limbs being mildly more affected
- *Diplegia:* spasticity involving all four limbs, with the lower extremities being significantly more affected

Extrapyramidal forms of cerebral palsy have wide clinical variability. Hypertonicity, when present, tends to have the quality of rigidity rather than spasticity, showing a steady increase and decrease in flexion and extension, as opposed to the sense of "give" often seen in spasticity. Abnormal movements such as chorea, dystonic posturing, athetosis, and, uncommonly, tremor and ataxia are often reported. Facial grimacing, drooling, and dysarthria may also be present.

The diagnosis of cerebral palsy is primarily clinical, based largely on history and careful examination of the patient over a period of time. Its natural course is associated with the evolution of signs and symptoms so that reclassification as the child develops is often necessary, and "mixed" varieties are not uncommon.

Evaluation of the child with suspected cerebral palsy begins with careful review of the events relating to pregnancy, delivery, and the neonatal period. It is often helpful to review complete hospital records including obstetric records, delivery room and nursery records, as well as nurses' notes in all settings; potential risk factors should be sought. Information recalled by the parents as to the infant's behavior in the newborn period (e.g., abnormal levels of activity, unusual sleep patterns, feeding difficulties and hyperirritability) may provide early clues.

Frequently, the earliest parental concern relates to delayed motor development, such as failure to sit, crawl, stand, or walk at the expected time. Examination by the physician should include measurement of the child's length, weight, and head circumference, documentation of growth rate since birth, and scrutiny of dysmorphic features. Neurologic assessment may show increased or decreased muscle tone, exaggerated deep tendon reflexes (possibly associated with sustained clonus), asymmetry of motor activity in one or more limbs, or increased fisting of one or both hands in a child older than 3 months of age. Definite hand dominance noted prior to 12 months of age should lead to a suspicion of hemiparesis. Preferred toe-walking may be a sign of spasticity.

The persistence of primitive reflexes beyond their usual time of disappearance should be considered suspect. The tonic neck response should disappear by 4 months of age, and the Moro response should disappear by 6 months. An asymmetric Moro response at an earlier age may be an initial indication of hemiparesis.

In general, signs of choreoathetosis do not appear much before 12 to 18 months of age. Prior to this age, slow motor development, hypotonia, excessive drooling, and the retention of primitive reflexes may be noted. Additional clues may include the presence of opisthotonic posturing, poor suck reflex, difficulty chewing, and poor tongue control.

DIFFERENTIAL DIAGNOSIS

When a child younger than 12 to 18 months of age with motor developmental delay initially presents to the pediatrician, a wide variety of possible diagnoses are suggested. These include global nonspecific mental retardation; muscular weakness and hypotonia secondary to a myopathy or neuropathy; spinal cord abnormality secondary to injury, tumor, or congenital defect; abnormalities of the joints or tendons; inherited syndromes such as familial spastic paraplegia, some aminoacidemias, familial microcephaly, or one of the hereditary ataxias; other recognizable syndromes such as sporadic chromosomal defects or intracranial vascular malformations; possible degenerative disorders of the CNS; and maternal deprivation, malnutrition, or abuse. A definitive diagnosis may not be reached until the child has been repeatedly examined over a period of months and sometimes years and results of laboratory studies have ruled out other possibilities.

LABORATORY TESTS

The evaluation of the child with early motor developmental delay relies heavily on the obtaining of a good birth and developmental history and multiple physical and neurologic examinations over time. Laboratory studies may be useful in determining the possible causes of the child's motor disability. The appearance of dysmorphic features may suggest the need for chromosomal analysis. The presence of weakness and hypotonia may lead to evaluating thyroid function and nutritional status, obtaining serum muscle enzymes, serum iron, electromyography, nerve conduction studies, and occasionally muscle biopsy. Determination of serum and urine amino acid levels and urine studies for evaluation of organic acids may also be considered. If the lower extremities are primarily involved, roentgenograms of the spine should be performed. A skeletal survey may be useful if child abuse is suspected. Computed tomography (CT) or magnetic resonance imaging (MRI) may be useful in delineating hydrocephalus, porencephaly, subdural hematoma, leukodystrophy, or CNS or spinal cord vascular abnormality or tumor or in demonstrating evidence of intracranial calcification suggestive of possible cytomegalic inclusion disease, toxoplasmosis, or tuberous sclerosis.

Computed tomography findings in cerebral palsy may also be useful in suggesting the underlying neuropathogenetic events that resulted in the presenting clinical picture (e.g., central atrophy with ventricular enlargement). Infarction and hemiatrophy are significantly more frequent in patients with hemiplegia than those with other types of cerebral palsy.

Ultrasound examination of the CNS has also been reported. Findings delineated in children with cerebral palsy using this technique have included diffuse bilateral multiple periventricular cysts, bilateral asymmetric dilatation of the lateral ventricles following grade III intraventricular hemorrhage, and ventricular porencephaly following ipsilateral grade IV intracranial hemorrhage. The presence of moderate to severe periventricular echodensities with large cyst formation is a highly specific and sensitive predictor for the development of cerebral palsy in premature infants, regardless of the presence or absence of intracranial hemorrhage.

TREATMENT

By nature of the wide spectrum of handicaps with which the child with cerebral palsy presents, a multidisciplinary approach to therapy is needed. If available, the child should be referred to a *multidisciplinary clinic* where further diagnostic evaluation of the child's abilities and disabilities can be fully evaluated by a interdisciplinary team and a unified approach to therapy can be provided.

If the child is younger than 2 years of age, the most

obvious disability is usually a motor handicap, and evaluation and intervention by a *pediatric physical therapist* should be initiated as soon as the handicapping condition is identified. In some localities this service can be provided in the home for very young children; in other areas the child must attend a center-based facility. The aim of this therapy initially is to improve function in both upper and lower extremities, posture, and locomotion and to prevent contractures. To maximize the usefulness of the therapy, some exercises are taught to the parents that can be altered by the therapist as the child's condition evolves and needs change. The physical therapist also plays an important role in assisting with adaptive equipment for home and school use and in working closely with the orthopedic surgeon.

The *pediatric occupational therapist* generally works toward the improvement of function in the upper extremities, particularly as it relates to play skills and self-help skills such as feeding and dressing. The therapist may work on improved head and trunk control, adaptive toys, equipment, and clothing and, later, on modified equipment for school use.

Frequently, the *speech and language pathologist* will become involved in the therapy of the child with cerebral palsy when it becomes apparent that the function of the oral-motor musculature is poor and leads to difficulties with chewing, swallowing, and articulation. In addition, the child may exhibit delays in the ability to understand and express language, necessitating early intervention. Occasionally, alternative means of communication may need to be considered, usually in conjunction with the other therapists and physicians, such as the use of sign language, a communication board or book, and/or an adapted typewriter or computer.

Fifty to 70% of the children with cerebral palsy will show some intellectual impairment. This defect, combined with other handicapping conditions, necessitates the need for an educational program designed to meet the needs of the child while furthering independence, social and emotional growth, as well as academic and eventually vocational achievement.

Medically, the child will need to be evaluated by an ophthalmologist and audiologist to ensure adequate vision and hearing. Since it has been estimated that 30% to 60% of the cerebral palsy population has seizures, management and good seizure control become a major factor in the child's care and ability to function adequately. In some centers, medications are used to alter muscular tone and improve the ease of therapy and motor function. Dantrolene sodium has been used in both athetoid and spastic children; its use as a muscle relaxant appears to be helpful in approximately 50% of the cases. However, diazepam and lorazepam have been more widely used in both athetosis and severe spasticity.

Although oral baclofen has been generally ineffective in relieving spasticity, one study has shown that a single dose injection of intrathecal baclofen relieved spasticity, primarily in the lower extremities. Further studies are warranted,

with consideration of a trial of continuous infusion of baclofen using a programmable subcutaneous pump to provide more long-term relief.

Surgical procedures may be an important addition to the habilitation of the child with cerebral palsy. The purpose of orthopedic surgical intervention is to improve function, facilitate daily care, provide cosmetic improvement, and prevent deformity. Careful selection of patients for surgery as well as evaluation of the child's existing functions will increase the possibility of a beneficial outcome and prevent unnecessary or unsuccessful surgical intervention. Long-term results are variable and often depend on postoperative rehabilitation efforts.

In recent years, selective posterior rhizotomy, a neurosurgical procedure first used nearly 100 years ago, has become popular as an intervention designed to reduce spasticity. Briefly, the technique involves an L2–L5 laminectomy, followed by the division of selected posterior spinal rootlets, determined by electromyographic analysis. Most reports emphasize the importance of careful patient selection and the need for postoperative physical and occupational therapy to achieve a positive outcome. However, given the concern that the efficacy of the procedure has yet to be proven, further objective assessment of its effectiveness with carefully controlled studies is indicated.

ANNOTATED BIBLIOGRAPHY

Albright AL, Cervi A, Singletary J: Intrathecal baclofen for spasticity in cerebral palsy. JAMA 265:1418–1422, 1991. (Intrathecal baclofen may be an effective treatment for spasticity in children with cerebral palsy; it was effective in 13 of 17 children studied.)

Bennett FC, Chandler LS, Robinson NM et al: Spastic diplegia in premature infants. Am J Dis Child 135:732–737, 1981. (Prematurity carries a significant risk of cerebral palsy.)

Ellenberg JH, Nelson KB: Cluster of perinatal events identifying infants at high risk for death or disability. J Pediatr 113:546–552, 1988. (Full-term infants are at increased risk of cerebral palsy if clusters of symptoms, including seizures, are noted in the neonatal period.)

Freeman J et al: National Institutes of Health report on causes of mental retardation and cerebral palsy. Pediatrics 76:457–458, 1985. (Little is certain about the prenatal and perinatal causes of most cases of cerebral palsy.)

Landau WH, Hunt CC: Dorsal rhizotomy: A treatment of unproven efficacy. J Child Neurol 5:174–178, 1990. (Recommendation for further careful analysis of the efficacy of posterior rhizotomy.)

Lord J: Cerebral palsy: A clinical approach. Arch Phys Med Rehabil 65:542–548, 1984. (Discussion of diagnostic and therapeutic approaches to the child with cerebral palsy.)

Nelson KB, Ellenberg JH: Antecedents of cerebral palsy. N Engl J Med 315:81–86, 1986. (The cause of cerebral palsy is probably not known.)

Paneth N: Birth and the origins of cerebral palsy. N Engl J Med 315:124–126, 1986. (Birth asphyxia does not appear to play a central role as the cause of cerebral palsy.)

Peacock WJ, Staudt LA: Spasticity in cerebral palsy and the selective posterior rhizotomy procedure. J Child Neurol 5:179–185, 1990. (Review of the current status of posterior rhizotomy and its effectiveness in the management of spasticity.)

Pidcock FS, Graziani LJ, Stanley C et al: Neurosomographic features of periventricular echodensities associated with cerebral palsy in preterm infants. J Pediatr 116:417–422, 1990. (Discussion of abnormalities in cranial ultrasound that reliably correlate with the subsequent development of cerebral palsies with 90% accuracy.)

Torfs CP, VandenBerg BJ, Oechsli FW et al: Prenatal and perinatal factors in the etiology of cerebral palsy. J Pediatr 116:615–619, 1990. (Discussion of prenatal and perinatal risk factors is a large cohort of infants followed over a 5-year period.)

Vining EPG, Accardo PJ, Rubenstein JE et al: Cerebral palsy. Am J Dis Child 130:643–649, 1976. (Discussion of classification of the cerebral palsy disorders and a therapeutic approach to the patient.)

155

Febrile Seizures

Eileen M. Ouellette

Febrile seizures are convulsions that typically occur between 6 months and 5 years of age, in the context of a febrile illness, without evidence of intracranial infection or other defined cause. It is estimated that 500,000 children in the United States have had febrile seizures. By 5 years of age, 2% to 4.2% of children have had febrile seizures. Although most studies report that boys have a higher incidence of febrile seizures than girls, two longitudinal studies have reported no sex differences.

Younger children are more likely to have a febrile seizure: 1% to 2% are younger than 6 months of age; 50% are younger than 2 years of age; and 90% are younger than 3 years of age at the time of the first febrile seizure. One to 6% of first febrile seizures occur after 5 years of age. There is often a positive family history of febrile seizures. A simple autosomal dominant inheritance with incomplete penetrance is postulated as the form of transmission.

PATHOPHYSIOLOGY

The control of body heat depends on the integrity of the anterior hypothalamus and preoptic area, which contains temperature-sensitive neurons. With infection, bacterial products, known as exogenous pyrogens, activate phagocytic leukocytes. When released into the bloodstream and cerebral ventricular system, they exert an effect on the anterior hypothalamus that results in fever. Interactions between viruses and monocytes also result in the release of exogenous pyrogens. Exogenous pyrogens are a variety of chemicals that act as mediator substances in the production

of fever, and they are not believed to be normal products of thermal regulation (see also Chap. 183).

Neurotransmitters of the cholinergic and monoaminergic systems are also important in temperature regulation. In addition, the fever process is mediated in part by the release of a prostaglandin of the E series in the brain. Seizures are believed to be produced by the effects of neurochemicals involved in the production of fever acting on other parts of the brain; however, evidence for this hypothesis is lacking.

CLINICAL PRESENTATION

The source of the fever must lie outside the central nervous system (CNS) for a seizure to be classified as a febrile seizure. Therefore, seizures in children with meningitis, encephalitis, or lead encephalopathy or associated with marked dehydration are not considered febrile seizures, although a fever may be present.

Febrile seizures are of two types. *Simple febrile seizures* are brief, last less than 15 minutes, and are generalized. Only one seizure occurs with each febrile illness. *Complex febrile seizures* are prolonged, focal, or multiple within each febrile episode. Most febrile seizures occur early in the febrile illness and are often the first sign that a child is ill. They occur generally within the first 6 hours and rarely occur later than 24 hours after the onset of fever.

Most febrile seizures are simple and brief. Forty percent last less than 5 minutes; 75% last under 30 minutes; only 2% last more than 1 hour. Seizures that last longer than 30 minutes are called *febrile status epilepticus,* and they carry the same risks as afebrile status epilepticus. The peak age for a first febrile seizure is 13 months. The overall recurrence rate is 33%, but it is higher if the first seizure occurs before 13 months of age. Prolonged seizures are more common in children younger than 18 months of age and in girls. About 15% are focal, and 16% of children have more than one seizure in 24 hours.

Many children experience a postictal state of obtundation or sleep for several hours after a seizure. Focal signs, such as hyperreflexia or an extensor plantar response, may be present.

DIFFERENTIAL DIAGNOSIS

Two considerations are important in the differential diagnosis of febrile seizures: (1) to exclude disease of the CNS as a cause of the seizure and (2) to determine the cause of the fever.

Bacterial and viral meningitis, encephalitis, Reye syndrome, acute hemiplegia of infancy, and intracranial hemorrhage are all acute disorders of the CNS that may present as fever and seizures. More chronic diseases of the CNS may manifest initially as a seizure in the context of a febrile illness. These diseases include hypoxic ischemic encephalopathy, congenital infections such as cytomegalovirus infection and toxoplasmosis, chronic subdural effusions, tuberous sclerosis, porencephaly, and other developmental defects of the brain.

Most febrile seizures are associated with common infections of childhood: pharyngitis, otitis media, tonsillitis, and diarrhea. Bronchitis, pneumonia, and pyuria are less common but are also associated with febrile seizures. Fifteen percent of children with pyuria younger than 5 years of age have febrile seizures. Metabolic disorders, which include hypoglycemia, hypocalcemia, hyponatremia, other electrolyte disturbances, and renal disease, must also be considered. Roseola and *Shigella* infections have a particularly high association with febrile seizures, probably as a result of the very high fevers that occur with roseola and secondary to an endotoxin associated with *Shigella* infections.

WORK-UP

History

Historical information should include a description of the seizure type, duration, and possible focal component. Parents generally find seizures frightening and tend to overestimate their duration. Many parents also include the postictal state in their timing of the seizure; therefore, specific questions about the actual events witnessed are important. Many parents do not witness the onset of the seizure; thus, the presence of a focal component cannot be firmly established. A history of the pregnancy and perinatal period and a developmental history of the child should be obtained to assess whether a prior neurologic abnormality was present. A history of possible trauma should be sought. A family history of seizures, both febrile and afebrile, should also be obtained.

Physical Examination

A complete general physical and neurologic examination should be performed. Signs of increased intracranial pressure should be sought by an evaluation of the level of alertness, a funduscopic examination, and the fullness of the fontanelle, when appropriate. Nuchal rigidity may indicate meningitis or intracranial hemorrhage, but its absence does not preclude these diagnoses, particularly in children younger than 2 years of age. Focal neurologic signs should be noted. Cranial auscultation for bruits is important in diagnosing vascular malformations. In infants, transillumination of the skull may lead to the diagnosis of chronic subdural effusions, porencephaly, or other brain malformations. The skin should be examined by observation and by Wood's lamp examination for the presence of hypopigmented "ash-leaf spots" seen in tuberous sclerosis.

Laboratory Tests

Cerebrospinal fluid (CSF) should be examined at the time of the first febrile seizure and whenever meningitis cannot

be ruled out, particularly in children younger than 2 years of age. In one study, 13% of 325 children with meningitis lacked meningeal signs, 50% of whom were found to have bacterial meningitis. Some children were older than 2 years old. CSF pressure should be recorded and the fluid should be examined for bacteria, the number and types of cells, and the protein and glucose levels. Bacterial cultures of CSF should be obtained.

A simultaneous blood glucose level should be obtained. CSF glucose should be one half to two thirds of blood glucose. Lower levels suggest meningitis or encephalitis. A white blood cell count and a differential count should be obtained. In the highly febrile child without a known source of the fever, blood cultures, urinalysis, and urine culture should also be obtained to determine the etiology of the fever. Serum calcium and electrolyte values are often determined, but this is probably not cost effective because of their low yield, particularly if the sample is drawn without a specific indication, such as dehydration. Liver function tests should be performed and blood ammonia levels should be obtained when Reye syndrome is a possibility.

Computed tomography or magnetic resonance imaging of the brain need not be routinely obtained. These scans may be indicated in the presence of increased intracranial pressure, focal symptoms or signs, a history of trauma, an abnormal neurologic examination, or persistent seizures.

Electroencephalograms (EEG) obtained during the acute febrile illness are often abnormal and are generally not helpful when performed then. Either a fever or a seizure may produce slowing of the EEG for up to 10 days. Asymmetric or focal slowing may be present in the absence of a focal component to the seizure and is of little diagnostic or prognostic value. The EEG generally returns to normal 10 days after a simple febrile seizure. Persistent slowing beyond that time may be helpful in distinguishing simple from complex febrile seizures when the history is not clear or when the seizure was not witnessed.

TREATMENT

Acute treatment consists of a reduction of fever, treatment of the underlying cause of the fever, and treatment of the seizure(s). Elevated temperatures can be reduced by antipyretics and sponging. The cause of the fever should be treated appropriately. During the seizure, an adequate airway must be maintained and the child should be placed in a semiprone position to reduce the risk of aspiration.

Acute anticonvulsant therapy should be given intravenously to a child who is actively experiencing a seizure. Phenobarbital up to 15 mg/kg can be given slowly by intravenous drip. An alternative regimen is to give diazepam, 0.3 mg/kg, at a rate of 1 mg/min, or lorazepam, 0.05 to 0.1 mg/kg, slowly intravenously. No more than 1 to 2 mg of Valium or ½ to 1 mg of Ativan should be given to children less than 2 years of age. Phenobarbital has the added advantage of having an antipyretic effect. Diazepam and phenobarbital should not be routinely used together parenterally because respiratory arrest may occur.

Long-term management of a single or even several simple febrile seizures with continuous or intermittent anticonvulsant therapy is no longer advocated. Patients who have febrile seizures longer than 15 minutes, or who have other risk factors, may be candidates for long-term therapy. Treatment is generally given for 2 years or 1 year after the last seizure, whichever is longer.

Phenytoin has been demonstrated to be ineffective in the prevention of recurrence of febrile seizures. Controversy exists as to whether the risk of recurrence of febrile seizures can be lessened by long-term continuous treatment with phenobarbital and whether phenobarbital has an adverse effect on cognition. Phenobarbital is known to produce behavioral changes in a significant number of children. Because of the high risk of idiosyncratic hepatoxicity in children younger than the age of 2 years, the use of valproate is not recommended in this age group. These factors must be considered when assessing patients for long-term therapy.

The frequency of recurrent febrile seizures may be reduced with the prompt rectal use of diazepam at the onset of a febrile illness. Intermittent use of oral phenobarbital, however, has been shown to be ineffective in preventing febrile seizures because therapeutic levels of the drug are not achieved by this route for several days. An important preventive measure is to initiate prompt and vigorous fever control with antipyretics and sponging (see Chap. 183).

The prognosis for children with febrile seizures varies with the type of seizure and with the previous state of the child. Normal children with no history of febrile seizures have a risk of 0.9% of developing epilepsy by 7 years of age. Previously normal children with a simple febrile seizure have a 1.1% to 2% risk of developing afebrile seizures by that age. If the seizure was complex, the risk is 1.7% to 3.5%. Children with a prior neurologic abnormality have a 2.8% to 3.1% risk of developing epilepsy by 7 years of age following simple febrile seizures and a 9.2% to 12.3% risk if the febrile seizure was complex.

INDICATIONS FOR REFERRAL OR ADMISSION

Children in whom CNS disorders cannot be excluded should be hospitalized. Children who have complex febrile seizures should generally be admitted to the hospital to facilitate their evaluation and treatment. Children who have simple febrile seizures, whose cause of fever has been established, and who have families who are competent to care for their illness need not be hospitalized.

A consultation with a pediatric neurologist may be indicated for children who have abnormal neurologic examinations or when questions arise regarding diagnosis and treatment, particularly with reference to possible involvement of the CNS.

ANNOTATED BIBLIOGRAPHY

Consensus Statement, Conference on Febrile Seizures, NIH. Pediatrics 66:1009–1012, 1980. (Consensus statement of the significance, evaluation, and treatment of febrile seizures.)

Farwell JR, Young JL, Hirtz DG et al: Phenobarbital for febrile seizures: Effects on intelligence and on seizure recurrence. N Engl J Med 322:364–369, 1990. (Comparison of IQs and recurrent febrile seizure in patients who were treated with phenobarbital as compared with those who received no treatment.)

Nelson KB, Ellenberg JH: Predictors of epilepsy in children who have experienced febrile seizures. N Engl J Med 295:1029–1033, 1976. (Comprehensive review of 1706 children with febrile seizures registered in the Collaborative Perinatal Project between 1959 and 1966.)

Nelson KB, Ellenberg JH: Prognosis in children with febrile seizures. Pediatrics 61:720–726, 1978. (Frequency of adverse outcomes and risk factors in 1706 children with febrile seizures registered in the Collaborative Perinatal Project between 1959 and 1966.)

Ouellette EM: Febrile seizures. In Browne TR, Feldman RG (eds): Epilepsy Diagnosis and Management, pp 315–323. Boston, Little, Brown, & Co, 1983. (Comprehensive review of febrile seizures, their pathophysiology, types, management, and prognosis.)

Stores G: When does an EEG contribute to the management of febrile seizures? Arch Dis Child 66:554–557, 1991. (Thoughtful review of pros and cons of electroencephalograms in children who have febrile convulsions; the author does not recommend this test.)

Verity CM, Butler NR, Golding J: Febrile convulsions in a national cohort followed up from birth: I. Prevalence and recurrence in the first five years of life; II. Medical history and intellectual ability at 5 years of age. Br Med J 290:1307–1315, 1985. (Report of a series of 303 of 13,135 English children followed from birth to age 5 years.)

Wolf SM et al: The value of phenobarbital in the child who has had a single febrile seizure: A controlled prospective study. Pediatrics 59:378–385, 1977. (Comparison of daily, intermittent, and no long-term phenobarbital therapy on the recurrence rate of febrile seizures.)

156

Seizures and Epilepsy

Mohamad Mikati and Thomas R. Browne

A *seizure disorder* is a relatively nonspecific term that includes patients with any one of the following disorders: febrile seizures, epilepsy, single seizures, or seizures secondary to metabolic, infectious or other etiologies. *Epilepsy* is a chronic disorder in which seizures recur without any external cause. Thus, patients with single seizures, febrile seizures, or seizures secondary to metabolic disorders do not have epilepsy. An *epileptic syndrome* is a disorder that manifests the following: (1) one or more specific seizure types, (2) specific electroencephalographic (EEG) manifestations, (3) a specific age of onset, and (4) a relatively predictable clinical course and prognosis.

The modern approach to the diagnosis and management of epilepsy in children requires familiarity with the International League Against Epilepsy classification of epileptic seizures (1981) and its most recent revised classifications of epileptic syndromes (1989). The International Classification of Epileptic Seizures divides epileptic seizures into two major categories: partial seizures and generalized seizures. Partial seizures are seizures in which the first clinical and EEG changes suggest initial activation of a system of neurons limited to part of one cerebral hemisphere. Generalized seizures are those in which the first clinical and EEG changes indicate involvement of both hemispheres.

Simple partial seizures occur without impairment of consciousness and may involve one of the following: motor, sensory, autonomic, or psychic symptoms. *Complex partial seizures* impair consciousness. These seizures may occasionally start as simple partial seizures (an aura) and progress into complex partial seizures. Sometimes simple partial seizures and complex partial seizures may progress into secondarily generalized seizures.

In children, childhood absence epilepsy, epilepsy with grand mal seizures on awakening, West syndrome and Lennox-Gastaut syndrome are examples of generalized epilepsies. Partial epilepsies are represented by idiopathic partial epilepsies such as benign childhood epilepsy with centrotemporal spikes and by symptomatic localization-related epilepsies such as temporal lobe, frontal lobe, parietal lobe, and occipital lobe epilepsies.

PATHOPHYSIOLOGY

The final common pathway of many epileptic seizures is a sudden electrical depolarization of cortical neurons that is usually seen on the surface EEG as a negative spike. This is frequently followed by a sustained inhibitory hyperpolarization usually seen as a slow wave on the surface EEG. In certain types of seizures the discharges are believed to originate from single or multiple groups of *epileptic neurons*. If such a group of neurons is located in one of the cerebral hemispheres, the result is an epileptic focus with focal (partial) seizures. If, however, there is no primary unilateral epileptic focus and the epileptic discharge is manifested simultaneously in both hemispheres, a primarily generalized seizure results.

CLINICAL PRESENTATION

Generalized Epilepsies

Childhood Absence Epilepsy (Pyknolepsy, Petit Mal Epilepsy). This familial seizure disorder presents between the ages of 5 to 15 years with repeated episodes of unre-

sponsiveness. Typically, there is an abrupt interruption of activity with a blank stare with unresponsiveness lasting for a mean of 10 seconds that is followed by an immediate return of full consciousness and a resumption of previous activity without a postictal period. It is associated occasionally with repeated three-per-second (Hz) blinks or small clonic movements of the extremities. There may also be mild changes in tone (decrease or increase), automatisms (e.g., chewing), or autonomic changes. Absence status is rare, and, because it can manifest as a confusional state with or without blinking, it may be difficult to diagnose without the help of the EEG. The EEG of patients with absence status shows the typical generalized 3-Hz spike slow-wave discharges. In contrast to Lennox-Gastaut syndrome, the EEG background is typically normal. Approximately 30% of patients have a positive family history of absence seizures. Most children have normal intelligence and normal neurologic examinations, but they may have significant problems in maintaining attention. Prior neurologic damage and, rarely, brain tumors, may coexist with the absence seizures. These, however, are believed to act as triggers of the seizures rather than as primary etiologic agents. Approximately 50% of patients with absence seizures also manifest generalized tonic-clonic seizures. These patients generally have a less favorable prognosis than those with absence seizures alone. Ninety percent of the patients with normal IQs, no tonic-clonic seizures, and a negative family history of seizure disorder outgrow their seizures completely. The overall remission rate, however, is approximately 50%.

Tonic-Clonic (Grand Mal) Epilepsy. Generalized tonic-clonic seizures are the most common type of seizure in childhood and may begin at any age. Unlike adults, most children with this disorder have primary rather than secondary generalized seizures. These children frequently have a positive family history and may manifest other associated generalized seizure types such as absence seizures or myoclonic seizures. A typical generalized tonic-clonic seizure consists of an initial short cry followed by generalized stiffening of the body (tonic phase), falling down, suppression of respiration, and cyanosis. Biting of the tongue, frothing at the mouth, and vomiting may occur, and these are followed by repeated clonic jerks with intervening relaxation of muscles. This may last for a few minutes, and generalized hypotonia and incontinence of urine or stools may occur. A gradual return of consciousness with varying degrees of postictal confusion, exhaustion, or sleep ensues. At least 50% of the patients eventually experience remissions. The interictal EEG may be normal but typically shows bilaterally synchronous 2- to 6-Hz spike and slow-wave discharges. These frequently do not have the well-formed 3-Hz morphology of an absence seizure.

Based on the most recent International League Against Epilepsy Classification of Epileptic Syndromes, patients who manifest epilepsy with grand mal seizures may be divided into two categories. The first is the syndrome of epilepsy with grand mal seizures on awakening. The other category includes all other patients with generalized grand mal idiopathic epilepsy as described above. The epilepsy with grand seizures on awakening starts in the second decade of life and manifests exclusively, or predominantly, with seizures occurring shortly after awakening in the morning or after awakening at any time in the day. Many patients also have evening seizures at the time of relaxation. Sleep deprivation frequently precipitates the seizures, and the EEG shows one of the patterns of idiopathic generalized epilepsy. Many patients have EEG features of juvenile myoclonic epilepsy, and many manifest other seizure types seen in juvenile myoclonic epilepsy such as juvenile absence or juvenile myoclonic seizures.

Some generalized tonic-clonic seizures are secondary from specific unilateral seizure foci. The clinical symptoms are essentially similar except that they may be preceded by an aura that tends to localize the seizure focus. These seizures are more difficult to control than primarily generalized seizures and frequently occur in patients who also have simple or complex partial seizures.

Juvenile Myoclonic Epilepsy (Impulsive Petit Mal Epilepsy of Jantz).

This syndrome usually starts in adolescence with bilateral myoclonic jerks of the neck and shoulder muscles and with clonic-tonic-clonic seizures shortly after awakening. These patients show multiple-spike slow-wave discharges (4–6 HZ) on EEG. These discharges are frequently precipitated by photic stimulation. The patients have normal intelligence and normal results on neurologic examination. About 37% have associated juvenile absence seizures. Juvenile absence seizures should be distinguished from childhood absence by the age at onset (in teenage years rather than childhood) and by EEG criteria (4- to 6-Hz spike or polyspike wave discharges instead of the 3-Hz spike wave). Patients with juvenile myoclonic epilepsy respond well to treatment with valproate and usually have a good prognosis.

West Syndrome (Infantile Spasms, Salaam Seizures, Flexor Spasms).

This is an age-dependent seizure syndrome that presents between the ages of 2 months and 1 year. The seizures consist of sudden flexion of the extremities, head, and trunk that last usually for only a fraction of a second but rarely up to 1 minute. They frequently occur in clusters of 10 to 60 spasms. Extension spasms may also occur. Accompanying phenomena may include cries, laughs, smiles, autonomic dysfunction (e.g., flushing, sweating, and tachycardia), abnormal eye movements, and postictal exhaustion. Consciousness is not clearly impaired during the spasms. The disorder is relatively common and occurs in one of 4000 to 6000 births, with a male predominance of 2:1.

Patients who have infantile spasms are divided into two etiologic groups: the symptomatic group (80%) and the idiopathic group (20%). The symptomatic group includes pa-

tients with known causes for their seizures, such as prenatal infections, cerebral malformations, chromosomal abnormalities (e.g., trisomy 21), neonatal hypoglycemia or hypoxia, kernicterus, aminoacidopathies, organic acidurias, meningitis, encephalitis, hemorrhages, phakomatoses, lysosomal disorders, neuronal ceroid lipofuscinosis (NCL), mitochondrial disorders, and, rarely, Aicardi's syndrome. About 10% of the infants with infantile spasms have tuberous sclerosis. Patients in the idiopathic group generally present later and tend to do better than the symptomatic group. Up to 30% of these patients have a normal outcome, in contrast to the 10% of the symptomatic group. Untreated infantile spasms can subside within 1 to 4 years of onset but are usually replaced by other forms of seizures.

The EEG picture most frequently seen in infantile spasm is hypsarrhythmia, defined as high-voltage arrhythmic slow waves with multifocal spikes in waking and a burst suppression pattern in sleep. Clinical seizures are usually associated with synchronous slow waves followed by low-voltage fast activity (beta seizures).

Lennox-Gastaut Syndrome (Petit Mal Variant Epilepsy, Astatic or Astatic-Myoclonic Epilepsy, Minor Motor Seizure Syndrome).

This is a seizure syndrome that typically starts between 1 to 7 years of age and manifests the following: (1) atypical absence, myoclonic, tonic and atonic seizures in various combinations; (2) EEG findings of slow (1.5 to 2.5 Hz) spike wave discharges superimposed on an abnormal and slow background.

Unlike *typical absence seizures* (typical petit mal) that have less prominent changes in tone during their staring spells, patients who have Lennox-Gastaut syndrome have *atypical absence seizures* (petit mal variants) in which the staring and blinking episodes may be associated with pronounced tone changes, gradual rather than abrupt onset and resolution of the spells, and slow (1.5 to 2.5 Hz rather than 2.5 to 3.5 Hz) spike and slow-wave discharges. Atonic, tonic, or myoclonic seizures also occur independently. *Atonic seizures* include a loss of tone of the head (head drops) or of the whole body (drop attacks), which may result in limb or skull fractures and may therefore require protective helmets. *Tonic seizures* frequently occur in sleep. *Myoclonic seizures* may manifest as sudden generalized synchronous jerks (massive myoclonus), frequently preceding falls, or as asynchronous, arrhythmic, asymmetric involuntary jerks of various muscle groups (polymyoclonia). This latter form is frequently associated with CNS degenerative disease as the underlying cause of Lennox-Gastaut syndrome.

The etiology includes all the causes cited for infantile spasms. In addition, one third of the patients who develop Lennox-Gastaut syndrome have had infantile spasms. Children who have cerebral malformations, severe mental retardation, preceding CNS insults, or preceding infantile spasms have a poorer prognosis with persistent seizures and retardation. Patients who have no known etiology (approximately 30% of cases), minimal initial retardation, and late onset of the syndrome tend to have a better, although still a very guarded, prognosis.

Other Generalized Epilepsy Syndromes. There are several less common epilepsy syndromes that have become increasingly important in the past few years. *Benign neonatal familial convulsions* usually start during the second or third day of life, but several patients have seizures beyond the neonatal period or even into childhood. Inheritance is autosomal dominant, and the disorder is inherited on a gene located on the long arm of chromosome 20. The *early myoclonic encephalopathy* and *early infantile epileptic encephalopathy* with burst suppression are two syndromes that manifest with predominantly myoclonic (the former) or with tonic seizures (the later) in the first 2 months of life. Both syndromes usually have a very bad prognosis. The *severe infantile myoclonic encephalopathy* patients manifest focal febrile seizures in the first year of life followed by myoclonic seizures in the second year of life. These patients have a guarded prognosis. In contrast, patients with a *benign infantile myoclonic encephalopathy* usually present with myoclonic seizures in the first year of life. These patients have spike wave on their EEGs, but the background is otherwise normal. They have normal results of neurologic examinations and normal development and a favorable prognosis for seizure control.

The *"epilepsy with myoclonic astatic seizures"* and the *epilepsy with myoclonic absences* are two syndromes that start during childhood and have features similar to those of Lennox-Gastaut syndrome, but neither shows the usual EEG features of Lennox-Gastaut syndrome. Both have a guarded prognosis that is usually only slightly better than that of Lennox-Gastaut syndrome.

Partial Epilepsies

Localization related (partial) epilepsies are divided into idiopathic partial epilepsies and symptomatic partial epilepsies. The prototype for *idiopathic* partial epilepsies is benign childhood epilepsy with centrotemporal spikes. The *symptomatic* partial epilepsies usually occur because of specific focal brain lesions such as focal sclerosis, post-traumatic scarring, tumor, or arteriovenous malformation. They are distinguished by the location of the focal seizure focus. Hence, they are divided into temporal, parietal, frontal, and occipital lobe epilepsies. They also could be discussed in terms of whether the seizures are simple partial or complex partial.

Sylvian Seizures Syndrome (Benign Rolandic Epilepsy). This syndrome starts between the ages of 5 and 10 years and almost always disappears by the age of 15 years. A family history is frequently positive (15% of the siblings have the same syndrome). The seizures occur predominantly (75%) during sleep, usually in the early hours of the morning, and typically consist of an initial oral and perioral sensation with

speech arrest (when awake), salivation, and tonic or clonic movements of one side of the face and the limbs. A progression of the seizures into a full-blown generalized tonic-clonic seizure frequently occurs. The EEG shows frequent spike discharges of a characteristic morphology over one or both sylvian and rolandic areas (central, midtemporal). The EEG background is normal. These seizures often alternate sides over the course of the illness. Prognosis is excellent. Most of these children outgrow their seizures by puberty or shortly thereafter. The seizures are generally benign, and many authorities believe that treatment may not be necessary in many of these cases.

Childhood Epilepsy With Occipital Paroxysms. These patients have occipital spike waves on their EEG and are neurologically normal otherwise. Onset is in later childhood with frequent migraine headaches and complex partial seizures with visual aura. Response to medications is favorable. Prognosis is excellent since virtually all patients outgrow their seizures during their teenage years.

Simple Partial Seizures Syndrome (Focal Seizures). These seizures may be seen at any age and are restricted to one side of the body without impairment of consciousness. A motor seizure may sequentially involve the face, the arm, and then the leg (motor march, jacksonian seizure) or may involve one or more of these sites at the same time. Tonic and adversive movements can also occur. Postictal (Todd's) paralysis, for minutes and rarely hours, can occur after focal motor seizures. Simple partial seizures need not be motor. Sensory phenomena such as tingling sensation, olfactory, gustatory, and visual hallucinations (e.g., flashing lights in one visual field) as well as vertigo, psychic phenomena, and automatic behavior with preservation of consciousness can also occur. The location of the seizure focus determines the nature of the seizures observed. Prenatal infections, hypoxia, CNS malformation, Sturge-Weber syndrome, meningitis, cerebrovascular accidents, brain tumor, arteriovenous malformations, lead encephalopathy, and head trauma can all cause focal seizures. The prognosis of simple partial seizures is related to the etiology.

Partial Complex Seizures Syndrome. These seizures were previously called *temporal lobe* or *psychomotor seizures.* Although most complex partial seizures originate from the temporal lobe, it is now apparent that they can also originate from foci in other sites (e.g., the frontal or occipital lobes) and do not always have psychic or motor phenomena. They are distinguished from simple partial seizures by an impairment of consciousness. A typical attack may start with a motionless stare or with an aura (a simple partial seizure) that frequently gives a clue as to the site of the seizure focus (e.g., olfactory: temporal lobe; visual: occipital lobe). A "rising" uncomfortable abdominal sensation is probably the most common aura. The patient may have déjà-vu experiences, hallucinations, confusion, or fear. During the seizure the patient experiences impairment of consciousness and may have automatisms such as chewing, lip smacking, running in circles, fumbling with clothing, stereotyped speech, or, rarely, complex behavior like riding a bicycle. Pallor and tachycardia are common. Postictally, there is amnesia, frequent exhaustion, and a gradual return to full consciousness. Partial complex seizures can also be distinguished from absence seizures by the presence of an aura, by their more gradual onset, by the presence of a postictal period, and by their usually longer duration (more than 60 seconds). Automatisms can occur in both. The EEG is distinctive and shows focal spikes and sharp waves over the involved area. The causes of partial complex seizures are essentially the same as simple partial seizures. Personality and psychiatric disorders may coexist with partial complex seizures. Epidemiologic proof for such an association, however, is still lacking and in most, if not all, such cases the psychiatric disorder is independent of the seizure disorder and should be managed accordingly. Probably more than half of the patients with partial complex seizures continue to have seizures into adulthood.

Chronic Progressive Epilepsia Partialis Continua of Childhood (Kojewnikow Syndrome). This is a condition characterized by refractory partial seizures and/or focal myoclonus resistant to therapy. This may occur secondary to focal lesions (e.g., tumor, infarct, or cat-scratch fever encephalitis); mitochondrial encephalopathy; or chronic progressive idiopathic encephalitis with associated chronic slowly progressive hemiparesis on the side of the seizures (Rasmussen's syndrome).

DIFFERENTIAL DIAGNOSIS

Many disorders can mimic seizures. Vasovagal syncope, postural hypotension, and cardiac disrhythmias may produce a loss of consciousness followed by generalized tonic-clonic seizures due to brain hypoxia. These seizures do not necessarily imply the diagnosis of epilepsy. Breath-holding spells occur between the ages of 6 months and 6 years. These episodes often follow crying or minor painful stimuli (see Chap. 212). Narcolepsy may be misdiagnosed as a seizure disorder, and cataplexy can mimic atonic seizures. EEG (multiple sleep latency test) shows a disturbed sleep pattern with frequent rapid-eye-movement onset sleep periods in narcolepsy and cataplexy. A migraine may be episodic and may mimic focal sensory seizures (e.g., tingling sensations, flashing lights) or may present as a confusional state mimicking a partial complex status or an absence status. Apnea in the newborn, sleep apnea, and night terrors may be difficult to distinguish from nocturnal seizures and may require prolonged EEG recordings. Ketotic hypoglycemia (typically presenting between 1½ and 5 years of age), hypocalcemia, hypomagnesemia, and hyponatremia may also present as seizures. Infantile spasms are frequently initially misdiagnosed as spasms due to colic. Abdominal epilepsy (a rare form of partial seizures) can present as recurrent abdominal pain of unknown etiology. Pseudoseizures are seizure-like episodes of a nonorganic nature but with a normal EEG. Simultaneous monitoring with video and EEG recordings may be required to make the diagnosis. A complicating factor, however, is that many patients with pseudoseizures also have a real seizure disorder. Other disorders that can mimic or be misdiagnosed as epilepsy include spasmus nutans, benign paroxysmal vertigo, alternating hemiplegia of childhood, paroxysmal dystonia and choreoathetosis, tics, hyperactive startle response, shuddering attacks, sleep myoclonus and benign myoclonus of infancy.

WORK-UP

History

The history should identify the seizure type, its severity, and possibly its etiology. The age at onset is important because many seizure syndromes (e.g., infantile spasms) are age dependent. The presence of developmental delay should be investigated. If the child's development had always been delayed, a prenatal insult, a CNS malformation, or rarely a peroxisomal disorder (e.g., Zellweger syndrome) is suggested. A progressive loss of developmental milestones after an initial normal period suggests a progressive storage or degenerative disease. A detailed description of the seizures including the time of occurrence, precipitating factors, fever, the presence of aura, focal or generalized involvement of the body, cyanosis, incontinence, duration of the postictal period, frequency of the seizures and how they vary, whether there is more than one type of seizure, and associated sleep disturbances should all be documented. The physician should determine the presence or absence of prenatal distress or teratogenicity, perinatal anoxia or hemorrhage, hypoglycemia, meningitis, head trauma, and exposure to toxins and poisons, including lead encephalopathy. It is often problematic to establish which came first—the seizure or the head trauma.

A family history of seizures, febrile seizures, or degenerative storage diseases should be sought. The ethnic background is relevant because of the predisposition of certain storage diseases to specific groups (e.g., Tay-Sachs disease in Ashkenazi Jews). The social background is important in terms of assessing the ability of the family to cope with the diagnosis and to comply with the treatment. Special attention should be given to ruling out other entities that may mimic seizures (e.g., syncope, breath-holding spells, narcolepsy, febrile seizures, migraine, CNS infections, and pseudoseizures).

Physical Examination

A developmental assessment to determine the presence or absence of a developmental delay is important. The use of the Denver Developmental Scale or other screening tests is helpful. Macrocrania may suggest the diagnosis of hydrocephalus or other CNS disorders. Microcephaly may be primary or secondary to an early brain injury (e.g., perinatal hypoxia). In infants, transillumination of the head may suggest the presence of a porencephalic cyst.

Congenital malformations may suggest a chromosomal or malformation syndrome (e.g., trisomy 21). A hemifacial hemangioma may suggest Sturge-Weber syndrome, and café-au-lait spots (six or more measuring at least 1.5 cm in diameter) strongly suggest neurofibromatosis. Ash leaf spots, shagreen spots, and hypopigmented lesions (seen best with Wood's lamp) are associated with tuberous sclerosis. An intracranial bruit may signify an underlying arteriovenous malformation. A heart examination may reveal a cardiac etiology. An extremely elevated blood pressure may signify hypertensive encephalopathy. Organomegaly may suggest storage diseases such as Tay-Sachs disease.

A complete neurologic examination should be performed. Papilledema may suggest a brain tumor, and other funduscopic abnormalities (e.g., cherry-red spots) may indicate degenerative diseases. Lateralizing signs such as homonymous hemianopsia, unilateral facial weakness, hemiparesis, reflex asymmetry, facial asymmetry, limb and thumb asymmetry, or dystonia and Babinski's sign should be sought. Subtle hemiparesis may sometimes be uncovered by having the child perform rapid movements of the hand or hop on one foot. Hyperventilation in the office may precipitate an absence spell. In acute situations, signs of meningitis, head trauma, intracranial hemorrhage, increased intracranial pressure, and possible drug intoxication should be carefully sought.

LABORATORY TESTS

Following the child's first seizure, blood chemistries (e.g., glucose, electrolytes, calcium, magnesium, liver and kidney function tests) and a CT scan or magnetic resonance imaging (MRI) usually should be done. The CT scan should be contrast enhanced if a brain tumor or an arteriovenous malformation is suspected.

Magnetic resonance imaging scanning is usually superior to CT scan in detecting anatomical malformations or CNS tumors. However, it is less sensitive in detecting subtle calcification and bone pathology. MRI enhanced with the injection of gadopentate dimeglumine is safer than the contrast-enhanced CT scan but is rarely needed. MRI is a more prolonged procedure, more expensive, more difficult, and frequently necessitates significant sedation or even anesthesia. Additionally, it is contraindicated in patients with cardiac pacemakers and intracranial magnetic metal implants.

A spinal tap should be performed if encephalitis, meningitis, subarachnoid hemorrhage, or a degenerative storage disease is considered. The fundi should always be checked for papilledema before the tap because herniation can occur if increased intracranial pressure is present. A sleep-deprived EEG done in waking and sleep is essential. An EEG may need to be repeated because the initial EEG is occasionally normal in a patient with true epilepsy. Depending on the age, the type of seizures, and the clinical situation, an additional evaluation may include lead level, toxic screen, urine and serum amino acid chromatography, biotinidase deficiency screen, blood for lysosomal enzyme assays, an electroretinogram, skin biopsy to look for intracytoplasmic inclusions of neuronal ceroid lipofuscinosis, liver or muscle biopsy to look for Lafora bodies, porphyria screen, and karyotype.

TREATMENT

The child who has had a first seizure and who has a normal neurologic examination and a normal EEG may have a relatively low risk of recurrence of seizures, particularly if the seizure occurred in the context of an acute illness such as electrolyte imbalance, toxic encephalopathy, or recent head trauma. Because only a minority of these children have further seizures (20% to 30% if both EEG and neurologic examinations are normal versus 50% to 60% if either is abnormal) it may be appropriate to delay chronic antiepileptic treatment until the second seizure occurs. Most experts would initiate therapy if either the neurologic examination or the EEG is abnormal. Parents, however, should be informed of the risks and benefits of initiating or withholding treatment.

Drug treatment should be based on the type of seizure. Infantile spasms are probably best treated with nonsynthetic adrenocorticotropic hormone (ACTH). The dose may vary, but one regimen is 110 units/M^2/d for 3 weeks followed by 70 units/M^2/d for 2 weeks followed by 50 units/M^2/d on alternate days for 3 weeks. Side effects including hypertension, electrolyte imbalances, and infections should be carefully monitored. ACTH is generally believed to offer an added advantage over prednisone, other corticosteroids alone, or the more traditional antiepileptic drugs. There is frequently an amelioration of the seizures and the EEG. Most patients, however, have a poor prognosis despite ACTH.

In Lennox-Gastaut syndrome, which is one of the most difficult seizure syndromes to control, treatment may vary according to the preponderant type of seizures that the patient is manifesting. For tonic seizures, phenytoin with or without phenobarbital is effective and may also control the other types of seizures that the patient may have. For those patients with Lennox-Gastaut syndrome who have a preponderance of atypical absence, myoclonic, and atonic seizures, valproate or ethosuximide should be the first drugs to try.

Absence seizures are treated initially with ethosuximide, which is as effective as valproate but usually less toxic. Patients whose seizures are resistant to ethosuximide may still respond to valproate or to the combination of the two. Acetazolamide has probably fewer side effects and may be tried initially, but it has the least chance of controlling the seizures and its effects are often transitory. Other medications that could be used include clonazepam, methsuximide, trimethadione, and phensuximide. Benign myoclonic epilepsies are often best treated with valproate, particularly when patients have associated grand mal seizures.

Medications effective for partial, primary, and secondary generalized tonic-clonic seizures include carbamazepine, phenytoin, phenobarbital, valproate, and primidone. In children, definitive comparative studies of these medications are lacking. In adults with partial or secondarily generalized seizures, carbamazepine and phenytoin have been shown to be more effective than phenobarbital and primidone. Carbamazepine has not been approved by the Food and Drug Administration for use in children younger than 6 years of age, although there is a significant body of literature documenting its use in younger children. Phenytoin is approved for this age group but has frequent untoward cosmetic side effects (e.g., hirsutism, gingival hyperplasia).

It is reasonable to start treatment in all children younger than 1 year of age who have partial, primarily, or secondarily generalized seizures with phenobarbital because it has been the medication most used in this age group. If it is ineffective or if side effects (e.g., hyperactivity) prohibit its use, then alternative medications such as phenytoin should be used. In children older than 1 year, it is probably best to start treatment with carbamazepine or phenytoin or (less frequently) phenobarbital. Valproate is used as a secondary drug because of its potential hepatotoxic side effects, but it

may be the preferred drug in patients who have a combination of grand mal and absence or myoclonic seizures. Primidone is also only used as a secondary medication because of its frequent sedative side effects (Table 156-1).

Therapeutic levels should be monitored and maintained. After starting the maintenance dose or after any change in the dosage, a steady state is not reached until at least five half-lives, which for most antiepileptics is about 1 week; for phenobarbital, it is 2 to 4 weeks. To achieve the therapeutic level faster, loading with twice the dose per elimination half-life may be done (see also Chap. 173). Only one drug should be used initially, and the dose should be increased until complete control is achieved or until side effects prohibit further increases. Another drug may then be added, and the initial medication should be tapered. Control with one drug (monotherapy) should be the goal, although some patients may need to take more than one drug. The levels should be checked periodically and on addition (or discontinuation) of a second drug because of potential drug interactions. During follow-up, repeating the EEG may be helpful to evaluate changes in the seizure pattern. Free antiepileptic drug levels should be taken in cases of hypoalbuminemia and in cases in which certain drug interactions are suspected (e.g., interaction of phenytoin with valproate).

Before starting treatment, baseline complete blood cell count, liver function tests, kidney function tests, and urinalysis should be performed and usually are repeated periodically, particularly in multiply handicapped and retarded children. For carbamazepine, the complete blood cell count and platelet count should be monitored more often than with other drugs, especially initially. It is not uncommon (10%

Table 156-1.   Doses and Indications of Commonly Used Antiepileptic Drugs

DRUG	DOSE	INDICATIONS	THERAPEUTIC RANGE OF SERUM CONCENTRATE
Phenobarbital	3–6 mg/kg/d	Partial, primary and secondary generalized tonic-clonic seizures	15–40 μg/mL
Phenytoin	4–7 mg/kg/d	Partial, primary and secondary generalized tonic-clonic seizures; status epilepticus	10–20 μg/mL
Carbamazepine	10–30 mg/kg/d	Partial, primary and secondary generalized tonic-clonic seizures	6–12 μg/mL
Valproate	10–60 mg/kg/d	Combination of absence and generalized tonic-clonic seizures, resistant absence, myoclonic seizures; some cases of partial seizures	50–150 μg/mL
Ethosuximide	20–40 mg/kg/d	Absence seizures (first choice)	40–100 μg/mL
Acetazolamide	15–30 mg/kg/d	Absence seizures	
Clonazepam	0.01–0.2 mg/kg/d	Resistant absence seizures, myoclonic seizures	5–70 ng/mL
Diazepam	0.10–0.80 mg/kg/d	Status epilepticus*	0.6–1.0 μg/mL
Primidone	10–25 mg/kg/d	Partial, primary and secondary generalized tonic-clonic seizures	5–15 μg/mL

*Note that the dosages are not for the treatment of status epilepticus, which is beyond the scope of this chapter.

of patients) to encounter reversible, dose-related relative leukopenia in patients who take carbamazepine. This responds to decreasing the dose or to discontinuing the medication and should be distinguished from the much less frequent idiosyncratic aplastic anemia. Gingival hyperplasia that occurs with phenytoin therapy necessitates good oral hygiene and in some cases may be so severe as to warrant a surgical reduction and a change of medication. An idiosyncratic allergic rash may occur with any medication but is probably most common with phenytoin. A Stevens-Johnson syndrome may occasionally develop. Other potential side effects are rickets from phenytoin, phenobarbital, and carbamazepine and hyperammonemia from valproate. Irreversible hepatic injury and death are particularly feared in young mentally retarded children who are taking valproate in combination with other antiepileptic drugs. The risk of hepatotoxicity from valproate is also increased in children whose seizures are caused by certain metabolic disorders. Almost all antiepileptic drugs can produce sleepiness, ataxia, nystagmus, and slurred speech with toxic levels.

If started, treatment should generally be maintained for a 2- to 4-year seizure-free period. Medications should be tapered gradually and not abruptly discontinued. Prognostic factors reported to predict a poor outcome after stopping antiepileptic drugs include an abnormal EEG, diffuse chronic encephalopathy and retardation, long duration of seizure disorder, and difficulty in initial seizure control. The overall risk of recurrence after a seizure-free period of 2 years is about 25% the first 2 years and is usually only minimally increased over the general population after that.

An important aspect of the management of a patient with epilepsy is the education of the family and the child about the disease, its treatment, and its limitations. Bathtub bathing is prohibited. Restriction of swimming and driving (in adolescents) is frequently necessary but is not usually needed for other sports, particularly in children with good seizure control. Swimming in a pool under direct lifeguard supervision is permissable in well-controlled patients. Counseling may frequently be helpful to support the family and to educate them about the resources available in the community. Educational and occasionally psychiatric evaluations may be necessary to evaluate possible learning disabilities or behavioral abnormalities that may coexist with the epilepsy.

INDICATIONS FOR REFERRAL OR ADMISSION

Every patient with a new onset of seizures should have an initial neurologic consultation. Day-to-day follow-up is usually best managed by the pediatrician in conjunction with the neurologist who may examine the child every few months, or yearly. Earlier follow-up may be necessary if adequate seizure control is not achieved or a change in the pattern of the seizure occurs. Hospitalization is frequently not necessary for the initial evaluation of the patient unless the child presents acutely with frequent seizures or status epilepticus or if etiologic factors such as acute bacterial meningitis, intracranial hemorrhage, or brain tumor are suspected and further inpatient work-up and treatment are needed. Patients who have poor seizure control and who need significant modification of their drug regimen frequently benefit from admission for close monitoring and documentation of their seizures. Patients who are being considered for seizure surgery (removal of a tumor or of a seizure focus) are hospitalized for the presurgical work-up as well as the subsequent surgery.

ANNOTATED BIBLIOGRAPHY

Browne TR, Feldman RG (eds): Epilepsy, Diagnosis and Management. Boston, Little, Brown & Co, 1983. (Comprehensive and well-referenced book containing detailed discussions of the choice, use, and pharmacology of antiepileptic drugs.)

Commission on Classification and Terminology of the International League Against Epilepsy: Proposal for revised classification of epilepsies and epileptic syndromes. Epilepsia 30:389–399, 1989. (Most recent international classification of epileptic syndromes.)

Dreifuss FE: Pediatric Epileptology, Classification and Management of Seizures in the Child. Boston, PSG Wright, 1983. (Comprehensive book covering all clinical aspects of pediatric epilepsy.)

Holmes GL (ed): Seizures. Pediatr Ann 2:1–52, 1991. (Comprehensive up-to-date review of various aspects of the diagnosis and management of single seizures, febrile seizures, and various epileptic syndromes.)

Levy RH, Dreifuss FE, Mattson RH et al: Antiepileptic Drugs, 3rd ed. New York, Raven Press, 1989. (Authoritative reference reviewing all aspects of antiepileptic drugs—their pharmacology, efficacy, toxicity, clinical use, and mechanisms of action.)

Mikati MA, Browne TR: Comparative efficacy of antiepileptic drugs: A review. Clin Neuropharmacol 11:130–140, 1988. (Review of definitive comparative studies establishing the preferred drug for various epileptic seizures.)

Mikati MA, Browne TR: Generalized tonic clonic seizures. Hosp Med 28:92–101, 1992. (Review of the presentation and clinical features of generalized tonic-clonic [grand mal] seizures and their emergency treatment.)

157

Tics

Peter B. Rosenberger

Tics, or *habit spasms*, are quite common in the adult population. We have all noted minor muscular twitches, usually about the face, at one time or another. Their precipitation or aggravation by stress or fatigue is usually obvious.

Tics, however, are far less common among normal children. Their appearance is frequently a cause for alarm among parents and teachers and provokes ridicule by friends and classmates. The practical problem for the pediatrician is usually not to decide whether tics are present but whether and how to intervene.

PATHOPHYSIOLOGY

Unlike epilepsy, myoclonus, or tremors, tics have yielded little to the formal physiologic study that was not apparent on careful observation. Like myoclonus, tics involve rhythmic contractions of agonist muscle groups followed by relaxation of both agonists and antagonists; tremor is characterized by alternating contractions of agonists and antagonists. Like chorea, tics are slightly slower than myoclonus. However, tics differ from chorea in two important respects. First, tics are stereotyped, repetitively involving certain muscle groups, whereas chorea moves about the body. Second, although not strictly under voluntary control, tics are subject to voluntary suppression, albeit sometimes only through considerable effort. It has been shown that tics differ in their electrical properties from voluntary movements, which are usually preceded immediately by a premovement negative potential in the electroencephalogram.

For many patients, having a tic is a compulsion comparable to scratching an itch. They report that "it makes something feel better." Consideration of this compulsive nature of tics has recently improved our understanding of their pathophysiology. The connection is most easily seen in *Gilles de la Tourette's syndrome*. This syndrome, which occurs most commonly in preadolescent boys, combines motor tics with explosive, compulsive vocalizations, which are usually unintelligible but are occasionally in the form of obscene or scatologic language (coprolalia). It is now generally accepted that tics and Tourette's syndrome form a clinical continuum and frequently appear together in families.

From its original description until recently, Tourette's syndrome was considered a primarily psychiatric disease. This view has been modified since the discovery that medications with a known effect on certain neurotransmitters are therapeutically useful. Nevertheless, there is a high incidence of premorbid psychiatric difficulties in patients with Tourette's syndrome. Furthermore, the coprolalia is not accidental but intentional, a response to the same sort of irresistible urge as the tic. The concept of tics as compulsions has been further strengthened by recent research showing a genetic linkage between Tourette's syndrome and obsessive-compulsive disorder (OCD).

As mentioned earlier, interest in the neuropharmacology of tics was greatly stimulated by the discovery that haloperidol, a potent antidopaminergic drug, can dramatically reduce the symptom frequency and severity in Tourette's syndrome. Further research has confirmed the hypothesis of dopamine hyperergy in this condition. Cerebrospinal fluid levels of homovanillic acid, a dopamine metabolite, are reduced in the pretreatment stage in patients with Tourette's syndrome and are elevated after the administration of haloperidol. These levels are also reduced by treatment with amphetamines, which are known dopamine agonists.

The genetic aspects of tic syndromes have also received much recent attention. Numerous studies have shown patterns of familial association. Twin studies have shown a difference in concordance between monozygotic and dizygotic twins. Although precipitating influences are numerous, the basic neurochemical imbalance that favors tics is at least partly inherited.

CLINICAL PRESENTATION

The clinical presentation of tics is often insidious and is clearly a threshold phenomenon. Many more cases exist than come to clinical attention, and estimates of the date of onset by patient or parent can often be pushed back in time by careful questioning. In the case of children, peer contact on the playground or in the classroom is frequently the deciding factor in seeking medical attention.

Although tics may occur in any muscle group, the face is most commonly involved, followed by the neck and upper extremities. The movement may reflect a simple contraction of motor units but is more often complex, frequently amounting to an expressive gesture, suggesting a deficit at a much higher level of motor integration. Movements are rarely distributed evenly in time, usually occurring in bursts. The relationship to emotional stress is usually so obvious as to favor the conclusion that stress is the direct cause. Since the tics themselves usually cause some degree of emotional upset, a "vicious circle" can ensue. The child will sometimes attempt to integrate the tic into a purposeful movement, such as scratching the face or grooming the hair.

The natural history of tics is highly variable. Although the tendency may be lifelong, the more severe forms are usually self-limited over a few years. Some change in their character (the preferred movement or gesture, or in the case of coprolalia, the word used) usually occurs eventually. This change can be insidious, with the new movement or word gradually increasing in frequency as the old one disappears.

DIFFERENTIAL DIAGNOSIS

The movement disorder with which tics are most confused is *chorea*. The stereotypy and voluntary suppression of tics are the most useful distinguishing features from chorea. Fortunately, Huntington's chorea is rare in children; when it does occur, it usually features rigidity and cerebellar deficits rather than chorea. Sydenham's chorea is usually more precipitous in onset and more rapidly progressive. Paroxysmal choreoathetosis, both familial and sporadic, can involve movements similar to tics but is usually less stereotyped and more widespread. Stuttering can include vocal mannerisms resembling Tourette's syndrome, especially when it involves precipitous changes in pitch or volume, which can also occur in chorea. Stuttering is also frequently accompanied by accessory facial motor mannerisms essentially indistinguishable from tics. There is reason at least to speculate that stuttering resembles tic disorders physiologically.

Focal motor seizures can resemble tics. They can usually be distinguished by their simpler nature, myoclonic speed, and greater frequency. Electroencephalographic abnormalities and response to anticonvulsant medications are helpful in the differential diagnosis.

WORK-UP

History

The history should focus first on what brings the problem to attention. Although the child can offer valuable information regarding the time of onset, it is usually the parent or teacher who is the source of the complaint. Major events affecting the child's emotional stability, such as a change in school situation, a move to a new home, or the birth of a sibling, should be noted. A careful developmental and adaptive behavioral history should be taken, since attention deficits and adjustment problems are well documented features of Tourette's syndrome. Finally, a family history of motor disorders must be included.

Physical Examination

The essential physical examination in the tic work-up will frequently be completed before the child is placed on the examining table, as a result of careful informal observation during the history taking. Note should be taken of the muscle groups involved, the degree of stereotypy, and the complexity of the movement. If the movements are sufficiently frequent, a test for voluntary suppression should be performed by asking the child to concentrate hard to remain perfectly motionless for a full minute. This test can have positive therapeutic value, demonstrating to the child that control is possible, as long as the clinician indicates an understanding that such suppression is usually not worth the effort. The neurologic examination will usually be otherwise unrevealing. It is important to look for other evidence of chorea, athetosis, or rigidity.

Laboratory Tests

No specific laboratory test is essential to the diagnosis of tics, and few are helpful in the differential diagnosis. If the clinical presentation is clearly ictal in nature, and especially if accompanied by some alteration in state of awareness, an electroencephalogram should be ordered. On rare occasions chorea may have an epileptic origin, and tics can occasionally be confused with focal motor seizures. If Sydenham's chorea is suspected, an electrocardiogram and an anti–

DNAase B titer may be helpful for the diagnosis of acute rheumatic fever.

TREATMENT

The two cornerstones of treatment for tics are behavior management and medications. Some form of behavior intervention and counseling will be necessary in every case, even if merely to explain to the child and family the essentially benign character of the condition. It is especially helpful in the relief of guilt for the parents to understand that tics have a neurophysiologic basis, although the clinician frequently makes the error of assuming an "either-or" dichotomy, thus ignoring important environmental precipitants. It is sometimes helpful to draw an analogy with asthma, explaining that "there is little or no asthma in Arizona, although there are plenty of asthmatics there."

The physician can explain to the child that while voluntary suppression frequently involves strenuous effort, it need not be practiced all the time. A concentration on suppression can be most helpful at times of maximum public exposure. Siblings, playmates, and teachers should be informed that the movements do not indicate a serious physical or emotional disorder. Their curiosity about strange behaviors is natural, and advice to "just ignore it" is often more easily given than followed. Most can understand, however, that undue attention to the symptom merely increases the child's discomfort and sets the "vicious cycle" in motion.

The most effective of the medications for tics impair alertness and attention, and thus learning ability, especially in classroom settings. They should be reserved for more serious cases but will usually need to be tried at some point when Tourette's syndrome is involved. Haloperidol is the drug of choice, and it is usually effective at much lower doses than needed for treatment of psychosis. The treatment is usually started at 0.5 mg once to twice a day and increased at weekly intervals by 0.5 to 1.0 mg/d to a maximum of 0.1 mg/kg/d. The side effects of haloperidol, particularly akathisia, are more bothersome in children than in adults.

Clonidine and pimozide are about equally preferred as drugs of second choice. Lithium carbonate, propranolol, clonazepam, imipramine, and, more recently, clomipramine, have all been reported effective.

The precipitation of tics, including full-blown Tourette's syndrome, by central nervous system stimulants is now well documented. Such symptoms can persist long after the offending agent is discontinued. Dextroamphetamine, methylphenidate, and pemoline have all been implicated. With methylphenidate, frequency is well under 1% at the usual therapeutic doses of 0.3 to 0.4 mg/kg but much higher at higher doses; in our experience, some form of dyskinesia is practically universal at 0.7 to 1.0 mg/kg. This can pose a serious dilemma for the clinician, since the attention deficits and hyperactivity for which stimulants are so effective are frequently encountered in children with tics. The possibility of tics as a side effect must be mentioned whenever stimulants are prescribed. In children who show tics in pretreatment, or who have a strong family history of tics, stimulants should be used only when absolutely necessary, and then with care and well-informed consent. A recent demonstration of the effectiveness of tricyclic antidepressants for attention deficit hyperactivity disorder makes these medications, particularly desipramine, a viable alternative for treatment of this disorder in children believed to be susceptible to tics.

INDICATIONS FOR REFERRAL

Referral resources to the pediatrician for the patient with tics will commonly include the neurologist and the psychiatrist. The neurologist should be consulted if there is doubt about the diagnosis, particularly if a progressive disease is suspected, if a simple medication trial is ineffective, or if a learning disorder or attention deficit is involved. The psychiatrist can be helpful when an associated psychiatric disease is recognized in the patient or immediate family, when behavioral or environmental precipitants are striking features of the history, or when adjustment difficulties are a prominent consequence of the motor disorder.

ANNOTATED BIBLIOGRAPHY

Cohen D, Shaywitz B, Caparuo B et al: Chronic multiple tics of Gilles de la Tourette's disease: CSF acid metabolites after probenecid administration. Arch Gen Psychiatry 35:245–250, 1978. (Neurotransmitter research showing a reduced function of inhibitory serotonergic mechanisms.)

Comings D, Comings B: Tourette syndrome: Clinical and psychological aspects of 250 cases. Am J Hum Genet 37:435–450, 1985. (Comprehensive clinical review of the largest personal sample on record.)

Golden G: Tics in childhood. Pediatr Ann 18:821–824, 1983. (Clinical review of the general problem of tics.)

Golden G: Tourette syndrome: Recent advances. Pediatr Neurol 2:189–192, 1986. (General review, including treatment.)

Kurlan R, Behr J, Medved L et al: Familial Tourette syndrome: Report of a large pedigree and potential for linkage analysis. Neurology 36:722–776, 1986. (Most recent in a long list of such reports, with complete references to previous studies.)

Obeso J, Rothwell J, Marsden C: Simple tics in Gilles de la Tourette's syndrome are not prefaced by a normal premovement EEG potential. J Neurol Neurosurg Psychiatry 44:735–738, 1981. (Convincing electrical demonstration that tics are physiologically distinct from voluntary movements.)

Pauls D, Leckman J, Towbin K et al: A possible genetic relationship exists between Tourette syndrome and obsessive compulsive disorder. Psychopharm Bull 22:730–733, 1986. (Recent evidence further confirming the compulsive nature of tics.)

Shapiro A, Shapiro E, Wayne H: Treatment of Gilles de la Tourette's syndrome with haloperidol: Review of 34 cases. Arch Gen Psychiatry 28:92, 1973. (Reporting the clinical experience that ushered in the "new age" of understanding of tics as biological phenomena.)

158

Ptosis

Elizabeth C. Dooling

Ptosis is defined as drooping of the upper eyelid. It may be classified as follows:

1. Hereditary
   a. Congenital (present at birth)
   b. Noncongenital
2. Congenital, nonhereditary
   a. Unilateral—due to birth injury
   b. Bilateral—isolated; associated with other defects (e.g., Turner syndrome)
3. Acquired
   a. Local or systemic disease—recurrent infection (e.g., diphtheria, trachoma, botulism)
   b. Neurologic—oculomotor or sympathetic nerve palsy
   c. Trauma
   d. Toxins—drugs (e.g., morphine, cocaine)

PATHOPHYSIOLOGY

Ptosis is caused by a defect in, or paralysis of, the superior levator palpebrae muscle, which is innervated by the superior division of the third cranial nerve, or, less commonly, by a defect in, or paralysis of, Müller's muscle, which is innervated by the cervical sympathetic system. Ptosis may result from lesions at various levels in the nervous system from the cerebral cortex to the levator muscle. Unilateral ptosis caused by a hemispheric lesion without associated partial herniation is rare. Mild bilateral ptosis may occur with frontal lobe lesions. Lesions of the levator portion or caudal end of the third nerve nucleus may produce a severe, symmetric ptosis. Lesions of the peripheral third nerve are usually unilateral and are often associated with mydriasis and extraocular muscle weakness. Mechanical disruptions such as penetrating orbital injuries, fractures, or operative procedures in the posterior superior area of the orbit may cause isolated ptosis. Congenital absence of a third nerve branch to the levator muscle may occur. Sympathetic nerve lesions may produce a partial unilateral ptosis as in Horner's syndrome. Ptosis due to dysfunction or disorders of the neuromuscular apparatus such as myasthenia gravis, infantile botulism, or organic pesticide poisoning is usually associated with clinical evidence of involvement of other muscles, including the ocular muscles, the orbicularis oculi, facial muscle, or skeletal muscles. *Pseudoptosis* is a term describing ptosis resulting from inflammation, hemorrhage, swelling, infiltration, or other mechanical barriers to lid elevation.

CLINICAL PRESENTATION

The child with congenital ptosis usually presents with bilateral drooping lids that cover the pupils. There may be associated paralysis of the superior rectus muscles or of all the ocular muscles supplied by the third nerve. When ptosis is hereditary, it is often associated with epicanthus (a fold of skin extending vertically downward from the inner end of the brow to the side of the upper part of the nose) and other defects. Some forms of hereditary ptosis are not obvious at birth but appear later in life. Acquired ptosis is usually unilateral and neurogenic in origin but may be related to trauma to the eyelids or levator muscle or to focal infection. When other muscles innervated by the third nerve are involved in addition to the superior levator palpebrae, the child may not be able to rotate the eye upward, downward, or medially and he or she may have difficulty reading because of mydriasis and weakness of accommodation. When ptosis results from paralysis or injury of the sympathetic nerve in the neck, it is part of the triad of *Horner's syndrome*, which includes ptosis (due to paralysis of Müller's tarsal muscle rather than the superior levator palpebrae), a constricted pupil, and slight enophthalmos. Patients with bilateral ptosis not only have upper eyelid droop but also have an exaggeration of the forehead wrinkles and elevation of the eyebrows as a result of their efforts to lift the eyelids by contracting the frontalis muscles. They may throw their heads back to try to see better under their lowered lids.

The course of ptosis varies. Congenital nonhereditary forms are usually nonprogressive, whereas hereditary forms generally are slowly progressive. Some acquired diseases are progressive; however, ptosis due to injury may improve partially or completely. Ptosis due to infantile botulism usually improves completely.

Ptosis is part of the uncommon jaw-winking phenomenon of Marcus Gunn. The eyelid will be raised when an infant sucks or a child opens the jaw maximally or moves the jaw from side to side. The disorder is attributed to anomalous pterygoid-lingual-levator innervations that make the levator hypofunctional unless the jaw or tongue muscles are contracted.

DIFFERENTIAL DIAGNOSIS

The differential diagnosis of unilateral ptosis includes a contralateral facial weakness that causes a widening of the opposite palpebral fissure; myasthenia gravis; encephalitis; neurofibromas of the eyelid; neoplasms of the temporal lobe, midbrain, sella, or base of brain; diabetic ischemic neuropathy; demyelinating disease; trauma; and infection.

Myotonic dystrophy should be considered if ptosis is bilateral. If bilateral ptosis is progressive and nonhereditary, mitochondrial myopathies such as Kearns-Sayre syndrome or congenital fiber-type disproportion should be excluded (by muscle biopsy).

WORK-UP

History

The key points to establish are whether the ptosis (1) is present at birth versus apparent later in life; (2) is static versus progressive (check old photographs); (3) is unilateral versus bilateral; (4) changes with exercise or fatigue; (5) is associated with other anomalies or third nerve dysfunction; (6) is noted in any of the child's relatives.

Physical Examination

The following observations should be emphasized during the complete physical examination: an inspection of the eyelids for discharge, redness, or evidence of infection; an assessment of oculomotor, trochlear, and abducens nerve functions in each eye; an inspection of the face and facial movements, including gag reflex, swallowing, chewing, voice quality, and salivation; and examination of bulk, alignment, and motility of the tongue. The muscle strength and tone and the tendon reflexes should be checked. The skin should be examined for hemangiomas of the face and café-au-lait spots.

Laboratory Tests

No testing may be necessary in the cases of congenital unilateral, nonprogressive ptosis. When a congenital myopathy or dystrophy is suspected, muscle enzyme studies and electromyography will be helpful. A contrast-enhanced computed tomographic scan may exclude a mass lesion. Blood glucose determination and urinalysis should be obtained if diabetes may be an underlying cause. Rectal swab on stool for *Clostridium botulinum* assay should be obtained when infantile botulism is suspected.

TREATMENT

Children in whom ptosis obstructs vision should have surgery to prevent amblyopia because of a lack of use of the ptotic eye. A child with acquired unilateral or bilateral ptosis without a history of trauma to, or infection of, the eye should be tested with edrophonium chloride (Tensilon), the dose is 1 mg if the child weighs $\leq$ 75 lb or 2 mg if he or she weighs $\geq$ 75 lb, and the drug is injected slowly intravenously. An obvious decrease in ptosis should be evident within 30 seconds and should persist for 3 to 4 minutes. Alternatively, neostigmine (Prostigmin), 0.75 mg, can be injected intramuscularly and should produce an elevation of the eyelid within 20 to 30 seconds. An electromyogram of extraocular muscles may be diagnostic. There is a progressive fallout or tiring as the muscle fatigues after a few voluntary contractions of the involved muscles. No improvement of ptosis occurs if the patient has myotonic dystrophy, a mitochondrial myopathy, traumatic or infectious process, or hereditary disorder. When the clinical findings are consistent with Horner's syndrome, it is appropriate to instill one drop of 10% phenylephrine into the affected eye. The pupil will dilate dramatically, and the ptosis will be eliminated within 15 minutes.

INDICATIONS FOR REFERRAL OR ADMISSION

A referral to an ophthalmologist is indicated when the ptosis is so severe that vision is obscured and there is a potential for loss of functional vision in the eye(s) with ptosis. If other muscles innervated by the third nerve are affected and strabismus is present, surgical correction can be performed concomitantly. A referral to a neurologist is indicated for an initial evaluation and treatment of myasthenia gravis, a myopathy, or a dystrophy. Respiratory monitoring and assisted ventilation may be necessary for infants with botulism.

ANNOTATED BIBLIOGRAPHY

Liebman SD, Gellis SD (eds): The Pediatrician's Ophthalmology, pp 182–184. St. Louis, CV Mosby, 1966. (Basic introduction to eye pathology in children.)

Miller NR: Solitary oculomotor nerve palsy in childhood. Am J Ophthalmol 83:106–111, 1977. (Reviews most common causes of third nerve palsies in children.)

Miller NR: Walsh and Hoyt's Clinical Neuro-ophthalmology, pp 936–945. Baltimore, Williams & Wilkins, 1985. (Comprehensive discussion of the pathogenesis of ptosis.)

Swaiman KF, : Pediatric Neurology, St. Louis, CV Mosby, 1989. (Excellent description of normal and abnormal eyelid innervation and function in children.)

159

Nystagmus

Elizabeth C. Dooling

Nystagmus designates involuntary rhythmic oscillating movements of one or both eyeballs and may occur on vertical or horizontal gaze or in both directions. It is defined by the direction of its fast component and may be rotatory, horizontal, vertical, oblique, or mixed. It may be classified as congenital or acquired and as physiologic or pathologic.

PATHOPHYSIOLOGY

Physiologic

Nystagmus can be induced in normal individuals with certain stimuli. *Voluntary* nystagmus consisting of rapid, low-amplitude, conjugate, pendular eye movements represents an exaggeration of the normal saccadic eye movements. It is likely to be seen in hysterical patients who may complain of diplopia. *Opticokinetic* nystagmus (OKN) is elicited by moving a series of objects (on a drum or strip of cloth) from side to side or up and down in front of the patient. The slow component results from following the objects out of the field of vision, and an opposite fast component results from fixating on the succeeding object. Opticokinetic nystagmus is usually equal in both directions. *Vestibular* nystagmus is obtained by stimulating the semicircular canals by rotation of the patient or irrigation of the ear canal (if the drum is intact) with warm or cold water (caloric testing). *Terminal* nystagmus results at the extremes of horizontal gaze when the testing object is moved out of the patient's binocular field of vision. It is more obvious in the abducting eye, and the fast component is in the direction of the patient's gaze.

Pathologic

These types of nystagmus result from a dysfunction of normal mechanisms of ocular control of fixation and gaze, and also from vestibular dysfunction. *Pendular* or *sensory defect nystagmus* is due to structural abnormalities that affect central vision. If a child develops a severe visual defect interfering with fixation before 6 years of age (e.g., from trauma, infection, tumor, or a congenital disorder such as cataracts, glaucoma, albinism, or retrolental fibroplasia), pendular nystagmus characterized by almost equal oscillations in both directions, but more marked when fixation is attempted, may occur. If the visual deficit is acquired after 6 years of age, such nystagmus rarely develops. Diseases of the labyrinth from ototoxic drugs such as gentamicin, the vestibular portion of the eighth cranial nerve, or the pontine vestibular nuclei will produce nystagmus. Nystagmus of vestibular origin is usually jerky, characterized by eye movements alternating between a slow oscillation in one direction and a fast corrective oscillation in the opposite direction. Labyrinthine and eighth-nerve lesions produce a rotatory nystagmus. Disorders of gaze mechanisms most commonly result from toxic levels of phenytoin, barbiturates, tranquilizers, or antihistamines. Cerebellar and brain stem tumors, Chiari Type I malformation with low-lying cerebellar tonsils, infections, and demyelinating or vascular diseases are less frequently the cause of gaze palsies. Convergence nystagmus may be accompanied by retraction nystagmus in children with pineal tumors.

CLINICAL PRESENTATION

The child with nystagmus may have ocular instability at rest or with intentional movement of the eyes. The younger child may be noted to have difficulty in fixating on faces or toys; poor visual acuity may be suspected and detected. The older child may complain of blurred vision or nausea. The child's schoolwork may deteriorate, and he or she may be less steady when walking or riding a tricycle or bicycle. Head tilt to one side to avoid diplopia may be noted. A child with a brain stem or cerebellar mass lesion may appear to have developed a squint, which actually represents a sixth-nerve palsy from mass effect or infiltration. Disorders of gaze may precede other signs of increased intracranial pressure, such as drowsiness, vomiting, lethargy, personality changes, or gait changes.

DIFFERENTIAL DIAGNOSIS

Congenital

- Dominant
- X-linked dominant or recessive
- Albinism
- Aniridia
- Cataracts
- Glaucoma
- Bilateral macular defects
- Neonatal myasthenia gravis
- Retrolental fibroplasia
- Total color blindness
- Arnold–Chiari malformation

Acquired

Spasmus nutans associated with head nodding and head tilt starts by 18 months of age and disappears by 3 years of age. This pendular nystagmus does not persist in sleep. On rare occasions, spasmus nutans has been associated with hypothalamic tumors.

1. Drug intoxication
   a. Phenytoin
   b. Barbiturates
   c. Tranquilizers including benzodiazepines
   d. Antihistaminics
   e. Alcohol
   f. Aminoglycosides
   g. Dihydrostreptomycin
2. Infections
   a. Viral mesencephalitis or encephalitis
3. Tumors
   a. Cerebellar or brain stem tumors including medulloblastoma, glioma, ependymoma, acoustic neuroma
   b. Hypothalamic or diencephalic tumors including hamartoma, glioma, craniopharyngioma
   c. Neuroblastoma in association with myoclonus
4. Neuromuscular disorders
   a. Myasthenia gravis
   b. Botulism

WORK-UP

History

The onset of the ocular motor disturbance must be determined as accurately as possible. Contributing factors must be ascertained, such as prematurity, associated somatic abnormalities such as Sturge–Weber syndrome and glaucoma due to buphthalmos, Wilms' tumor and aniridia, storage disease of the mucopolysaccharide type, and a family history of similar defects. The physician must ascertain if there is a history of treatment of seizures, allergies, or psychiatric disease.

Physical Examination

The child's eyes must be examined carefully, and the color of the irides, the opacity of the cornea and lens, and the size of the eyes should be noted. The type of nystagmus should be described: pendular, jerky, rotatory, horizontal, vertical, latent (a jerk horizontal nystagmus present only if one eye is covered), monocular, or binocular. Other signs of neurologic disability should be sought, such as hearing defects, disequilibrium or ataxia to indicate vestibular dysfunction, and level of consciousness, respiratory status, and pupil size in a patient with suspected drug intoxication.

Laboratory Tests

Drug screening of blood and urine should be obtained in an afebrile child with acutely acquired nystagmus. If the child is febrile or has had an infectious contact, an examination of the cerebrospinal fluid should be made to assess encephalitis or mesencephalitis. Formal hearing tests should be obtained if ototoxic drugs were administered. A computed tomography scan with contrast may show a mass lesion in the posterior fossa, optic tracts, or optic chiasm. A magnetic resonance imaging scan with gadolinium will allow visualization of the level of the cerebellar tonsils or a syrinx.

MANAGEMENT AND REFERRAL

The infant who has congenital nystagmus should be examined by an ophthalmologist. A pediatric neurologic assessment should be obtained if there is any associated developmental problem that is suspected or apparent and if there is any acquired nystagmus of unclear etiology.

ANNOTATED BIBLIOGRAPHY

Adams RD, Victor M: Principles of Neurology, pp 217–220. New York, McGraw-Hill, 1989. (Good review of nystagmus.)

Cogan DG: Neurology of the Ocular Muscles, pp 184–226. Springfield, IL, Charles C Thomas, 1956. (Comprehensive discussion of abnormal eye movements in children.)

Liebman SD, Gellis SD (eds): The Pediatrician's Ophthalmology, pp 190–192. St. Louis, CV Mosby, 1966. (Introduction to eye pathology in children.)

160

Ataxia

G. Robert DeLong

PATHOPHYSIOLOGY

Ataxia may be defined as incoordination of movement. It is associated with a dysfunction or disease of the cerebellum, although it may also result from a disease of afferent systems (*sensory ataxia*).

Ataxia appears in different guises in different systems: *appendicular or limb ataxia* (as demonstrated by tremor and dysmetria in finger-to-nose testing); *truncal ataxia* (with inability to support the trunk stably when sitting); and *gait ataxia* (inability to walk with a narrow base, as in tandem walking). Truncal and gait ataxia may be called *axial ataxia* and result from midline cerebellar disease, as opposed to *appendicular ataxia* (affecting the appendages or limbs) resulting from disease of the ipsilateral cerebellar hemisphere. Ataxia is commonly accompanied by dysarthria or nystagmus, which may be considered ataxia of buccolingual function and of gaze mechanisms, respectively. Ataxia of sensory (afferent) systems, either peripheral nerves or dorsal columns of the spinal cord, has a dysmetric wavering quality; that associated with cerebellar outflow systems may approximate myoclonus or chorea.

Ataxia must be differentiated from chorea, which has a more writhing or dancing and quasipurposeful or organized character; and from myoclonus or polymyoclonus, which consist of brief, irregular jerky muscle movements. Weakness may simulate ataxia, whether caused by muscle disease, Guillain–Barré idiopathic polyneuropathy, or disease of cerebral hemispheres. Finally, vestibular or brain stem disease may cause dysequilibrium that simulates ataxia.

Ataxia is classified conveniently into acute, intermittent, and chronic forms. *Acute* ataxia is a common response of the young nervous system to many insults, especially toxic, metabolic, infectious, or epileptic. Thus, ataxia often appears before other specific neurologic dysfunctions become apparent in acute illness. *Chronic* ataxia presents a different clinical problem. If progressive, it is usually caused by genetic, metabolic, or degenerative systems diseases. Stable chronic ataxia may be the result of congenital encephalopathy (ataxic cerebral palsy) or brain injury (head trauma or hypoxic–ischemic insult).

Acute ataxia is a relatively common pediatric problem. Many acute ataxias will resolve spontaneously or after the withdrawal of the offending agent. Others may signal major problems other than ataxia, such as brain tumors, neuroblastoma, or metabolic disease.

CLINICAL PRESENTATION

The typical presentation of acute ataxia with unstable, veering, wide-based gait, falling, and wavering unsteadiness of arm movements will not be mistaken. On more careful examination, dysarthria and nystagmus may be evident. Other presentations in young children may be less obvious, however, and may cause ataxia to be overlooked. Toddlers with severe acute ataxia may refuse to attempt to walk or sit up, as may the child with associated lethargy, obtundation, or increased intracranial pressure. Children with posterior fossa tumors with incipient herniation may assume a fixed position (e.g., prone in bed with the head turned to one side), refusing to move, thus masking ataxia. Truncal or axial ataxia may give no clue to its presence in a child examined lying in bed; it is necessary to have the child attempt to sit, stand, and walk to reveal the ataxia. Similarly, ataxia is difficult to demonstrate in young infants until they can sit or stand holding on to something. Children who have brain tumors or increased intracranial pressure may have intermittent ataxia; thus, a parent's report describing ataxia should not be dismissed if the physician finds a normal examination at first.

Chronic ataxia presents in two forms: nonprogressive and progressive. *Nonprogressive ataxia* may be present from early life, if caused by congenital encephalopathy, cerebellar dysgenesis, or cerebral palsy; or it may be the late residual of a known insult such as a head injury or hypoxic–ischemic, or rarely hyperthermic, insult. The distinction between a stable and progressive ataxia may occasionally be obscure until the course unfolds over time. *Progressive ataxia* may be divided into those conditions with known genetic biochemical disorders (e.g., metachromatic leukodystrophy, presenting usually in the second year) and those system degenerations with obscure causes (e.g., the hereditary ataxias typified by Friedreich's ataxia, which has an insidious onset during the first decade).

DIFFERENTIAL DIAGNOSIS

Acute Ataxia

Acute ataxia is commonly encountered in the child as a secondary or incidental consequence of a known disease process. The most common examples are ataxia from excessive levels of medications, especially anticonvulsants; ataxia following seizures, especially minor motor, in the young child; ataxia following meningitis; and ataxia in the older child or adolescent from an overdose of drugs or alcohol.

Ataxia is a prominent symptom of many intoxicants, including drugs (e.g., anticonvulsants, tranquilizers, sedatives, phencyclidine, and rarely lithium). The effects of these are self-limited and reversible. (Exceptions are rare intoxications with heavy metals such as lead, organic mercury, and thallium, which may have severe permanent residua.)

Tumors of the posterior fossa must be considered in every case with a recent onset of ataxia. Papilledema, a history of headache or vomiting, or head tilt indicates a posterior fossa tumor. Sixth-nerve palsy or hemiparesis suggests a brain stem tumor (pontine glioma). A posterior fossa cyst or hematoma, angioma, or Arnold–Chiari malformation occasionally presents as acute or intermittent ataxia.

The most characteristic acute ataxia of childhood is acute parainfectious cerebellar ataxia, a form of parainfectious encephalomyelitis associated with patchy central nervous system demyelination. Manifestations may be essentially limited to cerebellar functions, as in the familiar postvaricella cerebellitis; or additional cerebral hemisphere, brain stem, and spinal cord involvement may occur. Severe or subacutely evolving cases may be associated with increased intracranial pressure, and a computed tomography (CT) scan may demonstrate cerebellar swelling. Patchy multifocal areas of demyelination are better seen by magnetic resonance imaging (MRI).

Multiple sclerosis with protean, multifocal deficits, including ataxia, is rare in prepubertal children. The diagnosis can be suspected during the first attack, but definitive diagnosis depends on recurrence. Diagnosis is aided by MRI, as well as typical cerebrospinal fluid (CSF) changes (oligoclonal bands, mild lymphocytosis, elevated gammaglobulin).

A syndrome presenting as postinfectious ataxia may be produced occasionally by a mild or slowly evolving postinfectious polyneuropathy (Guillain–Barré). This occurs in young children who cannot report sensory symptoms reliably and in whom weakness is minimal for a time. The Miller–Fisher syndrome (ataxia, ophthalmoplegia, and areflexia) is regarded as a variant of the Guillain–Barré syndrome. It often follows a viral illness and is self-limited.

Severe acute cerebellar encephalopathy may result in a rare syndrome of polymyoclonus and opsoclonus, which may be considered a severe form of cerebellar ataxia. This striking syndrome, which has been called *myoclonic encephalopathy* or *dancing eyes, dancing feet syndrome*, is seen under three circumstances: (1) associated with neuroblastoma, which may be inapparent at the time the patient is first seen; (2) as a form of congenital encephalopathy; or (3) in older children in relation to an acute viral illness. In such cases, it may be equivalent to severe acute parainfectious cerebellar ataxia.

A basilar migraine may cause acute ataxia. It typically presents as a florid syndrome with headache, drowsiness, visual symptoms, and brain stem signs and should be differentiated from a hemorrhage or other major structural disease.

Several metabolic disorders may cause an intermittent cerebellar ataxia, which is often precipitated acutely by an infectious illness that sometimes progresses to a stu-por or coma. Reye's syndrome may be an example of such a process, although the ataxic stage is brief and inconspicuous. Conditions producing such intermittent metabolic ataxias include amino acid disorders, urea cycle disorders with hyperammonemia, organic acidoses, and disorders of lactate and pyruvate metabolism. Suspected cases of recurrent metabolic ataxia should be carefully evaluated with studies of serum electrolytes, acid–base status, glucose, ammonia, lactate, pyruvate, and ketones. More specific metabolic studies should then include amino acids and organic acids. Reports describe intermittent cerebellar ataxia in an inherited biotinidase deficiency resulting in multiple carboxylase deficiencies. Affected children show immunologic defects, rash, frequent infections, acute intermittent ataxia, and lactic acidosis. The clinical manifestations are improved by pharmacologic doses of biotin. There have been rare reports of kindreds with paroxysmal intermittent ataxia without an identified metabolic basis, with autosomal dominant inheritance. In one such family, attacks were completely prevented by treatment with acetazolamide.

Thiamine deficiency is an unusual cause of acute ataxia and nystagmus in children. It may occur in children with chronic illness receiving long-term intravenous therapy in which vitamin supplementation had been neglected. There is a prompt, although not always total, response to thiamine administration.

Chronic and Progressive Ataxia

Chronic progressive ataxia constitutes a problem different from that of acute ataxia. Several rare disease entities will be considered by the neurologist. Their elucidation requires a detailed clinical examination, family history, or search for specific enzymatic or metabolic disorders. The system degenerations (spinocerebellar degeneration) may present, in addition to ataxia, some combination of spasticity, peripheral nerve disease, ocular disease, and dementia. Friedreich ataxia, the prototype of this group, is an autosomal recessive disorder with an onset in the first decade, with ataxia, areflexia, pes cavus, and variable mental changes and heart disease. Ataxia telangiectasia has the onset of ataxia in the first 3 years of life, and later there are oculocutaneous telangiectasias and sinopulmonary infections. Some neurologic degenerative and storage diseases with known biochemical disorders may present with progressive ataxia; these include Wilson's disease and some lipid storage disorders. Wilson's disease, should never be overlooked because it can be treated.

Vitamin E deficiency may produce ataxia, in addition to acanthocytosis, neuropathy, retinitis pigmentosa, and spinal cord degeneration. This condition, caused by steatorrhea or liver disease with impairment of vitamin E absorption, may be halted or reversed by adequate administration of vitamin E.

WORK-UP

History

The history should elucidate the following: duration, onset, previous occurrences, drug or toxin ingestion or exposure, infection, seizures, head injury, hypoxic–ischemic or hyperthermic episode, family history, migraine, and chronic illness (e.g., steatorrhea, vitamin deficiency).

Physical Examination

A complete examination should be performed, and particularly important aspects of the physical examination should include gait; sitting posture; arm and leg coordination (finger–nose, heel–knee–shin, rapid alternating movements; looking for intention tremor, dysdiadochokinesia, dysmetria, decomposition of movements); hypotonia, decreased tendon reflexes; scanning dysarthria; nystagmus; papilledema, neck stiffness; head tilt; other neurologic abnormalities; spasticity; hemiparesis; Babinski reflexes; areflexia; weakness; obtundation; stupor; sensory deficits; hearing; retinopathy; and cranial nerves. Breath odor (e.g., alcohol, ketosis, musty) and somatic anomalies such as shelved posterior skull, oculocutaneous telangiectasias, and pes cavus should also be noted.

Laboratory Tests

A complete blood count (CBC), urinalysis, electrolytes, bicarbonate, BUN, blood sugar, and ammonia should usually be included in the initial laboratory evaluation of acute ataxia. Lactate, pyruvate, toxic screen, amino acids, organic acid screen, anticonvulsant levels, and electroencephalogram are ordered as indicated. Lumbar puncture should be considered if there is no papilledema. A CT scan is indicated in any patient with acute cerebellar ataxia, except if a toxic or metabolic cause is suspected and ataxia promptly resolves after the cause is corrected.

In addition, for chronic progressive ataxia, ceruloplasmin, immunoglobulins, vitamin E, arylsulfatase, phytanic acid, lipoprotein electrophoresis, hexosaminidase, and nerve conduction velocities (NCV) should be obtained. A peripheral nerve biopsy should be considered if the NCV are abnormal. The work-up of any chronic ataxia, whether static or progressive, should include an MRI because of its superior capability to image the posterior fossa and its superb delineation of many disease processes and structural abnormalities.

TREATMENT AND MANAGEMENT

An understanding of etiology—and thus differential diagnosis—is essential for the consideration of treatment. No specific treatment for ataxia as such exists in most cases. Many acute ataxias are self-limited or will resolve after the removal of the offending agent, such as a drug or toxin. Some will prove to be major problems other than ataxia (e.g., brain tumor).

The question of treatment often arises in cases of parainfectious encephalomyelitis. Corticosteroids may be beneficial in these cases (dexamethasone 0.5 mg/kg/day for 7 to 10 days), and they should probably be used in severe or subacutely evolving cases. With increased intracranial pressure, corticosteroids and possibly mannitol are urgently indicated. In the dancing eyes, dancing feet polymyoclonus syndrome, the movement disorder may respond well to ACTH. (A vigorous search for neuroblastoma should also be made.)

Epilepsy may be associated with ataxia in the young child, especially with minor motor seizures, as an ictal or postictal phenomenon. Proper treatment of the seizure disorder with valproate or clonazepam is indicated. Excess levels of anticonvulsants, of course, may also cause ataxia in the setting of epilepsy.

No useful neuropharmacologic treatment exists for ataxia. Specific agents may be useful in certain instances, such as in the treatment of thiamine deficiency or biotin in the treatment of biotinidase deficiency. A discussion of the management of the rare metabolic disorders that produce ataxia is beyond the scope of this chapter. In established severe ataxia, the use of weights on the wrists or ankles to reduce the amplitude of movements may benefit some patients.

INDICATIONS FOR REFERRAL OR ADMISSION

It is easier to state the indications for *not* referring or admitting a child with acute ataxia: if the cause is evident and is self-limited, such as a medication overdose; if it is a postictal ataxia in a child with a known seizure disorder; or if it is a mild postinfectious ataxia. Hospitalization is indicated when the diagnosis is uncertain or when ataxia is severe or associated with other symptoms. A neurologic or neurosurgical consultation should be obtained, and neuroimaging with CT scan or MRI should be performed.

ANNOTATED BIBLIOGRAPHY

De Negri M, Rolando S: Child ataxias: A developmental perspective. Brain Dev 12:195–201, 1990. (Review.)

Menkes JH: Textbook of Child Neurology, 4th ed. Philadelphia, Lea & Febiger, 1990. (Standard reference.)

Pasternak JF, DeVivo DC, Prensky AL: Steroid-responsive encephalomyelitis in childhood. Neurology 30:481–486, 1980. (Good discussion of encephalomyelitis.)

Rowland L: Molecular genetics, pseudogenetics and clinical neurology. The Robert Wartenberg lecture. Neurology 33:1179–1195, 1983. (Best listing of metabolic diagnostic considerations in ataxia.)

Telander RL, Smithson WA, Groover RV. Clinical outcome in children with acute cerebellar encephalopathy and neuroblastoma. J Pediatr Surg 24:11–14, 1989. (Outcome in ten patients with this entity.)

Weiss S, Carter S: Course and prognosis of acute cerebellar ataxia in children. Neurology 9:711–721, 1959. (Classical clinical description of this entity.)

Weiss S, Guberman A: Acute cerebellar ataxia in infectious disease. In Vinken PJ, Bryn GW (eds): Handbook of Clinical Neurology, Vol 34, p 619. Amsterdam, North-Holland, 1978. (Comprehensive discussion of causes of ataxia in this group.)

161

Bell's Palsy

Elizabeth C. Dooling

Facial weakness of acute onset, known as *Bell's palsy* or *peripheral facial palsy*, affects approximately 1% of the population ranging in age from several months to the elderly. It sometimes occurs on a familial basis, and, in rare circumstances, a person may have recurrent facial palsy or bilateral involvement at different times.

PATHOPHYSIOLOGY

The pathogenesis of this disorder is not completely understood. Multiple hypotheses have been proposed to explain the appearance of unilateral facial weakness after an acute infectious process such as otitis media or pneumonia. Acute swelling of the facial nerve and congestion of the facial canal occur with minimal inflammatory reaction. The predilection for either of the facial nerves may be attributed to the deposition of immune complexes; the demyelinating process differs from similar illnesses such as Guillain–Barré syndrome, where there is typically symmetric bilateral weakness and a different lymphocytic response. Subclinical involvement of the trigeminal and auditory nerves, determined by evoked potential testing, indicates that the process is a polyneuropathy.

CLINICAL PRESENTATION

Before the facial paralysis, the child may complain of pain in the ear or over the cheek near the ear. The patient with acute facial weakness has drooping of one side of the face and a wider palpebral fissure on the affected side. When asked to frown or look upward, the child cannot crease the forehead or elevate the eyebrow. (In contrast, with central facial weakness the forehead is not involved because of bilateral innervation.) There may be excessive tearing resulting from weak closure of the eye. Taste may be affected, and the patient may be hypersensitive to noise. Pain is usually temporary, and sensory disturbances do not occur, although the child may state that the affected side of the face feels stiff or heavy. At rest, the degree of facial weakness may not be apparent. As soon as the child begins to talk, laugh, or cry, the weakness is obvious. Incomplete paralysis is a good prognostic sign. Symptoms may develop over 2 to 5 days. Recovery usually starts within 1 to 6 weeks and is maximum by 9 to 24 weeks, depending on the extent of denervation.

DIFFERENTIAL DIAGNOSIS

Acute facial palsy in children may occur with various infections, including cellulitis, mastoiditis, Lyme disease, varicella, enteroviral encephalitis, infectious mononucleosis, Guillain–Barré syndrome, mumps, herpes simplex, and herpes zoster. It is essential to consider neoplasms of the brain stem and to look for involvement of other cranial nerves, especially the sixth, either ipsilaterally or contralaterally. Tumors of the head and neck such as cystic hygromas, retropharyngeal rhabdomyomas, parotid or salivary gland tumors, chordomas, and acoustic neuromas and pseudotumor cerebri may cause facial nerve dysfunction.

WORK-UP

History

When the symptoms and signs of an acute infectious illness, with or without fever or trauma, precede or accompany the onset of hemifacial weakness, the diagnosis is not equivocal. The child occasionally states that his or her eyes feel gritty, as if there is sand in them, often complains of auricular or periauricular pain, may tear profusely, and may complain that food tastes differently. During forceps deliveries, accidental pressure of a forceps blade over the infant's face may result in a facial nerve palsy. A family history of neurofibromatosis suggests that a slowly growing tumor may be responsible for the onset of facial weakness. Enlarging masses in the face and neck may affect the child's appetite or voice. Brain stem or posterior fossa tumors are associated with diplopia, weakness, and ataxia.

Physical Examination

The findings of facial weakness include sagging of the affected side of the face, lack of expression, inability to close the eye completely or partially, excess tearing on the affected side, inability to wrinkle the ipsilateral forehead, asymmetric retraction of the corner of the mouth on the weak side when the child is asked to smile or show the teeth, and drooling from the weak side of the mouth. Facial sensation is intact. Taste over the anterior two thirds of the tongue may be diminished when it is tested with sugar or quinine. Also, the child may complain of hyperacusis. Inability to wrinkle the forehead and raise the eyebrow on the affected side distinguishes a *peripheral* or lower facial palsy from a *central* facial palsy due to a supranuclear or hemispheral lesion.

A careful general physical examination is necessary. In particular, the child's skin should be scrutinized for ticks or the typical lesion of erythema chronicum marginatum (the pathognomonic "bull's-eye" lesion of Lyme disease), the vesicular lesions of varicella or zoster, and evidence of trauma. Also, the presence of café-au-lait spots and cutaneous neurofibromas may signify that the child has neurofibromatosis and might be at risk for acoustic neuromas.

Laboratory Tests

A Lyme titer should be obtained when there is a history of tick bite or a possible exposure. A heterophil titer should be ordered in a patient with symptoms consistent with infectious mononucleosis. If there has been a gradual onset of the facial weakness and accompanying neurologic signs of cranial nerve dysfunction or hemiparesis, an enhanced CT or MRI brain scan should be ordered. Electrophysiologic testing (i.e., electromyography and evoked potentials) may be helpful in ascertaining the degree of facial nerve involvement and thus might be useful in postulating how long it could take for recovery of normal facial nerve function.

TREATMENT

There is controversy about treatment of acute facial weakness. In most cases there is excellent recovery. Antibiotics are indicated when there is exudative tonsillitis, suppurative otitis media, or Lyme disease. It is common practice to use a short course of steroids for treating "idiopathic" Bell's palsy if the patient seeks medical attention 48 to 72 hours after weakness develops and if there are no contraindications. Prednisone, 2 mg/kg/day, is given orally for 1 week, then 1 mg/kg/day for 1 week. To avoid corneal scarring from drying of the cornea in the absence of normal blinking, artificial tears should be used three to four times daily. When the child sleeps, the eye should be taped closed with paper tape that does not adhere to the eyebrow. If the tongue is involved, the child should be cautioned to bite foods carefully.

INDICATIONS FOR REFERRAL

When facial weakness is severe and little spontaneous recovery has occurred, or tumors of the facial nerve or head and neck are identified, referral to an otolaryngologist is indicated. Surgery may be effective in restoring partial facial nerve function. If a child is found to have central facial weakness of acute or subacute onset, neurologic referral is needed. When intracranial masses are diagnosed, a neurosurgeon should be consulted.

ANNOTATED BIBLIOGRAPHY

Devriese PP, Schumacher T, Schiede A, DeJongh RH, Houtkooper JM: Incidence, prognosis and recovery of Bell's palsy. A survey of 1000 patients (1974–1983). Clin Otolaryngol 15:15–26, 1990. (Retrospective study from Holland; older age of onset was associated with less complete recovery.)

Hughes GB: Prognostic tests in acute facial palsy. Am J Otolaryngol 10:305–11, 1989. (Electroneurography [ENOG] and the maximal stimulation test [MST] have proved to be most helpful in prognosticating the degree of recovery.)

Markby DP: Lyme disease facial palsy: Differentiation from Bell's palsy. Br Med J 299:605–606, 1989. (Patients with Lyme disease had swelling erythema of the face resembling cellulitis before developing facial weakness.)

Menkes JH: Textbook of Child Neurology, pp 451–453. Philadelphia, Lea & Febiger, 1990. (Good discussion of Bell's palsy.)

20

RESPIRATORY PROBLEMS

162

Apnea of Infancy

Dorothy H. Kelly

The sudden unexpected and unexplained death of infants has been reported since biblical times. In recent years, many researchers have investigated numerous hypotheses of the causes of such deaths. As a result of these investigations, it seems probable that the *sudden infant death syndrome* (SIDS) is due to multiple causes. There are population studies from several countries linking SIDS with how an infant is put to sleep. Babies positioned on their backs or sides had a lower incidence of SIDS than babies placed prone. Although these data are inconclusive, the American Academy of Pediatrics issued a statement in May 1992 advising that infants who do not have lung disease or evidence of gastroesophageal reflex be put to sleep on their backs or sides. If, however, they roll over, infants need not be repositioned.

One of the factors that can result in the sudden death of infants is an abnormal control of ventilation or heart rate. Apnea was first documented in 1972 by a report of the sudden death of two infants in one family who were SIDS siblings and who had prolonged apnea. Since that time, others have reported sudden and unexpected deaths in some infants with *idiopathic apnea of infancy* (AOI). It is a clinical challenge for the primary care physician to evaluate and manage infants with apnea.

PATHOPHYSIOLOGY

Numerous physiologic studies of infants with apnea have documented abnormalities in the control of ventilation in some of these infants, including a decreased ventilatory re-

sponse to breathing carbon dioxide, mild hypoventilation in quiet sleep, prolonged sleep apnea, excessive short apnea, periodic breathing, and obstructive sleep apnea. Others have failed to document such abnormalities. Many of these abnormalities were present in infants with AOI who subsequently died. However, the cause(s) of these abnormalities remain(s) unknown. Only two autopsy studies on infants with AOI have been reported. In the first study, increased muscularity of the pulmonary vasculature was reported in five infants, and in the second, gliosis in the brain stem was described in one infant. Both findings can be associated with chronic hypoxia either as a cause or as an effect.

CLINICAL PRESENTATION

There are three typical presentations of infants with AOI. The first is the occurrence of apnea during sleep, usually associated with a change in color and tone. Frequently, there is a history of some degree of stimulation that is used by the care-giver to terminate the episode and return the infant to normal breathing, color, and tone. The second presentation is that of an infant who experiences an episode of apnea while awake. Such episodes frequently follow choking or regurgitation and are commonly associated with stiffening, redness, and a frightened look. The mouth is often opened as if trying to breathe. If uninterrupted by care-givers, the event can proceed to cyanosis, limpness, unconsciousness, and central apnea in some infants. Finally, infants may present for an evaluation because of a history of color change during sleep with shallow or irregular breathing or because the care-giver has observed numerous episodes of sleep apnea without a change in tone or color.

DIFFERENTIAL DIAGNOSIS

The following diseases must be considered in the differential diagnosis of apnea of infancy: *congenital*—anatomic airway abnormalities, vascular abnormalities causing airway obstruction, congenital heart disease and cardiac arrhythmias; *infectious*—sepsis, meningitis, pneumonia, and respiratory syncytial virus (RSV) infection; *toxic*—botulism, sedative drug use or overdose; *metabolic*—hypoglycemia, hyponatremia, hypothermia, and some inborn errors of metabolism; *neoplastic*—tumors in or around the airway, leading to an obstruction, or in the brain causing seizures resulting in apnea; and *other*—gastroesophageal reflux, seizures, hypoxemia, anemia in the preterm infant, and abnormalities in the control of ventilation.

WORK-UP

History

An evaluation of an apneic event should include a meticulous history taken from every person who observed the infant during the event or immediately following the episode (Fig. 162-1). The detailed history is necessary to help the clinician determine the severity and possibly the cause of the episode as judged by the manner of presentation as well as by the type, duration, and appropriateness of the intervention used to terminate the event. A thorough past history and family history should also be obtained.

Physical Examination

A careful physical examination should be performed to determine if signs of partial airway obstruction, congenital anomalies, intercurrent illness, or metabolic or neurologic abnormalities are present.

Laboratory Tests

Laboratory tests should be performed to attempt to identify a cause for the event, based on the history, the physical examination, and the differential diagnosis. Such an evaluation generally includes a complete blood count, differential

---

Name _____

HISTORY OF EVENT (leading to evaluation): Please circle features and complete as needed.

Date: _____ ; Age: _____ ; # hours after feed: _____

Last Immunization (specify date / type): _____ ; Medications; _____

Recent illness: _____

OBSERVER	LOCATION	INFANT POSITION	STATE	COLOR	COLOR CHANGE
Parent	Holding infant	Prone	Asleep	Cyanotic	Entire body
MD	Same room	Supine	Awake	Grey	Extremities
RN	Audible distance	Upright	Drowsy	Pale	Face
Other _____	In car	Infant seat	Feeding	Red	Perioral
	Other _____	Other _____	Other _____	Purple	Lips
				Normal	Other _____

BREATHING	TONE	EYES	NOISE	FLUID	HEART RATE
No effort	Limp	Closed	Cough	Milk	Bradycardia @ ____bpm
Shallow	Stiff	Dazed	Choke	Vomitus	Tachycardia @ ____bpm
Struggling	Tonic/clonic	Scared	Stridor	Mucus	Normal
Rapid	Normal	Rolled	Gasp	Blood	Unknown
Normal	Other _____	Staring	Cry	None	
Other _____		Normal	None	Other _____	
		Other _____	Other _____		

STIMULATION	DURATION OF EVENT:	ABNORMALITIES FOLLOWING EVENT
None	_____ sec / min	Abnormal breathing x _____ min / hrs
Gentle		Color change x _____ min / hrs
Vigorous		Behavior _____
MTM: # breaths _____		None
CPR: # cycles _____		

EMT/ER Observations:

Figure 162-1.   History form that is used as a guide in obtaining a complete history of the apneic event.

white count, serum sodium, potassium, chloride, glucose, urea nitrogen, urinalyses, arterial blood gases, chest radiograph, electrocardiogram, electroencephalogram, and a barium esophagram with fluoroscopy. Other studies such as cultures, lumbar puncture, bronchoscopy, and computed tomography scan or magnetic resonance imaging may be indicated in some cases.

If no cause can be identified by a careful history, physical examination, and the usual laboratory examinations, tests to identify abnormalities in the control of ventilation, including polysomnography, pneumogram, and studies of ventilatory responses to hypercarbia and hypoxia, are appropriate to consider. This usually necessitates a referral to a center specializing in the evaluation and management of infants with AOI.

MANAGEMENT

Specific treatment is indicated in those infants in whom a cause of the apneic episode has been identified during the evaluation. For those infants who have idiopathic AOI, the treatment approach is based on the infant's gestational and chronologic age as well as his or her clinical presentation.

Preterm infants who have idiopathic apnea, documented clinically as well as in the laboratory by an abnormal polygraphic or pneumographic recording, are usually treated with theophylline (5 to 7.5 mg/kg/day) given every 6 to 8 hours. A loading dose is generally not used because this often results in irritability, tachycardia, and regurgitation. At 48 hours after the medication has been started, serum peak and trough levels of theophylline are measured, and, if these are in the therapeutic range (≥ 10 μg/ml and <20 μg/ml), a pneumogram is obtained. If this recording is normal and the symptoms have resolved, the infant is discharged on theophylline, increasing the dose/kg weekly for weight gain and liver maturation in order to maintain serum theophylline levels within the therapeutic range. Between 48 and 52 weeks postconceptional age, the infant is readmitted to determine if the apnea has resolved. At this time, the medication is discontinued and the infant is studied by a pneumogram or polygraph. The drug is then permanently discontinued if the infant remains asymptomatic and the study is normal. If, however, the infant becomes symptomatic or the study is abnormal, theophylline is continued in the therapeutic range for an additional 4 to 8 weeks, at which time the medication is again discontinued and the study is repeated. This method for discontinuing theophylline may be carried out in the home with the infant monitored continually by a cardiorespiratory monitor.

If the infant improves initially but does not resolve the clinical or laboratory abnormalities during theophylline treatment, then he or she is discharged on the medication in addition to a home monitor when the clinical apnea or bradycardia has resolved. Following discharge with the home cardiorespiratory monitor when the clinical and laboratory

abnormalities have resolved, the drug is withdrawn gradually while home monitoring is continued until the criteria to discontinue home monitoring are met.

Finally, if no improvement in the clinical or laboratory abnormalities occurs during theophylline treatment, then the search for a cause of the disorder must be repeated, with special emphasis on gastroesophageal reflux, seizure, hypoxemia, anemia, and a congenital central hypoventilation syndrome (Ondine's curse).

Full-term newborns (<1 month of age) with *idiopathic* AOI who have abnormal pneumographic recordings are managed with theophylline as outlined for preterm infants. Those full-term newborns who have no pneumographic or polygraphic abnormalities and no explanation for the apneic event are managed as outlined below for the older infant with idiopathic apnea.

The older infants (≥ 1 month of age) with *idiopathic* AOI are routinely discharged with a cardiorespiratory monitor to be used at home because they may not be completely controlled with theophylline alone. In addition, medication is recommended based on the following criteria:

1. Medication for a specific abnormality such as gastroesophageal reflux or a seizure disorder
2. Theophylline if there are:
   a. Major abnormalities on testing (prolonged apnea >20 seconds), episodes of prolonged bradycardia (lasting 10 seconds or longer) for which no cause can be found, or marked hypoventilation (average P_ACO_2 ≥ 50 mm Hg during quiet sleep)
   b. Continued symptoms of apnea or bradycardia

If theophylline is instituted and the infant has been asymptomatic for 1 month, the medication is gradually discontinued. If signs or symptoms recur, it is reinstituted.

When a decision is made to institute electronic surveillance at home with a cardiorespiratory monitor, the parents are trained to use the equipment. They are also instructed in the use of techniques of observation and intervention as well as infant cardiopulmonary resuscitation as outlined in our handbook (Haight BF, Kelly D, McCabe KC) and recommended by the American Academy of Pediatrics. During the course of monitoring, the infants and families should be followed carefully by medical, nursing, and social service staff. The use of a monitor at home for idiopathic AOI is generally associated with acceptable stress and family disruption if accompanied by a strong support system. Without such support, home monitoring can be stressful and disruptive to all family members.

The symptoms of apnea often increase initially with the stress of upper respiratory tract infections or sleep deprivation. However, in most infants, the signs and symptoms of AOI resolve usually within 1 to 3 months. For many infants there is no recurrence of symptoms after the initial episode. We, therefore, recommend that monitoring be discontinued when all the following criteria are met:

1. No apnea or bradycardia requiring vigorous stimulation for 3 months (4 months if 12 to 18 months of age and 6 months if older than 18 months of age)
2. No apnea requiring gentle or no stimulation for 2 months
3. Two normal pneumograms or documented monitoring recorded at home
4. Normal polygraphic recording if previously abnormal
5. Resolution of physical abnormalities often present in infants with AOI, such as bradycardia in response to ocular pressure or nasal occlusion, neck and shoulder hypotonia, or lack of oral breathing during nasal occlusion

These criteria are reviewed with the parents during each follow-up visit. Using this method, ~95% of the parents can comply with the recommendation to discontinue monitoring within 2 weeks of the time that it is made. Increased support by the nursing staff is necessary at that time.

INDICATIONS FOR ADMISSION OR REFERRAL

All infants who have had an episode of apnea accompanied by a color change should be admitted for continual cardiorespiratory monitoring by medical personnel trained in infant monitoring and cardiopulmonary resuscitation, while the infant is being evaluated for the cause of the event. Infants requiring tests (other than a pneumogram) to determine abnormalities of ventilation are best referred to centers specialized in the evaluation of AOI. A referral and possibly a transfer is recommended in those infants who are in the high mortality rate groups. These include (1) siblings of SIDS victims who have had at least one episode of sleep apnea that resolved following mouth-to-mouth resuscitation (25% mortality rate) and (2) infants who presented initially with an episode of sleep apnea requiring resuscitation (13.2% mortality) and those who have had at least one subsequent severe episode of sleep apnea requiring either vigorous stimulation or resuscitation (28% mortality rate). If these infants with severe AOI develop a seizure disorder during the course of home monitoring, their mortality rate is even higher (4/7; 57%). Because of these high mortality rates, a referral of such infants to a center specializing in the evaluation and management of infants with AOI is strongly recommended.

OUTCOME

For many infants who experience an apneic episode, the etiology can be discovered with careful searching. For those with idiopathic AOI, treatment with theophylline, home monitoring, or both, with appropriate teaching and support, is usually successful. However, depending on the type and severity of their initial episode, between 30% and 50% will have a subsequent significant sleep apnea episode during home monitoring. Ninety-two percent of infants are well by 12 months of age. However, some infants with severe AOI have died during home monitoring, and half of these

deaths occurred when intervention was incorrectly performed or was delayed. Meticulous investigation and management of these high-risk infants will result hopefully in improved control of the symptoms and a decreased mortality rate.

ANNOTATED BIBLIOGRAPHY

American Academy of Pediatrics Task Force on Prolonged Infantile Apnea: Prolonged Infantile Apnea: 1985. Pediatrics 76:129, 1985. (Official statement of the AAP on the evaluation and management of infants with apnea.)

Guntheroth WG, Spiers PS: Sleeping prone and the risk of sudden infant death syndrome. JAMA 267:2359–2362, 1992. (Their critical review of the literature concludes that babies should not sleep in the prone position for the first 6 months of life unless there is a medical reason prohibiting sleeping otherwise.)

Haight BF, Kelly D, McCabe KC: A Manual for Home Monitoring, 1980. (Summarizes the specifics of the training program for the infant's care-givers, which is necessary before an infant can be discharged with a monitor.)

Kelly DH, Shannon DC: Treatment of apnea and excessive periodic breathing in the full-term infant. Pediatrics 68:183, 1981. (Demonstrates that pneumogram abnormalities in full-term infants normalize with theophylline.)

Oren J, Kelly DH, Shannon DC: Identification of a high risk group for sudden infant death syndrome among infants who were resuscitated for sleep apnea. Pediatrics 77:495–499, 1986. (Identifies the characteristics of the infants with AOI who have a high mortality rate [13% to 57%] and suggests methods of managing those infants to decrease mortality.)

Steinschneider A: Prolonged apnea and the sudden infant death syndrome. Clinical and laboratory observations. Pediatrics 50:646, 1972. (Report of the first two cases of sudden and unexplained death during sleep of two infants [siblings] who had apnea.)

163

The Common Cold

Robert A. Dershewitz

There have been no major breakthroughs for the treatment of the common cold. The term "cold" is a subset of, but is not synonymous with, "upper respiratory tract infection." Colds are the most common infectious disease entity, and in children, about 50% of upper respiratory infections (URIs) are common colds. Most children develop three to eight colds per year, but some children are prone to more frequent respiratory infections. Colds are more common in boys than in girls and are most prevalent in winter. Day care and preschool programs increase the risk of "catching" a cold.

Preschoolers are usually responsible for household spread, and the risk of acquiring colds is inversely related to age.

PATHOPHYSIOLOGY

Over 200 viruses cause the common cold, although occasionally nonviruses (e.g., mycoplasma) may produce "coldlike" illnesses. Rhinoviruses, with over 100 serotypes, are the most common causative agents and are responsible for 30% to 50% of all colds. Coronaviruses are the next most common, accounting for 10% to 20% of colds. Parainfluenza, respiratory syncytial (RS) virus, enterovirus, and influenza viruses are other frequent causes. Any of these viruses may intermittently colonize or infect the upper respiratory tract.

Hand contact of contaminated objects is probably the most important mode of transmission. Infection is also spread by inhalation of large and small airborne droplets, which may then replicate on nasal or other respiratory epithelium. Cold symptoms usually appear 2 to 4 days later, but viral shedding may occur 1 to 2 days before the onset of clinical symptoms. Viremia is unusual. Infection is acute, and it spreads locally on respiratory epithelium. The belief that nasal symptoms result from destruction of nasal mucosa is questioned. Impaired mucociliary transport resulting from cellular injury and release of chemical mediators (e.g., lysyl bradykinin and bradykinin) may account for the nasal discharge and stuffiness. Interferon is produced locally after 3 to 5 days. Chilling, wet feet, and drafts play no role in "catching a cold."

CLINICAL PRESENTATION

There are no distinctive clinical characteristics unique to any of the viruses. All causative viruses produce similar symptomatology, although influenza and RS viruses typically cause more serious illnesses than rhinoviruses and coronaviruses. Nasal irritation with a scratchy feeling in the throat is usually the first sign of infection. Within a few hours, sneezing and watery nasal discharge develop. Mild nasal congestion may precede a watery rhinorrhea. The child may also have a fever, general malaise, conjunctivitis, headache, and myalgias. Symptoms in infants tend to be more variable, as is a febrile response. Low-grade fevers are most common, but fevers of 103° to 104°F are not rare. Nasal obstruction can interfere with eating and sleeping. After about the second day of illness, the nasal discharge typically becomes mucopurulent and less copious. Symptoms usually persist for at least 2 more days, with the rhinorrhea often becoming more purulent. Symptoms usually resolve by the fifth to seventh day, although they may last longer than 10 days. A nocturnal cough attributable to a postnasal drip is often present. Occasionally, the rhinitis and cough may linger for weeks. Although colds are self-limited, complications or spread of the disease frequently occurs, with acute otitis media being the most common.

DIFFERENTIAL DIAGNOSIS

Colds should be distinguished from other upper respiratory tract illnesses (e.g., pharyngitis, sinusitis, and obstructive airway disease). A coldlike illness may be the prodrome for other diseases such as measles and pertussis. Streptococcal infection in infancy may be clinically indistinguishable from the common cold.

Allergic rhinitis is probably the most common and difficult entity to differentiate from the common cold, particularly when symptoms first occur. A strong family history of atopia and seasonal recurrence incriminate allergies. Violaceous, edematous nasal mucosa, itching eyes, and allergic facies (e.g., nasal increase, allergic shiners, and the allergic salute) are signs strongly suggestive of an allergic etiology. Although more commonly seen in adults, vasomotor rhinitis should also be considered (see Chap. 46).

A thick (i.e., purulent) nasal discharge is usually indicative of a resolving cold, but it may be due to a bacterial primary infection or superinfection. Other relatively common causes of purulent rhinitis include allergy (although a thin nasal discharge is more common), sinusitis, adenoiditis, nasal polyps, septal deviations, and systemic illness such as cystic fibrosis. Sinusitis and adenoiditis are common causes of chronic rhinitis (see Chap. 80). A unilateral, thick, foul-smelling or bloody discharge is strongly suggestive of a foreign body.

Rhinitis secondary to chronic medication use (e.g., topical decongestants), drug abuse (e.g., cocaine), and leakage of cerebrospinal fluid is thin. The use of a bulb syringe for more than 5 days may result in mechanical trauma to the nasal turbinates, causing mucopurulent rhinitis.

WORK-UP

History

Is there a history of seasonal or perennial rhinitis? Allergic children obviously get colds, but an abrupt onset of nasal symptoms suggests an infectious etiology. Pale blue and swollen turbinates suggest an allergic etiology. Is the child otherwise healthy and thriving? If the child has been symptomatic for several days, is the rhinorrhea becoming less copious and thicker? Purulent rhinitis for more than 10 days suggests sinusitis. Is the discharge bilateral? Are there other likely causes of rhinitis (e.g., forced hot air heating without humidification, or prolonged use of a bulb syringe)? Chronic rhinitis in the adolescent without a history of nasal problems may be caused by cocaine use.

Physical Examination

A child with rhinitis warrants a complete examination of at least the respiratory tract, including ears. In addition to the requisite nasal findings, there may be conjunctivitis and pharyngitis. The tonsils may be enlarged, and lymphoid hyperplasia may be seen in the posterior pharynx. Often, the cervical lymph nodes are mildly enlarged and slightly tender. Although bilateral purulent rhinitis is more likely caused by bacterial infection than is mucopurulent or thin rhinorrhea, bacterial primary and secondary infections are uncommon. At least for the first several days, it is of little clinical significance to place importance on the color and thickness of the nasal discharge. As already mentioned, a foul-smelling or unilateral discharge suggests the presence of a foreign body.

Laboratory Tests

No laboratory test ought to be considered routine, and none "rule in" or "rule out" a cold. Throat cultures are neither helpful nor indicated. Flora from a nasopharyngeal (NP) culture, even if a pure growth is recovered, is difficult to interpret because it may reflect colonization rather than infection. Nasopharyngeal cultures should be obtained only selectively (e.g., if pertussis is suspected). Wright or Hansel staining of nasal secretions to look for eosinophils is useful: large numbers of eosinophils suggest allergy and large numbers of neutrophils suggest infection. Because the peripheral white blood cell count is usually normal, but may be elevated, it should not be routinely ordered. Sinus x-rays may help diagnose sinusitis, but the radiation exposure, age of the child (the younger the child, the more difficult the x-rays are to interpret), and duration of symptoms must be considered prior to ordering sinus films.

Viral cultures are expensive and usually not helpful, in part because results are not available for 4 to 7 days. Rapid diagnostic tests are available for RS virus, parainfluenza virus, and influenza virus. These are not recommended for routine use by the practitioner but may be useful for community surveillance.

TREATMENT AND MANAGEMENT

Currently, there are no commercially available antiviral agents against viruses that cause the common cold. Hundreds of cold preparations are marketed for the symptomatic treatment of the common cold. Parents should be told that none are curative or of proven benefit. All may have side effects potentially worse than the cold symptoms themselves and may be dangerous to use in children under 6 months of age. Moreover, it is unknown whether these products shorten the duration of the cold or prevent bacterial complications.

Most preparations contain a decongestant. Topical decongestants are vasoconstrictors and probably provide symptomatic relief as great as or greater than that of other classes of medications by decreasing nasal secretions and mucosal edema. Although they generally have fewer side effects, they must be used cautiously because systemic absorption may cause the same troublesome side effects as the oral de-

congestants. In young infants, a rebound effect may result in obstructive apnea. If used for longer than 4 days, rebound congestion may develop, which may then lead to rhinitis medicamentosa. The most widely used topical decongestants are phenylephrine (e.g., Neo-Synephrine) and oxymetazoline (e.g., Afrin). Oral decongestants do not cause rebound but have more side effects.

Most oral cold preparations also contain an antihistaminic, which may be useful to counter the stimulatory side effects of the decongestants or control an allergic component (if suspected), or it may be useful for sedation (e.g., at bedtime). Manufacturers claim, although they have not proved, that the anticholinergic effects of antihistamines reduce nasal secretions, sneezing, and nasal itchiness. The efficacy of all five classes of antihistamines is probably comparable, although they are often ineffective. One study found chlorpheniramine somewhat effective in reducing cold symptoms.

Oral terfenadine, a selective H_1 antihistamine, has no beneficial effects on cold symptoms.

The main goal of supportive care is to relieve nasal obstruction and promote nasal drainage. Beneficial nonpharmacologic approaches include isotonic saline followed by bulb syringe suctioning for rhinorrhea or congestion. The saline may be useful in liquefying the nasal secretions. To avoid rebound swelling, suctioning should be gentle and discontinued after 4 consecutive days. If rhinitis persists, suctioning may resume in 1 to 2 days. Rest in general and hydration to relieve a dry or scratchy throat are probably as effective as any medication. Candy, gum drops, or lozenges can also relieve an irritated throat. Because dry air can mimic or exacerbate cold symptoms, humidification—either central or bedside—may be helpful. Several studies have shown that inhaling humidified air at 43°C relieves nasal symptoms and shortens the duration of the cold. However, a well-conducted double-blind, randomized clinical trial refuted these findings.

Antibiotics should be used only for presumed bacterial complications and never for treatment of the common cold or to prevent complications. The use of vitamin C to prevent colds or to shorten their clinical course has largely been disproved. Acetaminophen may be used for malaise or high fevers. Aspirin should be avoided because it increases viral shedding and may cause Reye syndrome.

Prevention

With all the causative viruses and antigenic drifts, it is unlikely that a vaccine against "the common cold" will soon be developed. However, several experimental approaches at prevention are being investigated. Two of the more promising ones are virucidal paper handkerchiefs intended to reduce hand-to-hand transmission, and monoclonal antibodies to block the receptor sites to which the virus or group of viruses attach. Results of field trials using intranasal alpha$_2$-

interferon conflict. Even when shown to have a beneficial effect, it was active only against rhinoviruses and prevented a cold in only 40% of those who were exposed. It must be used only short term, for when given longer than 1 to 2 weeks, unacceptable side effects such as bloody mucus and nasal mucosal erosion may develop.

In practical terms, the best means of prevention remains the standard advice: hand washing and avoiding an environment contaminated with nasal secretions.

COMPLICATIONS AND REFERRALS

In addition to acute otitis media, the other most common complications of colds include sinusitis, adenitis, pneumonia, croup, and bronchitis. Major complications from the common cold are unusual. When hospitalization is required, it is usually due to pneumonia from extension of the virus to the lower respiratory tract or to asthma in those children with hyperreactive airways. Referral to an allergist for the initial evaluation of chronic rhinitis is common, although it is frequently unnecessary if the primary physician takes a thorough history and performs a baseline work-up. Referral, however, is warranted if the rhinitis is unresponsive to environmental control and appropriate medications.

ANNOTATED BIBLIOGRAPHY

Cherry JD: The common cold. In Feign RD, Cherry JD: Textbook of Pediatric Infectious Diseases, 2nd ed, pp 155–161. Philadelphia, WB Saunders, 1987. (Complete and authoritative discussion with exhaustive bibliography.)

Douglas RM, Moore BW, Miles HB et al: Prophylactic efficacy of intranasal alpha$_2$-interferon against rhinovirus infections in the family setting. N Engl J Med 314:65–70, 1986. (Study showing that intranasal interferon reduces both the number of colds and the duration of symptoms, especially from rhinoviruses.)

Gwaltney JM Jr: The common cold. In: Mandell GL, Douglas RG Jr, Bennett JE (eds): Principles and Practice of Infectious Diseases, 3rd ed. New York, Churchill Livingstone, 1990. (Excellent review.)

Howard JC, Kantner TR, Lilienfield LS et al: Effectiveness of antihistamines in the symptomatic management of the common cold. JAMA 242:2414–2417, 1979. (Controlled clinical trial showing that chlorpheniramine significantly improved cold symptoms.)

Macknin ML, Mathew S, Medendorp SV. Effect of inhaling heated vapor on symptoms of the common cold. JAMA 264:989–991, 1990. (In contrast to previous studies, this randomized clinical trial showed that the Rhinotherm, an ultrasonic heater that delivers heated mist intranasally, had no beneficial effect on common cold symptoms.)

Simons FER: Chronic rhinitis. Pediatr Clin North Am 31:801–819, 1984. (Excellent presentation of this elusive entity.)

Sperber SJ, Levine PA, Sorrentino JV et al: Ineffectiveness of recombinant interferon β_{serine} nasal drops for prophylaxis of natural colds. J Infect Dis 160:700–705, 1989. (This randomized clinical trial did not demonstrate a prophylactic efficacy of interferon.)

164
Stridor

Ellen M. Friedman

Stridor is a nonspecific term that means noisy breathing. Stridor, in itself, is not pathognomonic or diagnostic of any disease process and may not even be related to otolaryngologic abnormalities. An initial consideration of stridor in the newborn should include congenital cardiac malformations, neurologic disorders, or general toxicity. If these etiologies are ruled out, the physician should look to the airway as the most likely source of difficulty.

PATHOPHYSIOLOGY

Stridor is caused by an increase in turbulence when air passes through a narrow inlet. Because of the small size of the infant and the pediatric airway, even a small amount of airway narrowing may result in a significant obstruction. The prolonged and tubular curved omega shape of the infant epiglottis and the redundant aryepiglottic folds may further compromise the airway. The elastic cartilage of the pediatric larynx is flexible and, therefore, may partially obstruct the airway with the dynamic changes associated with respiration. By determining if the stridor is present on inspiration, expiration, or both, the physician should be able to approximate the anatomic location of the obstruction.

Stridor will occur on inspiration if a narrowed area is in the nasopharynx, pharynx, or supraglottis. This is the result of the increased negative pressure on inspiration that causes the supraglottic structures to collapse into the airway. Expiration will force these structures open and allow unobstructed airflow; therefore, there will be no audible sound on expiration with supraglottic obstruction. The subglottic space is encompassed by the circumferential cricoid ring, which is inflexible; therefore, changes in the phase of respiration will not alter the stridor. An obstruction in this region will result in noisy breathing on both expiration and inspiration, or biphasic stridor. Stridor associated with pathology of the lower trachea, such as tracheomalacia, will be present on expiration only. The relative positive pressure associated with expiration will further infringe on the already narrowed tracheal lumen, resulting in a low-pitched expiratory wheeze. Inspiration will be unobstructed.

CLINICAL PRESENTATION AND EVALUATION

Stridor may or may not be associated with respiratory distress. Frequently, loud inspiratory stridor may occur in a very pink, happy child without a significant obstruction. If

Table 164-1.   Signs and Symptoms Associated with Lesions

	SUPRAGLOTTIC	SUBGLOTTIC	TRACHEAL
Stridor	Inspiratory	Biphasic	Expiratory
Dysphagia	Present	Absent	Absent
Cry/voice	Muffled	Normal	Normal
Retractions	Mild	Present	Present

air hunger and significant obstruction are present, however, it is essential for the physician to proceed promptly and aggressively to alleviate the obstruction. The degree of respiratory distress can be estimated by assessing certain parameters: color, retractions, respiration rate, air entry, and state of consciousness. Pulse oximetry is used increasingly in ambulatory settings. It can supplement the physical exam by providing objective data on the severity of the obstruction and on monitoring clinical changes. When actual respiratory distress is absent, stridor may be evaluated with leisure. Questions regarding birth history, mode and age of onset, and the presence of associated symptoms will be most helpful. Associated symptoms such as feeding difficulties, quality of cry/voice, and the presence or absence of retractions may complete the clinical picture and will help elucidate the final diagnosis. A summary of the signs and symptoms associated with lesions in the different anatomic areas is listed in Table 164-1.

DIFFERENTIAL DIAGNOSIS

Most cases of stridor (~60%) are secondary to problems at the level of the larynx. *Laryngomalacia* is a frequent diagnosis that causes low-pitched, fluttering inspiratory stridor. This diagnosis is a benign, self-correcting condition and is thought to represent immaturity of the laryngeal cartilages. Some cases may result from a neuromuscular disorder. The stridor gradually improves as the soft cartilage matures. This condition usually resolves without any intervention between the ages of 12 and 18 months. Lists of common lesions in specific locations are given in Tables 164-2, 164-3, and 164-4.

Table 164-2.   Supraglottic Stridor

CONGENITAL	INFLAMMATORY	NEOPLASMS	TRAUMA
Choanal atresia	Adenotonsillar	Benign	Postoperative
Nasal septal deviation	hypertrophy/infection	Dermoid	Caustic ingestion
Epiglottic cyst	Retropharyngeal	Cystic hygroma	
Laryngomalacia	abscess	Malignant	
	Supra(epi)glottitis	Lymphoma	
		Rhabdomyosarcoma	

Table 164-3.   Subglottic Stridor

CONGENITAL	INFLAMMATORY	NEOPLASM
Web	Croup	Benign
Stenosis	Angioneurotic	Papillomatosis
Vocal cord	edema	Hemangioma
paralysis		Malignant
		Rhabdomyosarcoma

Table 164-4.   Tracheal Stridor

CONGENITAL	INFLAMMATORY	NEOPLASM	TRAUMA
Tracheoesophageal fistula	Bacterial tracheitis	Benign	Foreign body
		Papillomatosis	
		Adenoma	
Tracheomalacia		Malignant	Stenosis
		Chondrosarcoma	

TREATMENT

Overzealous handling or investigations of the child with respiratory distress may exacerbate the situation. The ensuing work-up, therefore, should be determined by the degree of toxicity and respiratory distress of the patient. Observation of the patient in various positions and during feeding is helpful. Radiographic studies, including fluoroscopy of the airway and barium swallow, are helpful in determining dynamic changes associated with respiration and the possibility of an extratracheal cause for obstruction, such as a vascular ring.

In general, no further blood tests or laboratory studies are routinely indicated. However, in specific cases special tests (e.g., C-reactive protein or pulmonary function tests) may be required. The diagnosis is established most commonly by laryngoscopy and bronchoscopy. The airway of the neonate and premature infant can be evaluated with use of the magnifying telescope. The rigid ventilating bronchoscope allows for a relatively leisurely inspection of the entire length of the larynx, trachea, and upper bronchi.

Controversy arises concerning the role of diagnostic flexible bronchoscopy because of both its advantages and disadvantages. Although flexible laryngoscopy and bronchoscopy can be performed without anesthesia, there are significant limitations. Without the benefit of an endotracheal tube, the airway control is not assured, which limits the duration of a safe examination. Many of the more complex situations are difficult to assess with only brief visualization. The small size of the pediatric flexible endoscopes allows limited capability for suctioning and secretion removal, and no possibility of removing a foreign body or obtaining a biopsy. The significant advantage of flexible endoscopy is the ability to view the larynx and trachea in the dynamic state of spontaneous respirations without an obstructed view due to an endotracheal tube.

A referral to an otolaryngologist should be based on the degree of stridor and associated airway obstruction. An unusual history or progressive clinical course should alert the physician that a consultation is needed. Laryngoscopy and bronchoscopy should be performed by an experienced pediatric endoscopist with the aid of an experienced pediatric anesthesiologist.

ANNOTATED BIBLIOGRAPHY

Cotton R, Reilly JS: Stridor and airway obstruction. In Bluestone CD, Stool SE (eds): Pediatric Otolaryngology. Philadelphia, WB Saunders, 1983. (Excellent general reference.)

Holinger LD: Etiology of stridor in the neonate, infant and child. Ann Otol 89:397, 1980. (Good review of differential diagnosis.)

Holinger PH, Brown WT: Congenital webs, cysts, laryngoceles and other anomalies of the larynx. Ann Otol Rhinol Laryngol 76:744, 1976. (Good overview of the various congenital anomalies.)

165
Foreign Body Aspiration

Victor C. Baum

Accidental aspiration of foreign matter into the airway is a major cause of childhood morbidity and mortality and results in several hundred deaths each year in children in the United States. Approximately 10% of children with foreign body aspirations are less than 1 year of age; 50% to 75% are 1 to 3 years of age; and 15% to 30% are over 3 years of age. The most commonly aspirated material is food, with nutmeats accounting for 50% of all aspirations (peanuts are the most common). About half of the children who seek care do so within the first 48 hours of aspiration; up to 20% may not develop symptoms or may have their symptoms overlooked for over 1 month.

PATHOPHYSIOLOGY

Foreign objects in the airway can do damage either by partial or complete occlusion of a portion of the tracheobronchial tree or by direct trauma to the mucosa. Although it has been stated that aspirated material is typically aspirated into the right lung, a review of several large series reveals that this predilection does not occur often enough to be clinically useful. Indeed, in one series, a preponderance of foreign bodies was located in the left main stem bronchus. The final resting place is determined by the size of the aspirated material in relation to the size of the airways. The main stem bronchi are the site of impaction in 75% to 80% of cases; the trachea (typically the distal trachea) in about 10%; and the larynx in ~4% of cases. The onset of symptoms, the nature of symptoms, and the radiologic findings depend on three factors: (1) *Type of object*: sharp or irritating objects may result primarily in hemoptysis and blood-tinged sputum, unlike organic or other objects that cause damage primarily by airway obstruction. (2) *Location of the object*: resulting in upper (extrathoracic) or lower (intrathoracic) airway obstruction. (3) *Complete or partial obstruction*: because airway diameters vary with changes in airway pressure during the respiratory cycle, aspirated objects either may completely obstruct airways to produce atelectasis or may allow air entry during inspiration, but obstruct during exhalation, resulting in localized air trapping.

CLINICAL PRESENTATION

Over 90% of children present with some respiratory distress, usually dyspnea and cough. As mentioned, the clinical presentation is determined by the type of foreign object, the location of the object, and whether aspiration has resulted in a partial or complete obstruction of that portion of the airway. Obstruction of the larynx by a large object results in immediate cessation of effective ventilation and progresses rapidly to cyanosis and syncope (*cafe coronary*). Impaction in the upper, extrathoracic airway results primarily in difficulty during inspiration with retractions and inspiratory stridor. Intrathoracic partial obstruction results primarily in a cough and in difficulty during exhalation with expiratory wheezing. Smaller aspirated particles may not produce symptoms for several weeks, at which time an afebrile chronic cough or a lower respiratory tract infection develops. Only a few, however, present with a chronic infection or bronchiectasis. Few patients present with hemoptysis from excoriation of the airway mucosa by a sharp or rough object.

DIFFERENTIAL DIAGNOSIS

The differential diagnosis of foreign body aspiration includes all causes of upper and lower airway obstruction. Congenital abnormalities causing airway obstruction typically present with chronic obstruction; these may develop acute exacerbations mimicking foreign body aspiration. Because foreign body aspiration can have a chronic, indolent course, causes of chronic pulmonary infiltrates, such as pulmonary sequestration, should be considered.

A partial list of causes of acute airway obstruction includes asthma, massive tonsillar enlargement, peritonsillar or retropharyngeal abscess, croup (laryngotracheobronchitis), epiglottitis, bacterial tracheitis, diphtheria, subglottic stenosis, laryngomalacia and tracheomalacia, anaphylaxis, craniofacial anomalies with macroglossia or mandibular hypoplasia, subglottic hemangioma, laryngeal papillomatosis, and vascular anomalies such as vascular rings and pulmonary artery sling. In addition, because the trachea of children is softer than the adult trachea, impaction of large hard objects such as coins in the esophagus can cause tracheal compression.

WORK-UP

History

A history of foreign body aspiration is usually elicited. Various series, however, report a positive history in only 50% to 90% of cases, leaving a sizable minority in whom clinical suspicion is a major factor in instituting further evaluation. With a positive history and appropriate symptoms, a foreign body can be found on bronchoscopy in 90% of cases.

Physical Examination

The physical findings depend on the location of the object and the degree of airway obstruction. A partial obstruction of the upper, extrathoracic airway results primarily in in-

spiratory difficulty with inspiratory stridor. Lower, intrathoracic airway obstruction results primarily in expiratory difficulty. The location in lobar or segmental bronchi produces unilateral findings of asymmetric breath sounds, focal wheezing, or localized decreased air entry. Aspiration of a foreign body may also result in the findings of a chronic infiltrate with a chronic cough, crackles, and fever.

Laboratory Tests

Although most aspirated foreign bodies are radiolucent, radiologic imaging procedures are commonly employed diagnostic tests. Routine radiographs are suggested to document passage of ingested coins through the esophagus into the stomach. Although somewhat controversial, this recommendation prevents asphyxiation caused by a coin dislodged into the airway and a late complication of coins impacted in the esophagus, even after an asymptomatic interval. Fluoroscopy of the chest can demonstrate evidence of an aspirated foreign body in up to 90% of bronchial foreign bodies and 30% of laryngotracheal foreign bodies. Most laryngeal foreign bodies, however, will be missed. Laryngeal obstruction from any cause can produce a dilated hypopharynx. Signs on fluoroscopy include an inspiratory shift of the mediastinum, mediastinal widening on inspiration, and air trapping with reduced expiratory diaphragmatic excursion on the affected side. Plain chest radiographs can produce evidence for foreign body aspiration in ~75% of cases. The most common findings are unilateral hyperaeration, infiltrates, and atelectasis. Less common findings (<10%) are a radiopaque foreign body, a narrowed tracheal lumen, bronchiectasis or lung abscess, pneumomediastinum, or pneumothorax. A film obtained at end-exhalation will make unilateral hyperexpansion more apparent. If the child cannot cooperate, obtaining bilateral decubitus films or pushing up on the epigastrium with a gloved hand will also demonstrate unequal lung volumes. Compared with bronchoscopy, inspiratory and expiratory films have only 68% sensitivity and 67% specificity. The subglottic tracheal lumen should be evaluated for evidence of croup (*pencil point* or *church steeple* sign) (see Chap. 166).

THERAPY

The current consensus for life-threatening airway obstruction in children older than 12 months and adults is to deliver six to ten abdominal thrusts (*Heimlich maneuver*) until the foreign body is expelled. If unsuccessful, four sharp blows should be delivered to the victim's back between the shoulder blades, and, if still necessary, the Heimlich maneuver should be repeated.

The current recommendation for the choking infant younger than 1 year old is to support the prone infant on one arm of the rescuer with the head lower than the trunk and to deliver four back blows. If unsuccessful, the infant is turned to the supine position, supported between two hands, and four chest thrusts are delivered. These thrusts are identical to external cardiac compressions and they are delivered to the chest rather than to the abdomen because of the relatively large size of the liver in infants. If the infant is unconscious and the airway cannot be opened with the aforementioned maneuvers, an attempt should be made to ventilate mouth-to-mouth following correct positioning of the neck and jaw and removal of any foreign body visualized in the oropharynx.

Bronchoscopy is indicated if there is a history of foreign body aspiration; the urgency is determined by the location and degree of respiratory distress. This should be done, if at all possible, by a bronchoscopist/anesthesiologist/operating room team experienced in pediatric endoscopy. A rigid bronchoscope is preferred, and these objects can be removed by various instruments and manipulations. The removal of one foreign body does not exclude the presence of another. In one series, 15% of patients required a second examination because of a second foreign body missed during the first procedure or incompletely removed. A thoracotomy is rarely required (<1%). Postbronchoscopy complications include laryngeal edema that responds to racemic epinephrine and steroids. Most patients are rapidly discharged from the hospital. One series reported that 88% of their patients were discharged within 24 hours of admission and 36% were discharged home directly from the recovery room.

Postural drainage alone is not indicated as a primary therapy. It may not be successful and may relocate a foreign body from one bronchus to the other, resulting in a foreign body in one bronchus and an edematous airway on the other side. The foreign body may also be dislodged, producing laryngeal obstruction. Postural drainage may be indicated if bronchoscopy does not identify a foreign body, suggesting small fragments.

INDICATIONS FOR REFERRAL

Any history of foreign body aspiration deserves further evaluation, and a documented foreign body in the airway requires referral to a skilled endoscopy team. A history of unexplained cough, wheeze, or decreased air entry also provides a reason for referral, as do unexplained hemoptysis and a chronic localized infiltrate.

PATIENT EDUCATION

Appropriate foods for age should be part of routine well-child discussions with parents because most aspirated material is food matter. Food should be cut into age-appropriate pieces rather than offered uncut. Children should be taught to eat just one piece of food at a time rather than stuffing their mouths, and they should never leave the table with food still in their mouths.

ANNOTATED BIBLIOGRAPHY

Blazer S, Naveh Y, Friedman A: Foreign body in the airway. Am J Dis Child 134:68, 1980. (Series of 200 cases of foreign body aspiration in children.)

Cotton E, Yasuda K: Foreign body aspiration. Pediatr Clin North Am 4:937, 1984. (General review of foreign body aspiration.)

Foods and Choking in Children. Conference Report to the FDA, U.S. Department of Health and Human Services, and U.S. Department of Agriculture. Elk Grove Village, IL, American Academy of Pediatrics, 1983. (AAP recommendations including parental education.)

Svedstrom E, Puhakka H, Kero P: How accurate is chest radiography in the diagnosis of tracheobronchial foreign bodies in children? Pediatr Radiol 19:520, 1989. (In a series of children with suspected foreign body aspiration, inspiratory/expiratory chest radiographs, when compared to bronchoscopy, had a sensitivity of 68% and a specificity of 67%.)

166

Inflammatory Illnesses of the Pediatric Airway

Ellen M. Friedman

As discussed in Chapter 164, because of the anatomy of the pediatric airway, a small amount of edema may lead to significant airway obstruction. Inflammatory conditions are second only to congenital anomalies as the most common cause of airway obstruction. The three most common inflammatory illnesses of the pediatric airway are supraglottitis (epiglottitis), croup, and bacterial tracheitis. Each of these entities has a fairly distinctive clinical presentation and requires specific intervention. Because these illnesses can progress rapidly to complete respiratory obstruction, it is imperative that the physician be familiar with the diagnosis and treatment of each disease.

SUPRAGLOTTITIS

Supraglottitis is a true pediatric emergency. The clinical progression from partial to complete airway obstruction is rapid and requires prompt intervention. The morbidity and mortality associated with supraglottitis has decreased with the use of antibiotics and endotracheal intubation.

Pathophysiology

Supraglottitis is a bacterial infection that is most commonly secondary to *Haemophilus influenzae* type b. The bacterial invasion causes inflammation of the lingual surface of the epiglottis, the aryepiglottic folds, the ventricular bands, and the paraglottic space. The involvement of all of these structures has supported supraglottitis as the preferred name for the entity previously known as epiglottitis. Because of the massive supraglottic edema, inspiratory stridor is a predominant clinical feature. Swelling in the area of the esophageal inlet results in difficulty with secretions and subsequent drooling.

Children with supraglottitis are usually between 3 and 5 years old and in previous good health. A consistent male predilection is demonstrated with this disease, as in many airway ailments. The clinical picture rapidly evolves from a mild sore throat to severe respiratory distress, with inspiratory stridor and drooling. The child becomes increasingly toxic within hours, developing a high fever and a rapidly increasing respiratory rate. The frightened child will sit upright, with head extended, jaw thrust forward, and mouth open in an attempt to maintain a patent airway. The child will become limp and will relinquish this posture only when he or she is completely exhausted and is hypoxic. Such a change in position indicates collapse and impending respiratory arrest.

Because of the fragile nature of the compromised airway in supraglottitis, a physical examination of the child should be minimized. Overzealous handling of a child in this condition can be disastrous. Although some physicians feel that direct visualization of the epiglottis with a tongue depressor in the emergency department will confirm or rule out the diagnosis, the serious possibility of inducing laryngospasm and subsequent respiratory arrest does not warrant such an examination. The patient should remain with the parent and must not be alarmed or disturbed. Blood tests should not be performed and intravenous lines should not be established. All attempts should be directed at the prompt establishment of a secure artificial airway.

Supraglottitis is a clinical diagnosis and does not require a confirmatory radiogram. The possibility of a sudden complete respiratory obstruction in the radiology suite is real. Although there is a diagnostic radiographic appearance of supraglottitis, it does not warrant delay in the establishment of a secure airway. In cases where the possibility of supraglottitis is raised but considered unlikely, a radiogram may be useful in ruling out the diagnosis. In this setting, the patient must be sent for a radiogram accompanied by resuscitation equipment and experienced staff if intubation becomes necessary.

In general, hospitals with a well-defined protocol for the management of supraglottitis have lower morbidity and mortality rates. The team approach has proved most successful. Team members include a pediatrician, an otolaryngologist, an anesthesiologist, and an intensive care unit staff member. It is important for each member to be familiar with the procedure in order to minimize confusion and to smoothly organize the management of the patient.

Supraglottitis was previously treated by either intubation, tracheotomy, or close observation in the intensive care unit. The option of monitored observation should be highly discouraged. The progression of this illness is rapid and may be unpredictable. There is a 6% mortality rate in patients who are closely monitored without airway support, but this rate decreases to less than 1% with the establishment of an artificial airway. Such data reemphasize the need to establish an artificial airway and highlight the fact that observation is an unacceptable practice.

The decision to intubate rather than to establish a tracheotomy depends on the clinical facilities available. Certain hospital personnel are more comfortable with the postoperative care and management of the tracheotomized patient. The complication rate associated with pediatric tracheotomies has been reported to be between 10% and 19%. Complications include hemorrhage, pneumothorax, and subglottic stenosis. A general preference for nasotracheal intubation in this illness has emerged because it is highly effective and has fewer inherent risks. When nasotracheal intubation is selected, it is important to use an endotracheal tube that is ~1 mm smaller than the normal tube size. Because of the smaller tube size, attentive nursing care and frequent suctioning will alleviate the possibility of mucous plug obstruction. Meticulous taping of the tube will avoid an accidental extubation. The nasotracheal tube can be removed immediately when the supraglottic edema has resolved. Because there is no need to await tracheotomy decannulation, shorter hospitalization has been the rule.

Because supraglottitis is usually due to *H. influenzae* type b, intravenous antibiotic therapy directed against this organism should be started immediately. The increasing incidence of amoxicillin-resistant *Haemophilus* influenza nationwide has altered the choice of appropriate antibiotic therapy. Current recommendations are ceftriaxone, cefuroxime, or chloramphenicol and oxacillin.

It is postulated that the *H. influenzae* B vaccine (HIB) will decrease the incidence of supraglottitis.

CROUP

Croup is a term that is used interchangeably to describe various respiratory illnesses. Three specific entities constitute the croup syndromes: spasmodic croup, laryngotracheitis, and laryngotracheobronchitis. Characteristics common to each of the diseases include a varying degree of respiratory obstruction, barking cough, and toxicity. Each entity is discussed separately, although in practice they may not always be distinguishable.

Spasmodic Croup

Spasmodic croup usually begins with difficulty in breathing at night and the sudden onset of a barking cough. It occurs throughout all ages of childhood and may recur. The children are usually afebrile and nontoxic. A mild upper respiratory infection may precede the development of spasmodic croup.

The etiology is undetermined, but spasmodic croup is

currently believed to reflect an allergic phenomenon or a low-grade viral infection. Symptoms resolve quickly when treated with humidity (e.g., running the shower or going out in the night air) and reassurance. Other medications that have been used with varying responses include corticosteroids, syrup of ipecac, diphenhydramine elixir, and subcutaneous epinephrine. Airway intervention in the form of intubation or tracheotomy is rarely necessary.

Laryngotracheitis

Laryngotracheitis is a viral infection in which submucosal edema is present in the subglottic space. Because of the inflammation and swelling, there is destruction of the ciliated epithelium with poor mucous transport. Without increased humidification, the fibrinous exudate will dry out and become hardened crusts, which will further compromise the airway.

Laryngotracheobronchitis

Laryngotracheobronchitis refers to a viral infection that extends further and involves the entire respiratory tract. The most common viruses are parainfluenza and respiratory syncytial viruses. When the respiratory tract is extensively involved, a bacterial suprainfection may occur. When there is a bacterial component, it is usually secondary to streptococcus, staphylococcus, or *H. influenzae* type b.

The children involved are usually less than 3 years of age. They appear ill but not toxic. They have the characteristic croupy cough and biphasic stridor. Laryngotracheitis and laryngotracheobronchitis are most common during the winter. Significant yearly variations are determined by the virulence of the specific viruses.

The history is fairly straightforward. A mild preceding upper respiratory infection usually occurs. The symptoms may intensify at night and then wane during daytime. Most commonly, croup will resolve within 3 to 7 days. Prolonged or recurrent episodes of croup should alert the physician to the possibility of an underlying congenital malformation (e.g., congenital subglottic stenosis), the presence of a foreign body, or a bacterial infection.

An anteroposterior radiogram of the airway will reveal the characteristic narrowing of the subglottic space: this is referred to as the *steeple sign* or the *pencil point sign* (Fig. 166-1). No other studies are useful in the work-up.

Most patients with any of the croup syndromes do not require hospitalization. Humidification is crucial and is effective in reducing the airway obstruction, and it may be implemented at home. It is helpful to use a croup score or another established criterion to evaluate the child who has croup. A suggested croup scoring symptom includes the following parameters: stridor, retraction, air entry, color, and level of consciousness.

Children who do not respond to humidification and oxygen administration will require racemic epinephrine. The

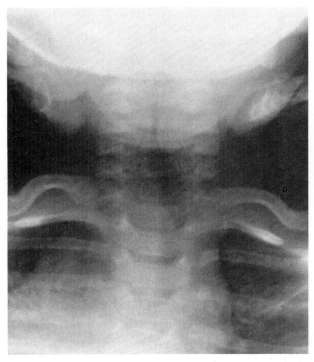

Figure 166-1. Anteroposterior view of the neck demonstrating the "steeple sign" in croup.

response to racemic epinephrine should be dramatic; however, this response may not be long-lived. After one administration of racemic epinephrine in the emergency department or in a physician's office, the patient should be admitted to the hospital for observation. A deterioration of the clinical status or actual pharmacologic rebound may occur following even one dose of racemic epinephrine.

Airway support should be considered in those few patients with an increasing croup score, a decreasing response to epinephrine, decreasing arterial oxygen saturation (determined, for example, by pulse oximetry), or the need for more frequent epinephrine injections. Controversy surrounds the decision to intubate children who have an inflamed, narrowed subglottis. The fear is that the foreign body response to an endotracheal tube will heighten the subglottic irritation and will result in an acquired stenosis. Tracheotomy has been suggested as an alternative.

The role of steroids remains controversial in the management of croup, but the weight of current evidence favors their therapeutic efficacy. Reports in the literature are difficult to analyze because frequently in the various papers the specific croup syndrome is not defined and there are significant differences in dosages and dosage schedules. It appears that a significant dose (i.e., 1.5 mg/kg, up to 20 mg) of dexamethasone may decrease the amount and the duration of subglottic inflammation. Even a single dose of dexamethasone (0.6 mg/kg) has been shown to significantly reduce the severity of moderate to severe croup in hospitalized children. In all but the most mild outpatient cases of croup, where any type of intervention is likely to be unnecessary, it is also reasonable to administer this dose of dexamethasone to the child.

Most children who have croup can be managed at home with humidification and reassurance. Close patient follow-up must be maintained. In cases where the clinical symptoms of airway obstruction are progressing, the child should be evaluated in an emergency department. Signs of increasing obstruction are patient fatigue, increasing stridor, retractions, and cyanosis. Pulse oximetry is useful in detecting hypoxemia or documenting deterioration. A referral for an endoscopy should be made to a pediatric otolaryngologist if croup recurs more than three times a year, if it is prolonged beyond reasonable expectation, or if it does not clear between recurrences.

BACTERIAL TRACHEITIS

Bacterial tracheitis is an acute infectious disease of the airway in infants and children and has features common to both croup and epiglottitis. It is felt that bacterial tracheitis represents a true infection of the trachea and not merely a suprainfection of viral croup.

Pathophysiology

Bacterial tracheitis is characterized by subglottic edema and copious mucopurulence in the trachea. The bacterial infection impedes mucociliary flow and there is stasis of the secretions. Bronchoscopy reveals thick mucus with a disruption and sloughing of the tracheal mucosa.

The most common causative organism is *Staphylococcus aureus,* although *H. influenzae* type b and streptococcus have also been isolated. The blood cultures are uniformly negative, although the blood count will show an elevated white blood cell count with a shift to the left.

Clinical Presentation

The age of children who have bacterial tracheitis ranges from several months old to early adolescence. A preceding mild upper respiratory infection usually occurs with an 8- to 10-hour deterioration of clinical status. During this period, there is a progressive hoarseness, a brassy cough, and inspiratory or biphasic stridor. Cardiopulmonary arrest has been reported with increasing obstruction.

On physical examination, the patient with bacterial tracheitis will appear to have a varying degree of respiratory distress. Stridor, cough, retractions, and cyanosis are also present. The patient is frequently febrile and may have concomitant pneumonia. A lateral neck x-ray shows cloudiness of the tracheal air column, with an irregularity or scalloping of the tracheal wall. The sloughed tracheal mucosa sometimes gives the radiographic impression of a foreign body and may be misread as such.

Many centers recommend inserting an artificial airway in patients with bacterial tracheitis. Most series, even with intubation or tracheostomy, report a significant number of cardiac arrests and death. These occurrences have been related to plugs of sloughed mucosa, which may obstruct the artificial airway or the bronchi. Thus, meticulous suctioning of the airway is the key to successful management of these patients. Bronchoscopy will be not only diagnostic but also therapeutic in that it will allow for direct visualization as well as for complete removal of debris. Further management involves humidity, appropriate intravenous antimicrobial therapy, and close monitoring in the intensive care setting. Intubation or tracheotomy is reserved for those patients in whom adequate ventilation is impossible without such intervention.

ANNOTATED BIBLIOGRAPHY

Davis HW, Gartner JC, Galvis AG et al: Acute upper airway obstruction, croup and epiglottitis. Pediatr Clin North Am 4(28), 1981.

Fried MP: Controversies in the management of supraglottitis and croup. Pediatr Clin North Am 4(26):931–942, 1979.

Jones R, Santos JI, Overall JC Jr: Bacterial tracheitis. JAMA 242: 721–726, 1979. (This reference and the ones above provide good overviews of the topics indicated by their respective titles.)

Kairys SW, Olmstead EM, O'Connor GT et al: Steroid treatment of laryngotracheitis: A meta-analysis of the evidence from randomized trials. Pediatrics 83:683–693, 1989. (Combined results of nine randomized clinical trials involving 1286 patients; showed that steroids significantly improve the severity of croup.)

Super DM, Cartelli NA, Brooks LJ et al: A prospective randomized double-blind study to evaluate the effect of dexamethasone in acute laryngotracheitis. J Pediatr 115:323–329, 1989. (Prospective, randomized study; showed that a single parenteral dose of dexamethasone [0.6 mg/kg] reduced the severity of croup.)

Waisman Y, Klein YW, Boenning DA, et al: Prospective randomized double-blind study comparing L-epinephrine and racemic epinephrine aerosols in the treatment of laryngotracheitis. Pediatrics 89:302–306, 1992. (The readily available and far less expensive L-form of epinephrine is as effective as racemic epinephrine in treating croup in children.)

167

Bronchiolitis

Henry L. Dorkin

Bronchiolitis is one of the more prevalent respiratory illnesses encountered by pediatricians who treat young infants. It is usually the result of a viral infection, and the more common causative agents in this age group are respiratory syncytial virus (RSV), parainfluenza type III, adenovirus, and, occasionally, enteroviruses.

PATHOPHYSIOLOGY

The exact immunologic nature of the host–virus interaction is not fully understood, but the resultant pathophysiology is well described. A necrotizing desquamation occurs along the epithelium of the bronchioles. This results in the deposition of luminal debris, which both increases airway resistance and leads to air trapping in alveoli behind the partially obstructed airway lumina. Because of the air trapping and hyperinflation, much more negative pressure must be generated by the muscles of inspiration in order to move the same tidal volume of air. Such large negative pressures in the pulmonary interstitium upset the hydrostatic forces that keep interstitial fluid content low. The increased interstitial fluid that results adds to the work of breathing not only by increasing airflow obstruction but also by further decreasing pulmonary compliance. The respiratory rate increases to minimize this work of breathing and maintain respiratory function.

CLINICAL PRESENTATION

Bronchiolitis usually begins as a mild upper respiratory tract infection with rhinitis or cough. There is usually little or no fever, although a high fever may occur. After 1 or 2 days, there is onset of a wheeze and tachypnea. The child is somewhat irritable and often has less interest in feeding. The child's color may be normal or slightly cyanotic. The nares are often flared, and the child may be using accessory muscles of respiration. The chest is, to some degree, hyperinflated with intercostal or subcostal retractions. Abdominal organs are often easily palpated below the costal margins. Wheezes are prominent on auscultation, but crackles and rhonchi may also be heard diffusely throughout the lung fields.

DIFFERENTIAL DIAGNOSIS

In a child under 2 years of age, bronchiolitis is one of the most common causes of episodic airflow obstruction. Asthma can be difficult to differentiate from bronchiolitis; in fact, some physicians will not try to separate borderline cases, referring to them only as *wheezing-associated respiratory illness (WARI)*. In clear-cut cases with a strong family history of asthma, a marked response to bronchodilators, and clinical symptoms in the absence of a predisposing viral respiratory tract infection, the physician can feel more confident about diagnosing asthma in an infant (see Chap. 47). Cystic fibrosis often presents in a child as repetitive episodes of bronchiolitis. A recurrent presentation outside of the epidemic time frame, or the presence of other complicating cystic fibrosis symptoms (e.g., diarrhea, failure to thrive, meconium ileus), warrants sending the child to a cystic fibrosis center for a sweat test (see Chap. 171). Anatomic abnormalities such as vascular rings or tracheo-

malacia do not remit during the standard bronchiolitis time course. Chest fluoroscopy with barium swallow may reveal the defect. Gastroesophageal reflux is often a confounding factor in the differential diagnosis of bronchiolitis. All infants reflux to some degree, and this may be enhanced secondarily as a result of the hyperinflation of bronchiolitis. Nevertheless, the presence of recurrent symptoms associated with emesis, acid reflux on a pH probe, and esophagitis on biopsy all suggest that there may be a contribution of reflux to the recurrent wheeze. This is important in the differential diagnosis because many of the drugs that are used for bronchodilation will decrease lower esophageal sphincter tone and hence exacerbate the reflux (see Chap. 102). Aspiration of a foreign body must be considered in a child who wheezes for the first time, especially if otherwise well. The wheezing, however, is usually paroxysmal in onset and can often be related to a choking episode with feeding or play (see Chap. 165). Numerous other diagnoses, including immunodeficiency, dysmotile cilia syndrome, and alpha$_1$-antitrypsin deficiency, can occur but are less likely in the absence of a positive family history. In addition, congestive heart failure in a child with congenital heart disease may present with wheezing and respiratory distress.

Work-Up

History

Several features of the history are important. The physician should ascertain if the baby has been active and playful or has merely been lying in the crib or stroller interacting little with the environment. The physician should determine if the child has been fed relatively normally or with great difficulty, or if the child is breathing so quickly that he or she can nurse only for a few moments before coughing and choking. Both the intake over the previous 24 hours and determination of whether the baby has been urinating as frequently as usual should be noted. The child's temperature should be taken, and the physician should observe how prolonged the temperature elevation has been. A history of apnea or cyanosis with the current illness is particularly worrisome. The mother's experience in dealing with illness in small children should also be determined. Evidence suggests that bronchiolitis occurring before 3 months of age and a gestational age of less than 34 weeks are associated with more severe disease.

Physical Examination

The physical examination can confirm or refute some aspects of the history. It is important to unclothe the child so that only a diaper remains. A complete assessment of respiratory function cannot be performed adequately in a dressed infant. In particular, the respiratory rate and child's color should be noted. The presence of pallor or cyanosis indicates hypoxemia. A tachypneic child who has any degree of nasal flaring, cervical accessory respiratory muscle use, or intercostal or subcostal retractions has the potential for developing respiratory failure. The inferior liver margin should be palpated and the upper border percussed. It is important to ascertain whether the liver edge is depressed secondary to lung hyperinflation or whether the liver is enlarged possibly because of congestive heart failure. In any event, careful measurements are useful in following the course of the child's illness. The physician should pay particular attention to chest wall and abdominal motion. As the diaphragm tires, the abdomen no longer moves outward with inspiration but rather moves inward and toward the thorax; such breathing is an ominous sign.

Laboratory Tests

Pulse oximeters, standard equipment in hospital emergency rooms, are now used in some private offices and may be helpful in determining the child's degree of hypoxemia. Relying on visual cyanosis alone may be inaccurate; in one study, half of those children whose room air hemoglobin saturations were less than 95% were not identified as hypoxic by their skin color. Other than oximetry, there is little in the standard office laboratory that will help the physician discern the severity of the illness. If urine can be collected, a urine specific gravity can be useful in determining hydration status. In children old enough to concentrate their urine, dilute urine (specific gravities below ~1.008) suggests that the child is adequately hydrated. Concentrated urine (specific gravities greater than ~1.015) suggests that the child is preserving his or her intravascular status. Other laboratory data helpful in assessing the child may be available at the local hospital. Oximetry, helpful for measuring the degree of hypoxemia, does not reveal if the child is retaining carbon dioxide. Historically, the arterial blood gas has been the standard method for determining the level of hypoxemia and hypercarbia. This information, if carefully gathered, is invaluable, but the agitation of arterial puncture may produce spurious results. (The physician can sometimes administer local Xylocaine, allow the child to fuss briefly, and then obtain the arterial sample through the anesthetized region when the child has calmed down.) A specimen obtained by venipuncture can be used if the pH and pCO_2 are corrected. Usually, venous pH is 0.04 pH units lower and venous pCO_2 is 6 mm Hg higher than the corresponding arterial values. Syringes with dry heparin should be used because liquid heparin will dilute the sample. Although this will have little effect on the pH, it can severely affect the pCO_2 results, falsely suggesting that the problem is predominantly one of acidemia secondary to metabolic acidosis and not to carbon dioxide retention. Information from poorly obtained blood gases and improperly attached oximeters can lead to incorrect therapeutic decisions, reminding us that bad data are worse than no data.

MANAGEMENT

Management of patients with a severe or mild disease is relatively straightforward. Oxygen, critical monitoring of vital signs and oxygen/carbon dioxide levels, ventilatory support, intravenous nutrition, antiviral agents where appropriate, antibacterial agents where superinfection has been proved, and bronchodilators where a response has been established are the standard approach in the hospital for the severely ill child. Reassurance, nasal suctioning as necessary, judicious feedings, and appropriate use of antipyretics suffice for the limited illness in most children. The remaining group, those who are borderline between outpatient care and hospitalization, tax the physician's medical acumen. Close observation and family contact are important in outpatient management. A follow-up phone call in a few hours or even a return office visit allows the physician to develop a perspective on the child's illness and the progression or resolution of incipient respiratory failure. It must be remembered that there is little warning when children with bronchiolitis begin to tire out. Retractions will lessen and the child may appear not to work as hard as earlier in the illness. This is an ominous sign when coupled with lack of playfulness, decreased interest in feeding, and persistent tachypnea.

The usefulness of beta-2 bronchodilators is controversial. Theoretically, smooth-muscle bronchospasm does not play a large role in the pathogenesis of bronchiolitis. These drugs also have little effect on luminal debris and mucus plugging. Moreover, despite relative airway specificity, even the most selective beta-2 agonist may have some cardiac chronotropic effect. Nevertheless, studies continue to be published both supporting and refuting a clinical response in bronchiolitis with beta-2 agents. The clinical data on methylxanthines are also unclear.

Retrospective studies and clinical impressions are somewhat at variance and no conclusive data support the use of corticosteroids in this illness. One recent, well-conducted double-blind study of steroids found no improvement in pulmonary function in the treated group when compared to the saline control population.

It is reasonable to try a beta agonist or methylxanthine in the treatment of these children. Clinical observation, however, is important. Failure to document a clinical response to a medication trial would argue for the cessation of such therapy before problems developed from drug side effects. It is also important not to develop a false sense of security because a wheezing child has been placed on bronchodilators. Chest physiotherapy and large-particle mist are often considered adjunct care. With regard to chest physiotherapy, the benefits of helping expectoration of luminal debris must be balanced against the agitation and possible oxyhemoglobin desaturation that may result. If begun, the child should have adequate time to rest between sessions. Large-particle mist has little chance of getting to the lower respiratory tract and may theoretically increase airway resistance. Careful suctioning of the nasopharynx, with saline nose drops just prior to suctioning, may be much more useful. Mist tents hide the child from care-givers and make it more difficult to perceive deterioration.

Future trends in control of infection and management of disease can be extrapolated from current knowledge. Simple hand washing by family members and care-givers, as well as preventing cohorts with respiratory infection from attending day-care centers, may decrease the incidence of the disease. Previous attempts at immunization were unsuccessful, but newer vaccines or temperature-sensitive viral mutants may play a future role in prevention. Although the use of aerosolized antiviral agents such as ribavirin is currently limited to hospital administration for proven viral infection in the compromised host (e.g., chronic lung disease, congenital heart disease, immunodeficient patient), further investigation may lead to outpatient administration for the general population at risk. However, concerns about toxic exposure of care-givers and teratogenesis make this drug inappropriate for mild, outpatient disease therapy. At present, the physician's best weapon in caring for the infected child is to understand the pathophysiology and to anticipate the individual patient's course so that intervention can prevent respiratory failure.

ANNOTATED BIBLIOGRAPHY

Denny FW, Collier AM, Henderson FW et al: The epidemiology of bronchiolitis. Pediatr Res 11:234–236, 1977.

Hall CB: The shedding and spreading of respiratory syncytial virus. Pediatr Res 11:236–239, 1977. (This and the above reference detail the natural history of RSV infection.)

Outwater KM, Crone RK: Management of respiratory failure in infants with acute viral bronchiolitis. Am J Dis Child 138(11):1071–1075, 1984. (Logical approach to progressive respiratory failure in infants; certain therapies such as the use of theophylline are suggested, although supporting data are predominantly by clinical impression.)

Schuh S, Canny G, Reissman JJ, Kerem E, Bentur L, Petric M, Levinson H: Nebulized albuterol in acute bronchiolitis. J Pediatr 117(4):633–637, 1990. (Supports the use of albuterol in bronchiolitis; contrast with the paper by Sly et al.)

Shaw KN, Bell LM, Sherman NH: Outpatient assessment of infants with bronchiolitis. Am J Dis Child 145(2):151–155, 1991. (Study designed to determine at the initial outpatient evaluation the historical, physical, and laboratory clues that may predict more severe disease.)

Sly PD, Lanteri CJ, Raven JM: Do wheezy infants recovering from bronchiolitis respond to inhaled salbutamol (albuterol)? Pediatr Pulmonol 10(1):36–39, 1991. (Finds no response to inhaled beta agonist; compare to Schuh et al.)

Springer C, Bar-Yishay E, Uwayyed K, Avital A, Vilozni D, Godfrey S: Corticosteroids do not affect the clinical or physiological status of infants with bronchiolitis. Pediatr Pulmonol 9(3):181–185, 1990

Webb MS, Martin JA, Cartlidge PH et al: Chest physiotherapy in acute bronchiolitis. Arch Dis Child 60(11):1078–1079, 1985.

Wohl ME: Bronchiolitis. In Kendig EL Jr, Chernick V (eds): Disorders of the Respiratory Tract in Children, pp 360–370. Philadelphia, WB Saunders, 1990. (Extensive reviews of the subject with good discussions of the pathophysiology of postulated immunologic interaction.)

168
Persistent Cough

Robert A. Dershewitz

A cough is not an illness but a sign for which a cause should be sought. The term "persistent cough" is synonymous with "chronic cough" and is usually defined as lasting for at least 3 weeks. Some use the term "persistent cough" interchangeably with "the chronic bronchitis complex in children," but there are many etiologies other than bronchitis that may result in chronic coughing. It is often difficult to differentiate a persistent cough from a recurrent cough.

Coughing is largely a host defense mechanism to expectorate foreign matter from the respiratory tract and to clear secretions already there. Once this function is explained, much parental concern can be allayed, and parents can accept the fact that a cough does not necessarily (or frequently) require suppression. Cough receptors located primarily throughout the pharynx to the bronchioles, but also in the extrapulmonary sites of the external ear canal and stomach, constitute the afferent limb of the cough reflex. Once the receptors are stimulated, impulses travel along the vagus nerve to the brain stem. Efferent fibers then travel to the larynx, intercostal muscles, diaphragm, and muscles of the abdomen and pelvis, and they trigger a cough. There is, however, some voluntary control over coughing.

CLINICAL PRESENTATION AND DIFFERENTIAL DIAGNOSIS

Most children with persistent coughs appear healthy. Indeed, those children who are thriving and active and who are without fever, tachypnea, and clubbing usually have a benign etiology for their cough. The history and physical exam often suggest the etiology. At times, the cause of a persistent cough is obvious, but it is not uncommon for a proven etiology to be elusive, even after an extensive workup. The two most common causes of persistent cough are viral bronchitis and hyperactive airway disease (i.e., asthma or asthma-variant). Upper respiratory tract infections are the most common cause of recurrent coughs, but they may also trigger asthmatic attacks. Viral etiologies of bronchitis are much more common than bacterial superinfections. Some children are prone to recurrent bouts of bronchitis, a tendency that decreases by 8 to 9 years of age.

Table 168-1.   Major Causes of Persistent Cough

Reactive airway disease (e.g., asthma, allergy)
Bronchitis (e.g., viral, bacteria, mycoplasma)
Physical irritants (e.g., tobacco smoke, GE reflux)
Foreign body aspiration
Congenital abnormalities (e.g., tracheoesophageal fistula,
   tracheobronchomalacia, aberrant mediastinal vessels)
Postinfectious (e.g., pertussis, bronchiolitis)
Mediastinal or pulmonary masses (e.g., tumors, cysts, nodes,
   hemangiomas)
Suppurative lung disease (e.g., tuberculosis, cystic fibrosis,
   bronchiectasis)
Psychogenic
Chronic upper airway disease (e.g., sinusitis)

The major causes of persistent coughs are listed in Table 168-1. Often, special characteristics of the cough point to an etiology (see Table 168-2). Some common causes of persistent coughing have no age predilection, including dry air, passive smoking, irritants (e.g., from wood-burning fireplaces), air pollution, asthma, and atelectasis from suppurative lung disease. Although any cause may be present at any age, it is useful to consider the age of onset when formulating differential diagnoses.

Infancy

A young infant with a chronic cough has an increased likelihood of congenital malformations such as tracheoesophageal fistula, cysts, and vascular rings. A perinatal infection must also be considered if the cough started within the first few weeks of life. Chlamydial pneumonia with its characteristic staccato cough occurs in the young infant. Bronchiolitis is another disease of infancy, and pertussis is more common in young children. In both, as with any infection of the lower respiratory tract, coughing may persist for weeks after the infectious process has resolved. Pulmonary manifestations of cystic fibrosis (CF) and AIDS may occur in this age group (see Chaps. 52 and 171). Recurrent coughing is a well-known manifestation of symptomatic gastroesophageal (GE) reflux, and when it is symptomatic, it is more likely to be diagnosed in infancy. In addition, chemical irritation of the lungs may result from overfeeding and dyskinetic swallowing. The child whose cough results from congestive heart failure should not be difficult to recognize.

Preschool Age

Toddlers are at greatest risk of foreign body aspiration. Because a history of choking is not always elicited, the diagnosis may require a high index of suspicion. Breath sounds may be asymmetric. Hyperinflation or air trapping on inspiratory/expiratory chest x-rays is strongly suggestive of aspiration (see also Chap. 165).

The preschooler with cystic fibrosis often looks frail, and he or she may have associated gastrointestinal (GI) problems such as steatorrhea and increased appetite. Cystic fibrosis, AIDS, immunodeficiencies, and bronchiectasis must always be considered in a child with a chronic, suppurative cough, especially if the child is not growing well.

Table 168-2.   Clues to Etiology

IF THE COUGH IS	THINK OF
Nonproductive	Reactive airway disease, bronchitis, irritants
Productive	
Purulent	CF, bronchiectasis
Clear or white	Asthma
Blood-streaked	Tuberculosis, bronchiectasis, CF, hemosiderosis
Nocturnal	Asthma, postnasal drip, GE reflux
Absent with sleep	Psychogenic
On awakening	Postnasal drip, CF, bronchiectasis
Seasonal	Asthma, allergies
Paroxysms	Foreign body, pertussis, chlamydia
With feeding	Aspiration, GE reflux
With exposure to cold	Asthma
With exercise	Asthma
With excitement/laughing	Asthma
With wheezing	Asthma
With stridor or voice changes	Glottic pathology
With cyanosis	CF, pertussis, foreign body, aspiration
With failure to thrive/malabsorption	CF

Chronic upper airway disease, such as sinusitis and allergic rhinitis, is often associated with reactive airways. Although it is debatable whether a postnasal drip by itself causes a chronic cough, it is common practice to attribute the cough to a postnasal drip in a child who coughs only when supine. Children with GE reflux may also cough when supine.

School Age

Mycoplasma pneumoniae infections peak in school-age children, and coughing may persist 1 to 3 months after other symptoms resolve. A psychogenic cough is more common in older children. The cough may be honking, sounding like a Canadian goose, or it may sound bizarre. The cough disappears during sleep and is exacerbated at times of stress. Tourette's syndrome should be considered if tics or other mannerisms are present. Cigarette smoking may also cause a persistent cough.

WORK-UP

History

The following questions should be asked: Has the child ever had a persistent cough? If there were previous episodes, were medications used? Which ones were used and what was the response? Asthma is suggested if the cough is nocturnal, precipitated by exercise, improved by bronchodilators, exacerbated in the spring or summer, or if there is a strong family history of asthma. Is there a family history of cystic fibrosis or malabsorption? A chronic cough during winter suggests recurrent or persistent viral bronchitis, although asthma and irritation (e.g., from fireplaces and dry air) may be causative.

What is the nature of the sputum? A productive cough from asthma and chronic infectious bronchitis is clear, mucoid, or tenacious. A dry, harsh, or hacking cough is characteristic of tracheal irritation. Purulent sputum suggests CF and bronchiectasis, and if either are advanced, hemoptysis may be present. A progressive cough that becomes productive and perhaps blood-streaked is consistent with tuberculosis (TB). A "wet-sounding" cough is usually from pneumonia or asthma. A history of aspiration is difficult to elicit in young children. Was the cough preceded by feeding or a choking episode? Is the child drooling and does he or she sound hoarse?

Paroxysms of coughing suggest pertussis, a pertussis-like syndrome, CF, and chlamydial infection. A recent bout of pertussis or measles may cause bronchiectasis, which in turn may result in a chronic cough. The cough that disappears at night may be psychogenic.

Physical Examination

The complete physical exam should concentrate on the following:

General. Does the child appear robust or wasted? Are the height and weight age-appropriate, and are the growth parameters being maintained? Cystic fibrosis, bronchiectasis, and immunodeficiency disorders must be considered in children who fail to thrive. If the neurologic development is abnormal, aspiration must be suspected.

Chest. What is the respiratory rate, and is cyanosis present? An increased chest circumference suggests CF or other causes of chronic air trapping secondary to pulmonary disease. Generalized wheezing, crackles (rales), or prolonged expirations point to asthma, while focal crackles, if coarse and low-pitched, suggest bronchiectasis. Decreased aeration suggests a foreign body. Viral or mycoplasma pneumonia is the likely diagnosis if only fine inspiratory crackles are heard, and less commonly, a fibrotic process in the lungs.

The auscultatory exam is usually normal in children with bronchitis, but rhonchi may be heard. Children 5 years and older can usually cough on demand. One should listen for post-tussive wheezes and see if the cough is productive. A chronic cough with stridor suggests an anatomic lesion in the larynx, subglottic region, or upper trachea (see Chap. 164).

Other. Finger clubbing suggests CF; tracheal deviation suggests a mediastinal mass or foreign body aspiration; and purulent rhinitis may be a sign of sinusitis. One should look also for other evidence of atopia, such as the allergic salute and allergic rhinitis.

Laboratory Tests

With few exceptions, a tuberculin skin test, chest x-ray, and sweat chloride test should be part of the initial evaluation in all children who have unexplained persistent coughs. A chest x-ray is the most helpful test because it can detect many causes of a persistent cough. In addition to masses and infiltrates, hyperinflation suggests obstruction, especially from asthma and CF. Inspiratory and expiratory films often detect a foreign body. A complete blood count (CBC) may show eosinophilia (indicating asthma), neutrophilia (suggesting a bacterial infection), anemia (suggesting pulmonary hemosiderosis), lymphocytosis (suggesting pertussis or a viral infection), and decreased polymorphonuclear leukocytes or lymphocytes (suggesting an immunodeficiency). Eosinophilia may also be seen in chlamydia infections. If the cough is productive, one should obtain Wright and Gram stains of the sputum, and it should be cultured. Eosinophils suggest asthma, while bacteria and pus cells indicate infection. A barium swallow is often helpful if structural lesions causing compression (either congenital or acquired masses), GE reflux, tracheoesophageal fistula, or foreign body aspiration is suspected.

Spirometry is a simple office test to detect airway obstruction. Asthma may be diagnosed if bronchodilators reverse the airway narrowing. If the cough does not improve or respond to initial therapy, other tests should be considered. These include TORCH titers if the cough began in early infancy, serologic testing for mycoplasma, alpha$_1$-antitrypsin levels, immunologic or allergic work-up, and a sinus roentgenogram.

TREATMENT

Treatment is based on the diagnosis or diagnostic probabilities revealed by the work-up. Often, simple recommendations such as home air humidification, keeping the throat moist, or eliminating cigarette smoking at home eliminate the cough.

A chronic, dry, irritative cough, especially if it keeps the child or family awake at night, exhausts the child, or is socially disruptive (e.g., at school), may be suppressed by either codeine or dextromethorphan. A 3- to 4-day, or bedtime only, course may relieve the cough cycle. Both are centrally acting antitussives. Codeine is more effective, but drawbacks include its addiction potential and respiratory depression. It should never be given to young infants. The dose is 1 mg/kg/day in four divided doses, not to exceed 60 mg/day. Dextromethorphan is considerably safer, and the dose is the same as or slightly higher than that for codeine. A purulent cough should never be suppressed because the cough reflex is valuable in protecting the lungs. Other productive coughs constitute relative contraindications for prescribing antitussive medications.

A diagnostic (and therapeutic) trial of a bronchodilator is appropriate before prescribing antitussives if airway reactivity is suspected, and it may be used in the absence of atopia. Beta-adrenergic medications such as metaproterenol and albuterol are less toxic than and probably superior to theophylline. A poor initial clinical response does not rule out the diagnosis. Because the etiology of the reactive airways may be inflammatory, it would be worthwhile to next try inhaled corticosteroids or cromolyn. (Many authorities now recommend that an inhaled antiinflammatory such as beclomethasone be the initial medication.) The child who fails this approach should be given a 10- to 14-day course of erythromycin for presumptive bacterial bronchitis. It is, however, reasonable to use erythromycin initially if infectious bronchitis is the more likely diagnosis. The dose of theophylline must be reduced by approximately 25% if given with erythromycin because theophylline's half-life is prolonged by erythromycin.

Expectorants and mucolytic agents such as guaifenesin (glyceryl guaiacolate) are usually ineffective and, indeed, have not been shown to be beneficial in controlled clinical trials. Antihistamines may be prescribed if a postnasal drip is thought to cause or contribute to the cough. Diphenhydramine has been used as an antitussive, but it is not as effective as codeine or dextromethorphan, and if given in effective doses, it usually causes drowsiness.

It is axiomatic that the child should be well-hydrated, but overhydration should be avoided because it may compromise pulmonary function. Sinusitis should be treated with an antibiotic such as amoxicillin (see Chap. 80), and erythromycin should be prescribed for mycoplasma and chlamydial infections. Unless there is a suppurative pulmonary infection or secondary atelectasis, chest physical therapy and postural drainage are usually unnecessary.

INDICATIONS FOR REFERRAL OR ADMISSION

Most children with persistent coughs who are worked up systematically by their primary care physician do not need to be referred to a specialist. Consultation may be indicated if the etiology of the cough remains unclear, if the clinical response to therapy is unsatisfactory, if the disease is rare or complex, or if the primary physician or parents want "a second opinion." An allergist, pulmonologist, immunologist, or surgeon (e.g., to correct GE reflux) may be consulted. Bronchoscopy is indicated if a foreign body aspiration is suspected. Finally, all children with CF should be referred to a CF center.

ANNOTATED BIBLIOGRAPHY

Dolovich J, Ruhno J, O'Bryne P et al: Early/late response model: Implications for control of asthma and chronic cough in children. Pediatr Clin North Am 35:969–979, 1988. (Makes a strong argument that controlling the inflammatory response by inhaled steroids or cromolyn is the best way to treat a chronic cough.)

Hotaling AJ: Cough. In Bluestone CD, Stool SE (eds): Pediatric Otolaryngology, 2nd ed, pp 1078–1084. Philadelphia, WB Saunders, 1990. (In-depth discussion, especially strong on differential diagnosis.)

Morgan WJ, Taussig LM. The child with persistent cough. Pediatr Rev 8:249–253, 1987. (Good, practical overview.)

169

Pneumonia

Kenneth M. Boyer

Pneumonia is a potentially serious respiratory infection often encountered by the pediatrician practicing in an ambulatory setting. Incidence ranges from 40:1000 children/year at ages less than 5 to 7:1000 children/year at ages 12 to 15. Although pneumonia at present generally has an excellent prognosis with treatment, the pediatrician should remember that this diagnosis may engender fear on the part of parents because of its frequent fatal outcome in the preantibiotic era.

PATHOPHYSIOLOGY

The usual first step in the pathogenesis of pneumonia is damage to the mucociliary clearance mechanism induced by viral respiratory infection. This damage may be more severe in patients with preexisting clearance abnormalities such as bronchopulmonary dysplasia or cystic fibrosis. Particularly in the young infant, involvement of terminal airways leads to bronchiolitis, air trapping, and segmental atelectasis. Extension into peribronchial tissues leads to interstitial pneumonia. Alveolar inflammation (lobar pneumonia) usually represents a superimposition of bacterial infection on previously damaged terminal airways as the result of minor aspiration.

Complications of nonbacterial pneumonia include atelectasis, bronchospasm, apneic spells, and respiratory failure. Complications of bacterial pneumonia include septicemia, pleural extension (effusion or empyema), and lung abscess.

CLINICAL PRESENTATION

The clinical presentation of pneumonia varies with age and with infecting agent. A young baby with pneumonia generally has minimal systemic signs but obvious respiratory distress. On general inspection, tachypnea, retractions, grunting, and nasal flaring are usually apparent. A cough may or may not be present. The older child or adolescent generally has more obvious signs of systemic illness, including fever and prostration. Rather than respiratory distress, pulmonary involvement is usually manifested by cough, chest pain, or sputum production. All of these manifestations may be present in the older infant, toddler, or preschooler with pneumonia.

Nonbacterial pneumonia generally has a gradual onset that correlates with the gradual progression of disease from the upper to the lower airways and interstitial tissues. Bacterial pneumonia often presents as a sudden change in a previously mild respiratory illness, usually with a recrudescence of fever or chills. Common nonbacterial and bacterial causes of pediatric pneumonia are summarized in Table 169-1, with clinical clues that may suggest specific etiologies in an individual patient.

DIFFERENTIAL DIAGNOSIS

The major categories of disease that need to be differentiated in patients with pneumonia are (1) bacterial etiologies that require specific antimicrobial therapy, (2) nonbacterial etiologies that may require antiviral or broad-spectrum antimicrobial therapy, (3) noninfectious conditions that may simulate pneumonia but for which other forms of therapy may be essential, and (4) unusual or "exotic" infections. Additional considerations that enter into differential diagnosis include the status of the host, whether compromised or normal, the age of the patient, the exposure history, and the season of the year.

Pneumonias caused by bacteria characteristically are lobar in distribution and exhibit consolidation on chest radiograph. Atelectasis is common in nonbacterial pneumonia and must be distinguished from a true consolidation. Pleural effusions, circular infiltrates, consolidations with convex margins, and pneumatoceles all favor a bacterial etiology. Because of the association of bacteremia with high fever and significant leukocytosis in the young child, these clinical features also favor bacterial etiology. Positive cultures of blood, pleural fluid, or lung aspirates establish etiology in bacterial pneumonia.

In certain settings, nonbacterial pneumonia may be diagnosed with relative certainty based on the clinical presentation, season, and age. Viral pneumonias characteristically appear as bronchopneumonia on chest roentgenogram, with hyperinflation, segmental atelectasis, or interstitial infiltrates. Despite recent advances in techniques for rapid viral diagnosis, however, in most instances this category of pulmonary infection remains a diagnosis of exclusion. Mycoplasma pneumonia is usually lobar in distribution, but not densely consolidated. Serologic tests usually permit diagnosis in the acute phase.

The list of noninfectious conditions that may simulate pneumonia should be kept in mind and is provided in the display entitled "Noninfectious Conditions That May Simulate or Underlie Acute Pneumonia in Children." The line of demarcation between infectious and noninfectious conditions is not always sharp. In the child with sickle cell anemia, for example, a pulmonary vascular occlusive crisis presents with fever, leukocytosis, and patchy pulmonary infiltrates. Differentiation from pneumococcal, hemophilus, or mycoplasmal pneumonia, to which the child with sickle cell anemia has increased susceptibility, may be difficult or impossible. Early recognition of noninfectious conditions either mimicking or underlying pneumonia may prevent a recurrence or improve prognosis. Asthma, for example, is the most frequent cause of recurrent pneumonia. Treatment with bronchodilators or cromolyn may prevent recurrences. Similarly, early recognition and treatment of cystic fibrosis as an underlying condition are clearly beneficial in slowing irreversible pulmonary damage.

The more unusual infectious conditions that may present as acute pediatric pneumonia include mycobacterial, fungal, and parasitic infections. Tuberculin testing is an important consideration in the initial evaluation of a patient with pneumonia and is especially important for children residing in urban areas, recent immigrants, and native Americans. Fungal pneumonia, particularly coccidioidomycosis, blastomycosis, and histoplasmosis, should be considered in children residing in or visiting endemic areas. A suggestive exposure history may often be elicited, such as backyard swimming pool excavations, clean-up chores in old barns or sheds, or exposure to dust storms. Other fungal pneumonias, such as aspergillosis and cryptococcosis, occur almost exclusively in the setting of immunosuppression. Pneumocystis pneumonia implies a major defect in cell-mediated immunity and may be the presenting problem in congenital immunodeficiency or pediatric AIDS.

Table 169-1. Nonbacterial and Bacterial Agents Causing Pediatric Pneumonia, According to Age*

AGE GROUP, INFECTING AGENT	CLINICAL CLUES	AGE GROUP, INFECTING AGENT	CLINICAL CLUES
Young Infant (≤ 3 Months)		**Older Infant/Toddler/Younger Child (4 Months–5 Years)** (*continued*)	
Nonbacterial agents		Bacteria	
Chlamydia trachomatis	Afebrile, "staccato cough," conjunctivitis	*Streptococcus pneumoniae*	Lobar consolidation antigenuria
RS virus†	Low-grade fever, wheeze, apnea, winter season	*Haemophilus influenzae*	Lobar consolidation, pleural effusion, antigenuria, amoxicillin Rx failure, immunization history
Cytomegalovirus†	"Blueberry muffin," transfused premie		
Parainfluenza viruses†	Sibling or parental URIs or LTB, fall or spring season	*Staphylococcus aureus*†	Pneumatoceles empyema
Influenza viruses†	Parental or sibling "flu" illness, winter season community epidemics	*Bordetella pertussis*	Immunization history, lymphocytosis, pertussoid cough
Bacteria		Group A streptococci†	Empyema, scarlatiniform rash
Group B streptococcus†	Amniotic fluid infection, antigenuria	Oral anaerobes†	Aspiration secondary to neuromuscular or anatomic abnormality
Staphylococcus aureus†	Skin pustules, empyema, pneumatoceles	**Older Child/Adolescent (6–16 Years)**	
Klebsiella pneumoniae†	Nosocomial pneumonia in a premie	Nonbacterial agents	
Oral anaerobes†	Aspiration secondary to neuromuscular or anatomic abnormality	*Mycoplasma pneuoniae*	Cold agglutinins, no coryza, subacute course
Older Infant/Toddler/Younger Child (4 Months–5 Years)		Influenza viruses	Parental or sibling "flu" illnesses, winter season, community epidemics
Nonbacterial agents			
RS virus	Wheeze, winter season	*Chlamydia pneumoniae*	No cold agglutinins, subactue course
Parainfluenza viruses	Sibling or parental URIs or LTB, fall or spring season	Measles virus	Rash, immunization history
Influenza viruses	Sibling or parent "flu" illness, winter season, community epidemics	Bacteria	
		Streptococcus pneumoniae	Lobar consolidation, antigenuria
Adenoviruses†	Severe, may involve liver, CNS, skin	*Staphylococcus aureus*†	Pneumatoceles, empyema
Measles virus	Rash, immunization history	Group A streptococci†	Empyema, scarlatiniform rash
Human immunodeficiency virus	Blood transfusion, maternal drug abuse or STDs		
Mycoplasma pneumonia	Cold agglutinins, no coryza, subacute course		

*Agents in each category in approximate order of frequency. Clinical clues may suggest a specific etiology but are not definitive.
†Inpatient management mandatory.
URI = upper respiratory infection; LTB = laryngotracheobronchitis, CNS = central nervous system; STD = sexually transmitted disease

WORK-UP

History

Key elements in the history of a child with pneumonia are the family history, the past medical history, and a history of unusual exposures. Family history may uncover relatives with genetic diseases that may affect the lungs (e.g., cystic fibrosis) or an atopic tendency (e.g., asthma, eczema, or hay fever). A factor that is frequently overlooked but is perhaps more important than these is a history of recent infectious illnesses in the family, such as flu-like illnesses, upper respiratory infections, or croup. Such a history makes an infectious process, usually viral, more likely than a nonin-

Noninfectious Conditions That May Simulate or Underlie Acute Pneumonia in Children

Technical
Poor inspiratory chest radiograph
Underpenetrated chest radiograph

Physiologic
Prominent thymus
Breast shadows

Chronic Pulmonary Disease
Asthma
Cystic fibrosis
Bronchiectasis
Bronchiolitis obliterans
Pulmonary sequestration
Congenital lobar emphysema
Pulmonary hemosiderosis
Desquamative interstitial pneumonitis

Recurrent Aspiration
Gastroesophageal reflux
Tracheoesophageal fistula
Craniofacial defect
Neuromuscular disorders
Familial dysautonomia

Allergic Alveolitis
Dusts (farmer's lung)
Molds (allergic aspergillosis)
Excreta (pigeon breeder's lung)

Atelectasis
Cardiomegaly
Mucous plug
Foreign body

Damage by Physical Agents
Bronchopulmonary dysplasia
Lipoid pneumonia
Kerosene pneumonia
Near drowning
Smoke inhalation

Iatrogenic Pulmonary Damage
Drugs (nitrofurantoin, bleomycin)
Radiation pneumonitis
Graft-*vs*-host disease

Pulmonary Infarction
Sickle vaso-occlusive crisis
Fat embolism

Miscellaneous
Congestive heart failure
Adult respiratory distress syndrome
Systemic lupus erythematosus
Sarcoidosis
Neoplasms (lymphoma, teratoma, neuroblastoma)
Pleural effusion or reaction
Bronchogenic cyst
Vascular ring
Histiocytosis

fectious condition. As a clue in their medical history, a low-birth-weight premature infant may have a higher probability of having nosocomial bacterial pathogens or a greater predisposition to apnea (and hence a stronger indication for hospitalization) during viral pneumonia. Gaps in immunization may indicate a susceptibility to measles, pertussis, or

Haemophilus influenzae type b infection. Previous hospitalizations for pneumonia should alert the physician to the possibility of an underlying anatomic or immunologic disease. Patients known to have chronic diseases, such as cystic fibrosis, bronchopulmonary dysplasia, asthma, sickle cell disease, or congenital heart disease, may have unusual pathogens or an unusual severity of illness. A history of "choking" should suggest the possibility of foreign body aspiration. Recent travel, exposure to pets, or unusual activities may increase the possibility of fungal disease, psittacosis, Q fever, or unusual bacterial pathogens.

Physical Examination

A physical examination is usually sufficient to indicate a strong probability of pneumonia (and thus the need for laboratory confirmation). More important, it identifies the child with respiratory decompensation (which may require hospitalization for oxygen therapy or mechanical ventilation) or dehydration (which may require other forms of supportive therapy most appropriate in a hospital setting). General appearance is the most important aspect of the physical examination, particularly in the infant or young child. By inspection of the child at rest, the physician can best estimate the severity of respiratory involvement and the presence of tachypnea (especially a respiratory rate >50/minute), grunting, flaring, or retractions. The experienced clinician often recognizes pneumonia on the basis of these findings alone. Findings on auscultation may vary and range from a normal examination to localized diminished breath sounds to the more classic findings of rales, tubular breath sounds, or egophony.

Laboratory Tests

The basic laboratory work-up of pediatric pneumonia includes a PA and lateral chest radiograph, a white blood cell count and differential, a tuberculin test, and cold agglutinins. The Gram stain and culture of sputum, standard in the adult work-up, are generally not practical in pediatrics. Blood culture, although a "low-yield" test, is an appropriate one for the highly febrile child less than 2 years of age with a markedly elevated white count. Ten to twenty percent of these children are bacteremic. Establishing a specific etiology in those with positive blood cultures is worth the expense. Tests for bacterial polysaccharide antigens in urine may help in diagnosing bacterial pneumonia, but unfortunately they are not sufficiently sensitive to permit a bacterial process to be completely ruled out in an individual patient. The reagents for these tests are best for *H. influenzae* type b and group B streptococcus. Viral cultures, previously considered to be an academic exercise, are becoming increasingly important in the hospital management of young infants with pneumonia because of the recent availability of the antiviral drug ribavirin. Rapid diagnosis of infection by respiratory syncytial virus (RSV) by means of immunofluorescence microscopy or enzyme-linked immunosorbent assay (ELISA) now makes it possible to identify patients who would benefit from this inhalational drug therapy. Such tests are particularly appropriate for the young baby with underlying cardiopulmonary disease who is at high risk for serious consequences of RSV pneumonia. With the exception of tests for mycoplasmal or chlamydial infection, serologic tests are futile.

In the patient with cyanosis or significant respiratory distress, blood gas determinations or oximetry is indicated. The latter, with the use of simple noninvasive instruments, is a real advance in the hospital management of the sick infant with pneumonia. Finally, for immunocompromised hosts, whose range of possible pathogens is wide and who are particularly susceptible to a progressive disease, invasive diagnostic procedures such as bronchoalveolar lavage or open lung biopsy are usually indicated.

TREATMENT

Although most textbooks conveniently describe the most appropriate therapeutic regimens for specific etiologic agents of pneumonia, the reality of clinical practice is that most children with acute pneumonia must be treated as having pneumonias of unknown cause. The patient's age, radiographic findings, and white count may be guides to probable etiologies. However, the goal of diagnostic efforts should be to replace empiric with specific treatment.

In the baby 5 days old or younger, major considerations for treatment are early-onset infections due to perinatally acquired bacteria. An appropriate combination therapy for such babies is ampicillin and gentamicin. The premature infant who has had a prolonged hospitalization is susceptible to nosocomial pneumonia with hospital pathogens. Under these circumstances, the parenteral combinations of nafcillin/gentamicin and vancomycin/ceftriaxone are reasonable empiric treatments. Normal babies who develop pneumonia in the first 3 months of life are most likely to have either chlamydial or respiratory syncytial viral infections. Erythromycin is a reasonable oral regimen for such babies (see also Chap. 196).

In the older baby and young child between 4 months and 5 years of age, about two thirds of pneumonias are due to viruses and one third are due to bacteria. For the child who can be treated as an outpatient and in whom a bacterial etiology appears likely, or cannot be excluded, treatment with

Table 169-2. Oral Antimicrobial Agents for Outpatient Treatment of Pediatric Pneumonia

DRUG	EFFECTIVE AGAINST	DOSAGE (MG/KG/24 HOURS)
Amoxicillin	S. pneumo, group A strep* Some H. flu	40 ÷ q8H
Amoxicillin/clavulanic acid	S. pneumo, all H. flu, group A strep*, S. aureus,* oral anaerobes*	40 ÷ q8H
Cefactor	S. pneumo, all H. flu, group A strep*, S. aureus*	40 ÷ q8H
Cefixime	S. pneumo, all H. flu, group A strep*	8 ÷ q12–24H
Cephalexin	S. pneumo, group A strep*, S. aureus*	25–50 ÷ q6H
Clindamycin	S. aureus*, oral anaerobes*, group A strep*	20–30 ÷ q8H
Dicloxacillin	S. aureus*, S. pneumo, Group A strep*	25–50 ÷ q6H
Erythromycin	S. pneumo, M. pneumo, B. pertussis, C. trachomatis	40 ÷ q6H
Erythromycin/sulfisoxazole	S. pneumo M. pneumo, B. pertussis, C. trachomatis	40 ÷ q6H (erythromycin component)
Penicillin	S. pneumo, group A strep*	25–50 ÷ q6H
Trimethoprim/sulfamethoxazole	All H. flu, S. pneumo, P. carinii*	10–20 ÷ q12H (trimethoprim component)

*Initial therapy should be parenteral (inpatient).

oral amoxicillin or amoxicillin/clavulanic acid is reasonable. The use of inhalational ribavirin is now recommended for the child with preexisting cardiopulmonary disease and an apparent viral pneumonia. In the child who requires hospitalization for an apparent bacterial pneumonia, parenteral antibiotic regimens with broad activity against the most likely pathogens (e.g., pneumococci, *Haemophilus,* and *Staphylococcus aureus*) are indicated. Cefuroxime or the combination of nafcillin and ceftriaxone is a good initial empiric regimen. The child older than 6 years of age with pneumonia is most likely to have mycoplasma or pneumococcal pneumonia. In that setting, erythromycin should be considered the preferred oral drug, with the combination of erythromycin and cefuroxime for hospitalized patients.

Most children with mild to moderate disease can be managed satisfactorily with oral antimicrobial agents outside the hospital. Commonly used oral agents are summarized in Table 169-2, with their "coverage" and recommended dosages. (Initial therapy with these agents would be inappropriate for some pathogens, such as *S. aureus,* but they may be used judiciously during convalescence.) The child managed as an outpatient should be seen within 72 hours of initiation of therapy to document improvement; parents should be instructed to return with the child earlier if there are signs of a progression of disease. Children who require hospitalization are those with severe disease at onset or who appear to be deteriorating on outpatient management, those with underlying pulmonary or cardiac problems, and those whose families lack the ability to reliably provide therapy and supportive care. Special concern is needed for infants under 1 year of age whose signs of respiratory disease may initially be subtle, who may progress rapidly, and who are experiencing their first major infectious illness and have unproven immunologic competence.

Durations of treatment vary with etiology. A 10-day course is recommended for outpatient antimicrobial therapy of most pneumonia cases. For viral disease being treated in the hospital with ribavirin, a brief duration of 3 to 5 days is generally considered adequate. For the complicated case (e.g., a child with *S. aureus* pneumonia, empyema, and prolonged chest tube drainage), 3 to 6 weeks of treatment (parenteral followed by oral) may be necessary. Follow-up chest roentgenograms are not mandatory but are a reasonable way to document the resolution of disease at 6 to 8 weeks after onset. They should always be performed on hospitalized children and should be performed selectively in children managed as outpatients who have a persistent cough or who fail to return to normal activities or weight gain.

INDICATIONS FOR REFERRAL

The indications for outpatient referral are primarily a failure to clear the first episode of pneumonia or recurrent disease.

Indications for inpatient consultation or transfer include a failure to respond to parenteral regimens (in terms of fever and toxicity) within 48 to 72 hours of admission, respiratory failure necessitating intensive respiratory therapy or mechanical ventilation, development of empyema, or suspicion of a foreign body or airway impingement, indicating the need for bronchoscopy.

ANNOTATED BIBLIOGRAPHY

Beem MO, Saxon E: Respiratory-tract colonization and a distinctive pneumonia syndrome in infants infected with *Chlamydia trachomatis*. N Engl J Med 296:306, 1977. (Exemplary study of the afebrile pneumonitis syndrome of infancy that established *C. trachomatis* as a common etiologic agent.)

Cherian T, John TJ, Simoes E et al: Evaluation of simple clinical signs for the diagnosis of acute lower respiratory tract infection. Lancet 2:125, 1988. (Third-World study that demonstrates the value of simple physical findings, particularly tachypnea, in the diagnosis and empiric treatment of pneumonia.)

Dennehy PH, McIntosh K: Viral pneumonia in childhood. In Weinstein L, Fields BN (eds): Seminars in Infectious Disease. Vol 5: Pneumonias, p 173. New York, Thieme-Stratton, 1983. (Scholarly review of the pathogens and clinical features of pneumonias caused by viral agents in children.)

Denny FW, Clyde WA Jr: Acute lower respiratory tract infections in nonhospitalized children. J Pediatr 108:635, 1986. (Most recent in an outstanding series of studies of respiratory infection in a Chapel Hill, NC, group practice that have defined patterns of illness associated with common respiratory viral pathogens.)

Grossman LK, Wald ER, Nair P et al: Roentgenographic follow-up of acute pneumonia in children. Pediatrics 63:30, 1979. (Prospective study of 129 children with acute pneumonia demonstrating that follow-up chest x-rays may be done selectively based on persistent respiratory symptoms or failure to thrive.)

Hall CB, McBride JT, Gala CL et al: Ribavirin treatment of respiratory syncytial viral infection in infants with underlying cardiopulmonary disease. JAMA 254:3047, 1985. (Comparative trial of ribavirin aerosol treatment versus placebo in 53 infants with respiratory syncytial virus infection and underlying bronchopulmonary dysplasia or congenital heart disease; treated infants did significantly better, establishing a role for ribavirin treatment in this high-risk patient group.)

Long SS: Treatment of acute pneumonia in infants and children. Pediatr Clin North Am 30:247, 1983. (Comprehensive review of pediatric pneumonias, with an emphasis on epidemiologic, clinical, and laboratory features that aid in diagnosis, and a rational approach to antimicrobial and supportive therapy.)

Seto DSY, Heller RM: Acute respiratory infections. Pediatr Clin North Am 21:683, 1974. (Review of classic pneumonia syndromes in pediatrics, according to specific etiology, with representative radiographs.)

Turner RB, Lande AE, Chase P et al: Pneumonia in pediatric outpatients: Cause and clinical manifestations. J Pediatr 111:194, 1987. (Comprehensive microbiologic evaluation of 98 pediatric outpatients with pneumonia, demonstrating the similarities between bacterial and viral cases and the frequency of dual etiology.)

170

Tuberculosis: Screening and Prophylaxis

L. Gerard Niederman

The screening of asymptomatic children for tuberculous infection, a traditional part of pediatric office care, is based on three premises: (1) tuberculous disease (i.e., the presence of symptoms or clinical signs consistent with tuberculosis) is curable; (2) asymptomatic tuberculous infection progresses to symptomatic tuberculous disease; and (3) the progression from infection to disease is preventable with chemoprophylaxis. Recent recommendations focus screening and control measures on high-risk populations and suggest that this strategy, coupled with technologic developments, can result in the elimination of tuberculosis in the United States by the year 2010.

In 1987, there were 22,201 cases of active tuberculosis reported in the United States; 1177 were in children less than 15 years old, and 674 were in children less than 5 years old. The ongoing transmission of tuberculosis in children emphasizes the continuing need for vigorous comprehensive control programs.

WHO SHOULD BE SCREENED?

All children should have a careful history to ascertain increased risk for tuberculosis. In most areas of the United States, the prevalence of tuberculous infection in children is well below 1% (often between 0.1% and 0.5%), making general screening with tuberculin skin tests an inefficient method of finding infection and disease. Nonetheless, some authorities recommend that even children at low risk for tuberculosis be screened three times during childhood: at 12 to 15 months of age, before entering kindergarten, and around 14 to 16 years of age. A multipuncture skin test such as the Mono-Vacc is adequate for this purpose, rather than purified protein derivative (PPD). Children at risk, however, should be identified and screened yearly, usually with the Mantoux (PPD) skin test (see Table 170-1).

Asymptomatic children who are contacts of proven or suspected cases of tuberculosis should be tested, and if they were recently exposed they may need repeat testing after an interval appropriate for delayed hypersensitivity to develop. Contact children who have signs or symptoms that suggest tuberculous disease should be thoroughly evaluated regardless of skin test results.

Not all low-income populations are at risk for tuberculosis, and local public health departments should set county or municipal guidelines for practitioners. Blacks, Hispan-

ics, and native Americans have a higher incidence of tuberculosis, as do children who are homeless and children immigrating from most countries in Africa, Asia, and Central and South America. Annual screening is recommended for these groups.

HOW TO SCREEN—SKIN TESTING AND INTERPRETATION

Delayed (cellular) hypersensitivity to *Mycobacterium tuberculosis* usually develops within 2 to 10 weeks of infection and is manifested by a positive tuberculin skin test. The Mantoux test is the preferred method of testing. PPD (0.1 ml) containing 5 tuberculin units (TU) is injected intracutaneously on the volar aspect of the forearm with a short-bevel, 26- or 27-gauge needle. With proper administration, a discrete 6- to 10-mm wheal is produced. The Mantoux test should be read on the second or third day after injection, when induration is usually most evident. Significant induration, however, may persist for 5 to 7 days. The margins of induration (not erythema) should be determined by palpation or by using a ball-point pen and should be measured in millimeters transversely to the long axis of the forearm.

Induration measuring 10 mm or more is frequently considered the definition of a positive Mantoux test. Interpretation of tuberculin skin tests, however, should be done in the clinical context of why the test was performed. Induration measuring 15 mm or greater is almost always due to *M. tuberculosis* infection or disease, and reactions less than 5 mm usually exclude tuberculosis. Induration between 5 mm and 15 mm may be more difficult to interpret.

False-positive tuberculin tests are most often reactions to nontuberculin mycobacteria. In the southeastern United States, as well as other areas of the world where infection with nontuberculous mycobacteria is common, cross-reactions may outnumber reactions to *M. tuberculosis*. This is particularly true when there is no history of tuberculous exposure and the population has a low prevalence of tuberculosis. In such areas, preventive treatment might be reserved for children with reactions greater than 15 mm. On the other hand, reactions between 5 mm and 10 mm should be considered due to *M. tuberculosis* if there is a history of contact with an infectious case of tuberculosis, if there is radiographic evidence of present or past tuberculosis, or if there is HIV infection. Induration between 10 mm and 15 mm should be considered evidence of tuberculous infection if the child has any risk factor listed in Table 170-1.

The interpretation of tuberculin skin tests in children vaccinated with bacillus Calmette–Guerin (BCG) may be confusing. The intensity and duration of positive tuberculin skin reactions following BCG vaccination are variable, and there is no completely reliable way to distinguish reactions due to *M. tuberculosis* from those due to BCG. The child with a positive skin test reaction and a history of vaccination with BCG should be managed on the basis of the clinical

Table 170-1. Populations at High Risk for Tuberculosis

Table 170-1. Populations at High Risk for Tuberculosis

Close contacts (home or classroom) of persons known or
suspected to have tuberculosis

Medically underserved low-income populations

Children born in, or immigrating from, countries with high TB
prevalence

Children with medical factors known to increase the risk of
disease if infection has occurred

Children infected with the human immunodeficiency virus (HIV)

Residents of long-term care facilities

Local risk factors as defined by local health departments

risk of tuberculous infection and disease. Most reactions
due to BCG are <10 mm if BCG was given more than
12 months previously. Prophylactic therapy with isoniazid
is indicated if there is a history of tuberculous exposure and
there is a reasonable chance of transmission to the child,
particularly since BCG vaccination is not completely
protective.

As alternatives to the Mantoux test, various multipuncture tests are currently in widespread use. Concentrated tuberculin (old tuberculin [OT] or PPD) is introduced into the
skin with coated applicator (e.g., Tine Test®) or by a puncture through a liquid film (e.g., Mono-Vacc® test). The dose
introduced is imprecise and often exceeds 5 TU. The Mono-
Vacc is a more reliable screening test than the Tine Test.
These tests are not intended to be diagnostic but rather are
for screening asymptomatic persons. After 48 to 72 hours,
induration of the largest single papule or induration of coalescence of papular reactions should be measured and recorded. Induration of 2 mm or more needs verification by
the standard Mantoux test. If vesiculation is present, the test
is interpreted as positive. Induration of less than 2 mm is
considered a negative reaction.

False-negative skin tests occur, and reasons for their occurrence are listed in Table 170-2.

PREVENTIVE MANAGEMENT OF TUBERCULOUS INFECTION AND CONTACT

Preventive treatment with isoniazid (INH) reduces the progression of tuberculous infection to tuberculous disease.
The highest risk of developing disease occurs in the first
2 years after infection, and the risk of disease and its complications increases with decreasing age. Other risk factors
for developing tuberculous disease include diabetes (particularly poorly controlled insulin-dependent diabetes), corticosteroid or immunosuppressive therapy, malnutrition,
acquired or congenital immunodeficiency diseases, and malignancies of lymphoid tissue.

Preventive treatment is indicated for children with positive tuberculin skin tests who have no evidence of clinical

disease, and also for tuberculin-negative children with close
contact to an infectious (or presumed infectious) case of
tuberculosis.

A child or adolescent with a positive tuberculin skin test
and no history of tuberculosis exposure should be evaluated
with a chest roentgenogram. If it is normal and no previous antituberculous treatment has been received, preventive
therapy with isoniazid should be initiated.

Household contacts and other close contacts of a proven
or potentially infectious case of tuberculosis should also receive preventive therapy. If the Mantoux test is positive
(5 mm or more induration in this clinical situation), or if
there is clinical suspicion of tuberculosis, a chest radiograph
should be obtained. If the tuberculin test is negative, treatment for 10 to 15 weeks should be given, particularly for
infants and children. The tuberculin test should be repeated
at the end of this treatment period, and, if it is positive,
treatment should be continued for 1 year. If, after 3 months,
the skin test is negative and the risk of transmission has
been eliminated, INH can be discontinued. If compliance
with prophylaxis is questionable or INH is contraindicated,
and exposure to tuberculosis cannot be avoided, BCG vaccination should be considered, particularly for newborns.

INH is given in a single daily dose of 10 mg/kg/day,
not to exceed 300 mg/day. Twelve months of treatment is
recommended, although there is evidence to suggest that
6 months may be as effective. Future guidelines may recommend a shorter duration of treatment. Alternatively, if
compliance with daily administration of INH cannot be assured, INH can be administered in a dose of 20 to 40 mg/
kg/day (not to exceed 900 mg/day) twice a week. Prophylaxis with rifampin (10 mg/kg/day, up to 600 mg/day)
should be given for 12 months if there is proof that infection
has occurred with an isoniazid-resistant organism or if INH

Table 170-2. Causes for False-Negative
Tuberculin Reactions

Factors Related to the Person Being Tested
Infections that cause temporary anergy
Live virus vaccinations (e.g., measles, mumps, polio)
Metabolic and nutritional derangements
Diseases affecting lymphoid organs
Corticosteroid and immunosuppressive drugs
Age (newborns, elderly patients with "waned" sensitivity)
Recent infection with *M. tuberculosis*

Factors Related to the Tuberculin Used
Improper storage and dilution
Chemical denaturation and adsorption
Contamination

Factors Related to Administration and Interpretation
Injection errors (e.g., too little antigen, subcutaneous)
Inexperienced or biased reader
Error in recording

(Adapted from American Thoracic Society: The tuberculin skin test. Am
Rev Respir Dis 124:356–363, 1981.)

cannot be tolerated. Combined INH and rifampin treatment may be given pending sensitivity results if resistance is suspected.

Hepatotoxic reactions to INH are rare in children and adolescents, and routine monitoring of liver enzymes is not indicated. Monthly personal or telephone contact should be made with parents or patients receiving INH, and they should be instructed to report symptoms suggesting hepatitis (e.g., fever, anorexia, nausea, vomiting, malaise, jaundice, dark urine, or right upper quadrant pain). Peripheral neuritis may occur, particularly in malnourished children receiving INH, and it may be prevented by concurrent administration of daily pyridoxine (1 mg per 10 mg of INH).

ANNOTATED BIBLIOGRAPHY

American Thoracic Society: The tuberculin skin test. Am Rev Respir Dis 124:356–363, 1981. (This and the following two references provide current, comprehensive guidelines for the office management of tuberculosis [and much more!].)

American Thoracic Society/CDC: Diagnostic standards and classification of tuberculosis. Am Rev Respir Dis 142:725–735, 1990.

American Thoracic Society/CDC: Treatment of tuberculosis infection in adults and children. Am Rev Respir Dis 134:355–363, 1986.

Donaldson JC, Elliott RC: A study of co-positivity of three multipuncture techniques with intradermal PPD tuberculin. Am Rev Respir Dis 118:843–846, 1978. (Mono-Vacc is the preferred multipuncture tuberculin skin test.)

Snider DE: Bacille Calmette–Guerin vaccinations and tuberculin skin tests. JAMA 253:3438–3439, 1985. (Sound, practical advice on this confusing clinical problem.)

Snider DE, Rieder HL, Combs D, Bloch AB, Hayden CH, Smith MHD. Tuberculosis in children. Pediatr Infect Dis J 7:271–278, 1988. (Current epidemiology of TB in the United States and succinct recommendations for management of tuberculous infection and disease.)

171

Cystic Fibrosis

Allen Lapey

Cystic fibrosis (CF) is the most common lethal genetic disease of Caucasians. Although early recognition and effective therapy have brightened prospects over the past 20 years, the disease continues to cause substantial morbidity and mortality in affected patients. Nonetheless, anticipated mean survival for a child born today with CF is 28 years.

Inherited as a Mendelian autosomal recessive trait, CF affects ~1 individual in 2500 live births, corresponding to a carrier rate of 4%.

The identification of the CF gene in 1989 represents one of the monumental achievements of twentieth-century genetics. The gene is a huge, 250,000 base pair region residing on the long arm of chromosome 7 near the centromere. By 1992, over 80 different mutations had been documented. The most common, ΔF508, is responsible for 68% of all mutations and is due to a specific deletion of three base pairs, which results in the loss of a phenylalanine residue at amino acid position 508 of the resultant protein. This gene product, termed the cystic fibrosis transmembrane conductance regulator (CFTR), has been identified and cloned; its specific function is debated. Presumably, CFTR functions as the epithelial chloride channel; in CF, channel function is defective and cells fail to secrete chloride ions. In 1991, the defect was corrected in vitro by the addition of normal CFTR to malfunctioning cells.

With the genetic breakthrough, reliable carrier detection and prenatal diagnosis are available for essentially all CF families, using either direct DNA analysis for ΔF508 or indirect linkage analysis. It will be necessary to define most of the other CF mutations before reliable DNA-based genetic testing is available to the general population.

PATHOPHYSIOLOGY

Cystic fibrosis is characterized by an increased viscosity of exocrine secretions and an increased salt content of sweat. Defective Cl− ion transport in CF epithelial cells is likely to result in dehydration of the sol and gel layers lining the bronchial epithelium. This phenomenon is possibly accentuated in viral respiratory illnesses, thus explaining the difficulties with secretions seen with respiratory infections. The same chloride transport defect leads to faulty reabsorption of Na+ and Cl− in the sweat duct and elevated sweat electrolytes. This is the basis for the sweat test, which is still considered the most important diagnostic test for CF.

Viscid exocrine secretions underlie all the clinical features of CF: pancreatic duct obstruction with achylia and maldigestion; progressive obstructive airway disease beginning with a suppurative bronchiolitis, evolving to chronic bronchitis and ultimately bronchiectasis; chronic sinusitis, often with inflammatory nasal polyps; and various intestinal obstructive phenomena ranging from meconium ileus at birth to recurrent intussusception, intestinal impaction, cholestatic jaundice, and cirrhosis.

CLINICAL PRESENTATION

Over 60% of CF patients are diagnosed in infancy with the characteristic features of failure to thrive secondary to maldigestion as well as the chronic unremitting cough of suppurative bronchiolitis and bronchitis.

The multiple different mutations in the CF gene explain in part the striking phenotypic variation of this disease. For example, pancreatic-sufficient patients are never homozygous for the more severe ΔF508 mutation and often es-

Presenting Features of Cystic Fibrosis

Newborn
Meconium ileus, intestinal atresia
Prolonged neonatal jaundice

Infant
Failure to thrive
Chronic cough
Recurrent bronchiolitis, hyperinflation, persistent infiltrates, atelectasis
Chronic diarrhea, abdominal distention
Persistent vomiting, especially with cough
Chronic hypochloremic alkalosis
Hypovitaminosis A with pseudotumor cerebri

Child
Rectal prolapse
Steatorrhea
Nasal polyposis
Clubbing
Hyperinflation, infiltrates, rales, ronchi, and wheeze
Sputum culture: *Stapylococcus aureus or Pseudomonas aeruginosa*

Adolescent, Adult
Sterility in males
Portal hypertension
Growth failure, delayed puberty
Pansinusitis, nasal polyposis
Chronic pulmonary disease

cape clinical detection until later in childhood. Presumably, milder mutations allow for persistence of CFTR function.

The more typical presenting features of CF are listed in the display entitled "Presenting Features of Cystic Fibrosis." Given the variability and at times subtlety of early clinical features, the clinician should maintain a high index of suspicion and obtain a sweat test when indicated. *A child is never too well to have CF.*

Although usually colonized with *Staphylococcus aureus, Haemophilus influenzae,* and eventually *Pseudomonas aeruginosa,* the CF patient is rarely acutely ill with pneumonia or sepsis. Rather, the process is insidious and is typically endobronchial. Unlike the infant or toddler with reactive airway disease who is generally free of cough between episodes of illness, CF results in an unremitting chronic cough, at times with cough-induced emesis that clears only following prolonged antimicrobial therapy. The ravenous appetite with a large oral intake secondary to pancreatic insufficiency often also leads to emesis and additional coughing.

Airway obstruction is usually reversible early in the course. It is not surprising that patients will appear to have asthma, with symptomatic improvement following theophylline, adrenergic agonist, or steroid therapy. Wheeze, dyspnea, and retractions following respiratory viral infections are as much a part of the clinical spectrum of CF as they are of childhood asthma. In general, however, patients with CF are slower to recover and may require prolonged antibiotic therapy for superimposed bacterial bronchiolitis. The hy-

perinflation on a chest roentgenogram and physical examination rarely reverses entirely.

At least 15% of patients have normal or adequate pancreatic function. The presentation in this group, as expected, is more subtle, with better growth, normal appetite, and normal bowel function. Chronic or recurrent respiratory symptoms may be the only hints of disease. Even with pancreatic insufficiency and malabsorption, many otherwise healthy CF children maintain normal growth by a voracious appetite with phenomenal caloric intake. Generally, however, malabsorption results in bulky, foul stools; a marked increase in gaseous distention and fecal mass with a protuberant abdomen; and a tendency to rectal prolapse. Protein malabsorption, in its extreme, can result in hypoalbuminemia and edema. In addition, there can be hypocarotenemia, vitamin A deficiency with xerophthalmia and pseudotumor cerebri, and hypoprothrombinemia with bruising. Any one or combination of these consequences of pancreatic insufficiency can be present.

The pulmonary features in some patients are sufficiently mild to escape detection in childhood. Patients who are diagnosed in adolescence or adulthood characteristically demonstrate pansinusitis, *S. aureus* or *P. aeruginosa* on sputum culture, and chronic changes on chest film associated with hyperinflation. On history, there is usually only a cough, which is often productive. Digital clubbing evolves early in the course of bronchiectasis in CF and helps to differentiate such patients from those with asthma. Nasal polyposis is another important clinical feature. The allergic child will rarely demonstrate polyps prior to age 10. In CF, polyps are not unusual early in childhood. Their presence should alert the physician to the possibility of CF, and a sweat test should be ordered. Aspermia in the adult male may also be a presenting manifestation of CF.

DIFFERENTIAL DIAGNOSIS

With a respiratory presentation, respiratory syncytial virus, bronchiolitis, chlamydia pneumonitis, gastroesophageal reflux with aspiration, asthma, ciliary dysmotility, and immune deficiency are frequently considered. Respiratory syncytial virus is usually epidemic and is diagnosed readily by an analysis of nasal washings. Chlamydia has a typical history of conjunctivitis, onset weeks after birth, eosinophilia, and lack of hyperinflation on chest film. The child with reflux and aspiration may be a spitter; he or she has an abnormal pH probe or barium swallow study and typically responds to positioning, thickened feedings, antacids, and metoclopramide. Ciliary dysmotility is rare; it can be associated with dextrocardia and situs inversus and early on results primarily in rhinosinusitis and serous otitis. Pulmonary symptomatology occurs most often later in the course. These patients are not particularly ill and they thrive. IgG-deficient children suffer from recurrent sinopulmonary infections typically due to the encapsulated organisms *S. pneumoniae, H. influenzae* type b, and *Streptococcus he-*

molyticus. The infections are apt to be acute, with hyperpyrexia and possible septic complications. The pulmonary presentation is not one of dyspnea, cough, and hyperinflation; rather, consolidation with localized changes on chest examination and x-ray is the rule. Other than tachypnea, symptoms are more likely to be systemic than pulmonary. A prompt response to appropriate antibiotics and laboratory evidence of IgG or IgG-subclass deficiency confirm the diagnosis. The infant with congenital acquisition of HIV can present a difficult and differential diagnosis. Failure to thrive and persistent pneumonitis due to opportunistic infection may suggest CF. Recognition of risk factors and appropriate HIV serology are essential to the diagnosis if suspicion exists.

Asthma in early childhood is the pulmonary illness most easily confused with CF; it coexists in many patients. The cough is a helpful differential feature and should be analyzed carefully. The cough of hyperactive airways is typically tight, nonproductive, and responsive to bronchodilators. The CF cough is unique; it is deep, resonant, and strenuous enough in the extreme to result in rib fractures and cough emesis.

Only 10% of CF patients present with isolated pancreatic insufficiency. In infancy, the only unusual feature is persistent diarrhea. Older patients demonstrate more typical steatorrhea (i.e., frequent, bulky, greasy, foul-smelling stools). The differential diagnosis includes chronic nonspecific diarrhea, gluten-induced enteropathy, intestinal lymphangiectasia, parasitism, and milk protein allergy. Although rare, pancreatic insufficiency not due to CF can be seen in Schwachman–Diamond syndrome and isolated deficiencies of lipase, trypsinogen, and enterokinase.

WORK-UP

The current standard diagnostic test for CF is the sweat test. With rare exceptions, it is abnormal in all CF patients at all times. Sweat chloride values over 60 MEq/L are generally considered diagnostic of CF, with mean values of over 100 MEq/L compared to 20 MEq/L in controls. Unfortunately, although many have been tried, no reliable screening tests are available.

Reliable sweat testing requires a rather laborious procedure known as the quantitative pilocarpine iontophoretic test (QPIT). This procedure is required for a definitive diagnosis at all accredited CF centers in the United States. Sweat is stimulated at two sites (forearm) by iontophoresis of a cholinergic drug. The samples are collected on preweighed gauze; they are weighed and the sweat is eluted. Concentrations of sodium, chloride, or both are measured by standard methods. Preferably over 100 mg sweat is collected from each site, because smaller volumes are inadequate for a determination. The testing of the neonate is usually deferred until 1 month of age, when adequate sweat volumes can be reliably obtained.

A positive sweat test in the presence of a positive family history or clinical features of CF establishes the diagnosis. Although other conditions have been reported associated with elevated sweat electrolytes, they are rare. Malnutrition, nephrogenic diabetes insipidus, and adrenal insufficiency are probably the most important entities associated with a mild elevation of sweat electrolytes.

An evaluation of the child suspected of having CF should also include a chest x-ray, a sputum culture, and, when indicated, a quantitative 72-hour stool collection for fecal fat. Early chest roentgenographic changes include hyperinflation and increased peribronchial markings that do not clear completely with therapy. There is a predilection for involvement of the upper lobes, a feature of CF that is yet to be explained. Lobar or segmental atelectasis, in particular involving the right upper or middle lobes, is common in infancy. While the disease progresses, bronchiectasis inevitably develops and is seen on a roentgenogram as parallel bronchial markings (tram lines) extending to the periphery, often associated with hilar adenopathy.

The laboratory assessment of pancreatic function is cumbersome. In most patients, maldigestion and steatorrhea are evident by a history and physical examination. On the other hand, chronic pulmonary suppuration alone can result in inadequate intake, malnutrition, and growth failure. A direct examination of the stool for fat is helpful; however, a positive Sudan stain for fat is normal in infants up to 6 months of age. Quantitation of fecal fat on a 72-hour stool collection is still the most reliable means of assessment, assuming an adequate fat intake (3 g/kg/day in infants, 50 to 100 g/day in older children).

TREATMENT AND MANAGEMENT

The therapeutic goals of CF management are the following:

- Prevent bronchial obstruction and control infection.
- Optimize nutrition with adequate caloric intake and replace pancreatic enzymes and fat-soluble vitamins.
- Identify and correct pulmonary and gastroenterologic complications promptly.
- Provide a healthy, positive psychosocial climate that will allow the patient and his or her family to lead as normal a life as possible.

Prevention of Bronchial Obstruction and Infection

Excluding meconium ileus, ~90% of the morbidity and 98% of the mortality in CF relate to pulmonary disease.

The goal is to maintain clean and patent airways. Regular physical activity to stimulate cough is encouraged; the cough should never be suppressed. Chest physical therapy (gravity, percussion, vibration) is recommended for all patients with evidence of lung disease; families understand to intensify therapy with exacerbations. If there is clinical or physiologic evidence of reversible airway obstruction, bronchodilators are added, preferably by aerosol. Patients are followed at frequent intervals, and sputum or deep throat specimens are monitored for pathogens, which early in the course are likely to be *S. aureus* and *H. influenzae*. Patients are typically treated with dicloxacillin, erythromycin, sulfisoxazole, trimethoprim–sulfamethoxazole, or cefaclor. Chloramphenicol appears particularly effective for more serious involvement with *S. aureus* or β-lactamase producing strains of *H. influenzae*. Unfortunately, these drugs are ineffective against *P. aeruginosa,* which eventually colonizes all but a few patients.

Early in the course of pseudomonas involvement and before long-standing inflammation causes irreversible bronchiectasis, the new oral fluoroquinone agents such as ciprofloxacin can be very effective in reducing endobronchial inflammation and restoring lung function. These drugs, however, are not approved for use in children because of the potential for cartilage damage in growing bones. Other therapeutic strategies designed to prevent progression in relatively asymptomatic patients are currently under study by the Cystic Fibrosis Foundation. These include long-term alternate-day oral prednisone and high-dose aerosolized tobramycin for early exacerbations. Both offer considerable promise but cannot be recommended until possible adverse effects are clarified.

Patients who have an acute exacerbation of lower respiratory disease respond best to hospitalization for high-dose intravenous (IV) antibiotic therapy. For *P. aeruginosa,* or if the pathogen is unknown, a β-lactamase—resistant penicillin and aminoglycoside are used. Second-generation cephalosporins such as cefuroxime and third-generation cephalosporins such as ceftriaxone are highly effective against *S. aureus* and *H. influenzae*. Serum antibiotic levels are monitored as indicated. Treatment is continued until the improvement in chest examinations, sputum production, weight gain, and pulmonary function tests reaches a plateau, presumably representing the best achievable therapeutic response. The usual course is 10 to 14 days.

Patients who have established chronic bronchiectasis in a slow decline are often admitted to the hospital for antibiotic administration in an effort to improve their well-being and pulmonary function. Such admissions are now increasingly replaced by home IV antibiotic therapy.

End-stage CF is characterized by chronic hypoxemia and oxygen dependency with lungs destroyed by bronchiectasis. In the past, such patients followed a predictably downward course of malnutrition, increasing hospitalization for IV antibiotics, cor pulmonale, and respiratory failure. The future is now more hopeful because of nocturnal gastrostomy feeds to maintain nutrition and strength and the increasing successes of double lung transplantation. Limited donor availability remains a problem.

What is the role of "prophylactic" antibiotic administration in healthy patients with no definable sputum pathogens? There are no long-term controlled studies to answer this question. However, both intuition and available data suggest an accelerated rate of colonization with *P. aeruginosa* in patients thus treated.

Optimal Nutrition

The availability of enteric-coated pancreatic enzyme capsules has dramatically improved the nutritional management of CF. Coated enzymes escape gastric breakdown and deliver their product to the small bowel. This has allowed considerable liberalization of the CF diet so that patients can eat with minimum restriction and enjoy the enhanced variety and flavor that dietary fat allows. Nonetheless, caloric intake continues to be deficient in a significant proportion of CF patients; this is not so much a function of fecal loss as it is of persistent high basal energy requirement related to the work of breathing and chronic infection. Every effort must be made to increase caloric intake with food that the patient enjoys, rather than with rigid unpalatable supplements. Parents will quickly learn that the CF child usually prefers to eat from dawn to dusk (i.e., he or she "grazes")! Appropriate nutritious snacks with enzymes must be available at home and on the go.

Infants with CF are generally started on a formula that is predigested (Pregestimil or Portagen) and supplemented with medium-chain triglycerides or glucose polymers. Pancreatic enzymes are given with each feeding. The diet is liberalized as tolerated, and parents are given free reign to adjust enzyme dosage depending on the nature of the stool and change in diet. Generally, by 2 years of age, the child is switched to cow's milk, gradually moving from skim to whole milk.

Fat-soluble vitamins A, D, and E are provided in twice the recommended daily dose, whereas vitamin K is generally supplemented weekly for the first 2 years of life.

INDICATIONS FOR REFERRAL

Every child with cystic fibrosis **should** be followed by an accredited CF center, part of the network established almost 40 years ago by the Cystic Fibrosis Foundation. Through the center, patients have the advantage of financial backup through state crippled children programs, educational and psychological input through center support groups, and access to expert pulmonary and nutritional consultation. Nonetheless, the interested and involved generalist can and should provide primary care and should be alert to complications.

A list of multiple complications of CF includes every organ system of the body. A thorough discussion is beyond the scope of this presentation. The major pulmonary complications necessitating a referral include atelectasis for aggressive medical management and consideration of bronchoscopy; pneumothorax for tube thoracostomy and possible pleurodysis; massive hemoptysis for close observation and possible bronchial artery embolization; and cor pulmonale. Intestinal complications include meconium ileus, intussusception, rectal prolapse, biliary cirrhosis and portal hypertension, malnutrition, and intestinal impaction with bowel obstruction. The pancreatic complications of diabetes mellitus and acute pancreatitis are common and serious. All of these complications, if recognized and referred, can be corrected or controlled; herein lies the art of the management of CF.

ANNOTATED BIBLIOGRAPHY

Boat TF, Welsh MJ, Beaudet AL: Cystic fibrosis. In Scriver CL, Beaudet AL, Sly WS, Valle D (eds): The Metabolic Basis of Inherited Disease, 6th ed, pp 2649–2680. New York, McGraw-Hill, 1989. (The definitive review, stressing pathophysiology and basic science; an exhaustive bibliography.)

Collins FS, Tsui L-C, Riordan JR et al: Identification of the CF gene (three articles). Science 245:1059–1080, 1989. Accompanying editorial p 1029. (The milestone in CF research; immediately increases accuracy of diagnosis and accelerates progress in therapy—all subsequent breakthroughs in CF will be possible because of this work.)

Lloyd-Still JD (ed): Textbook of Cystic Fibrosis. Littleton, MA, John Wright PSG, 1983. (Extremely readable, well-organized, and well-documented text that is particularly strong on the historical as well as psychosocial aspects of cystic fibrosis.)

Taussig LM (ed): Cystic Fibrosis. New York, Thieme-Stratton, 1984. (Comprehensive text that emphasizes pathophysiology with ample discussion of basic science; bibliography alone makes this book invaluable.)

172

Pulmonary Function Tests

Robert G. Zwerdling

Morbidity due to respiratory illness in childhood results in more loss of time at school than does any other cause. The physician who cares for children must, therefore, have the proper tools to evaluate the functional status of the respiratory tract in an objective and quantitative fashion.

An overview of techniques available for such evaluations is provided in this chapter. In most cases, such assessments can be accomplished in a noninvasive and cost-effective manner, and they are well suited to the ambulatory setting.

INDICATIONS FOR PULMONARY FUNCTION TESTS

Pulmonary function tests (PFT) are used to assess the degree and type of physiologic derangement, the responses to pharmacologic intervention, and the progress of various diseases. They are indicated for the evaluation of children having or suspected of having lung disease when the physician needs physiologic (functional) information. Children presenting with recurrent or chronic cough or dyspnea ("can't keep up," "won't keep up") are easily evaluated with the use of such tests. On the other hand, chest radiographs are used to visualize anatomic defects, but they are relatively insensitive and make quantitative physiologic abnormalities difficult.

TECHNIQUES FOR MEASURING PULMONARY PHYSIOLOGY

Respiratory Rates

The respiratory rate, although generally believed to be part of the physical examination, is a reproducible measure of pulmonary function. It is affected by virtually all severe derangements of pulmonary physiology. However, it varies with age, activity, and state of consciousness (Table 172-1). It is often useful to have parents keep a log of sleeping respiratory rates at home. Respiratory rates and assessment of oxygenation often constitute the only readily available measures currently obtainable for the young or uncooperative infant and child.

Arterial Blood Gases

Arterial blood gases (ABGs) reflect gas exchange and, with various transcutaneous measurements, are often one of a few measurements available for use in infants and young children. To properly evaluate the results, the physician must know the concentration of inspired oxygen; that the sample is composed only of arterial blood; and that excess heparin is not used (because it will falsely depress the PCO_2). Diseases that involve the lung in a diffuse manner virtually always result in hypoxemia if the patient is breathing room air. This becomes more pronounced with exercise. In addition, there may be a derangement of acid–base status most often caused by hyperventilation.

The pattern of blood gas abnormalities varies in a characteristic way depending on the type and severity of the problem (Table 172-2). Diffuse pulmonary disease such as bronchiolitis, cystic fibrosis, and pneumonia results in a mismatch of ventilation to perfusion (V/Q). Characteristically, the ABGs seen in such a situation are those of hypoxemia and hypocapnia, with the hypoxemia being correctable by oxygen supplementation. Right-to-left shunts are produced by intracardiac or intrapulmonary shunting. These shunts also produce hypoxemia and hypocapnia. In this case, however, oxygen supplementation only minimally corrects the resultant hypoxemia. Hypoventilation, most often a manifestation of neuromuscular disease, drug overdose, or obstruction of the upper airway, produces hypox-

Table 172-1. Respiratory Rates by Age and Sex

AGE (YEARS)	BOYS (MEAN ± SD)	GIRLS (MEAN ± SD)
0–1	31 ± 8	30 ± 6
1–2	26 ± 4	27 ± 4
2–3	25 ± 4	25 ± 3
3–4	24 ± 3	24 ± 3
4–5	23 ± 2	22 ± 2
5–6	22 ± 2	21 ± 2
6–7	21 ± 3	21 ± 3
. . .	. . .	. . .
17–18	16 ± 3	17 ± 3

Active children have rates that are considerably higher. (Iliff A, Lee VA: Pulse rate respiratory rate, and body temperature of children between two months and eighteen years of age. Child Dev 23:237, 1952.)

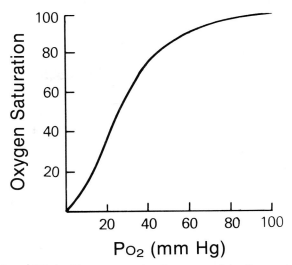

Figure 172-1. The oxygen saturation curve relates the percent saturation of oxygen to the partial pressure of oxygen.

emia correctable with oxygen supplementation and also produces hypercapnia (see also Chap. 194).

Pulse Oximetry

Pulse oximetry is now becoming a widely available method for the measurement of oxygen saturation. It is noninvasive, accurate, and suitable for office and even home measurements. The reading is of oxygen saturation rather than the more familiar partial pressure of oxygen (PO_2). The relationship between oxygen saturation and PO_2 is shown in Figure 172-1. For example, an oxygen saturation of 90% corresponds to a PO_2 of 60 mm Hg. It must be noted that the curve is shifted to the left by alkalosis, hypothermia, and fetal and other unusual types of hemoglobin, and it is shifted to the right by acidosis, hyperthermia, hypercapnia, and certain other abnormal hemoglobins. Keeping these factors in mind, oximetry is simple, rapid, and easier than transcutaneous oxygen measurements. It may be useful to obtain readings under a variety of circumstances, such as during feeding, during sleeping, and following exercise. The increasing numbers of children on home oxygen because of cystic fibrosis, bronchopulmonary dysplasia, and other less common respiratory diseases make this measurement particularly attractive.

Movement artifact and failing to sense the pulse will produce false low readings. In addition, the probe size is based upon the weight of the patient. Manufacturers of these units will not guarantee the accuracy of a reading unless it is done according to their specifications.

Pulse oximetry is beginning to be used as a parameter in the determination of the need for admission. A concern is that once unrecognized mild hypoxemia will result in inappropriate hospitalization. Unfortunately, data assessing the reliability of this modality are scanty.

Lung Volumes

Lung volumes refer to the amount of gas in the lungs at varying degrees of inspiration (Fig. 172-2). Total lung capacity (TLC) is the amount of gas contained at a full inspiration; residual volume (RV) is the amount of gas left in the lung after the patient expires completely. The vital capacity (VC) is the amount of gas that the patient can expel and is the most widely measured value. The office-based pediatrician will most commonly measure VC either as part of

Table 172-2. Causes of Abnormal Arterial Blood Gases

	Po₂		
	RA	100%	Pco₂
V/Q mismatch	↓	↑	↓
Diffusion def	↓	↑	↓
Hypoventilation	↓	↑	↑
R to L shunt	↓	↓	↓

RA = room air; V/Q = ventilation/perfusion; R = right; L = left.

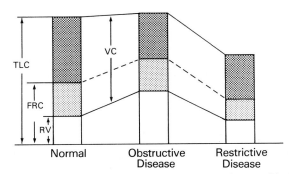

Figure 172-2. The expected changes in lung volumes with obstructive and restrictive defects are demonstrated.

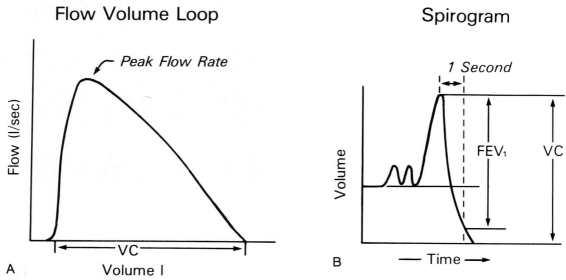

Figure 172-3. (**A**) An expiratory flow volume curve (flow versus volume) is illustrated. (**B**) An example of spirometry (volume versus time) is given.

a complete pulmonary function evaluation or when following a child with neuromuscular weakness, such as Guillain–Barré syndrome. The measurement of VC requires the cooperation of the child; therefore, it is rarely accurate for a child under 5 years of age.

Flow Rates

Flow rates are the most widely used and useful measurement of pulmonary function in the ambulatory setting (Fig. 172-3). This is because of the high prevalence of asthma and other airway diseases in childhood. These are generally measured as volume versus time or flow versus volume, as demonstrated in Figure 172-3. Flow rates can also be measured before and after bronchodilators, exercise, cold air, and occasionally antigen challenge to evaluate the degree and nature of airway reactivity (see the section on challenge testing). These tests also require the child's cooperation. Simple measurements of peak expiratory flow can often be performed at 3 years of age, although more extensive testing usually requires that the child be over 5 years of age.

Peak Expiratory Flow Rates

The peak expiratory flow rate (PEFR) is a simple, inexpensive, and reproducible gauge of obstruction. It is a measurement of the highest expiratory flow rate achieved and is generally reported in liters/minute. The child blows into a mechanical device and the reading is taken directly off of a meter. Because this study is effort-dependent, one must be sure that the effort is maximal. This may be confirmed if

the patient's readings are within 5 to 10 L/min on at least two occasions. With practice, children 3 years of age and older are readily tested.

Interpretation is based on comparing the patient's reading with normal values, which, in childhood, are generally based on height. It is also useful to compare the patient's own previous values with those of the current study. In addition, if there is an indication that the patient has an obstructive defect, the child should be retested after receiving a bronchodilator (see challenge testing). Although the PEFR is one of the least sensitive of the PFTs, it is significantly more sensitive than the physician using a stethoscope. The PEFR will drop to 50% to 60% of predicted before the physician or patient detects obstruction. It is, therefore, an excellent early warning system for airway obstruction, allowing for the early institution or modification of therapy.

The use of PEFRs in the home allows the patient and family to determine when to institute additional therapy, to call the physician, or to visit the emergency room. The result is a significant decrease in anxiety for all concerned.

GUIDELINES FOR THE PERFORMANCE AND ANALYSIS OF PULMONARY FUNCTION TESTS

Standards for the performance of PFTs in childhood have been established. It is the responsibility of the primary care physician to ensure that the laboratory to which these patients are referred adheres to these standards.

Pulmonary function tests report the patient's observed value, the predicted value (variously based on height, sex, age, and race), and the percent of the predicted value. The latter is the observed value divided by the predicted value. In addition, an interpretation is usually provided by the pulmonologist directing the laboratory. That individual also evaluates the technical aspects of the test as part of the interpretation.

Outside of a formal pulmonary function laboratory, the primary care physician is most successful using a simple measure of obstruction such as the PEFR in a consistent way rather than becoming involved with complete testing. Pressure from the vendors of pulmonary function equipment who paint rosy clinical and economic pictures should be resisted.

PATTERNS OF PULMONARY FUNCTION ABNORMALITIES

Three patterns of pulmonary function abnormalities are seen: restrictive, obstructive, and mixed obstructive and restrictive defects.

Restrictive patterns result in a decrease in most lung volumes while preserving the ability to empty gas from the lung rapidly (Table 172-3). Thus, the percent of the vital capacity that is emptied in the first second (FEV_1/VC) is normal or elevated. Space-occupying lesions such as tumors, pleural effusions, interstitial fluid, and neuromuscular weakness are common causes for such findings.

Obstructive patterns (Table 172-3) result in decreased air flow, an elevation of residual volume, functional residual capacity, and an elevation of total lung capacity. The amount of the vital capacity emptied in the first second (FEV_1/VC) is decreased. Common diseases such as asthma, chronic obstructive lung disease, and cystic fibrosis usually produce such findings.

Mixed patterns are seen in situations such as a patient who has an airway obstruction with mucous plugging and atelectasis.

INHALATION CHALLENGE TESTING

Any measure of lung volume or flow rate can be determined after the patient is given a challenge of bronchodilator, methacholine, histamine, cold air, exercise, or antigen. As a result, the dynamic properties of the lung are readily assessed. For practical purposes, one usually needs to measure only the FEV_1 and perhaps vital capacity after a par-

Table 172-3. Patterns of Lung Function Abnormalities

	OBSTRUCTIVE	RESTRICTIVE
VC	↓	↓
FEV_1	↓	↓
FEV_1/VC	↓	↑

VC = vital capacity; FEV_1 = forced expiratory volume in 1 second.

ticular challenge. Patients who are obstructed should receive an inhaled bronchodilator and have a repeat FEV_1. An increase of 15% to 20% or greater indicates bronchodilator responsiveness. Patients who have normal flow rates are often retested after exercise, breathing cold air, or inhalation of progressive concentrations of methacholine. This enables the physician to determine the degree of airway reactivity, which is helpful in the analysis of complaints of chronic cough, dyspnea, and unexplained recurrent pneumonia. Such studies should be performed only in laboratories directed by physicians experienced in such testing. This is important because there is a small but real danger of significant airway obstruction associated with these studies. It is strongly urged that the guidelines for inhalation challenge testing provided by the American Thoracic Society (Cropp) be followed.

BIBLIOGRAPHY

Cropp GJA, Bernstein IL, Boushey HA et al: Guidelines for bronchial inhalation: Challenge with pharmacologic and antigenic agents. ATS News, Spring 1980.

Hess D, Kochansky M, Hassett L et al: An evaluation of the Nellcor N - 10 Portable Pulse Oximeter. Respir Care 31:796, 1986.

Hsu KHK, Jenkins DE, Hsi BP et al: Ventilatory functions of normal children and young adults—Mexican-American, white, and black. I: Spirometry. J Pediatr 95:14, 1979.

Kerem E, Canny G, Tibshirani R et al: Clinical-physiologic correlations in acute asthma of childhood. Pediatrics 87:481–486, 1991.

Ruppel G: Manual of Pulmonary Function Testing. St. Louis, CV Mosby, 1979.

Schnapp LN, Cohen NH: Pulse oximetry: Uses and abuses. Chest 98:1244–1250, 1990.

Taussig LM, Chernick V, Wood R et al: Standardization of lung function testing in children. J Pediatr 97:668, 1980.

West J: Respiratory Physiology. Baltimore, Williams & Wilkins, 1985.

21

TOXICOLOGIC PROBLEMS

Michael A. McGuigan, Section Editor

173

Therapeutic Drug Monitoring in Pediatric Practice

Algis K. Rasymas

Therapeutic drug monitoring (TDM) provides valuable, objective information essential to the provision of optimal medical care. This chapter focuses on the principles of pharmacology and therapeutic monitoring necessary in the practice of ambulatory pediatrics. In general practice, it is frequently impractical to obtain multiple blood samples over time to completely characterize the pharmacokinetics of a drug in a particular patient. Therefore, a basic approach with emphasis on practical dosage adjustments for orally administered drugs is presented. Following a discussion of principles, individual attention is given to theophylline, the anticonvulsants, digoxin, and aspirin. The aminoglycosides are mentioned briefly because of the frequency with which these drugs are used even by office-based pediatricians. The adjustment of dosage in renal or hepatic failure and the existence of important drug interactions are outlined when appropriate. Illustrative examples are provided at the end of the chapter. The general pediatrician should be aware that TDM has important applications in the use of anti-infective, psychotropic, antineoplastic, and antiarrhythmic drugs whose infrequent use does not warrant inclusion in this chapter.

INDICATIONS FOR THERAPEUTIC DRUG MONITORING

Before deciding to use therapeutic drug monitoring in a particular clinical situation, one must consider the nature of the drug and the use of the derived information.

First, there must be a specific and reproducible assay available, and second, there must be a clinically meaningful relationship between the response to the drug (therapeutic or toxic) and the serum concentration. If these two requirements are not met, therapeutic monitoring of the drug is useless. Next, the response to the drug should be examined. If the response is easily measured through routine patient assessment, TDM is probably not necessary. However, TDM would be indicated if verification of the presence of a drug was necessary (i.e., to assess compliance or if toxicity or overdose was suspected). When response is not easily measured, TDM can provide the most benefit.

TDM is indicated when:

1. Objective monitoring parameters are limited. TDM can be helpful in instances where clearly defined therapeutic end points are lacking. A good example is the need to achieve a sufficient concentration of an anticonvulsant to prevent the occurrence of a seizure.
2. There is a high probability of encountering a failure in therapy because of:
   a. A narrow therapeutic range—TDM would help to adjust drug dosage to maintain concentrations below those usually associated with toxicity yet above those concentrations needed for minimal efficacy. Digoxin is an excellent example.
   b. A poor relationship between dose and concentration—The serum concentration of a patient may be subtherapeutic because of poor drug absorption or rapid drug elimination. It may be helpful to measure serum concentrations following a witnessed dose to characterize absorption and elimination, to help determine why the patient is not responding as would be expected for a particular dose.
   c. Nonlinear pharmacokinetics of the therapeutic agent—This is discussed later in this chapter.
   d. Predictable drug interactions—TDM can be used to assure therapeutic serum concentrations in the face

of predictable interactions between drugs or between a drug and other environmental factors.

e. Disease states—Many disease states affect drug absorption and elimination. TDM is particularly useful when patients have renal or hepatic disorders.

f. Noncompliance—TDM can be helpful in determining whether the patient is taking the medicine as prescribed or whether the treatment is ineffective despite compliance.

When interpreting drug concentrations for all these applications, it is important to recall that some patients will respond only with concentrations well into the purported "toxic" range, whereas others will be unable to tolerate even marginally "therapeutic" serum concentrations. Using clinical assessment and the laboratory ranges as a guide, the physician must always seek the patient's own optimal therapeutic range. Finally, when the patient has had the desired clinical response without developing unacceptable toxicity, the physician should not feel obligated to perform TDM simply to document "therapeutic" levels.

PRINCIPLES OF PHARMACOKINETICS

An understanding of basic pharmacokinetics is essential in order to interpret and apply the results of therapeutic monitoring. This section will attempt to impart a basic understanding of pharmacokinetic terminology and principles, and to make useful generalizations about drug pharmacokinetics.

Linear Pharmacokinetics (First-Order)

Linear pharmacokinetics adequately describes the disposition of most drugs when serum concentrations are in the usual therapeutic range. Exceptions include aspirin, phenytoin, procainamide, and sometimes theophylline. The term *linear pharmacokinetics* implies that only a constant *fraction* of the drug is removed per unit of time (e.g., one third of the drug in the body is removed each hour), regardless of the actual amount of drug in the body. In effect, the rate of elimination increases and decreases exactly in proportion to rising and falling serum concentrations. For convenience, the rate of removal is usually expressed as the time needed to remove half the drug from the body—the *half-life* (t½). A drug is usually assumed to distribute into a hypothetical volume, the *volume of distribution* (Vd), expressed in liters per kilogram of body weight. The measure of the drug removal rate and capacity is known as the *clearance* (Cl) and is expressed as the volume of blood that is completely cleared of drug per unit of time (liters per minute). The half-life is dependent upon both the volume of distribution and the clearance.

Several important generalizations can be made about first-order pharmacokinetics.

1. A continuous infusion will achieve a constant serum drug concentration. The serum concentration is determined only by the rate of drug administration and the body clearance. This concentration is directly proportional to the dose in a particular patient (i.e., doubling the dose doubles the concentration).

2. If an infusion is started with no drug in the body, it will take approximately four to five half-lives to reach this constant serum concentration, which is known as the *steady state concentration*. During this state of equilibrium, the amount of drug that is administered is equal to the amount of drug eliminated by the body in a given time interval.

3. Intermittent IV or oral doses will achieve the same *average* concentration as a continuous infusion of the same dose over the same interval. As doses are given further apart, the size of the dose must be increased to obtain the same average concentration, and the amount of fluctuation in the concentrations increases.

4. With intermittent dosing, the serum concentrations at any time remain proportional to the dose (i.e., if 1 mg given every 6 hours gives a certain level 2 hours after the dose, then 2 mg every 6 hours will give twice that concentration at the same time after dosing).

5. Whenever a drug dose or infusion is changed, it again takes five half-lives (not five doses) to reach a new steady state.

6. After a dose, the highest concentration is called the *peak* and the lowest concentration (just prior to the next dose) is called the *trough*. The peak (mg/L) after any dose may be estimated by dividing the dose (mg) by the volume of distribution (L) and adding the previous trough level (mg/L). This may also be done by extrapolating (on semi-log paper) the concentration versus time line back to the time of drug administration.

7. Slow-release drugs do not have a longer half-life. Like a continuous infusion, they slowly release the drug into the body, giving less fluctuation of concentrations between doses. Five half-lives (not five doses) are still required to reach steady state. The timing of "peaks" and "troughs" is erratic with these preparations, and a half-life cannot be calculated with concentrations obtained between doses.

Nonlinear Pharmacokinetics (Zero-Order)

Nonlinear pharmacokinetics is used to describe the behavior of some medications such as aspirin, phenytoin, and procainamide. Theophylline also behaves in this way when serum levels are high. Zero-order pharmacokinetics is much more complex than linear pharmacokinetics, and a direct prediction of serum concentrations over time is difficult.

With nonlinear pharmacokinetics, the body is not able to increase the amount of drug eliminated in proportion to the serum concentrations. This results in an apparent slowing of elimination as serum concentrations increase. It is important to remember that the amount excreted per unit of time is not actually diminished at high concentrations but simply approaches a plateau at which it is impossible for the body to further increase elimination (*saturation*). As a result, the fraction of the total drug in the body excreted per unit of time becomes smaller as serum concentrations rise. It is often stated that nonlinearly excreted drugs have a longer half-life at higher serum levels. Although this is conceptually useful, it is not mathematically correct, because *half-life* is a derived term applicable only to linear pharmacokinetics.

Important generalizations about nonlinear pharmacokinetics are as follows:

1. A constant infusion produces a constant steady-state concentration.
2. The volume of distribution of a nonlinear drug is still useful for calculating initial concentrations (using level = dose/volume of distribution) after a loading dose.
3. It may take a long time (weeks) to reach equilibrium following a change in dosing regimen.
4. Changes in blood concentrations are disproportionately large compared to changes in dose or infusion rate. Small changes in the dosage of a drug may result in a dramatic change in serum concentrations.

Drug Dosage in Renal and Hepatic Failure

The elimination of almost all drugs is affected to some degree by alterations in hepatic or renal function. In cases of altered drug excretion, it is important to remember that the initial or *loading dose* needed to achieve a therapeutic level generally remains the same because the volume of distribution for the drug *is not usually altered*. Rather, it is the dosage used or the frequency with which the drug is administered to maintain a therapeutic concentration that must be altered in the face of organ dysfunction.

Many renally excreted drugs are eliminated in direct proportion to the glomerular filtration rate (GFR) (e.g., aminoglycosides) and hence can be easily adjusted once the GFR has been estimated. When there is some renal dysfunction, the interval of the dosage regimen has to be prolonged. For hepatically eliminated drugs and for drugs with substantial tubular reabsorption and tubular secretion, no simple method is available for dosage adjustment.

MONITORED DRUGS

Theophylline

Although the use of theophylline is declining, it still remains one of the most frequently monitored drugs. There are a variety of preparations, including several slow-release formulations that are designed to provide more stable serum concentrations. In general, the absorption from all of these preparations is complete and, for the standard preparations,

rapid. In certain individuals, the absorption of slow-release preparations may be poor, irregular, or both. Despite this, the convenience, improved compliance, and more stable blood concentrations seen in most patients using slow-release preparations generally outweigh this unpredictability.

Theophylline has a volume of distribution of about 0.5 L/kg. The drug is eliminated by hepatic metabolism with a variable half-life. In term infants, half-lives range from 14 to 26 hours, whereas in children over 1 year of age, the mean half-life is 3 hours. Half-lives tend to increase as the children grow older, and approach the nonsmoking adult mean of 8.2 hours. Therapeutic levels are 55 to 110 μmol/L (10–20 μg/ml).

When serum concentrations exceed 110 μmol/L, the ability of the patient to eliminate theophylline may be limited. Caution should be used in adjusting dosages upward when the serum concentration is at or near 110 μmol/L, because changes in concentration that are larger than expected may occur.

Age-specific dosage recommendations, with adjustment for smoking habits in older patients, are widely available and should be used for the initiation of therapy when no other patient data are available. With rapid-release forms, dosage adjustment can be made based on peak and trough levels obtained after five half-lives (~24 hours in a typical child). Peak levels should be obtained 2 hours after dosing to allow for complete absorption. With slow-release (SR) dosage forms, a single predose concentration in the mid-therapeutic range is often all that is necessary to assure that the patient is within the therapeutic range. If a patient is responding poorly to SR therapy or shows signs of toxicity, it may be worth obtaining one or more serum drug concentrations 2 to 10 hours after dosing in order to document the patient's absorption profile. The "peak" concentration may occur at any time following SR dosing, although 4 to 6 hours is typical. Because there is diurnal variation with theophylline absorption (less theophylline absorbed at night), repeated serum concentration determinations should be obtained at the same time each day. No adjustment of theophylline dosage is required in renal failure. The drug should be used cautiously in hepatic disease. A large number of drugs interfere with theophylline metabolism. Rifampin can increase the clearance of theophylline, whereas erythromycin can decrease the clearance. Viral illness may also significantly impede elimination in some patients.

Phenobarbital and Primidone

Phenobarbital (PB) has a volume of distribution of 0.6 L/kg in children over 1 year of age. The bioavailability of oral tablets is over 90%. It is eliminated primarily by hepatic metabolism with an average half-life of 62 hours in children and over 100 hours in adolescents. This long half-life allows once-a-day dosing with minimal fluctuation in serum concentrations. Once the patient has reached a steady state, which may take 8 to 14 days, a single blood level obtained at any time is adequate to allow dose adjustment. After adjusting the dose, one should remember that steady state will be reached in ~five half-lives. The generally accepted therapeutic range is 65 to 170 μmol/L (15–40 μg/ml).

Primidone is converted into two active metabolites—PB and phenylethylmalonamide. The latter is not usually measured, but primidone and PB concentrations should both be measured whenever primidone is used. Primidone has a variable volume of distribution ranging from 0.4 to 1 L/kg and a half-life of 4.5 to 11 hours. Therapeutic primidone serum concentrations are 23 to 55 μmol/L (5–12 μg/ml). Plasma phenobarbital:primidone ratios are generally ~1:1, but there may be wide variation depending on the rates of phenobarbital production and elimination. The time of blood sampling can also affect the ratio because the half-lives of the two compounds are different. Therefore, when comparing concentration ratios from different regimens, blood sampling must be done at precisely the same time after the dose. When evaluating concentrations, sufficient time should be given for both drugs to achieve steady state. Because phenobarbital generally has the longer half-life, this will require 8 to 14 days. Poor compliance with primidone can create a confusing picture in which the patient has a substantial phenobarbital concentration at a time when there is little primidone present.

Phenobarbital and primidone concentrations can be easily adjusted with the use of first-order pharmacokinetics because the serum concentrations are directly proportional to the dose.

Phenobarbitol enhances the metabolism of many drugs, including other anticonvulsants. In hepatic disease, the elimination of both drugs is diminished to a variable extent.

Carbamazepine

Carbamazepine (CBZ) is rapidly becoming the preferred drug for many seizure disorders in the pediatric age group because of its effectiveness and lack of unacceptable cosmetic and behavioral side effects. The drug is very well absorbed with a volume of distribution of 1 to 2 L/kg. The half-life is generally in the 5- to 12-hour range. The therapeutic range is 17 to 50 μmol/L (4–12 μg/ml). The monitoring of carbamazepine is complicated by two considerations. First, the drug induces its own metabolism (i.e., it causes an increase in enzymatic activity that increases the elimination of the drug). Current dosage recommendations reflect this phenomenon in the fact that CBZ is begun at a low dose and gradually increased at biweekly intervals. Second, a portion of the activity of CBZ is due to the presence of a metabolite. Fortunately, the concentrations of the metabolite, which are not generally measured, are proportional to the concentrations of the parent compound.

The simple first-order rules for dosage adjustment apply to CBZ if one recalls that a true steady-state concentration can be measured only after enzymatic induction is complete, usually 1 to 2 weeks after a change in dose. Increases in serum concentration may be less than predicted after an increase in dosage because of enzyme induction. In addition, slow absorption makes it difficult to obtain a peak concentration or to estimate half-life. A single predose trough concentration can be used to determine whether the patient is within the therapeutic range. In the child with rapid metabolism, it may be helpful to obtain two or more concentrations between doses in order to define a plasma concentration curve.

The addition of CBZ will generally accelerate the metabolism of other anticonvulsants. Similarly, the addition of anticonvulsants other than valproic acid will accelerate the metabolism of CBZ. The use of CBZ is not recommended in patients who have liver disease. Use in renal disease has not been extensively studied, but dosage probably requires adjustment only in the severely uremic patient.

Valproic Acid

Valproic acid (VPA) is a unique anticonvulsant whose pharmacology differs significantly from that of the other anticonvulsants. The drug is well absorbed in all dosage forms and by all routes, including rectal administration. The enteric-coated tablets are completely absorbed, but delays of up to 6 hours may occur before peak concentrations are reached. Food may significantly delay the absorption of standard preparations. The pharmacokinetics of VPA vary widely among individuals, as indicated by the wide dosing range of 10 to 60 mg/kg/day. Determination of half-life following initial dosing has been shown to be advantageous in achieving therapeutic concentrations rapidly. It may be helpful to establish a dosing regimen using a nonenteric dosage form and then change to an enteric-coated form if the patient develops gastric intolerance.

The volume of distribution of VPA is only 0.2 L/kg, and half-lives in children range from 4 to 17 hours. Therapeutic concentrations are 350 to 700 μmol/L (50–100 μg/ml).

Samples for half-life determination should ideally be taken 4 to 8 hours after an oral dose of nonenteric valproic acid, either at steady state or after a single dose. Because absorption is slowed with food or enteric coating, monitoring of a predose concentration will be most helpful in the uncontrolled clinical situation.

The metabolism of VPA is enhanced by other anticonvulsants. VPA generally slows the metabolism of other anticonvulsants (and many other hepatically excreted drugs). VPA displaces phenytoin from protein-binding sites, which may lead to acute phenytoin intoxication.

Ethosuximide

Ethosuximide (ESX) is less commonly used and less well studied than the other anticonvulsants. Ethosuximide follows first-order pharmacokinetics, with a volume of distribution of 0.7 L/kg and a half-life of 30 hours in children (60 hours in adults). The therapeutic range is 280 to 710 μmol/L (40–100 μg/ml). In general, a single daily dose is satisfactory, and random concentrations will reflect steady-state values because daily fluctuations will be fairly small. The occasional rapid metabolizer may require twice-daily dosing.

The pharmacokinetics of ethosuximide in hepatic and renal failure is inadequately studied, and caution is needed when ESX is combined with other anticonvulsant drugs. Interactions have been reported anecdotally but have not been studied systematically.

Phenytoin

Phenytoin (diphenylhydantoin [DPH]) is a commonly used anticonvulsant, and therapeutic problems are frequently encountered because of nonlinear pharmacokinetics and substantial protein binding. The drug is about 80% absorbed, with a substantial variation among individuals. Nasogastric feedings can nearly abolish absorption. The volume of distribution ranges from 0.6 to 0.8 L/kg. The time needed to eliminate 50% of the drug from the body (t_{50}) in children is 4 to 12 hours. During puberty, the t_{50} increases toward the adult range of 20 to 40 hours. Therapeutic trough concentrations are 40 to 80 μmol/L (10–20 μg/ml). It is not infrequent for children to require up to twice the maximal recommended starting dosage for phenytoin.

Many days may be required to achieve a steady state. For this reason, a loading dose may be needed to establish therapeutic concentrations. Serum concentrations can be measured after a loading dose to determine if a therapeutic concentration has been reached. Dosage adjustment is largely empirical, but it should be more conservative than estimates based on linear pharmacokinetics.

Phenytoin variably affects other anticonvulsants. Valproic acid displaces phenytoin from protein-binding sites and may cause phenytoin toxicity. Dosage adjustments are required for patients with hepatic and/or renal dysfunction.

Digoxin

The therapeutic monitoring of digoxin is plagued by several problems. The drug suffers from erratic absorption, with a bioavailability of about 70% for digoxin tablets, 80% for the elixir, and 90% for the capsules. Following absorption there is a prolonged distribution/equilibration phase of 6 to 12 hours during which digoxin slowly enters the body tissues. The apparent volume of distribution is about 10 L/kg. Because of the prolonged distribution phase, peak concentrations are meaningless, and a half-life cannot be determined from peak and trough values. Practical monitoring of digoxin is restricted to the measurement of trough concentrations, which should be in the range of 1 to 2.5 nmol/L

(0.8–2 ng/ml). It can generally be assumed that trough concentrations will be proportional to daily dosage, and adjustment can be made accordingly. The half-life of digoxin in children ranges from 16 to 40 hours, so steady-state concentrations may not be achieved for 1 week or more. For newly digitalized or unstable patients, it may be necessary to check concentrations prior to steady state in order to ensure that excessive accumulation is not occurring. Dosage adjustment is required in both hepatic and renal failure as well as for many disease states and drug interactions.

The presence of endogenous "digoxinlike immunoreactive substances" (DLIS), particularly in the newborn or fluid-overloaded patient, makes interpretation of the reported digoxin concentration difficult. However, newer assay systems are more specific for digoxin, and plasma samples may be pretreated in the laboratory before the assay to remove the DLIS.

Aminoglycosides

The therapeutic monitoring of aminoglycosides has become a matter of routine practice. After intravenous or intramuscular administration, the aminoglycosides have a volume of distribution of 0.5 L/kg and a half-life of about 2 to 3 hours. Effective mathematical methods for dose adjustment are available. Detailed examples of gentamicin dosage adjustment are given at the end of this chapter and can be applied to the other aminoglycosides. It is important to modify the dosing interval as well as the dose when adjusting aminoglycoside dosages for rapid or slow elimination. Therapeutic concentrations of gentamicin and tobramycin are peaks of 5 to 10 μg/ml and troughs of less than 2 μg/ml. Recommended peaks for amikacin are 20 to 35 μg/ml and troughs are 2.5 to 10 μg/ml. The aminoglycosides are eliminated renally, and maintenance dosage adjustment based on creatinine clearance is required in renal dysfunction. No adjustment is required in hepatic failure.

Salicylates

The monitoring of salicylate (ASA) concentrations is necessary only when the drug is used in high doses. Monitoring is critically important because therapeutic concentrations are close to toxic concentrations.

The absorption of ASA is rapid and complete. The volume of distribution is roughly 0.16 L/kg, but it changes with concentration. Elimination is largely by hepatic metabolism with urinary excretion of metabolites. A steady-state concentration is usually established within 2 weeks. Typical initial doses for JRA, pericarditis, Kawasaki's disease, and rheumatic fever are 60 to 100 mg/kg/day, divided into four doses. The goal of therapy is to establish trough concentrations of 1.1 to 2.2 mmol/L (15–30 mg/dl) by gradually increasing the dosage. Because of the marked nonlinearity of salicylates, increases should be limited to increments of 10 to 20 mg/kg/day. Doses in excess of 130 mg/kg/day are rarely required. Once therapeutic serum concentrations are established, salicylates are often continued for months to years, and periodic monitoring is recommended.

Caution is required in the presence of hepatic or renal failure.

EXAMPLES

Example 1. Phenobarbital

Q. A 4-year-old patient has been chronically on 6 mg/kg/day of PB. Following an isolated seizure, you check a random serum concentration and obtain a value of 80 μmol/L. How would you increase this serum concentration to 120 μmol/L?

A. Because levels of phenobarbital are proportional to dose (follows first-order pharmacokinetics), you increase the dose to 120/80, or 1.5 times the original dose. The patient does well on 9 mg/kg/day.

Example 2. Valproic acid (approach could apply equally well to theophylline)

Q. Your patient has not responded well to a dose of 30 mg/kg/day of VPA. You suspect noncompliance; thus, you obtain concentrations 2 and 8 hours after a witnessed dose. The 2-hour serum concentration is 550 μmol/L and the 6-hour concentration is only 270 μmol/L. The patient has a brief seizure in your office. How do you interpret the results? What do you do to improve therapy?

A. You examine the concentrations obtained and calculate a half-life of approximately 4 hours (the concentration dropped from 550 μmol/L to 270 μmol/L, about half, in 4 hours). You conclude that the patient is compliant but is a rapid metabolizer and thus requires a dose increase and (more importantly) a q6h dosing schedule. He responds well to 40 mg/kg/day divided every 6 hours.

Example 3. Gentamicin

Q. Your patient is on standard doses of gentamicin—2.5 mg/kg every 8 hours. Serum concentrations are obtained 1 hour after the dose (peak) and immediately before the next dose (trough). Assuming that the patient is at steady state, what would you do with the following concentrations:

    a. trough = 3 μg/ml, peak = 15 μg/ml
    b. trough = <1 μg/ml (lower limit of detection), peak = 13 μg/ml
    c. trough = 3.1 μg/ml, peak = 10 μg/ml

    a. Both peak and trough concentrations are about 1.5 times too high, and the half-life is typical of gentamicin. You decrease the dose proportionately to two thirds of 2.5 mg/kg, or 1.6 mg/kg q8h.

    b. Trough concentrations are low and peaks are too high. The half-life is short. The best solution is to shorten the dosing interval to q6h, keeping the same daily dose. Because each dose will be three quarters as large as before, peaks will be roughly two thirds of 13, or about 10.

    c. The half-life obtained from these data is prolonged—about 4 hours. You elect to increase the interval to q12h without changing the size of the dose. This gives a smaller total daily dose; thus, the peak should be less than 10 μg/ml. Twelve hours later (~three half-lives), the trough should be $\frac{1}{2} \times \frac{1}{2} \times \frac{1}{2} \times 10$ μg/ml, which is less than 2 μg/ml.

Example 4. Aspirin

Q. You start a patient on ASA for rheumatoid arthritis, beginning with a dose of 80 mg/kg/day. One week later, a predose concentration is 0.8 mmol/L. What do you do?

A. If ASA had linear pharmacokinetics, you would increase the dose by 1.1/0.8, or 1.4 times, to 120 mg/kg/day. This initial calculation is helpful because it places an upper limit on the size of dose adjustment needed. You know, however, that ASA has nonlinear pharmacokinetics. You opt for the maximum recommended dose increase of 20 mg/kg/day (to 100 mg/kg/day).

Example 5. Phenytoin

Q. A colleague asks you what to do with a 5-year-old patient who "can't get a concentration above 14 μmol/L" on the maximum recommended dose of phenytoin. What do you suggest?

A. If phenytoin had linear pharmacokinetics, you would have to triple the dose just to get into the low therapeutic range. Because you know that the pharmacokinetics is nonlinear, you suggest increasing the dose by 10% and checking trough concentrations in 1 week in order to determine the new steady-state concentration. You point out that toddlers often require large doses of phenytoin.

ANNOTATED BIBLIOGRAPHY

Brodie MJ, Feely J: Practical clinical pharmacology—Therapeutic drug monitoring and clinical trials. Br Med J 296:1110–1114, 1988. (Brief reports on the TDM of various drugs with suggestions on how to critically assess clinical trials.)

Dettli L: Drug dosage in renal disease. In Gibaldi M, Prescott L: Handbook of Clinical Pharmacokinetics, pp 261–276. New York, ADIS Health Sciences Press, 1983. (Practical approach to dosage adjustment in renal disease.)

Evans WE, Oellerich M (eds): Therapeutic Drug Monitoring Clinical Guide. Irving, TX, Abbott Diagnostics, 1984. (This comprehensive, concise pocket handbook is available to physicians free of charge through Abbott Laboratories.)

Evans WE, Schentag JJ, Jusko WJ (eds): Applied Pharmacokinetics, 2nd ed. San Francisco, Applied Therapeutics, 1986. (Rigorous yet practical text on the state-of-the-art application of pharmacokinetic methods, pharmacodynamic principles, and relevant data to optimize patient therapy.)

Gilman JT: Therapeutic drug monitoring in the neonate and pediatric age group. Clin Pharmacokinet 19:1–10, 1990. (Problems and clinical pharmacokinetic implications of TDM in children.)

Hendeles L, Weinberger M: Theophylline—A state of the art review. Pharmacotherapy 3:2–44, 1983. (Up-to-date review of all aspects of theophylline therapy.)

MacKichan JJ, Comstock TJ: General pharmacokinetic principles. In Taylor WJ, Cavines M (eds): A Textbook for the Clinical Application of TDM. Irving, TX, Abbott Laboratories, 1986. (Excellent review of pharmacokinetics and TDM; other chapters in this textbook concentrate on the TDM of individual drugs.)

Pippenger CE, Massoud N: Therapeutic drug monitoring. In Benet LZ, Massoud N, Gambertoglio JG, et al (eds): Pharmacokinetic Basis for Drug Treatment. New York, Raven Press, 1984. (Excellent review of the theory and concepts of TDM.)

174

Cough and Cold Medications

Michael A. McGuigan

Prescription and over-the-counter cough and cold preparations are common in households with young children. Not only are children encouraged to take them, but the medications are designed specifically to be attractive in color and flavor. It is no wonder that cough and cold preparations are involved commonly in accidental ingestions.

Cough and cold medications form a heterogenous group of pharmacologic agents. Medications used to treat nasal congestion include sympathomimetics (decongestants) and antihistamines. Those agents used for the treatment of coughing include suppressants (opiates and opiate derivatives, including dextromethorphan) and expectorants (usually guiafenesin). Many commercially available preparations also include aspirin, acetaminophen, or both.

This chapter will discuss the clinical toxicology of the three main classes of cough and cold medications: antihistamines, decongestants (phenylpropanolamine), and cough suppressants (opiate derivatives). The reader is referred to Chapter 163 for a discussion of the common cold.

ANTIHISTAMINES

Pathophysiology

Literally dozens of chemically different antihistamines are currently available. Although there are subtle differences in the effects produced by each of these antihistamines, for

practical purposes it is reasonable to consider them as a single group.

Antihistamines, in general, are absorbed rapidly from the gastrointestinal tract and are distributed widely throughout the body. These compounds are excreted by way of the hepatic metabolism with an elimination half-life following an overdose of up to 8 hours. The exact mechanism of toxic effect is uncertain but is believed to be related to peripheral antagonism of histamine at the H_1-receptor and direct central nervous system (CNS) effects.

Clinical Presentation

Nearly one third of young children who ingest excessive amounts of one of the standard formulations of antihistamines will demonstrate signs of toxicity within 2 hours. Clinical effects may not begin for 6 to 8 hours if a slow-release preparation has been ingested. Evidence of CNS stimulation was noted in nearly 85% of the reported cases of overdoses involving antihistamines. Common excitation manifestations include insomnia, restlessness, nystagmus, ataxia, tremor, hyperreflexia, myoclonic jerks, and hallucinations. Convulsions occurred more commonly with large ingestions; seizures were reported in ~70% of pediatric antihistamine overdoses in the literature. Central nervous system depression also occurs (60% of reported cases) and is manifest as drowsiness or lethargy, or coma. Anticholinergic (or atropinelike) effects occur, but their frequency has not been documented. Findings may include dilated pupils, xerostomia, tachycardia, low-grade fever, and flushed dry skin. Multifocal premature ventricular contractions are an uncommon complication of a severe antihistamine overdose. Clinical evidence of toxicity may last as long as 12 hours.

Differential Diagnosis

The differential diagnosis of a child who overdoses on an antihistamine that was being used to treat his or her upper respiratory infection includes Reye syndrome and encephalitis or meningitis. Other toxins that may produce a clinical picture similar to that caused by an antihistamine overdose include chronic salicylate intoxication and the acute ingestion of phenothiazines, lithium, tricyclic antidepressants, sympathomimetics (e.g., cocaine, phenylpropanolamine, amphetamines), and plants containing belladonna alkaloids (e.g., deadly nightshade). Thyrotoxicosis (either endogenous or from ingestion of thyroid hormone) and hypoglycemia should also be considered in the differential diagnosis.

Work-Up

The correct identification of the product is essential. Each active ingredient and its concentration should be identified, and the maximum quantity ingested should be estimated.

The time of ingestion must be estimated in order to determine whether or not therapeutic intervention would be reasonable. If symptoms are present, they should be detailed with regard to the time and sequence of onset. In products in which several different antihistamines are combined, it is reasonable to add all antihistamines together in calculating a single ingested dose. The toxic dose of antihistamines is not well established. However, single acute ingestions of more than three times the usual maximum daily dose may be considered to be potentially toxic.

A careful physical examination may reveal the anticholinergic signs as well as evidence of drowsiness, CNS excitation, or hallucinations. Laboratory investigations are not useful in antihistamine overdoses except in eliminating other causes of similar syndromes. Documentation of antihistamines in the blood or urine is confirmatory but not beneficial in managing the acute overdose. Many liquid antihistamine preparations contain ethanol; thus, measurement of blood ethanol and blood sugar levels is an important consideration.

Treatment

Treatment should consist of the administration of ipecac to an asymptomatic child at home within 1 hour of an overdose. Activated charcoal will bind unabsorbed antihistamine within the gastrointestinal tract, and its use is recommended. Symptomatic supportive care should be used to treat most of the clinical effects. Intravenous diazepam, phenytoin, or barbiturates may be used to control convulsive activity. Hallucinatory activity often responds to non-pharmacologic treatment: quiet reassurance in a normally lit room. If the hallucinations do not respond to such therapy and are becoming disruptive, a small dose of a short-acting benzodiazepine (e.g., lorazepam) may be beneficial.

Physostigmine has been used to treat serious complications of antihistamine overdose, but because physostigmine itself is potentially toxic and its duration of action is short, it should not be used unless the effects of the antihistamine overdose are potentially life threatening. If it appears that physostigmine is necessary, a discussion with a regional poison center is recommended.

Indications for Admission or Referral

A medical evaluation is recommended for any child who has ingested an unknown or potentially toxic amount of an antihistamine. Admission to a hospital is recommended for any patient who is symptomatic within 4 hours of an overdose.

DECONGESTANTS

Available oral sympathomimetics include drugs such as ephedrine, orciprenaline, pseudoephedrine, phenylephrine,

and phenylpropanolamine (PPA). Toxicity resulting from ingestion of any of these drugs is rare, except for PPA.

Pathophysiology

PPA is readily absorbed through the stomach and exerts its toxic effects both by direct stimulation of α-adrenergic receptors and by causing the release of stored epinephrine. If PPA is ingested in conjunction with the antihistamine chlorpheniramine, the duration of toxicity may be prolonged because the antihistamine inhibits the re-uptake of catecholamines by the nerve endings.

Clinical Presentation

Ingestion of excessive amounts of PPA results most commonly in headache, hypertension, and bradycardia. Other less commonly reported symptoms of PPA overdose include dizziness, nausea, sweating, agitation, and various cardiac arrhythmias.

Differential Diagnosis

The differential diagnosis of PPA overdose should include previously unrecognized causes of hypertension (e.g., renal, vascular, and adrenal) or the ingestion of other sympathomimetic drugs such as amphetamines or cocaine, or hallucinogenic drugs such as phencyclidine. Certain combinations of symptoms and signs may suggest hypoglycemia or the effects of nicotine or insecticides.

Work-Up

In any case of PPA overdose, not only must the quantity of PPA be estimated but efforts must also be made to identify other ingested drugs that may interact adversely (e.g., chlorpheniramine or caffeine). Acute doses of PPA in excess of 1.5 mg/kg may result in toxicity. A physical examination should be directed primarily at the central nervous system and cardiovascular system. No specific laboratory tests are available to confirm a PPA overdose or to help evaluate its severity. Routine laboratory tests may be used to help eliminate renal disease and hypoglycemia.

Treatment

The early induction of vomiting may be useful, but the administration of ipecac should be considered in light of the rapidity with which PPA is absorbed from the stomach and the vomiting-induced delay in the administration of activated charcoal. In any event, treatment should include the administration of activated charcoal to patients who have ingested toxic doses of PPA. The use of activated charcoal is especially important because many preparations are mixtures of different drugs. Dividing the amount of PPA ingested by the patient's weight can be used to estimate the expected toxicity. Physical examination should include a careful look for narcotic symptoms and signs as well as an evaluation of the respiratory function (at rest).

No specific guidelines are available for the treatment of hypertension associated with PPA ingestion. Recommendations include treatment of blood pressure in excess of 180/100 or at lower levels if the patient has a headache, signs of encephalopathy, or a blood pressure that rises over 30 minutes of observation. Patients who have a congenital heart disease that may be adversely affected by hypertension should receive antihypertension therapy at lower levels of hypertension. The initial treatment of PPA-induced hypertension consists of placing the patient in a head-elevated position because PPA-induced hypertension appears to be more severe in the supine position. If this does not reduce the blood pressure, the preferred pharmacologic agent is nitroprusside (see also Chap. 56).

Acidification of the urine will increase the renal clearance of PPA, but this therapy should be reserved only for severely affected patients. Convulsions secondary to PPA should be treated with rapidly acting intravenous anticonvulsant drugs, such as diazepam.

Indications for Admission or Referral

Patients with ingestions of PPA alone in quantities exceeding the minimum toxic dose (1.5 mg/kg) should be observed for 4 to 8 hours for symptoms of sympathetic stimulation. Patients who are objectively toxic need to be admitted to the hospital for observation and care.

Opiate Derivatives
Pathophysiology

Codeine, hydrocodone, hydromorphone, and dextromethorphan are the opioid drugs most commonly used as cough suppressants. In overdose, they all exert similar effects: miosis, and central nervous system and respiratory depression to a variable degree. Dextromethorphan overdose has been associated with convulsions in rare instances.

Clinical Presentation

The triad of CNS depression, miosis, and respiratory depression is characteristic of opioid drugs. Head trauma secondary to a fall may result when an ingestion of a depressant results in neuromuscular unsteadiness.

Differential Diagnosis

A similar clinical picture may result with a pontine hemorrhage (a rare occurrence) or from the ingestion of large quantities of ethanol, barbiturates, phenothiazines, or clonidine. An overdose of benzodiazepines may produce CNS depression and miosis without respiratory depression.

Work-Up

A work-up must include identification of the drug ingested and its formulation (liquid versus tablet, regular versus sustained-release) as well as any other ingested drugs. The timing is important; thus, establishing when the ingestion occurred is critical. The milligram quantity of the drug ingested divided by the patient's weight can be used to estimate the expected toxicity (see the section on admission). A physical examination should include vital signs as part of a careful look for narcotic symptoms and signs as well as an evaluation of the respiratory function (at rest). No definitive laboratory tests are useful in diagnosing or assessing the degree of toxicity. When a patient requires hospitalization, a qualitative identification of the drug in question should be done for purposes of documentation. Liquid preparations of cough suppressants may contain ethanol; thus, measurements of blood sugar and blood ethanol concentrations may be warranted.

Treatment

Activated charcoal effectively binds the opioid drugs and should be used. Patients with clinical toxicity to the point of respiratory compromise (as documented by cyanosis or abnormal blood gas values) should be treated with ventilatory support and perhaps endotracheal intubation. Naloxone (0.03 mg/kg intravenously) may be used to reverse the signs of a narcotic overdose. It may be repeated at 2- to 3-minute intervals. If a dramatic response in the level of consciousness and respiratory effort does not occur following a naloxone dose of 0.1 mg/kg, the diagnosis of opiate overdose should be reconsidered.

Indications for Admission or Referral

Medical evaluation is indicated for children who, by history, ingest toxic doses of the common opioid cough suppressants: dextromethorphan >10 mg/kg; codeine >1.5 mg/kg; hydrocodone >0.2 mg/kg; and hydromorphone >0.1 mg/kg. Admission to a hospital is recommended for any child who demonstrates symptoms and signs compatible with opioid overdose within 6 hours of ingestion. If respiratory support or naloxone therapy is required, the child should be cared for in a hospital that is capable of providing pediatric intensive care.

ANNOTATED BIBLIOGRAPHY

Bernstein E, Diskant BM: Phenylpropanolamine: A potentially hazardous drug. Ann Emerg Med 11:311–315, 1982. (Pathophysiology and clinical presentation of PPA overdose.)

Committee on Drugs: Use of codeine and dextromethorphan-containing cough syrups in pediatrics. Pediatrics 62:118–122, 1978. (Excellent review of both the therapeutic and toxic sides of the subject.)

Hooper RG, Conner CS, Rumack BH: Acute poisoning from over-the-counter sleep preparations. JACEP 8:98–100, 1979. (Good presentation of a large series of patients; useful frequency data.)

Howrie DL, Wolfson JH: Phenylpropanolamine-induced hypertensive seizures. J Pediatr 102:143–145, 1983. (Interesting report that implies possible interaction with caffeine.)

Krenzelok EP, Anderson GM, Mirick M: Massive diphenhydramine overdose resulting in death. Ann Emerg Med 11:212–213, 1982. (Case presentation with a good discussion of pathophysiology.)

Shaul WL, Wandell M, Robertson WO: Dextromethorphan toxicity: Reversed by naloxone. Pediatrics 59:117–119, 1977. (One of the few cases of serious toxicity from dextromethorphan.)

vonMuhlendahl KE, Scherf-Rahne B, Krienke EG et al: Codeine intoxication in childhood. Lancet 2:303–305, 1976. (Good discussion of the likelihood and timing of symptoms following acute codeine overdose.)

175

Salicylate, Acetaminophen, and Ibuprofen Poisoning

L. Gerard Niederman

Preparations containing salicylates, acetaminophen, or ibuprofen are widely used by children and adolescents as analgesics, antipyretics, and anti-inflammatory agents. Aspirin (acetylsalicylic acid) and acetaminophen are present in numerous over-the-counter preparations, as well as in many combination prescription medications. Ibuprofen, available since 1974 by prescription, became available as over-the-counter tablets in 1984 and as a nonprescription suspension in 1989 in the United States. Other salicylates may be found in analgesic ointments and liniments (methyl salicylate), sunscreens (homomenthyl salicylate), and keratolytic agents (salicylic acid). Toxicity from acetaminophen, salicylates, and ibuprofen may follow accidental or intentional ingestion. Accidental ingestion usually occurs in younger children, whereas intentional ingestion is more common in adolescents. Chronic salicylate poisoning occurs in all ages, though more commonly in young children and most commonly in infants, whereas chronic poisoning from ibuprofen or acetaminophen has not been described. The association of salicylate exposure with Reye syndrome has markedly reduced its use in infants and children.

SALICYLATE POISONING

Pathophysiology

When salicylates are taken in therapeutic doses, they are rapidly absorbed in the stomach and small intestine. However, with larger doses, absorption may be prolonged by delayed tablet dissolution and by delayed gastric emptying. Enteric-coated tablets are even more erratically absorbed in overdosage. Aspirin is rapidly hydrolyzed to salicylic acid, which at low serum concentrations is largely bound to plasma proteins, primarily albumin. Salicylate, with a pKa of 3.5, is present primarily in the ionized fraction, which penetrates biologic membranes poorly and remains largely in the blood. As blood concentrations increase, albumin binding is saturated, and if acidemia occurs, the nonionized fraction of salicylate will also increase. Both of these factors facilitate passive diffusion across cell membranes, increasing tissue drug levels and toxicity. Alkalemia, on the other hand, increases the proportion of ionized salicylic acid, thus impeding tissue penetration.

The symptoms of salicylism are related to the direct stimulating effect on the central nervous system, particularly the respiratory center of the brain; the uncoupling of oxidative phosphorylation with increased oxygen consumption, carbon dioxide accumulation, and heat production; the alteration of Krebs' cycle enzymes with resultant accumulation of organic acids; and, in severe poisoning, central nervous system (CNS) depression.

One of the complex manifestations of salicylism is derangement of acid–base balance. Early in its course, direct respiratory center stimulation results in hyperventilation and respiratory alkalosis, which, if present for any duration, will be compensated by renal bicarbonate excretion. This may be the only alteration in acid–base balance. However, with more severe toxicity, metabolic acidosis may occur. The acidosis is not the result of accumulated salicylic acid but rather is due to the accumulation of organic acids (lactate and pyruvate) secondary to salicylate-induced derangements of Krebs' cycle function. Underlying caloric deprivation and dehydration coupled with stimulation of lipid metabolism also result in the production of ketoacids. Further adding to the acidosis is the accumulation of CO_2 and depletion of O_2 resulting from the uncoupling of oxidative phosphorylation.

Significant alteration in fluid and electrolyte balance often accompanies the acid–base derangements described above. Increased heat production from uncoupled oxidative phosphorylation, hyperpnea, and hyperventilation all increase insensible water loss and result in some salt loss through perspiration. Early renal compensation for respiratory alkalosis results in sodium and potassium loss, as hydrogen ion is initially conserved. Later, renal excretion of organic acids in acidemic patients results in further water and salt depletion. Vomiting and poor oral intake aggravate the fluid balance, particularly in the young child. The sum of these effects may be considerable water, sodium, and potassium depletion, particularly with chronic salicylism. Rarely, the syndrome of inappropriate antidiuretic hormone has been reported, probably a direct effect of salicylate on the hypothalamus.

Either hypoglycemia or hyperglycemia may be present

with salicylism. Although blood glucose measurements may be normal or high, central nervous system "hypoglycemia" may occur and may cause mental status changes. Bleeding phenomena rarely occur with salicylate poisoning, although platelet function is altered and prothrombin time may be prolonged.

At relatively low blood concentrations, salicylate is conjugated in the liver, but at toxic concentrations these enzymes are saturated and salicylic acid accumulates. The half-life for salicylate at low blood levels is between 2 and 3 hours, whereas at toxic levels the half-life may be as long as 30 hours. Salicylate and its conjugates are primarily excreted in the urine. Urinary alkalosis enhances salicylate excretion severalfold.

Clinical Presentation

Early symptoms include nausea and vomiting, tinnitus (described by older children), confusion, hyperpyrexia, and, most commonly, hyperpnea and hyperventilation. Lethargy, convulsions, and coma may occur with increased toxicity. For reasons not entirely clear, children and particularly infants are more likely to develop serious acidemia. Chronic intoxication, rather than a single-dose ingestion, also results more commonly in acidemia.

Differential Diagnosis

The differential diagnosis of salicylism can be organized around the central nervous symptoms (confusion and lethargy); the respiratory symptoms (hyperpnea and hyperventilation); and the metabolic acidemia. Head trauma, Reye syndrome, CNS infections, and other intoxicants such as alcohol may present with changes in mental status similar to those seen with salicylate toxicity. Children with head trauma may also manifest central neurogenic hyperventilation, although history and other physical signs usually preclude confusion with salicylism. Anxiety attacks with hyperventilation and respiratory illness such as asthma may also be initially confused with salicylism. Metabolic acidosis is seen in diabetes mellitus, gastroenteritis with dehydration, hypoperfusion, severe renal disease, ethylene glycol and methanol intoxication, and rare metabolic diseases. A careful history and clinical suspicion are needed to recognize the child with gastroenteritis or diabetes who concomitantly has been given aspirin for fever or analgesia.

Evaluation and Treatment

Salicylate intoxication can usually be suspected by a history of acute ingestion, a history of repeated therapeutic overdosage, or recognition of the characteristic symptoms. Salicylism should be suspected in any child with unexplained metabolic acidosis or nonfocal neurologic signs. Single-dose ingestions of greater than 150 mg/kg of salicylate may result in toxic symptoms. Chronic salicylism may occur at

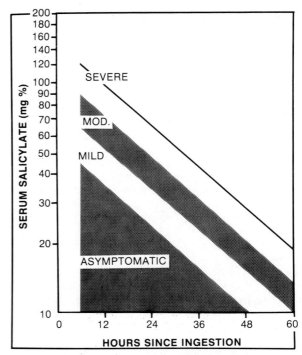

Figure 175-1. This nomogram relates serum salicylate concentration and expected severity of intoxication at varying intervals following the ingestion of a single dose of salicylate. (Done AK: Salicylate intoxication: Significance of measurements of salicylate in blood in cases of acute ingestion. Pediatrics 26:800, 1960. Reproduced by permission of Pediatrics, 1960.)

therapeutic dosage (80–100 mg/kg/day), although it more commonly occurs with higher daily intakes.

Urine ferric chloride testing is a simple bedside test that can confirm the presence of salicylic acid in the urine, although it has no quantitative value. A few drops of 10% ferric chloride solution is added to about 5 ml of urine, and a stable purple color, persisting after heating the urine to boiling (which removes ketones), indicates a positive test for salicylic acid. Testing plasma or serum with a Phenistix is a bedside test with semiquantitative value. A tan reaction approximates a serum salicylate value of less than 40 mg/dl (2.9 mmol/L); a deeper brown to purple color indicates a level of 40 to 90 mg/dl (2.9–6.5 mmol/L); and a pure purple color indicates a level of greater than 90 mg/dl (6.5 mmol/L). Although these tests are helpful, a serum salicylate level will confirm the diagnosis. The Done nomogram is useful in predicting the severity of an acute single-dose exposure (Fig. 175-1). It is not useful following ingestion of enteric-coated salicylates or for managing chronic salicylism, where the toxicity correlates less with serum levels and more with salicylate tissue distribution. Serial salicylate determinations are necessary to determine when peak levels occur and to assess the need for therapeutic intervention.

A careful evaluation of the acid–base and fluid and electrolyte manifestations of salicylism requires frequent determinations of arterial blood gases and serum electrolytes. A clinical pitfall to be avoided is reliance on only an arterial or venous *p*H to gauge the significance of these disturbances. Not infrequently, the *p*H may be normal or almost normal in a child with mixed respiratory alkalosis and metabolic acidosis. Other appropriate studies, especially in the hospitalized child, include measurements of glucose, prothrombin time, and hepatic enzymes.

The initial treatment of salicylate poisoning includes ipecac-induced emesis, or gastric lavage in the unresponsive patient, followed by the administration of activated charcoal in a dose of 1 to 2 g/kg. Both of these attempts to prevent absorption are most effective if performed within 4 hours of ingestion. Osmotic cathartics (e.g., magnesium citrate or sorbitol) may also prevent absorption, particularly with enteric-coated aspirin preparations.

Careful correction of water, electrolyte, and glucose deficits are crucial, particularly with chronic salicylism. Hypoglycemia should be treated aggressively. Seizures should be treated with anticonvulsants and, if unresponsive, a trial of intravenous glucose.

The brain is the most vulnerable organ in salicylate poisoning, and therapy is aimed at reducing the amount of salicylate that enters the central nervous system. Systemic alkalinization prevents tissue penetration of salicylate and enhances urinary excretion of unbound plasma salicylic acid. Alkalinization can usually be achieved with intravenous bicarbonate. The goal of therapy is to maintain a normal or slightly alkalotic serum *p*H (7.35–7.45) while producing an alkaline urine. Care must be taken to provide adequate potassium, because a sudden shift in the *p*H from acidemic to alkalemic may precipitate arrhythmias in the child with intracellular potassium depletion. Paradoxical aciduria may also occur despite adequate systemic alkalinization in the potassium-depleted child.

Hemodialysis has been shown to remove salicylate more rapidly than alkaline diuresis and should be considered with severe acidemia, with salicylate levels over 80 mg/dl (5.8 mmol/L), or with clinical deterioration despite adequate bicarbonate therapy.

ACETAMINOPHEN POISONING

Pathophysiology

Acetaminophen (N-acetylpara-aminophenol), when ingested, is rapidly absorbed in the upper gastrointestinal tract. With therapeutic doses, peak serum levels are achieved approximately 0.5 to 2 hours after ingestion; following toxic quantities, peak levels may be delayed up to 4 hours.
tion resulting from acetaminophen poisoning. In therapeutic doses, acetaminophen is metabolized by the liver primarily into conjugates of glucuronic and sulfuric acid, with smaller amounts being oxidized by the mixed-function oxidases. With increasing dosages, the capacity to conjugate aceta-

minophen is exceeded, resulting in the oxidation of larger amounts of acetaminophen. A reactive intermediate metabolite of acetaminophen oxidation is, under normal conditions, conjugated with glutathione to acetaminophen-mercapturate, which is excreted in the urine. Following larger doses of acetaminophen or under conditions where the mixed-function oxidases are induced, glutathione becomes depleted, resulting in the direct covalent binding of this intermediate reactive metabolite to intracellular proteins, with resultant centrilobular hepatic necrosis.

Clinical Presentation

Although severe toxicity may occur, children generally tolerate larger overdosage without hepatotoxicity than do adolescents and adults. Toxic ingestions of acetaminophen cause only mild symptoms during the first 24 hours. Nausea, vomiting, abdominal pain, anorexia, and malaise may occur several hours after ingestion. Diaphoresis may be seen in adolescents and adults, but rarely in children. These symptoms cease within 24 hours of ingestion. For the next 24 to 48 hours, the child appears well. During this silent period, however, laboratory evidence of hepatic necrosis and dysfunction is present in the untreated patient. Transaminase levels (SGOT [AST], SGPT [ALT]) and bilirubin begin to rise, and prothrombin time (PT) is prolonged. Evidence of hepatic injury becomes clinically apparent 2 to 4 days postingestion. Jaundice, malaise, nausea, vomiting, and, in severe cases, symptoms of fulminant hepatic necrosis and hepatic encephalopathy occur. The recovery of hepatic function usually occurs 6 to 8 days after ingestion and does not result in cirrhosis.

Differential Diagnosis

Acetaminophen toxicity may be confused with various forms of hepatitis, particularly when there is no history of ingestion. Infectious causes include viral hepatitis (A, B, C, Epstein–Barr) as well as hepatitis due to toxoplasmosis. Toxic hepatitis may occur from trichloroethylene, carbon tetrachloride, yellow phosphorus, the mushroom *Amanita phalloides,* and medications such as halothane, isoniazid, valproic acid, and methyldopa. Reye syndrome should be distinguished from acetaminophen intoxication by its different clinical presentation and by the characteristic fatty infiltration without significant inflammation seen on histologic appearance of the liver.

Evaluation and Treatment

When one is faced with the child who may have ingested acetaminophen, it is important to obtain an accurate history, including the time of ingestion and the amount ingested. With an intentional overdosage, one should assess if additional drugs have been taken. A single, acute acetaminophen ingestion of 140 mg/kg is potentially toxic and re-

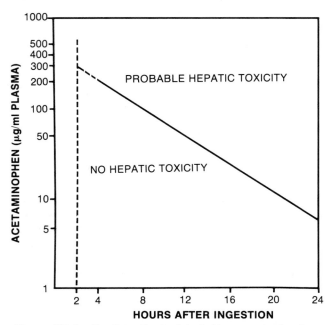

Figure 175-2. Semilogarithmic plot of plasma acetaminophen levels versus time (Rumack BH, Matthew H: Acetaminophen poisoning and toxicity. Pediatrics 55:871, 1975. Reproduced by permission of Pediatrics, 1975.)

quires careful evaluation. A plasma acetaminophen level should be obtained at least 4 hours postingestion. The Rumack–Mathew nomogram is useful for predicting the severity of a single, acute ingestion of acetaminophen (Fig. 175-2). A level of 200 μg/ml (1300 μmol/L) at least 4 hours after ingestion indicates risk for hepatic injury and that treatment should be initiated. Multiple acetaminophen levels obtained to calculate the plasma half-life rarely add helpful information to the assessment or management of the child.

The successful treatment of acetaminophen toxicity requires removal of unabsorbed acetaminophen and early treatment with oral N-acetylcysteine (NAC). Syrup of ipecac or gastric lavage should be used within 4 hours, and preferably within 90 minutes of ingestion. Activated charcoal is effective in binding acetaminophen and should be administered within 4 hours of the ingestion. Although NAC is bound to activated charcoal, it is probably still effective in preventing hepatotoxicity.

Oral N-acetylcysteine is, in the United States, the current preferred treatment of potentially hepatotoxic acetaminophen poisoning. Treatment should be initiated as soon as possible after ingestion and, to be maximally efficacious, should be started within 8 hours of ingestion. If the time of ingestion is uncertain, the initial loading dose of NAC can be given while awaiting further history and laboratory confirmation of ingestion. Treatment initiated more than 24 hours after ingestion probably does not prevent hepatotoxicity. The initial loading dose of NAC is 140 mg/kg, and

the treatment is continued with 70 mg/kg given every 4 hours for 17 additional doses. NAC can be diluted in water, juices, or sodas to increase palatability. If not tolerated orally, it can be administered through a gastric or duodenal tube. Experimental protocols using intravenous N-acetylcysteine can be obtained from regional poison information centers.

Tests to evaluate hepatocellular necrosis (SGPT [ALT], SGOT [AST]) and hepatic function (PT, bilirubin) should be performed daily. Hepatic coma and encephalopathy should be anticipated with severe ingestions and appropriate supportive care initiated.

IBUPROFEN POISONING

Pathophysiology

Ibuprofen [2-(4-isobutylphenyl)propionic acid] is rapidly absorbed in both therapeutic and toxic amounts—80% within 1 to 2 hours. The elimination half-life is approximately 2 hours, and there is no accumulation with repeated dosing. Ibuprofen is about 99% bound to plasma proteins. After hepatic metabolism, more than 90% of ingested ibuprofen is excreted in the urine.

Ibuprofen is a direct gastrointestinal irritant, particularly at higher than therapeutic dosage. A potent cyclooxygenase inhibitor, ibuprofen reduces prostaglandin synthesis. Inhibition of kidney prostaglandin synthesis results in altered renal blood flow, hyperkalemia, and acute interstitial nephritis. Ibuprofen and its metabolites are weak acids, which in overdosage may cause mild and transient metabolic acidosis with an increased anion gap.

Clinical Presentation

Although most ingestions are asymptomatic or result in mild symptoms, significant morbidity and rarely mortality have been reported from ibuprofen poisoning. Clinical symptoms, if present, usually develop within 4 hours of ingestion. The most common symptoms are gastrointestinal (nausea, vomiting, and abdominal pain) and neurologic (drowsiness and lethargy). In severe ingestions, coma and generalized seizures may occur. Apnea (probably centrally induced) was reported in one 16-month-old child who subsequently died from aspiration pneumonia and its complications. Acute oliguric renal failure, generally reversible with supportive care, also occurs. Less common symptoms include hypotension and bradycardia, metabolic acidosis, nystagmus, and blurred vision. Rarely, entrapment of ibuprofen in the esophagus has resulted in esophageal stricture with subsequent swallowing symptoms.

Differential Diagnosis

Unexplained lethargy and coma of acute onset may be caused by other ingestions, including phenothiazines, antihistamines, ethanol, salicylates, opiates, barbiturates, phencyclidines, and tricyclic antidepressants. Trauma, hypoglycemia, and the postictal state should be considered. The differential diagnosis of the gastrointestinal symptoms includes infectious gastroenteritis, ingestion of plants (see Chap. 177), or ingestion of iron (see Chap. 176).

Evaluation and Treatment

The management of children with toxic ingestions of ibuprofen is symptomatic. The rapid absorption and short half-life result in the early appearance and rapid disappearance of symptoms. Ingestion of less than 100 mg/kg is unlikely to cause toxicity and requires only home observation. Children ingesting between 100 and 200 mg/kg should receive syrup of ipecac to induce emesis, and they should be observed. Children ingesting greater than 200 mg/kg should be managed under physician observation, having emesis induced (unless contraindicated by obtundation or convulsions). They should receive activated charcoal (1–2 g/kg) with cathartic and if asymptomatic 4 hours after ingestion may be discharged home. Ibuprofen levels are available in some settings but usually are not necessary for guiding therapy.

Symptomatic children should be observed in a hospital setting with seizure and apnea precautions provided. Renal function (urinalysis, BUN, creatinine, and urine output) should be monitored carefully. Metabolic status should be determined with arterial blood gases. Further therapy is based on the clinical course. Although experience is limited, it is unlikely that repeated charcoal administration (to reduce absorption from enterohepatic circulation) or alkaline diuresis will prove efficacious.

ANNOTATED BIBLIOGRAPHY

Done AK: Salicylate intoxication: Significance of measurements of salicylate in blood in cases of acute ingestion. Pediatrics 26:800, 1960. (Clinical study in which the Done nomogram was developed.)

Done AK, Temple AR: Treatment of salicylate poisoning. Mod Treat 8:528, 1971. (Still an excellent clinical review.)

Hall AH, Smolinske SC, Conrad FL et al: Ibuprofen overdose: 126 cases. Ann Emerg Med 15:1308, 1986. (Good clinical review of spectrum of ibuprofen toxicity.)

Hill JB: Salicylate intoxication. N Engl J Med 288:1110, 1973. (Provocative animal research supporting bicarbonate therapy and extracorporeal removal of salicylate in severe poisoning.)

Mitchell JR, Jollow DJ, Potter WZ et al: Acetaminophen induced hepatic necrosis. I. Role of drug metabolism. J Pharmacol Exp Ther 187:185, 1973. (First of a series of four consecutive papers in the same issue providing experimental evidence for the pharmacopathology of acetaminophen-induced hepatic injury and its treatment.)

Rumack BH, Peterson RC, Koch GG, Amara IA: Acetaminophen overdose: 662 cases with evaluation of oral acetylcysteine treatment. Arch Intern Med 141:380, 1981. (Clinical study from which standards for treatment with oral N-acetylcysteine were developed.)

176
Iron Overdose

Pierre Gaudreault

Iron is present in a large number of over-the-counter medications. The accidental ingestion of these products is relatively common in childhood. Most iron poisonings result from the ingestion of multivitamin preparations or prenatal vitamins containing iron. In 1989, 21,230 cases of iron poisoning were reported in the United States. Most of these cases (85%) involved children less than 6 years old. Although rarely fatal (only three deaths were reported), the ingestion of a substantial amount of iron may lead to serious sequelae. Iron preparations are usually dispensed as ferrous sulfate, fumarate, or gluconate. The amount of elemental iron ingested determines the severity of the intoxication. The percentage of elemental iron varies with each salt, ranging from 33% for the fumarate salt to 20% and 12% for the sulfate and gluconate salts, respectively.

PATHOPHYSIOLOGY

The pathophysiology of iron intoxication has not been clearly elucidated. The morbidity and mortality result from the toxic effect of the iron on several systems, including gastrointestinal irritation with hemorrhage, cardiovascular depression with hypotension, hepatic injuries, and metabolic changes such as acidosis and coagulation defects. Ferrous iron is absorbed primarily by the duodenum and jejunum, oxidized to its ferric state, and bound to ferritin, which is an iron-storage protein. The ferric iron is then released into plasma where it is bound to transferrin. Transferrin becomes attached to sites in the bone marrow and releases the iron necessary for erythropoiesis. The iron content of the body is mainly regulated by the absorptive mechanisms. Indeed, there are no specific excretory mechanisms. Approximately 1 mg of iron is lost each day from the intestine, skin, or urinary tract. This phenomenon explains the accumulation of iron that occurs following an overdose. With an overdose, transferrin's binding capacity is exceeded and the remainder of the iron circulates in the free form. It is the unbound iron that causes systemic toxicity.

Gastrointestinal symptoms such as vomiting, hematemesis, and bloody diarrhea result from a direct toxic effect of iron on the mucosa. The mucosa, submucosa, and basement membrane cytoplasm and nuclear tissue show heavy iron staining. Hemorrhages and necrotic lesions to the stomach and the proximal small bowel may result, and segmental infarctions characterized by marked mucosal congestion and submucosal venous thrombosis in the distal small bowel have also been described. The large intestine is usually not affected. Although the loss of blood and fluids from the damaged structures is usually not sufficient to result in death, these losses contribute to the severity of the shock.

Shock appears rapidly in animals given lethal doses of iron. The exact mechanism of action has not been clearly elucidated. The circulatory failure may be induced by a direct action of iron on blood vessels. The circulating free iron damages the vessels, inducing an increase in the capillary permeability and a postarteriolar vasodilation. These changes result in a decrease of the effective circulatory blood volume as well as of the total blood volume, which leads to a decrease in the cardiac output. It has also been noted in animals that plasma concentrations of ferritin, serotonin, and histamine are elevated following an iron overdose. These substances are well-known vasodilators that may play a role in the generation of hypotension.

The liver damage results from the uptake of iron by hepatic cells once plasma transferrin has been saturated. Iron is localized primarily in the area of the mitochondria, which causes alterations in several hepatic cell oxidative processes. Hepatic necrosis may result and is usually limited to the periportal parenchymal cells. In humans, hepatocellular damages have not been incriminated as a causative factor in death.

The release of hydrogen ions resulting from the conversion of ferrous iron to its ferric form is the main factor responsible for the metabolic acidosis. The accumulation of organic acids, such as lactic and citric acid, from anaerobic metabolism may also contribute to acidosis. The inhibition of enzymatic processes in the Krebs cycle aerobic metabolism may be secondary to a direct action of iron or to cardiovascular insufficiency.

The coagulation defects are secondary to a direct action of iron on the various proteins involved in blood coagulation. Animals poisoned with high doses of iron (700 mg/kg) developed prolongation in clotting time, thrombocytopenia, hypoprothrombinemia, and qualitative changes in fibrinogen. Coagulation defects, however, are not a major factor in the lethality of iron overdose.

CLINICAL PRESENTATION

The severity of an acute iron intoxication is proportional to the amount of elemental iron ingested. Although the oral lethal dose is generally accepted to be ~200 to 250 mg/kg of elemental iron, doses in excess of 20 mg/kg may lead to toxicity. The clinical presentation usually evolves through phases.

First Phase

Following an acute oral overdose, signs and symptoms appear ½ to 6 hours after the ingestion. Nausea, vomiting, hematemesis, abdominal pain, melena, and bloody diarrhea may occur. In severe cases, the decrease of effective circu-

latory volume as well as total blood volume results in hypotension with reflex tachycardia.

Central nervous system manifestations range from lethargy and hypotonia to seizures and coma secondary to decreased cerebral perfusion or a direct effect of iron on the central nervous system. Laboratory findings may include metabolic acidosis, hyperglycemia, and leukocytosis. Shock or coma during this period usually indicates a grave prognosis.

Second Phase

The patient may experience a period of relative stability following the first phase. The appearance and duration of this period are probably related to the severity of the intoxication. Because the patient's status may deteriorate, it is imperative to pursue adequate treatment during this phase. Following this period of quiescence, the patient may develop shock, coma, or seizures, and he or she may die. Elevated levels of hepatic enzymes and hypoglycemia may be seen.

Late Phase

Pyloric or antral strictures may develop 2 to 5 weeks after the ingestion. Diffuse fibrosis of the liver with fatty degeneration has been reported.

WORK-UP
History

The physician should determine the type of iron preparation and the maximal amount of elemental iron that has been ingested. Ingestion of multivitamins with iron (~4–5 mg of elemental iron/pill) rarely causes serious morbidity.

In contrast, iron preparations (60–65 mg elemental iron/pill) used as supplemental intake during pregnancy are responsible for most serious intoxications.

Physical Examination

The physical examination should be directed toward the evaluation of the clinical signs expected with this intoxication.

Laboratory Tests

The severity of an iron intoxication correlates with serum iron concentrations as long as the blood sample is obtained within a few hours of the ingestion. Indeed, the rapid clearance of iron from the plasma may be responsible for deceptively low serum iron concentrations within a few hours of a substantial ingestion. Serum iron concentrations should be determined 3 to 5 hours after the ingestion. Normal serum concentrations range from 100 to 125 μg/dL. Concentrations less than 300 μg/dL are usually associated with no or mild symptoms such as nausea, vomiting, or melena. Abdominal cramps, bloody diarrhea, and lethargy may occur with concentrations between 300 and 500 μg/dL. Patients who have concentrations above 500 μg/dL may develop mild hypotension as well as gastrointestinal manifestations. Concentrations of more than 750 to 1000 μg/dL may be associated with hypotension, shock, metabolic acidosis, coma, and death.

Hematocrit, hemoglobin level, serum electrolytes, and acid–base status should be monitored.

A flat plate of the abdomen may reveal the presence of ingested iron tablets. It can usually detect prenatal iron preparations but not multivitamin preparations with iron. An x-ray can also document the success or failure of the gastrointestinal decontamination.

TREATMENT

Because the severity of the intoxication is proportional to the amount of iron absorbed, measures to prevent its gastrointestinal absorption should be undertaken. The removal of iron from the stomach can be accomplished with emesis induced by syrup of ipecac or gastric lavage with the largest orogastric tube possible. However, more and more physicians favor whole bowel irrigation. This procedure hastens the passage of toxic substances through the gastrointestinal tract, thereby reducing their absorption. Whole bowel irrigation is the treatment of choice if iron pills are located in the intestine. This technique consists on the administration of a polyethylene glycol electrolyte solution through a nasogastric tube. The rate of administration for toddlers and preschoolers is 0.5 L/hr and for adolescents and adults is 2 L/hr. Vomiting can be a problem. For some patients it can be controlled by slowing the rate of infusion and then gradually increasing it to the recommended rate. If the patient continues to vomit, antiemetic agents such as metoclopramide (0.1–0.3 mg/kg in children and 10 mg in adults) have been used intravenously with success. The end point of this intestinal irrigation is a clear rectal effluent, which usually takes 4 to 6 hours. Significant gastrointestinal hemorrhage, ileus, and obstruction are contraindications for whole bowel irrigation. Activated charcoal does not adsorb heavy metals and therefore should not be administered.

Once iron has been absorbed, measures should be taken to reduce the free toxic fraction. Deferoxamine is a chelating agent that binds the free iron and competes with transferrin and ferritin for the iron. It removes only a small amount of the iron from transferrin and does not bind the iron in the cytochrome system or hemoglobin. Deferoxamine may be given intramuscularly (IM) or intravenously (IV) to chelate the absorbed iron.

A deferoxamine provocative chelation challenge (dose of 50 mg/kg with a maximum of 1 g IM or IV) should be given to patients with a history of a large ingestion (>50 mg elemental iron/kg), signs or symptoms of more than mild gastrointestinal upset, or a serum iron concentration above 300 μg/dL. It should also be given to patients with a history of a potentially toxic ingestion when serum iron concentrations cannot be determined.

If the patient passes a vin rosé–colored urine within 2 hours of the administration of deferoxamine, it signifies that free iron was chelated to deferoxamine and that therapy should be continued (negative results do not prove that there is no free iron). The patient should be given 50 mg/kg (maximum 1 g) every 4 hours IM or as a constant IV infusion until signs of toxicity have subsided, serum iron concentrations are less than the total iron-binding capacity, and the vin rosé–colored urine has stopped for 4 to 6 hours.

The IV infusion rate should usually not exceed 15 mg/kg/hr to avoid the risk of inducing hypotension. The IV route should be used in patients with hypotension or metabolic acidosis and those who have a severe ingestion. Patients remaining asymptomatic 6 hours after the ingestion without vin rosé urine and with an abdominal roentgenogram demonstrating no residual iron tablets can be safely sent home.

There are no efficacious procedures to increase the elimination of free iron. Dialysis and exchange transfusion do not remove the free fraction and remove only a small portion of the iron–chelate complex. Dialysis should be used only in patients with renal failure.

Finally, adequate supportive care should be instituted to correct fluid losses, hypotension, and metabolic acidosis.

ANNOTATED BIBLIOGRAPHY

Robotham JL, Lertman PS: Acute iron poisoning. A review. Am J Dis Child 134:875, 1980. (Very good review of the pathophysiology and treatment of iron overdose.)

Tenenbein M: Whole bowel irrigation as a gastrointestinal decontamination procedure after acute poisoning. Med Toxicol 3:77, 1988. (Excellent review of whole bowel irrigation.)

Westlin WF: Deferoxamine as a chelating agent. Clin Toxicol 4:597, 1971. (Very good review of deferoxamine.)

Whitten CF, Brough AJ: The pathophysiology of acute iron poisoning. Clin Toxicol 4:585, 1971. (Pathophysiology of iron poisoning is reviewed.)

177

Plants

Michael A. McGuigan

Plants, as a group, account for one of the most common ingestions in childhood. Potentially dangerous plants are available to children nearly every day of their lives. Poisonous plants grow wild but are often cultivated and even brought into the home as ornamental plants. Although every

Nontoxic Plants

African violet	Prayer plant
Begonias	Rubber plant
Coleus	Schefflera
Dracena	Spider plant
Ferns	Swedish ivy
Jade plant	

plant contains toxic chemicals, the concentration of these toxins is generally so low as to render most plants nontoxic (see the display entitled "Nontoxic Plants"). Certain plants do contain quantities of chemicals that may pose a toxic hazard. An important factor is that the concentrations of the toxic elements in any plant will vary with the season, climate, age of the plant, and degree of cultivation, among other variables. Some plants have small amounts of toxins that have a high "scare potential," such as cyanide or cardiac glycosides. This chapter will discuss the clinical toxicology of plants containing oxalates, gastrointestinal irritants, cyanogenic glycosides, and cardiac glycosides.

The prevention of plant poisoning can be accomplished by taking the following simple precautions:

1. All plants in and around the home should be identified.
2. Plants and related parts (e.g., seeds, fruit, bulbs) should be kept away from young children.
3. Children should not drink out of flowers or use leaves, seeds, or berries to make "tea."
4. Do not make children's playthings from unknown plants or trees.

OXALATE

Pathophysiology

Crystals of calcium oxalate are found in all parts of house plants such as dieffenbachia, dumbcane, elephant's ear, and philodendron as well as in the leaves of outdoor plants such as rhubarb, jack-in-the-pulpit, wild cala, and skunk cabbage. Although the exact mechanism of the toxicity of these plants is uncertain, it is presumed that chewing the appropriate part of the plant results in mucosal lesions from chemical irritation caused by the plant juice and mechanical damage from the calcium oxalate crystals. Proteolytic enzymes have also been found in the sap of the dieffenbachia plant.

Clinical Presentation

Topical symptoms and signs develop within minutes of chewing or sucking on these plants. Typical symptoms include a burning sensation and irritation of the mucous membranes, edema and inflammation of the lips and tongue, and excessive drooling. Dysphagia is common. Rarely, mucous membrane bullae may develop. Facial edema may occur in

areas that have come in contact with the sap. Systemic symptoms do not result from insoluble calcium oxalate crystals. Acute symptoms generally last only a few hours, although necrotic areas resulting from severe irritation may take longer to heal.

Differential Diagnosis

The differential diagnosis should include the causes of urticarial reactions, viral or bacterial stomatitis/pharyngitis, and the ingestion of caustic or corrosive products. The inflammation of the oral mucous membranes and excessive drooling may mimic epiglottitis, although coughing and fever are usually absent in oxalate-induced inflammation.

Work-Up

The evaluation of the child who ingested a plant containing oxalate should include a proper identification of the plant. If the care-giver does not know the name of the plant, a nursery, florist, or local botany department may be able to identify it based on a telephone description. The main focus of the physical examination is to evaluate the possibility of the inflammation obstructing the airway. Laboratory investigations are not helpful in the diagnosis or assessment of severity. Hypocalcemia and oxalate crystaluria have occurred following the ingestion of plants (e.g., rhubarb) containing soluble oxalate salts. The use of soft-tissue x-ray examinations of the neck has not been reported.

Treatment

Plant debris in the mouth should be removed immediately. Administration of cool, soothing substances such as water, milk, popsicles, or ice cream may bring symptomatic relief. The use of ipecac syrup or activated charcoal is not recommended. Prophylactic intubation should be considered if airway obstruction is a possibility.

INDICATIONS FOR ADMISSION OR REFERRAL

Most cases may be managed at home or in an ambulatory setting. Hospitalization may be necessary if the oral lesions are severe, if the child is unable to tolerate fluids, or if there are symptoms or signs of airway compromise.

GASTROINTESTINAL IRRITANTS

Pathophysiology

Many plants contain substances that cause gastrointestinal irritation. The gastroenteritis may be due to any of a variety of substances, such as saponins (e.g., horse chestnuts, amaryllis, wisteria), resins (e.g., iris), or irritant oils (e.g., buttercup). The exact mechanism of action of these substances is uncertain, although the effect is believed to occur at the gastrointestinal level with, perhaps, some stimulation of the vomiting center in the brain.

Clinical Presentation

The time interval between ingestion and the onset of gastrointestinal effects is highly variable, ranging from a few minutes to several hours. The severity of the presenting symptoms or signs may also vary considerably, ranging from minor abdominal discomfort to severe vomiting, abdominal cramps, and explosive diarrhea. Oral irritation may also occur as a sole finding.

Differential Diagnosis

The differential diagnosis should include viral or bacterial gastroenteritis and ingestion of other toxins that cause gastroenteritis, such as iron or arsenic. Staphylococcal food poisoning should be considered. Oral lesions must be differentiated from viral or bacterial stomatitis or ingestion of caustic substances (e.g., lyes or acids).

Work-Up

A work-up should include a thorough history of events preceding the onset of the symptoms; it is especially important to identify where the child was playing and what potential toxins might have been available. A physical examination may reveal signs of irritation of the oral mucous membranes or findings compatible with dehydration secondary to severe diarrhea. No specific diagnostic or laboratory tests are available for this type of poisoning. Laboratory investigations, therefore, should be aimed at assessing the severity of the effects rather than at trying to identify the cause. Renal and hepatic function tests may be indicated in patients who are severely symptomatic.

Treatment

The "toxic dose" of any of these plants is unknown, so if a child has ingested one of these plants but no symptoms have occurred, a "wait and watch" approach is recommended.

The efficacy of gastrointestinal decontamination procedures has not been investigated. Emesis or lavage is not indicated. Although activated charcoal theoretically *may* be beneficial, its use in practice is difficult; prophylactic use is not recommended, and toxin-induced vomiting may preclude its administration. Cathartics should not be used if the child has diarrhea. Fluid and electrolyte replacement may be required to prevent or correct imbalances and shock. The use of antiemetics and antidiarrheal agents is not indicated.

Indications for Admission or Referral

The indications for admission depend on the severity of the symptoms, the presence of dehydration, and the ability of the child to take adequate oral fluids.

CYANOGENIC GLYCOSIDES

Pathophysiology

Cyanogenic glycosides are contained in a number of fruit pits or seeds such as apple, wild cherry, elderberry, and peach and apricot kernels. The products of cultivated apricot plants may contain as little as $\frac{1}{25}$ the concentration of cyanogenic glycosides found in the wild plants. Following ingestion, the glycosides are hydrolized within the gut to liberate cyanide, which is absorbed into the body. Cyanide, once absorbed, distributes to the cells, where it binds to and inhibits cytochrome oxidase activity, thus blocking cellular respiration.

Clinical Presentation

Patients who ingest large quantities of the appropriate fruit material may present $\frac{1}{2}$ to 2 hours later with symptoms and signs of cyanide poisoning: malaise, vomiting, weakness, unsteadiness, confusion, tachypnea, and coma.

Differential Diagnosis

The differential diagnosis of acute collapse may include central nervous system hemorrhage, convulsions, or exposure to toxic gases such as hydrogen sulfide or carbon monoxide.

Work-Up

A history may identify the suspected fruit and the circumstances. The toxic dose of each fruit pit or seed is difficult to establish. However, it has been estimated that for cultivated peaches, the toxic dose of peach pit kernels is ~one kernel/kg. A physical examination will reveal an unconscious or deteriorating child with hypotension and bradycardia but not cyanosis. The bitter almond smell of cyanide may be noted. Laboratory investigations may document elevated cyanide levels as well as metabolic (lactic) acidosis.

Treatment

If a large quantity of seeds or pits has been ingested, it is reasonable to use ipecac syrup followed by activated charcoal. Ipecac may be used within 2 hours of the ingestion. Unless the diagnosis is certain, treatment should be symptomatic and supportive. Ventilatory assistance with supplemental oxygen is indicated, as is support of circulation with the use of volume expanders and pressor agents. Acidosis should be corrected with sodium bicarbonate. Once the diagnosis of cyanide poisoning has been made, standard therapy consists of the intravenous administration of sodium nitrite followed by sodium thiosulfate.

Indications for Admission or Referral

Indications for admission include any child with a positive history and compatible symptoms.

CARDIAC GLYCOSIDES

Pathophysiology

Many attractive plants contain cardiac glycosides. Lily-of-the-valley, foxglove, and oleander are all popular flowering plants that contain variable quantities of cardiac glycosides as well as gastrointestinal irritants. Following ingestion of these plants, the digitalislike glycoside is absorbed and exerts an effect on the myocardium similar to that produced by digoxin.

Clinical Presentation

Symptoms usually become evident within 2 hours of ingestion. Vomiting is the most common presenting complaint. Topical or oral irritation may be present, as well as salivation, abdominal pain, and diarrhea. Cardiac symptoms may begin 1 to 6 hours after the ingestion and consist of bradycardia, hypotension, and cyanosis.

Differential Diagnosis

The differential diagnosis includes acquired cardiac disease of other causes and ingestion of pharmaceutical digitalis preparations.

Work-Up

A history of exposure or availability of these plants is important, but the reliable "toxic dose" has not been established. No documented cases of lily-of-the-valley poisoning have been reported in children. A physical examination may document oral irritation and an atrioventricular block. An electrocardiogram may demonstrate conduction defects compatible with digitalis cardiotoxicity: exaggerated sinus arrhythmia, sinus bradycardia, and second- or third-degree block. Hyperkalemia may occur.

Treatment

Treatment is not necessary for accidental ingestion of lily-of-the-valley. Ingestion of wild oleander or foxglove should be treated with ipecac syrup or gastric lavage, followed by activated charcoal. Atropine has been useful in the treatment of oleander-induced bradyarrhythmias. Other therapy should follow the guidelines established for the treatment of digoxin overdose (e.g., electrical pacing for atropine-resistant heart block). Fab antibody fragments have been used successfully for the treatment of this type of cardiac glycoside poisoning.

Indications for Admission or Referral

Patients who ingest lily-of-the-valley do not need to be admitted to the hospital. For patients who have ingested wild oleander or foxglove, admission is recommended if any symptoms or signs occur within 6 hours of ingestion. Patients with cardiac abnormalities should be hospitalized in a center capable of monitoring and treating them.

ANNOTATED BIBLIOGRAPHY

Ansford AJ, Morris H: Fatal oleander poisoning. Med J Aust 1:360–361, 1981. (Case history and clinical presentation.)

Arditt J, Rodriguez E: Dieffenbachia: Uses, abuses and toxic constituents: A review. J Ethnopharmacol 5:293–302, 1982. (Scientific more than clinical review.)

Haynes BE, Bessen HA, Wightman WD: Oleander tea: Herbal draught of death. Ann Emerg Med 14:350–353, 1985. (Case history and clinical presentation.)

Lasch EE, El Shawa R: Multiple cases of cyanide poisoning by apricot kernels in children from Gaza. Pediatrics 68:5–7, 1981. (Clinical case presentations.)

Rubino MJ, Davidoff F: Cyanide poisoning from apricot seeds (letter). JAMA 241:359, 1979. (Clinical case presentations.)

Shaw D, Pearn J: Oleander poisoning. Med J Aust 2:267–269, 1979. (Case history and clinical presentation.)

178

Hydrocarbon Ingestion

David W. Johnson and
Michael A. McGuigan

Accidental exposure to a hydrocarbon product occurs commonly in children and is potentially fatal. More than 58,000 exposures and 31 deaths were reported in 1989 by Poison Centers in the United States, making hydrocarbons the ninth leading cause of death due to toxic ingestion. Hydrocarbons have been classified or divided in many ways: aromatic versus aliphatic, petroleum distillate versus nonpetroleum distillate, high viscosity (thick) versus low viscosity (thin), halogenated versus nonhalogenated, and, finally, hydrocarbons with toxic additives versus those without additives.

Aromatic hydrocarbons are aromatic ring structures and they include such compounds as benzene, toluene, turpentine, and xylene. The aromatic ring is important because it appears that the aromatic hydrocarbons are absorbed from the gastrointestinal tract in quantities sufficient to cause systemic toxicity. Aliphatic hydrocarbons are formed from the distillation of crude petroleum.

Viscosity is important only with respect to the risk of developing widespread aspiration pneumonitis. Most hydrocarbons are of low viscosity and, therefore, pose a risk of aspiration pneumonitis. High-viscosity hydrocarbons such as greases, petroleum jelly, or tar are hazardous only as a foreign body and have no toxic effects.

Halogenated hydrocarbons (e.g., carbon tetrachloride, trichloroethane) and hydrocarbons with toxic additives (e.g., pesticides) are unique entities and are not discussed. It is important to remember, however, that the therapeutic approach to the patient who ingested one of these products may depend on the *additive* and not on the hydrocarbon.

This chapter discusses only the low-viscosity, nonhalogenated, additive-free, aliphatic petroleum distillate hydrocarbons: gasoline, kerosene, lighter fluid, lubricating oils, furniture polish (mineral seal oil), mineral spirits, and naphthas. These compounds are dealt with as a group and are referred to as petroleum distillate hydrocarbons (PDH).

PATHOPHYSIOLOGY

Drinking a PDH results in mild irritation of the mucous membranes of the mouth. These substances are not significantly absorbed through the gastrointestinal tract and, therefore, will produce no pulmonary or nonpulmonary (systemic) disease as a result of an uncomplicated ingestion. Chemical pneumonitis arises only as a result of pulmonary aspiration of the hydrocarbon liquid. Following aspiration of significant quantities of PDH, central nervous system (CNS) depression may develop secondary to hypoxemia or from the CNS effects of PDH absorbed through the lung.

CLINICAL PRESENTATION

Most patients present shortly after the exposure has been discovered. The commonest symptom resulting from the ingestion of PDH is vomiting, which occurs in 50% of ingestions. Coughing occurs in 40% of children, but ~20% of the children present with no respiratory complaints. Drowsiness is an unusual presenting complaint, occurring in 10% of cases. Stupor or seizures are rare, occurring in less than 1% of cases. Dyspnea (6%) and abdominal pain or diarrhea (3%) are unusual. Fever and leukocytosis within 4 hours of exposure have >80% positive predictive value for the development of pneumonitis, whereas the absence of tachypnea has >80% negative predictive value.

DIFFERENTIAL DIAGNOSIS

The correct diagnosis is usually not difficult to make because PDHs have a distinct petroleum smell and an accurate history is volunteered. Poisoning with insecticides (e.g., organophosphates or carbamates) that inhibit the enzyme cholinesterase will produce a clinical picture similar to that caused by PDH ingestion and aspiration: vomiting, excess salivation, tachypnea, drowsiness, and chest findings. Other diagnoses to consider in a child who presents with an acute onset of vomiting and abdominal pain are infectious gastroenteritis (bacterial or viral) and ingestion of other substances such as acetaminophen, salicylates, caffeine, iron, digitalis products, theophylline, and tobacco. The differential diagnosis of an acute consolidation on a chest roentgenogram includes viral or bacterial infections and foreign body aspiration.

WORK-UP

History

The most important questions to answer are "What was the product?" and "Did the child aspirate?" The correct identification of the product as a pure PDH is essential; estimates of the volume ingested are less important. In assessing whether or not the child aspirated, the presence or absence of respiratory *symptoms* can be a useful guide. If the episode was observed by a reliable witness and there is no history of coughing, choking, gagging, vomiting, or burping, then the likelihood that the child aspirated is negligible.

Physical Examination

A careful examination of the respiratory tract should be emphasized. A low-grade fever may be noted. During the physical examination, the physician should attempt to detect the smell of PDH in the child's mouth and to look for irritated oral mucous membranes. Procedures that might induce gagging or choking, such as depression of the tongue with a tongue-blade, should be avoided. The respiratory rate and depth should be documented. The chest should be examined carefully. Although rhonchi and crepitations may be found, the physician should remember that an examination within a short time of aspiration may give false-negative results. The examination should thus be repeated several times over a period of 6 hours after the ingestion before the results may be considered reliable. The presence of any central nervous system depression should be noted. Finally, the skin around the mouth and on the neck, chest, abdomen, and groin should be examined for evidence of irritation.

Laboratory Tests

If the child is not severely ill, a chest roentgenogram should be delayed until 4 to 6 hours after the aspiration. In patients who eventually develop pneumonitis, a chest roentgenogram is positive in only 60% by 1 hour after the aspiration. Therefore, a negative chest roentgenogram 1 hour after aspiration may have to be repeated after several hours. The chest roentgenogram, when positive, demonstrates a unilobar infiltrate in 83% of patients and a perihilar pattern in only 9%. The white blood cell count may be elevated as high as 16,000 cells/mm² in patients with pneumonitis.

TREATMENT

Neither induced vomiting nor gastric lavage should be used to treat patients with PDH ingestion because PDHs are not absorbed to a significant degree through the gastrointestinal tract. Activated charcoal binds kerosene and turpentine, but its use is impractical because such large quantities are required. For children with no or mild symptoms, the best therapy consists of careful observation.

If the clothes or skin is contaminated, clothing should be removed and the skin gently washed with lukewarm water and a mild soap.

When aspiration pneumonitis has been documented, one should maintain close monitoring of ventilation and oxygenation with arterial blood gases (and, if available, transcutaneous CO_2 monitoring and pulse oximetry). If pO_2 cannot be maintained above 50 mm Hg with inspiration of 60% oxygen by face mask, or if pCO_2 exceeds 50 mm Hg, intubation with positive end-expiratory pressure may be necessary. Excessive crystalloid administration should be avoided. Extracorporeal membrane oxygenation (ECMO) has been used successfully in cases of severe pneumonitis unresponsive to standard ventilation. Corticosteroids have no place in either the prophylaxis or the treatment of hydrocarbon pneumonitis. The use of systemic antibiotics is indicated if secondary bacterial infections are suspected or documented.

INDICATIONS FOR ADMISSION OR REFERRAL

Patients who have severe pneumonitis should be admitted immediately to a hospital capable of providing adequate respiratory care. Patients presenting with symptomatology of a moderate degree should be admitted and observed for a progression of symptoms and signs. Patients with minor presenting complaints should be observed for 6 hours before a decision of whether or not to admit the patient is made. The patient may be sent home at the end of the 6-hour period if his or her physical examination *and* chest roentgenogram are normal. If, on the other hand, either the patient's physical examination *or* chest roentgenogram is abnormal, the patient should be admitted to the hospital for observation. Patients who have been entirely asymptomatic following ingestion can be observed at home, and their progress can be reevaluated in 2 to 4 hours by telephone.

The clinical course of aspiration pneumonitis is usually fairly benign unless the aspiration is severe. Fever, tachycardia, and tachypnea may last for less than 2 days. In one study, the mean duration of hospitalization was 4 days. Severe cases of aspiration pneumonitis may require intubation, ventilation, or even ECMO to maintain adequate arterial blood gas values. Residual pulmonary effects are unusual; there are rare reports of pneumatoceles that persist for up to several months postaspiration.

ANNOTATED BIBLIOGRAPHY

Anas N, Namasonthi V, Ginsburg CM: Criteria for hospitalizing children who have ingested products containing hydrocarbons. JAMA 246:840–843, 1981. (Retrospective review of 950 children exposed to hydrocarbons.)

Baldachin BJ, Melmed RN: Clinical and therapeutic aspects of kerosene poisoning: A series of 200 cases. Br Med J 2:28–30, 1964. (Excellent brief presentation of children with clinical toxicity.)

Dice WH, Ward G, Kelly J et al: Pulmonary toxicity following gastrointestinal ingestion of kerosene. Ann Emerg Med 11:138–142, 1982. (Experimental evaluation of the question of gastrointestinal absorption.)

Majeed HA, Bassyouni H, Kalaawy M et al: Kerosene poisoning in children: A clinico-radiological study of 205 cases. Ann Trop Paediatr 1:123–130, 1981. (One of the largest studies; a great deal of useful information is presented.)

Marks MI, Chicoine L, Legere G et al: Adrenocorticosteroid treatment of hydrocarbon pneumonia in children—A cooperative study. J Pediatr 81:369–369, 1972. (Excellent review, with duration of symptoms and hospitalization information.)

Wolfsdorf J: Kerosene intoxication: An experimental approach to the etiology of CNS manifestations in primates. J Pediatr 88:1037–1040, 1976. (Good presentation of the role of gastrointestinal absorption versus aspiration in the production of CNS findings.)

179

Caustic Ingestions

Pierre Gaudreault

The ingestion of caustic substances is a significant problem. In 1989, 54,182 cases of caustic poisonings were reported in the United States. Children less than 6 years old were involved in 43% of these cases. Although rarely fatal (23 adults [0.04%]), such ingestion carries serious immediate and long-term morbidity. The morbidity is greater in adolescents and adults who ingest these products in an attempt to commit suicide. The morbidity related to liquid or solid caustic substances results from perforation or stenosis secondary to severe esophageal or gastric injuries.

Lye was previously the alkali agent most frequently ingested. With the introduction of drain cleaners, sodium or potassium hydroxide has become more prevalent. Other alkali products encountered are laundry and dishwasher detergents (e.g., carbonate, phosphate), denture cleaners (e.g., bicarbonate, phosphate), and Clinitest tablets (sodium hydroxide).

The acidic compounds encountered most frequently are toilet-bowl cleaners (e.g., hydrochloric, phosphoric, and sulfuric acids), antirust compounds (e.g., hydrochloric, phosphoric, and sulfuric acids), automobile battery fluids (sulfuric acid), and slate cleaners (hydrofluoric acid).

Household bleach products (containing less than 8% of sodium hypochlorite) usually cause only a mild irritation to the esophagus; they rarely cause tissue necrosis and virtually never cause strictures. Most authorities, therefore, do not regard bleach ingestions as a caustic ingestion.

PATHOPHYSIOLOGY

Alkali products destroy tissues by partially dissolving tissue proteins, a process that is referred to as liquefaction necrosis. This destruction permits deep penetration into tissues. In contrast to alkali agents, acids are potent desiccants and coagulate tissues. This coagulation necrosis limits acid penetration and frequently results in damage only to the mucosa.

Factors that influence the severity of the tissue destruction and the development of complications include the pH, the concentration, and the quantity of the product ingested, the length of contact with the mucosa, and the relative tonicity of the pyloric sphincter. Alkali products with a pH greater than 12 are more likely to produce severe esophageal injuries.

Alkali and acid burns usually evolve through three stages. The acute phase is characterized by a marked inflammatory response with edema. This inflammation may extend through the muscle layer with severe burns, and perforation may occur.

Vascular thrombosis and hemorrhages can be seen. Cell death and necrotic tissue accumulation end 4 to 7 days after the insult. The necrotic tissue is sloughed, edema decreases, neovascularization begins, and granulation takes place. This second phase occurs between the second and third week postingestion. The last phase begins with the proliferation of fibroblasts and the formation of connective tissue. This cicatrization phase begins at the end of the third week. During this period, if the burn is deep, adhesions may form and narrowing or obliteration of the esophageal lumen may occur. Reepithelialization occurs between the third and sixth week postingestion.

CLINICAL PRESENTATION

The ingestion of caustic substances primarily induces burns to the gastrointestinal tract, particularly to the oropharynx, esophagus, and stomach. The severity of these burns and associated symptoms depend on several factors, such as the type of product (acid versus alkali), the nature of the product (solid versus liquid), the amount ingested, the concentration, and the pH of the substance.

The ingestion of solid products usually causes severe burns to the mouth, pharynx, or upper portion of the esophagus. Solid products may adhere to the mucosa, causing deeper burns. In contrast, because liquid substances are easier to swallow, they often cause less injury to the mouth but extensive damage to the esophagus or stomach. The extent of the burns ranges from slight erythema and edema to severe ulcerations with grayish pseudomembranes.

Alkali agents have traditionally been considered to damage mainly the esophagus, whereas acid products affect primarily the stomach. However, in a review of 378 cases of caustic ingestion treated in our hospital, we found that the incidence of esophageal lesions was similar with acid or alkali agents.

Injuries to the oral or esophageal mucosa may be accompanied by excessive salivation, drooling, dysphagia, painful swallowing, and retrosternal pain. Nausea, vomiting, hematemesis, epigastric or abdominal pain, or tenderness may be experienced. Substernal or back pain and abdominal pain with rigidity may also indicate mediastinitis or peritonitis. The presence of hoarseness, aphonia, stridor, or dyspnea suggests laryngeal, tracheal, or pulmonary involvement secondary to aspiration.

The major clinical questions with caustic ingestion are to determine the location of the burn (if it occurred in the esophagus or the stomach) and the extent and the depth of the injury. Several studies have demonstrated that the presence of clinical manifestations cannot predict the presence or severity of esophageal lesions. However, patients who present with unprovoked vomiting, drooling, or stridor are more likely to have severe esophageal lesions.

The acute manifestations last 1 to 3 days, depending on the severity of the intoxication. The patient is at the highest risk for perforation during the first 72 hours following the ingestion. This period is followed by a latent phase that lasts for several weeks. Delayed complications such as stricture formation may occur toward the end of this phase. Progressive dysphagia secondary to stricture formation may be noted 3 to 4 weeks after the ingestion but may take months to appear, again depending on the severity of the mucosal burn.

Several classifications of esophageal injury have been proposed. These classifications are based on the depth of the burn. The absence of an esophageal lesion is termed grade 0. Burns that are limited to the mucosa and are characterized by the presence of edema or erythema are classified as grade 1. Grade 2 burns penetrate beyond the mucosa and are characterized by the presence of ulcerations or whitish membranes. Finally, the presence of perforation is classified as grade 3. Burns that are circular or penetrate the muscular layer carry the greatest risk of inducing a stricture formation.

WORK-UP

History and Physical Examination

The clinician should determine the type of product involved and, as best as possible, the quantity ingested. One should particularly look for the appearance of respiratory distress or signs of perforation as well as the presence of signs or symptoms (e.g., vomiting, stridor, drooling) that suggest an increased risk of serious esophageal or respiratory involvement.

Laboratory Tests

Esophagoscopy is the most accurate way to evaluate the involvement of the esophagus and stomach following the ingestion of caustic substances. Therefore, an esophagoscopy is recommended for all patients who have ingested a caustic substance regardless of the presence or absence of clinical signs or symptoms. To avoid risk of perforation, the esophagoscope should not be advanced beyond the first area of ulceration. This procedure carries a low risk of morbidity when performed by an experienced endoscopist using a flexible endoscope.

Children who have a questionable history of ingestion without oropharyngeal burns, dysphagia, stridor, drooling, or vomiting should be observed for 3 to 4 hours. They may be discharged without esophagoscopy if they remain asymptomatic. Other laboratory tests should be performed as dictated by the clinical status of the patient.

An esophagogram (barium swallow) is not as accurate as an esophagoscopy in determining esophageal involvement in the acute phase. Indeed, because there is no clear correlation between esophaphagraphic findings during the acute stage and the final outcome, this study should be reserved for documenting a perforation or observing the progress of a stricture.

TREATMENT

The initial treatment should consist of immediate washing with water to remove the caustic substance from the esophagus, unless the patient demonstrates signs of airway swelling, obstruction, or gastrointestinal perforation. Neutralizing agents such as vinegar to neutralize acid agents are not useful and may increase the esophageal injury by producing an exothermic reaction.

Emesis induced with syrup of ipecac is contraindicated because it would subject the esophagus to further exposure to the caustic agent. Gastric lavage is also contraindicated because the blind passage of a nasogastric tube may cause an iatrogenic esophageal perforation. Some authors recommend the insertion of siliconized rubber nasogastric tubes to prevent the obliteration of the esophageal lumen secondary to strictures. However, the efficacy and safety of this procedure have not been adequately evaluated and are controversial. If nasogastric tubes are used, they shouldbe positioned under direct visualization during an esophagoscopy.

Results from an esophagoscopy enable the clinician to rapidly discharge patients without esophageal involvement and to start the appropriate treatment in other patients. The esophagoscopy should be performed within 48 hours of the ingestion, when the risk of perforation is low.

The role and efficacy of steroids in the prevention of stricture formation following a caustic ingestion in patients with grade-2 esophageal burns remain unclear, because the number of randomized controlled studies that evaluate the efficacy of steroids in such patients is limited. Some authors have reported beneficial effects of steroids in reducing the incidence of stricture formation following alkali ingestions, whereas others have not found any beneficial effects. Patients with grade-0 or grade-1 lesions do not require treat-

ments. Patients with grade-3 lesions need surgical intervention and do not benefit from steroids.

There are no data evaluating the best dosage. Until data are available, a dose of 1 to 2 mg/kg/day of prednisone (maximum 50 mg/day) or its equivalent should be sufficient. This dose should be tapered after 21 days, a time period adequate to reduce the inflammatory response during the acute-injury and early-reparative phases. Treatment should be started as soon as possible in patients with grade-2 esophageal burns in order for them to benefit from the antifibroblastic action of steroids. If an esophagoscopy cannot be performed soon after an alkali ingestion, steroids should be started immediately and their necessity reevaluated after the esophagoscopy.

The use of prophylactic antibiotics in patients treated with steroids is controversial. Their use is based on animal studies in which an increased mortality rate was noted in animals treated with steroids but without antibiotics. These data are not supported by human data. In our experience with more than 100 children treated with steroids but without antibiotics, none developed complications. Prophylactic antibiotics, therefore, should not be used. Antibiotics should be reserved for patients who develop signs of secondary infection or who experience esophageal or gastric perforation.

Adequate nutrition is essential because inadequate calorie intake inhibits appropriate healing and increases susceptibility to infection. Parenteral nutrition should be started early in patients with severe esophageal lesions. If oral intake is delayed for a long time, a gastrostomy for the placement of a gastrojejunal feeding tube may be indicated.

After 3 to 4 weeks, the status of esophageal injuries should be reassessed. An esophagogram or esophagoscopy should be performed. A contrast esophagogram will depict the functioning of the esophagus,while the esophagoscopy will give the physician a visual image of the healing process.

If stricture formation has begun, dilation and bougienage should be started. The success of these techniques relates in part to the severity of the stricture and the presence of an esophageal lumen. As mentioned earlier, some physicians recommend the early insertion of a siliconized rubber nasogastric tube in order to maintain a lumen that can be dilated later. Patients who do not respond to dilation or who develop a complete obliteration of their esophageal lumen may need a colon interposition. Patients who develop stricture with lye may have an increased risk of developing esophageal carcinoma.

PREVENTION

Prevention of caustic ingestions remains the best way to avoid serious sequelae in children. Corrosive materials should be kept out of the reach of children in locked cabinets and in their original containers with child-resistant closures. Furthermore, physicians should provide parents with adequate anticipatory guidance so that they may provide a safe environment for their children.

ANNOTATED BIBLIOGRAPHY

Anderson KD, Rouse RM, Randolph JG: A controlled trial of corticosteroids in children with corrosive injury of the esophagus. N Engl J Med 323:637, 1990. (Study evaluating the efficacy of steroids in the prevention of esophageal strictures. Steroids did not reduce the incidence of strictures in patients with corrosive-induced esophageal burns when compared to controls. However, the small number of patients studied does not warrant the conclusion that the two treatments are equivalent.)

Appelquist P, Salmo M: Lye corrosion carcinoma of the esophagus. A review of 63 cases. Cancer 45:2655, 1980. (Study reviews a possible association between esophageal lye burns and esophageal carcinoma. Among agents causing esophageal strictures, lye is the one most commonly associated with the development of esophageal carcinoma. The authors found a lye corrosion incidence of 2.6% in patients developing an esophageal carcinoma.)

Crain EF, Gershel JC, Mezey AP: Caustic ingestions. Symptoms as predictors of esophageal injury. Am J Dis Child 138:863, 1984. (Good study evaluating symptoms as predictors of esophageal lesions.)

Friedman EM, Lovejoy FH Jr: The emergency management of caustic ingestions. Emerg Med Clin North Am 2(1):77, 1984. (Good review of the subject.)

Gaudreault P, Parent M, McGuigan MA et al: Predictability of esophageal injury from signs and symptoms. A study of caustic ingestion in 378 children. Pediatrics 71:767, 1983. (Study of signs and symptoms as predictors of esophageal injuries.)

Hawking DB, Demeter MJ, Barnett TE: Caustic ingestion: Controversies in management. Laryngoscope 90:98, 1980. (Excellent article on the treatment of caustic ingestions.)

Wasserman RL, Ginsburg CM: Caustic substance injuries. J Pediatr 107:169, 1985. (Very good review of the subject.)

180

Food Poisoning

Milton Tenenbein

The patient or the care-giver often wonders if it was something that the patient ate recently that was responsible for an acute onset of illness. Indeed, the recognition of food as a vector of illness and disease is a basic requirement for human survival. Safe foods and preparation practices have been learned through the process of trial and error. These include sanitation and food preservation through the processes of heating, freezing, fermentation, and treatment with chemical additives.

Food poisoning can be considered an acute onset of ill-ness caused by the consumption of a particular food. This concept of food-induced illness, however, is too broad because it includes the abdominal pain and diarrhea following the consumption of a glass of milk by an individual with lactase deficiency. It is better to think of *food-borne disease,* recognizing that the food is a vector for the agent responsible for the symptoms and that the presence of the agent (the poison) is unexpected. This excludes naturally toxic "foods" such as poisonous plants, mushrooms, fish, and shellfish.

It is generally agreed that food-borne disease is common but underreported. The agent may be biologic (e.g., bacteria, viruses) or chemical (e.g., heavy metals, pesticides). One epidemiologic survey reported that 24% of outbreaks of food-borne disease are caused by chemical agents. The food may become toxic prior to, during, or after its processing. Most cases (70% in one series), however, are caused by errors in food-handling practices, either in restaurants or in homes. In the same series, only 3% of the total outbreaks were traced to commercial food processing establishments. An overview of the clinical features of food poisonings from multiple organisms is presented in Table 180-1. For food poisoning due to chemical agents, the clinical features are dependent on the toxin that has contaminated the food.

CLINICAL PRESENTATION

The patient with a food-borne illness usually presents with an acute onset of gastrointestinal illness. The most common symptoms are abdominal pain, nausea, vomiting, and diarrhea. Fever may be present if there is an infectious etiology. Depending on the responsible agent, alternative presentations may include neurologic symptoms such as headache, paresthesias, weakness, and paralysis.

DIFFERENTIAL DIAGNOSIS

The most common clinical presentation of food poisoning is an acute onset of gastrointestinal symptoms, including abdominal pain, nausea, vomiting, and diarrhea. The differential diagnosis of this presentation is reviewed in Chapters 101, 103, and 105. Whether or not these symptoms are a result of food-borne disease, they are usually due to a microbiologic agent. Although the management of the patient with gastrointestinal illness is usually the same regardless of whether the etiology is a primary gastrointestinal infection or an infection acquired from food, there are specific preventive and public health concerns that make this distinction important.

WORK-UP

History

If the patient or the care-giver is concerned that the illness is associated with food, it is important to inquire about the

Table 180-1. Food Poisoning: Differential Diagnosis of Gastrointestinal Presentation

ORGANISM	PATHOGENESIS	INCUBATION PERIOD	SYMPTOMS	FOODS
Staphylococci	Ingestion of enterotoxin	1–6 hours	Nausea, vomiting, diarrhea, and abdominal cramps; no fever; several hours' duration	Cream-filled desserts, cold meats, salads
Clostridium perfringens	Formation of enterotoxin in vivo	8–12 hours	Watery diarrhea and abdominal cramps; fever and vomiting are uncommon; several hours' duration	Cooked meats
Bacillus cereus I	Ingestion of enterotoxin	1–6 hours	Nausea, vomiting, diarrhea, and abdominal cramps; no fever; less than 24 hours' duration	Rice, starches, vegetables, meats
Bacillus cereus II	Formation of enterotoxin in vivo	8–12 hours	Watery diarrhea and abdominal cramps; no fever; less than 24 hours' duration	Rice, starches, vegetables, meats
Shigellae	Bacterial invasion of colonic mucosa	24–96 hours	Diarrhea (often bloody), abdominal pain, and fever; dehydration, meningismus, and seizures can develop	Water supply
Salmonellae	Bacterial invasion of intestinal mucosa	12–48 hours	Diarrhea (may be bloody); nausea, vomiting, and abdominal pain less common; fever; up to 5 days' duration	Poultry, egg products, water
Vibrio	Uncertain	12–24 hours	Explosive diarrhea; occasionally cramps, nausea, and vomiting; ~3 days' duration	Seafood
Campylobacter	Bacterial invasion of intestinal mucosa	48–120 hours	Diarrhea (may be bloody), abdominal pain, and fever; vomiting uncommon; several days' duration	Water supply

presence of symptoms in others who have eaten the same foods. If it is the physician who is considering food poisoning as the cause of an illness, he or she should inquire if any unusual, esoteric, or tainted foods have recently been eaten. The physician should also determine if the patient has recently altered his or her normal routine and has eaten a meal, for example, at a school picnic or on a camping trip. Preparation of food in advance, improper storage, and inadequate cooking, cooling, and reheating are the most common factors contributing to food poisoning. The interval between food consumption and onset of symptoms is important. Rapid onset (within a few hours) supports the ingestion of a bacterial toxin or chemical food poisoning. Later onset (many hours to a few days) is consistent with an enteric infection.

Physical Examination

The patient with a gastrointestinal presentation should be assessed for dehydration. The remainder of the physical examination usually contributes little except in the patient with botulism.

Laboratory Tests

Depending on the clinical severity, a complete blood count, serum electrolytes, creatinine, and BUN may be necessary. Samples of vomitus and stool for culturing and toxin analysis should be taken. This often requires the involvement of the local public health agency. Any suspected food should be submitted for testing.

MANAGEMENT

Clinical management of food-borne illness is dependent on its etiology, which can be divided into bacterial and chemical agents.

Bacterial Food Poisoning

Food poisoning caused by bacteria is due to an infection by the agent or to the effects of a toxin elaborated by the agent. The clinical features of bacterial food poisonings presenting with gastrointestinal symptoms are described in Table 180-1. Botulism, a neurologic disease, is discussed separately.

Staphylococci, *Clostridium perfringens,* and salmonellae are the most common causes of food poisonings. The gastrointestinal food poisoning syndromes due to toxins (staphylococci, *C. perfringens,* and *Bacillus cereus*) usually do not last a long time and thus require no specific therapy. Dehydration is uncommon, as is the need for hospitalization. Those syndromes due to direct invasion of gastrointestinal mucosa (shigellae, salmonellae, and *Campylobacter*) have longer courses, and symptoms can be more severe. Dehydration may result, especially in infants. Hospitalization, therefore, may be required for intravenous therapy. Those with moderate to severe illness due to shigellae or *Campylobacter* should also receive antibiotics (either ampicillin or trimethoprim-sulfamethoxazole for the former and erythromycin for the latter).

Botulism

The toxin of *Clostridium botulinum* is the most toxic substance known to man. It is elaborated under anaerobic conditions at a *p*H greater than 4.5. Ingestion of the preformed toxin produces botulism (except for infant botulism). This consists of anticholinergic symptoms because the toxin irreversibly binds to the peripheral neuromuscular junction, blocking transmission by preventing acetylcholine release. Initially there may be gastrointestinal symptoms such as nausea, vomiting, and abdominal pain. Neurologic symptoms and signs develop within several hours to a few days. Cranial nerve involvement appears early. Thus, patients may present with dry mouth, diplopia, dysarthria, dysphagia, and third- and sixth-nerve palsies. The severity of ocular symptoms may be of prognostic value. Systemic skeletal muscle paralysis follows cranial nerve involvement, with death being due to respiratory failure.

The differential diagnosis is large and may include myasthenia gravis, Guillain–Barré syndrome, tick paralysis, poisonings (e.g., carbon monoxide, atropine, organophosphate insecticides, and soluble barium salts), and trichinosis. Most cases of botulism are caused by foods canned at home.

Botulism should be suspected in any patient with a recent onset of cranial nerve palsies and a history of eating home-canned foods. Confirmation of the diagnosis requires demonstration of the organism or toxin in the food, vomitus, or stool. Serum can be tested for toxin. All of these tests are time-consuming, and a specific therapy should be instituted if there are reasonable clinical grounds to suspect the diagnosis. This involves the administration of specific trivalent antitoxin. Mechanical ventilation may be required if respiratory failure develops. Penicillin therapy is not indicated because botulism is an intoxication and not an infection. Guanidine therapy is controversial.

Infant botulism differs from classical botulism in that the toxin is elaborated from organisms growing within the gastrointestinal tract. This entity is limited to infants under 12 months old with a peak incidence from 3 to 26 weeks of age. They present with constipation followed by lethargy, weakness, and poor feeding. Generalized weakness and hypotonia ensue, which can be followed by respiratory failure. Diagnosis can be confirmed by a demonstration of organisms or toxin in the stool. Serum is negative for the toxin. The treatment consists of meticulous respiratory and nutritional support. The roles for antitoxin, penicillin, and guanidine are unclear. Honey is implicated as a source of *C. botulinum* organisms, and it should not be fed to infants less than 1 year of age.

Chemical Food Poisoning

There are many reports of food-borne illness due to chemicals. Examples include insecticide poisoning from cucumbers, tin poisoning from tomato juice, solanine poisoning from potatoes, and methemoglobinemia from meats. Food poisoning due to chemicals is characterized by the rapid onset of symptoms (within 1 to 2 hours) and multiple victims. Cases of food poisoning involving a single victim are usually not recognized as such. The chemical may contaminate the food during the production, processing, distribution, or preparation. The management of cases depends on the specific toxin and the degree of illness.

PUBLIC HEALTH CONCERNS

When one is faced with a single case of acute gastrointestinal illness, food poisoning is difficult to confirm. When the history identifies multiple victims, the pediatrician should ensure that implicated foods are saved, and should initiate specimen collection (vomitus, stool). The local public health authority should be notified so that these samples and specimens can be tested. They will investigate the situation with the goals of preventing additional cases and correcting improper food-handling practices.

ANNOTATED BIBLIOGRAPHY

Brown LW: Commentary: Infant botulism and the honey connection. J Pediatr 94:337–338, 1979. (Honey as a risk factor for infant botulism and a recommendation not to feed it to infants.)

Cooke EM: Epidemiology of foodborne illness: UK. Lancet 336:790–793, 1990. (Review of the more common and current causes of foodborne illness.)

Donadio JA, Gangarosa EJ, Faich GA: Diagnosis and treatment of botulism. J Infect Dis 124:108–112, 1971. (Review of classical botulism with a good discussion on its differential diagnosis.)

Hughes JM, Merson MH: Fish and shellfish poisoning. N Engl J Med 295:1117–1120, 1976. (Good general review of poisoning due to toxic fish and shellfish.)

Johnson RO, Clay SA, Arnon SS: Diagnosis and management of infant botulism. Am J Dis Child 133:586–593, 1979. (General review of infant botulism and its management.)

Roberts D: Factors contributing to outbreaks of food poisoning in England and Wales 1970–1979. J Hyg Camb 89:491–498, 1982. (Analysis of those factors contributing to food poisoning.)

Sours HE, Smith DG: Outbreaks of foodborne disease in the United States, 1972–1978. J Infect Dis 142:122–125, 1980. (Review of the epidemiology of food poisoning.)

Waites WM, Arbuthnott JP: Foodborne illness: An overview. Lancet 336:722–725, 1990. (Introduction and overview of a 16-article series in this journal on foodborne illness.)

181

Alcohol Intoxication

Steven M. Marcus

Calls to U.S. poison centers for exposure to alcohol represent 5% of the total call volume. The source of the ingested alcohol varies widely and includes alcoholic beverages, mouthwashes, cosmetics, windshield-wiper fluid, and even innocent-appearing "glo-sticks." Most of the accidental ingestions produce few, if any, symptoms. The potential, however, for serious toxicity from alcohol-containing products varies greatly and depends on the nature of the offending alcohol and the dose ingested. The dose ingested is, in turn, related to the mixture involved, the taste, and the age of the patient.

Patients ingesting alcohol-containing products range in age from infancy on up. The cause of the ingestion ranges from accidental ingestion in a child to intentional suicidal ingestion in the adolescent age group. In intentional or suicidal ingestions, alcohol is frequently the second or third substance ingested rather than the primary one.

All alcohols depress central nervous system (CNS) function; they all cause stupor, coma, and, in excessive quantities, even death. Death may occur from respiratory depression or the direct toxic effect on neurons. Many of the alcohol effects occur outside the CNS and can produce serious morbidity and mortality.

Alcohol is absorbed rapidly from the gastrointestinal tract. Absorption begins in the mouth and may be delayed by food in the stomach or by high concentrations of consumed alcohol. Peak blood levels after ingestion are achieved within 20 minutes on an empty stomach. Alcohols diffuse rapidly throughout the body and, because of their solubility in water, are distributed throughout total body water.

The CNS effects of alcohol frequently appear more rapidly than elevations in venous blood alcohol determinations. Arterial concentrations of alcohol rise more rapidly than venous concentrations and, hence, result in the rapid onset of lightheadedness and stupor after the ingestion of alcohol. Alcohols are metabolized in the liver by alcohol dehydrogenase. The elimination of ethanol by the kidneys, lungs, and sweat glands represents only 2% to 5% of the total ingested dose. The rate of alcohol oxidation by alcohol dehydrogenase is relatively constant at 100 mg/kg/hr of ethyl alcohol. This represents a mean of 16 mg/dl/hr when expressed as a decline in blood alcohol concentrations.

Because all alcohols are osmotically active, significant overdoses may predispose to a hyperosmolar state. This property can also be used to approximate blood alcohol concentrations if levels are unavailable. A blood ethanol concentration of 100 mg/dl increases the serum osmolarity by 22 mOsm/L. Alcohol intoxication is unlikely if osmolarity is only slightly increased or normal.

ETHANOL

Ethanol is the index alcohol for discussion. Ethanol, which is contained in beverages, mouthwashes, cosmetics, pharmaceuticals, elixirs, solvents, some brands of medicinal rubbing alcohol, and cooking products such as vanilla extract, is found in almost every household in the United States.

Experimental data suggest that most individuals with blood ethanol levels over 100 mg/dl will show signs of inebriation. As a "rule of thumb," 1 ml/kg of absolute ethanol results in blood alcohol levels above this value. Many individuals, however, particularly small children, will begin to show signs of insobriety, particularly stupor and even coma, at considerably lower levels.

The most common source of alcohol exposure is alcoholic beverages. Concentrations of ethanol in alcoholic beverages are reported in *proof*, which expresses approximately double the alcohol concentration in percent volume. Thus, a beverage that contains 80 proof contains 40% alcohol by volume. Because ethanol is less dense than water, the quantity of alcohol in weight is slightly less than the volume.

Adolescents frequently "experiment" with alcoholic beverages. Frequently abused are wine coolers, which are mixtures of fruit juices and alcohol. Fortified fruit wine coolers have recently been introduced. Ingestion of such fortified fruit coolers with alcohol concentrations of over 20% has resulted in outbreaks of serious adolescent toxicity. The use of "jello shots," jello made with vodka in lieu of water, by adolescents has similarly produced serious toxicity. Adolescents frequently ingest large quantities of such alcoholic beverages and lose consciousness prior to the complete absorption of such alcohol. Thus, these newer alcoholic beverages may act as virtual "time bombs."

Pathophysiology

Reports of hypoglycemia leading to convulsions, brain damage, and death have been reported as serious complications of acute ethanol ingestions in small children. The hypoglycemic effect of ethanol appears to be related to the impair-

Table 181-1.   Ethanol Intoxication

BLOOD ETHANOL LEVEL	CLINICAL SYNDROME
40–50 mg/dl	Inebriation, excessive laughter, hyperactivity or lethargy, slurred speech, blurred sensory input, relaxed inhibitions
100 mg/dl	Considered as presumptive evidence of impairment in most states
200 mg/dl	Marked muscular incoordination, blurred vision, stupor
300 mg/dl	Profound lethargy or stupor, hypoglycemia common, hypothermia not uncommon
500 mg/dl	Coma, depressed vital signs—potentially fatal

ment of gluconeogenesis as a result of an increased NADH/NAD ratio.

Some patients with ethanol overdose have a mild to moderate metabolic acidosis, which appears to be a true lactic acidemia secondary to the metabolism of the ethanol, the enhanced release of free fatty acids, and the accumulation of acetone and β-hydroxybutyrate. Vasodilatation and depression of the cardiovascular centers of the brain may lead to pooling of blood in the periphery and an increased heat loss with subsequent hypothermia.

Ethanol is a competitor of antidiuretic hormone (ADH). Acute intoxications have produced a diabetes insipidus–like syndrome with excessive fluid losses. The metabolism of ethanol also requires seven molecules of water for every molecule of ethanol metabolized. These fluid losses, when combined, can represent substantial fluid shifts and can produce serious dehydration (Table 181-1). Aside from symptomatic treatment, especially of hypoglycemia, no specific therapy is available. The recommendations for the severely intoxicated patient are:

- Protect the patient's airway. If the patient is not breathing, tracheal intubation should be provided to facilitate respiratory support.
- Provide intravenous fluids to counteract or prevent dehydration.
- Administer dextrose intravenously if the patient is hypoglycemic.
- Treat by aggressive use of fluid and bicarbonate if metabolic acidosis is present.
- Induction of emesis is rarely indicated. Absorption of alcohol is generally completed by the time the patient is seen.
- Activated charcoal fails to bind significant amounts of ethanol and, therefore, is of little use.
- Consider hemodialysis with potentially lethal concentrations of ethanol.

METHANOL

Methanol, also known as methyl alcohol, wood alcohol, acetone alcohol, and Manhattan spirit, is a well-known substance that is used frequently as an industrial solvent, antifreeze, and fuel. Common sources of methanol exposure in children are windshield-wiper fluid and phonographic record-cleaning fluid.

Methanol intoxication can present with significant CNS effects similar to those of ethanol. The more serious effects of methanol, however, are extraneurologic.

Oxidation, like that of ethanol, proceeds in the liver by way of the enzyme alcohol dehydrogenase. In the case of methanol, the metabolite formic acid is considerably more toxic than the metabolite of ethanol, acetaldehyde. Symptoms of methanol poisoning may be delayed for a long time because of the delay in metabolic production of the toxic product. Once the latent period is over, characteristic findings include a significant metabolic acidosis with swelling, edema, and redness of the retina and optic disc.

The early period of insobriety or inebriation is followed characteristically by an asymptomatic latent period. The characteristic symptoms and signs may appear between 6 and 30 hours after the ingestion. These signs consist of vertigo, vomiting, abdominal pain, diarrhea, back pain, shortness of breath, motor restlessness, blurring of vision, and hyperemia of the optic disc. The visual disturbance may proceed to optic atrophy, and pupillary light reflexes may be diminished or absent.

Data suggest that the prognosis in methanol overdose is more closely related to the delay in onset of therapy and to the presence of acidosis than to the concentration of methanol. The treatment of methanol intoxication depends on the preferential metabolism of ethanol by alcohol dehydrogenase. The administration of ethanol depresses the rate of oxidation of methanol and, hence, delays or prevents its metabolism to formic acid, blocking its biochemical and clinical effects.

Methanol is excreted only to a small extent by the lung, the sweat glands, and the kidneys. Treatment with hemodialysis is recommended if evidence of toxicity from methanol exists, or if there are significant elevations in methanol concentration. The following protocol is suggested:

- If a significant methanol ingestion is suspected, a blood determination of methanol concentration, electrolytes, and blood gases should be obtained. A measurement of serum osmolality and comparison with a calculated osmolality can be used to estimate the concentration of methanol in the blood if a blood methanol level cannot be obtained.
- Attention to the airway and to the circulatory volume is essential. Correction of any acidosis with bicarbonate is imperative.
- Ethanol should be administered in all cases of significant methanol intoxication to achieve and maintain a blood

ethanol concentration of 100 mg/dl. Once the concentration of methanol is available, a decision can be made regarding whether methanol should be removed by hemodialysis. It is generally accepted that when blood methanol levels are greater than 50 mg/dl, hemodialysis should be considered.

ISOPROPYL ALCOHOL

Isopropyl alcohol is found widely in the home and in industry, both as a solvent and as rubbing alcohol or as a sterilizing agent.

In the home, isopropyl alcohol is found in small quantities in various skin lotions, hair tonic, some after-shave lotions, window-cleaning solutions, and household detergents. Isopropyl alcohol is most commonly encountered as 70% solution, intended for use as rubbing alcohol. Not all solutions labeled as rubbing alcohol will contain isopropyl alcohol; some will contain denatured ethanol rather than isopropyl alcohol. Most of the preparations of rubbing alcohol are in pint containers without child-resistant packaging or child-resistant caps.

Isopropyl alcohol appears to be more toxic than ethyl alcohol but significantly less toxic than methanol. On a molar basis, it is about twice as potent as ethanol in producing insobriety. Isopropyl alcohol is absorbed rapidly and completely through the gastrointestinal tract and by inhalation. Isopropyl alcohol appears to be metabolized at a rate slower than that of ethanol.

The use of isopropyl alcohol in water to lower fever in children has been reported to cause stupor and even coma secondary to the absorption of isopropyl alcohol from both inhalation and transdermal absorption. It is thought, however, that the inhalation route is the more important route of absorption. The metabolism of isopropyl alcohol produces relatively large quantities of acetone without the production of appreciable quantities of acetoacetate, acetoacetic acid, or β-hydroxybutyric acid; thus, the diagnosis of isopropyl alcohol ingestion is made frequently on the basis of the presence of nonacidotic ketosis.

The ingestion of isopropyl alcohol frequently produces gastritis with vomiting and occasional hematemesis. Most emesis occurs early and is thought to be a local reaction. Systemic symptoms such as stupor and insobriety frequently occur within 30 minutes of ingestion.

Treatment

As with most ingested alcohol, absorption occurs so rapidly that gastric lavage or gastric emptying may not be efficacious. However, because isopropyl alcohol is frequently ingested in concentrated form and because high concentrations of alcohol lower the rate of absorption of alcohol, gastric emptying may remove significant quantities of isopropyl alcohol.

BENZYL ALCOHOL

The presence of benzyl alcohol as a preservative in many intravenous (IV) fluids leads to a syndrome of gasping in newborns. This appears to occur from the metabolism of benzyl alcohol by way of oxidation to benzoic acid and hippuric acid. In prematures with relatively low renal clearances, this leads to an accumulation of these compounds in the serum. Following the reports of illness in several infants in whom solutions of benzyl alcohol were used, a warning was released by the Food and Drug Administration alerting clinicians to the dangers of exposure in infancy. One must carefully consider the possibility that IV medications and heparin may contain benzyl alcohol if planning to use them in small infants or in patients with inadequate renal function.

ETHYLENE GLYCOL

Ethylene glycol is commonly found in permanent antifreeze and is available in many homes. In addition to its widespread use, it is frequently packaged as an attractive and colorful but odorless liquid. The liquid has a pleasant, warm, sweet taste; thus, ingestions are frequently in substantial quantities. Although it has a low toxicity, ethylene glycol is metabolized by alcohol dehydrogenase to oxalic acid, and this metabolite may cause cardiac and renal toxicity as well as significant and sometimes profound acidosis.

On presentation, the patient may appear to be inebriated as with all alcohols, although in this ingestion the absence of an alcoholic breath is characteristic. As in methanol overdose, there may be a time lag of several hours between the ingestion and the onset of toxicity because of the formation of a toxic metabolite. Many patients experience nausea, vomiting, and hematemesis; however, the major effects are those in the CNS, with the patient frequently presenting in coma. As with methanol, a latent period when the patient appears to be getting better is followed by progressive acidosis, flank pain, and oliguric acute renal failure.

Ethylene glycol poisoning must be suspected in patients who appear inebriated but who have no smell of alcohol on their breath. With a history of ingesting some form of antifreeze, ethylene glycol should be the primary consideration. The presence of oxalate crystals in the urine supports the diagnosis of ethylene glycol intoxication. An elevated measured serum osmolarity lends further support to the diagnosis of ethylene glycol intoxication.

Once the presumptive diagnosis of ethylene glycol intoxication is made, the further conversion of ethylene glycol must be blocked through the administration of ethyl alcohol. Hemodialysis or hemoperfusion may be necessary to remove the unmetabolized ethylene glycol.

ANNOTATED BIBLIOGRAPHY

Gershanik J, Boecler B, Ensley H et al: The gasping syndrome and benzyl alcohol poisoning. N Engl J Med 307:1384–1388, 1982.

(Describes the experience with 10 newborns and discusses the metabolism of benzyl alcohol.)

McCoy HG, Cipolle RJ, Ehlers SM et al: Severe methanol poisoning: Application of a pharmacokinetic model for ethanol therapy and hemodialysis. Am J Med 67:804–807, 1979. (Two case reports, with a general discussion and literature review.)

Moss MH: Alcohol-induced hypoglycemia in coma caused by alcohol sponging. Pediatrics 4:445–446, 1970. (Report of alcohol intoxication secondary to the absorption of inhaled ethyl or isopropyl alcohol vapor during sponge bathing.)

Ricci L, Hoffman S: Ethanol-induced hypoglycemic coma in a child. Ann Emerg Med 11:202–204, 1982. (Case report of ethanol-induced hypoglycemic coma in a small child after an accidental ingestion of ethanol; is also a nice review.)

Smithline N, Gardner KD: Gaps—Anionic and osmolal. JAMA 236:1594–1597, 1976. (Discussion of anionic and osmolar gaps with clinical implications.)

Stokes JB, Aureon F: Prevention of organ damage in massive ethylene glycol ingestion. JAMA 243:2065–2066, 1980. (Case report of massive ethylene glycol poisoning and brief discussion of therapy.)

22

SIGNS, SYMPTOMS, AND SYSTEMIC PROBLEMS

182

Identification of a Sick Child

Paul L. McCarthy

Children in the first 2 years of life have approximately four to six acute infectious episodes per year. The number of episodes each year lessens as the child grows older. Thus, the young child with an acute infectious illness is a common problem for pediatricians. This review concentrates primarily on the differentiation of the child with an acute illness that is minor or trivial from the child with an acute illness that is serious.

DIFFERENTIAL DIAGNOSIS

In the study of 1169 consecutive children of all ages with fever who presented to Yale-New Haven Hospital's pediatric emergency department, ~30% had otitis media and 50% had diagnoses of *viral syndrome, viral upper respiratory infection (URI), viral gastroenteritis,* or *flulike illness.* Approximately 18% had diagnoses of the more common serious infectious illnesses that the physician sees in pediatric patients: pneumonia (12%), bacteremia (4%), and urinary tract infections (UTIs) (1%). One patient in 300 had bacterial meningitis. Other diagnoses, such as varicella and DPT reaction, made up the remainder.

In another study, 330 consecutive children less than 24 months of age with a fever ≥104°F were evaluated extensively in the same emergency department and were followed carefully until they became well. The diagnoses in these children are shown in Table 182-1. Bacteremia, bacterial meningitis, and pneumonia were seen slightly more often than in the first series of 1169 unselected patients.

CLINICAL PRESENTATION

Do these common serious illnesses in febrile children represent a diagnostic challenge? In the study of 330 children with high fever, the examining physician was asked to list a diagnosis based on the history and physical examination and before laboratory data were obtained. Ninety-five percent of 20 instances of bacteremia without meningitis, over 50% of 52 episodes of pneumonia, and all three instances of urinary tract infection were not diagnosed by the initial history and physical examination. All four instances of bacterial meningitis were diagnosed by the initial history and physical examination. The 49 episodes of unrecognized serious illnesses occurred when the impression after the history and physical examination was either otitis media (7 patients with pneumonia and 9 patients with bacteremia) or a nonspecific febrile illness (20 instances of pneumonia, 10 of bacteremia, and 3 of urinary tract infection).

It is not surprising that these common serious illnesses may be clinically silent in the febrile child <24 months old. An optimal chest examination in the young child is difficult because of noncooperation and a respiratory rate more rapid than that of the adult. Bacteremia, especially that caused by *Streptococcus pneumoniae,* most frequently presents in the febrile child as a minor illness such as a URI, a fever without an apparent source, or otitis media. Most patients with a UTI may present with nonspecific findings such as fever, irritability, decreased feeding, or mild gastrointestinal symptoms. Bacterial meningitis may be an occult infection in a child. Samson found that 11 of 152 patients with bacterial meningitis did not have nuchal rigidity, Brudzinski sign, bulging fontanelle, or depressed sensorium. All of these children were less than 16 months of age and had had a febrile seizure. Therefore, meningeal signs may not be reliably present in the age group at greatest risk for meningitis. Serious illnesses are special diagnostic challenges in children less than 3 months of age. In this group, there is a

Table 182-1. Diagnosis in 330 Children <24 Months with Temperature ≥104°F

DIAGNOSIS	NUMBER*
Recognizable bacterial infection:	
Bacterial meningitis	4
Bacteremia	20
Urinary tract infection	2
Cellulitis	3
Shigellosis—other	2
Pneumonia	51
Otitis media	122
Recognizable viral illness:	
Exanthem—enanthem	19
Croup	5
Gastroenteritis	6
Aseptic meningitis	12
Nonspecific illness	84

*Children with two positive laboratory tests are classified under only one final diagnosis.

higher occurrence of sepsis and meningitis, and the organisms causing these infections are often group B streptococcus or gram-negative organisms. Pneumonia may be caused by *Staphylococcus aureus* or gram-negative bacteria. Finally, there is a higher occurrence of bacteremic UTIs in these patients.

WORK-UP

Information that the pediatrician has available for the diagnosis of the child with an acute infectious illness comes from several sources: observing the child, taking a history, performing a physical examination, assessing age and temperature risk factors, and using laboratory tests.

Observing a febrile child before the history and the physical examination is a key part of the diagnostic process. These observation data supplement the history and physical examination. The history has some limitations in evaluating febrile children because the child often cannot tell us what "hurts." For example, costovertebral angle pain in a child with pyelonephritis might present in the history only as the mother's perception of fever, crying, and decreased appetite. The two most frequently used observation variables to judge the degree of illness involve the use of the child's eyes (looking at the observer and looking around the room). Eye function or appearance can be described in many ways; for example, shiny, bright, looks at observer, glassy, stares vacantly into space. These descriptions probably reflect what pediatricians mean by the term *alertness*.

Other observation data that are also frequently used include the child's sitting, moving arms and legs on table or lap, lying limply on table, and not moving in mother's arms. These phrases describe and define what is often referred to as *motor ability*.

Several of the most commonly used observation variables, including vocalizing spontaneously, playing with objects, reaching for objects, smiling, and crying with noxious stimuli, are descriptions of data that are referred to as *playfulness* and severe impairment which is termed *irritability*.

Another commonly used observation variable is the response of a crying child to being held by the parent. A normal response is that the child stops crying when held by the parent. Severe impairment can be indicated, for example, by a continual cry despite being held and comforted. These data probably represent a more precise description of what is termed *consolability*. Most observation variables correspond to the child's response to stimuli rather than to "organic" variables such as petechiae and nasal flaring. Variables relating to eye appearance or function, for example, stimulus–response data about the eyes (e.g., looks at pen being offered), are noted much more often than are "organic" data about the eyes (e.g., sunken, red, glassy). More experienced pediatricians rely more heavily on stimulus–response data than do less experienced physicians. Thus, the judgment of the degree of illness by observation is based largely on the assessment of the interaction between the child and his or her environment. The extent of the interaction is often immediately apparent. The child smiles at the observer and reaches for the offered pen. At other times, the child cries and clings to the mother. The experienced examiner orchestrates the stimuli in an attempt to make the child act normally. To accomplish this, the pediatrician must know what is an appropriate stimulus for children of various ages and what is a developmentally appropriate response. Thus, observation of febrile children is a complex process involving both developmental skills and clinical skills. Pediatricians must assess the child's responses to multiple stimuli and must also be alert to clinical clues such as sunken eyes or cyanosis.

Observation data have been further examined to identify those criteria that are the key predictors of serious illness in febrile children. Six items have been identified, and each has a three-point scale: 1 = normal, 3 = moderate impairment, and 5 = severe impairment. The items and their scales are termed the *Yale Observation Scales* (Table 182-2). Note that four of six items concern the child's response to stimuli. When these six items and their scales are used in practice, the best possible score is 6 × 1 = 6; the worst possible score is 6 × 5 or 30. Nearly two of three children with acute illnesses have been found to have scale scores ≤10 (i.e., appear well), and less than 3% of these children have serious illnesses. On the other hand, severely ill–appearing children with a scale score ≥16 are relatively uncommon, but if such a child is seen, the chance of serious illness is high (92% in one study). Approximately one in four children appear moderately ill (scale score 11–15), and even here the chance of a serious illness is high (26% in the same study). The occurrence of serious illness in moderately or severely ill–appearing febrile children as defined

Table 182-2. Six Observation Items and Their Scales (Yale Observation Scales)

OBSERVATION ITEM	1 NORMAL	3 MODERATE IMPAIRMENT	5 SEVERE IMPAIRMENT
Quality of cry	Strong with normal tone OR content and not crying	Whimpering OR sobbing	Weak OR moaning OR high pitched
Reaction to parental stimulation	Cries briefly then stops OR content and not crying	Cries off and on	Continual cry OR hardly responds
State variation	If awake → stays awake OR If asleep and stimulated → wakes up quickly	Eyes close briefly → awake Awakes with prolonged stimulation	Falls to sleep OR will not rouse
Color	Pink	Pale extremities OR acrocyanosis	Pale OR cyanotic OR mottled OR ashen
Hydration	Skin normal, eyes normal AND mucous membranes moist	Skin and eyes are normal AND mouth is slightly dry	Skin doughy OR tented AND dry mucous membranes AND sunken eyes
Response (talk, smile) to social overtures	Smiles OR alerts (≤2 mo)	Brief smile OR alerts briefly (≤2 mo)	No smile Face anxious, dull, expressionless OR no alerting (≤2 mo)

by a scale score >10 is 13 times greater than the occurrence in well-appearing children (scale score ≤10).

What is the relation between data gathered by observation and the results of the history and physical examination? In one study, 36 of 350 children with acute infectious illness had a serious illness. Ill appearance, abnormal history, and abnormal physical examination were equally important in detecting serious illnesses. The history and physical examination together detected 78% (28 of 36) of children with serious illnesses. However, it was a combination of observation, history, and physical examination that had the highest sensitivity for serious illnesses and detected 86% (31 of 36) of children with such illnesses.

The abnormalities found on a history and a physical examination have also been analyzed. Findings relating to the pulmonary or central nervous systems represent most abnormalities; in addition, abnormalities of the pulmonary and central nervous systems have the strongest correlation with serious illnesses. This is not surprising because diseases of these systems represent 60% to 65% of serious illnesses in children with acute infectious illnesses.

Children with acute infectious illnesses can also be assessed for age or temperature risk factors. Selected serious illnesses occur in febrile children <3 months old (see Chap. 196). There is also an association between height of temperature and serious illness. As the degree of fever increases, so does the risk of bacteremia. The occurrence of bacteremia in young children is ~7% when the temperature is ≥104°F, 13% when the temperature is 105 to 105.9°F, and increases to 26% when the temperature is ≥106°F. In addition, there is a 10% occurrence of bacterial meningitis when the fever is ≥106°F (see Chap. 198).

Laboratory Tests

Screening laboratory studies may be helpful in identifying the child at increased risk for many of the common serious illnesses discussed. For example, a WBC ≥15,000 per mm³ or ESR ≥30 mm/hr in children ≤24 months with a fever ≥104°F places those children at five times the risk of bacteremia (15% versus 3%) compared to children in whom the WBC is <15,000 and the ESR is <30. A similar risk of bacteremia occurs with combinations of WBC ≥15,000 per mm³, PMN count ≥10,000 per mm³, and band count ≥500 per mm³. The risk of *any* serious illness in febrile children is approximately twice as great if the WBC is ≥15,000 per mm³ or the ESR is ≥30 mm/hr as it is if neither of these elevations is present. Thus, screening laboratory tests, though far from perfect in detecting serious illnesses in febrile children, can point toward an increased risk of these illnesses.

The foregoing considerations in this chapter have implications for ordering laboratory tests in children with acute infectious illnesses. Children at greatest risk for serious illnesses are those who have an ill appearance, abnormal history findings, or abnormal physical examination findings. Such patients constitute 20% to 30% of febrile children. The specific findings from observation, history, and physical examination dictate the laboratory evaluation. For example, if abnormal physical examination findings suggest pneumonia, a chest roentgenogram is indicated. An ill appearance, with or without other abnormal findings, warrants a laboratory evaluation. The studies ordered can be based on other associated findings. For example, an ill-appearing febrile child with rhinorrhea is a better candidate for blood culture, lumbar puncture, and chest roentgenogram than he or she is for a urine or stool culture. The history information may provide clues to the diagnosis; for example, the child with a history of bloody diarrhea with a nonspecific physical examination should have a stool culture performed. The interpretation of an ill appearance, abnormal history, or physical examination and the subsequent ordering of laboratory tests can be aided by a consideration of age and temperature risk factors. Ill appearance with a nonspecific physical examination in a child <3 months old warrants a full sepsis work-up. Fever ≥104°F in an ill-appearing febrile child, with or without abnormal history or physical examination findings, suggests a bacterial bloodstream invasion, and a blood culture is a minimal part of the laboratory evaluation.

A child with an acute infectious illness may, on the other hand, appear well and may demonstrate no abnormal history or physical examination findings suggestive of a serious illness. That is, the illness seems nonspecific or suggests that a minor illness such as otitis media may be present. Laboratory studies are not indicated if no age or temperature risk factors are present. The child may be followed expectantly, or the otitis media may be treated. The largest proportion of febrile children, perhaps 60% to 65%, meet these criteria. The risk for serious illness is low, and it is reasonable to forego a laboratory evaluation.

In well-appearing children with acute illness, without an abnormal history or physical examination, the implications of age <3 months or temperature ≥104°F for ordering laboratory tests are less clear. Some would argue that these risk factors alone are indications for a further work-up; others would argue that no work-up is indicated. Until data prove otherwise, it is prudent and reasonable to perform sepsis work-ups on febrile children <3 months old and to admit these patients to the hospital for observation. For febrile infants older than 28 days, some authors have advocated using IM ceftriaxone on an outpatient basis in lieu of hospitalization if the sepsis work-up is normal. Careful outpatient follow-up is mandatory. The use of expectant antibiotics once the infant is hospitalized and while awaiting cultures is a matter of judgment, but it is probably wise in children <6 weeks of age. If high fever (≥104°F) is detected in a child between 3 and 24 months old, a blood culture is indicated; a screening WBC or WBC/ESR may aid in the decision to obtain a blood culture (see also Chap. 198).

MANAGEMENT/ADMISSION

The decision to admit a child with an acute infectious illness to the hospital or to follow the child as an outpatient is based on several considerations:

- *Age*—The management and treatment of the febrile infant <3 months old should be handled as discussed above.

- *Appearance*—The child who appears ill, even in the absence of a specific diagnosis after the initial clinical and laboratory evaluation, should be admitted to the hospital. Antibiotics can be started once bacterial cultures have been obtained.

- *Diagnosis*—Certain diagnoses, such as bacterial meningitis, warrant admission and intravenous antibiotics. Other diagnoses, such as pneumonia, do not necessarily warrant admission. Factors such as the degree of distress, the extent of organ involvement (in this case, the extent of the pneumonia), and the ability of the parents to observe and care for the child and to keep follow-up appointments are critical considerations regarding admission.

If the decision is made to follow the child on an outpatient basis, then the follow-up evaluation can serve many purposes. The physician can ascertain if symptoms are resolving. If a serious illness, such as pneumonia, has been diagnosed, one can ascertain if the child is responding to therapy. Outpatient follow-up can become part of the diagnostic process when the diagnosis was not apparent at the initial visit. The follow-up visit can also serve as an opportunity to support and educate the parents.

ANNOTATED BIBLIOGRAPHY

Baron MA, Fink HD: Bacteremia in private pediatric practice. Pediatrics 66:171–175, 1980. (Discusses the use of screening laboratory tests in private pediatric practice to detect serious illness, such as bacteremia, in febrile children.)

Baskin MN, O'Rourke EJ, Fleisher GR: Outpatient treatment of febrile infants 28–89 days of age with intramuscular administration of ceftriaxone. J Pediatr 120:22–27, 1992. (Largest series to date concerning the use of ceftriaxone on an outpatient basis for febrile infants 28–89 days of age; outcome was excellent.)

McCarthy PL (ed): The Evaluation and Management of Febrile Children. Norwalk, CT, Appleton–Century–Crofts, 1985. (Concentrates on the use of clinical judgment in detecting the common serious illnesses in children with acute infections: meningitis, pneumonia, bacteremia, bacterial diarrhea, urinary tract infection.)

McCarthy PL, Jekel JF, Dolan TF: Temperature greater than or equal to 40°C in children less than 24 months of age: A prospective study. Pediatrics 59:663–668, 1977. (Reports on a large series of children ≤24 months old with high fever; discusses differential diagnosis and the value of screening laboratory tests.)

McCarthy PL, Jekel JF, Stashwick CA et al: Further definition of history and observation variables in assessing febrile children. Pediatrics 67:687–693, 1981. (Definition of the observation data on which pediatricians rely to make a judgment of toxicity.)

McCarthy PL, Sharpe MR, Spiesel SZ et al: Observation scales to identify serious illness in febrile children. Pediatrics 70:802–809, 1982. (Scales that can be used to judge, in a systematic way, the appearance of a child with an acute infectious illness.)

McCarthy PL, Sznajderman SD, Lustman-Findling K et al: Mothers' clinical judgment: A randomized trial of the Acute Illness Observation Scales. J Pediatr 116:200–206, 1990. (Describes the characteristics of mothers' clinical judgment.)

Samson JH: Febrile seizures and purulent meningitis. JAMA 210: 1918–1920, 1969. (Discusses the problem of a lack of selected clinical findings in children with bacterial meningitis.)

Wright PF, Thompson J, McKee KT et al: Patterns of illness in the highly febrile young child: Epidemiologic, clinical and laboratory correlates. Pediatrics 67:694–700, 1981. (Describes the value of a pediatrician's impression of toxicity in detecting febrile children with serious illnesses.)

183

Fever

Robert A. Dershewitz

Fever in children arouses much parental, and occasionally provider, concern. Its presence is one of the most common reasons for parents to seek medical care.

Because of circadian variations and the influence of multiple factors (e.g., activity) on the body's temperature, the healthy child's temperature fluctuates within a "normal" range. Body temperature is lowest between 2:00 and 6:00 AM and highest between 5:00 and 7:00 PM, and this diurnal pattern persists in the presence of a fever. If the temperature exceeds 38.0°C (100.4°F) rectally, 37.8°C (100°F) orally, or 37.2°C (99°F) axillary, the temperature is said to be elevated, and hence there is a fever.

The vast majority of fevers in children result from infection. The fever response is initiated when any of multiple agents, such as viruses and bacteria, are phagocytosed by leukocytes. Interleukin-1 (formerly called endogenous pyrogen) is produced and stimulates the production of prostaglandins, which act on the thermoregulatory mechanism in the hypothalamus. The body's thermostat is upwardly readjusted, and temperature becomes elevated by such mechanisms as increasing metabolism and peripheral vasoconstriction.

DETERMINATION OF FEVER

Although touch cannot yield a precise measurement of temperature, one can usually tell by touch when the child's temperature is high (i.e., above 103°F). Hands and feet should not be used to gauge fever because they may be cold from peripheral vasoconstriction. A glass mercury thermometer has been the traditional instrument to measure temperature, but for reasons of sanitation, comfort, and speed, electronic and tympanic membrane thermometers are increasingly being used. Tympanic membrane thermometers measure emitted infrared energy and have excellent correlation with glass mercury thermometers, even in children having acute otitis media. In a high-volume practice, advantages may offset the cost of the instrument. Rectal thermometers should not be used in neutropenic patients for fear of rectal trauma. Many pediatricians fear using oral thermometers in children under 4 to 5 years of age. The accuracy of axillary measurements is controversial. In clinical practice, it is usually used in newborn nurseries (to avoid risk of cross-contamination and rectal perforation), in the infant or toddler with diarrhea, in the uncooperative child, and in any child when simply knowing a fever exists, rather than obtaining an exact temperature, is desired. For reasons of ease, convenience, and safety, liquid crystal forehead strips have become popular. Unfortunately, they are unreliable.

Except for ear thermometers, all children must be still when their temperatures are taken. A lubricated rectal thermometer is gently inserted 3 to 6 cm and left inside for 1 to 3 minutes with the buttocks squeezed together. If inserted further, a higher core body temperature will be recorded. An oral thermometer should be placed on either side of the posterior sublingual pocket and left in place for 3 minutes. Parents should be cautioned not to give the child hot or cold food just before taking the temperature. For an axillary temperature, the thermometer should be left in a dry axilla for 4 minutes.

TO TREAT OR NOT TO TREAT

By itself, the presence of fever is not necessarily the marker of a child who is sicker than one who has the same symptoms but is without fever. In fact, hypothermia is usually much more ominous than hyperthermia. Although the majority of febrile children have trivial illness, fever should provoke high anxiety in certain conditions. These include: newborns (especially under 6 weeks of age), fever above 105°F (greater incidence of bacteremia), and the child who is immunodeficient, lethargic, or inconsolable. The febrile child with disorientation, meningismus, petechiae, or purpura constitutes a medical emergency. The identification of a sick child is covered in Chapter 182.

Clearly, all children with fevers do not need antipyretic medication. Most children are not made ill or uncomfortable by a temperature elevation per se. Children who appear to be uncomfortable by the fever, regardless of its height, should receive medication. Although brain damage does not occur with fever below 107°F (41.7°C), most clinicians recommend antipyretics in children whose fevers are 105°F (40.5°C) or greater to prevent temperatures from reaching dangerous levels (a rare event) and to prevent febrile seizures. Children with a history of febrile seizure and those in whom the side effects of a fever may be harmful (e.g., borderline dehydration, compensated cardiac disease) should have aggressive fever management.

The arguments against treating a fever appear to be less cogent. Although fever may enhance the body's ability to fight infection by several mechanisms, such as stimulating phagocyte mobility, this primarily laboratory effect has not been convincingly demonstrated in clinical practice. Allowing a fever to remain neither hastens resolution of the illness nor impairs natural defense mechanisms.

Under certain circumstances, it may be advantageous to chart a fever pattern, but in the ambulatory setting, concern about obscuring this pattern is usually unwarranted (see Chap. 184, "Fever of Unknown Origin"). The major reason for not treating a fever in an otherwise comfortable child is that temperatures under 106°F (but probably 107°F) are not harmful. Because antipyretic agents do not alter the course or duration of the disease causing the fever, therapeutic nihilists would argue against giving a medication if it would not be beneficial. Other reasons include the avoidance of overdose and untoward effects of the antipyretic.

DIFFERENTIAL DIAGNOSIS

The physical exam is far superior to lab tests at arriving at a diagnosis. The height of the fever, its duration, and its response to antipyretics are not helpful in differentiating viral from bacterial illness. Most fevers in children are of viral etiology. Typically, the fever does not exceed 104°F and resolves within 3 days, although it may last as long as 14 days. Most fevers above 107°F do not come from infection. Fever usually causes an increase in heart rate (10–15 beats per 1°C) and an increase in the respiratory rate. Their absence may be a clue to factitious fever, mycoplasmal infection, and typhoid fever. Malignancy, collagen-vascular disease, sickle cell disease, central nervous system (CNS) lesions, and hyperthyroidism usually cause signs and symptoms other than pyrexia to suggest the diagnosis. Fever in a child with gastroenteritis may be due to hypernatremia or dehydration. In a previously well child with a fulminant onset of hyperthermia, one should consider environmental causes (e.g., being overwrapped in blankets and sitting in a car parked in the sun with windows rolled up) and heat stroke. Other causes of acute onset of fever include immunization reaction, bites (e.g., ticks, spiders, snakes), and ingestions (e.g., salicylates and anticholinergics).

TREATMENT

All antipyretic agents act in the same way. They prevent prostaglandin synthesis, enabling the hypothalamic set-point to be lowered. The body then responds by dissipating heat by evaporation (perspiration) and vasodilation (flushed appearance). Acetaminophen has replaced salicylate as the mainstay of treatment because it has fewer side effects, is not associated with Reye syndrome, and is available as a liquid preparation. Both medications are equally effective antipyretics, and both have the same dose (i.e., 10–15 mg/kg/dose), given every 4 hours as needed. When given together, the temperature falls more than when either is given separately, and fever reduction lasts longer. In practice, this beneficial effect is usually unnecessary. Therapeutic efficacy has not been demonstrated by alternating aspirin and acetaminophen every 2 hours. Currently, there is little reason to use aspirin as an antipyretic.

Nonsteroidal anti-inflammatory agents (NSAIDs) are another therapeutic option to lower temperature. Ibuprofen 5 mg/kg/dose has an effect equal to acetaminophen 10 mg/kg. In children with temperatures of ≥102.5°F, ibuprofen 10 mg/kg/dose is more efficacious than either ibuprofen 5 mg/kg or acetaminophen 10 mg/kg. The duration of ibuprofen is 6 to 8 hours. Side effects are most often mild and gastrointestinal. It is not believed to be associated with Reye syndrome.

The choice of agents should be based on cost and safety. Acetaminophen currently holds the advantage. Ibuprofen is a good second-line drug and a good alternative for children who do not respond well to acetaminophen. With greater experience to establish its safety record and a price decrease, ibuprofen may become the antipyretic of choice.

Most children dislike being sponged. Sponging is not much more effective than undressing the child. Most often, sponging is unnecessary because it lowers the temperature only a little faster than does an antipyretic alone. If the temperature is extremely high or if aggressive fever management is indicated (e.g., to prevent recurrent febrile seizure and with overwhelming infection), children may be sponged, but only after the antipyretic medication is given. This is to lower the hypothalamic set-point (which sponging does not), thereby avoiding shivering from sponging, which may, in itself, raise the body temperature. The water should be lukewarm and the water temperature raised if the child shivers. The greater the exposure of skin to the water, the more rapid the body temperature will fall. Ice-water enemas and sponging with alcohol should be avoided. In special instances, sponging has a major role in reducing the temperature—such situations include children with severe liver disease; neurologic disorders in which the temperature regulatory mechanism is altered, thereby rendering the antipyretics ineffective; defective heat loss (e.g., heat stroke, ectodermal dysplasia), and excessive heat production (e.g., excessive environmental temperature, malignant hyperthermia). Only for these latter conditions may ice blankets or baths be used.

PARENT EDUCATION

Much of a pediatrician's illness management is devoted to mitigating or dispelling fever phobia. Parents should be taught that fever is a sign, not a disease, and that it is much more important to note how the child is acting rather than how high the fever is. Nevertheless, many parents will want firmer guidelines on when and how to treat their child's fever. Open lines of communication (including telephone) between doctor and parent should always be fostered. Parents should be told to call immediately if their newborn has a fever, if their child's fever is over 105°F, or if the child is twitching, lethargic, inconsolable, or has a stiff neck, a swollen joint, or a purplish rash. Less urgent indications for calling include a child whose fever has persisted for more than 3 days, a child who acts ill, or parents who want reassurance. If the child has had a febrile convulsion, prompt and aggressive fever management should be instituted for that and future episodes. Parents should be reassured that although febrile convulsions are to be avoided, they do not result in neurologic damage.

Parents should be taught to avoid overbundling or overdressing their febrile child. Finally, parents must administer the correct dose. As many as 25% of parents from all socioeconomic backgrounds may underdose with acetaminophen. One source of confusion may be that the dropper that comes with the bottle of infant drops is used in the less concentrated elixir form. A lack of fever response may result in undue anxiety and unnecessary office visits and lab tests.

ANNOTATED BIBLIOGRAPHY

Kenney RD, Fortenberry JD, Surratt SS et al: Evaluation of an infrared tympanic membrane thermometer in pediatric patients. Pediatrics 85:854–858, 1990. (Cost aside, this new technology in temperature taking is accurate and fast [less than 1 second].)

Robinson JS, Schwartz M-L, Magivene KS, et al: The impact of fever health education on clinic utilization. Am J Dis Child 143:698–704, 1989. (Audiovisual materials were effective in teaching parents fever management.)

Schmitt B: Fever in childhood. Pediatrics (Suppl) 74:929–936, 1984. (Good overall discussion, with excellent section on parent education.)

Walson PD, Galletta G, Braden NJ et al: Ibuprofen, acetaminophen and placebo treatment of febrile children. Clin Pharmacol Ther 46:9–17, 1989. (Double-blind study showing that ibuprofen is both safe and effective.)

Weisse ME, Miller GEA, Brien JF: Fever response to acetaminophen in viral vs bacterial infections. Pediatr Infect Dis J 6:1091–1094, 1987. (No correlation of fever response to etiology.)

184

Fever of Unknown Origin

Paul L. McCarthy

Fever of unknown origin (FUO) tests the diagnostic acumen of pediatricians. The array of laboratory tests that can be ordered is great; the clinician's goal should be to minimize the cost and trauma of studies while maintaining diagnostic accuracy.

DEFINITION AND PATHOPHYSIOLOGY

The differential diagnosis of FUO encompasses many disease entities. The pathophysiology of FUO is related to its etiology. For example, a fever due to an infection is different from that due to an autoimmune disorder. The duration of fever qualifies an illness to be termed *FUO*. Unfortunately, the definition of *duration* varies from one study to another. Pizzo and associates define FUO as fever $\geq 38.5°C$ on more than four occasions for at least a 2-week period. McClung's criteria are that the fever should last for 3 weeks and the cause should remain undiagnosed despite an active outpatient evaluation, or that the fever should last for longer than 1 week despite inpatient diagnostic efforts. It is unusual for fevers associated with most uncomplicated viral infections to last for more than 5 days. When a child has been febrile for 10 days or more and no cause is apparent, it is reasonable for the pediatrician to undertake the thorough evaluation mandated by the term *FUO*.

DIFFERENTIAL DIAGNOSIS

In their classical work of FUO, Petersdorf and Beeson reported on 100 adult patients and outlined an evaluative approach. However, the work done by Pizzo and associates and McClung raises many questions regarding the applicability of the adult experience with FUO (especially the differential diagnoses of FUO in adults) to children.

The occurrences of diagnostic categories in adults and children are compared in Table 184-1. The occurrence of infectious illnesses in adults and children is similar except for children less than 6 years of ago who, in Pizzo's series, had a higher incidence of infectious illnesses (65%). Infections in the adult series were unusual and included 11 patients with tuberculosis, 7 patients with hepatobiliary infections, and 4 patients with abdominal abscesses. Children, on the other hand, had other infections. In Pizzo's series, 34 of 100 children had bacterial infections and 18 children had viral illnesses. Of note, 22 of the 34 bacterial infections were those commonly seen in the pediatric age group: urinary tract infection (UTI) (4), pneumonia (4), tonsillitis (4), sinusitis (3), meningitis (3), septicemia (2), and streptococcosis (2). In McClung's series of 99 patients, 28 had bacterial infections and only 1 had a viral infection. Again, most bacterial illnesses (17 of 28) were not unusual infections: UTI (4), pneumonia (4), septicemia (3), tonsillitis (2), sinusitis (2), and meningitis (2).

Neoplastic disease is more common in adults: 19% versus 6% (Pizzo) and 8% (McClung). The types of tumors also differed. In adults, one half of tumors were solid tumors or disseminated carcinomas. In children, most were leukemias and lymphomas.

Collagen inflammatory diseases, most commonly systemic lupus erythematosus and acute rheumatic fever, were diagnosed in 13% of Petersdorf's patients. Collagen inflammatory diseases represented 20% of Pizzo's patients and

Table 184-1. Causes of FUO in Adults and Children

	ADULT PATIENTS (N = 100)*	CHILDREN (N = 100)†			CHILDREN (N = 99)‡
		<6 Yr	≥6 Yr	Total	
Infection	36%	65%	38%	52%	29%
Neoplastic	19%	8%	4%	6%	8%
Collagen	13%	8%	33%	20%	11%
Miscellaneous	25%	14%	6%	10%	10%
No diagnosis	7%	5%	19%	12%	11%
					30% (normal or resolving illness)

*Petersdorf RG, Beeson PB: Fever of unexplained origin: Report on 100 cases. Medicine 40:1, 1961.
†Pizzo PA, Lovejoy FH Jr, Smith DH: Prolonged fever in children: Review of 100 cases. Pediatrics 55:468, 1975.
‡McClung HJ: Prolonged fever of unknown origin in children. Am J Dis Child 124:544, 1972.

only 11% of McClung's patients, with juvenile rheumatoid arthritis causing approximately one half of the illnesses in both series. In Pizzo's series, 33% of children 6 years of age or older had juvenile rheumatoid arthritis (JRA). In Pizzo's series, 10% of children had miscellaneous diagnoses such as "CNS fever" (2%), dehydration (1%), Behçet's disease (1%), hepatitis (1%), ruptured appendix (1%), and other (4%). McClung had six patients in a miscellaneous category who had regional enteritis (3), thyroiditis (1), salicylate toxicity (1), and *erythroblastopenia* (1).

Twelve children remained undiagnosed in Pizzo's series; at least three continued to have symptoms for which an etiologic diagnosis was not established. In McClung's series, a total of 11 patients remained undiagnosed and continued to have symptoms such as arthralgias, abdominal pain, and fever.

WORK-UP

History

The most critical diagnostic maneuver in arriving at a diagnosis of a child with FUO is a carefully performed history and physical examination. In Pizzo's series, the history and physical examination could have diagnosed 62 of 100 patients. In McClung's series, the history and physical examination suggested the diagnosis in 87 of 99 patients.

It is necessary first to establish that the child does, in fact, have a fever. Dinarello and Wolff reported on over 400 patients who were said to have FUO and found that 18% actually did *not* have a fever. Most commonly, the fever was factitious (in 6%) or the technique of temperature taking or interpretation of temperature was erroneous (12%).

Physical Examination

Pizzo found the following signs and symptoms most useful:

- *Skin findings:* These include rash, pruritus, edema, and infection. Of the 24 patients with such findings, 6 patients had a malignancy and 8 patients had a fatal outcome.

- *Joint pain:* 14 patients had arthralgia, including 9 patients with a collagen-inflammatory disorder.
- *Joint findings:* Of the 9 patients with these findings, 6 had a collagen-inflammatory disorder.
- *Significant heart murmurs:* 4 of the 8 patients with a significant heart murmur had subacute bacterial endocarditis.
- *Chest pain, cyanosis, dyspnea:* 6 of 7 patients with these findings had a fatal outcome.
- *Hepatosplenomegaly:* This sometimes pointed toward malignancy.

Although Pizzo noted that fever patterns, anorexia, fatigue, chills, sweats, weight loss, abdominal pain, and adenopathy were unrelated to diagnosis or prognosis, the experiences of others are different. For example, the once-daily elevation of fever at the same time each day, often in association with abdominal and joint pain, may suggest juvenile rheumatoid arthritis (see Chap. 133). Weight loss and abdominal pain may indicate occult inflammatory bowel disease, whereas significant adenopathy may point toward malignancy or juvenile rheumatoid arthritis.

The physician should, therefore, carefully seek those signs and symptoms associated with the most common etiologies of FUOs in children. He or she should search carefully in particular for clues in a patient's history or physical examination that indicate bacterial infections that may present as FUOs (e.g., pneumonia, meningitis, UTI, sinusitis, tonsillitis, subacute bacterial endocarditis, and bacteremia-sepsis).

Laboratory Tests

A WBC, differential, platelet count, and erythrocyte sedimentation rate (ESR) should always be obtained. In McClung's series, four of five children with leukemia had abnormalities of the white blood count, differential, or platelet count. Pizzo found that anemia and elevated ESR indicated an active process; on the other hand, of 20 children with ESR <10 mm/hr, 18 had a fever secondary to a nonserious or viral illness. A shift to the left on the WBC suggests collagen-inflammatory disorders and bacterial infections.

The urinalysis is mandatory. In Pizzo's series, it helped establish the diagnosis in four patients with urinary tract infections, three with subacute bacterial endocarditis, and five with collagen-inflammatory disorders.

All children in Pizzo's series had chest roentgenograms performed, and 13 of these studies were abnormal.

Appropriate bacterial cultures of urine, blood, throat, cerebrospinal fluid, and stool are important for diagnosing common serious bacterial infections that can cause an FUO.

Because the occurrence of collagen-inflammatory disorders is high in children with FUO, investigating this possibility should be part of the initial laboratory evaluation and should include antinuclear antibodies, rheumatoid factor, quantitative immunoglobulins, and a serum complement.

A purified protein derivative (PPD) along with candida, mumps, and trichophyton controls should also be applied.

Consideration should be given to a bone marrow examination if the aforementioned studies do not result in a diagnosis. In Pizzo's series, 6 of the 14 bone marrow examinations were diagnostic: leukemia (4), lymphosarcoma (1), and agranulocytosis (1). An additional 6 of the 14 bone marrow examinations suggested either a collagen-inflammatory disease (with a plasma cell predominance) or an infectious process (with a *shifted-cell line*).

Other, more invasive biopsy, surgical, or radiologic procedures should be done only if the child continues to be symptomatic and no diagnosis has been established. These procedures may include an intravenous pyelogram (IVP), a GI series, a barium enema, a laparotomy, or biopsies (e.g., lymph node, liver). The yield from a liver biopsy and laparotomy in pediatric patients is far less than that in adult patients. A gallium scan is useful if the physician is concerned about an occult infectious focus that has not been identified by the bacterial cultures discussed previously. An abdominal computed tomography scan can sometimes identify a lesion that would not be apparent otherwise, such as an occult malignancy. Thus, these more invasive tests should be reserved for more perplexing patients with persisting symptoms that remain undiagnosed.

ADMISSION/TREATMENT

The decision to hospitalize a child should be based on several considerations. If the child does not appear severely ill and has no findings that suggest a serious illness, an outpatient work-up may be initiated. The technique of temperature taking should be reviewed with the parents and a fever diary should be kept. If, on the other hand, the child appears more severely ill, or has findings suggestive of a serious illness (e.g., hepatosplenomegaly), then inpatient care is warranted. Admission to the inpatient service may also be needed to document that the child has a fever. The temporal characteristics of the illness can also be appreciated better

while the child is an inpatient. For example, the child with systemic juvenile rheumatoid arthritis may have a fleeting *salmon* rash only once a day when the fever peak occurs, and these findings may be associated with severe joint achiness.

The therapy of FUO depends on the etiology. If it is established that the child has a fever, treatment with an antipyretic such as acetaminophen is reasonable. If the disease is a collagen-inflammatory process, an initial therapeutic trial of a nonsteroidal anti-inflammatory drug is warranted. In other circumstances, no antipyresis is warranted. These may include, but are not limited to, the following:

- Situations in which the fever has not been sufficiently documented or in which a purpose of the inpatient evaluation is to define the temperature pattern.
- Situations in which acute rheumatic fever is suspected and the physician wishes to establish whether the pattern of joint complaints is migratory. It may be wise to withhold salicylates because joint complaints in this disease often respond dramatically to aspirin.

Contraindications to using antipyretics include nonsteroidal anti-inflammatory drugs in a child with thrombocytopenia and acetaminophen in a child with liver disease.

ANNOTATED BIBLIOGRAPHY

Dinarello CA, Wolff SM: Pathogenesis of fever in man. N Engl J Med 298:607–612, 1978. (Discussion of mechanisms of fever with some comments on the NIH experience with FUO.)

McClung HJ: Prolonged fever of unknown origin in children. Am J Dis Child 124:544–550, 1972. (Value of the history and physical examination is clearly shown in this study.)

Petersdorf RG, Beeson PB: Fever of unexplained origin: Report on 100 cases. Medicine 40:1–30, 1961. (Classic article on FUO in adults.)

Pizzo PA, Lovejoy FH Jr, Smith DH: Prolonged fever in children: Review of 100 cases. Pediatrics 55:468–473, 1975. (Experience with FUO at a large children's hospital.)

185
Child with Recurrent Infections
Raoul L. Wolf

Recurrent infections are frequent in childhood, mainly as a consequence of exposure in nursery schools and other reservoirs of infection. The difficulty lies in determining when this problem indicates an underlying disorder, such as an immune defect. A careful history, noting the pattern of infections, and a planned clinical investigation can generally resolve this dilemma.

PATHOPHYSIOLOGY

Most recurrent infections occur within tubular structures, which are usually the middle ear, the lung, the nose and paranasal sinuses, and the kidney. The problem can be considered a result of either resistance of the organism to therapy or a defect in the host. Organisms, such as staphylococci, frequently become resistant to antibiotics. The choice of antibiotic may be incorrect or may lack specificity for the organism. However, the most common cause of antibiotic failure is failure to complete the course of treatment. Resistance to antibiotics and an inappropriate choice of antibiotic are also common causes for persistent infection. The host defects may be local or systemic. Local etiologic factors result in an obstruction of the lumen, causing stasis of air or fluid. Pathogenic organisms then persist in the lumen and become invasive. The infection responds to therapy, only to recur weeks or months later when stasis provides a medium in which pathogenic organisms can proliferate.

A wide range of systemic disorders cause recurrent infections by producing an immunologic dysfunction. Diabetes mellitus and sickle cell disease are examples. In diabetes, there is a reduction in lymphocyte function and a loss of tissue barriers. Patients with sickle cell disease suffer from a lack of opsonins in plasma and poor to absent splenic function. Immune defects can generally be considered as primary (congenital) or secondary. The primary defects involve either antibody production (humoral) or the interaction and function of lymphocytes and monocytes (cell mediated). These two processes are intimately linked. The lymphocytes are divided into two main groups: T cells and B cells. The T cells orchestrate the immune response, receiving signals from macrophages and other adherent cells. Macrophages process antigens and react to their presence, activating T cells during this sequence. The T cells pass information to and stimulate B cells, which proliferate, giving rise to plasma cells that secrete specific antibody binding. The antibody binds to the stimulating antigen, activating the complement pathway. This attracts polymorphonuclear cells to the site, where they ingest and destroy the complex. This intricate system can break down at many points.

The production of antibody may be defective, resulting in repeated otitis media, rhinosinusitis, and pneumonia, with rarer episodes of meningitis or sepsis. T-cell abnormalities result in severe infections or infections with unusual organisms such as *Pneumocystis carinii*. Growth retardation is prominent, and these children usually die at an early age. Associated anomalies are common. Defects in killing by polymorphonuclear cells result in an unusual condition called the *cold* abscess. This is the formation of an abscess without an inflammatory response that may involve the skin and viscera. Its presence is diagnostic of a functional defect in polymorphonuclear cells. The patient with recurrent *Neisseria* infectious organisms should be suspected of having a deficiency of the sixth or eighth component of serum complement.

CLINICAL PRESENTATION

Recurrent upper respiratory infections are common in childhood. Most of these are of viral etiology; only recurrent bacterial infections are likely to be associated with an immune defect. Several physical signs (e.g., high fever, rigors, purulent discharge, and sputum production) indicate bacterial infection. There are few physical signs that might indicate the need to work up a patient for an immune defect. The occurrence of three or more separate, presumed bacterial otitis media episodes within a 6-month period has been used as a guide by some centers. In such a patient, the absence or paucity of lymphoid tissue, especially tonsillar tissue, strongly suggests a B-cell deficiency. Arthritis involving large joints is often associated with immunodeficiency. Other features associated with immune defects may occur, such as thrombocytopenia, eczema, and cardiac defects; however, these occur in rare syndromes and are usually associated with severe infections.

A common problem (frequently frustrating to both patient and physician) is the question of recurrent boils and furuncles: these are rarely caused by an underlying immunologic or chronic systemic disease. Poor hygiene is more likely to be the reason for this type of persistent infection. The patient who has a deep abscess formation without an inflammatory response (cold abscess) is an exception. This is associated with an inability of polymorphonuclear cells to kill and is peculiar to the problem of *chronic granulomatous disease*.

Recurrent urinary tract infections are usually based on an underlying mechanical problem and are rarely associated with systemic diseases and immune defects.

DIFFERENTIAL DIAGNOSIS

There are two major differential considerations: the cause for recurrent infections lies with the organism or with the host.

Organisms

The infectious agent may be resistant to antibiotics, or the antibiotic may be incorrect or in a low concentration. The organism may become sequestered in an inaccessible area (e.g., renal parenchyma). The infection may be caused by an unusual or unexpected organism such as atypical mycobacteria. Another example could be a *Salmonella* species causing osteomyelitis.

Host Factors

Because most recurrent infections occur in hollow viscera, the causes can be considered in mechanical terms. These may lie in the lumen, in the wall, or outside the wall.

In the Lumen. Here one must consider the presence of a foreign body. This is one of the most common causes of recurrent infection in childhood. It may be a pea in a nostril or a peanut in a bronchus. A "check-valve" effect results in intermittent obstruction and also intermittent stasis. This cycle leads to clearing of infection followed by a recurrence of symptoms. Other causes in this category include deformities of the lumen such as congenital webs and strictures. Cystic fibrosis causes thickened mucus that traps organisms, allowing proliferation. Conditions in which there is a reservoir of infection are a related group of conditions. Bronchiectasis and chronic sinusitis are examples where seeding of infection to the lung is frequent. The infections are self-perpetuating because of an obstruction.

In the Wall. Distortions of the wall from tumors, benign or malignant, belong in this group. These masses may be carcinomata or hemangiomas. Inflammatory conditions can cause chronic thickening of the bronchial wall with an obstruction leading to poor drainage of secretions and repeated secondary infections. Granulomas, which occur in sarcoidosis, can obstruct drainage. Dysfunction of ureteral musculature causes poor peristalsis, with stasis then leading to a recurrent urinary tract infection.

Outside the Wall. Vascular anomalies often compress a bronchial lumen. Tumors may cause an obstruction of the ureters, bronchi, and sinuses. For example, granulomatous conditions such as Wegener's granulomatosis often present with repeated infections, particularly of the sinuses.

Several local conditions result from a combination of these three groups. *Dysfunctional cilia syndrome* is an unusual condition in which the cilia are abnormal and do not clear secretions. It results in recurrent sinusitis, bronchitis, pneumonia, and bronchiectasis. When a pneumonia recurs in the same lobe, usually the left lower lobe, the physician should consider a sequestration of that lobe or lobule. This is a congenital malformation in which the bronchi of the sequestered lobe do not communicate with the main bronchi. There is also no connection with the pulmonary vasculature. The blood supply is derived from the aorta by way of the bronchial vessels. Because of the poor communication with the rest of the lung, air stasis results in repeated infections and seeding to other parts of the lung.

SYSTEMIC CONDITIONS

Immunodeficiency

This group of diseases results from defects in humoral or cellular immunity; humoral defects are more frequent. These humoral disorders can be considered in two groups: selective defects and total or pan-hypogammaglobulinemia.

Humoral-Selective Deficiency. IgA deficiency is a selective defect and is the most common of the immune defects. It occurs with a frequency of $1:600$. Patients present with sinopulmonary infections and diarrhea. (Recently, several authors have questioned whether IgA deficiency is a disease or only a laboratory finding.)

Subclass IgG deficiency is usually a defect of IgG_2 but may be a defect of IgG_3 or IgG_4. There are four subclasses of IgG, and IgG_2 is concerned with the control of encapsulated organisms, such as *Haemophilus influenzae* and *Streptococcus pneumoniae*. These patients also develop sinopulmonary infections.

Humoral-Total Deficiency. Pan-hypogammaglobulinemia is best described by an X-linked disorder, known as *Bruton's agammaglobulinemia*. In this disorder, there is an absence of mature B cells, and antibody levels are low. Recurrent sinopulmonary infections are common, and meningitis occurs occasionally.

Another category of conditions is classified together as a *common variable immunodeficiency*. This group encompasses a variety of underlying problems, such as the inability to synthesize an antibody or to release it from cells.

Cellular Defects. Defects of cell-regulated immunity are much rarer. These patients develop severe systemic infections often with opportunistic organisms such as *P. carinii* and *Mycoplasma pneumoniae*. Many patients have associated abnormalities that may draw attention to the immunologic problem. Failure to thrive is common. Viremia and septicemia often cause an early demise. There is a wide range of underlying defects in this condition. The thymus may be absent, stem cells may not mature into T cells, or an arrest may occur in the development of T cells.

There are subclasses of T cells, predominantly helper and suppressor. Several conditions cause disturbances in the normal cell ratio of 2 helper: 1 suppressor. The most striking example of this problem is the acquired immunodeficiency syndrome (AIDS). This disease is caused by a virus, HIV, that destroys helper T cells. This results in excessive suppression, leading to overwhelming infection by cytomegalovirus, hepatitis B virus, and Epstein–Barr virus. Persistent candidiasis is often present. Malignancy is common. The condition occurs in children, usually associated with hemophilia and blood transfusions, or transmission of the virus by an infected mother (see also Chap. 52). Epstein—Barr virus may also cause severe immunologic disturbances.

Polymorphonuclear Cell Defects. Defects in the ability of polymorphonuclear cells to kill organisms cause recurrent abscess formation. The best known cause is chronic granulomatous disease. The cold abscess is typical of this deficit, and the lung is often involved. Neutropenia, on the other hand, is associated with septicemia rather than with localization to an abscess.

Chronic Diseases

Diabetes mellitus is associated with recurrent infections, especially of the skin, but all organs may be involved. This is due to a loss of the barrier function of the skin as well as reduced T-cell function.

Cardiac disease is another chronic problem that can

cause recurrent pneumonia because of persistent pulmonary edema.

Chronic renal disease is associated with systemic infections and pneumonia. In this condition there is an accumulation of toxic peptides that block T-cell function.

WORK-UP

History

A careful history is essential in the evaluation of patients with recurrent infections. The physician should ask the following questions:

- Has the child been well between infections? This will distinguish a persistent infection from repeated separate infections.
- Are the episodes associated with high fever? This implies a bacterial origin.
- Is the same organ involved (e.g., are the infections confined to the respiratory tract)? In this circumstance, a structural anomaly may be present, or an obstruction such as a foreign body.
- Do the infections occur in the same site (e.g., one lobe of the lung)? This may indicate an anomaly such as sequestration.
- Has the child been in any unusual areas or in rural areas or farmlands? Unusual organisms are possible, such as animal-borne diseases.
- Have other family members had a similar problem? This question will expose a possible hereditary or familial disorder.
- Have any siblings, cousins, or other relatives had repeated infections or died from overwhelming infections? This expands on genetic problems and immune defects.
- Are there symptoms that suggest an acute illness, or are the infections silent? Silent infections imply that the usual immune response with polymorphonuclear cell activation is not present.

Physical Examination

This is specific for the site of infection. In accessible areas, such as the nose, one should look for a foreign body if unilateral purulent rhinitis is present. Evidence of unequal respiration or breath sounds, or unilateral wheezing, may suggest a foreign body within the lung. The most notable sign in patients with recurrent upper respiratory tract infections is a lack of tonsillar tissue. This often indicates an underlying immune defect because tonsillar tissue has a high content of B lymphocytes, and one would expect the tonsils to be enlarged under these circumstances.

Laboratory Tests

The specific nature of the tests performed depends on the site and the type of infection. A complete blood count will indicate deficiencies of neutrophils, lymphocytes, or platelets. A left shift would suggest that the infection is bacterial. Cultures should be taken of sputum, nasal secretions, blood, and obviously infected tissues to determine the type of infection and the degree of sensitivity to antibiotics.

X-ray studies will be determined by specific needs. Persistent purulent rhinitis is an indication for sinus roentgenograms. Sinus scan by computed axial tomography may, at times, be indicated. They are often more helpful than x-rays when the ethmoid sinuses are involved. Chest roentgenograms taken at different times in the patient with recurrent pneumonia should be compared for the site of infection and evidence suggesting an obstructed bronchus. Infection occurring in one site is indicative of a sequestered lobe or an obstructive lesion.

A suspicion of an immune defect can be addressed by a two-step approach. The first includes a blood count and differential count to exclude numerical deficiencies in lymphocytes or polymorphonuclear cells. Serum quantitative immunoglobulins must be compared to age-appropriate controls because levels are low in the first few years of life. Isohemagglutinins (anti–blood group A or B substances) provide an easy measurement of endogenous antibody production. This can also be measured by specific antitetanus or antidiphtheria antibodies; if the child has had a booster shot, a rise in the titer can be expected. A low immunoglobulin level or a lack of response to tetanus or diphtheria is an indication of an immune defect. Skin testing for cell-mediated responses can be done with the use of intradermal injections of *Candida albicans* antigen, mumps, and streptokinase/streptodornase from streptococcal antigens. These are read at 72 hours. A measurement of serum complement is rarely indicated, because deficiencies are unusual. Complement defects are suggested by recurrent *Neisseria* infections and rheumatoid disease with recurrent infections. If the preliminary series of tests outlined is normal, one can assume that an immune defect is unlikely and can observe the patient over several months. However, if there is an abnormality, the patient should have a full immunologic work-up included in the second step. This should also be performed if there are signs and symptoms that suggest the presence of an acquired immunodeficiency syndrome. The basic procedures are an enumeration of T cells and B cells and the evaluation of their function in vitro. This type of testing can be done at a high level of sophistication, and it is often possible to precisely delineate a defect.

TREATMENT AND MANAGEMENT

Acute episodes of infection should be treated with the appropriate antibiotic, and resistant organisms should be detected by cultures. In case of persistent infection, unusual organisms can be considered and treated if found.

Structural defects can be treated where appropriate. A sequestered pulmonary lobe may be resected surgically; a foreign body can be removed from a bronchus or other obstructed site.

An underlying defect, such as an immune deficiency, requires an avoidance of risk situations. These children should avoid nursery schools and other known risk areas. Live vaccines should never be given because of the risk of disseminated viral infection. In patients with immunodeficiency, tetanus toxoid and diphtheria toxoid will not induce a response and should not be given. Whole blood must be avoided in patients with immune defects because of the risk of graft-versus-host disease. In this condition, the recipient who cannot develop an immune response is rejected by viable T cells that are infused with the whole blood. If blood must be given, only packed, washed red cells should be used.

Patients with panimmunoglobulin defects can be well controlled with replacement gamma globulin, given monthly by either the intramuscular (100 mg/kg) or intravenous route (400 mg/kg). Care must be taken even with new IV preparations, and blood pressure must be monitored because there is a risk of shock if the infusion is too rapid. Intravenous infusion is best administered in a specialized clinical hospital setting. With cellular immune deficiencies, transplantation of bone marrow or thymus may offer a cure, but these circumstances are rare.

Prophylactic antibiotics are used for patients with immune defects in whom replacement gamma globulin therapy is insufficient or for patients with other diseases that cause recurrent infections, such as cystic fibrosis. It is best to rotate the drugs on a 4-month cycle. Trimethoprim-sulfamethoxazole is efficacious, especially in patients with hypogammaglobulinemia (see also Chap. 199).

INDICATIONS FOR REFERRAL

When a physician suspects an underlying structural defect or an immunologic or other underlying disease such as cystic fibrosis, a referral to a specialist is appropriate.

ANNOTATED BIBLIOGRAPHY

Aytag A, Yurdakul Y, Ikizler C et al: Inhalation of foreign body in children. Report of 500 cases. J Thorac Cardiovasc Surg 76: 145–151, 1977. (Good discussion of the spectrum of foreign bodies in the airway.)

Blazer S, Naveh Y, Friedman A: Foreign body in the airway: A review of 200 cases. Am J Dis Child 134:68–71, 1980. (Good discussion of the spectrum of foreign bodies in the airway.)

Buckley RH: Immunodeficiency. J Allergy Clin Immunol 72:627–644, 1983. (Well-referenced review.)

Fraser RG, Paré JAP: Pulmonary abnormalities of developmental origin. In Fraser RG, Pare JAP (eds): Diagnosis of Diseases of the Chest, pp 602–628. Philadelphia, WB Saunders, 1977. (Excellent review of sequestration and lung abnormalities.)

Gallin JI, Wright DG, Malech HL et al: Disorders of phagocyte chemotaxis. Ann Intern Med 92:520–538, 1980. (Difficult reading, but a good discussion of the topic.)

Gotoff SP: The secondary immunodeficiencies. In Stiehm ER, Fulginiti VA (eds): Immunologic Diseases in Infants and Children, 2nd ed, pp 399–430. Philadelphia, WB Saunders, 1980. (Detailed review of diseases that cause infection by altering the immune function.)

Ross SC, Densen P: Complement deficiency states and infection: Epidemiology, pathogenesis and consequences of neisserial and other infections in an immune deficiency. Medicine 63:243–273, 1986. (Review of recurrent neisserial infections—good coverage of a difficult topic.)

Wilson CB: Immunologic basis for increased susceptibility of the neonate to infection. J Pediatr 108:1–12, 1986. (Discussion focused on group B streptococcus, herpes virus, and nonviral intracellular pathogens.)

186
Pain

Russell S. Asnes

Almost all children experience pain as a manifestation of an acute illness, and a significant number of children have chronic pain syndromes. By the time children enter early adolescence, 20% complain of frequent headaches, 10% to 15% complain of recurrent abdominal pain, and 15% experience intermittent limb pain.

Children, particularly young children, lack the ability to describe pain in adult terms. The evaluation of the pediatric patient with pain must often be assessed within the context of a developmental framework. A child's level of cognitive development directly influences or defines his or her perception of pain. The fetus responds to noxious stimuli by withdrawal, and the newborn exhibits several behavioral and physiologic responses when subjected to pain or discomfort. The pain reaction in infants between 3 and 12 months of age begins to become more localized, and by 1 year of age (some as early as 6 months) children can localize pain and have memories of painful experiences.

Recent evidence suggests that young infants may experience pain more acutely than older infants and children because of the immaturity of neuromechanisms that dampen the transmission of pain. The presence of irritability, restlessness, poor feeding, a particular cry, tachycardia, excessive sweating, and sleep disturbances may be the only indication that the infant or preverbal child is in pain. Preschool children are unable to relate their pain to their injury or illness and are incapable of understanding the reasons for their discomfort. When experiencing pain, particularly repetitive pain, they may become withdrawn, quiet, and clingy, and they may exhibit other evidence of regressive behavior. Children may view pain in terms of punishment. Many children may suffer in silence because they believe that their pain is a result of having been bad. With the development of the ability to recall painful experiences, there is the evolving ability to anticipate painful experiences. This accounts for the resistance of many children between 1 and 3 years of age in coming to the physician's office. The child between 4 and 7 years of age will frequently respond to pain with increased anxiety and aggressive behavior. The school-aged child may be fearful of bodily injury and may tend to exaggerate minor bruises and injuries. By 7 years of age, an age that corresponds to Piaget's concept of the origin of concrete thinking, children are capable of a greater understanding that their pain is the consequence of injury or illness. For children between 10 and 12 years of age, a major component of pain may be their anxiety and fear of the loss of control.

There are several critical biologic, social, and psychological variables that must be considered in the evaluation of a pediatric patient with pain. These variables include the child's age, sex, developmental stage, temperament, personality style, affective state, cultural background, past experiences with pain, and coexisting intrafamilial stresses. Most studies suggest that pain-prone families are more likely to have pain-prone children. Children tend to follow the family style of expressing and coping with pain. Thus, in some families, the children are encouraged to express pain and are provided with a "pain language" to express their symptoms. In other families, the expression of pain is considered a sign of weakness and the children are chided to "grin and bear it."

Children experiencing painful illnesses, injuries, or procedures are less likely to receive attention to and treatment for their symptoms of pain than are adults in similar situations. Children receive fewer analgesics, at longer intervals and for shorter periods of time, than do adults. In addition, children who are unable or unwilling to communicate the extent of their discomfort are least likely to receive relief. Many medical personnel continue to believe that children do not experience pain with the same intensity as do adults, that children quickly forget painful experiences, that children recover more quickly and do not need pain control, and that narcotic analgesics should be avoided in children because they become addicted more easily than do adults. These concepts have all been disproved. In fact, it is likely that the younger the child, the lower the pain threshold and the greater the sensitivity to pain.

Physicians and nurses need to determine if their pediatric patients are in pain, and they need to be aware of the physiologic alterations that accompany pain, such as increased heart rate, respiratory rate, blood pressure, and sweating. Each patient experiences pain as an individual, and assumptions regarding an individual's pain should not and cannot be inferred from the extent of tissue damage or the procedure he or she is undergoing. A guiding principle in the prevention and relief of pain in children is that any procedure, injury, or illness that is painful for an adult will be painful for a child.

NONPHARMACOLOGIC PAIN RELIEF

Children who have been provided with clear and realistic explanations about their illness and treatment have been shown to experience less pain and less anxiety. Most painful experiences that result from illness, injuries, and diagnostic studies can be anticipated. There are many excellent children's books available that describe common illnesses, what the child can expect in a visit to the doctor's office, and hospitalization procedures. In addition, permitting parents to be present during medical procedures may contribute to pain relief or make the pain more tolerable.

The application of local measures, such as using cold or warm compresses or hiding the injury with a Band-Aid, may relieve pain. A variety of cognitive–psychological measures have been reported to lessen the fear associated with expected and actual pain and thus help the child cope with the pain. Pain relief has been achieved through the use of relaxation imagery, guided imagery, biofeedback, hypnotherapy, and structured play activities. These techniques have been found to be extremely helpful, particularly if used in conjunction with appropriate analgesics and local anesthetics.

Relaxation imagery is a process involving relaxation and a focus on mental images that can lead to deliberate control of certain physiologic responses, such as responses to painful stimuli. Children love fantasy, and if they are included in the imagery of a story being told during a painful procedure, they will frequently become temporarily oblivious to that procedure.

Hypnosis is a specific behavioral method that has been used to reduce pain and anxiety experienced by children and adolescents during various medical procedures (e.g., dressing changes in burn patients, bone marrow aspirations, and recurrent injections). Hypnotherapy has also been successfully used to treat patients with a variety of medical illnesses such as sickle cell disease and migraine. Patients are taught how to narrow their attention, to limit awareness of peripheral stimuli, and to become so focused, concentrated, and relaxed that they are able to exclude pain stimuli.

Approximately 60% to 70% of the general population can be successfully hypnotized, and children have been shown to be more hypnotizable than adults. Children as young as 4 years of age can be taught the technique of self-hypnosis whereby they can learn to modify or ignore painful stimuli. Several excellent books and courses are available for those clinicians who wish to learn how to use hypnotic techniques in their practices.

PHARMACOLOGIC PAIN RELIEF

The usual prescribing practice of ordering analgesics pro re nata (p.r.n.) is both ineffective and impractical. Who is to determine when pain relief is needed? Children may lack the language facility to communicate that they are experiencing pain and to indicate the intensity of their pain. They may be unaware that relief is available or may be afraid that pain relief can be provided only by a "shot." Recent discussions of analgesic management have suggested the concept of an "analgesic ladder" that progresses from the simplest analgesic to the most complex technologic approaches to pain management. Progressing up each step in this therapeutic ladder is determined by the specific condition and needs of an individual patient. Simpler approaches are preferable to more complicated approaches whenever the simpler approaches are effective. Analgesics are more effective when given when the pain is slight rather than severe. This approach provides patients with some control over their treatment, which may have positive psychological benefits.

A relatively new approach to pain control in hospitalized patients involves the use of a computer-controlled infusion pump that permits the patient to self-administer medication by pushing a button. This method, called patient-controlled analgesia (PCA), has been successfully employed with adolescent patients. There are even reports from some pediatric centers of the routine use of PCA in children as young as 6 years of age.

Aspirin

Aspirin, which has both analgesic and anti-inflammatory properties, remains one of the most effective medications for the treatment of mild to moderate pain. It exerts its action by repressing the synthesis of prostaglandins, which are released in tissue as the result of injury or inflammation. Aspirin reaches a peak level 2 hours after oral administration and has a half-life of 3 hours. The usual therapeutic dose is 10 to 15 mg/kg/dose, and the therapeutic blood level is between 15 and 30 mg/dl. Aspirin suppositories have an unpredictable absorption. Until recently, aspirin was the analgesic most commonly used by parents for the treatment of pain. With the recent recognition of the association between aspirin use in children with influenza and chickenpox and the development of Reye syndrome, many health care providers have been reluctant to recommend, and parents have refused to administer, aspirin under any circumstance.

Acetaminophen

Acetaminophen is presently the most popular analgesic used for children with mild to moderate pain. It is also beneficial in the amelioration of more severe forms of pain when it is used in combination with opioid analgesics. Although it is as effective as aspirin with regard to its analgesic properties, it has no anti-inflammatory activity and is thus less useful in treating the pain associated with inflammatory conditions. Acetaminophen does not have the gastrointestinal side effects commonly encountered with aspirin; it is rapidly absorbed; peak levels are achieved within 30 to 60 minutes; and it has a half-life of 2 to 5 hours. The recommended dosages are 10 to 15 mg/kg PO q4h or 15 to 20 mg/kg by rectal suppository.

Nonsteroidal Anti-Inflammatory Agents

Nonsteroidal anti-inflammatory drugs (NSAIDs) have beneficial analgesic effects and are particularly useful in treating pain of inflammatory origin, bone pain, and pain from rheumatic conditions. As with aspirin, NSAIDs can produce gastritis and have to be used with caution in patients with bleeding problems. Nephrotoxicity and hepatotoxicity can occur with prolonged use. Naprosyn (5–7 mg/kg PO b.i.d. or t.i.d.) and Tolectin (5–7 mg/kg PO t.i.d. or q.i.d.) have FDA approval for analgesic use in children 2 to 12 years old. Although approved for use in young children only as an antipyretic, ibuprofen (5–10 mg/kg PO q6h) is being used with increasing frequency as an analgesic in children.

Codeine

Codeine is the preferred drug for the treatment of moderate pain not relieved by aspirin or acetaminophen. When codeine is used in combination with aspirin or acetaminophen, its analgesic effect is potentiated. Codeine is well absorbed. Peak levels are reached 1 to 1½ hours after oral administration, and it has a duration of action of 4 to 6 hours. The oral dosage for analgesia is 0.5 to 1 mg/kg q4h. Unfortunately, many physicians undertreat children with narcotic analgesics for fear of overmedicating them. There is significant individual variation in patient response to doses of opioids. The dose administered should be titrated to clinical effect, obviously monitoring for dose-related side effects such as drowsiness, lethargy, apathy, nausea, vomiting, and constipation. Prolonged use may produce physical dependence.

Morphine

Morphine is the most effective analgesic for the treatment of severe pain. At therapeutic doses, it produces selective analgesia without altering the other senses. Peak levels are attained within 30 minutes of subcutaneous (SQ) or intramuscular (IM) administration, and the half-life is 2 to 3 hours. The therapeutic dose is 0.1 to 0.2 mg/kg/dose administered IM or SQ every 4 hours. Paregoric, which is tincture of morphine, contains 0.4 mg morphine/ml and can be administered to infants and young children in a dose of 0.2 to 0.4 mg/kg q4h. Morphine should be used when control of severe pain is needed, but it should be used cautiously. Respiratory depression is a serious and potentially fatal side effect of overdosage in patients with compromised pulmonary function. The duration of treatment with morphine must be carefully monitored to avoid tolerance and physical dependency.

Meperidine

Meperidine (Demerol) was once considered an effective analgesic but is no longer recommended for treating children with pain. Meperidine is only one eighth to one tenth as potent as morphine, and seizures and dysphoric reactions have been encountered with its use.

INDICATIONS FOR REFERRAL OR ADMISSION

It is difficult to offer specific guidelines regarding when or to whom a child with persistent, recurrent, or chronic pain should be referred, or when he or she should be hospitalized. However, among the most important considerations in this decision-making process are (1) the degree to which the clinician is confident with his or her understanding or diagnosis of the etiology of the patient's pain, and (2) the degree of dysfunction that the child or the family is experiencing from his or her symptoms. If the findings from the history, physical examination, or initial laboratory screening suggest a specific diagnosis, referral to a "subspecialist" might be appropriate.

If there is a significant history of psychosocial problems that could be presenting as a somatic pain syndrome, referral to a psychiatric social worker, psychologist, or child psychiatrist could be of assistance to both the pediatrician and the patient (see also Chap. 26).

If the history is confusing, the physical findings inconsistent, and the results of laboratory studies inconclusive, a brief period of hospitalization for the purpose of observation might be helpful. We can frequently learn a great deal by following Gellis' dictum: "Don't just do something, stand there . . . and observe and think."

ANNOTATED BIBLIOGRAPHY

Olness K, Gardner GG: Hypnosis and Hypnotherapy with Children. Philadelphia, Grune & Stratton, 1988. (Comprehensive review of the application of hypnotherapeutic techniques to children.)

Report of the Consensus Conference on the Management of Pain in Childhood Cancer. Pediatrics 86:813–834, 1990. (Practical review of current approaches to the management of pain in the pediatric patient, with emphasis on pharmacologic treatment.)

Schechter NL (ed): Acute pain in children. Pediatr Clin North Am 36:781–794, 1989. (Comprehensive, up-to-date series of articles that cover neurophysiologic, developmental, and psychological aspects of pain, and nonpharmacologic and pharmacologic methods of pain management in both the ambulatory and inpatient settings.)

187
The Overweight Child

Evan Charney

We live in a society obsessed with fitness and a sleek body image. During child health supervision visits, the clinician may perceive medical or psychological problems related to the child's weight status that the family may or may not have considered to be a problem. In either case, the physician caring for children who are overweight has an important role to play. The first task is to identify those few children who have medical conditions associated with obesity and who need to be brought under therapy. For most of the remaining cases, the clinician needs to determine whether a problem exists, who the patient is, and how best to influence the body fat depot, the whole child, and the whole family.

PATHOPHYSIOLOGY

Obesity implies an excess of body fat rather than just increased body weight, which also reflects lean body mass. Ideally, the definition of what is excessive fat ought to be related to some pathologic condition that becomes manifest when the fat depot attains a certain mass. We could then comfortably identify which patient has the "disease" and proceed accordingly. In reality, there is no such point in overweight children short of morbid obesity, which may cause respiratory embarrassment. We are left with a statistical definition—those children at some arbitrary percentile or weight-for-height status are declared overweight or obese. Although there are many other biologic conditions that have a range of intermediate values bridging normality and disease (e.g., hemoglobin concentration, blood pressure), the condition of "overweight" is a good example of labeling by statistics. Children with greater-than-average body weight have no significant morbidity in childhood. Their "disease" is based on two factors: they deviate from a socially defined ideal weight, and their condition has a well-defined risk of tracking into adulthood, where the hazards of overweight appear to be real.

The underlying pathophysiology of obesity is not well defined at present. Genetic factors are clearly important and may be more potent than environmental influences: for example, studies suggest that adult weight status of adopted children correlates more strongly with their biologic parents than with their adoptive parents. Twin studies show double the concordance rate for overweight among monozygotic compared to dizygotic twins, independent of whether they were reared apart or together. The physiologic mechanism by which this genetic tendency becomes manifest is less evident. A host of studies have failed to clarify whether obese children eat more and exercise less than their normal weight peers, although the preponderance of data suggests both to be the case to some degree. Once an individual becomes obese, little additional caloric intake is required to maintain that status, because the fat depot is not metabolically active. Can some aberration in metabolism account for obesity over and above a simple imbalance between calories ingested and energy expended? Differences between obese and lean individuals (and animals) in carbohydrate metabolism and energy storage have been described, but we are not yet at a point where metabolic or biochemical factors in those destined to be obese can be identified, much less subject to alteration.

CLINICAL PRESENTATION AND DIFFERENTIAL DIAGNOSIS

"If he looks fat, he is fat" may be a workable definition of adult obesity, but it does not apply to children. Because the normal amount of subcutaneous fat and body muscle mass varies with age, the child who is at the 50th percentile for both height and weight looks quite different at different points in childhood. Thus, the premature infant appears thin because the bulk of body weight is gained in the third trimester. The 6- to 12-month-old child has more subcutaneous fat than at any point before puberty, and therefore the "Buddha" appearance of late infancy is normal. Toddlers appear progressively thinner as linear growth rates stabilize at 2 to 3 inches/yr while the rate of gain in weight progressively slows and the thickness of the subcutaneous fat layer actually diminishes. Children appear most lean at about 6 years of age, and the chubby-appearing child at that age is usually markedly overweight. From age 5 or 6 years to the time of the adolescent growth spurt, both muscle mass and subcutaneous fat increase rapidly, and the preadolescent boy or girl normally has a chubbier or at least a stockier build. Both the family and clinician should distinguish these physiologic variations in the child's appearance from true deviations from normal.

There is no universally accepted definition of overweight or obesity in childhood because, as indicated, there is no identified weight status or body fat distribution pattern that correlates with a clear disease state. Weight-for-length percentiles (or merely a weight percentile greatly in excess of length percentile) are simplest to use. Some experts suggest the use of skinfold calipers, because triceps and subscapular skinfold thicknesses correlate reasonably well with total body fat measured by more precise means such as densitometry, K40 analysis, or prompt gamma ray emission methods. However, *fatfold thickness* is difficult to measure reliably by caliper in infancy or early childhood and may add more apparent than real scientific precision to what is a clinical estimate. For practical purposes, *overweight* can be defined as a weight 110% to 120% above the comparable weight for the child's height percentile, and *obesity* can be defined as a weight in excess of 120% of that figure.

Plotting the child's weight and height on the National Center for Health Statistics Growth Chart is the first step. These most current growth standards can be applied in all American children if racial and genetic variations are taken into account. The rate of the child's weight gain and linear growth should track regardless of genetic factors between 2 years and adolescence.

Most obese children have a somewhat accelerated linear growth that parallels their weight gain. If the child is of short stature and is hypertensive, then Cushing's syndrome should be ruled out. If the child is both short and mentally slow, the Prader–Willi and Laurence–Moon–Biedl syndromes should be considered.

WORK-UP

History

The physician should determine who wishes the child to lose weight (e.g., one or both parents, the grandparents, or the child him- or herself). Because family weight status is a strong predictor of the child's ultimate weight status, it is important to assess both parents' current weight and height and, if they are obese, when that condition developed. A family history of hypertension, noninsulin-dependent (type II) diabetes, and cardiovascular disease should be obtained. The family's social class and educational level are worth noting because those factors correlate strongly with the child's ultimate weight status. Beginning just prior to adolescence in girls, there is a dramatic "sorting out" process: the prevalence of obesity increases among girls in the lower social class and diminishes among girls in the upper social class. That trend is both less marked and in the opposite direction for boys; richer boys (and their fathers) tend to be heavier; poorer boys (and their fathers) tend to be leaner. How are these data useful to the clinician? In the low-income family, if the overweight mother or adolescent girl who is rapidly gaining weight is not concerned about weight status or even considers heaviness a desirable social trait, intervention strategies are unlikely to succeed. Conversely, the thin, affluent parents of the newly chubby preadolescent girl can be reassured that she will probably lose weight during or after adolescence, without any externally imposed diet. In fact, emphasizing her "overweight" status may only encourage a tendency toward anorexia or bulimia, which may pose more important health risks for her than obesity. The clinician should be alert to the preadolescent whose weight is "socially dissonant"; that is, the fat child in an affluent family of thin adults or the thin girl in a family of poor obese women. The obese child in a thin, upper-income family will need support from the physician in the future to temper the alternating enthusiasm and despair associated with a series of dietary manipulations of varying degrees of rationality. Conversely, the slender girl in a low-income family with many obese adults may also need guidance and support regarding the normality of her body weight.

Physical Examination

A complete and careful examination is particularly important where weight and, by implication, health status are concerned. Both the parent and the child need to be reassured that all is well independent of weight, if that is the case. Blood pressure measurement and height and weight plotted on growth charts are essential. Further assessment of the obese child who is less than 50% for height or who is developmentally slow is indicated.

Laboratory Tests

If the child is of at least normal height for age and has had a normal growth velocity, endocrinologic abnormalities such as acquired hypothyroidism and Cushing's syndrome are excluded, and thyroid studies and serum electrolyte values do not need to be obtained. Serum cholesterol and triglyceride levels should be obtained in children whose families have a strong history of cardiovascular disease. Other screening laboratory tests are unnecessary without specific indication.

TREATMENT

"There is no known safe, effective, long-term treatment for obesity" is the summary of the 1981 Statement by the Committee on Nutrition of the Academy of Pediatrics. In 1985, the Committee concluded that "the long-term success rate for treatment of obesity is poor, and it remains to be seen whether efforts at prevention will be effective." No therapeutic modalities have been developed since then to alter the validity of those conclusions. Studies using behavioral techniques, particularly group programs involving the family, report encouraging weight reductions in children that are more likely to be sustained over time. There are no medications that will result in sustained weight loss in children (or adults). The use of thyroid hormone is both ineffective and potentially hazardous. Surgical techniques such as a gastric bypass or a jaw wiring carry serious risks and are contraindicated in all but the morbidly obese patient; even in those cases, hazards are likely to outweigh benefits.

The physician who is confronted with a family concerned about the child's weight status is in a difficult position. We would like our overweight patients to lose weight, and if we had safe and effective therapy we would be overjoyed to prescribe it. The reality, however, is that current intervention strategies are not efficacious in perhaps 80% of cases. At best, these strategies may "help" 20% and probably leave some patients more obese than before our intervention. In what other area of medicine do we recommend therapy for a clinical condition with unclear morbidity, where our intervention is usually ineffective and often leaves the child with the same problem but less self-esteem than he or she had prior to seeking our advice? Given this current reality, what help can we offer? The clinician can be an important resource in helping the child and his or her family cope with, if not "cure," the problem.

Primary Prevention

Birth weight correlates poorly with weight status in childhood or adulthood. Although the risk of early adult obesity is doubled if the infant exceeds the 90th percentile for weight in the first year of life, two thirds of heavy infants will be normal-weight adults. Because genetic factors are such a strong influence, the physician should consider offering anticipatory guidance when one or both parents are significantly overweight. Recommending breast-feeding, delaying the introduction of solids until 4 to 6 months of age, and, in bottle-fed infants, counseling the family against using the bottle as a pacifier seems reasonable advice, but it must be acknowledged that there is no good evidence that these strategies work. Skim milk formulas are contraindicated before 1 year of age, but a reduced fat milk thereafter is prudent for those at high familial risk of obesity. Counseling the family to offer the infant and toddler a balanced diet, with limited high-calorie snack foods, may help establish appropriate eating habits while the child's intake is under the family's control. If, however, the parents are serious about limiting the risk of evolving obesity, a change in the entire family's eating habits may then be necessary. They will need to consider essentially excluding high-calorie snack foods from the home and setting the habit of eating only at the dinner table and only at mealtimes. Eating while watching television is another "high-risk" habit that should be avoided, because long hours of television viewing have been associated with obesity in older children, probably from a combination of inactivity and increased snack food intake. Establishing patterns of regular family exercise (e.g., bicycle riding, swimming, walking, and hiking) may be particularly worth cultivating in the child who is at a high risk of becoming obese. We must, however, be cautious in giving this advice to families because no clinical trials demonstrate the efficacy of these interventions (logical though they appear to be) and because excessive zeal may alienate the family and child who will need our ongoing support. It would seem prudent to titrate the forcefulness of our primary prevention advice against the perceived risks. The family in which one or both parents are obese, particularly where early cardiovascular disease or type II diabetes is present, merits an attempt at intervention. Less advice is necessary or indicated when these conditions are not present. A cautionary note about excessive fear of obesity is in order: Some lean parents become concerned lest their normally growing child develops obesity, and they may interpret the appropriate chubby appearance of the 5- to 12-month-old child as pathologic. They need reassurance that their child is well.

Secondary Prevention

The age at which the child is obese is predictive of adult weight status. Perhaps one third of overweight infants are at risk (compared to 10%–15% of all infants); ~40% of obese 7-year-olds and ~70% of obese adolescents will be obese adults, with the powerful influence of family factors increasing or decreasing that risk. Mild to moderately obese children should have no dietary limitations beyond a reduction of dietary fat (e.g., use of low-fat or skim milk and a reduced intake of fried foods, gravies, salad dressings) and a restriction of high-calorie snacks. Family exercise patterns should be encouraged. At present, the physician must be cautious about casually prescribing more severe dietary interventions. They have not been successful, and the risk of beginning a lifetime habit of alternating diet and normal eating with weight swings is of little value and may be harmful. The early adolescent who has just become overweight, particularly in a normal-weight family, has the best prognosis, and no intervention is necessary. If more severe calorie-limiting diets are invoked, abundant daily protein intake (1–1.5 g/kg ideal body weight) is essential to limit the effect that all such diets have on linear growth. Family- and group-based programs and those involving behavior modification measures (eat only at designated times, in designated places, and eat slowly) are more likely to demonstrate short-term results. Weight control programs in middle school and high school involving dietary advice and exercise groups have been attempted in some communities. The physician should be alert to the possibility that such programs may add to the social labeling (and further lowering of self-esteem) that is already the plight of the overweight child. Vigorous aerobic exercise programs in schools, unless part of a family pattern, are inappropriate, and no long-term benefits have been documented. For most obese children, a reasonable goal is the maintenance of weight status and the avoidance of a super-obese state, which is even more refractory to intervention.

The clinician's role with the obese child and family therefore transcends diet and exercise advice. As outlined, a complete history and physical examination are sufficient to rule out an underlying medical disease or to suggest that specific diagnoses be pursued. If the child is over 6 years of age and is not motivated to lose weight, individual dietary advice is inappropriate and alterations in the family's caloric intake and energy output are more appropriate subjects for discussion. Is the family using the obese child as a scapegoat for parental conflict? If this is the case, that conflict should be addressed. Perhaps we can be of most help by resisting the scenario in which the overweight (but otherwise low-risk) child is labeled by the doctor as in need of treatment. Diet and exercise are prescribed, and the child is told to return periodically for "checkups". The high rate of failure of this approach means that the physician becomes one more authority figure, along with parents, friends, and gym teachers, who concludes that the child is abnormal. Moreover, when the child fails to lose weight or to sustain any weight loss, his or her inadequacy is further confirmed and a potentially supportive relationship with the physician is compromised. It may be more important to examine the children carefully, to reassure them of their basic normality and personal worth, and to offer to be available for guidance and advice over the years while they cope with the blizzard of advice on cures for their affliction. At present, the advice to "first do no harm" remains the most appropriate one in dealing with the overweight child.

ANNOTATED BIBLIOGRAPHY

Epstein L, Valoski A, Wing R et al: Ten-year follow-up of behavioral, family-based treatment for obese children. JAMA 264:2519–2523, 1990. (Longest follow-up study to date in children shows benefit among those provided a parent and child program with behavioral management as well as diet; children remained substantially overweight, although less so than controls.)

Freedman D, Burke G, Harsha D et al: Relationship of changes in obesity to serum lipid and lipoprotein changes in childhood and adolescence. JAMA 254:515–520, 1985. (Part of the Bogalusa Heart Study—analysis of 1598 5- to 12-year-olds suggests that an increase in obesity over this time is accompanied by an increasingly atherogenic lipoprotein profile.)

Garn S: Continuities and changes in fatness from infancy through adulthood. Curr Prob Pediatr 15:4–47, 1985. (Thorough discussion of the epidemiology of overweight by an authority and scholar of the field.)

Gortmaker S, Dietz W, Cheung L: Inactivity, diet, and the fattening of America. J Am Diet Assoc 90:1247–1252, 1990. (Identifies television viewing as a strong risk factor for childhood and adolescent obesity.)

Hammer L, Kraemer H, Wilson D et al: Standardized percentile curves of body-mass index for children and adolescents. Am J Dis Child 145:259–263, 1991. (Although visual inspection of disparity between height and weight percentiles is generally sufficient for most clinical purposes, this article provides useful body-mass index curves [weight in kg/height in m^2] for children based on national survey data.)

Lissner L, Odell P, D'Agostino R et al: Variability of body weight and health outcomes in the Framingham population. N Engl J Med 324:1839–1844, 1991. (In 3100 subjects, weight fluctuation over time—most likely due to loss and gain by repetitive dieting cycles—had adverse consequences for coronary heart disease, comparable to the risk of the maintenance of an obese state; results have important implications that require verification.)

Moses N, Banilivy M, Lifshitz F: Fear of obesity among adolescent girls. Pediatrics 83:393–398, 1989. (Pervasive among middle-class girls; 51% of underweight girls 13–18 years of age were extremely fearful of being overweight, and 20% were on diets, as were 50% of overweight girls.)

Rosenbaum M, Leibel R: Obesity in childhood. Pediatr Rev 11:43–55, 1989. (Thorough and balanced review of pathophysiology of obesity written for clinicians; see also more expanded treatise by same authors: Adv Pediatr 35:73–137, 1988.)

Stunkard A, Harris J, Pederson N et al: The body-mass index of twins who have been reared apart. N Engl J Med 322;1483–1487, 1990. (Correlation of body-mass index of monozygotic twins reared apart [0.70]—comparable to correlation of those reared together [0.74] and far higher than correlation of dizygotic twins reared apart [0.15] or together [0.33]: genetic influence on obesity is substantial.)

188

Failure to Thrive

Deborah A. Frank
and Donald M. Berwick

Failure to grow or to gain weight can be a consequence of most major physical and psychological problems of infancy and childhood. When it is the presenting problem, therefore, *failure to thrive* (FTT) is a formidable diagnostic challenge for the pediatrician. Evaluation and management are further complicated by the strong feelings that can easily come to surround the child who is growing poorly: guilt and a sense of failure in the parents, anxiety and accusatory impulses in the professional care-givers, and, often, irritability or emotional disturbances in the child. Because the long-term consequences of severe growth failure may include irreversible short stature, developmental delay, and impaired socio-emotional functioning, the diagnostic evaluation can easily be infused with a sense of urgency that poor growth is laying the seeds of more general future impairment.

Effective diagnosis and management of FTT depend on restrained, structured investigation and strict attention to maintaining an alliance with the child's parents. The pediatrician must also remember that FTT rarely has a single cause in a particular patient but rather results from many factors working together against adequate caloric intake and use. Rather than seeking to classify each child's growth failure as "organic" or "nonorganic" in origin, the physician should assess each child and family along four dimensions: (1) medical, (2) nutritional, (3) developmental–behavioral, and (4) psychosocial. The coordinated efforts of a multidisciplinary team, including at a minimum a health provider, a nutritionist, and a social worker or psychologist, provide the optimal approach to the diagnosis and management of children who fail to thrive.

PATHOPHYSIOLOGY

Failure to gain weight in children is usually due to problems in caloric balance: the child is either not being offered, not taking, or not retaining sufficient nutrients to grow to the potential limit set by his or her genetic endowment. Children who are losing weight or who are underweight for height are uniformly suffering from nutrition inadequate for their needs. Children who are symmetrically depressed in weight and height (but are within normal range of weight for height) may be manifesting the cumulative effects of chronic malnutrition, genetic short stature, achondroplastic dwarfism, or the effects of prenatal insults such as congenital rubella syndrome and fetal alcohol syndrome. However, even children with genetic or congenital constraints on growth should grow steadily and parallel to the usual growth curves. Weight loss or prolonged plateauing of growth must always be investigated.

Caloric intake may seem adequate or even excessive in certain states involving hypercatabolism, malabsorption, or occult loss of nutrients. In these conditions, the diagnosis rests on discovering the source of abnormally high calorie requirement or nutrient loss, such as chronic diarrhea or vomiting, celiac disease, cystic fibrosis, or congenital heart disease.

Once the cycle of poor growth begins, secondary physiologic abnormalities may develop that aggravate the problem and may even confuse the diagnosis. Pituitary insufficiency, depressed levels of growth hormone, abnormal glucose tolerance, elevated liver function tests, retardation of skeletal development, impaired immunocompetence, and anemia may appear as secondary conditions in children with FTT.

CLINICAL PRESENTATION

Despite its importance, FTT has no universally accepted clinical definition. Diagnosis may be made on the basis of attained growth or decreased growth velocity. Commonly, the label is applied to children below the third or fifth percentile of weight for age or with weights less than 80% of ideal (median) for age. Some physicians focus concern on children when slowed velocity of weight gain results in "crossing percentiles." Thus, a child who has moved from the 50th to the 15th percentile of weight for age may be said to be *failing to thrive*, particularly after 18–24 months of age, when changes in growth trajectories are rarely physiologic. The National Center for Health Statistics growth grids are considered by international consensus to be appropriate norms for infants and preschoolers regardless of ethnicity.

Among hospitalized children with growth failure of any cause, FTT is a secondary consequence of a prior known disease in 70% to 90% of cases. Cardiac, neurologic, and gastrointestinal diseases, along with cystic fibrosis, lead the list of the underlying causes. In severe cases, the underlying disease is rarely subtle. Children are often survivors of extremely low birth weight. With modern improvements in supportive technologies, the number of chronically ill children with special needs is increasing, and skill in managing nutrition, feeding strategies, and parental support and education is essential to good outcomes for these children. Approximately 40% to 50% of children admitted to the hospital specifically for an evaluation of FTT have a discharge diagnosis of "environmentally induced growth failure."

DIFFERENTIAL DIAGNOSIS

The differential diagnosis of FTT is virtually the same as the list of all serious diseases of infancy and childhood. The underlying disease is readily apparent by history and/or physical examination in most cases. Even for the child with an obvious major physical illness, such as a large ventricular septal defect, cerebral palsy, or multiple congenital anomalies, nutritional and psychosocial factors may be contributing to the growth failure, especially when the growth curve indicates a discontinuity in a child's usual growth pattern. When the trajectory of growth shows such an abrupt change, superimposed metabolic burdens such as infection; gaps in parents' skills such as feeding techniques and selection of foods; oral motor difficulties; superimposed social and emotional stresses in the family; and difficult developmental issues arising in the child around separation and individuation must also be considered.

The list of *occult* medical conditions that may present as failure to thrive is not nearly as extensive. In inpatient series of children admitted specifically to evaluate FTT, about one third eventually receive an organic diagnosis, and over three fourths of those are gastrointestinal disorders, such as chronic diarrhea, lactose intolerance, chronic gastroesophageal reflux, or malabsorption (primarily celiac disease). Giardiasis and other enteric pathogens may be implicated in the growth failure of immigrant children and children attending day care or living in shelters. Subtle oral motor difficulties, which sometimes interfere with the transition from liquids to solids, may be seen in children with otherwise subclinical neurologic difficulties. Multiple dental caries and abscesses may make eating and chewing painful and thus contribute to failure to thrive. Severe tonsillar–adenoidal hypertrophy may cause growth failure through mechanical feeding difficulties and hypoxia. Urinary tract infections and renal tubular acidosis may also be relatively occult. In recent years, the differential diagnosis of unexplained FTT has expanded to include perinatal HIV infection, a diagnosis that should always be considered in children whose mothers have a history of illicit substance use or are sexual partners of substance-abusing or bisexual men, or when mother, father, or child has had a blood transfusion (see also Chap. 52).

However, most cases of FTT, traditionally labeled as nonorganic, are manifestations of primary malnutrition. Malnutrition severe enough to produce growth failure may also impair immune function, particularly cell-mediated immunity and the production of complement and secretory IgA. Many children with FTT are trapped in the "infection malnutrition cycle," with recurring episodes of otitis media, respiratory illness, and gastrointestinal infection that lead to cumulative nutritional deficits followed by even more severe and prolonged infections and even less adequate growth. In addition, children with nutritional deficiencies show a heightened susceptibility to lead toxicity, which in turn has been implicated as a correlate of impaired growth.

WORK-UP

History

An evaluation of a child with FTT is best guided by specific clues from a history or physical examination, not by extensive laboratory screening. One should ascertain whether there is a family history of potentially growth-retarding illnesses such as cystic fibrosis or lactose intolerance. A family history may reveal a pattern of short stature, which can be highly reassuring if the child is short but not underweight for height. It is critical to assess whether the parents themselves were malnourished as children, as is often the case among immigrant and low-income families. In such cases, the parents' stature does not provide an accurate indication of the child's genetic growth potential.

A detailed perinatal history should include prenatal teratogen exposures and infections as well as the child's gestational age, birth weight, length, and head circumference. Unless growth parameters are corrected for gestational age in the early years of life, children born prematurely may be inappropriately labeled as FTT. However, if growth is truly impaired after correction for prematurity, it is unacceptable to defer a detailed search for potentially correctable causes of postnatal growth failure just because the child was "born small." Postnatal history should include intercurrent infections, lead exposure, and a detailed review of systems, including bowel movements, vomiting, dysphagia, and difficulties of chewing and swallowing.

A detailed nutritional history, including a 24-hour dietary recall, is essential. The strengths and weaknesses of the care-giving environment should be evaluated. Economic deprivation, with insufficient resources for food purchase, food storage, and food preparation, is the most common finding among children with FTT from primary malnutrition. Lack of knowledge regarding appropriate nutrition, particularly among immigrant, adolescent, and cognitively impaired care-givers, may also contribute to FTT. In all social classes, unusual dietary beliefs, such as adherence to a strict macrobiotic regimen, may result in inappropriate feeding practices (see Chap. 15). Failure to thrive has been described among children of economically privileged parents who overzealously enforce low-fat diets in the hope of preventing later heart disease. If the infant is exclusively breast-fed, a careful and supportive assessment of the nursing pattern is important, because a regimen of enhanced maternal nutrition, rest, and breast-feeding every 2 hours to build mother's milk supply (with or without supplemental formula feeding) can provide a dramatic improvement in growth.

In addition to evaluating the family's feeding practices,

nutritional knowledge, and material resources for feeding children, the clinician must assess the level of psychosocial resources available to nurture the child's growth. Marital discord, parental depression, a chronically ill child, and social isolation may deplete the family's affective resources for child care. Abuse of alcohol or of illicit substances may both divert financial resources from the care of the child and drastically compromise parenting abilities. The clinician should be aware that parents of children who fail to thrive often had eating disorders, were seriously deprived, or even abused themselves as children. Painful, unresolved emotional issues from their own childhood may impede parents' ability to recognize and respond to their children's needs.

A developmental history must be obtained in all cases because developmental impairment is more common among children with failure to thrive.

Finally, the clinician should evaluate the parent–child dyad for the presence of an interactive feeding disorder, ideally not only by history but by direct observation performed in the home by an experienced nurse or social worker. If this is not feasible, simply asking the parent to feed the child a snack in the office may be very revealing. The most common interactive feeding disorders are those that emerge in the second half of the first year when parents have difficulty in dealing with the child's efforts at separation/individuation.

Physical Examination

A physical examination must begin with the careful measurement of length, unclothed weight, and head circumference. These measurements must then be plotted on the National Center for Health Statistics growth grids, including a plot of weight for height. Children with genetic short stature will generally have concordant length and weight. Other specific clues to diagnosis can include multiple minor dysmorphic features suggestive of prenatal teratogen exposures or growth-retarding syndromes (particularly fetal alcohol syndrome), a murmur or cyanosis suggestive of cardiac disease, a protuberant abdomen (classically associated with celiac disease, malabsorption, or cystic fibrosis), or signs of chronic respiratory disease. A neurologic examination, including an oral motor evaluation, may suggest previously undiagnosed cerebral palsy or other central nervous system problems.

One general principle in the examination of the child with FTT is that, despite anecdotes to the contrary, most organic disease severe enough to cause FTT will yield clues in a careful physical examination. If an organic disease is an important cause of the child's growth failure, it is likely to be revealed in a history or a physical examination.

Laboratory Tests

When the cause of FTT is not apparent, the diagnostic evaluation should be guided by the history and the physical examination. Laboratory "fishing expeditions" are unlikely to reveal problems that are not suggested by the history and the physical examination, and they will often lead the pediatrician down costly and uncomfortable blind alleys. The hazard is compounded by the many secondary biochemical and hematologic abnormalities that may derive from FTT. Mild elevations of liver enzymes, for example, are a well-described concomitant finding of malnutrition, and workups are usually unrevealing.

Some basic laboratory studies are probably worthwhile in most cases and include complete blood count, lead and free erythrocyte protoporphyrin, urinalysis, urine culture, blood urea nitrogen or creatinine, serum electrolytes, and a tuberculin test. For children severely underweight for their height, an albumin and alkaline phosphatase, calcium, and phosphorus are indicated to assess protein status and rule out zinc deficiency or biochemical rickets. For short children whose weights are proportional for their heights, a bone age may be useful to discriminate children who are constitutionally short (bone age = chronologic age and greater than height age) from those with endocrine derangements or chronic malnutrition (bone age = height age and less than chronologic age) (see Chap. 85). HIV screening and sweat tests should be performed in at-risk children. The remainder of the laboratory investigation should be guided strictly by specific clues from the history, epidemiologic circumstances, and physical examination. It is critical to remember that organic disease is almost never discovered on the basis of laboratory testing alone.

MANAGEMENT

Three important philosophies should guide the management of the child with FTT. These apply equally well to FTT of organic and nonorganic origin:

1. Involve the parents in the process of diagnosis and treatment. The maintenance of this alliance is important whenever possible. Feelings of guilt in the parent and moral judgments by clinicians confound effective understanding and treatment. Pediatricians should be aware of possible countertransference reactions and impulses to judge apparently neglectful parents harshly.
2. Involve other disciplines and address the multiple areas of risk simultaneously. Medically, the clinician should seek to optimize management of chronic illness, identify and treat intercurrent infections, provide appropriate immunizations (including influenza vaccine in very underweight children), and treat lead intoxication if indicated. In consultation with a pediatric nutritionist, the physician should provide all children with high-calorie, high-protein diets to provide one and one half to two times the Recommended Daily Allowance for age, and they should be given a multivitamin supplement with iron and zinc to support the micronutrient needs of catch-up growth. Parents should be instructed to provide three

meals and three snacks a day and to omit low-calorie liquids such as juice, Kool-Aid, and carbonated beverages from the diet. If less than 3 years old, children should be referred to early intervention programs. If the older child is developmentally delayed, Head Start or public school special needs programs for assessment and intervention may also be helpful. Psychosocially, according to the assessed areas of risk, the family should be offered supportive and therapeutic intervention from social service or mental health agencies capable of addressing a wide range of issues from food shortages to family dysfunction.

3. Take the long view. Failure to thrive is a chronic problem and is rarely simply "cured." Children should be seen far more frequently to monitor growth and development than the frequency dictated by a routine schedule of health maintenance visits. Weekly visits are often necessary in the early stages of diagnosis and treatment. In follow-up studies, about one third of infants with FTT are physically small as long as a decade later. In addition, half of the children in hospital follow-up series have behavioral or psychoeducational difficulties during latency and afterward and therefore require ongoing developmental and psychosocial monitoring and referral.

INDICATIONS FOR REFERRAL OR ADMISSION

In some centers, the availability of interdisciplinary outpatient clinics for the assessment and management of FTT has greatly reduced the need for hospitalization. Any child who has not responded in 2 to 3 months to intensive efforts at management in a primary care setting should be considered for referral to such a clinic.

Hospitalization is indicated for severely malnourished children, for children with serious intercurrent infections, if the safety of the child is in question, or if a special combination of disciplines is required and can be assembled most efficiently inside the hospital. One theory, which is now outdated, suggests that organic FTT can be differentiated from nonorganic FTT by observing growth in the hospital; the child with an environmental deprivation will grow (according to the theory), while the child with an organic disease will not. In fact, children with organic illnesses grow as well as those with primary malnutrition if given adequate nutrition, so positive response to hospital management is a poor discriminant of organic disease, although it may be helpful in restoring the physiologic stability of the child.

On occasion, placement of a child with FTT outside of the home may be the only safe choice, especially if parents are active substance abusers, have inflicted injury on the child, are profoundly psychiatrically or cognitively impaired, or are seriously noncompliant with health care. When the child's physical condition causes parental emotional and logistic problems beyond their capabilities (even with outside support), outside placement in a medically specialized foster home or rehabilitation center may also be

necessary. The decision is, of course, difficult and is best undertaken only with the intensive involvement of appropriate social service agencies. Ideally, the goal of sustained interdisciplinary management is a thriving child in a thriving family.

ANNOTATED BIBLIOGRAPHY

Berwick DM, Levy JC, Kleinerman R: Failure to thrive: Diagnostic yield of hospitalization. Arch Dis Child 57:347–351, 1982. (In a case series of 122 infants aged 1 to 25 months, admitted to a teaching hospital for evaluation of FTT of obscure origin, 34% had no diagnosis even after evaluation, 32% received a social or environmental diagnosis, and 31% had a specific organic diagnosis. Organic disease usually offered a clue on history or physical examination.)

Bithoney WG, McJunkin J, Michalek J, Egan H, Snyder J, Munier A: Prospective evaluation of weight gain in both nonorganic and organic failure to thrive children: An outpatient trial of a multidisciplinary team strategy. J Dev Behav Pediatr 10:27–31, 1989. (Outpatient multidisciplinary assessment of 64 nonorganic and 22 organic FTT children showing excellent growth response to high-calorie feeding in both groups.)

Chatoor I, Schaeffer S, Dickson L, Egan J. Non-organic failure to thrive: A developmental perspective. Pediatr Ann 13:829–842, 1984. (Sophisticated description of the developmental diagnosis and treatment of eating disorders in infants and toddlers.)

Frank DA, Zeisel SH. Failure to thrive. Pediatr Clin North Am 35:1187–1206, 1988. (Comprehensive review stressing the importance of understanding malnutrition and its treatment in the management of FTT.)

Oates RK, Peacock A, Forrest D: Long-term effects of nonorganic failure to thrive. Pediatrics 75:36–40, 1985. (Long-term follow-up of 14 children with FTT showed significant behavioral and intellectual problems 12 years later; also contains an excellent review of the FTT follow-up literature.)

Sills RH: Failure to thrive: The role of laboratory evaluation. Am J Dis Child 132:967–969, 1978. (One of the largest and clearest published case series—185 children hospitalized for diagnosis of the reason for their FTT; 55% received a nonorganic diagnosis and 26% remained unexplained after evaluation.)

189

Dehydration

Victor C. Baum

Dehydration is a relatively common clinical problem in pediatric practice resulting usually as a complication of gastroenteritis. Infants and young children are at particular risk for dehydration because of their small size and restricted access to replacement fluids. The spectrum of dehydration ranges from mild dehydration, marked only by increased thirst and easily corrected with simple oral rehydration, to profound dehydration resulting in hypovolemic shock or major electrolyte abnormalities. In this latter state, there is a high risk of mortality or major morbidity either from the disease or from inappropriate management.

Over the past several decades, the general approach to moderate or severe dehydration in children has been hospitalization and intravenous therapy. However, with extensive experience developed in Third World nations, oral rehydration with carefully formulated oral rehydration solutions is becoming more accepted in current American practice.

PATHOPHYSIOLOGY

Dehydration is characterized by an excessive loss of fluid from the body. The pathophysiologic processes and clinical presentation depend on the net composition of the abnormal losses (i.e., the relative net loss of water and of solute [most importantly Na^+]). The net loss of these will result from the type of fluid lost (e.g., diarrhea, gastric, third space) and the type of oral fluids that have been given (balanced salt solutions, inappropriate hypertonic solutions, or hypotonic fluids). Other factors, such as small body size, an abnormal thirst mechanism, lack of appropriate renal water reabsorption, tachypnea, a hot, dry atmosphere, or limited water access, may contribute to excessive losses of water over solute. Abnormal sweat electrolytes or endocrinopathies involving the mineralocorticoids may cause excessive solute loss. With dehydration, the kidney attempts to reabsorb water by producing a concentrated urine, and oliguria results from decreased renal perfusion.

Dehydration is commonly classified as *hyponatremic* when the serum Na^+ is less than 125 mEq/L, *isonatremic* when losses of salt and water are balanced, and *hypernatremic* when the loss of water is greater than the loss of Na^+ and the resultant serum Na^+ is >150 mEq/L. The terms *hyponatremic, isonatremic,* and *hypernatremic* dehydration are often used interchangeably with the terms *hypotonic, isotonic,* and *hypertonic* dehydration, respectively. In actuality, if abnormal amounts of osmotically active agents, such as glucose or urea, or abnormal osmotic agents such as mannitol or radiologic contrast agents are not present, these terms may be roughly interchangeable, because Na^+ is the predominant osmotic agent in the extracellular fluid.

Isonatremic Dehydration

Isonatremic dehydration results in a loss of Na^+ and water in concentrations similar to those of the extracellular fluid. Thus, the fluid left behind will not be significantly altered in composition, although total body Na^+ and water will be depleted.

Hyponatremic Dehydration

Hyponatremic dehydration results primarily in depletion of extracellular fluid. Water, which can freely pass through the cell membranes, moves from the now diluted extracellular fluid to the intracellular fluid. Thus, early compromise of circulating blood volume occurs.

Hypernatremic Dehydration

Hypernatremic dehydration produces relative sparing of the extracellular fluid at the expense of intracellular fluid. With increased osmolality of the plasma and extracellular fluid, water moves out of the cells and into the extracellular fluid in order to try to equilibrate the differences in osmolality. With significant hypernatremia, cells generate *idiogenic osmols* that are thought to be primarily products of protein breakdown. These small molecules increase osmolality within the cells to help balance the osmolality differential and draw back the extracellular fluid.

Hypernatremic dehydration has a higher mortality rate and central nervous system morbidity (e.g., seizures, hemorrhage, thrombosis) than does hyponatremic or isonatremic dehydration. This may be due to decreased brain volume and rupture of blood vessels. In addition, if water is given too rapidly during attempted rehydration, water passes readily into brain cells that now have a higher osmotic load because of idiogenic osmol production. This results in swelling of these cells and cerebral edema. Pulmonary edema may also occur with rapid rehydration.

CLINICAL PRESENTATION

The best method of judging acute fluid losses is by serial weights or by comparison to a recent weight. Because these data are often unavailable, estimates of the extent of dehydration can be made based on the physical examination. For any degree of dehydration, the physical examination may be altered by hypernatremia or hyponatremia. It is important to understand that 1% = 1 ml fluid/100 g body weight. Therefore, 1% dehydration indicates that the individual has lost 10 ml fluid/kg. An individual who is 5% dehydrated has lost 50 ml/kg.

Traditionally, dehydration is estimated and expressed as follows:

- <5% loss in body weight: slightly increased thirst, no change in physical examination
- 5% to 10%: moderate thirst, decreased urine production, irritability, dry mucous membranes, decreased tearing (newborn infants do not cry with tears). There is also tenting of the skin. Skin turgor is determined by pinching up on anterior abdominal wall skin. Normally, this skin rapidly retracts to its normal position. In dehydrated states, it remains pinched up. Chronically malnourished children may have tenting in the absence of dehydration, and older children may not have tenting when dehydrated. The anterior fontanel may be depressed.
- 10% to 15%: intense thirst, irritability or lethargy, absent

tears, sunken anterior fontanel, decreased blood pressure, poor peripheral perfusion, pallor
- >15%: inability to maintain blood pressure

Because most of these physical findings result from decreased extracellular fluid, physical findings are greatest in hyponatremic dehydration for any degree of fluid loss. These patients may also have central nervous system symptoms with lethargy and seizures, but typically these do not occur until the serum Na^+ is <120 mEq/L.

Hypernatremic dehydration is primarily a loss of intracellular fluid; therefore, physical findings may not be as marked for any degree of loss of body weight. Because of the relative maintenance of circulating blood volume, these children may not be as oliguric as infants with isonatremic or hyponatremic dehydration, and shock is a late finding. These infants may be lethargic but when stimulated they become irritable with a shrill cry. They are hyperreflexic with increased muscle tone and may have seizures. The skin does not tent but rather has a thick "doughy" feel. An intense thirst is usually present. Approximately one half have hyperglycemia and 10% are hypocalcemic, but only rarely are these clinically significant. As with any small, stressed infant with decreased glycogen reserves, infants with dehydration may also present with hypoglycemia.

DIFFERENTIAL DIAGNOSIS

It must first be determined that the child is dehydrated. Hypernatremia without dehydration, for example, can be caused by salt poisoning (e.g., by incorrect preparation of powdered or concentrated formula or the feeding of inappropriate hypertonic fluids such as boiled skim milk). Water overload (pathologic water drinking or inappropriately diluted oral feedings) or excessive antidiuretic hormone (SIADH), a sequela of various pathologic processes, can cause hyponatremia without dehydration.

Once it is determined that the child has had adequate access to appropriate oral fluids, the cause of excessive fluid loss must be determined. Gastroenteritis with diarrhea and vomiting is the most common cause of excessive enteric losses. However, there may be other causes of excessive gastrointestinal losses, such as structural gastrointestinal abnormalities. Examples include hypertrophic pyloric stenosis in young infants, malrotation, and intussusception.

A renal concentrating defect in which the kidneys cannot reabsorb water appropriately is another potential source of excessive water loss. Examples are central or nephrogenic diabetes insipidus and renal tubular acidosis.

The most common endocrinologic disease that can present with dehydration is diabetic ketoacidosis. The various salt-losing endocrinopathies such as congenital adrenal hyperplasia, Bartter's syndrome, and Addison's disease produce hyponatremia. Hyponatremia can also occur in cystic fibrosis with excessive Na^+ losses in sweat, in renal diseases with salt wasting such as chronic renal insufficiency, and with chronic diuretic use.

WORK-UP

History

An accurate history is essential and should stress: (1) urinary frequency and volume (e.g., do the diapers need to be changed as frequently as usual, and when they are changed, are they as heavy as usual? Frequent diarrhea may make urine production difficult to evaluate, however.); (2) urinary concentration (e.g., does the urine smell stronger than usual?); (3) an estimate of stooling or emesis in terms of volume and frequency; (4) the child's mental status, and, most important, (5) what the most recent weight has been. In addition, the physician should determine what fluids the child has been offered and how much he or she has taken.

Physical Examination

All dehydrated children should be weighted both to objectively assess the dehydration and to establish a baseline should their clinical status worsen. Vital signs must be obtained in all patients. Hyperpnea and tachypnea suggest that decreased tissue perfusion has resulted in metabolic acidosis. Decreased circulating blood volume causes tachycardia, which can exceed 200 beats/min in infants. It is not uncommon for small, stressed infants to become hypothermic after lying unwrapped on an examination table. Blood pressures should be obtained with an appropriate-sized cuff in all children considered dehydrated. If an automatic or auscultatory blood pressure is not obtainable, a systolic blood pressure should be determined by palpation. The inability to obtain a blood pressure reading may suggest hypotension or poor peripheral circulation. The extent of dehydration (e.g., mental status, skin turgor, mucous membranes, anterior fontanel, peripheral perfusion, and peripheral pulses) should be evaluated. A careful examination of the abdomen should be performed to exclude signs of surgical disease, such as bowel obstruction and pyloric stenosis.

Laboratory Tests

The extent of laboratory investigation is largely based on the degree of dehydration. A urinalysis should be obtained. The specific gravity in the absence of glycosuria and proteinuria will indicate the severity of dehydration. Mild proteinuria may be present with significant dehydration. An alkaline urine with moderate to severe dehydration suggests renal tubular acidosis. Ketonuria and glycosuria are seen with diabetic ketoacidosis. Mild degrees of ketonuria are commonly seen in ill children who may not have been eating regularly. On microscopic examination there may be some cellular debris, but excessive cellular elements suggest the presence of renal disease. With moderate to severe dehydration, the physician should obtain blood for laboratory evaluation. Electrolytes, BUN, and creatinine should be determined to aid in evaluating the degree of dehydration (hemoconcentration will result in elevated BUN). Blood glucose can be evaluated initially by a semiquantitative indicator strip rather than waiting for a quantitative result from a laboratory. In infants with severe dehydration, an arterial blood gas should be obtained to determine if acidosis is present. If a renal concentrating defect is suspected, serum osmolality can be measured and compared to urine osmolality.

THERAPY

The approach to the management of dehydration is changing from the use of intravenous fluids in hospitals to an approach that encourages oral rehydration. As more experience is gained by American physicians, the oral approach will likely be increasingly used.

The first, and most critical, step in managing a patient with dehydration is to assure an adequate circulating blood volume. The evaluation is based on a history and a physical examination. Inadequate circulating blood volume requires urgent intervention with intravenous fluids. If there is adequate peripheral circulation, therapy can be by either the oral or the intravenous route (these will be discussed separately). It should be stressed that no matter which route is taken, clinical estimates of fluid and electrolyte requirements are only approximate, and that with adequate renal function, a general approximation of the degree of dehydration is sufficiently accurate.

Oral Rehydration

There has been a long and successful experience with oral rehydration solutions in Third World nations. Oral rehydration solutions combine glucose, sodium, potassium, and a buffer, taking advantage of the physiologic coupling of sodium and glucose transport in the gut. Current recommendations are that rehydration solutions contain 75 to 90 mEq/L sodium, 20 mEq/L potassium, 10 mmol/L base (usually citrate), and 2% to 2.5% glucose. The final osmolality is about 300 mOsm/L. Maintenance fluid is similar except that the recommended sodium concentration is 40 to 60 mEq/L. Several brands of oral rehydration solution are currently available. Maintenance oral rehydration solutions are adequate for acute rehydration of children with moderate dehydration and normal renal function. Commercially available flavored electrolyte solutions that are advertised for adults as sources of fluids and electrolytes are inadequate for oral rehydration in infants because they have excessive glucose and inadequate sodium, potassium, and alkali (see also Chap. 105).

Intravenous Therapy

The specific requirements of intravenous fluid therapy depend on the degree and the type of dehydration. However, the emergency therapy of all three types is similar. The ongoing intravenous rehydration of hospitalized patients is not discussed.

Emergency Considerations

An adequate circulating blood volume should be assured. Although the exact composition of the rehydration solution depends on the serum Na^+, isotonic fluids (normal saline or Ringer's lactate) can be given to any child with dehydration without worsening electrolyte imbalance. Thus, the initiation of therapy should not await the return of blood tests from the laboratory. Although adults often become hyperglycemic with stress, young children more commonly become hypoglycemic; thus, it is recommended that the first unit of fluid be D_5 normal saline or D_5 Ringer's lactate. Boluses of 10 ml/kg over 10 to 15 minutes can be given and repeated for a total of 20 to 30 ml/kg, depending on mental status, blood pressure, heart rate, and perfusion. As a rule, colloids (e.g., albumin, plasma, hetastarch) are not necessary in the absence of hypoalbuminemia.

Although acidosis will resolve spontaneously with adequate fluid repletion, profound metabolic acidosis (pH <7.0) should be treated with small amounts of bicarbonate (1 mEq/kg). Seizures may occur with hypernatremia or hyponatremia. Unlike hypernatremia, which needs to be corrected slowly, hyponatremia with seizures should be corrected rapidly with 3% saline (513 mEq Na^+/L). Approximately 5 mEq/kg/hr can be given to rapidly bring the serum sodium to safe (but still low) levels. The Na^+ deficit (correcting to 125 mEq/L) in mEq is calculated as follows: $(125 - $ patient's serum $Na^+) \times 0.6 \times$ patient's weight in kg. The number 0.6 is the apparent volume of distribution of sodium. In treating hypernatremic dehydration, one must be careful to avoid too-rapid declines in serum Na^+. As discussed earlier, rapid infusion of dilute solutions can result in cerebral edema. Normal saline or Ringer's lactate is also used for acute repletion of intravascular volume. However, with hypernatremia, Ringer's lactate may be a better choice because it provides a lower chloride load. A serum Na^+ of >180 mEq/L has a high incidence of central nervous system sequelae, and emergency peritoneal dialysis should be considered.

INDICATIONS FOR ADMISSION

The development of specific oral rehydration fluids has allowed for the oral therapy of many children with mild to moderate dehydration who previously would have been admitted to a hospital for intravenous therapy. It is anticipated that an increasing acceptance of oral rehydration by the medical community and the increasingly cost-effective approach by third-party payers will encourage oral outpatient therapy. There will always remain, however, a group of children in whom hospitalization will be indicated.

Hospitalization with intravenous therapy is indicated in the presence of shock, profound metabolic acidosis, and symptomatic hypernatremia and hyponatremia. Although oral rehydration has been used with adequate results for hypernatremic dehydration, until a further evaluation is available, intravenous therapy is probably indicated for moderate or severe hypernatremic dehydration. Serum Na⁺ at high levels requires dialysis. Hospitalization may also be indicated if oral fluids cannot be tolerated because of either emesis or exhaustion. Finally, the physician must be assured that the infant's care-givers are capable of caring for and rehydrating the infant.

ANNOTATED BIBLIOGRAPHY

Avery ME, Snyder JD: Oral therapy for acute diarrhea. N Engl J Med 323:891, 1990. (Well-referenced article strongly supporting oral rehydration therapy.)

Guzman C, Pizarro D, Castillo B, Posada G: Hypernatremic diarrheal dehydration treated with oral glucose–electrolyte solution containing 90 or 75 mEq/L of sodium. J Pediatr Gastroenterol Nutr 7:694, 1989. (Review of a series of infants with hypernatremic dehydration successfully treated with oral rehydration over a 12-hour period.)

Hirschhorn N: The treatment of acute diarrhea in children. An historical and physiologic perspective. Am J Clin Nutr 33:637, 1980. (Review of the historical and physiologic rationales for oral rehydration.)

Pizarro D, Posada G, Sandi L, Moran JR: Rice-based oral electrolyte solutions for the management of infantile diarrhea. N Engl J Med 324:517, 1991. (Comparison of rice-based and glucose-based rehydration solutions in the management of diarrhea with dehydration.)

Segar WE: Parenteral fluid therapy. Curr Probl Pediatr 3:1, 1972. (Thorough discussion of intravenous fluid therapy; particularly good for its explanation of maintenance fluid therapy.)

Snyder JD: Use and misuse of oral therapy for diarrhea: Comparison of U.S. practices with American Academy of Pediatrics recommendations. Pediatrics 87:28, 1991. (Good summary of AAP recommendations; argues that American pediatricians currently use oral therapy less than they should.)

190

Pallor

Paul G. Dyment

"Doctor, my child always looks so pale" is a refrain heard almost daily in a busy pediatric practice. Although frequently accompanied by other nonspecific complaints such as fatigue and listlessness, pallor may be the symptom of most concern to the parent because it is often considered synonymous with anemia and may indicate leukemia.

PATHOPHYSIOLOGY

A child may appear pale for many reasons. The manifestation of pallor can be affected by the state of vasoconstriction of the cutaneous blood vessels, by the presence of edema, and by anemia (i.e., an insufficient amount of circulating hemoglobin in the blood). Children frequently appear pale if they are tired, if they have an acute respiratory or gastrointestinal infection, if they have minimal exposure to sunlight, and if they have a chronic infectious or inflammatory disease, even in the absence of anemia. Acute causes of pallor are usually obvious, and patients generally have signs other than pallor that dominate the clinical picture.

CLINICAL PRESENTATION AND DIFFERENTIAL DIAGNOSIS

Probably the most common cause of pallor in pediatric practice is a fair complexion, which is frequently a familial trait. Food allergy ("the great masquerader") may be another common cause of pallor, along with fatigue and nervousness. The actual prevalence of this symptom complex has been the subject of great controversy because many consider it to be overdiagnosed and infrequently encountered. What is accepted, however, is that atopic individuals often appear pale.

Anemia is the most frequent serious cause of pallor. Classical symptoms of anemia in children and adolescents include headache, palpitations, light-headedness, fatigue, and irritability. However, because profound anemia can occur even without these symptoms, a hemoglobin or a hematocrit should be obtained in children who could be anemic.

Many other diseases can cause pallor. Among the more common ones are chronic inflammatory diseases (e.g., rheumatoid arthritis and inflammatory bowel disease) and chronic infectious diseases (e.g., chronic pyelonephritis, cystic fibrosis, nephrosis, malnutrition, juvenile diabetes mellitus, uremia, and hypothyroidism).

The causes of pallor of acute onset are varied. Pallor from closed head trauma and significant acute infectious processes such as acute pyelonephritis and bacteremia are commonly encountered in a busy pediatric practice. An acute blood loss or sudden hemolytic process even without shock causes pallor. Paroxysmal disorders such as seizures, breath-holding spells, and migraine often lead to, or have associated, pallor. Another common cause in an otherwise healthy child is a reaction to a DPT or DT immunization. This can be associated (but not necessarily) with screaming, fever, or hypotonia. In one British study of 10,000 children who received either of these immunization combinations, 10 children demonstrated an episode of acute pallor within 24 hours, from which they recovered quickly. Syncope, hypoglycemia, and intussusception are less common, though not rare, causes of pallor.

WORK-UP

The history should determine whether the pallor is acute or chronic; if the child is sick or well; and if the child has any of the aforementioned conditions associated with pallor. A complete physical examination should always be performed, with careful attention paid to the complexion and general appearance of the child. For an initial physical assessment of anemia, the physician may compare the lividity of his or her palm to that of the patient's palm to see if pallor is truly present and to carefully look at the degree of pallor of the inferior palpebral conjunctiva. One clue to the diagnosis of food allergy or other atopic conditions is the presence of dark circles under the eyes (*allergic shiners*).

If the child has always appeared pale, if he or she is healthy and growing well, and if the complete physical examination is normal (the usual scenario), then a basic hemoglobin or hematocrit to rule out anemia is the only laboratory test that is indicated. A history suggestive of, or positive for, a nonconstitutional etiology (e.g., failure to thrive), positive physical findings (e.g., edema, jaundice, chronic cough, arthritis, lymphadenopathy, splenomegaly), or a laboratory diagnosis of anemia necessitates a further work-up that should be directed by the suspected diagnosis.

TREATMENT AND INDICATIONS FOR REFERRAL

A child who is pale on the basis of constitutional makeup needs only parental reassurance. Unfortunately, in our culture there is an unwarranted association between vitality and good health and a skin tan. Adolescents and young adults believe they look better if tanned. Because of the alarming increase in skin cancer in this country due probably to increased exposure to the sun, physicians should discuss the need for sun-blocking lotions for all children. This is particularly important for those fair-skinned, "pale" persons who sunburn easily and who are believed to be at greater risk for developing skin cancer years later.

A pale complexion can also be seen in children who usually spend their after-school time indoors, perhaps watching television or playing with video games or a computer. The appropriate questioning can lead to the diagnosis of "exercise deficiency." It may need to be explained that exercising indoors (e.g., playing basketball and remaining "pale") and playing outdoor sports are equally beneficial. This is contrary to widely believed folklore.

The diagnosis of a milk allergy should be confirmed by the response of the symptoms to an elimination diet. Pallor immediately following minor closed head trauma and breath-holding spells may simply require reassurance, whereas other conditions may need to be treated as emergencies (e.g., neurologic signs or symptoms resulting from head trauma, severe blood loss, shock, and serious infectious disease). These children will likely require immediate hospitalization, and the primary care physician may elect to consult with an appropriate subspecialist. It is advisable to have a subspecialist participate in the management of children with more complex chronic conditions such as uremia, cystic fibrosis, and nephrosis. A surgeon should be consulted if a potentially surgical condition, such as intussusception, is suspected.

ANNOTATED BIBLIOGRAPHY

Crook WG: Food allergy: The great masquerader. Pediatr Clin North Am 22:227–238, 1975. (Written by a general pediatrician with many years of office-practice experience; the points he raises are reasonable, and perhaps most physicians do underdiagnose food allergy.)

Pollock TM, Miller E, Mortimer JY et al: Symptoms after immunizations with DPT and with DT vaccine. Lancet 2:146–149, 1984. (This large prospective study of 10,000 children who received either of these vaccines showed no difference in the rate of acute reactions; occur in 1 per 1000.)

Tunnessen WW Jr: Signs and Symptoms in Pediatrics, 2nd ed, pp 66–68. Philadelphia, JB Lippincott, 1988. (Excellent outline of the acute and chronic causes of pallor.)

191
Fatigue
Anita Feins

Beginning in utero, a sign of health is an active fetus. Activity heralds the growth and development of the normal baby. Toddlers explore and roam. As children enter school, activity varies; some children love sports activities, and others are sedentary. The sudden decrease in the "normal" activity of a child causes concern for both parent and pediatrician.

The approach to a child with sudden fatigue depends on the age of the child. Younger children are more likely to have an organic etiology causing fatigue. As a child matures and develops, psychological variables complicate the picture as the clinician tries to differentiate between fatigue that is organic and fatigue that is symptomatic of childhood depression or anxiety. Adolescents often complain of being tired. Do they have chronic fatigue, defined as lethargy lasting more than 2 months? Is this a child with a history of a recent viral illness, or is he or she developing chronic fatigue syndrome (CFS)? Chronic fatigue syndrome typically presents in females who are psychologically vulnerable and whose recovery from a viral illness is unusually protracted.

ACUTE FATIGUE

Clinical Presentation and Differential Diagnosis

Infants, toddlers, and school-age children differ in the clinical expression of acute fatigue. Babies begin life by sleeping irregularly, yet when awake are available for the activities of eating, fixing and following, babbling and smiling. Activity is the fuel that feeds normal development. The typically active baby who suddenly is too tired to eat, babble, and play needs to be evaluated. The dull infant concerns all who care for him or her. The baby who sleeps excessively, eats little, gaze averts, and cannot play may be a baby who is emotionally neglected and depressed. It is important to differentiate between the baby who is inactive because of fatigue and the baby who is hypotonic. Hypotonic infants have been inactive since conception. Congenital hypotonia, chromosomal abnormalities, congenital infection, hypothyroidism, inborn errors of metabolism, and Prader–Willi syndrome are important diseases to consider when working up the hypotonic child (see Chap. 146, "The Floppy Infant," for a complete discussion). Myasthenia gravis is one of the few muscle diseases that presents with lethargy. Infants who are withdrawing from drugs they were exposed to in utero tend not to be lethargic but hypertonic, lacking the "lazy" demeanor that characterizes the "tired" baby.

Infection, caused by any organism in any target organ, can cause fatigue and should be ruled out. Head trauma (resulting, for example, in a concussion or CNS bleed), lead poisoning, intussusception, ingestion, severe dehydration, respiratory insufficiency, anemia, severe hypoglycemia, and diabetic ketoacidosis are the most common causes of acute fatigue in this age group.

In addition to the organic causes stated above, the effect of school must be considered in the school-age child. With the psychological impact of school on the developing child, behavioral factors become increasingly important in considering the etiology of acute fatigue in childhood. Children who are having difficulty with peers or who are struggling academically may become excessively tired, perhaps even too tired to go to school. A recent history of fever or viral illnesses is also important to elicit, because postviral syndromes and chronic fatigue begin to emerge during this period.

Environmental toxins caused by gas leaks or faulty exhausts in cars may lead to carbon monoxide exposure, causing lethargy.

Competitive sports, overtraining for school teams, and extracurricular activities begin when children enter school. A busy academic schedule followed by daily sports practices and late bedtimes produces tired children. The illicit use of drugs, including cocaine, barbiturates, and alcohol, begins during this age. Many over-the-counter antihistamine drugs used to control cold or allergy symptoms may cause fatigue.

Work-Up

History. A careful history should include: onset of symptoms, development of symptoms (gradual versus sudden), associated factors (including fever, vomiting, and diarrhea), treatment given at home, medications in the house, recent travel, extracurricular activities, functioning at school, exposure to illnesses, growth and development, and accidents involving head injury.

Physical Examination. The physical exam must include vital signs and weight, and special attention should be paid to the head, ears, eyes, nose, throat, chest exam, abdominal exam, lymph nodes, and character of the skin. An evaluation of mental status and a complete neurologic exam in children of all ages enable the clinician to assess the extent of generalized fatigue on the central nervous system (CNS). Understanding the involvement of the central nervous system in the "fatigued" child will be critical in managing the patient.

Laboratory Tests. Initial laboratory evaluation must include those tests that will allow the clinician to diagnose serious or life-threatening illness. The work-up of a child with fatigue depends on the clinical situation, the child's history, and his or her physical finding. Children with acute fatigue and a history of fever will often require a complete blood count (CBC) with differential, a blood culture, urinalysis, urine culture for bacteria and cytomegalovirus (CMV), a heterophile titer, toxic screen, chest x-ray, and erythrocyte sedimentation rate (ESR). A lumbar puncture is indicated in the sleepy child who does not have focal findings on his or her neurologic exam. Any child who may have had a recent head injury or who has a focal neurologic finding needs an immediate CT scan or MRI scan to rule out an intracranial bleed. Work-up for metabolic abnormalities including thyroid disease, lead screen, electrolytes, BUN, creatinine, pH, and pregnancy test is also helpful if there is no indication of infection.

Management

Because infection is the most likely cause of acute fatigue in children of all ages, appropriate use of antibiotics may be life-saving in a child with a serious infection. The child with a serious infection, lethargy after a head injury, or a significant ingestion will need hospitalization and perhaps subspecialist consultation.

Most children who are tired because of a viral illness recover within several months. Fatigue that extends longer than 6 months is unusual and needs further evaluation focusing on particular characteristics of the child. Is the child overextended? Has he or she not received the adequate rest needed for recovery? Is fatigue a presentation of depression? Is the child receiving secondary gain in continuing to be tired? Consultation by a psychiatrist, therapist, or counselor may be helpful in understanding the role that continued fatigue may play in a child's life.

CHRONIC FATIGUE SYNDROME IN CHILDHOOD
Clinical Presentation and Differential Diagnosis

While fatigue is often a pervasive symptom with acute infection, the persistence of this symptom in the absence of fever becomes an entity in itself if it lasts longer than 2 months. *Chronic fatigue syndrome* (CFS), a state of debilitating fatigue described extensively in adults, may also be seen in the school-age child. Children aged 6 through 17 with CFS may present with complaints of fatigue, headache, and abdominal pain, which are very similar to the symptoms seen in adults. The etiology of CFS remains controversial and unclear. Brucellosis, Epstein–Barr virus (EBV), and chronic candidiasis have been implicated as causes of CFS. The typical patient with CFS is usually a female adolescent or young adult who has a history of previous psychological problems.

Prior viral infection with EBV predates the onset on the syndrome in many patients. Chronic enteroviral infections, coxsackievirus B, chronic brucellosis, chronic candidiasis, benign encephalomyelitis, vitamin B_{12} deficiency, sleep apnea, immunoglobulin deficiency in IgG_3 and IgG_1 subclasses, anemia associated with hypermenorrhea, and depression are also associated with syndromes of prolonged fatigue. Environmental toxins including carbon monoxide and radiation exposure, lead, sleep deprivation, allergies, and overtraining in athletics are factors leading to chronic fatigue that may be overlooked. The obese child, who tends to be inactive, often finds himself or herself in a cycle of fatigue–overeating–decreased activity. A youngster with a tired, depressed affect may have been a victim of sexual abuse. Fatigue is common in the first trimester of pregnancy.

Work-Up

A careful history focusing on the onset of symptoms, previous infections, associated symptoms, treatment to date, and environmental exposure is important in the initial evaluation of a patient who presents with chronic fatigue. Assessing the child's overall functioning in school, in extracurricular activities, and with his or her peers will allow the clinician to target a domain in which the child is having difficulty. Many children with CFS have had a history of psychiatric illness, particularly depression or acute anxiety, in addition to a recent viral illness. A complete physical exam is essential in the evaluation of a child with CFS because a positive physical finding allows the clinician to focus the work-up. The physical exam is often normal, however.

The laboratory work-up for the child with CFS must be complete without being excessive and unfocused. A complete blood count with differential, ESR, thyroid function studies, lead screen, screen for EBV (mono spot), culture for CMV, toxoplasmosis titer, BUN and creatinine, urinalysis and urine culture, liver function tests (e.g., SGPT, bilirubin), immunoglobulins with IgG subclasses if the child has had repeated infections, and a pregnancy test are reasonable initial screening tests.

Management

There is no treatment for children with CFS. Most symptoms improve within 6 months. Psychiatric referral is often indicated if fatigue persists in the presence of a continued normal physical exam and normal laboratory tests. Children with CFS need to be monitored closely, with particular attention to development of fever and patterns of fever, weight loss, and change in any aspect of the physical exam. Reassessment with or without laboratory tests (e.g., a CBC with differential, sedimentation rate, liver function tests, and urinalysis) should be repeated every 7 to 10 days. Children with CFS and behavioral problems may need psychotherapy while being followed medically. Unfortunately, the nonspecific nature of CFS and existing maladaptive functioning cause frustration in the clinician, the patient, and the family. The encouraging aspect of treatment is that fatigue usually resolves over time.

ANNOTATED BIBLIOGRAPHY

Bell K, Cookfair D, Bell D et al: Risk factors associated with chronic fatigue syndrome in a cluster of pediatric cases. Rev Infect Dis 13(Suppl 1):S32-S38, 1991. (Study of seven cases of CFS in rural New York showing that a combination of host and environmental factors, including infectious disease agents, contributes to the etiology of CFS in children.)

Hayden S: A practical approach to chronic fatigue syndrome. Cleve Clin J Med 58(2):116–120, 1990. (Outlines the approach to CFS in adults.)

Hotchin NA, Read R, Smith DG et al: Active Epstein–Barr virus infection in post-viral fatigue syndrome. J Infect 18(2):143–150, 1989. (Twenty percent of patients with postviral fatigue syndrome [PVFS] had serologic evidence of active infection with Epstein–Barr virus. The study suggests that there are multiple causes of PVFS, and that in the absence of an immunosuppressive agent that may in itself cause PVFS, EB virus may be an etiologic agent.)

Kruesi MJ, Dale J, Straus SE: Psychiatric diagnoses in patients who have chronic fatigue syndrome. J Clin Psychiatry 50(2):53–56, 1989. (Patients with CFS have a higher incidence of psychiatric disorders prior to their illness.)

Minden S, Reich P: Nervousness and fatigue. In Blacklow R: MacBryde's Signs and Symptoms: Applied Pathologic Physiology and Clinical Interpretation. Philadelphia, JB Lippincott, 1983. (Excellent and exhaustive chapter that discusses issues of fatigue and its differentiation from tiredness.)

Murray BJ: Complications following coxsackievirus B infection. Am Fam Physician 38(5):115–118, 1988. (Suggests that coxsackievirus B may be an etiologic agent in CFS.)

Sacks N, Van Rensburg AJ: Clinical aspects of chronic brucellosis. S Afr Med J 50(19):725–728, 1976. (Chronic brucellosis presents with fatigue, headache, muscle aches, and lymphadenopathy and should be considered an etiologic agent in CFS.)

Straus SE, Tosato G, Armstrong G et al: Persisting illness and fatigue in adults with evidence of Epstein–Barr virus infection. Ann Intern Med 102:7–16, 1985. (Study showing that fatigue following EB viral infection may last many months but eventually resolves.)

192

Syncope

Peter T. Heydemann

Syncope is a common, potentially serious symptom that occurs in all age groups and has been estimated to occur in more than one quarter of adolescents. The term *syncope* describes a rapid loss of consciousness and postural tone due to a sudden diminution in the brain's blood (or oxygen) supply. In addition to symptomatic treatment, the physician's major issues in evaluating a rapid loss of consciousness are determining whether the episode was due to a cause other than syncope (e.g., epilepsy, hypoglycemia, or behavior) and, if not, what specific factor predisposes the patient to syncope.

CLINICAL PRESENTATION AND PATHOPHYSIOLOGY

Because syncope is an intermittent phenomenon, the patient is usually without symptoms or signs in the doctor's office. Predisposing conditions may be apparent: heart disease, dehydration, anemia, or pregnancy (see the display entitled "Factors Predisposing to Syncope"). Orthostasis is a common element of many kinds of syncope.

There are four phases of syncope: a preceding event, the presyncopal symptoms, loss of consciousness and postural tone, and the recovery period. Syncope is commonly preceded by an event or activity that causes destabilization of autonomic function or cardiac output. Such factors include sudden standing, an overheated environment, hyperventilation, pain, and emotional shock. Often more than one of the preceding events will occur in combination. The early symptoms last a few seconds to several minutes. When they are brief, only a sense of lightheadedness and dimmed vision is noted along with pallor. If the early symptoms last longer, there is a sense of apprehensiveness accompanied by clammy perspiration and epigastric discomfort similar to nausea (but often distinct). Pallor is prominent because of peripheral vasoconstriction, and is associated with an initial tachycardia and pupillary dilation (similar to the "fight or flight" reaction). An urge to urinate or defecate is often noted. The patient may feel the need to lower his or her head to aid cerebral blood flow. Visual blurring and clouded consciousness occur as the tachycardia gives way to a slowing of the heart rate. If the attack is not interrupted, a loss of postural tone and consciousness ensues. The unconsciousness commonly lasts only 10 seconds and ends when the blood pressure and cerebral blood flow are re-established. Awakening is accompanied by pallor, mild confusion, and unsteadiness, which lasts seconds to minutes. This should

be distinguished from the more prolonged postictal state following a generalized seizure.

If cerebral blood flow is not reestablished quickly, convulsive syncope may occur. A loss of postural tone is protective in syncope because the patient falls, which lowers the head and allows the low systemic blood pressure to reach the cerebrum more easily. Thus, convulsive syncope is more likely to occur when the patient is prevented from falling because he or she is seated in a chair (or on a toilet), standing in a phone booth, or being held upright by a parent or bystander. The convulsion has all the typical characteristics of a grand mal seizure and may be associated with incontinence of the bowel or the bladder and a more prolonged postictal state.

The pathophysiology of syncope relates directly to the effects of decreased arterial blood flow on the cerebrum. There are three major mechanisms of diminished blood flow: (1) cardiac disease including arrhythmias and outflow obstruction, (2) vascular disorders generally resulting in inadequate venous return to the heart, and (3) reflex syncopes, most commonly vasodepressor syncope. With cardiac syncope, a decreased rate or stroke volume results in syncope when effective circulation to the brain cannot be maintained. Exercise is frequently the stimulus that brings on cardiac syncope.

Vascular disorders causing syncope are predominantly arteriolar and venous but may rarely involve the great arteries. When there is ineffective venous return to the heart, due to either hypovolemia or overexpansion of the peripheral vascular bed, syncope may result from the consequent diminished cardiac output. The act of rising to a standing position is frequently the final event that aggravates the already diminished venous return and results in orthostatic syncope. Hypovolemia should never be overlooked because it is common and easily treated. An unusual arterial vascular disease is known as *subclavian steal syndrome*. It is due to proximal obstruction of the subclavian artery and consequent shunting of blood from the brain to the arm by way of the ipsilateral vertebral artery, especially during arm exercise.

Vasodepressor or vasovagal (sometimes called "neurocardiogenic") *syncope* is the most common of the reflex syncopes. The actual reflex arc is complex. An emotional shock or surprise is interpreted rapidly by the limbic system and results in a vasomotor outpouring that causes marked peripheral vasodilation, particularly in the mesenteric and skeletal muscle beds. Thus, total systemic peripheral resistance suddenly drops. Cerebral perfusion cannot be maintained because cardiac output does not increase appropriately to compensate. Although increased vagal input to the heart may be the reason that a compensatory tachycardia does not occur, atropine does not abolish vasodepressor syncope. Like all other syncopes, it is aggravated by the upright posture. Other reflex syncopes, with varying mechanisms, include cough, micturition, and defecation

Factors Predisposing to Syncope

VASCULAR—DECREASED VENOUS RETURN

Pregnancy
Anemia
Dehydration
Hypovolemia
Obstructive venous disease
Poor autonomic reflexes (e.g., dysautonomia, neuropathy)
Spinal cord disease
Medications (e.g., diuretics, phenothiazines)

VASODEPRESSOR SYNCOPE

Pain
Emotional shock

OTHER REFLEX SYNCOPES

Breath-holding spells (see Chap. 212)
Cough syncope
Micturition syncope
Defecation syncope
Carotid sinus stimulation

VASCULAR—ARTERIAL DISEASE

Subclavian steal syndrome

CARDIAC DISEASE—OBSTRUCTIVE

Hypertrophic aortic stenosis
Mitral stenosis
Cardiac tamponade
Tetralogy of Fallot

CARDIAC DISEASE—ARRHYTHMIC

Tachyarrhythmias
    Paroxysmal atrial tachycardia
    Prolonged QT syndrome
    Recurrent ventricular tachycardia
Bradyarrhythmias
    A-V conduction block (Stokes–Adams)
    Sick Sinus Syndrome (bradycardia–tachycardia syndrome)

syncopes, in addition to pallid breath-holding spells of infancy.

The common orthostatic syncope of adolescence is due to faulty compensation of normal cardiovascular reflexes in this age group. Instead of appropriate mild tachycardia upon standing, the affected adolescent ultimately develops bradycardia after standing for a few minutes.

DIFFERENTIAL DIAGNOSIS

When a patient faints, syncope is only one of several diagnostic possibilities. Epilepsy, hypoglycemia, basilar artery migraine, hyperventilation spells, and hysteria are the primary alternatives. In addition, vertigo may be confused with presyncopal lightheadedness.

Akinetic seizures and complex partial seizures may produce a sudden loss of postural tone and a clouding or loss of consciousness. These spells are not consistently related to activity or postural changes. Like syncope, akinetic seizures (or drop seizures) may have a minimal postictal state; however, akinetic spells seldom have premonitory symptoms such as lightheadedness. Complex partial (psychomotor) seizures may include such premonitory symptoms (though rarely the whole group of "presyncopal symptoms"), but sudden loss of postural tone is a rare occurrence. In addition, primary grand mal seizures must be differentiated from seizures secondary to syncope. In one series, more than 50% of original diagnoses of primary epilepsy were later changed to syncope (see also Chap. 156).

Just as syncope results from an inadequate supply of the substrate oxygen, hypoglycemic attacks result from inadequate supply of the substrate glucose. Hypoglycemic attacks share certain characteristics with syncope: pallor, perspiration, abdominal discomfort, lightheadedness, confusion, unconsciousness, and seizures may occur in both. Hypoglycemic attacks are more gradual in onset and recovery (unless glucose is administered, in which case recovery is more rapid); they do not occur during or soon after meals; and the presyncopal symptoms do not improve with supine or Trendelenburg posture.

Basilar artery migraine, a variant of classic migraine, may occur with abdominal discomfort, dizziness, visual symptoms including "blackout," and a loss of postural tone. The nonsyncopal symptoms of tinnitus, scotomata, vomiting, and true vertigo may occur during the early attack. Postural changes do not affect symptoms. After the early symptoms, a headache is prominent (though not necessarily in each individual attack), and most patients prefer to sleep. A family history of migraine is common (see also Chap. 151).

Hyperventilation spells may lead to syncope because intense cerebral vasoconstriction is part of the pathophysiologic process. The typical spell consists of a feeling of apprehensiveness with deep sighing respirations that are often unnoticed by the patient. Such spells are similar to slow-onset syncopal attacks in that patients may note abdominal discomfort, palpitations, lightheadedness, and (rarely) loss of consciousness. The same emotional situations that sometimes produce syncope may also result in hyperventilation spells. Supine posture may improve symptoms in hyperventilation attacks primarily because lying down helps a patient to relax and reverse the anxiety–hyperventilation cycle.

Episodic behavior simulating fainting may occur as a conscious act or as a subconscious conversion symptom (hysteria). The pace of onset of symptoms varies but is often faster than typical syncope and without the usual premonitory findings. Pallor and hypotension are not part of the attack. Because most presyncopal symptoms are subjective, a sophisticated teenager may give an accurate syncopal history; however, the history is often accompanied by an indifferent affect. The spells generally last longer than brief syncopal spells, and there may be unusually good recall of events during the period of "unconsciousness." These spells occur typically in an emotionally charged setting; they do not relate consistently to postural changes; and they are rare before 10 years of age. Diagnosis is often difficult and may require hospitalization with EEG, cardiac, and video monitoring.

Vertigo and the presyncopal symptom of lightheadedness are often confused. A postural change may bring on either of these symptoms, and pallor, unsteadiness, and nausealike symptoms may accompany both. Vertigo consists of a sensation of the room moving around the patient; in addition, any movement may aggravate the vertiginous feeling, not simply movement to an upright posture as is common in lightheadedness. Children are often unable to make such a distinction, and the diagnosis of vertigo in preschool children is difficult.

WORK-UP

History

A detailed history surrounding the syncopal event is the key to a proper diagnosis. Crowds, overheated environments, emotionally loaded settings, prolonged prior bed rest, medicines, illicit drugs (especially cocaine), and the physical activity and posture of the patient are critical points. Most syncope occurs either with prolonged immotile upright posture or with a change to an upright posture. If the spells occur during vigorous exercise, a cardiac origin of the syncope should be thoroughly evaluated. The patient's sequential sensations at the onset of the spell should be elucidated with special reference to dizziness, lightheadedness, confusion, awareness of surroundings, tingling, palpitations, involuntary movements, abdominal discomfort, perspiration, and aberrations of the special senses (auditory, visual, and olfactory). With regard to the period of apparent unconsciousness, questions should focus on the length of the spell, awareness of surroundings and ongoing events, posture, skin color, body movements, incontinence, and self-injury such as biting. After the period of unconsciousness, the nature and time course of the recovery period should be evaluated. It is often important, in fact critical with small children, to speak to the most reliable person who observed the spell, such as a school teacher. This may necessitate making several telephone calls to get the most accurate history.

Physical Examination

The physical examination is usually normal. Nevertheless, a careful search must be made for abnormalities to help define a specific cause of syncope. An evaluation for cardiac disorders is particularly important because of the possibility of sudden death. It is essential to examine the pulse quality,

rate, and rhythm as well as blood pressure for orthostatic changes. Orthostasis is evaluated after 5 to 10 minutes supine, again after standing still for 15 seconds, and sequentially up to 10 minutes. A drop of more than 15 points in systolic pressure is abnormal, especially if there is a failure to increase heart rate in compensation. An excessive sustained rise in pulse rate (over 40%), pallor, or lightheadedness indicates a predisposition to syncope. "Tilt table testing" is a more sophisticated form of orthostatic blood pressure measurement (see Thilenius reference for details of the test). Observation of the general body habitus is important in looking for the asthenia of adrenal insufficiency, along with the associated increased palmar pigmentation. Mucous membranes and skin turgor must be checked for hydration status. Pallor of the lips or palpebral conjunctivae indicates anemia. The examination for cardiac disease is important. Conditions that decrease stroke volume such as aortic stenosis, pulmonary stenosis, carditis, and pericardial effusion should be carefully evaluated. Weakness of peripheral pulses may indicate focal obstructive vascular disease, such as the subclavian steal syndrome, which is characterized by an ipsilateral decreased radial pulse. Particular attention should be paid to the possibility of pregnancy, a common predisposing condition for syncope. Evidence of neuropathy, spinal cord disease, bulbar disease, or movement disorder must be sought by an observation of gait and movements and an examination of cranial nerves and deep tendon reflexes. Thus, muscle wasting, hyporeflexia, hyperreflexia, and gait or postural abnormalities may indicate an underlying neurologic disease.

Laboratory Tests

The laboratory work-up may range from minimal to extensive. In the case of an otherwise healthy teenager who faints immediately after becoming emotionally upset, an ECG may be the sole laboratory evaluation if the physical examination suggests no clues to an underlying disorder. When an otherwise healthy teenager, who is mildly dehydrated, faints when standing, it is reasonable to perform no laboratory evaluation and simply suggest rest and oral rehydration. At the other extreme, if the teenager has fainted many times during exercise, an exhaustive laboratory search for cardiac disease must be made. When the spells are repetitive and their nature is unclear, it may be necessary to perform detailed testing to differentiate syncope from the alternative causes of brief spells listed above. A detailed first-visit laboratory work-up might include: ECG, chest roentgenogram, electrolytes, fasting blood sugar, drug screen, hemoglobin, EEG, and tilt table test. The tilt test (with or without isoproterenol infusion) is a highly successful procedure used to evoke common "neurocardiogenic" syncope symptoms. A subsequent work-up becomes more detailed and directed toward particular suspicions. Along with a cardiac consultation, Holter monitoring, exercise testing, cardiac echogram, and cardiac catheterization (for

His-bundle study or angiogram) may become necessary. In the differential diagnosis of epilepsy, 24-hour ambulatory EEG may be helpful if a spell can be elicited; prolonged simultaneous video-EEG-ECG monitoring is even better. A neurologic consultation will be helpful. A further neurologic work-up may include a computed tomography or magnetic resonance imaging (MRI) scan of the brain and, less commonly, spine roentgenograms, nerve conduction study, electromyogram, MRI of the spine, myelogram, and measurement of blood catechols.

MANAGEMENT

The treatment for simple vasovagal (neurocardiogenic) syncope is patient education and reassurance. The patient must be well hydrated, have adequate salt intake, and avoid obvious predisposing circumstances, such as prolonged standing in an overheated environment or rising rapidly from a warm bathtub. While keeping in mind that exercise syncope may suggest cardiac disease, susceptible athletes and others prone to dehydration should focus on preventive fluid and salt intake. When the early presyncopal symptoms are noted, it is essential not to ignore them, as the self-conscious teenager is likely to do. The head must be lowered by lying down or flexing the head and body forward in an effort to increase cerebral blood flow. The patient with a history of syncope during venipuncture should always have the procedure performed supine. Tensing one's muscles provides further protection against syncope because vascular resistance in the skeletal muscle bed is increased.

Other treatment depends on individual circumstances, and correctable primary disorders must be addressed. For instance, anemia, dehydration, and cardiac arrhythmia have specific treatments. Predisposing medications may be withdrawn or substituted. Cough syncope may be controlled by treating the causes of a chronic cough, such as asthma.

Beta blocker therapy, such as atenolol 25 or 50 mg, is effective therapy for the teenager with neurocardiogenic syncope who has not responded to simpler measures. In frequently recurring pallid breath-holding spells, atropinic agents may be used. The patient who faints because of hyperventilation must be taught to consciously slow the respiratory pattern, to relax, and to use a paper bag for rebreathing. Propranolol may be effective for hyperventilation when simple measures fail.

When syncopal episodes persist with no obvious cause despite these simple measures, symptomatic management to increase venous return to the heart is indicated. Elastic stockings aid venous return from the legs. In addition, fluorinated mineralocorticoids are used to expand plasma volume.

ANNOTATED BIBLIOGRAPHY

Beder SD, Cohen MH, Riemenschneider TA: Occult arrhythmias as the etiology of unexplained syncope in children with structurally normal hearts. Am Heart J 109:309, 1985. (Emphasis on the diagnosis of arrhythmias as a cause of syncope.)

Boudoulas H, Weissler A, Lewis R, Warren J: The clinical diagnosis of syncope. Curr Probl Cardiol 7:1–40, 1982 (Thorough discussion of syncopal mechanisms with emphasis on cardiovascular mechanisms.)

Gastaut H: Syncopes: Generalized anoxic cerebral seizures. In Vinken and Bruyn (eds): Handbook of Clinical Neurology, Vol 15, pp 81–835. Amsterdam, North-Holland, 1974. (Discussion of syncope with focus on neurologic aspects and pathophysiology.)

Manolis A, Linzer M, Salem D, Estes N: Syncope—Current diagnostic evaluation and management. Ann Intern Med 112:850–863, 1990. (Broad discussion of syncope with over 200 references.)

Ormerod AD: Syncope. Br Med J 288:1219, 1984. (Presents an interesting algorithm to the approach of syncope.)

School S, Nelson S, Boudoulas H et al: Syncope. Curr Probl Cardiol 17:207–264, 1992. (Good algorithm for the work-up and management of syncope.)

Sledge W: Psychological factors in the onset of vasovagal syncope. Psychosom Med 40:568, 1978. (Discusses psychological circumstances in individuals who have recurrent vasovagal syncope.)

Thilenius O, Quinones J, Husayni T, Novak J: The tilt test for diagnosis of unexplained syncope in pediatrics. Pediatrics 87:334–338, 1991. (Explains the protocol and usefulness of the tilt test and documents the success of beta blockers in common neurocardiogenic syncope.)

193

Edema

Jody R. Murph
and Jerold C. Woodhead

Edema represents an abnormal accumulation of fluid within the interstitial space resulting from either excess fluid and water retention or increased fluid movement across capillary membranes. It may be *generalized* or *localized* to one region of the body and may be indicative of several disease states.

PATHOPHYSIOLOGY

Fluid volumes within the intravascular and interstitial compartments maintain equilibrium when capillary membrane permeability is intact and a balance exists between plasma oncotic pressure and intravascular hydrostatic pressure. Interstitial fluid accumulates when oncotic pressure decreases or when capillary membrane permeability or hydrostatic pressure increases. Edema forms as fluid escapes from the intravascular space to the interstitial space within the capillary bed.

In healthy children, colloid oncotic pressure, produced by plasma proteins, is exceeded by hydrostatic pressure at the arterial end of the capillary bed and causes movement of fluid into the interstitium. The reverse occurs at the venous end of the capillary bed where hydrostatic pressure is less than oncotic pressure and fluid is reabsorbed. Excess fluid filtered into the interstitial space is returned to the circulation through the lymphatic system. Normally, fluid movement remains balanced and there is no net change in fluid volumes. A shift in this equilibrium causes localized or generalized interstitial fluid accumulation; edema then develops.

Increased hydrostatic pressure accompanies several disease states, including congestive heart failure, constrictive pericarditis, and portal hypertension. In these situations, edema forms because the force driving fluid out of the vascular compartment is greater than the oncotic force that promotes fluid reabsorption. Decreased oncotic pressure occurs in illness characterized by protein loss, such as nephrotic syndrome or protein-losing enteropathy.

Increased capillary permeability may play a role in the formation of edema, occurring as a result of allergic reactions, hereditary angioedema, chemical or thermal injury, and certain infections such as Rocky Mountain spotted fever. Localized edema may occur more commonly in diseases associated with altered capillary permeability than in those associated with altered hydrostatic or oncotic pressures.

Impaired lymphatic flow may produce edema in children with Milroy disease, Turner syndrome, lymphoma, intestinal lymphangiectasia, and filariasis.

Renal handling of sodium and water also plays a role in the development of edema. Approximately two thirds of the glomerular filtrate undergoes obligatory reabsorption in the proximal tubule. Excretion or reabsorption of the remainder of the filtrate is regulated by the action of aldosterone and antidiuretic hormone in the distal tubule. Excretion of these hormones is altered in certain disease states such as congestive heart failure, cirrhosis, and the nephrotic syndrome, thereby contributing to edema formation.

DIFFERENTIAL DIAGNOSIS

Localized edema is much more common than generalized edema and may result from discrete areas of altered capillary permeability (e.g., an insect bite) or may be one of the first manifestations of a systemic illness that produces generalized edema (e.g., nephrotic syndrome). The periorbital area is particularly predisposed to edema formation because of the low tissue tension that allows the ready accumulation of interstitial fluid. Acute glomerulonephritis, nephrotic syndrome, Rocky Mountain spotted fever, angioedema, serum sickness, congestive heart failure, and hypothyroidism may cause periorbital or more generalized edema. Periorbital edema, as a localized reaction, may also occur with sinusitis, scarlet fever, infectious mononucleosis, roseola, conjunctivitis, orbital or periorbital cellulitis, conjunctival

foreign body, insect sting or bite, and local allergic reaction. Other forms of localized edema include mumps-related edema of the anterior chest wall; pretibial edema of hypothyroidism; edema of the hands and feet in newborns with Turner syndrome or Milroy disease, and in older children with sickle cell anemia (hand–foot syndrome) or Kawasaki disease; and edema of the forehead or scrotum in Henoch–Schönlein (anaphylactoid) purpura.

Generalized edema or *anasarca* (edema plus ascites) may occur at any age and may result from disease processes in several organ systems. Cardiovascular causes of generalized edema include congestive heart failure, pericardial effusion, and constrictive pericarditis. Gastrointestinal disorders may produce edema by protein malabsorption (e.g., cystic fibrosis) or protein loss (e.g., protein-losing enteropathy, celiac disease, ulcerative colitis, regional enteritis (Crohn's disease), and chronic infection or infestation, such as giardiasis, with severe or chronic diarrhea). Hepatic causes include biliary atresia, Chiari's syndrome, cirrhosis, hepatitis, hepatic failure, and portal hypertension. Nutritional deficiencies of protein (kwashiorkor), vitamin C (scurvy), and vitamin B_1 (beriberi) produce generalized edema. The infant with severe anemia may develop edema, and edema is the primary clinical feature of the newborn with hydrops fetalis. Possible causes of fetal hydrops include cardiovascular disease (malformations, arrhythmias, neoplasia, cardiomyopathy, or high output failure), anemia secondary to isoimmunization or parvovirus B19 infection, chromosome abnormalities, twin transfusion, intrauterine infection (cytomegalovirus, toxoplasmosis, rubella, herpes, or bacterial pathogens), and thoracic abnormalities. Collagen vascular diseases and systemic allergic reactions may also produce generalized edema, as may drugs such as oral contraceptives and other steroids. Generalized edema has also been described in children with type 1 diabetes in association with the institution or alteration of insulin administration. Excessive parenteral fluid and sodium administration is an important cause of edema among hospitalized children. Fluid management may be particularly problematic in children with multiple organ system dysfunction due to trauma, surgery, or disease.

Renal protein loss causes the form of edema most commonly seen in childhood. The combination of massive proteinuria plus edema, hypoalbuminemia, and hypercholesterolemia constitutes the *nephrotic syndrome* and represents the end result of various different pathologic processes within the kidney. Minimal change nephrotic syndrome (MCNS), also called idiopathic nephrotic syndrome, is the most common form of nephrotic syndrome in children. Features that distinguish minimal change nephrotic syndrome include (1) age of onset between 1 and 9 years (most commonly between 3 and 6 years), (2) normal serum complement, (3) absence of *persistent* hematuria, hypertension, or reduced renal function, and (4) response to prednisone therapy. Other causes of nephrotic syndrome in children include acute glomerulonephritis (including poststreptococcal), focal glomerulosclerosis, and membranoproliferative glomerulonephritis. Secondary nephrotic syndrome may also occur in association with such systemic disorders as systemic lupus erythematosus, Henoch–Schönlein purpura, sickle cell disease, and infections such as malaria, subacute bacterial endocarditis, hepatitis B, varicella, AIDS, and shunt infections.

WORK-UP

History

It is important to characterize edematous states with respect to onset, duration (persistent versus intermittent), and extent of the edema (generalized versus localized). In addition, the history should focus on associated signs or symptoms; chronic or acute intercurrent illnesses; exposure to possible allergens, toxins, drugs, chemicals, or environmental factors; and any precipitating events or conditions.

Parents may not be able to identify the onset of edema unless the physician focuses attention on rapid changes in clothing size, such as shoes, belts, or pants that have suddenly become too small. Complaints of puffiness of the eyes, protuberant abdomen, or swollen labia or scrotum may be the presenting feature in a child with generalized edema.

Localized edema should prompt consideration of trauma, insect bite, burn, foreign body, infection, allergy, and angioedema. Hereditary angioedema usually presents during adolescence and is often accompanied by a positive family history.

A comprehensive history is particularly important in determining the cause of generalized edema. A family history of renal or systemic disorders should be solicited. Diarrhea or other alteration in stool quantity or quality may suggest a gastrointestinal disease. A change in urine volume or color may suggest a renal etiology. Rapid heart or respiratory rate, decreased exercise tolerance (often noted by parents as fatigue or inability to keep up with peers), shortness of breath, or a persistent cough may indicate congestive heart failure. In infancy, however, congestive heart failure is more likely to present with irritability, tiring during feeding, and restlessness than with edema. A history of rash may suggest an infectious, allergic, or collagen-vascular etiology. Drug use, either prescribed, over-the-counter, or recreational, may be associated with edema secondary to idiosyncratic, allergic, or toxic reactions or infection from contaminated needles. The history should also include questions regarding an adolescent's menstrual cycle, sexual activity, and use of birth control. Adolescent girls may develop edema secondary to oral contraceptive use or may complain of cyclical edema related to premenstrual fluid retention. Dependent edema may also occur in pregnant adolescents in the second and third trimesters.

Physical Examination

Although localized edema would appear to result from a truly local phenomenon, the physician should be alert for findings that suggest a more generalized process, such as periorbital edema without obvious local irritation. Bilateral involvement of extremities also suggests a more generalized process. Generalized edema, especially anasarca, is easily detected. Evaluation of a child with this degree of edema must include careful attention to weight and vital signs, including pulse and respiratory rates, temperature, and blood pressure. Recent weight change is often the best indication of fluid retention. Orthostatic changes in blood pressure suggest serious depletion of intravascular volume and potential for shock. Hypertension may occur in some edematous states in response to the disease process or as a response to contracted intravascular volume. The presence of pulsus paradoxus of more than 12 mm Hg suggests pericardial tamponade or constriction. Fever must prompt a thorough search for infection, and likewise for local areas of tenderness and erythema. Tachypnea and respiratory distress, rales, wheezes, and areas of diminished breath sounds may indicate pneumonia or pulmonary edema. Abdominal fluid is obvious when a fluid wave can be produced in a distended abdomen. Lesser degrees of ascites present as dullness to percussion. Abdominal tenderness suggests peritonitis, but rebound tenderness may be absent, delayed, or difficult to elicit when ascites is present. Scrotal and labial edema may cause marked enlargement and discomfort. When edema is present, cyanosis, jugular venous distention, hepatomegaly, and petechiae or purpura may be ominous signs.

Laboratory Tests

The history and physical examination suggest a differential diagnosis, which determines the laboratory evaluation. Suspicion of a cardiac etiology should prompt a chest roentgenogram that may demonstrate an enlarged heart, pulmonary edema, the "bag of water" silhouette associated with hemodynamically significant pericardial effusion, or calcifications in the cardiac shadow suggestive of constrictive pericarditis. The electrocardiogram may reveal arrhythmias or may support the diagnosis of pericardial effusion with low-voltage QRS complexes. Echocardiography is the preferred diagnostic tool for the rapid evaluation of cardiac function and the detection of cardiac anomalies and pericardial effusion.

Because renal disease is the leading cause of generalized edema in children, a urinalysis is mandatory. The finding of proteinuria greater than 1+ (30 mg/dl) on dipstick evaluation of a random urine specimen from an edematous child should be followed by a timed 12- to 24-hour urine collection for protein quantification. More than 150 mg protein in 24 hours is generally considered abnormal, although some growing adolescents may spill up to 300 mg protein in 24 hours during their rapid growth spurt. Children with edema caused by renal protein loss typically have proteinuria >50 mg/kg/24 hours (usually more than 2 g total in 24 hours). A urine protein-to-creatinine ratio (Upr/Ucr in mg/dl) on a random urine sample has been shown to correlate with 24-hour protein excretion as a semiquantitative test of significant proteinuria. Levels ≥ 0.2 are generally considered abnormal, although children with nephrotic syndrome commonly have urinary protein-to-creatinine ratios of ≥ 3.5. Because protein loss decreases oncotic pressure, intravascular fluid depletion may occur, and reduced circulating volume may cause diminished renal perfusion. Renal function may consequently decline. Endogenous creatinine clearance should be determined whenever 24-hour urine collections are made so that renal function may be assessed (see Chap. 115 for a detailed discussion of proteinuria). Although up to 20% of children with MCNS have microscopic hematuria at presentation, macroscopic hematuria, when associated with proteinuria and edema, suggests other causes. Serum total protein and albumin, electrolytes, creatinine, urea nitrogen, cholesterol, triglycerides, complete blood count, and sedimentation rate should be performed. All children with generalized edema should also be screened for immune complex-mediated diseases by having C_3 and C_4 complement determinations performed. If hematuria is present, laboratory evaluation should include antinuclear antibody and antistreptolysin O titer (or similar streptococcal antibody screen) determinations. If hereditary angioedema is suspected, levels and function of C_1 esterase inhibitor should be measured. Sickle cell screening, renal ultrasound, and renal biopsy may be selectively indicated.

Other laboratory tests such as liver enzymes; cultures of blood, urine, stool, wounds, and pharynx; sweat chloride evaluation; viral studies; tests of gastrointestinal function; and evaluation for red cell antibodies are reserved for specific clinical indications.

MANAGEMENT

The therapy for edema should, if possible, be directed toward resolution of the underlying disease state. Edema caused by localized processes may respond to topical measures such as the application of ice, heat, or steroid cream, or the elevation of an edematous extremity. Antihistamines, aspirin, nonsteroidal anti-inflammatory agents, or antibiotics may be indicated. When localized edema results from systemic illness, therapy aimed at the illness may reduce the edema.

The management of generalized edema must be directed at its cause, but some basic treatment strategies apply. In general, *activities should not be restricted,* and children should be encouraged to attend school and enjoy their usual routines. *Fluid restriction is unnecessary in most instances* and is difficult to enforce outside of the hospital. When fluid must be restricted, water intake should be reduced to a volume equal to the child's daily insensible water loss plus urine output. Insensible water loss is age dependent, approximately 30 ml/kg/24 hours in the 1- to 5-year-old child, 20 ml/kg/24 hours in the 3- to 10-year-old child, and 15 ml/kg/24 hours in the child over 10 years. Fever and elevated respiratory rate increase insensible water loss.

Salt restriction greatly aids in the control of edema. However, severe restriction leads to poor dietary compliance and promotes "cheating." Compliance is best with a *no-added-salt diet.* Parents should be instructed to cook family meals without added salt, to remove salt shakers from the table, and to avoid foods high in salt, such as processed meats, pickles, soup, certain cheeses, and snack foods such as salted potato chips, pretzels, and nuts.

Diuretics may provide some relief of generalized edema but cannot be considered a definitive therapy and must be used cautiously. Diuretics may actually be detrimental when edema results from decreased plasma oncotic pressure. Because interstitial fluid accumulates at the expense of intravascular volume, diuresis may not occur with standard doses of diuretics, prompting an increase in subsequent doses. Continued high-dose diuretic therapy in this situation may produce a severe depletion of intravascular fluid with resultant shock. Cautious use of diuretics requires a prior assessment of serum proteins and an estimation of intravascular depletion. In general, when serum albumin is below 2.5 g/dl, and when anasarca is present, the intravascular fluid volume will be depleted and the use of potent diuretics will be dangerous unless accompanied by intravenous colloid. In situations such as nephrotic syndrome refractory to steroid therapy, the combination of furosemide plus intravenous salt-poor albumin produces effective diuresis and temporary reduction of edema. Such therapy requires hospitalization and close supervision.

Because MCNS represents one of the most common causes of generalized edema seen in an office-based practice, the subsequent discussion of the management of edema is directed toward this entity. The details of management for other causes of generalized edema are beyond the scope of this text because most require referral to specialists or hospitalization.

Corticosteroids are the mainstay of therapy for MCNS. Children who meet the clinical criteria discussed in the section on differential diagnosis may be started on corticosteroid therapy without a prior renal biopsy and without a referral to a pediatric nephrologist. For this form of nephrotic syndrome, the management of the disease process is synonymous with the management of edema.

Minimal change nephrotic syndrome typically responds to prednisone therapy within 4 weeks. Diuresis, cessation of proteinuria, and resolution of edema occur in 90% to 95% of children treated with steroids. The initial treatment is usually with prednisone, 60 mg/m²/day (or 2 mg/kg/day) with a maximum daily dose of 80 mg. Prednisone is divided into two equal doses daily and is continued for 4 weeks. At the end of 4 weeks, if the nephrotic syndrome has resolved, prednisone should be switched to an every-other-day schedule with 60 mg/m²/day of prednisone (maximum 80 mg/day) given as a single, morning dose on alternate days for an additional 4 weeks. Finally, prednisone should be tapered over a 3-week period at a maximum rate of 20 mg/week.

Relapse occurs in approximately 80% of cases and is often associated with a mild, intercurrent infection. A relapse is defined as proteinuria >2+ (100 mg/dl) on dipstick of random urine specimens for 3 consecutive days and is usually accompanied by the recurrence of edema.

To treat a relapse, prednisone (60 mg/m²/day, maximum 80 mg/day) should be given in divided doses until edema has resolved and urine is protein free (or has, at most, trace protein on dipstick) for *7 consecutive days.* Alternate-day prednisone as a single morning dose is then given for 1 week, followed by a slow tapering at a rate of 10 mg/week.

The child with generalized, persistent edema has an increased risk of infectious complications. Immunoglobulin loss in addition to altered cellular host–defense mechanisms caused by increased interstitial fluid and ascites predisposes to soft-tissue or intraperitoneal infection.

Infection may be difficult to detect and may have a serious outcome in children with anasarca. Signs of the inflammatory process may be blunted and thus delay the identification of an infection. A history of fever in an edematous child should prompt an evaluation for potentially serious infection. Abdominal pain and erythema, or increasing pain or discomfort at sites of minor trauma, may also indicate infection. Peritonitis caused by many different types of bacteria, including *Escherichia coli, Streptococcus pneumoniae,* and *H. influenzae* type b, occurs with increased frequency in patients with anasarca. This is a serious complication that requires the identification of the infecting organism by abdominal paracentesis, with culture and Gram stain of peritoneal fluid. A child with anasarca and peritonitis should be hospitalized in a center with pediatric intensive care facilities where intravenous antibiotics can be administered and the patient can be carefully monitored for evidence of overwhelming sepsis.

INDICATIONS FOR REFERRAL

Indications for referral to a pediatric nephrologist include (1) failure to respond to initial or relapse treatment after 1 month of high-dose daily prednisone, (2) frequent relapses (defined as three or more relapses/year), (3) inability to maintain a remission without steroid therapy, (4) signs of steroid toxicity (e.g., growth failure, cataracts, hypertension, marked cushingoid changes), (5) other signs of renal disease not compatible with MCNS (i.e., persistent hematuria or hypertension, decreased renal function, hypocomplementemia), and (6) children for whom the cause of

edema is not obvious or whose clinical presentation is complicated. Such patients may require renal biopsy or treatment with cytotoxic medications such as cyclophosphamide or immunoregulatory drugs such as cyclosporin. In addition, children with serious infectious complications of nephrotic syndrome, such as peritonitis, may require referral to a center with pediatric intensive care facilities.

ANNOTATED BIBLIOGRAPHY

Boyer JL, Lewy JE: Pathogenesis and treatment of edema in infancy and childhood. In Moss AJ (ed): Pediatrics Update: Reviews for Physicians, pp 281–292. New York, Elsevier Science Pub. Co., Inc., 1984. (Review of pathophysiology of edema and mechanism of action of commonly used diuretics.)

Haycock G: Clinical disorders of sodium, chloride, and water. In Holliday MA, Barratt TM, Vernier RL (eds): Pediatric Nephrology, 2nd ed, pp 95–113. Baltimore, Williams & Wilkins, 1987. (Excellent reference for renal diseases, overview of edema.)

Kher KK, Sweet M, Makker SP: Nephrotic syndrome in children. Curr Probl Pediatr 18(4):197–251, 1988. (Pathogenesis, evaluation, and management of nephrotic syndrome, with extensive references.)

Machin GA: Hydrops revisited: Literature review of 1,414 cases published in the 1980s. Am J Medical Genetics 34:366–390, 1989. (Review of hydrops fetalis, including prenatal diagnosis and management.)

Nash MA, Edelmann CM, Bernstein J, Barnett HL: The nephrotic syndrome and minimal change nephrotic syndrome, diffuse mesangial hypercellularity, and focal glomerular sclerosis. In Edelmann CM (ed): Pediatric Kidney Disease, 2nd ed, pp. 1247–1290. Boston, Little, Brown, & Co., 1992. (Detailed description of nephrotic syndromes, including diagnosis and treatment.)

Paller MS, Schrier RW: Pathogenesis of sodium and water retention in edematous disorders. Am J Kidney Dis 2:241–254, 1982. (Extensive review of edematous disorders.)

Radhakrishna B, Lewy JE: Pathogenesis and treatment of edema. Pediatr Clin North Am 34(3):639–648 1987. (Discussion of the differential diagnosis and treatment of various causes of edema.)

194
Cyanosis
Victor C. Baum

Cyanosis, derived from the Greek *kyanos* or blue substance, results from an excess of desaturated hemoglobin. Cyanosis depends on the presence of a critical absolute amount (not percent) of desaturated hemoglobin. This is often said to be 5 g/dl desaturated hemoglobin. However, with careful observation, cyanosis can be detected in the presence of only 3 g/dl desaturated hemoglobin. Cyanosis is usually categorized as *central* or *acrocyanosis.* With central cyanosis, there is excessive desaturated hemoglobin in arterial blood in all areas of blood flow that can be observed (e.g., skin, lips, tongue, and oral mucosa). Acrocyanosis is the result of an excessive removal of oxygen from localized distal areas of the circulation (e.g., hands, feet, and perioral area).

PATHOPHYSIOLOGY

The hemoglobin level and the oxygen–hemoglobin dissociation curve may affect whether cyanosis is present at any particular arterial PO_2.

Hemoglobin Level. A lower blood hemoglobin requires a higher percent desaturation in order to result in a total of 5 g/dl desaturated hemoglobin. A higher blood hemoglobin level can have 5 g/dl desaturated hemoglobin with a higher percent saturation. For example, a profoundly anemic individual with a total blood hemoglobin of 5 g/dl (hematocrit about 15%) might never be visibly cyanotic, no matter how desaturated the blood became. On the other hand, a polycythemic individual with a hemoglobin of 20 g/dl (hematocrit about 60%) could have an oxygen saturation of 75% to 85% and be cyanotic.

Oxygen–Hemoglobin Dissociation Curve. This curve relates oxygen saturation of hemoglobin (in percent) on the y-axis to PO_2 on the x-axis and results in the well-known sigmoid-shaped curve. A left-shifted curve results in a higher hemoglobin saturation for any given PO_2. Thus, cyanosis will become apparent only at a lower PO_2. Factors that shift this curve to the left include decreased PCO_2, decreased temperature, decreased levels of, or affinity for, 2,3-DPG, and the presence of fetal hemoglobin. Neonates will become cyanotic at lower PO_2 levels than will older individuals with predominantly hemoglobin A.

Although decreased oxygen saturation of arterial blood can be the result of a variety of factors, cyanosis results from one of the following five pathophysiologic mechanisms:

1. Alveolar hypoventilation: While decreased ventilation of the lungs can result in hypoxemia, the primary effect of alveolar hypoventilation is an increase in arterial carbon dioxide content (hypercarbia).
2. Right-to-left shunt: In right-to-left shunting, systemic venous blood bypasses ventilated alveoli and returns to the left side of the heart or to the aorta without being oxygenated. The site of shunting can be intracardiac (e.g., tetralogy of Fallot), at the great vessel level (e.g., pulmonary hypertension with shunting through a patent ductus arteriosus), or intrapulmonary with perfusion of nonventilated areas of the lung. The individual responds to hypoxemia with hyperventilation in an attempt to maintain arterial PO_2. The arterial PCO_2 is usually lower than normal.

3. Ventilation/perfusion ($\dot{V}/\dot{Q}$) mismatch: Normally, within the lung, areas of decreased ventilation are matched with decreased blood flow. Abnormal oxygen saturation can result if this relationship is altered.
4. Impairment of diffusion: Before hemoglobin can be oxygenated, oxygen molecules must diffuse from the alveoli into the pulmonary capillaries. Anything that interferes with this diffusion will affect oxygenation of hemoglobin.
5. Decreased affinity of hemoglobin for oxygen: Because cyanosis depends on the presence of desaturated hemoglobin, the presence of an abnormal hemoglobin with decreased affinity for oxygen at any given PO_2 can result in cyanosis. Oxygenation of hemoglobin can occur only when the iron atom is in its ferrous (Fe^{2+}) state. Hemoglobin with iron in the ferric (Fe^{3+}) state is unable to bind with oxygen and is termed *methemoglobin*. This is produced normally and is reduced to the ferrous state by the enzyme *methemoglobin reductase*. An excessive production of methemoglobin results in cyanosis and may occur by exposure to various agents, including nitrobenzene, aniline dyes, acetanilid, chloral hydrate, amyl nitrite, and even "exposure" to carrot juice and other sources of dietary nitrites. A functionally abnormal methemoglobin reductase can be inherited as an autosomal recessive trait. Certain abnormal hemoglobins, referred to as the *hemoglobins M,* in which a specific amino acid substitution in either the α or β globin chain prevents the return from the ferric to the ferrous state, result in methemoglobinemia. In addition, several other rare hemoglobins have decreased oxygen affinity. Because infants normally have a low level of methemoglobin reductase, they are particularly prone to the induction of methemoglobinemia when exposed to potentially toxic agents.

Acrocyanosis is typically due to pooling of blood in the extremities with increased local extraction of oxygen from hemoglobin. Thus, it can be the result of any factor that slows blood flow through the affected tissues, such as poor cardiac output, vasoconstriction, or peripheral vascular disease. Increased venous pressure can also result in decreased local blood flow with venous suffusion and cyanosis.

CLINICAL PRESENTATION

The presence of central cyanosis is always pathologic. Acrocyanosis may be a normal finding. Newborn infants typically have cyanotic hands and feet during the first day of life. Infants may have cyanosis of the hands and feet when cold and may have a bluish color in the perioral moustache and goatee areas with crying.

Dark skin or lip color can sometimes make a diagnosis of cyanosis difficult at marginal levels of desaturated hemoglobin. The tongue and oral mucosa should always be examined in children with heavily pigmented skin.

The clinical presentation depends on whether cyanosis is acute or chronic. The age at onset depends on the underlying lesion. Children with acute cyanosis may present with tachypnea and metabolic acidosis from decreased oxygen delivery. They have normal hematocrits. Children with chronic cyanosis are often well compensated and stable. They become polycythemic as a response to the decreased oxygen saturation of their hemoglobin. Children with chronic cyanosis typically develop clubbing (hypertrophic osteoarthropathy) of the fingers and toes after 1 to 2 years of age. Clubbing can, however, be due to noncyanotic causes and can be familial. Children with chronic cyanosis can grow and develop surprisingly well, particularly if they do not have congestive heart failure. However, right-to-left shunting predisposes to two potentially catastrophic complications: cerebral thrombosis (stroke) and brain abscess. Cerebral thrombosis occurs most often in children less than 2 years of age. The viscosity of blood increases markedly above a hematocrit of ~65%, resulting in the sludging of blood in small vessels. This hyperviscosity is exacerbated by anything that makes red blood cells stiffer, such as iron deficiency. Brain abscesses occur in ~2% of children over 18 months of age with cyanotic congenital heart disease. Although children with chronic cyanosis are frequently thrombocytopenic, this is rarely severe enough to result in nonsurgical hemorrhagic complications.

Many children with cyanotic congenital heart defects present in the newborn nursery with cyanosis. Others present with a later onset of cyanosis. There may be adequate shunting through a patent ductus arteriosus to prevent visible cyanosis until the ductus arteriosus closes at about 7 to 14 days of age, at which time the infant becomes profoundly cyanotic. Other cyanotic congenital heart defects, such as tetralogy of Fallot or Eisenmenger's syndrome, may not develop enough right-to-left shunting to result in cyanosis until several years of age.

Because of their relative frequency, the cyanotic spells associated with tetralogy of Fallot deserve special mention. These "tet spells," in which children frequently squat down, can be the first symptom in a child with tetralogy of Fallot who has not previously been cyanotic. They often first occur in the early morning after awakening. These children develop anxiety, hyperpnea, cyanosis, and a softening of their murmur. If allowed to progress, irritability, lethargy, loss of consciousness, and even death can ensue. When the episode resolves, the child returns to his previous state without any changes in cardiac or mental status.

DIFFERENTIAL DIAGNOSIS

Although cyanosis is usually a consequence of cardiac or pulmonary disease, disorders in other organ systems must be considered in the differential diagnosis. Numerous specific pulmonary diseases and cardiac malformations can result in cyanosis (see Chap. 54 for a more complete discussion on cardiac causes).

The various diagnoses that should be considered derive from the pathophysiologic mechanisms discussed earlier:

1. Alveolar hypoventilation: Airway obstruction, either congenital or acquired (e.g., aspiration of a large foreign body, morbid obesity, massively hypertrophied tonsils), space-occupying thoracic lesions (e.g., pneumothorax or diaphragmatic hernia), decreased lung volume (e.g., congenitally hypoplastic lungs), decreased pulmonary compliance (e.g., pulmonary edema), neuromuscular disease resulting in weakness of the respiratory muscles, central nervous system abnormalities affecting control of respiration (e.g., seizure activity, infection, trauma, depressant drugs, breath-holding spells)
2. Right-to-left shunt: Congenital heart disease, pulmonary hypertension with a ductal shunt (e.g., persistent fetal circulation also termed persistent pulmonary hypertension), pulmonary disease with atelectasis, pulmonary arteriovenous fistula
3. Ventilation/perfusion mismatch: Respiratory distress syndrome, asthma, pulmonary aspiration, drugs that abolish pulmonary hypoxic vasoconstriction (e.g., isoproterenol, dopamine)
4. Impairment of diffusion: Pulmonary edema, certain uncommon pulmonary alveolar diseases, central nervous system diseases resulting in neurogenic pulmonary edema
5. Decreased affinity of hemoglobin for oxygen: Exposure to toxic substance as described under pathophysiology, absent or functionally abnormal methemoglobin reductase, presence of an abnormal hemoglobin

The age of development of cyanosis with the hemoglobinopathies depends on the specific defect. Abnormalities of the α-globin chain present with cyanosis at birth. Infants with β-globin defects may not develop cyanosis until the β-chain becomes predominant over the fetal γ-chain during the first year of life. Methemoglobinemia results in a more grayish blue or slate gray color than does typical cyanosis.

A useful mnemonic to remember the major cyanotic cardiac lesions is the five T's: *T*etralogy, *T*ransposition of the great vessels, *T*runcus arteriosus, *T*otal anomalous pulmonary venous return, and *T*ricuspid atresia. With the addition of pulmonary atresia, most of the cyanotic lesions are represented.

Sepsis, polycythemia, hypoglycemia, and hypocalcemia must also be considered in the cyanotic newborn.

The differential diagnosis of acrocyanosis includes any cause of decreased cardiac output as well as cold and polycythemia. Acrocyanosis is typical on the first day of life.

Although cyanosis is almost always due to organic illness, breath-holding spells in young children can result in cyanosis. These children have violent crying followed by apnea, cyanosis, and hypotonia. There is a prompt resolution without sequelae, and these episodes are rare after 3 years of age (see also Chap. 212).

WORK-UP

History

It should be determined whether the cyanosis is of chronic or recent onset. A full prenatal and neonatal history should be obtained. A congenital heart defect that results in a murmur in the neonatal period may be responsible for the development of cyanosis many months later. A history of squatting or early morning cyanosis suggests the possibility of tetralogy of Fallot. Evidence of a pulmonary infection should be investigated. The possibility of drug ingestion or foreign body aspiration should be considered. A family history is also important. A family history of congenital heart disease raises the likelihood of congenital heart disease as an etiology, and a family history of chronic cyanosis may suggest a hemoglobinopathy.

Physical Examination

Acrocyanosis and central cyanosis should be differentiated by evaluating the extremities and oral mucosa. In acrocyanosis, the blood that immediately refills a compressed extremity will not be cyanotic. Children with borderline contents of desaturated hemoglobin have a plethoric look before frank cyanosis develops. The physician should consider a shunt at the level of the ductus arteriosus if there is differential cyanosis in the young infant (upper versus lower extremities), which may be made more obvious by having the infant breathe supplemental oxygen. Methemoglobinemia results in a more slate gray color rather than the typical blue of cyanosis. Evidence of respiratory distress (e.g., nasal flaring, grunting, retractions, crackles, wheezing, or stridor) suggests airway or pulmonary disease, whereas tachypnea without dyspnea suggests a cardiac or metabolic etiology. The presence of a murmur may be helpful, but serious cyanotic congenital heart disease may not be associated with a murmur, and children may develop very loud functional murmurs when stressed (Fig. 194-1).

Laboratory Tests

Any child in whom a diagnosis of congenital heart disease is considered should have an electrocardiogram and a chest roentgenogram. However, the electrocardiogram may be normal for age in newborns with certain congenital heart defects. The chest roentgenogram should be evaluated for cardiac size and shape, the presence of increased or decreased pulmonary blood flow, and evidence of abnormal situs (dextrocardia or abnormal shape or position of the liver or stomach). The lung fields should be examined for evidence of space-occupying lesions, pneumothorax, infiltrates, and foreign body aspiration. Because lateral chest roentgenograms are only rarely helpful in newborn infants, an anteroposterior view alone is usually adequate.

Arterial blood gases will document hypoxemia. Crying infants, however, may spuriously lower oxygen saturation compared to samples obtained at rest. The use of pulse oximetry will help obtain a reasonable estimate of arterial oxygenation in the resting infant. Elevated Pco_2 suggests lung disease. The Pco_2 will typically be normal or low in the presence of right-to-left shunting. A *hyperoxia test* in which an infant breathes 100% oxygen is often used in newborns to differentiate cyanosis due to pulmonary disease from cyanosis due to cardiac disease. Because blood that has not been shunted is normally fully saturated, arterial Po_2 will increase minimally in the presence of a right-to-left shunt (e.g., cyanotic congenital heart disease). When the infant is breathing 100% oxygen, an arterial Po_2 of less than 150 torr strongly suggests a cardiac etiology. Three points, however, must be remembered: (1) the physiology of cyanotic heart lesions may be complicated by associated pulmonary disease (e.g., total anomalous pulmonary venous return with obstruction to pulmonary venous flow and pulmonary edema); (2) cyanotic lesions associated with a markedly elevated pulmonary blood flow may have a significant increase in arterial Po_2 when the infant is breathing oxygen; (3) severe pulmonary disease can also result in hypoxemia while the infant is breathing oxygen-enriched gas. Pulmonary disease of this severity is, however, readily apparent on a chest roentgenogram. Capillary Po_2 is often measured in newborns but it is not as reliable beyond the newborn period. It is also unreliable in the presence of poor cardiac output. Venous Po_2 does not correlate with arterial Po_2. The blood of patients with methemoglobinemia and the other cyanotic hemoglobinopathies will have an appropriate Po_2 but an inappropriately low hemoglobin saturation because the problem is one of oxygen binding to hemoglobin. Hemoglobin saturation must be measured, however, and must not be derived from the Po_2 level. Blood containing methemoglobin becomes brownish after standing in room air. Pulse oximeter measurements will be spurious in the presence of methemoglobin. Significant methemoglobinemia will force the oximeter reading to 85%, independent of the true hemoglobin saturation.

MANAGEMENT

Cyanosis is most commonly treated in the hospital by various subspecialists, most often cardiologists. Although the therapy of cyanosis depends on the specific etiology, several general principles apply. Cyanosis of acute onset at any age is an absolute indication for hospitalization. If there is not an obvious pulmonary etiology, a referral to a pediatric cardiologist is indicated. Pulmonary disease producing cyanosis is an absolute indication for referral to a skilled bronchoscopist (for airway obstruction) or to a pediatric critical care unit for therapy of severe pulmonary disease. Dehydration increases the risk of thrombosis in polycythemic patients and should be avoided. Because of the large red blood cell production in polycythemic patients, an adequate iron

CYANOSIS

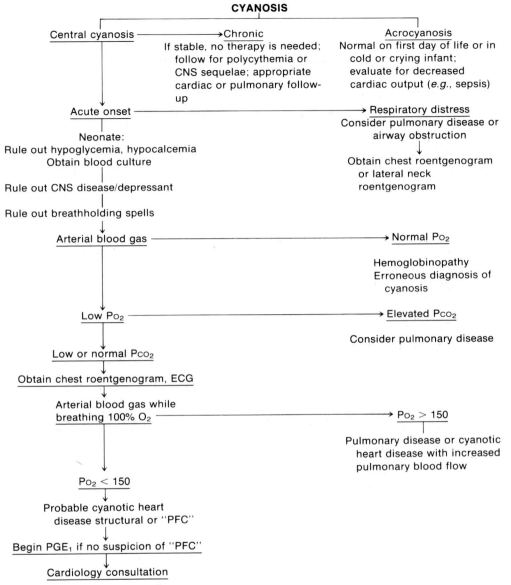

Figure 194-1. The work-up of cyanosis.

and folate intake should be assured, particularly because an iron deficiency may be partially masked by the elevated hematocrit, and iron-deficient blood is more viscous than normal blood. Scrupulous care must be taken to assure that no air is introduced into intravenous lines in the presence of right-to-left shunting because of the potential of air emboli traveling to the systemic arterial circulation.

An acute reduction in the hematocrit in symptomatic polycythemic patients with hematocrits greater than 65% should be done by an isovolemic exchange transfusion rather than by phlebotomy in order to avoid hypovolemia. This is best done by exchanging aliquots of blood with 5%

albumin in saline (5 g albumin/100 ml saline). The total amount exchanged equals:

$$\frac{\text{Initial hematocrit—desired hematocrit}}{\text{Initial hematocrit}}$$
$$\times \text{body weight (kg)} \times \text{blood volume}$$

Blood volume varies from 85 ml/kg in newborns to 60 ml/kg in adults. In severe cyanotic conditions, the hematocrit should be kept at Σ55% to 65% if possible. Persistently higher hematocrits are an indication for surgical correction or palliation of the cardiac defect.

In the immediate newborn period, cyanosis usually precedes a specific cardiac diagnosis. Because this can be life threatening, therapy should not be delayed until a complete diagnosis is made. As discussed above, supplemental oxygen typically does not raise the arterial Po_2 very much. However, additional oxygen is useful because even a small increase in arterial oxygenation is helpful. The maintenance of ductal patency is crucial because many cyanotic lesions depend on blood shunting across the patent ductus arteriosus to bring deoxygenated blood to the lungs or oxygenated blood to the aorta. This is accomplished by a continuous infusion of prostaglandin E_1 (PGE_1) in the newborn, which is diluted and infused at a constant rate of 0.05 μg/kg/min. This can be given through any vascular access. If the infant is later shown not to have a ductal-dependent defect, the prostaglandin can be stopped without adverse effect.

The "tet spells" of tetralogy of Fallot can be treated by various therapies. Initial approaches include oxygen (which will not have a major impact), flexing the legs at the hips and knees to simulate the knee–chest position of squatting, and giving the child morphine 0.2 mg/kg IM (or morphine 0.15 mg/kg IV). Other therapies include propranolol 0.1 mg/kg IV, an α sympathomimetic such as phenylephrine (Neo-Synephrine 1–4 mcg/kg IV), and the calcium channel blockers, all of which decrease right-to-left shunting. Calcium channel blockers are contraindicated in infants. Bicarbonate can be given if acidosis is severe, and transfusions should be given for a hemoglobin less than 15 g/dl. Emergency surgery (a palliative shunt or complete correction) should be performed if all these methods fail.

Acquired methemoglobinemia is treated with methylene blue, 1% solution, 1 to 2 mg/kg IV followed by daily oral doses of 2 mg/kg. The cyanotic hemoglobinopathies do not respond to methylene blue therapy.

Chronic cyanosis is well tolerated. These children, if stable, are readily followed as outpatients with referral only as required for diagnosis or management.

ANNOTATED BIBLIOGRAPHY

Chernick V (ed): Kendig's Disorders of the Respiratory Tract in Children, 5th ed. Philadelphia, WB Saunders, 1990. (General pediatric pulmonology text that elaborately discusses the numerous pulmonary causes of cyanosis.)

Feig SA: Methemoglobinemia. In Nathan DG, Oski FA (eds): Hematology of Infancy and Childhood, 3rd ed. Philadelphia, WB Saunders, 1987. (Detailed discussion of methemoglobinemia.)

Lees MH: Cyanosis of the newborn infant. Recognition and clinical evaluation. J Pediatr 77:484, 1970. (Discussion of the diagnosis and pathophysiology of cyanosis, specifically in the newborn.)

Lombroso CT, Lerman P: Breathholding spells (cyanotic and pallid infantile syncope). Pediatrics 39:563, 1967. (Detailed discussion of cyanotic breath-holding spells.)

Rudolph AM: Congenital Diseases of the Heart. Chicago, Year Book Medical Publishers, 1974. (Superb source for more reading on the pathophysiologic processes underlying the structural congenital heart diseases.)

195
Jaundice
Glenn T. Furuta and Colette Deslandres–Leduc

An overview of bilirubin metabolism is important in understanding the pathophysiology and differential diagnosis of jaundice in the pediatric population. Bilirubin is the principal degradation product of heme in humans. The major source of heme (80%) is hemoglobin from senescent erythroid cells, which is degraded in the reticuloendothelial system of the spleen, liver, and bone marrow. The other sources of bilirubin (10% to 20%) derive from nonerythroid sources, such as hepatic cytochrome P-450. Once heme is dissociated from the globin, it is converted to biliverdin, which is then reduced to bilirubin. This free (unbound to plasma protein) unconjugated bilirubin is a potential toxin. After binding to albumin in the systemic circulation, bilirubin is transported to the hepatocyte, where it is released from albumin and taken up by the hepatocyte. In the hepatocyte, the unconjugated (indirect) bilirubin is conjugated to glucuronide, a polar molecule, by the action of UDPglucuronyl transferase. The conjugated (direct) bilirubin is not toxic and is secreted in the bile. More than 97% of the bilirubin arriving in the gastrointestinal (GI) tract is in this form.

In the GI tract, direct bilirubin is reduced by bacterial action to mesobilirubin, stercobilinogen, and urobilinogen. The latter two are colorless and are oxidized to the colored pigments urobilin and stercobilin. These oxidized compounds may contribute part of the brown color to normal feces. Fuscins are responsible for most of the color of stools. About 75% of the urobilinogen and stercobilinogen is reabsorbed in the ileum by way of the portal circulation and is excreted in the urine.

The differential diagnosis of hyperbilirubinemia (jaundice) can be related to the pathways of bilirubin metabolism. Excessive degradation of red blood cells, displacement of indirect bilirubin from albumin by drugs, abnormal uptake of indirect bilirubin by the hepatocyte, and abnormalities of conjugation by a lack or deficiency of UDPglucuronyl transferase lead to unconjugated or indirect hyperbilirubinemia (Table 195-1). Abnormalities after the conjugation step will lead to a direct hyperbilirubinemia, which is also called *cholestasis*.

CLINICAL PRESENTATION

Jaundice may present with a constellation of symptoms depending on its cause. A newborn may appear ill, vomit, and fail to thrive, as with galactosemia, tyrosinemia, or sepsis, or may be healthy in the first month of life, as with breast

Table 195-1. Differential Diagnosis of Jaundice in Infancy

AGE	INDIRECT HYPERBILIRUBINEMIA	AGE	DIRECT AND MIXED HYPERBILIRUBINEMIA
1–14 days	Physiologic jaundice* Rh and ABO incompatibility Breast milk jaundice Lucey–Driscoll syndrome Crigler–Najjar types I and II	1 day–3 months	Infections: Neonatal hepatitis* E. coli sepsis Urinary tract infection TORCH
2 weeks–3 months	Breast milk jaundice* Lucey–Driscoll syndrome Crigler–Najjar types I and II Congenital hypothyroidism Pyloric stenosis		Anatomic: Choledochal cyst Extrahepatic biliary atresia Inspissated bile syndrome Alagille syndrome Metabolic: Galactosemia Fructosemia Tyrosinemia α_1-antitrypsin deficiency
Postneonatal period	Hemolytic diseases: Gilbert's disease* G6PD deficiency Congenital spherocytosis Autoimmune	Postneonatal period	Viral hepatitis* Wilson's disease Rotor syndrome Dubin–Johnson syndrome

*Most frequent cause in the specific age group.

milk jaundice or extrahepatic biliary atresia. Viral hepatitis may be accompanied by fatigue, fever, anorexia, and vomiting, along with jaundice. Pallor, right upper quadrant pain, poor weight gain, pruritus, arthritis, clay-colored stools, and dark urine are commonly associated with jaundice in a variety of different disorders.

DIFFERENTIAL DIAGNOSIS

The age of the patient and the type of hyperbilirubinemia (direct versus indirect) are major considerations in an evaluation of a child with jaundice.

Birth to 14 Days of Age

In this age group, indirect hyperbilirubinemia is the most frequent cause of jaundice, and physiologic jaundice is the leading diagnosis in this category. In the term infant, the peak rise in bilirubin occurs at 3 days of age and rarely exceeds 15 mg/dl. The preterm infant tends to have earlier and higher peaks, and the duration of jaundice is longer. Numerous hypotheses exist to explain the causes of physiologic jaundice. These hypotheses include immaturity of uptake and conjugating pathways, excessive heme from red cells and muscle, and shunting around the liver by a persistently patent ductus venosus.

Hemolytic diseases such as ABO incompatibility are the second most common cause of indirect hyperbilirubinemia in the first week of life. In this case, the quantity of indirect bilirubin overwhelms the hepatocyte's capacity to conju-

gate. Rh incompatibility is less frequent but more dramatic. A failure to control high peaks of indirect bilirubin in the neonatal period may lead to kernicterus. The hemolytic diseases usually present in the first 36 hours of life.

Toward the end of the first and the beginning of the second week of life, *breast milk jaundice* should be considered in a breast-fed infant with indirect hyperbilirubinemia. This benign condition often recurs in siblings. A substance(s) contained in breast milk apparently inhibits UDPglucuronyl transferase. The bilirubin usually is below 15 mg/dL. Jaundice typically resolves by 3 months of age, even when breast feedings are continued. Breast milk jaundice has not been known to cause kernicterus. The Lucey–Driscoll syndrome is a dramatic situation seen rarely in breast-fed infants in which kernicterus may be a serious complication of high indirect serum bilirubin levels occurring during the first few days of life.

Rarer causes of indirect hyperbilirubinemia in the first 2 weeks of life are the Crigler–Najjar types I and II syndromes where UDPglucuronyl transferase is lacking or deficient, and peaks of indirect bilirubin may be high. Congenital hypothyroidism should also be considered in a newborn with prolonged indirect hyperbilirubinemia. Finally, an abdominal obstruction and pyloric stenosis may be responsible for indirect hyperbilirubinemia.

Between 2 Weeks and 3 Months of Age

Jaundice is usually cholestatic after 2 weeks of age, and a differentiation between *hepatocellular* and *extrahepatic* causes is mandatory. Among the hepatocellular causes, metabolic, anatomic, infectious, and toxic possibilities must be excluded. In most newborns with hepatocellular cholestasis, no cause is found (see Chap. 110). Infectious disorders are the second largest category. Toxoplasmosis, rubella, cytomegalovirus, herpes, enteroviruses, syphilis, hepatitis B, *Listeria monocytogenes,* group B streptococcus, and *Escherichia coli* are the most common offending agents.

Toxic etiologies include parenteral nutrition, particularly in premature infants who received only this form of nutrition for a prolonged time. Metabolic causes are much rarer and include galactosemia, fructosemia, α_1-antitrypsin deficiency, and tyrosinemia. Anatomic causes include inspissated bile syndrome, which follows severe hemolysis and is characterized by plugs of bile in the hepatic canaliculi. The intrahepatic bile ducts may be hypoplastic as part of *Alagille syndrome* (syndromic paucity of interlobular bile ducts) or as an isolated finding. Finally, cystic fibrosis may also be a cause for cholestasis in a newborn.

Extrahepatic obstructive causes of cholestasis must be recognized quickly because they may have a surgical cure. Extrahepatic biliary atresia is a rare disorder occurring in 1:8000 to 1:14,000 live births. Early intervention (before 2 months of age) with a portoenterostomy gives some hope for survival. A choledochal cyst may also be responsible for an obstruction of the biliary tree and may require early surgical intervention.

Postneonatal Period

After the first 3 months of life, the appearance of jaundice in a previously well child is most frequently secondary to a viral hepatitis: HAV; HBV; hepatitis C; cytomegalovirus (CMV); and Epstein–Barr virus (EBV) should all be considered as possible causal agents. Hemolytic diseases such as glucose-6 phosphate dehydrogenase (G6PD) deficiency may manifest when a susceptible toddler is given an oxidizing agent. Severe anemia and indirect hyperbilirubinemia may develop. Although the following disorders may be encountered in other age groups, they are more frequent in late childhood and adolescence. *Gilbert's disease* occurs in up to 5% of whites, and it is the most frequent cause of indirect hyperbilirubinemia in this age group. This disease is a benign condition and presents as mild, intermittent, indirect hyperbilirubinemia. Jaundice is exacerbated with fasting or intercurrent illness. Gallstones may obstruct the biliary tree and produce jaundice (direct type) with severe right upper quadrant pain, nausea, and vomiting. In this age group, specific attention should be given to a hemolytic disease, such as congenital spherocytosis and sickle cell disease, as the cause of the gallstones. Autoimmune hemolytic diseases are seen in systemic lupus erythematosus (SLE) disease, *Mycoplasma* infection, and drug ingestion (e.g., α-methyldopa), or they may be idiopathic. Anemia and jaundice may be acute and impressive. Wilson's disease may also present as an acute hemolytic anemia with acute hepatitis and jaundice (mixed hyperbilirubinemia). Rotor's syndrome and Dubin–Johnson syndrome rarely present in the pediatric population. They are benign syndromes and present with cholestasis secondary to abnormalities in conjugated bilirubin excretion pathways from the hepatocyte.

WORK-UP

History

In the neonatal period, special attention should be given to the age at the time the jaundice was first noticed; the history during pregnancy to determine the role of intrauterine infection, preeclampsia, diabetes, or hypothyroidism; complications at delivery; and the weight at birth. Important antecedents post natum include the type of feeding, blood group incompatibility between mother and child, intolerance to feedings, failure to thrive, age when first stool appeared, and color of stools and urine.

After the neonatal period, special attention should be given to the mode of onset and the duration of jaundice. A history of contact with viral hepatitis, day care attendance, blood transfusions, IV drug abuse, travel in foreign countries, and drug or shellfish ingestion should be sought. A family history of hepatic or hemolytic disease, and a history of early onset of cholelithiasis in siblings, may also be important clues.

Physical Examination

The initial appearance of the patient, including congenital malformations and dysmorphism (Alagille syndrome), should be noted. The skin color may be yellow, greenish, or pale. The skin examination may reveal xanthomas, spider angiomas, palmar erythema, or hematomas.

Upon examination of the eyes, chorioretinitis, seen in toxoplasmosis or cytomegalovirus infections, or the typical Kayser–Fleischer ring of Wilson's disease, may immediately indicate the cause of jaundice. Conjunctivae will become icteric at a bilirubin over 2.5 mg/dl.

The physical examination of the liver should include an appreciation of the size, firmness, and texture of the surface. An acutely enlarging liver is often painful. The gallbladder will be palpable only if it is inflamed or if the outflow of bile is obstructed. Ascites and collateral circulation over the abdomen may also be noted. Splenomegaly may be an important sign in hemolytic disease or long-standing liver disease.

Among other important findings, the auscultation of the heart may reveal the murmur of pulmonary artery hypoplasia that accompanies paucity of intrahepatic bile ducts. Clubbing of the extremities indicates an intrapulmonary right-to-left shunting, which is often seen with cirrhosis.

Table 195-2.   Laboratory Work-Up of Hyperbilirubinemia*

INDIRECT HYPERBILIRUBINEMIA	DIRECT (CHOLEASTATIC) HYPERBILIRUBINEMIA	
	Neonatal Period	
CBC	5'nucleotidase	Serum α_1-antitrypsin
Reticulocyte count	Serum cholesterol	Pi typing of α_1-antitrypsin
Red blood cell smear	Blood, urine culture	Galactose-1-uridyl transferase
Platelet count	VDRL test	activity in RBC
Direct and indirect Coombs'	TORCH antibody titers	Amino acid screen of urine
test	HB_sAg in mother and child	and blood
Serum haptoglobin	Reducing substances in urine[†]	Sweat test
Cold agglutinins	*Postneonatal Period*	
Antinuclear antibodies (ANA)		
G6PD activity in RBC	5' nuceleotidase	CMV antibody titers
Thyroid function tests	Serum cholesterol	Serum ceruloplasmin
Urine culture	HB_sAg + IgM antiHB_cAg	24-hr collection of urine for
	IgM anti-HAV	copper
	Monotest	Toxin screen
		Serum α_1-antitrypsin level

*Serum bilirubin (total and direct), SGOT, SGPT, alkaline phosphatase should be the initial studies. Other tests should be performed selectively.
[†]Galactose and fructose are both reducing substances in the urine: They are Clinitest (+) and Clinistix (−). They may not be detected in urine unless ingested in sufficient quantities.

Laboratory Tests

The first step in evaluating jaundice is to differentiate between direct and indirect hyperbilirubinemia by obtaining a total and direct serum bilirubin (by the van den Bergh reaction). SGOT, SGPT, alkaline phosphatase, and 5'nucleotidase are useful indicators of hepatocellular or bile ductular disease. A general classification of appropriate laboratory tests according to the type of hyperbilirubinemia is presented in Table 195-2.

Imaging Techniques. Ultrasonography of the gallbladder and the portal structures will help detect a choledochal cyst. The presence of a gallbladder *does not* exclude extrahepatic biliary atresia. Hepatobiliary scintigraphy is a safe and important tool in the evaluation of neonatal cholestasis. It is done with iminodiacetic acid (IDA) derivatives labeled with technetium 99m. A 5- to 7-day treatment with phenobarbital is recommended before the scintigraphy.

TREATMENT

Jaundice may be part of a disorder that is curable through medical or surgical means. Frequently, however, palliative measures may be all that can be offered to alleviate the complications of the primary disease.

Diet

In most cases, nursing may continue with breast milk jaundice. If the hyperbilirubinemia is high, cessation of nursing for 2 to 3 days (while substituting formula) results in a dramatic lowering of the bilirubin. The level may rise again once nursing resumes, but not as high as the peak level.

Special dietary manipulation may be useful in the treatment of metabolic disorders such as galactosemia or fructosemia. In prolonged cholestasis, medium-chain triglycerides (MCT) should be the major source of lipids because they are less dependent on bile salts for absorption. In a newborn with cholestasis, formulas such as Portagen, which contains 87% MCT, can be used. Fat-soluble vitamins, especially vitamin E, must be supplied in adequate amounts to compensate for losses. Adequate protein of either animal or vegetable origin must be supplied to maximize the growth potential without causing hyperammonemia. Micronutrient repletion, including calcium, phosphorus, and magnesium, is also essential for growth.

Drugs

Phenobarbital has been used to promote bile secretion and alleviate pruritus, thereby improving the quality of life. Bile acid–binding resins such as cholestyramine may accomplish the same purpose. Both of these agents may have adverse metabolic effects. Recently the synthetic bile acid ursodeoxycholic acid has been used to promote choleresis and relieve cholestasis. The efficacy of this orally administered agent is promising and the drug is being studied in several centers to further determine its use. Pruritus has also been treated with a wide range of antihistamines, although severe cases are often refractory to standard therapies.

Phototherapy

Indirect bilirubin in the skin absorbs light energy and is transformed into nontoxic products excreted by the liver and kidney. The spectrum of light at which phototherapy is most effective corresponds to the maximum absorption peak of bilirubin: 420 nM to 460 Nm, which is the blue light range. The management of hyperbilirubinemia depends on the age (in days) of the patient and the levels of serum indirect bilirubin.

Indications for phototherapy are controversial and beyond the scope of this discussion. Many nurseries have their own policies of treating hyperbilirubinemia, and books on neonatology offer tables or graphs plotting the age of the newborn against the serum bilirubin to determine when phototherapy should be instituted. In general, phototherapy should begin whenever there is a rapid increase in the bilirubin level (i.e., more than 0.5 mg/dl/hr), *or* whenever a further increase in the bilirubin would be hazardous or would require an exchange transfusion. This prophylactic phototherapy might include premature infants with bilirubin greater than 10 mg/dl; healthy, term babies less than 3 days of age with levels of 10 to 15 mg/dl and levels of 15 to 20 mg/dl on day 4; and at lower levels if there is a hemolytic disease of the newborn. Medical problems, hydration, fluid intake, and urine and stool output are important criteria to consider when deciding at what point phototherapy should be started. If begun, babies should be monitored closely for dehydration, and their eyes and gonads should be covered. Alternatively, a fiberoptic mat (e.g., Bili-Blanket, Wallaby) may be used to treat the jaundice. It is wrapped around the torso, thus enabling the baby to be handled, fed, etc. without special precautions such as eye shields. The Wallaby is well-suited for home phototherapy (see also Chap. 213 and Table 213-1). Enteral feeding should be instituted in an effort to increase excretion of bilirubin. Phototherapy is not useful in lowering direct hyperbilirubinemia.

Exchange Transfusion

An exchange transfusion is performed when phototherapy is ineffective in lowering the rapidly rising levels of indirect bilirubin that occur with brisk hemolysis or when the level of bilirubin is believed to place the baby at risk of kernicterus.

Surgery

Surgical intervention is indicated to relieve an obstruction to the bile flow, as with obstructive gallstones and a choledochal cyst. A portoenterostomy (Kasai procedure) is usually the preferred surgery for extrahepatic biliary atresia, and an early operation (before 2 months of age) is associated with a better outcome.

INDICATIONS FOR REFERRAL

When a newborn presents with persistent cholestasis and no hepatocellular causes have been found, he or she should be referred to a tertiary center for an abdominal ultrasound and hepatobiliary scintigraphy. A liver biopsy (percutaneous or during a laparotomy) is mandatory if these tests are inconclusive. Because the Kasai procedure is more successful in a newborn under 2 months of age, there should be *no delay* in referral. Unexplainable jaundice in older pediatric patients is an indication for referral to a pediatric gastroenterologist. Finally, a baby may need to be admitted to the hospital if home phototherapy fails and the baby requires either standard phototherapy with fluorescent lamps or exchange transfusion.

ANNOTATED BIBLIOGRAPHY

Alpert G, Plotkin SA: A practical guide to the diagnosis of congenital infection in the newborn infant. Pediatr Clin North Am 33: 465–479, 1986. (Excellent resource for evaluating a patient with suspicion of infection.)

Altman RP: The portoenterostomy procedure for biliary atresia: A five year experience. Ann Surg 188:351–362, 1978. (Outcome of 43 patients with extrahepatic biliary atresia who underwent a Kasai procedure.)

Butler DA, MacMillan JP: Relationship of breast feeding and weight loss to jaundice in the newborn period: Review of the literature and results of a study. Cleve Clin Q 50:263–268, 1983. (Review of the literature on breast milk jaundice and report on a study of 588 newborns.)

Cashore WJ, Stern L: The management of hyperbilirubinemia. Clin Perinatol 11(2): 339–357, 1984. (Review of the management of hyperbilirubinemia in the newborn.)

Cloherty JP: Neonatal hyperbilirubinemia. In Cloherty JP, Stark AR (eds): Manual of Neonatal Care, 3rd ed. Boston, Little, Brown, & Co., 1991. (Detailed yet practical discussions of this subject; contains many tables for specific guidelines on when to institute phototherapy.)

Fitzgerald JF: Cholestatic disorders of infancy. Pediatr Clin North Am 35:357–373, 1988. (Good review of cholestasis and its management.)

Gollan JL, Schmid R: Bilirubin update: Formation, transport, and metabolism. Prog Liver Dis VII: 261–283, 1982. (Update on bilirubin metabolism.)

Kirks DR, Coleman RE, Filston HC, Rosenberg ER, Merten DF: An imaging approach to persistent neonatal jaundice. Am J Radiol 142:461–465, 1984. (Sonography and radionuclide scintigraphy studies in 15 patients with persistent neonatal jaundice; a diagnostic approach.)

Newman TB, Maisels MJ. Evaluation and treatment of jaundice in the term newborn: A kinder, gentler approach. Pediatrics 89:809–818, 1992. (Very thoughtful and practical guidelines. Argues that we should be less worried about jaundice in a healthy, term baby. In the absence of hemolytic disease, follow-up visits and lab studies are usually unnecessary. Phototherapy should not be started until the bilirubin is between 17.5 to 22 mg/dl, and exchange transfusion not considered until the bilirubin is at ≥25 mg/dl.)

Reichen J: Familial unconjugated hyperbilirubinemia syndromes. Semin Liver Dis 3:24–35, 1983. (Review of Gilbert's disease and the Crigler–Najjar syndrome.)

23

OTHER COMMON INFECTIONS

196

Neonatal Infections

Samuel P. Gotoff and
Mark A. Ward

Congenital and neonatal infections include all infections acquired during gestation, the perinatal period, and the first month of life. Most of these infections are inapparent, some are symptomatic during the neonatal period, and others produce clinical manifestations later in childhood. Infections in the first months of life may be localized or systemic. Systemic infections, such as meningococcemia, occur at any age, but systemic infections with less invasive organisms, such as gram-negative enterics, are more likely to occur in the very young infant. The premature infant, whose defense mechanisms are even less well developed, is more likely to be at risk for septicemia. A disruption of normal barriers to infection and an introduction of foreign bodies (central lines or ventriculoperitoneal shunts) increase the risk of infection at any age.

The localization of infection by clinical and laboratory examinations permits a more restricted consideration of etiologic agents than does the situation in which one encounters a sick infant with a suspected systemic infection. Selected localized and systemic infections in the infant are discussed in this chapter because they may differ significantly in etiology and management when compared to those in older children. However, it is important to remember that most of the infections seen in older children may occur in the young infant, depending on exposure and the status of transplacental immunity.

PATHOGENESIS

The transplacental passage of infectious agents may occur at any time during gestation. An intrauterine infection may result in abortion, stillbirth, prematurity, symptomatic neonatal infection, delayed manifestations, or inapparent infection depending on the etiologic agent, timing of infection during gestation, dosage, and host factors. In each case of congenital infection, there is maternal bacteremia, viremia, or parasitemia, and the placental barrier fails to prevent fetal infection. Early in gestation, infection may affect organogenesis, with resulting congenital malformations. Later in gestation, inflammatory responses lead to pathologic manifestations at birth or later in life. The spectrum of signs resulting from congenital syphilis illustrates this problem. Only a single organ may be involved, leading to deafness, ocular manifestations, cerebral damage, or hepatitis. In other cases, multiple organ systems may be involved.

Late in pregnancy, the ascending amniotic infection syndrome is the principal route of infection. Usually with ruptured membranes, but occasionally with presumably intact membranes, organisms inhabiting the birth canal invade the amniotic fluid and are aspirated or ingested prior to, or during, delivery. Perinatal infection may be signaled by fetal distress, or symptoms may be delayed until after birth. The duration of ruptured membranes correlates with the risk of amnionitis and neonatal infection. If maternal fever, attributed to endometritis, is present, the risk of infection in the newborn is greatly increased. In the nursery, the newborn may be exposed to pathogenic microbial flora from other infants, hospital personnel, and fomites. The mother, other members of the family, and community contacts are also sources of postnatally acquired infection.

OPHTHALMIA NEONATORUM

There are multiple etiologies of neonatal conjunctivitis. These include both infectious and noninfectious causes. To some extent, the various etiologies may be distinguished by time of onset. However, there is a substantial overlap in time of onset, making this an inadequate criterion for definitive diagnosis.

Chemical conjunctivitis is a routine manifestation of silver nitrate prophylaxis, occurring within hours of instillation. Complete resolution occurs within 1 to 2 days, and no therapy is required. Because of this effect, many centers now use topical tetracycline or erythromycin for eye prophylaxis.

Gonococcal ophthalmia typically appears 2 to 5 days after birth, but it has been reported at birth and weeks later as a result of postnatal acquisition. *Neisseria gonorrhoeae* usually produces an acute purulent conjunctivitis, but the spectrum of infection ranges from asymptomatic cases to panophthalmitis. Treatment includes parenteral antibiotics (penicillin G 100,000 U/kg/day; cefotaxime or ceftriaxone if penicillin resistant) and frequent irrigation of the eyes with normal saline (see also Chap. 92, "Ophthalmia Neonatorum").

Chlamydia trachomatis is currently the most commonly identified infectious cause of neonatal conjunctivitis. Onset is usually 5 to 14 days after birth, but the range of reported cases extends from 2 days to weeks after birth. The inflammatory response, which typically involves the tarsal conjunctivae, may be mild or severe, unilateral or bilateral, and may persist for weeks. Symptoms usually appear when the child is between 5 and 14 days old, although the range of reported cases extends from 2 days to weeks after birth. Standard gonococcal eye prophylaxis (including tetracycline and erythromycin) is ineffective in preventing chlamydial conjunctivitis. Treatment of established infection with topical antibiotics will suppress the infection but will not eradicate nasopharyngeal colonization, leaving the infant at risk for subsequent chlamydial pneumonia. Therefore, all infants with conjunctivitis due to chlamydia should be treated with oral erythromycin (40 mg/kg/day for 2 weeks).

Other agents that have been implicated in neonatal conjunctivitis include herpes simplex virus (HSV), *Staphylococcus aureus, Streptococcus pneumoniae,* and haemophilus species. With the exception of HSV, these infections may be treated with topical antibiotics unless signs of systemic infection are present. HSV requires parenteral acyclovir therapy.

RESPIRATORY INFECTIONS

Otitis media, ethmoid and maxillary sinusitis, and pneumonia are the major respiratory tract infections in the newborn. Infections that present in the first few days are due to bacterial pathogens acquired from the birth canal. Group B streptococcus is currently the most common organism producing perinatal pneumonia. Postnatal infections with *S. aureus, Haemophilus influenzae,* and *S. pneumoniae* also contribute to late-onset respiratory tract infections. Postnatal pneumonias may also be due to respiratory viruses (respiratory syncytial virus), and the most common agent is *C. trachomatis.*

Chlamydial pneumonia may appear as early as 2 weeks of age but occurs typically between 4 and 11 weeks. The infant is usually afebrile with tachypnea and a paroxysmal staccato cough. Other respiratory tract signs, such as conjunctivitis, nasal obstruction, and abnormal tympanic membranes, are common. A chest x-ray shows bilateral interstitial infiltrates and air trapping. A diagnosis is made by culturing *Chlamydia* from the respiratory tract or demonstrating a serologic response, rising titers, or IgM antibody to *C. trachomatis.* Treatment is the same as for chlamydial conjunctivitis (see above). Because infection results from vertical transmission, treatment of the infant's mother and her sexual contacts is indicated.

GASTROENTERITIS

Gastroenteritis in the newborn, presenting as diarrheal disease, is caused by the same agents that produce symptoms in older children. The etiologic agents may be divided into those that produce inflammation, characterized by fecal leukocytes, and those that do not. Inflammatory diarrhea is caused by *Salmonella, Shigella, Campylobacter,* invasive *Escherichia coli, Vibrio parahaemolyticus, Yersinia enterocolitica, Entamoeba histolytica,* and others. Noninflammatory diarrhea is usually caused by rotaviruses, enterotoxigenic *E. coli,* and, less commonly, enteroviruses and other agents. A bacteriologic culture and tests for rotavirus antigen will usually define the problem. Several noninfectious causes of neonatal diarrhea must also be considered (see also Chap. 105).

URINARY TRACT INFECTIONS

Neonatal urinary tract infection (UTI) is more common in males than in females. Circumcision reduces the incidence in males, presumably by reducing periurethral colonization with potential pathogens. UTI may occur by the ascending route or via hematogenous spread from a systemic infection. As in older children, *E. coli* causes the large majority of UTIs in newborns. Signs of UTI may be nonspecific, ranging from low-grade fever and failure to thrive to more acute signs of sepsis. If jaundice is a manifestation of UTI, it is usually associated with bacteremia. Diagnosis of UTI is by examination and culture of urine. Although pyuria is often present, as many as 25% of proven UTIs in newborns are associated with a normal urinary sediment. Dipstick methods for detection have been insufficiently studied in newborns to be relied upon for diagnosis. Culture remains the "gold standard." Unfortunately, collection of uncontaminated specimens is problematic. A negative bag specimen is useful in excluding a UTI, but a positive urine culture must be confirmed by a clean-voided urine specimen or one obtained by suprapubic bladder aspiration or by catheterization.

Empiric treatment for suspected UTI should include coverage for *E. coli,* enterococcus, as well as other enteric gram-negative organisms. Once the causative organism is identified and susceptibility testing is done, appropriate adjustments in antibiotic coverage can be made.

CUTANEOUS INFECTIONS

Skin and subcutaneous infections may be localized or they may occur as manifestations of systemic infections. They may result from a hematogenous spread of bacteria, viruses, or *Candida* or from injury to the skin due to circumcision, birth trauma, or fetal monitoring. The umbilical cord is a common focus for local or systemic bacterial infection. The source of a local skin infection is frequently not determined.

The type of skin lesion may suggest the etiology. Characteristic skin lesions include the staphylococcal scalded skin syndrome and ecthyma gangrenosum due to *Pseudomonas aeruginosa.* More often, the cutaneous manifestation suggests a limited number of possibilities that must be confirmed by Gram's stain, culture, or histologic examination. *Staphylococcus aureus* is the most frequent cause of skin infections in the newborn, presenting as impetigo, pustules, bullae, and abscesses. A large number of bacteria, viruses, and, less commonly, fungi may produce skin lesions early in infancy. Skin lesions, such as petechiae or vesicles from herpes simplex, may be the initial manifestation of a systemic infection (see also Chaps. 65 and 68).

EARLY-ONSET AND LATE-ONSET SEPSIS IN THE NEWBORN

Systemic neonatal infections may be classified by the age at onset into early- and late-onset disease. Early-onset disease is that occurring within the first week of life. Late-onset disease includes all cases following the first week.

Although somewhat arbitrary, this distinction is valid for several reasons. Early-onset disease results from in utero or intrapartum transmission from the mother. The source of infecting organisms in late-onset disease is less clear. Vertical transmission may also be important, but nonmaternal sources are responsible in at least some cases. A number of obstetric factors, including prematurity, prolonged rupture of membranes, amnionitis, and twinning, are associated with an increased risk of early-onset infection. These factors are less clearly associated with late-onset disease. Finally, as noted below, the manifestations of early- and late-onset disease are somewhat different.

Invasive bacterial infections must be considered in the differential diagnosis of any infant who becomes ill in the nursery. The clinical signs are often vague. Poor feeding, vomiting, abdominal distention, lethargy, temperature changes, respiratory distress, jaundice, hepatomegaly, sei-

zure activity, and petechiae are significant clues that should lead to a diagnostic evaluation and presumptive therapy. Most infants with early-onset disease have a respiratory tract focus and are bacteremic. Some will have meningitis or involvement of other organs (e.g., liver, kidneys, musculoskeletal system) or will be overwhelmingly ill because of high-level bacteremia (septicemia) manifested by septic shock (apnea, hypotension, and disseminated intravascular coagulation).

Late-onset infections may present with the same spectrum found in early-onset disease but are more often localized to the lungs, meninges, bones, or joints. Fever, without localizing signs, may be the initial presentation.

When an invasive bacterial infection is suspected in the newborn, blood, cerebrospinal fluid (CSF), and urine should be obtained for culture, and the CSF and urine should be examined. Group B streptococci, *E. coli,* and *Listeria monocytogenes* are the most common etiologic agents, but a large number of bacterial species may produce disease. Several viruses, fungi, and protozoa may also lead to systemic infections in the newborn. A laboratory diagnosis is essential.

If the physician makes a presumptive diagnosis of systemic bacterial infection or even considers this possibility, then antibiotics should be administered immediately. If there are no clues to the etiologic agent from an examination of biologic fluids (CSF, urine, joint aspiration, pus), broad-spectrum treatment is begun with a penicillin and an aminoglycoside. If a staphylococcal infection is suspected, a penicillinase-resistant penicillin should be included. Because of their superior penetration into spinal fluid, certain third-generation cephalosporins may be preferred for the treatment of gram-negative bacillary meningitis. However, no definitive studies exist demonstrating their superiority over aminoglycosides in this situation. When bacteriologic cultures are negative in infants with a syndrome consistent with septicemia, the physician should consider other nonbacterial etiologies, such as HSV, enteroviruses, rubella, CMV, and toxoplasmosis, and should obtain appropriate specimens for diagnosis. The management of these serious infections frequently requires consultation with an expert in infectious diseases.

SPECIFIC AGENTS

Cytomegalovirus

Cytomegalovirus is the most common congenital infection in the United States, affecting approximately 1% of all newborns. Congenital infection results from transplacental transmission of virus. Fetal infection may result from either primary maternal infection during pregnancy or reactivation of latent maternal virus. However, the risk to the fetus is quite different in these two circumstances. With primary maternal infection there is a 40% risk of transmission. Only

10% of such infected infants will be symptomatic at birth. However, 10% to 15% of the asymptomatic infants may also develop subsequent problems. On the other hand, infection due to reactivated maternal virus is rarely, if ever, symptomatic at birth. The precise risk for subsequent problems is unclear but appears to be very low.

Transmission can occur via breast milk or blood transfusion and horizontally in the nursery. Postnatally acquired CMV infection is generally associated with few or no symptoms. The exception is the premature infant who may develop pneumonitis, hepatitis, and other manifestations. Therefore, all transfusions in newborns should be with CMV antibody–negative blood.

Diagnosis of congenital infection is best made by viral isolation from urine or respiratory secretions obtained within the first week of life. Demonstration of a specific IgM antibody response is another way of establishing the diagnosis, but it lacks high sensitivity and specificity.

There is no proven therapy available for congenital CMV infection. Ganciclovir, which has proved useful in some other CMV-associated diseases, has not been adequately studied in congenital infection. Prevention of congenital CMV infection is problematic. There is no vaccine available, and screening of pregnant women is not useful because no intervention is available should infection be documented.

Rubella

Rubella is a mild febrile exanthem that has major consequences if infection occurs during pregnancy. Rubella-associated abortions, miscarriages, stillbirths, fetal anomalies, and the *congenital rubella syndrome* have been greatly diminished by the rubella immunization program. In the 1980s, less than 20 cases of congenital rubella syndrome (CRS) were reported annually in the United States, with only 6 cases total from 1987 to 1989. However, the number of CRS cases increased to 11 in 1990 alone, reflecting the increase in rubella activity seen in the general population.

The range of disease manifestations is extensive. Cardiac, ophthalmologic, auditory, and neurologic anomalies are well described. In addition, newborns may have growth retardation, hepatosplenomegaly, interstitial pneumonia, thrombocytopenia purpura, and radiolucent bone disease. Although major abnormalities are easily recognized in the neonatal period, mild cases with cardiac disease, deafness, developmental problems, and endocrinopathies may not be detectable for months or years. The so-called "silent" rubella infections in young infants are more common than are those that are symptomatic. The most common sequelae are auditory and are often associated with problems in language development.

If infected infants born to women with first-trimester rubella are monitored for at least 2 years, up to 80% will be affected. The congenital rubella syndrome occurs in 20% to 25% of infants born to women who acquire rubella during the first trimester. Subclinical rubella infection, detected by IgM radioimmunoassay (RIA), occurs in over 50% of infants whose mothers acquired rubella between the 12th and 16th week of gestation. Although fetal infection can occur at any stage of pregnancy, defects rarely occur after infection beyond the 20th week.

Congenital rubella infection is best diagnosed by culturing the virus from pharyngeal or conjunctival secretions, cerebrospinal fluid, or urine. A serologic diagnosis is made by a demonstration of rubella-specific IgM antibodies or the persistence of rubella antibodies for more than 3 months at a level beyond that expected from passive transfer of maternal antibodies. The hemagglutination inhibition (HI) test is now being replaced by a number of more sensitive antibody assays.

The diagnosis and management of rubella during pregnancy are not discussed here. There is no established treatment for congenital infection. Active immunization affords a method to prevent congenital rubella infection and is clearly attainable.

Herpes Simplex Virus (HSV)

An estimated 300 to 1500 cases of neonatal herpes occur in the United States each year. Transmission most commonly occurs intrapartum in association with maternal shedding of virus. Unfortunately, most of these women are asymptomatic for genital herpes and are without a history of genital herpes or a sexual partner with a vesicular rash (see also Chaps. 68 and 200). Transmission is more likely if the mother has primary infection during pregnancy. Reactivation of latent maternal infection, even if it occurs at delivery, is associated with a low risk to the newborn. Transmission may also occur in utero or postpartum. In utero infection is uncommon. The exact contribution of postpartum transmission is difficult to ascertain. Recent studies show a 30% incidence of type 1 HSV neonatal infection with only a 5% to 15% incidence of type 1 maternal genital infection.

In contrast to CMV, neonatal HSV is almost always symptomatic and is frequently associated with significant morbidity and mortality. The disease may be limited to the portal of entry (eye, mouth, skin), progress to the CNS, or have widespread dissemination. Congenital lesions may be noted at birth, but most natal infections present at the end of the first week. Postnatally acquired infections may appear even later. Vesicles are typical and frequently cluster, but the lesions become pustular and scab with evolution and may be mistaken for impetigo. Skin lesions typically recur. Occasionally, newborns with what appear to be only skin lesions may ultimately develop ocular or CNS sequelae. Eye findings include keratoconjunctivitis and chorioretinitis, which may appear later. The disseminated disease frequently resembles septicemia, with temperature alterations, lethargy, and involvement of the liver, lungs, and adrenal glands. The brain is involved in 70% of HSV infections; about one third of children have localized CNS infections. The mortality rate is about 80% in untreated disseminated disease and 50% in localized CNS disease.

When skin, conjunctival, or oral lesions are present, a presumptive diagnosis may be established by a cytologic examination and may be confirmed by cell culture. Intranuclear inclusions and multinucleated giant cells are typical of HSV and varicella-zoster (VZV) infection. The sensitivity of cytology is only about 60%; thus, viral culture is preferred. Other sites for virus culture include the nose, throat, conjunctivae, urine, CSF, and stool. Serology is generally not helpful, except to document maternal seroconversion.

Treatment should be instituted with an effective antiviral agent. Vidarabine and acyclovir have been shown to decrease morbidity and mortality, but residual neurologic abnormalities remain a problem. Because of ease of administration, acyclovir is currently the recommended treatment.

Women with clinically apparent genital HSV (whether primary or reactivated) should be delivered by caesarean section. Routine C-section is not indicated for women with a history of HSV who are asymptomatic at delivery. Serial prenatal genital cultures of women with a history of genital herpes are not indicated because they have not been found useful in predicting viral shedding at delivery. Viral culture at the time of delivery to look for viral shedding is reasonable. However, the management of infants delivered vaginally to women with documented viral shedding (whether symptomatic or not) remains controversial. Although antiviral treatment of clinically infected infants has not eliminated death and neurologic residua from neonatal herpes, earlier therapy may further improve the outcome. Some experts now recommend cultures of infants delivered vaginally to mothers with active genital herpes between 24 and 48 hours after delivery. Positive cultures would reflect the proliferation of virus in the infant, an indication for antiviral therapy prior to clinical signs.

Women with active herpes need not be isolated from their infants if careful hand washing is performed. Breast-feeding is contraindicated if breast lesions are present. Individuals with herpes labialis should wear masks.

Toxoplasmosis

The incidence of congenital infections with *Toxoplasma gondii* is approximately 1:1000 live births in the United States. Most of the infections are asymptomatic at birth with sequelae manifested after the neonatal period. Congenital toxoplasmosis refers to the disease. The classical findings in congenital toxoplasmosis are hydrocephalus, chorioretinitis, and intracranial calcifications. Neurologic signs such as seizures, increased intracranial pressure, and nystagmus are common. Approximately one third show signs of systemic infection, including fever, jaundice, hepatomegaly, splenomegaly, lymphadenopathy, anemia, and abnormal spinal fluid. Pneumonitis, abnormal bleeding, and eosinophilia are less common.

The common sequelae of congenital infections are chorioretinitis, which may not become apparent until adolescence, retardation, seizures, and other neurologic abnormalities.

A diagnosis is established easily by the demonstration of organisms or antigens in tissues or body fluids. The placenta should be examined, if it is available. The interpretation of serologic tests may be more difficult. Nonspecific laboratory clues to diagnosis are eosinophilia and high spinal fluid protein values.

Several serologic tests for the diagnosis of *Toxoplasma* infection are available. These include the Sabin–Feldman dye test, complement fixation, ELISA, indirect fluorescent antibody (IFA), and indirect hemagglutination. Interpretation of the results of these tests is often difficult.

The diagnosis of acquired toxoplasmosis in the mother is established by the demonstration of a significant increase in antibody titers. Because high titers may persist for years following infection, a single high titer is not diagnostic. A screening dye test during pregnancy will establish whether the woman is susceptible (negative test). A positive dye test and a negative IgM antibody test (IFA or ELISA) indicate prior infection. The duration of IgM antibody is variable, depending on the assay; thus, a negative IgM antibody test late in pregnancy may not exclude infection in the first trimester.

Serologic diagnosis in the newborn is even more complicated. The antibody in cord blood or neonatal sera may reflect IgG passed transplacentally from the mother. While the presence of IgM antibodies to *Toxoplasma* is diagnostic of congenital infection, the IgM IFA test is negative in 75% and the IgM ELISA is negative in 20% of newborns with congenital toxoplasmosis. Subsequent testing will show the decline of maternally derived antibody in uninfected infants; however, antibody synthesis in some infected infants is delayed until 3 or 4 months of age.

Unfortunately, there is a considerable variation in antigen preparations, relative contributions of IgG and IgM antibodies to titers, and the assays used in different laboratories. In questionable cases, it is best to consult a reference laboratory.

Treatment is recommended for all cases of congenital toxoplasmosis because of the late manifestations. Although an evaluation of therapy is difficult, the morbidity and mortality are sufficiently serious to warrant treatment. Several chemotherapeutic agents have been used for therapy, but the experience is limited. Spiramycin appears to be most promising but is not presently available in the United States. In this country, the combination of pyrimethamine and sulfadiazine is recommended for a 3-week course. With evidence of inflammation (meningitis, chorioretinitis), prednisone is added. Folinic acid is recommended during pyrimethamine therapy.

Hepatitis

Maternal hepatitis A during pregnancy appears to pose little risk to the newborn. If the mother is jaundiced at delivery, prophylaxis of the newborn with immune serum globulin (0.02 ml/kg) may be given. Proper hygiene should be stressed, but breast-feeding need not be discontinued.

Hepatitis B is a greater risk to the newborn. Although transplacental transmission may occur, neonatal infection usually occurs at the time of delivery. Although clinical manifestations are rare in the newborn period, newborns of women with hepatitis B are at risk for acute or chronic active hepatitis and hepatocellular carcinoma many years later. Asymptomatic hepatitis B antigenemia is more frequent in certain high-risk groups (women of Asian, Pacific Island, or Alaskan Eskimo descent; women born in Haiti or Sub-Saharan Africa; women who have histories of liver disease or contact with hemodialysis or institutionalized mentally retarded patients; women who are frequently exposed to blood; women who have had multiple episodes of venereal disease; and women who use illicit drugs percutaneously). However, universal screening of pregnant women is recommended because up to 50% of infected infants are born to women who do not fall into an identified high-risk group.

Effective prophylaxis is now available for hepatitis B. HBIG (0.5 ml) and hepatitis B vaccine (0.5 ml) should be given IM at separate sites, preferably within 12 hours of birth. The vaccine may be delayed as long as 7 days and should be repeated at 1 and 6 months of age. While HB_sAg is found in breast milk, breast-feeding is not contraindicated if infants are given HBIG prophylaxis. In the absence of prophylaxis, the risks and benefits of breast-feeding must be weighed on an individual basis (see also Chaps. 14 and 110).

Administration of hepatitis B vaccine to all newborn infants has recently been recommended as a strategy to prevent hepatitis B and its sequelae in children and adults.

The risk of hepatitis C to the newborn of an infected woman has not been extensively studied. Limited data suggest that vertical transmission may occur. However, the precise risk of transmission and nature of sequelae have yet to be defined. No prophylactic regimen has been proved effective, but some authorities recommend administration of immune serum globulin (0.06 ml/kg) to exposed newborns.

Varicella

Early intrauterine infection may result in cicatricial skin lesions, hypoplastic limbs, cortical atrophy, and ocular abnormalities. Neonatal varicella usually presents with a limited vesicular rash but can involve multiple organs and the central nervous system. The severe form of the disease may be complicated by disseminated intravascular coagulation, and fatality rates up to 30% have been reported.

A diagnosis is apparent when typical skin lesions are noted in the mother and infant. A presumptive diagnosis of a herpes virus (VZV or HSV) infection is made by an examination of Tzanck preparations of vesicles. Varicella antigen in fluid or culture of virus from the vesicle provides diagnostic confirmation. Infection may also be documented by a fourfold or greater rise in V-Z antibody or specific IgM antibody in a single specimen.

Although there are no published studies, a serious infection in the newborn should be treated with acyclovir, 30 mg/kg/day for 7 to 10 days. Congenital varicella may be prevented or modified in newborns born to mothers who acquired chickenpox less than 5 days before delivery by administration of varicella-zoster immune globulin (VZIG) or ZIG in a dose of 1.25 ml IM. No deaths have been reported in infants whose mothers had rash 5 or more days prior to birth, because transplacental antibody appears at this time. Newborns whose mothers have chickenpox postnatally are susceptible and may have infection. They should probably be given VZIG, although supportive data are lacking (see also Chap. 204).

Syphilis

The incidence of congenital syphilis has increased dramatically in recent years from a low of 108 cases in 1978 to 2867 cases (72/100,000 live births) in 1990. Although some of this increase is only apparent, because of changes in case definition, much of it is real. A diagnosis may be difficult because of the timing of the infection and interpretation of serologic tests, and management of the infant with a reactive test for syphilis on a cord blood specimen is a repetitive problem for the pediatrician.

The fetus is infected transplacentally. The placenta is large because of inflammation, and *Treponema pallidum* is usually demonstrable. Systemic spread may involve liver, spleen, lung, kidney, gastrointestinal tract, nervous system, and bones.

At birth, infants with congenital infection are usually asymptomatic. Late manifestations of infection may be delayed for a few months to years. Signs of early congenital syphilis include various mucocutaneous lesions, persistent rhinitis (snuffles), generalized lymphadenopathy, hepatosplenomegaly, jaundice, Coombs' negative hemolytic anemia, hydrops fetalis, various ocular and central nervous system abnormalities, nephrotic syndrome, osseous lesions that are usually asymptomatic but may result in pseudoparalysis, pneumonitis, and changes in peripheral blood (thrombocytopenia, anemia, leukemoid reaction).

The signs of late congenital syphilis include Hutchinson's triad (abnormal permanent central incisors, interstitial keratitis, and eighth-nerve deafness), mulberry molars, saddle nose, rhagades, and residual central nervous system and skeletal abnormalities.

The diagnosis of congenital syphilis is made by dark-field or histologic examination, or by a combination of epidemiologic, clinical, roentgenologic, and serologic criteria.

The Venereal Disease Research Laboratory (VDRL) and rapid plasma reagin (RPR) tests measure antibody to cardiolipin. These tests are usually used for screening, and reactivity depends on the duration and status of infection. The test may be positive in nonsyphilitic conditions and may be negative in maternal and cord blood if infection occurred late in gestation.

Several tests have been developed to detect specific antibodies to *T. pallidum*. The fluorescent treponemal antibody absorbed with nonpallidum treponemes (FTA-ABS) test is usually available in health department laboratories. FTA-IgM and FTA-IgG tests have been developed to differentiate fetal and maternal antibody in cord blood and neonatal sera. Unfortunately, not all infants with congenital syphilis make IgM antibody, and a positive FTA-IgM test may be due to an IgM anti-IgG antibody to *T. pallidum* analogous to a rheumatoid factor.

The management of a newborn with suspected syphilis depends on several considerations. If maternal syphilis is treated correctly with penicillin during pregnancy, the risk to the infant is minimal. The infant should be monitored clinically and serologically, with a demonstration of falling titers, to assure the effectiveness of maternal therapy on fetal infection. If maternal treatment is inadequate, if an alternative treatment such as erythromycin is employed, or if the infant cannot be properly monitored, then the infant should be treated with penicillin.

Every infant with suspected congenital syphilis should have a lumbar puncture. Neurosyphilis may be difficult to ascertain clinically because most infants have no neurologic abnormalities. A diagnosis of neurosyphilis usually rests on cerebrospinal fluid abnormalities. A positive VDRL on CSF indicates neurosyphilis, but a negative test does not exclude it. Elevated CSF protein and pleocytosis are compatible with neurosyphilis but are not diagnostic. A 10-day course of either aqueous crystalline or procaine penicillin G is recommended for all cases of congenital syphilis regardless of whether there is CNS involvement (see also Chap. 200, "Sexually Transmitted Disease," for a further discussion on syphilis).

ANNOTATED BIBLIOGRAPHY

Alford CA, Stagno S, Pass RF, Britt WJ: Congenital and perinatal cytomegalovirus infections. Rev Infect Dis 12(S-7):745, 1990. (Recent review.)

Arvin AM, Hensleigh PA, Prober CG: Failure of antepartum maternal cultures to predict the infant's risk of exposure to herpes simplex virus at delivery. N Engl J Med 315:706, 1986. (Antepartum cultures fail to predict viral shedding at delivery.)

Dorfman DH, Glaser JH: Congenital syphilis in infants after the newborn period. N Engl J Med 323:1299, 1990. (Explores factors responsible for missing diagnosis at birth.)

Feigin RD, Cherry JD (eds): Textbook of Pediatric Infectious Diseases, 2nd ed. Philadelphia, WB Saunders, 1987. (Detailed reference.)

Hammerschlag MR, Cummings CC, Roblin PM, Williams TH, Delke I: Efficacy of neonatal ocular prophylaxis for the prevention of chlamydial and gonococcal conjunctivitis. N Engl J Med 320:769, 1989. (Lack of efficacy of the three standard eye prophylaxis regimens against *Chlamydia*.)

Remington JS, Klein JO (eds): Infectious Diseases of the Fetus and Newborn Infant, 3rd ed. Philadelphia, WB Saunders, 1990. (Detailed reference.)

Whitley RJ, Corey L, Arvin A et al: Changing presentation of herpes simplex virus infection in neonates. J Infect Dis 158:109, 1988. (Decreased frequency of disseminated disease in more recent cases.)

Wiswell TE, Roscelli JD: Corroborative evidence for the decreased incidence of urinary tract infections in circumcised male infants. Pediatrics 78:96, 1986. (One of the major studies that have prompted a reevaluation of the risks/benefits of routine circumcision.)

Zenker EN, Berman SM: Congenital syphilis: trends and recommendations for evaluation and management. Pediatr Infect Dis 10:516, 1991. (Most recent recommendations for diagnosis and treatment.)

197
Infections in Day-Care Centers

Colin D. Marchant

As a result of economic and social pressures, the number of children receiving care entirely in their own homes is lower than that of a decade ago. Day-care centers, broadly defined as facilities that provide regular care to two or more children from different homes, have increased exponentially to meet the needs for child care. When infants and children from different homes are brought together in day-care settings, there are increased opportunities for the spread of contagious diseases. Physicians face new challenges when caring for these children and when asked to provide advice and assistance to day-care centers. To meet these challenges, physicians must appreciate the modes of transmission of infectious agents and the risks of contagion so that preventive measures and strategies for the management of outbreaks can be instituted.

The most common modes of transmission of infection are fecal–oral and respiratory. From their fecal and respiratory origins, pathogens are spread by hand contact to toys, playing surfaces, playmates, and care-givers. Some pathogens may survive on inanimate surfaces for hours, days, or longer. Contact with saliva or urine and direct skin-to-skin contact are additional modes of transmission that are important in the day-care setting. Infectious diseases that are sexually transmitted or acquired by intravenous inoculation are extremely rare in day-care centers. Occasionally, biting or direct contact with blood from cuts and scrapes may pose a theoretical hazard for transmission of these agents.

The risks of infection are increased in day-care centers compared with the risks in at-home care. The incidence of clinically defined respiratory disease and diarrheal disease is increased in infants and children in day-care settings. Increased risk of disease due to specific pathogens can generally be assumed when there are cases with active coughing or diarrheal illnesses in a day-care center. More caution is required in assuming that children or staff with asymptomatic carriage of a pathogen pose a risk in the day-care setting. In further contrast, the risk of hepatitis B or human immunodeficiency virus (HIV) in day-care centers is remote. Without documentation of increased risk for a given pathogen, we may do a disservice if we take strong measures in the face of imagined risks.

Those at risk in day-care centers include not only the children but also the adult care-givers. For example, cytomegalovirus infections are common and asymptomatic in children in day-care settings, and it is the fetuses of seronegative pregnant women who are at risk. Also, children with decreased respiratory or cardiac reserve may be at special risk of respiratory disease, while children with underlying gastrointestinal disease may be less able to tolerate infectious diarrhea. Those with immunodeficiency, such as symptomatic HIV infection, are also potentially vulnerable to a variety of infections.

To meet the health needs of children, prevention of infection and the management of both general and specific conditions are required. National performance standards for day-care settings have been developed jointly by the American Academy of Pediatrics and the American Public Health Association. The Committee on Infectious Diseases of the American Academy of Pediatrics has outlined guidelines for the prevention and management of infections in day-care centers. Physicians are urged to consult these sources. The general principles and the discussion of specific diseases outlined below are consistent with these guidelines. Physicians may also confront novel situations in which increased risks of contagion are suspected. At these times, it is important to ask whether there is any evidence of increased risk of contagion and whether proposed remedial action is effective or merely presumed to be effective. Consultation with public health authorities is often helpful.

PREVENTION

Sound practices for prevention of infection in day-care centers include written health care policies for staff and children, good communication between parents and day-care staff regarding signs and symptoms of potentially infectious illnesses, good sanitary practices, and appropriate immunization of children and care-givers.

Sanitary Practices. Physicians providing advice or guidance to day-care centers should be aware of the newly developed national standards for child care settings cited above. Briefly, sanitary practices include: Waterproof disposable diapers should have the capacity to contain urine and feces so as to minimize contamination of other children and the environment. Diaper changing surfaces should be sanitized after each use, and diapers should be disposed of in secure containers. Food handling should be completely separated from diaper-changing activities. Hand-washing facilities should be available and hand washing routinely practiced after diaper changing. Child-size flush toilets should be provided whenever possible. Playing surfaces should be cleaned regularly, and spills of body secretions should be cleaned appropriately with disinfectant solution (¼ cup household bleach per gallon of water).

Immunizations. Before admission to day care, all children should have received age-appropriate immunizations against diphtheria, tetanus, pertussis, polio, *Haemophilus influenzae* type b, measles, mumps, and rubella. Each child should have received a primary series of DTP, Hib, and polio immunizations by age 7 months, MMR vaccine by age 16 months, and booster immunizations with DTP, Hib, and polio by 19 months. If children have not been appropriately immunized, they may be allowed to attend day care if there are no cases of vaccine-preventable illnesses in the day-care setting and if every effort is made to bring immunization status up to date. Written records of immunization should be maintained. The adult staff of day-care centers should also be appropriately immunized against diphtheria, tetanus, polio, measles, mumps, and rubella.

MANAGEMENT

General methods for management of disease outbreaks in day-care centers include exclusion of ill and infected children or staff, implementation of strict hygienic practices, cohorting of infected and exposed individuals, and, in extreme situations, closure of the facility. Because minor illnesses are extremely common, it is neither feasible nor desirable to exclude all children for minor degrees of illness. In general, children should be excluded if they cannot be safely or comfortably cared for, if care makes excessive demands on the staff, or if they pose a risk to others. Children with signs of potentially severe illness such as fever should be excluded until the nature of their illness is defined and they can be safely returned to the day-care center. Children with a rash and either fever, lethargy, or irritability may have a contagious disease and should be excluded until it has been determined that they are not a risk to others. Rash without fever or other symptoms is unlikely to be the onset of a severe contagious disease.

Diseases Transmitted by the Fecal–Oral Route

Day-care centers are important foci for diarrheal diseases and hepatitis A. Large day-care centers and those with diapered children are at higher risk of outbreaks. Rotavirus, shigellosis, and giardiasis are common in day-care settings. Enteroviruses, calcivirus, *Clostridium difficile,* campylobacter, cryptosporidium, salmonella, and a number of strains of *Escherichia coli* have been documented in specific outbreaks.

General Measures. Because microbiologic diagnosis of diarrheal diseases is rarely established, general guidelines for management are required for all episodes of gastroenteritis. Additional measures may be required for infections caused by specific pathogens. A child with diarrhea (defined as increased frequency and water content of that child's stool) that is not contained within the child's diaper or toilet should be excluded from day care until diarrhea ceases. Children with minor degrees of diarrhea should not be excluded, but strict hand washing should be stressed. Hand washing programs have been clearly shown to reduce the incidence of diarrhea in day-care centers.

Rotavirus. Diarrheal disease caused by rotaviruses occurs in annual outbreaks during cool seasons in the United States. A minimal number of organisms are infective, and attack rates in day-care settings may be as high as 70%. Rotaviruses may be carried by asymptomatic persons for several weeks and remain viable on environmental surfaces for prolonged periods, so there is ample opportunity for spread. Specific therapy is not available, but vaccines are under development.

Shigellosis. Children with symptomatic shigellosis should receive specific antimicrobial therapy based on the results of antimicrobial susceptibility testing. Treatment usually eliminates fecal excretion promptly, and intestinal carriage beyond a month is rare. Children should have completed therapy and be free of diarrhea before returning to day care.

Salmonellosis. *Salmonella* species very rarely cause outbreaks of enteric disease in day-care settings, and specific antimicrobial therapy is not usually indicated, even for those with symptoms. Treatment of the carrier state is not effective, and exclusion of the asymptomatic carrier from day care is not warranted.

***Campylobacter* Enteritis.** *Campylobacter jejuni* rarely causes infections in day-care settings. Erythromycin eliminates this pathogen after approximately 3 days of therapy. Children should be excluded from day care until 3 days of erythromycin therapy have been completed and there is cessation of diarrhea.

***Escherichia coli* Infections.** Outbreaks of severe and protracted diarrhea due to enteropathogenic *E. coli* have been reported in day-care centers. When a serotype of *E. coli* known to be pathogenic is isolated, and after the results of antimicrobial susceptibility testing are known, patients should be treated with nonabsorbable drugs such as neomycin (100 mg/kg/day in three or four divided doses for 5 days) or colistin (10–15 mg/kg/day in three or four divided doses). Trimethoprim-sulfamethoxazole may be used in difficult cases.

Outbreaks of diarrhea followed by the hemolytic–uremic syndrome (HUS) due to *E. coli* 0157:H7 have also occurred in day-care settings. Specific antimicrobial therapy is not indicated because the pathogen clears spontaneously from the stool within a week. However, isolation and cohorting of affected individuals are required to prevent additional cases of HUS. There should be no new admissions to a day-care center during an outbreak of HUS.

Clostridium difficile. Diarrhea results from overgrowth of toxigenic strains of *C. difficile* in the colon. Antibiotic therapy is the most common reason for overgrowth of *C. difficile,* and increased use of antibiotics in day care is responsible for many cases. Specify therapy is not usually required. Control measures are those used for diarrhea of any cause.

Giardiasis. *Giardia lamblia* is a common enteric pathogen in day-care centers. Cysts survive for long periods on environmental surfaces, and prolonged asymptomatic carriage is common. Because some children have protracted diarrhea, the stools of symptomatic subjects should be cultured and antibiotic therapy prescribed for symptomatic cases. Children may return to day care when diarrhea ceases. Treatment of asymptomatic carriers is not recommended, and these children should not be excluded from day care.

Cryptosporidiosis. *Cryptosporidium* is protozoan that causes self-limited diarrhea in nonimmunocompromised hosts. No specific therapy is required. Excretion of cysts, although often prolonged, requires no specific measures, and children should not be excluded from day care after diarrhea ceases.

Hepatitis A. Day-care centers are a major source for the spread of hepatitis A in the community. Transmission rates are highest in large day-care centers and in those with diapered children. Many infants and children with hepatitis A are asymptomatic, and because fewer than 10% develop jaundice or dark urine, hepatitis is rarely suspected. The long incubation period of 2 to 7 weeks often makes it difficult to link cases with nonspecific diarrhea, vomiting, or abdominal discomfort. Typically, hepatitis A is suspected only when an adult staff member or household contact of a child develops jaundice. To further complicate matters, peak fecal excretion of the hepatitis A virus occurs before the onset of symptoms, and hepatitis A virus can survive on environmental surfaces for up to a month. The diagnosis should be confirmed in suspected cases by anti–hepatitis A IgM antibody testing.

Important control measures include strict hand washing and cleansing of potentially contaminated environmental surfaces with bleach solution (¼ cup of sodium hypochlorite per gallon of water). Cases with jaundice should be excluded for 1 week after the onset, or until contacts have received prophylactic immune serum globulin (ISG). If given within 2 weeks of exposure, ISG will prevent clinical disease in the majority of cases, but it is not known whether it reduces viral transmission. Intramuscular ISG (0.02 ml/ kg) should be administered to all children and staff in day-care centers with children 2 years of age or younger. When only older children are present, prophylactic ISG can be limited to those children and staff members who are in regular contact with each other in the same room. Prophylaxis of household contacts of a case is also indicated. If hepatitis occurs in three or more families of day-care attenders, but has not yet been diagnosed in the day-care center, prophylactic ISG should be administered to children and staff of the day-care center (see also Chap. 110, "Hepatitis").

Diseases Transmitted from the Respiratory Tract

Children in day-care centers have an increased incidence of respiratory infections during the first 2 years of life, and day-care attendance is an important risk factor for recurrent acute otitis media. Infections that are transmitted from the respiratory tract, but do not produce respiratory symptoms, are also important in day-care settings. The list of respiratory pathogens documented in day-care settings is long and includes all the common respiratory viruses, *Mycoplasma pneumoniae,* and *Streptococcus pneumoniae.* Specific control measures are not indicated for these pathogens, but other agents transmitted by the respiratory route require particular measures. While some pathogens are transmitted by aerosolized droplets, many are transmitted by hand contact or from contaminated environmental surfaces. Again, hand washing is an important method of preventing transmission.

Neisseria meningitidis. Contacts of cases of all ages with serious meningococcal infections may harbor the organism in their nasopharynxes and are at risk of systemic disease. Because of the often rapidly progressive nature of meningococcemia, chemoprophylaxis with rifampin (20 mg/kg/ day, up to a maximum of 600 mg divided b.i.d. for 2 days) within 24 hours of exposure should be administered to all day-care and household contacts. Nasopharyngeal cultures are not helpful because they do not provide timely results. A single oral dose of ciprofloxacin is effective in adults but is not recommended for children. A single intramuscular injection of ceftriaxone (125 mg in children, 250 mg in teenagers and adults) has been shown to be more effective than rifampin in a single study and may eventually become the method of choice (see also Chap. 199, "Antimicrobial Prophylaxis").

Haemophilus influenzae **type b.** There is an increased primary risk of meningitis and other invasive diseases due to *H. influenzae* type b in day-care centers, while it is unclear whether there is an increased risk of secondary cases. Specific control measures are controversial in day-care centers

after a single case, although prophylaxis of households with rifampin (20 mg/kg/day, up to a maximum of 600 mg once daily for 4 days) is recommended to eradicate nasopharyngeal colonization in households where there are children less than 4 years of age. Some authorities recommend chemoprophylaxis after a single case of *H. influenzae* for day-care centers with children less than 2 years of age and 25 or more contact hours per week. Chemoprophylaxis is recommended for centers with two cases of invasive disease within a 60-day period. Universal immunization against *H. influenzae* type b beginning at 2 months of age began in late 1990 and should make these issues moot (see also Chap. 199).

Streptococcal Pharyngitis. Group A streptococcal pharyngitis is spread by close contact with respiratory secretions; fomites are not highly infectious. Confirmed cases should be excluded from day care until 24 hours after starting antimicrobial therapy.

Pertussis. Although clinical pertussis is rarely suspected in immunized children, there is potential for unrecognized disease in day-care centers. All day-care and household contacts should receive erythromycin (40–50 mg/kg/day, max. 2 g, in four divided doses for 14 days) regardless of immunization status. Children with laboratory-confirmed pertussis or contact with a laboratory-confirmed case should be excluded from day care until 5 days of erythromycin therapy have been completed (see also Chap. 201, "Pertussis").

Tuberculosis. Primary tuberculosis in children is not contagious, but infection is commonly spread by adults with active secondary tuberculosis. Children with primary tuberculosis can return to day care as soon as chemotherapy has been instituted. Adults with tuberculosis should be excluded until they are deemed noninfectious by health authorities. Tuberculin testing should be performed on all children and adults if a staff member is diagnosed with tuberculosis (see also Chap. 170, "Tuberculosis: Screening and Prophylaxis").

Varicella. Chickenpox is spread by aerosolized droplets up to 2 days before and 5 days after the appearance of characteristic skin lesions. The skin lesions themselves can transmit infection by direct contact. All children who have not had varicella previously are susceptible. In addition, approximately 5% of adults with a prior history of varicella and 15% of those with negative histories are susceptible. Compared to varicella in healthy children, immunocompromised persons of all ages and healthy adults are at increased risk of complications. Pregnant women have been known to develop severe pneumonia, and their fetuses are at risk of congenital anomalies with infection in the first trimester. If varicella is contracted by a woman near the time of delivery, her newborn infant is at risk for severe varicella. Accordingly, all parents and staff members should be notified of a day-care outbreak so that they can receive timely advice regarding the advisability of varicella-zoster immune globulin (VZIG). Immunoprophylaxis is not recommended for healthy children. Children with chickenpox should be excluded from day care until 6 days after the onset of skin lesions (see also Chap. 204, "Chickenpox").

Parvovirus B19 Infection. Infection may be asymptomatic, may manifest as a nonspecific respiratory infection, or may manifest as *erythema infectiosum* with the characteristic "slapped cheek" rash and/or a truncal rash. Because parvovirus B19 is present in respiratory secretions before the appearance of the rash and is unlikely after the onset of the rash, exclusion of children with erythema infectiosum from day-care centers is not an effective measure. The most feared risk of parvovirus B19 infection is infection during pregnancy leading to fetal hydrops and death. However, most infections in pregnancy are mild and without consequence to the fetus, with fetal hydrops and death developing in fewer than 10% of cases. Because outbreaks of parvovirus B19 infection cannot be recognized in a timely manner, and serologic testing is not readily available, it is difficult to prevent exposure to most adult women by excluding them from child care or other settings.

Diseases Spread by Direct Contact

Conjunctivitis. Purulent conjunctivitis may be due to *H. influenzae* or other bacterial pathogens. Cases of purulent conjunctivitis should be excluded from day care until they are examined by a physician and appropriate antibiotic treatment is instituted. Those with red conjunctivae and clear discharge only (i.e., nonbacterial conjunctivitis) may be allowed to remain in day care.

Impetigo. Spread among children by direct contact is well documented. Children should be excluded until 24 hours after treatment has been initiated.

Herpes Zoster. The lesions of zoster contain live virus and are potentially infective by direct contact, but the risks of transmission are lower than for varicella (see above). Persons with zoster should be excluded from day-care settings if the lesions cannot be completely covered with a suitable dressing.

Scabies. Children with scabies should be excluded from day care until treatment has been completed.

Head Lice. Children with head lice may be readmitted after treatment.

Diseases Spread by Contact with Saliva, Urine, and Blood

The risks of transmission in day-care centers of diseases in this category vary widely, from cytomegalovirus where the chances of acquisition are high, to hepatitis B and HIV infections where the risks of transmission are remote.

Cytomegalovirus (CMV). Infants and children in day care are at increased risk for CMV acquisition, with a peak period of infection between 1 and 3 years of age. Infection is almost always asymptomatic, and because the virus is excreted in saliva and urine for a year or more, there is ample opportunity for transmission of infection. The fetus is at risk of severe neurologic impairment and other organ system disease when a seronegative pregnant woman contracts primary infection. Seronegative women who work in day care will benefit from protection from transmission. Specific diagnosis requires viral culture of urine and saliva, which is costly. Because infection is common, detection of asymptomatic children who pose a risk to pregnant women is neither feasible nor desirable. The only option is serologic testing of women who work in day-care centers and become pregnant, followed by counseling of those who are found to be seronegative. These women face a difficult decision: to remain and accept the risk or to end their employment in day care. If a child is known to be excreting CMV, excluding that child from day care is not warranted.

Herpes Simplex Virus (HSV). Persons who are chronically infected with HSV1 intermittently secrete virus in saliva, either with or without the appearance of active, visible lesions. These infections are common in day-care centers, and while there is potential for spread, disease due to HSV1 is not life threatening in this setting. Pregnant women are primarily at risk for transmission of genital strains of HSV2 to their newborns. Herpes simplex type 1 is rarely involved. In day-care centers, only children with stomatitis who cannot control their secretions should be excluded. Open lesions on the lips or skin should be covered with appropriate bandages in order to reduce transmission.

Hepatitis B. A few cases of hepatitis B infection have been documented in children who appear to have no source of infection other than an asymptomatic carrier in the same day-care center. In contrast, other studies have failed to demonstrate hepatitis B transmission despite long-term contact with a hepatitis surface antigen–positive playmate in the day-care setting. Furthermore, epidemiologic surveillance data indicate that acquisition of hepatitis B by children after the perinatal period is rare and that day-care attendance is not a risk factor for hepatitis B. Thus, the risks of hepatitis B transmission in day care are remote, and in general, children with hepatitis B infection should not be excluded from day-care centers. Routine testing for hepatitis B surface antigen (HB_sAg) or immunization of other children in day care with hepatitis B vaccine is not required. With the implementation of the Centers for Disease Control's recommendation for universal immunization against hepatitis B, children in day care will then be at even less risk.

The particular situation in which there is potential for hepatitis B transmission in day care is children who are HB_sAg positive and who bite other children or staff members. Although transmission of hepatitis B by biting has occurred, the magnitude of this risk is not known. Exclusion of such children from day care must be individualized. If a person is bitten by a child who is a known carrier, prophylaxis with hepatitis B immune globulin (HBIG) (0.06 ml/kg IM) should be administered and immunization with hepatitis B vaccine should be initiated (first dose administered simultaneously with HBIG at a different site, followed by a second dose 1 month later and a third dose 6 months later). The risk of transmission when a child who is negative for HB$_s$Ag bites a child who is positive is unknown. If there is an indication that there has been substantial contact with blood, then prophylaxis might be considered. Bites involving children of unknown HB$_s$Ag status do not require immunoprophylaxis.

In other settings, hepatitis B is spread by blood and blood product transfusion, inoculation by contaminated needles, sexual transmission, or prolonged close personal contact. The viral inoculum in saliva does not appear to be adequate for transmission through intact mucous membranes. However, because transmission is theoretically possible, reasonable preventive measures should be employed when a child infected with hepatitis B virus is present in a day-care setting. These include the use of separate toothbrushes, avoidance of contact with blood-contaminated body fluids, prompt cleansing with bleach (¼ cup of sodium hypochlorite per gallon of water) of any surfaces contaminated with blood or body fluids containing blood, and careful disposal of any contaminated materials (see also Chap. 110, "Hepatitis").

Human Immunodeficiency Virus (HIV).   Transmission of HIV infection in day-care centers has not been documented, and HIV-positive children should not be automatically excluded from day care. The most important issue, in fact, is not the risk of transmission to others but the risks of infection faced by the HIV-positive child when he or she becomes immunocompromised. Similarly, HIV-infected adults without open skin lesions do not pose a risk to children but may become at risk for secondary infections themselves. Physicians are urged to carefully consider each situation individually and to consult with public health authorities so that decision making is based on expertise and the latest information rather than on hypotheses and hysteria.

Once an HIV-positive person is present in a day-care setting, the precautions for avoiding exposure to blood or body fluids containing blood, as outlined above for hepatitis B, should be followed (see also Chap. 52, "Acquired Immunodeficiency Syndrome [AIDS] in Children").

ANNOTATED BIBLIOGRAPHY

American Public Health Association and the American Academy of Pediatrics: Caring for Our Children—National Health and Safety Performance Standards: Guidelines for Out-of-Home Child Care Programs. Washington, DC, American Public Health Association, 1991. (Newly developed guidelines for day care—can be obtained from: The American Public Health Association, 1015 15th St. N.W., Washington, DC 20005.)

Bartlett AV, Moore M, Gary GW et al: Diarrheal illness among infants and toddlers in day-care centers: I. Epidemiology and pathogens. II. Comparison with day care homes and households. J Pediatr 107:503, 1985. (Etiology and risks of enteric infections in day-care centers.)

Black RE, Dykes AC, Anderson KE et al: Handwashing to prevent diarrhea in day-care centers. Am J Epidemiol 113:445, 1981. (Hand washing comes through again!)

Committee on Infectious Diseases, American Academy of Pediatrics: Report of the Committee on Infectious Diseases: 1991. Elk Grove Village, IL, American Academy of Pediatrics, 1991. (Excellent source for current recommendations and for the prevention and management of specific diseases.)

Wald ER, Guerra N, Byers C: Frequency and severity of infections in day care: Three year follow-up. J Pediatr 118:509, 1991. (Prospective study of the risks of infection in day-care centers.)

198

Bacteremia

Robert A. Dershewitz and Sonia Lewin

Children may have bacteria in their blood at any age. Bacteremia may be primary (i.e., occult or unsuspected) or secondary to a focal infection (e.g., pneumonia or otitis media). Although definitions, risk factors, and management strategies are somewhat controversial, this chapter offers a reasonable clinical approach to this problem.

Children between 3 and 24 months of age are at greatest risk for unsuspected bacteremia. It is uncommon in children older than 36 months. Newborns represent a special category. Most recommendations require any febrile newborn under 2 months old and any "septic-looking" or "toxic" child to be hospitalized, to have a full sepsis work-up, and to be started on parenteral antibiotics. Children between 2 and 3 months of age do not have as great a risk as newborns; hence, they may be managed less conservatively if no risk factors other than fever are present. The number of "at risk" infants hospitalized now is lower than that in the past because of the great expense, the risk of nosocomial infections, the complications such as drug toxicity, the stress to the family, and, most important, no demonstrable improved outcome.

In addition to age (3–24 months), elevations in fever and white blood cells (WBC) constitute the classic triad of risk factors for occult bacteremia. In one representative study, only 0.9% of children less than 24 months of age who had fevers less than 38.9°C (102°F) were bacteremic; 4.1% were bacteremic if the fever was between 38.9° C and

39.4° C, and the incidence rose to 8.0% when it was greater than or equal to 40° C. Similarly, the higher the WBC, the greater the incidence of bacteremia; a fivefold increased risk of bacteremia exists if the WBC is greater than 15,000. The presence of both temperature elevation and leukocytosis increases the likelihood of bacteremia. Race, socioeconomic status, and sex are not risk factors.

Septicemia is an entity different from bacteremia; a septic (i.e., toxic) child represents a much more serious problem. These children require immediate hospitalization and aggressive management. In most instances, however, the highly febrile infant does not appear toxic, and management decisions should be individualized based on various factors, such as clinical judgment, reliability of the parents, and availability of follow-up care. Clinical judgment, however, is not highly accurate. Pediatric residents, attending physicians in emergency departments, and private practitioners are usually incorrect when they are asked to predict if the febrile infant they examined has bacteremia. On the other hand, physicians are more accurate in predicting specificity (i.e., identifying children who are not bacteremic). The ultimate goal, however, is not to diagnose bacteremia but to prevent its complications, such as sepsis and meningitis.

PATHOPHYSIOLOGY

Bacteremia from any organism may resolve spontaneously, may respond to antibiotic therapy, or may result in fulminant disease, despite appropriate antibiotics. *Streptococcus pneumoniae* is the most common cause of bacteremia (65%). *Haemophilus influenzae* type b accounts for 20% to 25% of the cases, and *Neisseria meningitidis, Escherichia coli, Salmonella* species, *Enterobacter–Klebsiella* species, and group A β-hemolytic streptococci are other pathogens. Possible contaminants include *Staphylococcus aureus, Streptococcus viridans, Moraxella, Candida,* and mixed organisms. A determination of the pathogenicity, however, must be based on the clinical context. *Staphylococcus epidermidis,* alpha streptococci, diphtheroids, and bacillus species are probable contaminants.

Streptococcus pneumoniae is the least aggressive of the common pathogens; most bacteremias resolve promptly, with or without antibiotics. In contrast, *H. influenzae* type b bacteremia often leads to invasive sequelae. Common "metastatic" spread includes pneumonia, meningitis, epiglottitis, cellulitis, and septic arthritis. *Neisseria meningitidis* bacteremia results in the worst outcome. In one series, 4:12 cases (33%) of unsuspected bacteremia resulted in meningitis or death, compared to 7% of *H. influenzae* type b and 4% of *S. pneumoniae.*

Children with congenital or functional asplenia are at considerably increased risk of overwhelming sepsis from bacteremia, especially from *S. pneumoniae.* Children with sickle cell disease have a tenfold increased incidence of pneumococcal septicemia and meningitis. Immunocompromised children are also at an increased risk of septicemia, most commonly from gram-negative bacilli and staphylococci. Close contacts (siblings and day care) of children with serious invasive *H. influenzae* type b and meningococcal disease are also at increased risk.

CLINICAL PRESENTATION

In one study, 25 of 699 nonhospitalized children between 3 and 24 months old with temperatures of 39.5°C (103°F) or higher had occult bacteremia (3.5%). Twelve children presented with otitis media, two had upper respiratory infections (URIs), two had pneumonia, one had a urinary tract infection (UTI), one had purulent rhinitis, and seven had no focus of infection. The most common organism was *S. pneumoniae,* which presents typically as a relatively minor illness in the febrile child. At any point in the illness, even while seeming to recover, the child may develop complications such as meningitis. It should be reemphasized that the moribund child, the toxic child, or the child with a primary diagnosis of osteomyelitis, septic arthritis, or meningitis in whom secondary bacteremia is common presents an entirely different clinical situation. These children, regardless of whether or not risk factors for bacteremia are present, must be hospitalized, worked-up completely, and treated aggressively.

WORK-UP

The work-up of a febrile child is geared to help the clinician decide which children should be started on expectant antibiotic therapy.

History

How sick is the infant? Has the child been less playful or alert? Is the child irritable or inconsolable? Has there been a recent or concurrent exposure or an illness predisposing to bacteremia, such as pneumonia? Does the child have a medical condition such as malignancy, splenectomy, shunt, or in-dwelling catheter that would increase the likelihood and potential serious sequelae of bacteremia?

Physical Examination

Optimal observation is important. The observer must avoid haste. The physician should ensure that the child is comfortable. He or she should take note if the child is looking about, consolable, or playful. McCarthy and associates have stressed the importance of observation variables such as cry, reaction to parents, state variation, color, state of hydration, and response to social overtures (see Chap. 182 for a detailed discussion of identifying sick from nontoxic-appearing children). These variables, however, are not reliable for detecting serious illness in febrile infants under

8 weeks old. The physician should perform a complete physical examination to look for focal infection. He or she should test carefully for meningismus, although this is often a late finding and frequently not present in very young infants. Certain findings on physical examination are clues to etiology: pustules suggest *S. aureus;* ecthyma gangrenosum indicates a *Pseudomonas* infection; and petechiae or purpura, although not pathognomonic, are characteristic of meningococcemia. Purpura, however, may occur in as many as one third of cases of invasive *H. influenzae* type b infection.

The physician should reassess the child repeatedly, especially after the fever is lowered. Although the response to antipyretics does not predict etiology of the fever (i.e., bacterial versus viral), it may help limit the extent of laboratory investigation. If a child is irritable and not interactive when highly febrile but smiles and plays normally upon defervescence, then a lumbar puncture will not be necessary. However, if no source for the fever is found on exam, certain laboratory tests will still be indicated (as discussed below).

Laboratory Tests

No laboratory test should be considered routine but rather should be chosen based on the clinical situation. The clinician must decide why a test is ordered. Is it obtained as part of a sepsis work-up, or to reveal the source of a fever (e.g., pneumonia or UTI), or to help decide which children should receive expectant antibiotic therapy for occult bacteremia? If the child appears well, and particularly if he or she is to receive antibiotics for a focal infection such as otitis media, no laboratory studies are necessary if the infant is more than 8 weeks old. A WBC, blood culture, and sterile urine are recommended for highly febrile infants who look neither well nor toxic, who are without focal illness, or for whom careful follow-up is questionable. A chest x-ray should also be considered. The clinician should order a blood culture if the WBC is greater than 15,000 but should also realize that bacteremia may be present when the WBC is below this level. Many clinicians obtain a complete blood cell count because of evidence that the more abnormalities on the CBC (e.g., elevation in total WBC, bands, polys, or band-to-poly ratio), the greater the likelihood of bacteremia. Although data are inconsistent, the erythrocyte sedimentation rate (ESR) is probably as sensitive as any combination of tests. Other acute-phase reactants, such as C-reactive protein, are probably not more sensitive. Slide agglutination tests and counterimmunoelectrophoresis (CIE) have not been proved efficacious in screening for occult bacteremia. Vacuolization and toxic granulation in polymorphonuclear neutrophils and acridine orange stains of buffy coat smears are sensitive but not practical for office screening.

Infants who appear ill or toxic should be hospitalized and should have a full sepsis work-up, including an LP. There are no studies documenting that bacteria have been introduced into the cerebrospinal fluid (CSF) by performing a spinal tap in the setting of bacteremia. Thus, an LP should be performed whenever the procedure is indicated and not otherwise contraindicated (e.g., thrombocytopenia, unstable vital signs, or focal neurologic findings).

TREATMENT

Although there is no consensus, data and current opinion favor expectant antibiotic therapy in children at high risk for bacteremia. Studies have shown that children treated with antibiotics improve faster and may suffer fewer complications.

Any child who does not look well or who is less than 24 months old and has a temperature of at least 39.5°C (103°F) and/or a WBC of greater than 15,000 is a candidate for expectant therapy. Antibiotics should be started more readily in patients who are perceived as less compliant, who have poorer access to medical care, and whose parents are unlikely to observe subtle changes in their condition. Traditionally, this has been targeted at, but should not be limited to, an inner-city clinic population. The presence of a focal infection such as otitis media or pneumonia usually eliminates the decision of whether or not to initiate expectant antibiotic therapy for bacteremia. Amoxicillin, 50 mg/kg/day for 10 days, is the preferred antibiotic for outpatient therapy because it covers all major pathogens. However, increasing numbers of *H. influenzae* type b (20%–30% in some areas) and other bacteria such as *Branhamella catarrhalis* produce β-lactamase. Thus, where resistance is a major concern, amoxicillin/clavulanate is a reasonable alternative. If the child is allergic to penicillin, cefaclor, trimethoprim-sulfamethoxazole, or erythromycin-sulfisoxazole can be used.

Most physicians would agree that blood cultures should be drawn prior to the initiation of therapy. Antibiotics may be discontinued after 72 hours if the blood cultures are negative, providing that there is no concomitant focal infection. Most important, and regardless of whether or not expectant therapy is begun, the child must have close and careful follow-up. While expectant antibiotic therapy reduces the possibility of a metastatic spread of infection, it does not eliminate this risk. Patients must be told to notify their physician if their status worsens, because this may indicate the onset of complications such as meningitis, septicemia, septic arthritis, epiglottitis, endocarditis, pneumonia, cellulitis, or otitis media.

HOSPITALIZATION

Any toxic-appearing child, regardless of whether or not "risk" factors for bacteremia are present, should be hospitalized. Any child whose condition worsens while on expectant antibiotic therapy should also be hospitalized. The child should have a sepsis work-up and should receive intrave-

Table 198-1. Summary of Management of the Highly Febrile Infant

CLINICAL SITUATION	MANAGEMENT
Serious infection or looks toxic	Hospitalize; sepsis work-up; treat.
Nonwell, but "nontoxic" appearing without focal illness	Obtain WBC, B/C, U/C, ± CXR. Treat for presumptive bacteremia. Careful F/U mandatory. If questionable, hospitalize.
Nonwell, but "nontoxic" appearing with focal illness	Treat; if compliance is questionable, do a WBC and B/C. Careful F/U mandatory. If questionable, hospitalize.
Well-appearing without focal illness	Obtain WBC, B/C, and U/C. If WBC elevated or F/U questionable, treat for occult bacteremia. Careful F/U mandatory.
Well-appearing with focal illness.	No laboratory studies are necessary; treat; F/U.

B/C = blood culture; F/U = follow-up; U/C = urine culture;
WBC = white blood cell count; CXR = chest x-ray.

nous antibiotics. A dilemma may arise when blood cultures are positive in nonhospitalized children who are NOT receiving antibiotic therapy. All children should be reexamined and treated for 10 days, even if they are clinically well. The organism and condition of the child determine the need for hospitalization. Because of their high complication rate, infants with *H. influenzae* type b and meningococcal bacteremia, unless they are completely well or greatly improved, should be hospitalized. They should have a full sepsis work-up, including an LP to rule out meningitis, and they should receive parenteral antibiotics. With pneumococcal bacteremia, no laboratory studies other than repeating the blood cultures are necessary if the child is well. The child should be hospitalized for intravenous antibiotics if his or her condition remains unchanged, and a full sepsis work-up should be done. If the child is still sick, though improved, a repeat blood culture and LP should be performed. If the LP is negative, the patient may be either treated in the hospital or followed carefully as an outpatient on oral antibiotics. In the latter case, if no improvement is made in 18 to 24 hours, the child should be hospitalized for intravenous therapy (Table 198-1).

Combination therapy, such as ampicillin (200 mg/kg/day divided q6h) and chloramphenicol (75 mg/kg/day divided q6h), has been the standard treatment of sepsis; however, this treatment is rapidly being replaced by third-generation cephalosporins such as ceftriaxone (50 mg/kg/dose q12–24h) as a single medication. The physician should realize that this latter regimen does not cover Rickettsiae (Rocky Mountain spotted fever) and it is not the drug of choice for salmonellosis. Intravenous antibiotics should be given initially; when improvement occurs, they can be switched to oral therapy (based on sensitivities of the organism) to complete a 10-day course.

PREVENTION

Contacts of patients who have a serious invasive disease such as septicemia or meningitis must seek medical attention at the first sign of illness. Specific prophylactic measures are available to reduce the risk of secondary spread of *N. meningitidis* and *H. influenzae* type b infections. All household, day-care, nursery, and classroom contacts of patients with meningococcemia should receive rifampin chemoprophylaxis, 10 mg/kg/dose every 12 hours for four doses, with a maximum dose of 600 mg. All household contacts of children less than 4 years old with *H. influenzae* type b invasive disease should receive rifampin, 20 mg/kg/dose, once a day for 4 days, with a maximum dose of 600 mg. The treatment of day-care and classroom contacts of patients with serious *H. influenzae* type b disease is somewhat controversial. Whereas some recommendations call for chemoprophylaxis of all contacts, most experts recommend rifampin only after outbreaks of at least two cases in the same setting within a 60-day period. Because index cases may still harbor either organism in their nasopharynx (appropriate intravenous antibiotic therapy for the acute illness does not eradicate the carrier state), they should also receive rifampin prophylaxis prior to discharge from the hospital in order to avoid reintroducing the invasive strain into their households.

ANNOTATED BIBLIOGRAPHY

Baker MD, Avner JR, Bell LM: Failure of infant observation scales in detecting serious illness in febrile 4-to-8-week-old infants. Pediatrics 85:1040, 1990. (Prospective study applying the Yale Observation Scale showed that it was neither sensitive nor specific for diagnosing serious disease in this very young age group.)

Carroll WL, Farrell M, Singer JI et al: Treatment of occult bacteremia: a prospective randomized clinical trial. Pediatrics 72:608–612, 1983. (Data to support treating the high-risk infant with expectant antibiotic therapy for presumptive occult bacteremia.)

Dashefsky B, Teele DW, Klein JO: Unsuspected meningococcemia. J Pediatr 102:69–72, 1983. (Outcome data showing that *N. meningitidis* is the worst bacteria to have in the blood.)

Dershewitz RA, Wigder HN, Wigder CM et al: A comparative study of the prevalence, outcome and prediction of bacteremia in children. J Pediatr 103:352–358, 1983. (Major conclusions: (1) race and socioeconomic status are not risk factors for bacteremia; (2) clinical judgment is limited in the prediction of bacteremia; (3) because highly febrile infants treated for focal illness do well, most do not need laboratory studies.)

Downs SM, McNutt RA, Margolis PA: Management of infants at risk for occult bacteremia: A decision analysis. J Pediatr 118:11, 1991.

Lieu TA, Schwartz JS, Jaffe DM, Fleisher GR: Strategies for diagnosis and treatment of children at risk for occult bacteremia: Clinical effectiveness and cost-effectiveness. J Pediatr 118:21, 1991. (The two articles above used decision analysis based on data from published studies and concluded that it is advantageous to draw blood cultures and empirically treat all infants at risk for occult bacteremia.)

McCarthy PL: Controversies in pediatrics: What tests are indicated for the child under 2 with fever. Pediatr Rev 1:51–56, 1979. (Most of the controversies and uncertainties persist.)

McCarthy PL, Lembo RM, Baron MA et al: Predictive value of abnormal physical examination findings in ill-appearing and well-appearing febrile children. Pediatrics 76:167–171, 1985. (The Yale Observation Scale is useful in teaching, screening, and predicting which febrile infants are at greatest risk of serious illness.)

Newman TB: Options in occult bacteremia. Pediatric Trauma and Acute Care 4:12, 1991. (Concise editorial cautioning against widespread use of empiric oral antibiotic therapy.)

199

Antimicrobial Prophylaxis

Ellen R. Wald

The purpose of this review is to provide the pediatric practitioner with access to the rationale, indications, and recommendations for prophylactic antimicrobials to prevent bacterial and parasitic infections in office practice. Prophylaxis for surgical procedures or for the immunosuppressed patient is not discussed.

ESTABLISHED INDICATIONS FOR ANTIMICROBIAL PROPHYLAXIS

There are ten established indications for antimicrobial prophylaxis in pediatric patients that are accepted and noncontroversial. These indications include antimicrobial prophylaxis to prevent endocarditis in patients with structural cardiac disease who undergo procedures likely to be associated with bacteremia; penicillin prophylaxis to prevent rheumatic fever recurrences; penicillin prophylaxis for patients with asplenia or sickle cell disease; erythromycin prophylaxis after exposure to pertussis; ophthalmic antimicrobials to prevent neonatal conjunctivitis caused by *Neisseria gonorrhoeae*; prophylaxis after exposure to a sexual contact with gonorrhea or syphilis; prophylaxis to prevent recurrent urinary tract infections; isoniazid prophylaxis for household contacts of individuals with tuberculosis; and malarial prophylaxis for travelers to an endemic area. The preferred drugs and route of administration are shown in Table 199-1.

Endocarditis

Prophylaxis with amoxicillin for endocarditis is indicated in patients with congenital heart disease (except uncomplicated secundum atrial septal defect), rheumatic fever or other acquired valvular heart disease, idiopathic hypertrophic subaortic stenosis, and mitral valve prolapse syndrome. Patients with rheumatic fever who have been on penicillin prophylaxis to prevent a recurrent infection due to group A streptococci may harbor viridans streptococci that are resistant to penicillin. Accordingly, for these patients and for those who are penicillin allergic, erythromycin is preferred to penicillin for prophylaxis against infectious endocarditis.

Rheumatic Fever

After the patient is diagnosed as having rheumatic fever, he or she is started on prophylactic penicillin to prevent recurrent group A streptococcal pharyngitis that might lead to recurrent rheumatic fever (particularly rheumatic fever with carditis). Although recurrent episodes of rheumatic fever tend to mimic the initial episode with regard to the major manifestation, a crossover may occur (i.e., patients initially presenting with arthritis or chorea may develop carditis during recurrences). The most serious outcome is that children who initially present with carditis will develop recurrent carditis with severe sequelae, including early mortality. It is important to recognize that the twice-daily penicillin prophylaxis does not protect patients with rheumatic fever from endocarditis. Although the recommendations regarding prophylaxis against endocarditis have not been subjected to critical clinical evaluation, their use represents the current standard of care.

The duration of twice-daily penicillin prophylaxis to prevent streptococcal infections in individuals with rheumatic fever is controversial. The decision must be based on the likelihood of the index case having contact with others who may be infected with group A streptococci. Because these infections are endemic in the age group 5 to 15 years, an evaluation of the degree of contact with school-aged youngsters is critical. Accordingly, continued prophylaxis is indicated for parents of school-age children or teachers of primary and secondary grade schools who continue to be vulnerable. If one elects to use benzathine penicillin G in younger children, these injections should be spaced ~3 weeks apart.

Asplenia

The role of oral penicillin prophylaxis in preventing pneumococcal infection in patients with sickle cell disease or asplenia has been evaluated in a randomized, double-blind, multicenter trial. The risk of septicemia from *Streptococcus pneumoniae* was decreased by 84% and no deaths occurred in the group that received penicillin. Although compliance

Table 199-1. Established Indications for Prophylaxis

INDICATION	ANTIMICROBIAL AGENT	ADMINISTRATION	DOSE AND DURATION
Endocarditis	Amoxicillin	Oral	50 mg/kg (not to exceed 3.0 g) 1 hour before procedure and 25 mg/kg 6 hr later (max 1.5 g)
	Erythromycin	Oral	20 mg/kg (max 1.0 g) 1½ to 2 hr prior to procedure, then 10 mg/kg (max 500 mg) 6 hr later
Rheumatic fever	a. Benzathine penicillin G b. Penicillin V, G c. Sulfisoxazole d. Erythromycin	Intramuscular Oral Oral Oral	1.2 million units 250 mg b.i.d. 1.0 g/day 250 mg/day
Asplenia	Penicillin V	Oral	125 mg b.i.d.
Pertussis	Erythromycin	Oral	40 mg/kg/day in four divided doses for 14 days
Ophthalmia neonatorum Gonococcal	a. Silver nitrate b. Erythromycin 0.5% c. Tetracycline 1.0%	Topically Topically Topically	Once at delivery Once at delivery Once at delivery
Gonorrhea exposure	a. Ceftriaxone	Intramuscular	125 mg if < 45 kg 250 mg if ≥ 45 kg
	b. Spectinomycin	Intramuscular	40 mg/kg
Syphilis exposure	Ceftriaxone is effective for incubating syphilis.		
Urinary tract	SMX-TMP	Oral	10 and 2 mg/kg, respectively, at bedtime
	Nitrofurantoin	Oral	2 mg/kg at bedtime
Mycobacterium tuberculosis	Isoniazid	Oral	10 mg/kg/day
Malaria	Chloroquine	Oral	5 mg/kg once weekly starting 1 week before and for 6 weeks after leaving endemic area
	Mefloquine	Oral	15−19 kg: ¼ tab/wk 20−30 kg: ½ tab/wk 31−45 kg: ¾ tab/wk > 45 kg: 1 tab/wk Start 1 week before and continue for 2 weeks after leaving endemic area

with the oral regimen could not be adequately monitored, oral penicillin prophylaxis is an effective strategy when combined with neonatal screening for sickle cell disease, pneumococcal vaccine, and comprehensive health care. The dose of phenoxymethyl penicillin was 25 mg/kg/day in two divided doses. Prophylaxis should be continued until the tenth birthday.

Pertussis

Primary prevention of pertussis is accomplished with the use of a whole killed bacterial vaccine. The exposure of an unimmunized host to active illness is likely to cause disease. The exposure of partially immunized individuals also provides some risk of infection.

Limited data suggest that erythromycin is an effective prophylactic agent against pertussis if the exposure is recognized early in the incubation period. Erythromycin prophylaxis was provided for 1 immunized and 12 unimmunized children who were exposed to an active case of pertussis within the family; only 3 children developed mild respiratory symptoms. In a hospital outbreak of pertussis in Cincinnati, only one of six infected staff who received erythromycin prophylaxis developed the disease. Within a nursery setting, administration of erythromycin to seven infants exposed to a 6-week-old child with pertussis appeared to prevent the appearance of clinical disease. In contrast to these reports, there is ample documentation that once the paroxysmal stage of illness has evolved, antimicrobial agents are not effective in modifying the course of illness.

Although no prospective randomized controlled trials have systematically evaluated erythromycin prophylaxis for pertussis, the Committee of Infectious Diseases of the American Academy of Pediatrics recommends that infants who are exposed to pertussis should receive erythromycin prophylaxis as soon as possible at a dose of 40 mg/kg/day in four divided doses for 14 days.

Ophthalmia Neonatorum

This syndrome is usually due to infection with either *Chlamydia trachomatis* or *N. gonorrhoeae*. Topical therapy with an erythromycin ophthalmic preparation is effective in preventing gonococcal ophthalmia and is accordingly the preferred drug for this indication (see Chap. 92).

Exposure to Gonorrhea or Syphilis

The victim of sexual abuse or a known sexual contact of an individual infected with *N. gonorrhoeae* or *Treponema pallidum* should be provided with prophylaxis for these infections. The regimens shown in Table 199-1 are all effective for gonorrhea and likewise for incubating syphilis. If a nontreponemal test for syphilis shows reactivity, then an alternate treatment will be required for established or primary infection with *T. pallidum* (see Chap. 200). Infants born to mothers with untreated gonorrhea are at high risk of infection and should be treated.

Recurrent Urinary Tract Infection

The two categories of patients that are best managed with chemoprophylaxis are children with demonstrable vesicoureteral reflux and those without anatomic problems who are subject to closely spaced recurrent acute urinary tract infections. In the former category, the intention of prophylaxis is to prevent renal damage by maintaining the sterility of the refluxing urine. In the latter, the aim of prophylaxis is simply to reduce the morbidity associated with frequent infections. The efficacy of nitrofurantoin, sulfamethoxazole-trimethoprim (SMX-TMP), and methenamine mandelate as prophylactic agents in urinary tract infections is well established. The first two are most commonly used in childhood. The third requires acidification of the urine, which is often accomplished by the coadministration of ascorbic acid. An acid pH allows the disassociation of methenamine mandelate to formic acid, thereby providing an antiseptic intravesicular environment. Both nitrofurantoin and SMX-TMP are well absorbed from the gastrointestinal tract. Accordingly, little active drug reaches the colon to be exposed to coliforms (a population of microorganisms that is likely to ultimately colonize the periurethral area and to be introduced into the bladder urine). On the other hand, antimicrobial agents such as amoxicillin, sulfisoxazole, and cephalexin are only moderately well absorbed orally. Consequently, sufficient drug reaches the colon, thereby providing an opportunity for secondarily resistant coliforms to become predominant and to emerge ultimately as the infectious pathogen.

One concern regarding urinary tract prophylaxis is the safety of the recommended antimicrobial agents. Nitrofurantoin has been shown to be a cause of pneumonitis and hepatitis and therefore requires monitoring during chronic usage. SMX-TMP may cause bone marrow suppression and Stevens–Johnson syndrome. A half dose of either at bedtime is usually sufficient to maintain sterile urine. When prescribed for reflux, the prophylactic agent should be used until the reflux resolves. An assessment of the persistence of reflux should be undertaken every 6 to 12 months with a radionuclide voiding cystourethrogram. When the indication for prophylaxis is frequent acute infections, a 6-month trial of prophylaxis is appropriate. Repeated courses may be required if frequent infections recur after the prophylaxis has been discontinued (see also Chap. 112).

Mycobacterium tuberculosis

Prophylaxis for *Mycobacterium tuberculosis* is indicated for skin test–negative household contacts of active cases of pulmonary tuberculosis. The skin test is repeated after 3 months of treatment; no further medication is necessary if the skin test is still negative.

Another isoniazid treatment group is asymptomatic tuberculin skin test–positive patients. Although asymptomatic, these patients have an infection, and therefore the isoniazid is not a prophylactic but rather an appropriate treatment (see Chap. 170).

Malaria

Travelers to malaria-endemic areas are at risk of acquiring an infection. In areas of chloroquine-resistant *Plasmodium falciparum*, mefloquine is now recommended.

CONTROVERSIAL INDICATIONS FOR PROPHYLACTIC ANTIMICROBIALS

There are five controversial areas involving prophylactic therapy that are common clinical situations for the practitioner, and they deserve a more detailed discussion. These areas include prophylaxis for *Neisseria meningitidis* and *Haemophilus influenzae* type b, otitis media, animal bites and lacerations, and early-onset group B streptococcal sepsis.

Neisseria meningitidis and Haemophilus influenzae Type b

Intimate contacts of a patient with infection caused by either *N. meningitidis* or *H. influenzae* type b are at an increased risk of developing invasive disease caused by these two bacterial species. The risk for both infections is highest for children between the ages of 3 months and 4 years, a time when many children lack the protective antibody that is directed against the polysaccharide capsule of the organism (anticapsular antibody). The risk for secondary meningococcal infection extends into adulthood with a second peak in the 15- to 24-year age group, when crowding due to dormitory-style housing (military barracks or college campus) facilitates the transmission of the organism. In contrast, the risk of secondary illness due to *H. influenzae* type b is decreased dramatically beyond the fourth birthday and is virtually nil in adults.

Pharyngeal colonization with *N. meningitidis* or *H. influenzae* type b is not rare. In circumstances in which there has been no exposure to an individual with invasive disease caused by *N. meningitidis* or *H. influenzae,* the pharyngeal colonization rate with these two bacterial species is ~10% and 2%, respectively. When there has been a case of invasive disease due to either of these pathogens, the pharyngeal colonization rate among contacts is usually dramatically increased—in the range of 30% to 70%. The individuals who are at highest risk of developing illness after an exposure to a patient with invasive disease are those who are not colonized and are antibody negative. (There is a suggestion that those individuals who are carriers are actually at low risk of invasive disease, probably because many already possess anticapsular antibody.) When a susceptible (antibody-negative) noncolonized individual is exposed to the invasive pathogen, one of two outcomes can be anticipated: either the individual will become a healthy carrier of the organism or invasion and subsequent disease will evolve. Factors favoring the latter outcome have not been delineated but may include the development of, or exposure to, viral agents that cause an upper respiratory infection. Thus, to protect antibody-negative, noncolonized individuals from acquiring colonization with these pathogens, we try to create a *Neisseria-* or *Haemophilus*-free environment. This can be accomplished with rifampin, an antimicrobial capable of eradicating these pathogens from the throats of those who are colonized. Most secondary cases in the household environment occur within a few days of the primary case. Because conventional throat cultures for the identification of *N. meningitidis* and *H. influenzae* are time-consuming and insensitive, the strategy employed to protect the unidentified individual who is at highest risk is the use of rifampin for all contacts who may be colonized without obtaining prior throat cultures. This will create (at least temporarily) a pathogen-free environment, consequently protecting against acquisition of the bacterial species by a potentially susceptible individual.

Other important guidelines regarding prophylaxis are: (1) index cases have persistent pharyngeal colonization even after parenteral therapy for their primary infection, and (2) individuals less than 2 years of age may fail to develop protective antibody even after invasive infections. Thus, the following procedure is recommended:

a. All household and intimate contacts of children with invasive illness due to meningococcal disease should receive rifampin at a dose of 10 mg/kg twice daily for 2 days (not to exceed 600 mg twice daily). A household contact may be defined as someone who lives with the index case or is a nonresident who spends considerable time with the index case. Day-care contacts or close neighborhood friends may be included in this definition. The index case should also receive rifampin at the end of treatment for the primary infection.

b. All household and intimate contacts of children less than 2 years of age with invasive disease caused by *H. influenzae* type b should receive rifampin at a dose of 20 mg/kg/day (not to exceed 600 mg) as a single daily dose for 4 days.

c. If the index case with disease caused by *H. influenzae* type b is older than 2 years, the requirement to provide prophylaxis is contingent on there being an additional age-susceptible child in the household. If there are no other children less than 4 years of age, then prophylaxis for household members is not recommended. If there are children less than 4 years, the procedure is as in (b) (see also Chap. 197 for a further discussion of prophylaxis in a day-care setting).

Otitis Media

Antimicrobial prophylaxis has been recommended for children with recurrent episodes of acute otitis media. The objective of prophylaxis is to reduce the morbidity (otalgia and hearing loss) associated with these episodes. Although several studies have addressed this issue, they are imperfect in their design and do not provide conclusive evidence of the benefits of prophylaxis. Nonetheless, the consensus is that antimicrobial prophylaxis with an appropriate agent will prevent symptomatic episodes of acute otitis media. The suggested indications for initiating prophylaxis are three episodes of acute otitis media in 6 months or four episodes in a year. The best studied regimen is sulfisoxazole at 75 mg/kg in two divided doses; others recommend amoxicillin at 20 mg/kg/day as a single nighttime dose. Although symptomatic episodes of otitis media may be prevented by these regimens, their impact on the persistence of middle ear effusion has been less thoroughly evaluated. Consequently, it is recommended that patients on antimicrobial prophylaxis be examined at regular intervals (every 4 to 6 weeks) to evaluate the possibility of persistent effusion. Persistence of middle ear fluid beyond 3 months—particularly if associated with significant hearing loss—may require an alternative management strategy. The duration of prophylactic antimicrobial therapy depends on the length of the remaining respiratory infection season. For example, if a patient experiences three episodes of acute otitis media by November, it will probably be necessary to treat prophylactically for 6 months, or until the respiratory season is over. Alternatively, if prophylaxis is not initiated until March or April, it may be necessary to treat only for 1 to 2 months (see also Chap. 75).

Animal Bites and Lacerations

The role of prophylactic antibiotics in dog bites has not been settled. However, there is consensus that antibiotic prophylaxis is not indicated for nonfacial or nonhand dog-bite-inflicted wounds that are adequately cleaned, irrigated, and debrided. In contrast, a small study (11 patients) of prophylactic therapy with oxacillin for cat bites showed a significant decrease in the infection rate in the treated group (see also Chap. 144).

Early-Onset Group B Streptococcal Sepsis

Pregnant women with heavy vaginal colonization with group B streptococci may transmit this organism to their newborns. If other high-risk factors are present, such as prematurity, prolonged rupture of membranes, or maternal perinatal fever, the infant may develop early-onset sepsis with group B streptococci. Studies show that intrapartum antimicrobial therapy with ampicillin can effectively prevent colonization of and disease in the neonate. The strategic problem that has evolved is identifying the mother with heavy colonization in a timely fashion so as to selectively identify the mother–infant pair at risk and to minimize the use of intrapartum antimicrobials in those who do not require them.

ANNOTATED BIBLIOGRAPHY

Feder HM: Chemoprophylaxis in ambulatory patients. Pediatr Infect Dis 2:251, 1983. (Nice review of eight indications for prophylaxis.)
Scheifele DW: Prophylactic antibiotics in children. Pediatr Infect Dis 1:420–424, 1982. (Attempts to identify key elements of successful chemoprophylaxis.)

Endocarditis

Prevention of Bacterial Endocarditis. Recommendations by the American Heart Association. JAMA 244:2919–2922, 1990. (Standard recommendations for prophylaxis in patients with structural heart defects.) Copies of these recommendations are available from the American Heart Association, 7320 Greenville Ave., Dallas, TX 75231.

Urinary Tract Infections

Hellerstein S: Recurrent urinary tract infections in children. Pediatr Infect Dis 1:271–182, 1981. (Provides useful guidelines for the evaluation and management of children with urinary tract infections.)

Holmberg L, Boman G, Bottiger LE et al: Adverse reactions to nitrofurantoin: Analysis of 921 reports. Am J Med 69:733–788, 1980. (Detailed account of toxicity related to nitrofurantoin use.)

Malaria

Recommendations for the prevention of malaria among travelers. MMWR 39:1–10, 1990.

Otitis Media

Paradise JL: Antimicrobial prophylaxis for recurrent acute otitis media. Otol Rhinol Laryngol 905:53–57, 1981. (Analysis of studies concerning prophylaxis for otitis media reported before 1981. More recent studies suffer from similar methodologic flaws but purport the same result—apparent efficacy of sulfisoxazole in preventing symptomatic episodes of acute otitis media.)

Pertussis

Altemeier WA, Ayoub EM: Erythromycin prophylaxis for pertussis. Pediatrics 59:623–625, 1977. (Limited experience with erythromycin as a prophylactic drug for pertussis.)

Animal Bites and Hand Lacerations

Galloway RE: Mammalian bites. J Emerg Med 6:325–331, 1988. (Comprehensive review of mammalian bites, including dog, cat, rat, and human bites.)

Sexually Transmitted Diseases

STD treatment guidelines. MMWR 38:1–43, 1989. (Comprehensive updated recommendations for treatment of STD's.)

Prophylaxis for *H. influenzae* and *N. meningitidis*

Shapiro E: Prophylaxis for contacts of patients with meningococcal or *Haemophilus influenzae* type b disease. Pediatr Infect Dis 1:132–138, 1982. (Comprehensive review of presumed epidemiology and pathogenesis of secondary or associated cases of illness.)

Asplenia

Gaston MH, Varter JI, Woods G et al: Prophylaxis with oral penicillin in children with sickle cell anemia. N Engl J Med 314:1593–1599, 1986. (Reports an 84% reduction in episodes of sepsis in penicillin-treated patients compared to controls.)

Group B Streptococcal Sepsis

Boyer KM, Gotoff SP: Prevention of early-onset neonatal group B streptococcal disease with selective intrapartum chemoprophylaxis. N Engl J Med 314:1665–1669, 1986. (Presents an effective and practical strategy for reducing GBS sepsis; women at high risk received intrapartum ampicillin.)

200

Sexually Transmitted Diseases

Barry Dashefsky

The primary care pediatrician encounters sexually transmitted diseases (STDs) in newborn, prepubertal, pubertal, and postpubertal patients. Each practitioner must decide *a priori* whether his or her office practice will be inclined and equipped to provide appropriate questioning, physical examination (including pelvic examination), laboratory studies, confidential management, follow-up, contact tracing, reporting, and education of patients with STDs or be prepared to refer patients elsewhere for these services. Although consideration is usually given to STDs when symptomatology is overt and obvious, anticipation and vigilance are required to facilitate their diagnosis when the presentation is vague, subtle, or frankly asymptomatic or when the patient is unable or unwilling to direct our attention. Routine screening of high-risk populations, including sexually active adolescents, for the most common STDs is appropriate.

Despite the fact that only traditional venereal diseases (i.e., gonorrhea, syphilis, chancroid, granuloma inguinale, and lymphogranuloma venereum) and, recently, human immunodeficiency virus (HIV) are mandatorily reported to public health authorities, and even these conditions are grossly underreported, epidemiologic data indicate that the incidence of nearly all STDs and their complications has burgeoned to epidemic proportions in industrialized countries during the past 35 years, especially among women, adolescents, and homosexuals. It is estimated that of the approximately 12 million people who acquire an STD annually in the United States, two thirds are less than 25 years old.

Most adolescents with STDs, like adults, are unwitting victims of voluntary (although perhaps unacknowledged) sexual contact. The clinical manifestations and consequences of these infections are identical to those in adults. The changing physiology of the maturing female genitourinary tract may explain a greater predilection of adolescents to endocervical infection due to *Neisseria gonorrhoeae* and *Chlamydia trachomatis.*

Although nonvenereal transmission by fomites or close nonsexual contact with infected adults is a tenable, albeit rare, explanation of an STD infection in a prepubertal child, involuntary sexual contact (i.e., sexual abuse) must always be suspected and explored as the most likely cause.

Newborns and infants may present with protean features of STD infection incurred in utero (either by hematogenous transplacental transmission or by retrograde extension from the maternal genital tract), during parturition (by direct contact with an infected birth canal), or postnatally.

This chapter is not intended to provide a comprehensive listing of all the numerous agents now recognized to cause STDs and their most common clinical manifestations in children and adolescents. Rather, selected aspects of the clinical presentation, diagnosis, and management of four of the most common STDs (gonorrhea, chlamydia, herpes simplex virus, and syphilis) are presented. The reader is referred to the following chapters in this book where information regarding many of the STDs is presented according to the presenting clinical syndrome: Chapters 52 (Acquired Immunodeficiency Syndrome [AIDS] in Children), 67 (Warts and Molluscum Contagiosum), 92 (Ophthalmia Neonatorum), 110 (Hepatitis), 112 (Urinary Tract Infections), 113 (Dysuria and Frequency), 118 (Genital Pain), 119 (Vulvovaginitis), 121 (Pelvic Inflammatory Disease), and 196 (Neonatal Infections). Additionally, the reader is referred to related topics in Chapters 16 (Sexuality Education), 20 (Child Abuse), and 42 (Pregnancy Prevention). (For a more detailed discussion of STDs, the reader is referred to one of several references listed in the bibliography.)

A few general statements regarding the evaluation and management of STDs are germane: (1) Multiple STDs often coexist. Suspicion or diagnosis of one infectious agent should generally result in (laboratory) assessment for additional candidate pathogens, including HIV, which may alter the natural history and responsiveness to treatment of coinfecting STDs. (2) Sexual partners should be identified, evaluated, and (often presumptively, on the basis of a history of contact) treated for infection due to the agent(s) identified in the index case. (3) Follow-up tests for proof of cure should usually be routinely obtained; sexual activity should be strongly discouraged pending results of follow-up tests. (4) The value of properly used barrier contraception, especially condoms (used with spermicide), in lowering, but not eliminating, the risk of contracting and transmitting STDs should be stressed in patient education. (5) Hepatitis B virus (HBV) vaccine is recommended for all HBV-susceptible patients with STDs or multiple sexual partners.

GONORRHEA

Background

Infection due to *N. gonorrhoeae* is the most common reportable infectious disease in the United States. Age-specific rates indicate that teenagers and young adults are at highest risk for acquiring gonorrhea. Although the highest number of reported cases occurs in the 20- to 24-year-old age bracket, more than one quarter of all cases occur among pediatric patients less than 19 years old. Of this group, girls between the ages of 15 and 19 years have the highest rate of infection (1146/100,000 in 1989). Although gonorrhea is usually a mild disease, 10% to 20% of infected females develop salpingitis; a significant proportion of these females become involuntarily infertile (at least 13% after one episode of salpingitis, 36% after two episodes, and 75% after three or more episodes). At least 1% of infected individuals develop disseminated gonococcal infection.

Clinical Presentation

Pubertal and Postpubertal Adolescents. The clinical manifestations of gonorrhea in children who have undergone puberty are similar to those in adults. Most females and a significant proportion of males are asymptomatic.

Males. Although gonococcal urethritis is uncommon among prepubertal males, it is the most common form of gonococcal infection in males after puberty. Following an incubation period of 1 to 14 (average, 2 to 7) days, disease presents with the sudden onset of dysuria, urgency, frequency, and a purulent, often thick and yellow discharge. Edema and erythema of the penile meatus may occur. If left untreated, the majority will resolve spontaneously within weeks; persistent, asymptomatic urethral carriage is rare.

Females. Urogenital disease is the most common manifestation of gonococcal disease in pubertal and postpubertal females. In that age group, under the effect of estrogen, the vagina develops cornified epithelium and an acidic milieu that render it relatively resistant to gonococcal infection (in contrast to the prepubertal vagina). The primary site of infection is the endocervical canal; the urethra is also often colonized simultaneously. Although most women with gonococcal cervicitis are asymptomatic, within 10 days of infection those females who do develop symptomatic disease manifest mucopurulent vaginal discharge, dysuria, urgency, frequency, menstrual irregularities, and lower abdominal pain. A physical examination reveals mucopus emanating from the cervical os. The cervix may be inflamed, erythematous, friable, and tender on manipulation. There may also be an expressible urethral or periurethral gland exudate.

Pelvic inflammatory disease (PID), which is an infection of the endometrium, fallopian tubes, and possibly the ovaries and peritoneum, may develop in 10% to 20% of women with cervical infection due to *N. gonorrhoeae* following the ascent of infecting organisms through the uterine cavity to the endosalpinx. Tubo-ovarian abscess, peritonitis, and *perihepatitis (Fitz–Hugh–Curtis syndrome)* are possible complications. PID often occurs at or within a few days of the onset of menses. A vaginal discharge is present in ~60% of cases of PID, but its absence does not preclude the diagnosis. In addition to vaginal discharge, the onset of PID may be heralded by fever, chills, nausea, and vomiting. The major findings on physical examination are cervicitis, marked pain on cervical manipulation, and adnexal tenderness or masses. The specific microbiologic etiology of a particular episode of PID is difficult to determine. In addition to *N. gonorrhoeae,* suspect organisms include one or more of the aerobic and anaerobic genital flora, *C. trachomatis,* and *Mycoplasma hominis.* Cultures of the endocervix, or even cultures of material obtained by culdocentesis, fail to clearly identify the cause of PID; accordingly, empiric antimicrobial therapy must be broader than regimens only adequate to treat gonorrhea (see Chap. 121).

Pharyngeal gonorrhea is associated with orogenital sexual activity and is found in 10% to 20% of heterosexual women, 10% to 25% of homosexual men, and 3% to 7% of heterosexual men with gonococcal infection. It is usually asymptomatic but may produce pharyngitis and cervical adenitis. It is often difficult to treat effectively.

Anorectal gonorrhea is common in women with cervical infection (35%–50%) and homosexual males. It seldom produces symptomatic infection (less than 10%), but when it does, it presents as proctitis with pruritus, tenesmus, and purulent and often hemorrhagic rectal discharge.

Disseminated gonococcal infection (DGI) with gonococcal bacteremia occurs in 0.5% to 3% of infected patients. It is the leading cause of septic arthritis in sexually active populations and uncommonly causes endocarditis, meningitis, pneumonia, or osteomyelitis. DGI occurs mostly in females and presents usually during the first menses (7 to 30 days) after the onset of an asymptomatic genitourinary tract or other local infection. The illness varies in its severity. A typical course is manifested by migratory polyarthralgias involving large joints and a rash of varying description usually involving extremities and sparing the face and trunk (most often pustules on an erythematous base but sometimes papules, petechiae, or hemorrhagic bullae) during the first week of symptoms. Twenty-five percent of patients will have tenosynovitis. Blood cultures are frequently positive during the first week of illness. Subsequently, a portion of patients will develop septic arthritis in one or two joints (usually with positive synovial fluid cultures) with variable degrees of fever and toxicity.

Prepubertal Child. Beyond infancy, involuntary sexual contact is the most likely mode of gonococcal acquisition in prepubertal children aged 1 to 9 years. Rarely, it occurs through fomites or nonsexual transmission from infected close contacts. The infection is most often acquired within the household during the mother's absence. Accordingly, gonococcal infection in this age group necessitates an assiduous evaluation for neglect or abuse. In children aged 10 to 14 years, both voluntary and involuntary sexual activity figure significantly in the pathogenesis of gonococcal infection.

Most (up to 85%) prepubertal gonococcal infections occur among girls, and they present most often as vaginitis. Most cases of vaginitis in the prepubertal age, however, are not attributable to a specific etiology. This is because of the physiology of the prepubertal vagina, which, unlike the mature vagina, is characterized by unestrogenized, non–glycogen-filled, uncornified epithelium and has a relatively alkaline pH, factors that make it susceptible to gonococcal colonization and disease. Because the endocervix is not patent in the prepubertal girl, it is uncommon for an infection to produce endocervical infection or PID. Gonococcal vaginitis presents with variable amounts of vaginal discharge, itching, and occasionally dysuria, usually in the absence of features of systemic illness. Abdominal pain and fever may occasionally be present in the rare instance of associated salpingitis or peritonitis. Asymptomatic vaginal colonization may occur and should be sought when sexual abuse is suspected.

Newborns. Neonatal gonococcal infection is acquired from a symptomatically or an asymptomatically infected mother in utero (secondary to amnionitis), during delivery through an infected birth canal, or following intimate exposure postnatally. Ophthalmia neonatorum is the most common manifestation among newborns, usually appearing by the end of the first week of life (from 1 to 12 days). Formerly a highly virulent infection, gonococcal ophthalmia purportedly has a severity that is more variable at present. It presents clinically as an intense, bilateral inflammation with a profuse exudate. If left untreated, the infection may progress from a superficial infection of the conjunctiva to an invasion and necrosis of the cornea. Gonococcal ophthalmia was one of the most common causes of blindness prior to the widespread practice of prenatal screening and ophthalmic prophylaxis (see Chap. 92, "Ophthalmia Neonatorum").

Disseminated gonococcal infection occurs rarely in newborns. When it does occur, it presents most often at 1 to 2 weeks of age with constitutional features of illness (fever and irritability) and septic arthritis, often involving multiple joints.

Work-Up

The diagnosis of gonococcal infection usually depends on the isolation of *N. gonorrhoeae* from the site of infection (e.g., blood, cerebrospinal fluid [CSF], synovial fluid, vagina, endocervix, urethra, conjunctiva), which is often suggested by a Gram stain and is confirmed by a culture. Immunofluorescent antibody tests and immunologic or biochemical techniques for detection of gonococcal antigens or metabolic by-products are investigational modalities. Most practitioners will transport specimens to laboratories for culture diagnosis, although Gram stains can be assessed in the office.

Because of the fastidious growth requirements of *N. gonorrhoeae,* specimens for culture must be obtained and processed carefully. Warm water rather than a petroleum product should be used to lubricate instruments that come in contact with the specimen. Calcium alginate rather than cotton swabs should be used to sample urethral specimens. Culture and transport media should be warmed to room temperature before inoculation. Urethral specimens can be obtained by inserting the swab 2 to 4 cm into the urethra or collecting the first 10 to 20 ml of a voided urine specimen. Specimens from normally sterile sites (e.g., blood,

cerebrospinal fluid, synovial fluid, peritoneal fluid, petechial scrapings) can be cultured on nonselective chocolate agar. Cultures from sites that are normally colonized by various flora (e.g., conjunctiva, cervix, vagina, rectum, pharynx) require selective culture media such as Thayer–Martin, Martin–Lewis, or New York City agar, which consist of chocolate agar containing antibiotics that inhibit normal flora, including most nonpathogenic *Neisseria* species. Specimens must be plated immediately and must be incubated at 35°C (95°F) in 5% to 10% carbon dioxide or transported in an appropriate commercially prepared holding medium such as Transgrow (which contains modified Thayer–Martin agar in a carbon dioxide atmosphere).

Gram-stained smears of exudates from symptomatic individuals, which show typical intracellular organisms within polymorphonuclear leukocytes, are highly suggestive of gonococcal infection. For males with symptomatic urethritis, such a finding is 90% to 95% sensitive and 95% to 100% specific compared with culture results and is considered adequately diagnostic. Confirmatory cultures are required in almost all other circumstances. In postpubertal females, the finding of intracellular organisms on Gram stain of endocervical smears is only 50% to 70% sensitive, although it is 95% to 100% specific in expert hands.

Appropriate specimens for culturing are dictated usually by the presenting symptomatology. Rectal and pharyngeal cultures, however, should be processed routinely in addition to genitourinary specimens when evaluating homosexuals, sexually abused patients, patients with oral or anal exposure to *N. gonorrhoeae,* and patients who are assessed for DGI.

Treatment and Management

Recommended antimicrobial regimens for the several clinical syndromes associated with *N. gonorrhoeae* are outlined in Table 200-1. (For the treatment of pelvic inflammatory disease, see Chap. 121.) Other management issues are briefly considered below:

1. Because of the frequency of poor compliance and the substantial long-term morbidity associated with PID, the threshold for hospitalizing adolescents with PID should be low, and patients with PID treated as outpatients should be reevaluated within 48 to 72 hours.

   DGI, as well as septic arthritis, endocarditis, meningitis, and ophthalmia neonatorum due to *N. gonorrhoeae,* likewise requires hospitalization and parenteral therapy.

2. Because a decade-long increase in the rate of antibiotic resistance (95% of which is due to penicillinase-producing *N. gonorrhoeae* [PPNG]) reached 8% by 1989, the traditional role of penicillin, ampicillin, or amoxicillin as preferred empiric therapy has been supplanted by ceftriaxone or, alternatively, for urethral, cervical, rectal, or pharyngeal gonorrhea, by single-dose oral cefixime. In addition, because of the frequent poly-

Table 200-1. Treatment of Gonorrhea

TYPE OR STAGE	DRUG OF CHOICE	DOSAGE	ALTERNATIVES
GONORRHEA* Urethral, cervical, rectal, or pharyngeal	Ceftriaxone	125–250 mg IM once	Cefixime 400 mg orally once Ciprofloxacin 500 mg orally once Ofloxacin 400 mg orally once Spectinomycin† 2 g IM once
Ophthalmia (adults)‡	Ceftriaxone	1 g IM once plus saline irrigation	Ceftriaxone 1 g IV or IM daily × 5 days, plus saline irrigation
Bacteremia and arthritis§	Ceftriaxone	1 g IV daily × 7–10 days	Ceftizoxime or cefotaxime, 1 g IV q8h for 2–3 days or until improved, followed by cefixime 400 mg orally bid or ciprofloxacin 500 mg orally bid to complete 7–10 days total therapy
Meningitis	Ceftriaxone	2 g IV daily for at least 10 days	Penicillin G at least 10 million U IV daily for at least 10 days‖ Chloramphenicol 4–6 g/day IV for at least 10 days‖
Endocarditis	Ceftriaxone	2 g IV daily for at least 3 to 4 weeks	Penicillin G at least 10 million U IV daily for at least 3 to 4 weeks‖
Neonatal Opththalmia	Ceftriaxone	125 mg IM once, plus saline irrigation	Penicillin G 100,000 U/kg/day IV in 4 doses‖ × 7 days, plus saline irrigation
OR	Cefotaxime	25 mg/kg IV or IM q8–12h × 7 days plus saline irrigation	
Arthritis and septicemia	Cefotaxime	25–50 mg/kg IV q8–12h × 10–14 days	Penicillin G 75,000 to 100,000 U/kg/day IV in 4 doses × 7 days‖
Meningitis	Cefotaxime	50 mg/kg IV q8–12h × 10–14 days	Penicillin G 100,000 U/kg/day IV in 3 or 4 doses for at least 10 days‖
Children (under 45 kg) Urogenital, rectal and pharyngeal	Ceftriaxone	125 mg IM once	Spectinomycin† 40 mg/kg IM once Amoxicillin 50 mg/kg oral once plus probenecid 25 mg/kg (max. 1 g) oral once‖
Arthritis	Ceftriaxone	50 mg/kg/day (max. 2 g) IV × 7 days	Penicillin G 150,000 U/kg/day IV × 7 days‖
OR	Cefotaxime	50 mg/kg/day IV in divided doses × 7 days	
Meningitis	Ceftriaxone	100 mg/kg/day (max. 2 g) IV × 7 days	Penicillin G 250,000 U/kg/day IV in 6 divided doses for at least 10 days‖
OR	Cefotaxime	200 mg/kg/day IV for at least 10 days	Chloramphenicol 100 mg/kg/day IV for at least 10 days‖

*Since a high percentage of patients with gonorrhea have coexisting *C. trachomatis* infection, all patients should also receive a course of treatment effective for *Chlamydia.*

†Not effective for pharyngeal infection.

‡An oral fluoroquinolone, such as ciprofloxacin for 3–5 days, probably would also be effective, but experience is limited.

§If the infecting strain of *N. gonorrhoeae* has been tested and is known to be susceptible to penicillin or the tetracyclines, treatment may be changed to penicillin G 10 million U IV daily, amoxicillin 500 mg orally qid, doxycycline 100 mg orally bid, or tetracycline 500 mg orally qid.

‖If infecting strain of *N. gonorrhoeae* has been tested and is known to be susceptible.

(From Abramowicz M [ed]: Drugs for sexually transmitted diseases. Med Lett 33:119–124, 1991.)

microbial etiology of PID (difficult to document with specificity in a particular case), antimicrobial regimens should be empirically selected to be sufficiently broad to be effective against *C. trachomatis,* anaerobes, gram-negative enteric organisms, and *M. hominis,* as well as *N. gonorrhoeae.*

Thus, with the frequent coincidence of other STDs in genitourinary gonorrhea and PID, especially *C. tra-*

chomatis (present in 15%–25% of men and 30%–50% of women with acute urogenital gonorrhea), preferred antimicrobial regimens are selected to cover both *N. gonorrhoeae* and *C. trachomatis* (e.g., ceftriaxone and doxycycline).

3. Because treatment failure following combination ceftriaxone/doxycycline therapy is rare, it is not necessary to perform "test-of-cure" follow-up cultures if this regi-

men is used. Follow-up cultures should be obtained ~4 to 7 days after completion of other therapeutic regimens. However, "rescreening" cultures should be obtained 1 to 2 months after treatment, irrespective of the regimen employed, in order to detect reinfection.

4. All cases of gonorrhea should be reported to public health authorities to facilitate contact tracing.

5. Sexual contacts should be identified and evaluated for gonorrhea. The presumptive treatment of sexual contacts exposed to persons with gonorrhea should be implemented. Child victims of sexual abuse are thought to be at low but uncertain risk of contracting STDs and, therefore, need not be prophylactically treated unless the assailant is known to be infected, parents request treatment, or follow-up cannot be ensured.

6. At least a representative sample of all isolates of *N. gonorrhoeae,* as well as all isolates associated with treatment failure, should be tested for antimicrobial susceptibility in order to facilitate recognition of the emergence of resistance to recommended antimicrobials and to guide retreatment of treatment failures.

7. A serologic test for syphilis (STS) should be obtained for all infected patients to look for coexisting infection at the time of first evaluation. Incubating syphilis is adequately treated by regimens recommended for treatment of *N. gonorrhoeae,* which include penicillins, cephalosporins, and tetracyclines. (The effectiveness of single-dose cefixime in treating incubating syphilis has yet to be determined.) However, because spectinomycin and quinolones have not been shown to be similarly effective, if these agents are used to treat gonorrhea, an STS should be repeated 4 to 6 weeks later.

CHLAMYDIA

Background

Chlamydia trachomatis is the most common STD in the United States. Although not an officially reportable condition, it causes an estimated three to four million infections each year. Its high and increasing prevalence is most striking among young and poor single women, and it has been reported to be as high as 37% among pregnant inner-city adolescents. Young males are also affected more often than older males. The risk of disease varies with the number of sex partners. In many of its clinical presentations, disease produced by *C. trachomatis* resembles that produced by *N. gonorrhoeae,* and the two infections frequently coexist. Both of them usually produce superficial mucosal genital infections, but they are also capable of producing more invasive diseases.

This discussion does not include the disease produced by serotypes of *C. trachomatis* responsible for trachoma or lymphogranuloma venereum, which are uncommon problems in the United States.

Clinical Presentation

As with many STDs, the asymptomatic or mildly symptomatic infection due to *C. trachomatis* must be suspected and sought to be diagnosed. Chlamydial cervicitis and, in homosexual males, chlamydial proctitis are common, and up to 30% of heterosexual males with chlamydial urethritis are asymptomatic or mildly symptomatic.

Pubertal and Postpubertal Males. *C. trachomatis* is the major cause of nongonococcal urethritis (NGU) and acute epididymitis in males 35 years of age or younger in the United States and is responsible for ~50% of cases of each. *C. trachomatis* can be cultured from up to 11% of asymptomatic sexually active males. In ~15% to 30% of heterosexual and 5% of homosexual males with gonococcal urethritis, *C. trachomatis* can be concomitantly isolated. Treatment of the gonococcal urethritis may result in persistent, relapsing, or (because of its longer incubation period) belatedly manifest NGU (referred to in this instance as *postgonococcal urethritis* or PGU) due to *C. trachomatis.*

Nongonococcal urethritis due to *C. trachomatis* usually produces less dysuria and less purulent (clear to white) urethral discharge than does urethritis due to *N. gonorrhoeae,* but the differentiation cannot be made securely on clinical grounds. Presenting symptoms include urethral discharge, itching, or dysuria after an incubation period of 7 to 21 days. A physical examination may further reveal meatal irritation. The diagnosis of NGU is based on demonstration of urethritis and exclusion of gonorrhea by Gram stain and culture. The objective diagnosis of urethritis requires a demonstration of at least four polymorphonuclear leukocytes for each oil-immersion field on a Gram-stained smear of a urethral exudate or at least 10 to 15 polymorphonuclear leukocytes for each high-power field in the sediment of the first 10 to 15 ml of a voided urine specimen.

Epididymitis or epididymo-orchitis presents with unilateral scrotal pain, swelling, tenderness, and fever, usually with accompanying NGU. In addition to *C. trachomatis,* the differential diagnosis includes epididymitis due to *N. gonorrhoeae,* uropathogens such as Enterobacteriaceae, and testicular torsion.

Proctitis due to *C. trachomatis* should be considered in homosexual males presenting with mild to moderate rectal discharge, anorectal pain, tenesmus, or constipation. *C. trachomatis* is possibly implicated etiologically in some cases of prostatitis and Reiter's syndrome.

Pubertal and Postpubertal Females. Like gonorrhea, chlamydia frequently infects females asymptomatically. Mucopurulent cervicitis (objectively defined as the presence of 10 to 30 or more polymorphonuclear leukocytes per oil-immersion field in a smear of cervical exudate) is the most common symptomatic form of infection. *Chlamydia trachomatis* is isolated from 30% to 50% of women with mucopurulent endocervical discharge, including coincidental isolation from 25% to 50% of cases of gonococcal infection. In addition to a creamy endocervical discharge, physical examination often reveals hypertrophic ectopy. *Ectopy* refers to the ectopic presence of endocervical columnar epithelium on the exocervix, giving it a bright-red circumoral appearance. Hypertrophic ectopy appears as an area of ectopy that is edematous, congested, and prone to bleeding.

Chlamydia trachomatis is a frequent cause of PID, implicated in 25% to 50% of the one million cases seen annually in the United States. As previously discussed in the section on *N. gonorrhoeae*, PID is frequently of polymicrobial etiology; causative agents cannot be reliably distinguished from each other on clinical grounds. *Chlamydia trachomatis* purportedly presents with milder signs and symptoms, but this tendency may be deceiving because the consequences of chlamydial PID may be as severe as those of *N. gonorrhoeae*. The complications include peritonitis and perihepatitis (Fitz–Hugh–Curtis syndrome). Long-term sequelae include ectopic pregnancies and infertility (see Chap. 121).

Chlamydia trachomatis is also responsible for urethritis in women (producing the dysuria–pyuria syndrome); up to two thirds of women with pyuria and sterile bladder urine have evidence of chlamydial infection (see Chap. 113). Bartholinitis and endometritis may also be caused by *C. trachomatis*.

Prepubertal Females. Rarely, *C. trachomatis* is isolated from vaginal specimens of asymptomatic girls. More often, it is isolated in the context of symptomatic nongonococcal vaginitis and indicates sexual abuse.

Newborns and Young Infants. *Chlamydia trachomatis* is the most common cause of neonatal conjunctivitis and one of the most common causes of interstitial pneumonitis in the first 3 to 6 months of life. The frequency of neonatal chlamydial infection is a function of the rate of colonization among pregnant women. The rates vary from 2% to 37%, with most studies reporting rates of 6% to 12% in the United States. Although most colonized pregnant women are asymptomatic, an estimated 60% to 70% of their vaginally delivered offspring will be colonized, including 18% to 50% who will develop conjunctivitis and 8% to 20% who will develop afebrile pneumonia due to *C. trachomatis*.

Chlamydial conjunctivitis is the most commonly documented cause of ophthalmia neonatorum (13%–74%; mean, 29%) in the developed western countries where the frequency of gonococcal ophthalmia has declined because of effective prophylaxis and prenatal maternal screening. Eighteen to fifty percent of infants born to infected mothers will have conjunctivitis between 1 and 3 weeks (usually 5–12 days) of age. Infection usually presents with a unilateral mucoid discharge associated with eyelid edema, bulbar and palpebral conjunctival inflammation, and bilaterality within 1 week of onset. Severity is variable. Other causes cannot be distinguished clinically. Smears of ocular discharge reveal both polymorphonuclear and mononuclear leukocytes.

Intracytoplasmic inclusions are noted on Giemsa-stained smears of epithelial cells. The conjunctivitis usually resolves spontaneously within weeks to months without visual sequelae, but if it is untreated, a prolonged course including the development of scarring and micropannus may ensue (see Chap. 92).

Chlamydial pneumonia is one of the most common causes of pneumonia in the first 6 months of life. It usually presents between 3 and 11 weeks of age with tachypnea and a characteristic staccato cough in an afebrile child with a prior 1- to 2-week history of mucoid rhinorrhea. Fine rales, usually without wheezes, are noted on auscultation. Approximately 50% of infants have prior or concurrent conjunctivitis. A chest roentgenogram shows hyperinflated lungs with diffuse interstitial or alveolar infiltrates. The leukocyte count is usually normal, but a moderate degree of both eosinophilia and hyperimmunoglobulinemia is often present. In most instances, the course of disease is mild and the infant improves gradually over 5 to 7 weeks with or without the benefit of therapy. Hospitalization is usually not clinically indicated. The risks of long-term sequelae, including asthma, chronic cough, and abnormal pulmonary function tests, are incompletely elucidated (see Chap. 196).

A role for *C. trachomatis* in producing otitis media, gastroenteritis, or apnea in infancy is uncertain.

Work-Up

Cell culture coupled with Giemsa or iodine staining or fluorescent antibody identification of intracellular inclusions constitutes the "gold standard" for the diagnosis of infection due to *C. trachomatis* at any site. Antigen detection with use of either a direct fluorescent monoclonal antibody technique (FA) applied directly to a smear (available commercially as Microtrak, manufactured by Syva Diagnostics) or enzyme-linked immunosorbent assay (ELISA, available commercially as Chlamydiazyme, manufactured by Abbott Diagnostics) offers alternative, more rapid, though somewhat less sensitive methods for detecting the presence of *C. trachomatis*. Culture sites in adults are from the urethra or cervix; in children they are conjunctival or nasopharyngeal. Cross-reacting fecal flora obviate the reliability of these diagnostic methods for urethral, vaginal, or rectal specimens from children. Cell culture should be employed in assessing all cases of suspected sexual abuse in order to maximize the reliability of diagnosis. Designated transport media must be used for culture and ELISA studies. Prior to inoculation into cell culture, specimens may be stored at 4°C (39.2°F) for up to 12 to 24 hours but thereafter must be frozen at −70°C (−94°F).

Serologic diagnosis of *Chlamydia* is not useful in routine practice, although antichlamydial IgM antibody determinations may help in the diagnosis of acute invasive infection (e.g., pneumonia) in patients with prior antibiotic treatment.

Table 200-2. Treatment of *Chlamydia Trachomatis*

TYPE OR STAGE	DRUG OF CHOICE	DOSAGE	ALTERNATIVES
CHLAMYDIA TRACHOMATIS			
Urethritis, cervicitis conjunctivitis, or proctitis (except lymphogran- uloma venereum)	Doxycycline*	100 mg oral bid × 7 days	Erythromycin† 500 mg oral qid × 7 days‡ Ofloxacin 300 mg oral bid × 7 days Azithromycin 1 g orally once
Infection in Pregnancy	Erythromycin†	500 mg oral qid × 7 days‡	Amoxicillin 500 mg oral tid × 10 days Clindamycin 450 mg oral qid × 10 days Sulfisoxazole§ 500 mg oral qid × 10 days
Neonatal			
Ophthalmia	Erythromycin	12.5 mg/kg oral or IV qid × 14 days	
Pneumonia	Erythromycin	12.5 mg/kg oral or IV qid × 14 days	Sulfisoxazole‖ 100 mg/kg/day oral or IV in divided doses × 14 days

*Or tetracycline 500 mg oral qid
†Erythromycin estolate is contraindicated in pregnancy.
‡In presence of severe gastrointestinal intolerance, decrease to 250 mg qid and extend duration to 14 days.
§Or another sulfonamide in equivalent dosage; avoid all sulfonamides in the third trimester.
‖Only for infants more than 4 weeks old.
(From Abramowicz M [ed]: Drugs for sexually transmitted diseases. Med Lett 33:119–124, 1991.)

Treatment

Table 200-2 details recommended treatment regimens for chlamydial infections. Chlamydial urethritis and cervicitis are treated with either tetracycline or erythromycin 500 mg P.O. q.i.d. for 7 days or doxycycline 100 mg P.O. b.i.d. for 7 days or with a single 1 g oral dose of azithromycin. Both neonatal ophthalmia and pneumonia are treated with erythromycin 12.5 mg/kg P.O. or IV q.i.d. for 14 days or, alternatively, after 1 month of age, sulfisoxazole 25 mg/kg P.O. or IV q.i.d. for 14 days. Other issues pertinent to management follow:

1. Patients with symptoms compatible with the following *Chlamydia*-associated syndromes (even without diagnostic confirmation), as well as their identified sexual contacts of the prior 30 days, should receive presumptive antimicrobial therapy adequate for chlamydial infection: nongonococcal urethritis; mucopurulent cervicitis; pelvic inflammatory disease; and epididymitis in men who are 35 years of age or younger.
2. Mothers and sex partners of mothers of infants with neonatal conjunctivitis or pneumonitis confirmed to be due to *C. trachomatis* should be treated for presumed genital chlamydial infection.
3. Although neonatal ophthalmic prophylaxis, with either topical erythromycin (0.5%), tetracycline (1%), or silver nitrate (1%), instilled within 1 hour of birth is effective in preventing gonococcal conjunctivitis, its efficacy in preventing chlamydial conjunctivitis, especially cases with belated onset, is inconsistent. None of these regi-

mens prevents nasopharyngeal colonization by chlamydia and subsequent development of pneumonia.
4. Two weeks of systemic erythromycin therapy for chlamydial conjunctivitis without concomitant topical therapy is effective in both treating the ocular infection and reducing nasopharyngeal colonization. Although based on uncontrolled observations, 2 weeks of systemic erythromycin therapy is also recommended to decrease shedding and effect clinical improvement in established chlamydial pneumonia.
5. Post-treatment cultures are generally advised in pediatric populations (though not in adults). Although no chlamydial resistance to recommended antimicrobials has been reported, persistence of symptoms may be due to tetracycline-resistant *Ureaplasma urealyticum* infection. Positive post-treatment cultures usually reflect noncompliance or reinfection from an untreated infected sex partner, and repeat treatment should be initiated.
6. Patients should be advised to abstain from sexual activity or, at least, to use condoms or other barrier methods of contraception pending the completion of therapy and a follow-up assessment.

HERPES SIMPLEX VIRUS—GENITAL INFECTION

Background

There are two serotypes of herpes simplex virus (HSV): HSV-1 and HSV-2. HSV-1 usually produces primary herpetic gingivostomatitis, pharyngitis, or conjunctivitis, typically in young children during the first 5 years of life. HSV-

2 is responsible for most (70%–95%) of sexually transmitted herpetic genital lesions. Genital herpes is classified as (1) primary genital infection (disease due to the first experience with either HSV-1 or HSV-2), (2) nonprimary first infection (the first clinically apparent genital infection in a person with prior experience with either HSV-1 or HSV-2), and (3) recurrent infection (repeat genital infection[s] in an individual with prior manifest genital infection). Although not a reportable condition, genital herpetic infections are estimated to have increased tenfold between 1966 and 1981. This epidemic increase in frequency, coupled with both their propensity for recurrence from latent status (60%–70%) and their frequently asymptomatic status (50%–70%), helps explain the significance of genital herpes infections.

Clinical Presentation

HSV, mostly HSV-2, is responsible for 40% to 60% of all ulcerative genital lesions. Herpetic genital lesions are most commonly found among adolescents and young adults 2 to 7 days after exposure. Sometimes herpetic genital infection (due to either HSV-1 or HSV-2) may be transmitted by nonvenereal means, such as by contaminated hands (including autoinoculation from oral lesions) or fomites. Most often, however, it is sexually transmitted, and its diagnosis in nonvoluntarily sexually active individuals must raise concern for sexual abuse.

The characteristic genital herpetic lesion consists of a vesicle on an erythematous base that is found in males on either the penile glans or shaft and in women on the vulva, perineum, buttocks, cervix, or vagina. The exanthem typically begins with nonspecific papules and evolves through the characteristic vesicular stage, becoming sequentially pustular, ulcerated, and finally scabbed.

Primary herpetic genital infections tend to have both systemic and local clinical features that are more severe and more prolonged than other nonprimary first infections or recurrent genital infections. Women tend to be more symptomatic and tend to suffer more complications than men. First genital infections that are not true primary herpetic infections (i.e., the patient previously had a nongenital herpetic infection) tend to be milder than true primary genital infections.

Systemic features of primary genital herpetic infection include fever, headache, malaise, and myalgias, and they occur in 40% of infected males and in 70% of females. These symptoms peak in the first 3 to 4 days and resolve by the end of the first week. Local symptoms include pain, itching, dysuria, and vaginal or urethral discharge. Painful genital lesions occur in 95% of males and in 99% of females, and they have a mean duration of 10 to 12 days.

The ulcerative stage of lesions may persist for 4 to 15 days until crusting occurs. New lesions occur in more than 75% of cases during the fourth to tenth days of infection. The mean duration of viral shedding from lesions is 12 days, and shedding remains a concern until the completion of scabbing. Cervical lesions occur in 90% of women with genital lesions due to primary HSV-2 infection and in 70% of women with genital lesions due to primary HSV-1. Cervical lesions occur in only 12% to 20% of women with recurrent external genital herpetic lesions. Cervical involvement can be asymptomatic. If symptomatic, herpetic cervicitis is usually associated with mucopurulent discharge with or without a friable, red, and ulcerated exocervix (in contrast to the endocervical site of gonococcal and chlamydial infections). The differential diagnosis of the genital lesion includes chancroid, syphilis, excoriation, erythema multiforme, candidiasis, and Behçet's disease.

Dysuria occurs in 44% of males and in 83% of females. Urethral discharge tends to be clear or mucoid. Local pain tends to increase in severity during the first week of symptomatic disease and tends to peak and recede by the end of the second week. Tender inguinal lymphadenopathy occurs during the second and third weeks of the disease and then resolves slowly.

Other sites of primary herpetic infection include the pharynx, which occurs coincidentally in 11% of primary HSV-2 genital infections, and rectum, especially among homosexuals.

Secondary or recurrent genital herpetic lesions occur in 80% of those who suffer primary HSV-2 genital disease. The characteristic lesions are identical to those suffered in primary disease but there are usually few, if any, systemic features, and a particular episode tends to be less severe and shorter than in primary infection. Approximately 50% of patients suffer prodromal symptoms of local tenderness, burning, or tingling sensations hours before the presentation of genital lesions. Lesions are on the penis in males and most often on the labia minora and majora and perineum in females; only 15% to 30% of women suffer concomitant cervicitis. Dysuria occurs in only ~27% of females. Lesions are frequently unilateral; they involve only approximately one tenth the area of the primary attack. They are associated with viral shedding for ~4 days, and they heal over the course of 6 to 10 days.

Complications of primary herpetic disease include local genital extension, extragenital infections, aseptic meningitis, encephalitis (which is most often due to HSV-1), transverse myelitis, autonomic nervous system dysfunction, disseminated disease, and bacterial or fungal superinfection. Neonatal infection due to the retrograde extension of genital herpes infections or the passage of the newborn through an infected genital tract (more often but not exclusively in primary disease) occurs in 1 in 3000 to 1 in 30,000 live births. HSV-2 genital infection is a risk factor for the development of cervical carcinoma. Genital ulceration due to HSV-2 also is a risk factor for acquisition of HIV infection.

Work-Up

Viral tissue culture of vesicular fluid or specimens obtained from other infected sites is the preferred diagnostic method and requires the use of a specialized laboratory equipped to perform such tests. Typical cytopathic effects appear quickly (usually within 4 days). Specimens must be planted promptly or transported in an appropriate holding medium; they may be held at 4°C to 9°C (39.2°F to 48.2°F) for up to 4 hours or at −70°C (−94°F) if a longer delay is incurred. A rapid presumptive diagnosis may be made with a Tzank preparation of scrapings of skin or mucosa from suspect lesions that are smeared, air-dried, fixed (with ethanol or methanol), and stained with Giemsa or Wright's stain. The presence of ballooned and multinucleated giant cells indicates that the lesion is due to one of the Herpetoviridae, but this is an insensitive detection method. A Papanicolaou smear of cervical or vaginal secretions may demonstrate suggestive intranuclear inclusions. Other highly specialized techniques for rapid diagnosis include antigen detection by direct immunofluorescence, immunoperoxidase staining, and ELISA tests. Electron microscopy and DNA hybridization offer additional diagnostic modalities. Serologic determination is seldom helpful in the clinical assessment of possible HSV infection.

Treatment and Management

The efficacy of acyclovir in the treatment of genital herpes lesions has been studied only in adults. Because it has not been explicitly approved for this use in pediatric patients, it should be used selectively, if at all, in this population. Treatment regimens for adults are outlined in Table 200-3.

In adults with primary genital infection, oral acyclovir reduces the duration of systemic and local signs, symptoms, and viral shedding by ~3 to 5 days if initiated within 6 days of the onset of symptoms. It has no effect on the rate or severity of recurrences. The recommended dosage is 200 mg orally five times each day for 7 to 10 days. This regimen should be considered in pediatric patients only if they have no prior history of herpes infection, including oral lesions (i.e., if they have a true primary genital infection). Topical acyclovir produces a slight but inferior benefit in the reduction of clinical features and viral shedding and, in general, is not recommended. Intravenous acyclovir is reserved for severely infected or complicated hospitalized pa-

tients. Acyclovir is generally not recommended for use during pregnancy. Routine treatment of sex partners is not recommended.

Oral acyclovir offers a marginal benefit in the treatment of recurrent genital infections and, when given continuously to adults with frequent recurrences, has resulted in fewer recurrences during the period of therapy. It is not recommended for use in immunocompetent pediatric patients for either recurrent genital disease or suppressive therapy.

Patients are urged to abstain from sexual activity while symptomatic lesions are present, even if they are receiving acyclovir. The use of barrier methods of contraception (e.g., condoms) is recommended to reduce the risk of transmission, and, because the risk of transmission in the asymptomatically infected individual is unknown, they should be considered for routine contraceptive use in patients with a history of genital herpes.

Women with genital herpes should have yearly Papanicolaou smears and, when pregnant, should inform their obstetricians of this history.

SYPHILIS

Background

Syphilis is the third most commonly reported communicable disease in the United States, ranking after gonorrhea and varicella. In 1989, 44,540 cases of primary and secondary syphilis were reported, representing a rate of 18.5:100,000 population. These rates are higher than any during the prior 40 years. Minority heterosexual and drug-using populations are conspicuously represented in this increased rate. In 1989, 859 cases of congenital syphilis were reported, representing a decline of 95% since 17,600 cases were reported in 1941; however, the frequency of reported cases has increased alarmingly since the nadir of 108 cases reported in 1978.

Syphilis is a disease of protean clinical expression caused by the spirochete *Treponema pallidum*. Its natural course is divided into four stages: (1) primary syphilis, which is manifested by a nonpainful chancre (usually genital) and regional (usually inguinal) adenopathy after a mean

Table 200-3. Treatment of Herpes Simplex

TYPE OR STAGE	DRUG OF CHOICE	DOSAGE	ALTERNATIVES
HERPES SIMPLEX			
First Episode Genital	Acyclovir	400 mg oral tid × 7–10 days	Acyclovir 200 mg oral 5 times/day × 7–10 days
First Episode Proctitis	Acyclovir	800 mg oral tid × 7–10 days	Acyclovir 400 mg oral 5 times/day × 7–10 days
Severe (hospitalized patients)	Acyclovir	5 mg/kg IV q8h × 5–7 days	
Prevention of Recurrence*	Acyclovir	400 mg bid	200 mg oral 2–5 times a day

*Preventive treatment should be discontinued for 1 to 2 months once a year to reassess the frequency of recurrence.
(From Abramowicz M [ed]: Drugs for sexually transmitted diseases. Med Lett 33: 119–124, 1991.)

incubation period of ~3 weeks; (2) secondary syphilis, which is manifested by mucocutaneous or visceral lesions with lymphadenopathy following hematogenous dissemination; (3) latent syphilis, which is a period of subclinical infection; and (4) late or tertiary syphilis, which is manifested by ascending aortitis and involvement of the central nervous and other organ systems, including skin, bone, liver, and spleen.

Syphilis is most often transmitted sexually but may also be acquired through saliva, through blood transfusion, through direct inoculation from moist mucocutaneous lesions, or transplacentally. Most cases occur in patients between the ages of 15 and 30 years; one third of cases occur in homosexuals. Although it is uncommonly diagnosed in pediatric populations, it serves as an easily diagnosed useful marker of sexually transmitted diseases and should be considered and sought whenever another STD is diagnosed or suspected.

Clinical Presentation

Primary syphilis begins at the site of inoculation as a single, painless papule that evolves into a chancre (a nontender, eroded ulcer with a smooth, clean base and raised, firm margins). Multiple chancres may occur. The usual sites of chancres include the external genitalia, cervix, anal canal, perianal region, and oral cavity. Regional lymphadenopathy is usually moderately large, firm, nonsuppurative, and painless. Irrespective of treatment, chancres typically resolve in 2 to 6 weeks, whereas the lymphadenopathy persists longer. The differential diagnosis of genital chancres and inguinal adenopathy includes herpes simplex (typically clustered vesicles), chancroid (typically painful, exudative, indurated ulcers with suppurative adenopathy), early venereal warts, granuloma inguinale, lymphogranuloma venereum, tuberculosis, atypical mycobacteria, tularemia, sporotrichosis, anthrax, and rat-bite fever.

Secondary syphilis develops in the untreated patient 2 to 8 weeks after the onset of the primary chancre. Following hematogenous dissemination, highly contagious mucocutaneous lesions may develop. Skin lesions may be macular, maculopapular, papular, or pustular and typically involve the trunk and extremities, including the palms and soles. Painless, moist, gray-white to erythematous plaques called *condylomata lata* may occur in intertriginous regions. Mucous patches consisting of silvery gray superficial erosions with erythematous margins may also occur. In addition, any of the following systemic or local features may develop: fever; malaise; pharyngitis; laryngitis; anorexia; weight loss; arthralgia; generalized, painless lymphadenopathy (including epitrochlear nodes); aseptic meningitis (which is symptomatic only in 1% to 2% of cases); immune complex–mediated glomerulonephritis; hepatitis; splenomegaly; uveitis; synovitis; osteitis; or periostitis. Mucocutaneous lesions of secondary syphilis usually resolve within 2 to 12 weeks

irrespective of therapy, but patients are subject to relapses, most of which occur within the first 2 years. The differential diagnosis of skin lesions of secondary syphilis includes pityriasis rosea, measles, infectious mononucleosis, erythema multiforme, leukemia, lymphoma, tinea, sarcoid, granuloma annulare, and lichen planus.

Latent syphilis is defined as the stage in which there are no clinical manifestations of infection. A diagnosis requires serologic testing. During early latency (defined as the first 4 years), relapses, mostly mucocutaneous, may occur, but 90% occur within the first year.

During late latency or tertiary syphilis, untreated patients may manifest the slowly progressive inflammatory disease of neurosyphilis, cardiovascular, or gummatous syphilis. This stage is not encountered in pediatric-aged patients.

For a discussion of congenital syphilis, see Chapter 196.

Work-Up

The practitioner must utilize specialized, widely available laboratory facilities to make the diagnosis of syphilis.

In primary, secondary, and early congenital syphilis, a definitive diagnosis is made by a darkfield examination of serous transudate obtained from moist lesions such as chancres, condylomata lata, or mucous patches. Serologic tests for syphilis (STS) are the only means of diagnosing syphilis during the latent stage and often provide corroborative evidence for the diagnosis of primary, secondary, or congenital syphilis. STS include nontreponemal reaginic tests (e.g., rapid plasma reagin [RPR], Venereal Disease Research Laboratory [VDRL]) and specific treponemal tests (e.g., fluorescent treponemal antibody absorption [FTA-ABS], microhemagglutination assay for *T. pallidum* [MHA-TP], *T. pallidum* immobilization [TPI]).

Nontreponemal STS are 70% to 80% and 99% sensitive in detecting primary and secondary syphilis, respectively. These tests are not specific for *T. pallidum*, and a positive test requires a confirmation by a specific treponemal test. Nontreponemal STS have the virtue of being quantifiable and, therefore, can be repeated serially to gauge the response to therapy and to detect relapses or reinfections. Fourfold decrements and increments in titer reflect successful treatment and relapse, respectively. Tests typically revert to nonreactive within 1 year of successful treatment of primary syphilis and within 2 years of successful treatment of secondary syphilis. False-positive tests can occur in the context of acute bacterial or viral infection, immunization, drug addiction, collagen-vascular disease, hypergammaglobulinemic states, and pregnancy.

As the name implies, specific treponemal STS measure antibodies specific for infection due to *T. pallidum*, and they are used for serologic confirmation of the diagnosis of syphilis. They are 50% to 80% and 97% to 100% sensitive in detecting primary and secondary syphilis, respectively. These tests are not readily quantifiable, and a positive test does not revert to negative; therefore, they are not helpful for monitoring the response to therapy. False-positive tests are uncommon, but they can occur in other spirochetal diseases such as Lyme disease.

The diagnosis of neurosyphilis is in part established seralogically. VDRL (but not RPR) is performed on CSF; though not highly sensitive, it is quite specific. The FTA-ABS, performed on CSF, is highly sensitive, is less specific, is associated with a great negative predictive value, but generally is not used to make this diagnosis.

Western blot analysis and ELISA for IgG and IgM as well as fluorescent antibody tests (helpful in the diagnosis of congenital syphilis) are investigational tools at this time.

Treatment

The reader is referred to Table 200-4 for antimicrobial therapy for syphilis. Additional issues involving management include the following:

1. Penicillin is the preferred drug for treating syphilis at all stages and is the only proven therapy for treating patients with congenital, gestational, or neurosyphilis. Whenever possible, patients with these diagnoses who have penicillin allergy should be skin tested and/or desensitized and then treated with penicillin.
2. Currently recommended therapy for treating gonorrhea (i.e., ceftriaxone and doxycycline) is thought to be effective in treating incubating (STS-negative) syphilis, as are alternate regimens that employ beta-lactam or tetracycline agents. Spectinomycin, trimethoprim-sulfamethoxazole, ciprofloxacin, and ofloxacin, on the other hand, are not considered adequate for this purpose; the capabilities of erythromycin and cefixime are undetermined. Whenever a regimen with an unsubstantiated efficacy in treating incubating syphilis is used to treat gonorrhea, a repeat STS should be performed in 3 months.
3. Adequate treatment of primary, secondary, or early latent syphilis of less than 1 year's duration requires sustained blood levels of penicillin (of $\geq 0.3\ \mu l/ml$) for at least 7 days; this is best achieved by intramuscular (IM) benzathine penicillin G at a dose of 50,000 U/kg (maximum: 2.4 million units). Syphilis of more than 1 year's duration is best treated with IM benzathine penicillin G at a dose of 50,000 U/kg (maximum: 2.4 million units) weekly for 3 consecutive weeks. CSF examination is recommended to exclude asymptomatic neurosyphilis. Neurosyphilis is treated with aqueous crystalline penicillin G, 50,000 U/kg every 4 to 6 hours for 10 to 14 days, possibly followed by benzathine penicillin G 50,000 U/kg weekly for 3 weeks.

Penicillin-allergic patients 9 years of age or older can receive doxycycline or tetracycline. Those younger than

Table 200-4. Treatment of Syphilis

TYPE OR STAGE		DRUG OF CHOICE	DOSAGE	ALTERNATIVES
SYPHILIS				
Early (Primary, secondary, or latent less than one year)		Penicillin G benzathine	2.4 million U IM once*	Doxycycline† 100 mg oral bid × 14 days Ceftriaxone 250 mg IM once daily × 10 days‡ Erythromycin 500 mg oral qid × 14 days§
Late (more than one year's duration, cardiovascular, gumma, late-latent)		Penicillin G benzathine	2.4 million U IM weekly × 3 weeks	Doxycycline† 100 mg oral bid × 4 weeks
Neurosyphilis		Penicillin G	2 to 4 million U IV q4h × 10–14 days	Penicillin G procaine 2.4 million U IM daily plus probenecid 500 mg qid orally, both × 10–14 days
Congenital		Penicillin G	50,0000 U/kg IM or IV q8–12h for 10–14 days	
	OR	Penicillin G procaine	50,000 U/kg IM daily for 10–14 days	

*Some experts recommend repeating this regimen after 7 days, especially in patients with HIV infection.

†Or tetracycline 500 mg oral qid.

‡Limited experience; use only if compliance and follow-up are assured.

§Treatment with erythromycin is associated with an increased rate of relapse and should be used only if compliance and 12 months' follow-up are assured and other regimens are contraindicated.

‖Patients allergic to penicillin should be desensitized. Most authorities recommend following either the IV or IM penicillin regimen with benzathine penicillin G 2.4 million units IM weekly × 3 weeks.

(From Abramowicz M [ed]: Drugs for sexually transmitted diseases. Med Lett 33:119–124, 1991.)

9 years should be considered for penicillin desensitization or treated with erythromycin. Careful follow-up is necessary.

4. Repeat quantitative nontreponemal STS should be performed in congenital, primary, secondary, and early latent syphilis at 3, 6, and 12 months after treatment or until they become nonreactive. They should be repeated again at 24 months for syphilis of more than 1 year's duration prior to therapy. Repeat treatment should be given if there is failure of the titer to decrease fourfold within 1 year; CSF should typically be evaluated before retreatment.

5. The self-limited Jarisch–Herxheimer reaction of fever and generalized malaise within a few hours of beginning therapy for syphilis requires only an anticipatory warning to penicillin recipients and expectant observation of those who experience it.

6. Because the moist mucocutaneous lesions of primary and secondary syphilis are highly contagious, drainage and secretion precautions are necessary. Infants with proven or suspected congenital syphilis likewise require drainage, secretion, and blood precautions until therapy has been administered for at least 24 hours.

7. STS are recommended for all pregnant women in early and late pregnancy. They are also recommended for high-risk populations (especially prostitutes and homosexuals) and patients with other documented or suspected STDs and their contacts. HIV testing should be encouraged for patients with syphilis. Patients coinfected with HIV and syphilis require careful and frequent assessment of the adequacy of treatment and a low threshold for evaluating the CSF.

8. Recent sexual contacts (at least those with contact within the preceding 3 months) of individuals with acquired syphilis should be evaluated and presumptively treated for early syphilis.

ANNOTATED BIBLIOGRAPHY

Abramowicz M (ed): Drugs for sexually transmitted diseases. Med Lett 33:119–124, 1991. (Succinct and authoritative tabular presentation of preferred antimicrobial therapies for common STD agents.)

Bell TA: Major sexually transmitted diseases of children and adolescents. Pediatr Infect Dis 2:153–161, 1983. (Brief but useful discussion of STDs in the pediatric age group; both an overview of the topic and a review of specific clinical syndromes, their differential diagnosis, and management.)

Corey L: The diagnosis and treatment of genital herpes. JAMA 248:1041–1049, 1982. (Clinically oriented presentation of the elements of diagnosis and therapy for genital herpes.)

Emans SJ: Vulvovaginitis in the child and adolescents. Pediatr Rev 8:12–19, 1986. (Practical approach to the evaluation, differential diagnosis, microbiologic considerations, and management of dysuria and vaginal discharge in children and adolescents.)

Hart G: Syphilis tests in diagnostic and therapeutic decision making. Ann Intern Med 104:368–376, 1986. (Review of guidelines for diagnosing syphilis and the diagnostic capabilities of the various STDs.)

Holmes KK, Märdh PA, Sparling PF et al (eds): Sexually Transmitted Diseases, 2nd ed. New York, McGraw-Hill, 1990. (Definitive, comprehensive text including discussions of the general subject of STDs as well as current, well-referenced chapters on each of the specific agents and clinical syndromes.)

Hook EW, Holmes KK: Gonococcal infection. Ann Intern Med 102:229–243, 1985. (Recent review of the topic including current material on epidemiology, microbiology and pathogenesis, clinical manifestations, diagnosis, therapy [including issues of antimicrobial resistance], and prospects for prevention.)

Murphy DM: Office laboratory diagnosis of sexually transmitted diseases. Pediatr Infect Dis 2:146–152, 1983. (Review of the capabilities and limitations of the office laboratory in making at least a preliminary diagnosis of such STDs as Candida, Trichomonas, Gardnerella, and N. gonorrhoeae.)

Rettig PJ: Chlamydial infections in pediatrics: Diagnostic and therapeutic considerations. Pediatr Infect Dis 5:158–162, 1986. (Review of the diagnostic and therapeutic aspects of chlamydial infections in pediatric patients.)

Rettig PJ: Infections due to Chlamydia trachomatis from infancy to adolescence. Pediatr Infect Dis 5:449–457, 1986. (Review of the epidemiologic and clinical features of chlamydial infections of newborns, children, and adolescents.)

Straus SE (moderator): NIH conference: Herpes simplex virus infection: Biology, treatment, and prevention. Ann Intern Med 103:404–419, 1985. (Review of epidemiology, biology, diagnosis, treatment, and prospects for prevention of herpes simplex virus infection.)

U.S. Department of Health and Human Services/Public Health Service: 1989 STD treatment guidelines. MMWR (Suppl) 38(S-8):1–43, 1989. (Authoritative and specific management guidelines from the Centers for Disease Control for each STD agent, including advice concerning counseling, follow-up, and special considerations; same guidelines presented in somewhat abbreviated form in Pediatr Infect Dis 9:379–382, 1990.)

U.S. Department of Health and Human Services/Public Health Service: Sexually transmitted disease surveillance, 1989. Atlanta, Centers for Disease Control, October 1990. (Most current and historical epidemiologic data regarding reportable STDs in United States.)

201

Pertussis

Colin D. Marchant

Pertussis continues to occur even in highly immunized populations. At least four factors account for the persistence of this disease: Infants in the first few months of life have not yet received pertussis vaccine and have little or no immunity; the current whole-cell pertussis vaccine does not always provide protection until after the third or even fourth dose; some individuals or groups may refuse to have their infants and children immunized for personal or religious reasons; and although natural infection appears to confer life-long protection, immunity from whole-cell pertussis vaccine wanes after approximately 10 years, leaving many adolescents and adults again susceptible to pertussis and capable of transmitting the disease to infants and other non-immune contacts.

Even though it is estimated that state health departments receive notification of only 5% to 10% of pertussis cases, from 1986 through 1988, 10,468 cases of pertussis were reported to the Centers for Disease Control (CDC). The reported incidence appears to be slowly increasing in all age groups, particularly in adolescents and adults. However, morbidity remains greatest in early life. Infants less than 6 months of age account for 35% of reported cases and 66% of hospitalizations. Complication rates are highest in this age group: 17% develop pneumonia, 2.5% develop seizures, 1% develop encephalopathy, and 0.5% die.

The pediatrician has a central role in efforts to reduce this morbidity. Early diagnosis is important both for timely provision of supportive care and for prevention of secondary cases in households, child-care settings, and schools. Universal immunization with pertussis vaccine, beginning at 2 months of age, is critical for the prevention of pertussis epidemics. In countries such as Sweden, Great Britain, and Japan, epidemics of pertussis returned when universal pertussis immunization programs were abandoned or when large numbers of parents refused to have their children immunized.

PATHOPHYSIOLOGY

Pertussis is caused by infection of the respiratory tract with the bacterium *Bordetella pertussis*. Only rarely is *Bordetella parapertussis* or *Bordetella bronchiseptica* isolated from cases of suspected whooping cough. Adenovirus has been isolated from clinically typical cases but with negative cultures for *B. pertussis* and without detectable antibody response to the bacterium. In other instances, both adenovirus and *B. pertussis* have been isolated simultaneously, which suggests that adenovirus is a co-pathogen rather than the sole etiologic agent of the pertussis clinical syndrome. Co-infections of *B. pertussis* and respiratory syncytial virus are well described.

Humans are thought to be the sole reservoir of *B. pertussis*, and infection is usually spread by way of droplets produced by the coughing of infected persons. Although asymptomatic infection has been documented serologically, sustained respiratory tract colonization is uncommon and has not been shown to be important in the transmission of disease. Pertussis is highly contagious. More than 90% of susceptible household contacts become infected during epidemics. The incubation period typically is 7 to 10 days but may be as short as 3 days or as long as 20 days.

Bordetella pertussis possesses several surface adhesins that enable it to attach to the respiratory epithelium, where it further elaborates a number of toxins that disrupt ciliary function and inhibit local host defenses. The organism rarely invades tissues but produces the characteristic disease by toxin production. One such toxin, pertussis toxin, has systemic effects at distant sites and is believed to be responsible for the prolonged clinical disease. Pertussis toxin produces the characteristic lymphocytosis observed in many cases of pertussis and also induces histamine sensitization and islet cell activation in vitro. Inactivated pertussis toxin is the principal, but not the sole, component of new acellular pertussis vaccines that has now been licensed for booster immunization (see also Chap. 14, "Childhood Immunizations").

CLINICAL PRESENTATION

Whooping cough begins as an undifferentiated, typically afebrile, upper respiratory tract infection with coryza and cough. This so-called catarrhal stage offers no specific diagnostic clues. Unfortunately, it is also the phase of disease when the diagnosis is most easily made by culture or direct fluorescent staining of nasopharyngeal secretions, when the disease is most contagious, and when antibiotic therapy is most likely to alter the subsequent clinical course.

During the second week, the illness may progress to the characteristic paroxysmal stage. Paroxysmal cough should always alert the physician to the diagnosis of pertussis. These paroxysms occur at variable intervals, and between episodes the patient usually appears comfortable without signs of severe illness. Coughing may be accompanied by an inspiratory whoop, but this is often absent, particularly in young infants. Copious mucus production is often observed. Paroxysms of coughing may be further complicated by vomiting, cyanosis, apnea, or respiratory arrest. After severe paroxysms, the patient may perspire profusely and appear exhausted. Subconjunctival hemorrhages, petechiae, or epistaxis may result from severe spasmodic coughing. The severity and frequency of these paroxysms of cough usually peak during the second or third week of the illness. Then there is gradual improvement over several weeks, but coughing can persist for 3 months or longer.

Classical whooping cough is so distinct that it was clearly described in the sixteenth century, long before the causative organism had been discovered. However, atypical, mild, and even asymptomatic cases are common, so physicians should not expect to see the fully developed clinical picture. Infants often present with vomiting, cyanotic episodes, or apnea, and the role of coughing in their illness is not appreciated until later in their clinical course. Infants and children who are partially immunized are likely to have mild or atypical symptoms. Adolescents and adults usually do not present with classical symptoms. Prolonged nocturnal or episodic coughing may be the only manifestation. Careful microbiologic and serologic studies of household outbreaks have documented many mild and asymptomatic cases of pertussis.

COMPLICATIONS

The most serious complications (pneumonia, seizures, and encephalopathy) are more frequent and severe in unimmunized infants in the first 6 months of life. Pneumonia is usually limited to perihilar infiltrates, and the typical patient is afebrile. In 1% to 2% of hospitalized cases, there is secondary bacterial pneumonia with progression of pulmonary infiltrates and fever. Severe coughing episodes may result in pneumomediastinum or pneumothorax. Although it was thought that pertussis could lead to bronchiectasis in later life, more recent studies do not confirm this association, and there do not appear to be long-term pulmonary sequelae.

Seizures and encephalopathy complicate the most severe cases of pertussis and are thought to be due to anoxia from severe repeated paroxysms of coughing. The hypothesis that pertussis toxin acts directly on neural cells, or indirectly through hypoglycemia induced by islet cell activation, remains speculative. Most children recover from pertussis without any permanent sequelae; however, half of those with encephalopathy have permanent neurologic handicaps.

WORK-UP

History

Pertussis should be suspected in anyone with a paroxysmal cough, post-tussive vomiting, or prolonged unexplained cough. A history of exposure to family members or other close contacts with paroxysmal or severe coughing illnesses is suggestive. If there has been significant exposure to a laboratory-confirmed case of pertussis, then any respiratory symptoms should be deemed significant enough to pursue the diagnosis and institute antibiotic prophylaxis.

A child with a history of three or more immunizations with whole-cell pertussis vaccine is very unlikely to acquire pertussis, but those, particularly infants, who have received only one or two inoculations with pertussis vaccine may still be susceptible. Furthermore, immunity may have waned in adolescents and adults despite receipt of a complete series of immunizations in childhood. Thus, a positive immunization history should not prevent pursuing the diagnosis in an older patient with suggestive symptoms.

Infants in the first 6 months of life with pertussis are often attributed another diagnosis on admission to the hospital, and pertussis is considered only later when coughing is observed. Cough may not be the most striking symptom to parents, so the parents of infants who present with vomiting, cyanosis, or apneic episodes should be carefully questioned about coughing in both the infant and family members.

Physical Examination

Other than coryza, there are no physical findings unless a coughing paroxysm is witnessed. Then, a paroxysm of coughing, especially if it progresses to apnea, cyanosis, or vomiting, may enable a diagnosis to be made on clinical grounds. Similarly, there may be coughing with an inspiratory whoop.

Laboratory Tests

A culture of nasopharyngeal secretions for *B. pertussis* may confirm the diagnosis. A swab (Calgi swab, Colab Laboratory, Chicago Heights, IL) is passed through the naris and along the floor of the nasal passage (about 2 in) into the nasopharynx. If possible, it should be kept in place until the child coughs. Then the swab should be streaked directly onto culture medium. Freshly prepared Bordet–Gengou medium containing 20% fresh horse, sheep, or rabbit blood, starch, and either penicillin (0.2 U/ml) or methicillin (4 μg/ml) is the standard medium. Other media such as charcoal-horse blood agar with cephalexin (Regan–Lowe) may have longer shelf lives, but none have been shown to be consistently superior to fresh Bordet–Gengou medium. *Bordetella pertussis* grows slowly on culture media, and up to a week may elapse before the culture becomes positive. Culture media may be available on request from state laboratories.

Even under optimal conditions, cultures may be negative in clinically typical cases with household exposure to a proven case. The sensitivity of cultures for pertussis is 80% at best, so a negative result does not exclude the diagnosis. The yield is greatest during the catarrhal and early paroxysmal stages and declines progressively with increased duration of illness. Cultures are also less likely to be positive in those who were previously immunized as well as in those who have recently taken antibiotics such as erythromycin, tetracycline, and trimethoprim-sulfamethoxazole. Prior treatment with penicillin, amoxicillin, and first- and second-generation cephalosporins has little or no effect on *B. pertussis*. Antimicrobial susceptibility tests suggest that third-generation cephalosporins, such as ceftriaxone, may affect *B. pertussis*.

Direct fluorescent antibody (DFA) staining of nasopharyngeal secretions is the most widely used test for the diagnosis of pertussis. Nasopharyngeal secretions are obtained as described above and smeared on a glass slide. In the laboratory, antiserum is added to the slide. Such antisera contain antibodies to *B. pertussis* that are conjugated to a material that fluoresces under ultraviolet light. The slides are washed to remove antibody–conjugate complexes not attached to *B. pertussis* and are examined under a fluorescent microscope by trained technicians. Both false-positive and false-negative tests can occur, because the performance of the test is heavily dependent on the skill of the observer.

New serologic methods have been developed, and the most widely tested is antibody to pertussis toxin measured by enzyme-linked immunosorbent assay. Although these tests are promising, clinicians should be very cautious in the interpretation of serologic tests, because diagnostic criteria for interpretation have often not been established.

The white blood cell (WBC) count in pertussis may be elevated above 15,000/mm³ with 70% or more lymphocytes. This finding may be absent in many cases, particularly in young infants. Leukemoid reactions with WBC >50,000/mm³ have been observed.

DIFFERENTIAL DIAGNOSIS

In the catarrhal stage, pertussis may be confused with disease caused by a variety of respiratory pathogens. In infants, bacterial or viral pneumonias may begin as illnesses that are indistinguishable from pertussis. However, extensive pulmonary infiltrates, marked respiratory insufficiency, and high fever suggest an etiology other than pertussis. In the first few months of life, infections due to *Chlamydia trachomatis* and respiratory syncytial virus may present with prominent coughing and apnea. Conjunctivitis and interstitial pulmonary infiltrates on chest radiographs may be clues to disease caused by *C. trachomatis,* but specific microbiologic testing should be performed to confirm the diagnosis. In older children, persistent cough may occur in those with sinusitis, cystic fibrosis, bacterial pneumonia, aspirated foreign body, or tuberculosis.

TREATMENT

Erythromycin is the antibiotic of choice for the treatment of pertussis. Recent studies have confirmed earlier data demonstrating that if treatment is begun in the catarrhal stage of disease, the duration of illness is shortened. However, the disease is most often diagnosed after paroxysmal coughing has started, and erythromycin therapy has little or no effect on the subsequent course of disease. The most important effect of erythromycin therapy is to eliminate the organism from the nasopharyngeal mucosa and thereby decrease secondary spread. With erythromycin therapy, the duration of nasopharyngeal carriage is reduced from a mean of 12 days to less than 4 days. The erythromycin regimen is 40 to 50 mg/kg/day (maximum 2 g/day) in four divided doses for 14 days. Lesser dosages and shorter durations of therapy have been associated with bacteriologic relapses. On the basis of higher serum and sputum concentrations with the estolate ester, some authorities recommend erythromycin estolate as the preparation of choice. Superior microbiologic efficacy in comparative trials has not been tested, and the estolate ester may be associated with rare, but serious, hepatic toxicity. Trimethoprim-sulfamethoxazole

(8 mg TMP–40 mg SMX/kg/day in two divided doses for 14 days) is a reasonable alternative for patients with erythromycin allergy or intolerance.

Infants with pertussis may have serious paroxysms of coughing sometimes followed by periods of prolonged apnea and cyanosis. These infants may require intubation and ventilatory support to maintain adequate oxygenation. Thus, most infants less than 1 year of age with pertussis are admitted to the hospital at least until it is established that coughing paroxysms are of only mild severity. Supportive care includes suctioning of secretions, humidified oxygen, nutrition, and comfort. Often, paroxysms occur following stimulation, so it is best to keep infants as quiet and comfortable as possible. If suctioning is needed, it should be done only after a paroxysm when the infant appears to be less sensitive to stimuli. Nutritional support may include gavage or intravenous feeding. Cough suppressants and sedatives are not usually effective and should be discouraged. Additional antibiotic agents may be required to treat concurrent bacterial infections such as pneumonia or otitis media.

Other therapies that have been reported to be beneficial are corticosteroids and beta-adrenergic agents. Two reports claim that corticosteroids reduce the frequency and severity of paroxysmal coughing compared with selected, untreated controls. Beta-adrenergic agents, specifically salbutamol, have been found in some studies to reduce the number and severity of paroxysms. However, the evidence has not been sufficiently established to recommend either therapy.

PREVENTION

Secondary spread of pertussis should be prevented by prophylaxis of household and other close contacts with erythromycin (40–50 mg/kg/day [2 g/day maximum] in four divided doses for 14 days). All contacts, regardless of immunization status, should receive prophylaxis, because even fully immunized individuals may transmit the disease. Pertussis hyperimmune globulin is no longer available in the United States and was of dubious value (see also Chap. 199).

ctive immunization with whole-cell pertussis vaccine has led to a marked decline in the incidence of pertussis since the 1950s when the vaccine was widely administered. Although it is not possible to precisely define vaccine efficacy because effectiveness has varied widely with the study methods employed, it is clear that universal immunization with whole-cell vaccine has had dramatic results.

The major problem with pertussis immunization has been the frequent vaccine-related side effects. The current whole-cell vaccine, developed in the 1930s, is composed of inactivated whole *B. pertussis* organisms, a relatively crude preparation by today's standards. Whole-cell pertussis vaccine is combined with diphtheria and tetanus toxoids (DTP), but it is the pertussis component that is responsible for most of the side effects: pain, redness, and swelling at the injection site in more than 50%, fever ≥38°C (100.4°F) in more than 40%, fretfulness in more than 50%, and drowsiness in more than 30%. Although these reactions can be decreased by administering only half the recommended dose of DTP vaccine, this practice is not known to provide adequate immunity and therefore is not recommended. Prophylactic acetaminophen, 15 mg/kg/dose given every 4 hours for three doses while awake and then as needed according to the parent's discretion, will reduce the frequency of these common side effects. More severe but less common adverse reactions include: persistent, inconsolable screaming or crying in 1%, a distinctive high-pitched unusual cry in 0.1%, fever ≥40.5°C (104.9°F) in 0.3%, collapse with shocklike state in 0.6%, and convulsions (primarily benign febrile convulsions) in 0.6%. The evidence that pertussis vaccine causes these reactions is based on prospective studies of DTP and DT immunizations in infants (see also Chap. 14).

More controversial has been the association between pertussis vaccine and encephalopathy and the potential for permanent neurologic handicap that may follow. Despite the occurrence of neurologic illnesses that appear to begin following administration of pertussis vaccine, and the passionate claims of the parents of such children, the scientific evidence of a causal relationship is extremely weak. The only study with a control group that addressed this issue was the National Childhood Encephalopathy Study in Britain. This study did not demonstrate a distinct neurologic syndrome following pertussis immunization, and 95% of neurologic handicaps were not related temporally to pertussis vaccine. Thus, a causal relationship between pertussis vaccine and neurologic handicap was not established, and the study demonstrated that even *if* such a relationship does exist, it must be exceedingly rare. Most of the neurologic illness that is observed after pertussis immunization appears to result from underlying conditions unrelated to pertussis vaccine. Well-designed studies have also been unable to find a causal link between DTP immunization and the sudden infant death syndrome.

Nonetheless, tort claims for damages have been substantial and prompted the enactment of the National Childhood Vaccine Injury Act of 1986, which established a compensation program for infants and children who experience injuries temporally associated with vaccine administration. The program is expected to reduce claims against physicians for vaccine-associated injury.

Despite the lack of solid scientific evidence for a causal relationship between pertussis vaccine and neurologic injury, the physician may still be faced by parents and attorneys with beliefs to the contrary. The pediatrician can best deal with these situations with the following reminders: First, even if it is accepted that brain damage can result from pertussis vaccine, careful cost–benefit analyses demonstrate that the benefits of universal pertussis immunization greatly outweigh the costs of purported vaccine-related injury. Parents should be encouraged to have their infants and children immunized. Second, physicians should carefully follow the guidelines of the Committee on Infectious Diseases of the American Academy of Pediatrics and/or the Immunization Practices Advisory Committee (ACIP) of the U.S. Public Health Service, particularly with respect to contraindications to immunization with pertussis vaccine. Third, informed consent, careful record keeping, and a good doctor–parent relationship are further protection against litigation.

Use of pertussis vaccine is contraindicated in patients who experience any of the following reactions after a DTP immunization: encephalopathy within 7 days; a febrile or a febrile convulsion within 3 days; persistent, inconsolable crying for 3 hours or more, or a high-pitched unusual cry within 48 hours; hypotonic–hyporesponsive (collapse, shocklike) episodes within 48 hours; hyperpyrexia (≥40.5°C or 104.9°F) within 48 hours; or an immediate, severe allergic reaction. In addition, those with an evolving or poorly defined neurologic condition should have immunization deferred until the clinical course or etiology of the condition becomes clear. Physicians should then resume immunization if the benefits of immunization outweigh the risks.

The issue of neurologic damage and pertussis vaccine may never be resolved. It may, however, fade away if new acellular pertussis vaccines become licensed for primary vaccination and then completely replace the whole-cell pertussis vaccine. These vaccines produce fewer side effects than do whole-cell vaccines. At present, licensure of these vaccines appears to be awaiting convincing evidence that the new acellular vaccine(s) is also at least as effective as whole-cell vaccine as a primary vaccination for the prevention of pertussis.

ANNOTATED BIBLIOGRAPHY

Baraff LJ, Cody CL, Cherry JD: DTP-associated reactions: An analysis by injection site, manufacturer, prior reactions and dose. Pediatrics 73:31, 1984. (Detailed examination of DTP reactions.)

Bass JW: Pertussis: Current status of prevention and treatment. Pediatr Infect Dis J 4:614, 1985. (Good review of antimicrobial agents and other treatments for pertussis.)

Cody CL, Baraff LJ, Cherry JD, Marcy SM, Manclark CR: Nature and rates of adverse reactions associated with DTP and DT immunizations in infants and children. Pediatrics 68:350–360, 1981. (The classic paper on adverse reactions after DTP and DT immunizations.)

Committee on Infectious Diseases, American Academy of Pediatrics: Report of the Committee on Infectious Diseases: 1991. Elk Grove Village, IL, American Academy of Pediatrics, 1991. (Excellent resource for current immunization recommendations.)

Griffith AH: Permanent brain damage and pertussis vaccination: Is there an end in sight? Vaccine 7:199, 1989. (Full and interesting review of the tenuous relationship between pertussis vaccine and brain damage.)

Pertussis surveillance—United States, 1986–88. MMWR 39:57, 1990. (Recent data on the incidence of pertussis.)

Sotomayor J, Weiner LB, McMillan JA: Inaccurate diagnosis in infants with pertussis. Am J Dis Child 139:724, 1985. (Clinical presentation of pertussis in early infancy.)

202

Measles

Mark A. Ward

Measles is an acute febrile illness with exanthem and is associated with significant morbidity and occasionally mortality. It was once a universal disease of childhood, but routine immunization has reduced the incidence dramatically.

VIROLOGY/PATHOPHYSIOLOGY

The measles virus is a member of the family Paramyxoviridae, genus *Morbillivirus*. The primary site of infection is the respiratory epithelium. Local replication is followed by viremia. During this phase, virus is spread by leukocytes to the reticuloendothelial system. Following necrosis of white blood cells, a secondary viremia occurs. Infection of T lymphocytes with subsequent destruction may account for the depressed cell-mediated immunity observed in this disease.

With the development of specific antibody and cell-mediated responses, viremia is terminated and the illness resolves. These responses develop at the point in the illness when the rash appears. Although measles virus has been isolated from the rash in its early phase, some evidence indicates that the rash may be due primarily to a hypersensitivity phenomenon. Patients with impaired cell-mediated immunity may develop a severe pneumonitis in the absence of the exanthem.

EPIDEMIOLOGY

Prior to the introduction of vaccine, measles was an epidemic illness. Although peaks occurred each winter, some activity occurred year-round. It was estimated that 4 million individuals were infected each year in the United States, a number roughly equal to the total births for a year. Therefore, virtually all individuals had been infected by adulthood.

Subsequent to the introduction of vaccines in the 1960s, there was a dramatic decrease in the incidence of measles. In 1978, the Measles Elimination Program was announced with the aim of eliminating endemic measles by October 1, 1982. Unfortunately, this goal has proved more elusive than initially anticipated. In fact, there has been a significant rise in the incidence of measles in the past few years (over 27,000 confirmed cases in 1990). Despite this increase, the incidence is a small fraction of what it was in the prevaccination era.

The most recent United States outbreaks have been concentrated in two main population groups: unimmunized preschool children and immunized adolescents/young adults. This is in contrast to prevaccine days when most cases occurred in the early school years. Measles in very young infants is uncommon because of the protective effect of passively acquired maternal antibody. However, in recent outbreaks there has been an increased incidence of disease in infants aged 6 to 12 months.

CLINICAL PRESENTATION

The incubation period for measles is 10 to 14 days. During this time the patient remains asymptomatic. Following the incubation phase, a prodromal period occurs, lasting 3 to 5 days. It is at this time that the classic three "C's" of measles (cough, coryza, conjunctivitis) make their appearance. It is also at this time that patients are most contagious. The enanthem of measles occurs during the prodrome. These lesions are known as *Koplik's spots*, taking their name from the physician who originally described them. The lesions are small, bluish gray papules on a red base. They may be few in number or involve almost the entire oral mucosa. Koplik's spots usually disappear by the second day of the enxanthem. While virtually pathognomonic of measles, similar lesions have been described in association with enteroviral infections.

Following the prodrome, the exanthem begins. The initial lesions are noted on the forehead and face. They subsequently spread downward to involve the trunk and extremities. The rash consists of an erythematous maculopapular eruption; these are initially discrete lesions but tend to become confluent on the areas of initial involvement (i.e., face, upper trunk). Clearing begins on day 4 to 5 and progresses in the same fashion as the appearance of the rash. As the rash resolves, a fine brownish desquamation may occur.

In addition to the classical symptoms outlined above, measles may be associated with a number of other manifestations, both as a direct result of the virus infection and also as secondary complications. Acute laryngotracheitis (croup) may be seen and may be severe enough to require intubation for airway maintenance. Bronchiolitis with a clinical picture identical to that of respiratory syncytial virus may also be seen. Diarrhea, at times severe enough to cause dehydration, is common in infants. Encephalitis occurs in approximately 0.05% to 0.1% of reported measles cases. Giant-cell pneumonia may occur in patients with impaired cell-mediated immunity.

Measles may also be associated with a number of secondary complications. The most common of these is otitis media, which may be seen in up to 20% of cases. Pneumonia due to bacterial superinfection may also be seen. Gingivostomatitis due to reactivation of latent herpes simplex virus is also common. In patients with untreated tuberculosis, dissemination may result from intercurrent measles infection. Presumably, these manifestations result from impairment of immune function, at the level of both mucosal defenses and immune effector cells (especially T cells).

DIFFERENTIAL DIAGNOSIS

When measles presents in its typical form during an epidemic, recognition is easy. During the prodromal phase, the illness may be indistinguishable from other respiratory viral illnesses. With the appearance of Koplik's spots, however, the diagnosis becomes apparent. In the exanthem phase, the diagnosis is generally straightforward. The illnesses most likely to be confused with measles are Kawasaki syndrome and Stevens–Johnson syndrome. Other entities that are commonly considered in the differential diagnosis include infectious mononucleosis, roseola, adenovirus, enterovirus, Rocky Mountain spotted fever, and scarlet fever.

WORK-UP

The diagnosis is usually clinical, made on the basis of a compatible history and typical physical findings. The results of common laboratory tests are nonspecific and therefore not helpful in making the diagnosis. Although seldom necessary, confirmation of the clinical diagnosis can be made by viral culture or serology. Because viral isolation is technically difficult, confirmation of clinical diagnosis is usually made serologically. A number of different antibody tests are available; confirmation requires demonstration of a fourfold or greater rise in antibody titer or the presence of specific IgM antibodies.

MANAGEMENT

Treatment is supportive and includes adequate hydration and antipyretics as needed for fever. Although active in vitro against measles virus, ribavirin has not been thoroughly evaluated in patients with measles and is not recommended for routine use. Other currently available antiviral agents have no demonstrated beneficial role in this disease. Specific therapy is available for some of the secondary complications of measles (e.g., otitis media).

PREVENTION

Measles immunization has evolved since the early 1960s when the first killed vaccine became available. The current preparation is a live attenuated viral vaccine. It is routinely recommended for use at age 15 months in combination with mumps and rubella vaccines (MMR). Routine administra-

tion at age 12 months is recommended in high-risk areas. In communities experiencing a measles outbreak, the initial dose may be given as early as 6 months of age. An additional dose should be given at age 15 months if the initial dose is given before age 12 months. Recent outbreaks of measles have prompted recommendations for the routine administration of a second dose of vaccine either at age 4 to 6 years (Centers for Disease Control) or at 10 to 11 years of age (American Academy of Pediatrics). It is suggested that the second dose also be with the MMR vaccine, rather than the monovalent measles vaccine (see also Chap. 14, "Childhood Immunizations").

Postexposure prophylaxis with immune serum globulin (ISG) in a dose of 0.25 ml/kg (0.5 ml/kg in immunocompromised patients; in either instance, maximum dose 15 ml) may also prevent or modify disease. Concomitant administration of ISG and vaccine is contraindicated because ISG may inactivate the live vaccine. If ISG is given, active immunization should be delayed for 3 months.

ANNOTATED BIBLIOGRAPHY

Centers for Disease Control: Measles—United States, 1990. MMWR 40:369, 1991. (Summary of recent epidemiology of the disease.)

Cherry JD: Measles. In Feigin RD, Cherry JD (eds): Textbook of Pediatric Infectious Diseases, 2nd ed. Philadelphia, WB Saunders, 1987. (Detailed review of the disease and its manifestations; extensive references.)

Lennon JL, Black FL: Maternally derived measles immunity in era of vaccine-protected mothers. J Pediatr 5:671, 1986. (Documents lower levels of antibody in children born to mothers with vaccine-induced immunity compared with those born to mothers with disease-induced immunity.)

Peter G, Lepow ML, McCracken GH, Phillips CF (eds): Measles. In: Report of the Committee on Infectious Diseases (Red Book). Elk Grove Village, IL, Am Acad of Pediatrics, 1991. (Most recent recommendations regarding immunization and outbreak control.)

203

Mumps

Thomas G. DeWitt

Mumps is a highly contagious viral illness primarily affecting children and young adults. Parotitis is the principal presentation of this illness. The annual incidence of mumps in the United States has decreased from over 200,000 cases in 1967 to less than 6000 cases in 1989 since the introduction of a live attenuated virus vaccine. Sporadic outbreaks still occur, such as in 1987 when almost 13,000 cases were reported.

PATHOPHYSIOLOGY

The infectious agent in mumps is an RNA virus, *myxovirus parotiditis*. It belongs to a group of viruses that cause influenza, parainfluenza, and Newcastle disease. The mumps virus is pathogenic only in humans.

The virus is transmitted primarily through saliva, though it has been found in blood, urine, stool, and breast milk. Acquired through the respiratory tract, the virus proliferates locally and in regional lymph nodes. A viremia then occurs after an incubation period of 18 days (range, 14–25 days). During this viremia, the virus may be disseminated widely to an array of tissues, including salivary glands, pancreas, testes, ovaries, thyroid, breast, and meninges. The shedding of the virus in saliva tends to occur 2 to 3 days before, and persists for up to a week after, the onset of symptoms. After infection, antibodies develop to both the nucleoprotein core (soluble [S]) antigen and a hemagglutinin surface (viral [V]) antigen. An immunity to the disease correlates with the acquisition of antibody to the surface antigen and not to the core antigen. Both parainfluenza and Newcastle disease viruses can elicit antibodies that cross-react with the mumps virus.

CLINICAL PRESENTATION

General malaise, anorexia, and myalgia with a low-grade fever are the nonspecific prodromal symptoms of a mumps infection, followed, most commonly, by a high fever and parotitis. Other manifestations may include pancreatitis, oophoritis, orchitis, mastitis, myocarditis, meningoencephalitis, and cranial nerve involvement. These symptoms can occur singly, sequentially, or concurrently. One third of patients infected with mumps virus show no clinical symptoms.

The parotitis often presents initially as an earache with no tympanic membrane abnormalities. Parotid edema begins with erythema and tenderness above the angle of the mandible within 1 or 2 days of the onset of the earache. Edema increases over several days and then persists for ~1 week. Swelling may progress to above the eye, to the mastoid area, or to the chin and anterior neck. Typically, the edema obliterates the angle of the mandible, making palpation of it difficult, and it may also cause an upturning of the earlobe. An examination of the buccal mucosa often reveals erythematous and edematous orifices of Wharton's and Stensen's ducts. In approximately three quarters of the patients, the parotid edema is bilateral, with the involvement of one gland tending to precede that of the contralateral gland by 1 to 5 days. Concurrent with the increasing parotid involvement is an increase in fever, which may be as high as 40°C. The temperature subsides with the reduction in size of the glands.

When parotitis is the initial presentation of mumps and if other focal manifestations develop, they tend to occur 1 week or more after the onset of parotid edema. Although

rare in prepubertal males, orchitis may occur in as many as 30% of postpubertal males. In 25% of these affected males, the orchitis is bilateral. Symptoms include testicular edema and tenderness, nausea, vomiting, and fever. A testicle may increase to four times its normal size. Although the extreme pain tends to subside in a few days, the edema and tenderness may last for weeks. Mild atrophy of one testis may develop in many cases, but sterility is uncommon.

As with orchitis, oophoritis is found primarily in postpubertal patients. The incidence, however, is ~5%, and the clinical presentation often mimics that of an acute abdomen. Although mastitis is rare in prepubertal females, it has been described in as many as one third of postpubertal females.

One of the more significant manifestations of mumps is meningoencephalitis. White blood cells are found in the spinal fluid of over half the patients infected with mumps. Most patients, however, have subclinical involvement. Unlike many of the other manifestations of mumps, the meningoencephalitis commonly presents (25%–50%) without an associated parotitis. Males are affected more commonly than females by 3:1. If the principal manifestation is meningitis, the patient presents with the symptoms of fever, headache, nausea, vomiting, and nuchal rigidity. In mumps encephalitis, the patient may present with convulsions, focal neurologic signs, movement disorders, or marked changes in sensorium. One may occasionally find symptoms of muscular weakness and a loss of reflexes, indicating myelin involvement.

Unilateral deafness occurs in a small percentage of mumps cases. The onset may be sudden or gradual, and the hearing loss tends to be complete and permanent.

Mumps may affect other organs and glandular tissues. Pancreatitis may be a manifestation presenting with upper abdominal pain and tenderness in the epigastrium. The incidence of subclinical pancreatitis may be as high as 5%. Myocarditis and pericarditis occur primarily in adults, presenting with ECG changes consistent with a prolonged atrioventricular conduction time. Joint, thyroid, renal, and prostate involvement may also occur.

DIFFERENTIAL DIAGNOSIS

Because most patients presenting with mumps have parotitis, the differential diagnosis must focus principally on other causes of parotid swelling. However, because the mumps virus may infect many glandular tissues, the general considerations that follow also pertain to other glandular involvement.

The most common causes of parotid swelling other than the mumps virus are infections. The viral agents, parainfluenza types 1 and 3, coxsackievirus A, Epstein–Barr virus (EBV), cytomegalovirus (CMV), and echovirus, may all cause parotitis. *Suppurative parotitis,* most often caused by staphylococcus, pneumococcus, or gram-negative bacilli, should be strongly considered when the patient presents with systemic toxicity. The expression of purulent material from Stensen's duct may help delineate this condition.

Noninfectious causes of parotid enlargement include obstruction, tumors (particularly lymphocytic), congenital or acquired cysts, and drugs such as iodides and phenothiazines. Malnutrition, or rapid refeeding after malnutrition, can be associated with enlarged parotid glands. Pneumoparotitis may occur in a child blowing up balloons or learning to play a musical instrument such as the trumpet.

Several systemic diseases can cause parotic enlargement, including diabetes mellitus, obesity, and cystic fibrosis. Parotid involvement, however, is an uncommon presentation in these conditions.

Other conditions in the area of the angle of the mandible may, on superficial examination, resemble parotitis. The most common one in children is cervical lymphadenitis. Typical and atypical mycobacteria, as well as cat-scratch fever, may affect preauricular nodes. Dental abscesses and severe otitis externa should also be considered. In the small child, infantile cortical hyperostosis (Caffey's disease) and a branchial cleft cyst may resemble parotitis.

WORK-UP

History

The most important history to obtain in a child who has parotid swelling or encephalitis is that of prior exposure to, or previous vaccination for, mumps. With an average incubation period of 18 days, exposure to a person with symptoms suggestive of mumps 2 to 3 weeks prior to the onset of the patient's symptoms may also be helpful. It is important to remember that although parotitis is the most common presenting symptom of mumps, other manifestations, such as pancreatitis, encephalitis, and orchitis, can occur without parotid involvement. Because the live attenuated virus vaccine is about 95% effective, a history of previous mumps vaccination would greatly decrease the likelihood of mumps virus as an etiology. However, a small percentage of patients can have mumps despite previous vaccination, and illnesses suggestive of recurrent mumps have been reported.

Physical Examination

In the child with suspected mumps, the physical examination should determine whether the child actually has parotitis, whether he or she has other tissue involvement, or whether he or she has abnormal neurologic signs.

The area of the parotid gland should be palpated to determine if the edema obliterates the angle of the mandible. An examination of Stensen's and Wharton's ducts for inflammation may help to confirm the diagnosis of parotitis. The neck should be palpated for thyroid enlargement and tenderness, and the abdomen for epigastric tenderness. In women, particularly postpubertal, the breasts and lower abdomen should be examined for evidence of mastitis and oophoritis. Likewise in postpubertal males, the testes should be examined. However, it should be remembered that involvement of these and other glands may occur 1 week or more after parotid involvement. Patients should be assessed neurologically for signs of meningeal irritation, sensory changes, or weakness.

Laboratory Tests

Because mumps is primarily a clinical diagnosis, laboratory tests are usually not helpful. Serum amylase may aid in differentiating between parotitis and other diseases that mimic it but will not confirm a diagnosis of mumps. Most laboratories are also not equipped to differentiate between parotid and pancreatic amylase. The presence of antibodies to the nucleoprotein core (S) antigen indicates a current or recent mumps infection, whereas the presence of antibodies to the hemagglutinin surface (V) antigen indicates a past history of mumps infection. These antibody assays are not readily available and are probably not indicated unless there are compelling epidemiologic or diagnostic reasons. A lumbar puncture is necessary in a patient with "hard" neurologic findings. The presence of only headache or photophobia makes the need for a lumbar puncture more of a clinical judgment. Other laboratory tests are indicated only if they may rule in, or out, other diseases mentioned in the differential diagnosis. In particular, an elevated white blood count with a left shift may be helpful in identifying suppurative parotitis.

TREATMENT AND MANAGEMENT

The optimal treatment is prevention, which is accomplished by the use of a live attenuated virus vaccine. Given intramuscularly to children older than 12 months of age, it provides an adequate immune response in over 95% of patients. Children younger than 1 year who receive the vaccine may have a poorer response because of the presence of maternal antibodies.

Because no mumps antiviral agent is available, the treatment of patients with mumps is symptomatic. Analgesics and antipyretics are helpful. Steroids and antibiotics have not been shown to be efficacious. Many state health departments require that mumps be reported as a communicable disease.

In cases of meningitis or meningoencephalitis, supportive therapy is again indicated, with particular attention to the complications of cerebral edema and seizures. The use of steroids does not seem to alter the course of these conditions, including the development of deafness.

INDICATIONS FOR REFERRAL OR ADMISSION

In the patient with mumps, the principal indications for referral or admission are significant neurologic involvement and metabolic derangements due primarily to nausea and vomiting. Most patients with mumps, regardless of the site of involvement, have a self-limited disease that with good supportive care and close follow-up resolves spontaneously without a need for hospitalization.

In the child or adolescent who has had mumps, the physician should be aware of some potential long-term effects. Deafness has been described in patients with mumps and may occur without meningitis or encephalitis. A follow-up hearing screen should be done on patients who have had mumps. In addition, although the association has not been clearly defined, there is some suggestion that diabetes mellitus may be associated with a previous mumps infection.

ANNOTATED BIBLIOGRAPHY

Brunell PA: Mumps. In Feigin RD, Cherry JD: Textbook of Pediatric Infectious Disease, 2nd ed, pp 1628–1632. Philadelphia, WB Saunders, 1987. (Comprehensive review of mumps with an extensive list of references.)

Centers for Disease Control: Mumps—United States, 1985–1988. United States Department of Health and Human Services. MMWR 38:101–105, 1989. (Good epidemiologic information with a focus on mumps vaccine and immunization.)

Jones GF, Ray CG, Fulginitti VA: Perinatal mumps infection. J Pediatr 96:912, 1980. (Good, brief review of perinatal mumps.)

Marcy SM, Kibrick S: Mumps. In Hoeprich PD: Infectious Diseases, pp 621–627. New York, Harper & Row, 1977. (Excellent listing of differential diagnoses.)

McDonald JC, Moore DL, Quennec P: Clinical and epidemiologic features of mumps meningoencephalitis and possible vaccine-related disease. Pediatr Infect Dis J 8:751–755, 1989. (Presents the spectrum of clinical presentation of mumps meningoencephalitis.)

204

Chickenpox

Janet L. Schwaner

Chickenpox (varicella) is a common, usually mild childhood disease caused by the varicella-zoster virus. The disease is highly contagious, and infection confers lifetime immunity; more than 90% of adults are immune. Adults and immunocompromised patients who develop chickenpox are more likely than normal children to develop severe disease or complications. After the disease subsides, the virus may remain dormant for decades and may then reappear as herpes zoster, a unilateral varicella-like eruption in the distribution of one to three sensory nerves of dorsal root ganglia or cranial nerve extramedullary ganglia.

CLINICAL PRESENTATION

The incubation period ranges from 10 to 21 days; most cases occur 14 to 17 days after exposure. The contagious period extends from 1 to 2 days before the rash erupts until all of the lesions have crusted. Chickenpox is spread person-to-person by direct contact or by the respiratory route. The prodrome, which may be mild or absent in young children but tends to be more severe in adolescents and adults, consists of 1 to 2 days of fever, headache, malaise, and anorexia.

The rash, often pruritic, begins as a macule and progresses rapidly through the stages of papule, vesicle, and crusted lesion. The spots first appear on the face or trunk and, at the height of the illness, are more numerous centrally than distally. The lesions erupt in crops for 3 to 4 days, and it is characteristic of the rash that lesions in different stages of development may be found in one area.

The vesicle is a 2- to 3-mm oval filled with clear fluid surrounded by an erythematous base. The fluid clouds and a crust forms within 1 day. Lesions occurring on the mucous membranes do not crust but form a shallow ulcer. Scars are unusual except at the site of secondary infections and where scabs have been pulled off rather than allowed to fall off. Inflamed skin such as the diaper area may have more lesions than other areas, and these lesions are more likely to be in the same stage of development.

The *congenital varicella syndrome* may develop in babies whose mothers have clinical varicella before 29 weeks' gestation. The percentage of such women who deliver affected babies is unknown. This rare and devastating syndrome includes hypotrophic limbs, cicatricial skin scarring, eye abnormalities, and severe psychomotor and growth retardation.

Maternal varicella 4 days or less before delivery may result in severe disseminated or fatal chickenpox in the newborn. Twenty percent of babies in these circumstances will develop varicella; death occurs in up to 30% to 35% of affected newborns. The development of neonatal chickenpox is probably related to the absence of maternal antibody. Varicella-zoster immune globulin (VZIG) may modify the course of newborns whose mothers develop chickenpox during the critical period. Infected newborns should be treated with acyclovir, 30 mg/kg/day for 7 to 10 days (see also Chap. 196).

COMPLICATIONS

Secondary bacterial infection of lesions, most often with staphylococci or β-hemolytic group A streptococci, is the most common complication. Systemic antibiotics may be necessary for infections, such as cellulitis, that do not respond to local care. Bullous varicella, which occurs usually in children under 2 years of age, is caused by phage group II toxigenic *Staphylococcus aureus* and is self-limited. Primary varicella pneumonia is uncommon in healthy children but affects immunocompromised patients and up to 35% of normal adults. The disease varies from mild to severe and may be fatal.

Encephalitis follows varicella in fewer than 1:1000

cases. The involvement of the cerebellum alone has an excellent prognosis, whereas cerebral involvement manifested as change in sensorium, convulsions, stupor, coma, or paralysis may result in permanent brain damage or death. Less common neurologic complications include Guillain–Barré syndrome, transverse myelitis, optic neuritis, and facial nerve palsy.

Along with influenza, chickenpox is one of the most common antecedents of Reye syndrome. Salicylate use in varicella has been associated with the development of Reye syndrome, and patients should be cautioned not to use it.

Idiopathic thrombocytopenic purpura, purpura fulminans, nephritis, appendicitis, gastritis, gangrene, myocarditis, and arthritis are rare complications.

DIFFERENTIAL DIAGNOSIS

Formerly, it was important to distinguish chickenpox from smallpox. The differentiation has been unnecessary since the eradication of smallpox in the 1970s. Early impetigo is vesicular and may be pruritic, but the rash is not widespread and has a predilection for the nasolabial area. Insect bites are papular and itchy but do not occur in crops; they are not vesicular; and they have no systemic symptoms. Scabies is often accompanied by burrows between the fingers or toes. Urticarial lesions are usually large and short-lived, and they do not develop vesicles. Patients who have eczema herpeticum have a history of eczema. The distribution of lesions is similar to that of the eczema, and the patients often appear toxic.

WORK-UP

Chickenpox is usually easy to diagnose, and laboratory tests are rarely needed. A mild leukocytosis may occur. Vesicle scrapings contain multinucleated giant cells, and vesicular fluid contains virus in the first several days of illness. The scabs do not contain virus. Virus grows in a number of human tissue culture cell lines. Acute and convalescent complement fixation titers confirm varicella-zoster virus infection.

TREATMENT AND MANAGEMENT

In most cases, only symptomatic treatment is necessary. Calamine lotion or a skin moisturizer containing menthol (e.g., Sarna) is helpful for pruritus, as are baths of pulverized oatmeal. More severe pruritus may respond to oral antihistamines such as diphenhydramine and hydroxyzine. The patient's fingernails should be cut short and the skin kept clean to prevent secondary infection from scratching. Acetaminophen is the preferred drug for fever control. Aspirin should *not* be used in children and adolescents because of its association in chickenpox and influenza with the development of Reye syndrome.

Oral acyclovir is safe and results in modest clinical benefit if begun at the onset of illness. On average, chickenpox may be expected to resolve one day earlier with acyclovir. But because of its limited efficacy, cost, and requirement that it be started early in the illness (which may result in undesirable office visits for case confirmation, or in unnecessary use if the diagnosis is incorrect), the routine use of oral acyclovir in uncomplicated cases of chickenpox is *not* recommended. However, the prescribing of oral acyclovir should be left to the discretion of the physician, since a variety of circumstances may or would justify its use. These include: immunocompromised children; children with chronic illnesses in whom varicella might have exaggerated untoward effects; a second child in whom the illness would be expected to be more severe; and parents for whom every day of work missed would be a burden.

Because of their potential seriousness, varicella infections in immunocompromised patients require more vigorous treatment, which usually occurs in the hospital. VZIG given as prophylaxis within 72 hours of exposure can attenuate the disease. Acyclovir (1500 mg/sq/m/day for 7 days in patients under 12 years of age; and 30 mg/kg/day for 7 days in adults) is the preferred drug for high-risk patients who develop varicella. Vidarabine is less effective and more toxic. Antiviral therapy is not required for high-risk patients who have received active or passive immunization and subsequently develop the disease, unless they are severely affected. VZIG is recommended for newborns whose mothers develop chickenpox between 5 days before and 2 days after delivery. The dose is 1.25 units/10 kg body weight; the minimum dose is 125 units and the maximum dose 625 units.

A live attenuated varicella vaccine has been developed and is undergoing clinical trials. It has been useful in preventing chickenpox in immunocompromised patients, but in recent trials some vaccine lots caused full-blown chickenpox in immunocompromised children. The vaccine has been reformulated, and trials have resumed. Questions about long-term persistence of antibody response and later development of herpes zoster in vaccinated individuals will not be answered for decades.

INDICATIONS FOR REFERRAL OR ADMISSION

Health care professionals can usually help the child's caregivers manage chickenpox with telephone contact alone. The patient should be evaluated in the office if he or she develops signs of bacterial infection, respiratory symptoms, central nervous system changes, or severe vomiting, or if he or she is immunocompromised. Patients requiring hospitalization include those with bacterial infections unresponsive to oral antibiotics, eczema herpeticum with systemic symptoms, severe respiratory disease, central nervous system signs, and Reye syndrome.

With eye involvement, it is prudent to have an ophthalmologic consultation within 24 to 36 hours to rule out infection of the cornea. A child with suspected keratitis (e.g., photophobia, tearing, or decreased vision) should be referred promptly. Herpetic corneal ulcerations constitute an emergency and usually require hospitalization.

ANNOTATED BIBLIOGRAPHY

Balfour H: Varicella zoster infections in immunocompromised hosts. Am J Med 85(Suppl 2A):68, 1988. (Thorough coverage of the topic.)

Brunell P: Varicella-zoster infections. In Feigin R, Cherry J: Textbook of Pediatric Infectious Diseases, 2nd ed, p 1602. Philadelphia, WB Saunders, 1987. (Concise, but thorough.)

Dunkle LM, Arvin AM, Whitley RJ et al: A controlled trial of acyclovir for chickenpox in normal children. N Engl J Med 325:1539–1544, 1991. (If begun early in the illness, acyclovir reduces the number of new lesions and the duration of the rash. Most authorities do not believe that this modest clinical benefit justifies the routine use of oral acyclovir.)

Fleisher G, Henry W, McSorley M et al: Life-threatening complications of varicella. Am J Dis Child 135:896, 1981. (Five years' experience in a large children's hospital.)

Gordon J: Chickenpox: An epidemiological review. Am J Med Sci 224:362, 1962. (The classic work; includes a section on history, beginning with the ninth century A.D.)

Hermann KL: Congenital and perinatal varicella. Clin Obstet Gynecol 25:605, 1982. (Clear presentation of a complicated topic.)

Starr S: Status of varicella vaccine for healthy children. Pediatrics 84:1097, 1989. (Contains a good explanation of the recent need for vaccine reformulation.)

Varicella-zoster infections. In Krugman S, Katz S, Gershon A, Wilfert C (eds): Infectious Diseases of Children. St. Louis, CV Mosby, Chap 33, p 433, 1985. (Complete; good diagrams and pictures.)

205

Influenza

Kenneth M. Boyer

Influenza is an acute respiratory infection caused by strains of the orthomyxoviruses. The first of the human respiratory viruses to be isolated and characterized, influenza viruses have also been studied the most extensively. Yet, despite great sophistication in our understanding of it as a disease, influenza continues to elude preventive measures. The pediatrician whose busy practice has been overwhelmed during an influenza epidemic is only too aware of this.

Influenza infections are seldom definitively proved by virus isolation in outpatient practice. Characteristic "influenzalike" illnesses with abrupt onset, fever, headache, myalgia, and respiratory symptoms are easily recognized, however. Influenza viruses are the most likely cause of such illnesses, although parainfluenza viruses, enteroviruses, and adenoviruses may also cause the syndrome.

MICROBIOLOGY AND PATHOPHYSIOLOGY

Influenza viruses are negative-strand RNA viruses of three major antigenic types—A, B, and C—and multiple antigenic subtypes. All have the property of hemagglutination and possess the enzyme neuraminidase. The World Health Organization system of nomenclature for influenza virus strains specifies type, host (for strains of animal origin), geographic source, strain number, and year of isolation, to which code designations of hemagglutinin and neuraminidase subtypes are appended. Thus, the original "Shope strain" of swine influenza virus is designated A/swine/Iowa/15/30 (H_{sw}N1); the 1989 epidemic influenza A strain is designated A/Beijing/353/89 (H3N2).

The biologic and antigenic diversity of influenza viruses is attributable partly to their unique, segmented RNA genome. Variation in hemagglutinin and neuraminidase specificity is the basis for antigenic *drift* and *shift* in prevalent viruses. Drift implies a minor change in either antigen, without a change in subtype; shift implies a major change in either or both antigens, with a change in subtype.

To establish infection, influenza viruses must penetrate the mucous blanket lining the respiratory tract and escape inactivation by nonspecific inhibitors as well as by specific local antibodies. The major site of infection is the ciliated columnar epithelial cell. Influenza pneumonia may occur as a result of primary viral infection, bacterial superinfection, or combined bacterial–viral infection. Diffuse encephalopathy and fatty degeneration of the liver (Reye syndrome) has been established as a potential complication of influenza, particularly type B, in children. It is now clear that the use of aspirin during the acute infection is a major cofactor in the pathogenesis of this syndrome.

Immunity against influenza results from a complex interplay of humoral, secretory, and cell-mediated mechanisms. Because of the brief incubation period of the disease, anamnestic stimulation of antibody affords little protection. Thus, some degree of preexisting antibody appears to be essential to prevent infection. The sequential antigenic changes that occur in the virus in the course of antigenic drift afford each new variant a selective advantage in establishing infection; the major antigenic changes that accompany antigenic shifts render larger populations susceptible and account for pandemic spread.

EPIDEMIOLOGY

Outbreaks of influenza may be localized, nationwide, or global; sporadic cases rarely occur. On the whole, other agents (e.g., respiratory syncytial virus, parainfluenza viruses, and *Mycoplasma pneumoniae*) account for most serious respiratory illnesses in childhood. During periods of epidemic or pandemic spread, however, respiratory infections by influenza viruses may exceed all other etiologies. In the peak month of a composite of 11 consecutive influenza A virus outbreaks observed in Washington, DC, influenza A virus was isolated from 68% of croup patients and 36% of all hospitalized children with respiratory disease.

Influenza infections have marked seasonality. In temperate climates, epidemics occur almost exclusively in winter months. Off-season infections are documented infrequently. Droplet spread, with inhalation of large airborne particles produced by coughing and sneezing, is generally accepted as the most common mode of natural influenza transmission. Once infection is established, peak virus shedding coincides with clinical symptoms. Virus may be recovered for 1 day prior to the onset of symptoms and for a variable period, usually less than 6 days, afterward. The incubation period of influenza ranges from 1 to 7 days but is commonly 2 to 3 days. This brief incubation period, coupled with the large amount of infectious virus in secretions and the relatively small amounts necessary for infection of susceptibles, accounts for the sharpness of influenza outbreaks.

CLINICAL PRESENTATION

Disease due to epidemic influenza A virus is unique in that persons of all ages in a population become ill with febrile respiratory complaints. In contrast, whereas other noninfluenzal respiratory viral agents may also cause community epidemics that involve both children and adults, the illness is different in the two age groups. Young children with primary viral infections with noninfluenzal agents have febrile illnesses. Older children and adults with similar infections most commonly have common colds and other upper respiratory involvement with no or minimal fever.

The symptoms and signs of "classic" influenza in older children and adolescents include abrupt onset, with fever and associated flushed face, chills, headache, myalgia, and malaise. The temperature range is from 39°C to 41°C (102°F–106°F), with a general inverse correlation with age. Systemic symptoms are generally more severe in the older patient. Although a dry cough and coryza are also early manifestations of influenza, these symptoms may go unobserved by the patients because of the severity of the systemic manifestations. A sore throat occurs in over half the cases and is usually associated with nonexudative pharyngitis. Ocular symptoms include tearing, photophobia, burning, and pain with eye movement (ophthalmodynia).

In uncomplicated illness, the fever usually persists for 2 to 3 days but may last up to 5 days. A biphasic temperature pattern may occur even without apparent secondary bacterial complications. By the second to the fourth days, respiratory symptoms become more prominent, and the systemic complaints begin to subside. The cough is dry and hacking and usually persists for 4 to 7 days; occasionally a cough, in association with some degree of general malaise, will persist for 1 to 2 weeks or longer after the rest of the illness has subsided.

In younger children, the manifestations of influenza viral infections are frequently similar to those resulting from other respiratory viruses. Laryngotracheitis, bronchitis, bronchiolitis, pneumonia, and the common cold all occur. Primary infection with influenza A in these age categories is typically seen as an undifferentiated febrile upper respiratory illness. Fever tends to be high and will exceed 39.5°C (103°F) in most patients. Affected children appear moderately toxic, with clear nasal discharge, cough, and irritability as almost constant findings. Pharyngitis is usually present, with diffuse erythema and boggy, enlarged tonsillar tissue. Between 5% and 10% of those infected will have some degree of pulmonary involvement; in hospitalized children, this percentage may be as high as 50%. Gastrointestinal symptoms have been noted in several studies of influenza infection in young children. Febrile convulsions, precipitated by fever of abrupt onset, have also been cited as common presenting complaints in several studies. Acute laryngotracheitis (croup) has been noted as a prominent feature of influenza A. Illness tends to be more severe than that in the croup syndrome induced by parainfluenza viruses. An increased severity of influenza should be anticipated in children with preexisting cardiac, pulmonary, and neuromuscular disease.

DIFFERENTIAL DIAGNOSIS

The differential diagnosis of influenza includes an extensive list of febrile conditions, most commonly caused by other respiratory viruses and group A streptococci. In common pediatric practice, influenza and other common respiratory viral illnesses are often grouped casually as viral URI. A definitive diagnosis of influenza in even a few children greatly increases the likelihood that other pediatric respiratory illnesses are caused by the same agent and may be useful in forecasting the development of serious influenzal infections in high-risk patients within a practice or community.

WORK-UP

Routine laboratory studies provide little help in the differentiation of influenza from other viral respiratory diseases. Hematologic manifestations are variable, with marked leukocytosis frequently observed in infants. Chest radiographs are useful primarily to determine the presence of complicating interstitial or lobar pneumonia.

A definite diagnosis of influenza depends on either virus identification in respiratory secretions or a significant rise in serum antibody during convalescence. In contrast to shedding of adenoviruses or herpes simplex from the respiratory tract, asymptomatic carriage of influenza viruses is rare. Thus, identification of virus by culture, immunofluorescence, or ELISA is considered conclusive evidence for an etiologic role in an illness. Serologic diagnosis may be accomplished with the use of complement fixation, hemagglutination-inhibition, or indirect immunofluorescence techniques, but it is not useful unless sera are paired.

TREATMENT

Symptomatic treatment is the cornerstone of management. Bed rest, adequate hydration with oral fluids, control of fever and myalgia with acetaminophen or ibuprofen, and maintenance of comfortable breathing by means of nasal decongestants and humidified air suffice in most cases. Prophylactic administration of antibiotics should be discouraged. A persistent irritative cough during convalescence can often be relieved with dextromethorphan or codeine.

Complicated illnesses demand the physician's clinical judgment in the use of other therapeutic modalities. Bacterial infections, suggested by a prolonged febrile course or recrudescence of fever during early convalescence, should be identified with regard to site, and appropriate cultures should be obtained. Antibiotic therapy is then indicated and should be guided and modified by the results of cultures.

Inhalation therapy is an integral part of the management of illnesses complicated by airway compromise (croup), apneic spells, or diffuse pneumonia. Such patients should be hospitalized and monitored carefully. Humidified oxygen is an important element in the management of croup, but endotracheal intubation is required in a high percentage of patients with croup due to influenza. Racemic epinephrine and dexamethasone are both useful in patients with severe croup and may avert the need for intubation. Hospitalized patients with apnea or pneumonia may also require supplemental oxygen or (if indicated by oximetry or blood gas analysis) intubation and mechanical ventilation.

The antiviral agent amantadine hydrochloride is active in vitro against influenza A viruses and has been shown to provide prophylactic and therapeutic benefit in adults. Amantadine lacks activity against influenza B viruses. During a documented community epidemic of influenza A, however, amantadine may be used to treat infants and children who present with fever and croup, bronchiolitis, or pneumonia. The drug may also be used in unvaccinated patients in high-risk categories either prophylactically or at the onset of a febrile upper respiratory illness under similar epidemic circumstances. The dosage is 4 to 6 mg/kg/day orally in two divided doses for 5 days. Dosage should not exceed 150 mg/day in young children. Children older than 10 years can take a 100-mg tablet twice a day.

PREVENTION

Immunization is the best method for the prevention of influenza. Prediction of the nature of new influenza virus variants and their potential for epidemic spread is the major difficulty. Vaccines must contain antigens identical or similar to those of the potential infecting agent in order to be effective. In years when a new variant arises and causes widespread outbreaks, the available vaccine may contain a previous variant with only modest heterologous immunizing potential. Conversely, in years in which new variants do not arise, vaccines may be formulated ideally, but the epidemic potential of virus strains that already have circulated may be minimal. Depending on the degree of "fit" between vaccine antigens and circulating virus strains, the protective efficacy of influenza immunization ranges from 50% to 95%.

Only inactivated (formalin-treated) influenza vaccines are licensed for use in the United States. Several improvements have been made in these vaccines since their introduction in the late 1930s. These innovations have included enhanced vaccine production with the use of recombinant virus strains that grow rapidly in eggs, exclusion of host antigens and other toxic impurities by zonal ultracentrifugation (current *whole virus* vaccines), and disruption of viral particles with ether or detergents (current *split-product* vaccines). Split-product vaccines, by virtue of their minimal reactogenicity, are preferred for the vaccination of children. Reactions, when they occur, include mild fever, "flulike" symptoms of malaise and myalgia, and local tenderness at the site of inoculation.

Current recommendations for vaccination aim at protecting patients who are at highest risk of the life-threatening complications of influenza. This goal may be accomplished directly (by immunization of high-risk populations) as well as indirectly (by immunizing others who are most likely to transmit infection to those at high risk). Eligible high-risk patients include children ≥6 months of age with chronic pulmonary disease (e.g., bronchopulmonary dysplasia, asthma, cystic fibrosis, recurrent aspiration, or a history of extreme prematurity); hemodynamically significant heart disease; other chronic diseases requiring close medical follow-up or frequent hospitalization (e.g., diabetes mellitus, renal dysfunction, hemoglobinopathies, autoimmune disorders, or malignancy); and disorders requiring long-term aspirin therapy (e.g., juvenile rheumatoid arthritis or coronary aneurysms as sequelae of Kawasaki syndrome). Individuals who should be immunized in order to protect their contacts include medical personnel and the household members (including baby-sitters) of high-risk children.

Recommendations for influenza immunization include not only the concept of target groups but also the reminder that vaccine should be repeated on an annual basis in the fall months. First-time vaccinees less than 9 years of age need to receive two doses of vaccine separated by a 1-month interval in order to achieve an adequate primary immune response. Simultaneous administration of pneumococcal vaccine (although *not* annual revaccination) is appropriate for most children older than age 2 who are in high-risk categories.

ANNOTATED BIBLIOGRAPHY

Bryson YJ: The use of amantadine in children for prophylaxis and treatment of influenza A infections. Pediatr Infect Dis 1:44,

1982. (Clear summary of the available data on prophylactic and therapeutic use of amantadine, with prescribing guidelines for pediatricians.)

Centers for Disease Control: Prevention and control of influenza. Recommendations of the Immunization Practices Advisory Committee (ACIP). MMWR 40(RR-6), 1991. (Recommendations [updated annually] that are the definitive reference for American physicians using influenza vaccination.)

Couch RB, Kasel JA, Glezen WP et al: Influenza: Its control in persons and populations. J Infect Dis 153:431, 1986. (Review of the extensive surveillance studies of influenza infections and immunization conducted during the past decade by the Influenza Research Center in Houston.)

Hurwitz ES, Barrett MJ, Brogman D et al: Public Health Service Study on Reye's syndrome and medications. Report of the pilot phase. N Engl J Med 313:849, 1985. (Case-control study that provides the strongest evidence for the association of Reye syndrome and aspirin use.)

Jordan WS, Denny FS, Badger GF et al: A study of illness in a group of Cleveland families. XVII. The occurrence of Asian influenza. Am J Hyg 68:190, 1958. (Classic description of influenza A infections in the "Cleveland family study".)

Serwint JR, Miller RM, Korsch BM: Influenza type A and B infections in hospitalized pediatric patients. Who should be immunized? Am J Dis Child 145:623, 1991. (Eye-opening study of 99 children hospitalized at one hospital in 1988–89 for influenza; none of the 43 high-risk patients who experienced significant morbidity had received influenza vaccination!)

Wright PF, Ross KB, Thompson J et al: Influenza A infections in young children. Primary natural infection and protective efficacy of live-vaccine-induced or naturally acquired immunity. N Engl J Med 296:829, 1977. (Delineates the clinical features of influenza A in young children aged 6 weeks to 3 years.)

206

Lyme Disease

Kenneth M. Boyer

Lyme disease is a relatively uncommon tick-borne zoonosis caused by the spirochete *Borrelia burgdorferi.* It has protean manifestations. They are easily arrested with early treatment but can be debilitating and chronic if unrecognized and untreated. The description of this condition in the U.S. and the remarkable elucidation of its pathogenesis, diagnosis, and treatment—all within the past 15 years—have given it considerable public notoriety.

MICROBIOLOGY AND PATHOPHYSIOLOGY

The causative spirochete, *B. burgdorferi,* may be inoculated during the prolonged attachment of one of several vector tick species. Spirochetes proliferate locally in the skin and then, in the ensuing weeks, may spread systemically, giving rise to metastatic skin lesions and involvement of the synovium, myocardium, and central nervous system (CNS). Persistence of organisms in these remote sites and the host's immune response may give rise to late manifestations months to years after initial infection. These rough chronologic stages are termed early, early-disseminated, and late Lyme disease. Untreated, they bear a striking similarity to the pathogenetic evolution of another spirochetal disease, syphilis.

EPIDEMIOLOGY

Lyme disease is transmitted by ticks of the genus *Ixodes*— *I. dammini* (the deer tick) in the East and Upper Midwest, *I. pacificus* in the Far West, and *I. ricinus* in Europe. In the U.S., 94% of all reported cases come from nine states— New York, New Jersey, Connecticut, Pennsylvania, Rhode Island, Massachusetts, Wisconsin, Minnesota, and California. As adults, *Ixodes* are the size of a ball-point pen "clicker"; ticks in the larval and nymphal stages are smaller than a pinhead, and engorged adults may be as large as a split pea. The reservoirs of larval and nymphal ticks are small rodents such as mice and voles. Populations of adult ticks generally are maintained by feeding on deer.

Exposure to vector ticks is determined by their geography and ecology. The original description of the disease involved children whose homes were located in Old Lyme, Connecticut—a semi-rural area near Long Island Sound, contiguous to several state forests. Lyme disease is now known to be prevalent in both suburban and rural areas in endemic regions, with the population of deer bearing a rough correlation with incidence. Children may also be exposed to vector ticks for brief periods while on camping trips and vacations. An exposure history, compatible in both time and place, is extremely helpful in diagnosis.

CLINICAL PRESENTATION

After an incubation period ranging from 3 to 32 days, the characteristic skin lesion termed *erythema migrans* develops at the site of tick attachment. Inflammation spreads outward from a macular central lesion in an annular, geographic pattern with characteristic central clearing. Large lesions (more than 5 cm in diameter) are most specific for the diagnosis. After evolution of the initial lesion, similar but anatomically remote lesions may develop as a result of hematogenous spread. These lesions are generally smaller, often involve the malar region, and are more evanescent and pleomorphic. Concurrently, affected children usually have a subacute febrile illness with malaise, headache, mild neck stiffness, myalgia, and arthralgia.

The most characteristic early-disseminated manifestation of disease in untreated children is Lyme arthritis, which tends to attack large joints (especially the knees) asymmetrically. Episodes usually are brief and recurrent; in untreated cases they may evolve to chronicity. Other early-disseminated manifestations include unilateral or, more typically, bilateral Bell's palsy, aseptic meningitis (Bannwarth's syndrome), polyradiculoneuropathy, conjunctivitis, myocarditis, pericarditis, and heart block—most often a fluctuating atrioventricular block (first degree, Wenckebach, or complete). Manifestations of Lyme disease other than skin involvement may be presenting features in 20% to 40% of patients.

Few descriptions exist of late manifestations of untreated Lyme disease in pediatric patients. However, children with delayed initial treatment (delays ≥4 years) have been followed prospectively. During the 6 years of follow-up described in one study of 39 patients, 12 (31%) had brief, occasional attacks of joint pain; 2 (4%) had episodes of stromal keratitis; and 2 (4%) had a subtle encephalopathy associated with intrathecal production of specific antibody. No data exist on the degree of host resistance to reinfection in children who have been treated for Lyme disease. Recurrence and reinfection, therefore, remain difficult to distinguish.

DIFFERENTIAL DIAGNOSIS

Differential diagnosis depends on the presentation of the illness. Localized erythema migrans (pathognomonic if considered as a possibility) may be confused with erysipelas, erythema marginatum, or a local allergic reaction to an insect bite. Disseminated skin lesions may be similar in appearance to erythema multiforme, urticaria, and lupus erythematosus (with malar involvement).

Joint diseases that may be confused with Lyme arthritis include pauciarticular juvenile rheumatoid arthritis, lupus, ankylosing spondylitis, and a wide variety of reactive and postinfectious arthritides. Concomitant skin, joint, cardiac, and even neurologic abnormalities could be highly suggestive of acute rheumatic fever, but without evidence of antecedent streptococcal infection. Heart involvement may also resemble viral myocarditis or pericarditis. Conditions similar to the neurologic presentations of Lyme disease include enteroviral meningitis, leptospirosis, and the postinfectious radiculopathies.

In children with exposure to ticks, the other tick-borne conditions prevalent in the U.S., such as Rocky Mountain spotted fever, relapsing fever, tularemia, babesiosis, tick paralysis, and Colorado tick fever, should be considered.

WORK-UP

In a patient with an appropriate epidemiologic history, *erythema migrans is diagnostic of Lyme disease.* Spirochetes may be cultivated from a biopsy of the lesion with BSK (Barbour–Stoenner–Kelly) medium, but in most instances this is unnecessary. Serologic confirmation is difficult in cases that are diagnosed early because treatment may abort

Table 206-1.   Recommended Antimicrobial Therapy for Lyme Disease in Children

STAGE/SEVERITY AND MANIFESTATION OF DISEASE	AGE (YRS)	DRUG, DOSE, AND DURATION OF TREATMENT*
Early/Mild Erythema migrans	≥9	Doxycycline 100 mg/dose q12h × 10 days Tetracycline 250 mg/dose q6h × 10 days
	<9	Amoxicillin 50 mg/kg/day ÷ q8h × 10 days Penicillin V 50 mg/kg/day ÷ q6h × 10 days Erythromycin† 30 mg/kg/day ÷ q6h × 10 days
Early-Disseminated/Moderate Disseminated erythema migrans Acute arthritis Mild carditis Isolated Bell's palsy		Above oral regimens for 30 days
Late/Severe Chronic or recurrent arthritis Myocarditis, pericarditis, or complete heart block Meningitis or encephalitis		Ceftriaxone 100 mg/kg/dose q.d. × 21 days Penicillin G 300,000 U/kg/day ÷ q6h × 21 days

*In each category, regimens are listed in order of preference, based on efficacy and convenience of administration.

†Erythromycin is recommended for use only in young patients with clear-cut penicillin allergy.

the serologic response. Species identification of *Ixodes* ticks removed from children is useful to confirm a legitimate exposure; most pediatric infectious disease specialists have gained this skill in recent years.

In early-disseminated and late disease, serologic testing is required for diagnosis. Borderline "false-positive" tests are common and lead to much parental anxiety and unnecessary treatment. Indirect fluorescent antibody tests are most fraught with nonspecificity, primarily because of the subjectivity of end-point interpretation. The most reliable current test is enzyme-linked immunosorbent assay (ELISA). Confirmation of positive results with use of the immunoblot technique (Western blot) can be helpful, but specimens must be sent to a reference laboratory.

TREATMENT

Even before *B. burgdorferi* was identified as the cause of Lyme disease, antibiotic treatment with penicillin or tetracycline was shown to be associated with more rapid resolution of erythema migrans and prevention of late complications. Antibiotics currently recommended for use in children with Lyme disease include penicillin, amoxicillin, ceftriaxone, tetracycline, doxycycline, and erythromycin. All have proven efficacy at various stages of the disease, although the data supporting efficacy for erythromycin are weaker than those for the other drugs. The choice of drug and route is determined by patient age, stage and severity of disease at diagnosis, and history of penicillin allergy. Duration of treatment is determined by the stage and severity of disease at initiation of therapy. Clinical response, however, should also be taken into consideration. Recommendations for treatment are summarized in Table 206-1.

PREVENTION

Lyme disease is best prevented by avoiding its vectors. Tangled woods and high grass are most hospitable to ticks. Wearing trousers and long sleeves is helpful, as is the use of tick repellents containing DEET (N, N-diethyl-m-toluamide). However, in the peak seasons of tick activity (late spring and early summer) it may be difficult to get a child to wear protective clothing. A careful daily inspection for ticks at bath time is the most reliable measure for preventing Lyme disease.

For children who have been exposed to ticks, antimicrobial prophylaxis is often requested by parents. Decisions regarding this should take into account several facts: (1) Most ticks removed from children are *not Ixodes*. (2) Prolonged (>24 hours) attachment of infected *I. dammini* is required for infection of experimental animals. (3) Although there is regional variation, most *Ixodes* ticks are not infected with *B. burgdorferi*. (4) A controlled trial of penicillin prophylaxis in Connecticut (see bibliography) showed roughly equal (and low) risk versus benefit. These facts

should be communicated to parents. A short course of amoxicillin (50 mg/kg/day for 10 days) is the most innocuous approach when a significant exposure has been documented; indiscriminate use of prophylaxis should be discouraged.

ANNOTATED BIBLIOGRAPHY

Anderson JF, Duray PH, Magnarelli LA: *Borrelia burgdorferi* and *Ixodes dammini* prevalent in the greater Philadelphia area. J Infect Dis 161:811, 1990. (Describes the rapid development of an endemic focus of Lyme disease in Montgomery County, Pennsylvania.)

Barbour AG: The diagnosis of Lyme disease: Rewards and perils. Ann Intern Med 110:501, 1989. (Summary of the interpretation and misinterpretation of Lyme serologies.)

Burgdorfer W, Barbour AG, Hayes SF et al: Lyme disease—A tick-borne spirochetosis? Science 216:1317, 1982. (First description of the etiology and transmission of Lyme disease.)

Committee on Infectious Diseases (AAP): Treatment of Lyme borreliosis. Pediatrics 88:176, 1991. (Good, brief summary of preventive and therapeutic options.)

Costello CM, Steere AC, Pinkerton RE et al: A prospective study of tick bites in an endemic area for Lyme disease. J Infect Dis 159:136, 1989. (Among 56 patients with *I. dammini* tick bites, 27 received prophylactic penicillin and 29 a placebo; erythema migrans developed in 1 placebo recipient [4%], and an allergic reaction developed in 1 penicillin recipient [4%].)

Steere AC: Lyme disease. N Engl J Med 321:586, 1989. (Authoritative review of current knowledge.)

Steere AC, Malawista SE, Snydman DR et al: Lyme arthritis: An epidemic of oligoarticular arthritis in children and adults in three Connecticut communities. Arthritis Rheum 20:7, 1977. (The original description of Lyme disease.)

Szer IS, Taylor E, Steere AC: The long-term course of Lyme arthritis in children. N Engl J Med 325:159, 1991. (Long-term follow-up study of a group of children with Lyme arthritis who were diagnosed from 1976 to 1979, prior to the development of effective treatment.)

207

Cat-Scratch Disease

Hugh A. Carithers

Cat-scratch disease is an infection that has been recognized worldwide. It is associated with direct cat contact and has a benign course with a good prognosis in most patients. After obvious cutaneous infections and infections of the nose and throat, it is probably the next most common cause of unilateral regional adenitis in childhood. Complications and unusual manifestations sometimes make the diagnosis imperative, such as when a malignancy of the lymph nodes is considered.

PATHOPHYSIOLOGY

The cause of cat-scratch disease (CSD) is a pleomorphic, small, gram-negative bacillus. The organism causing CSD is thought to be transmitted directly or indirectly only by the domestic cat. In those few patients in whom cat contact is strongly denied, inoculation by an object with which the cat was in contact may have resulted in an infection. The organism causing the disease enters the body through a break in the skin, which rarely may be a bite or other injury caused by another animal.

Cats that transmit the disease are usually immature and not ill, and they have no distinctive features. The length of time in which they are capable of transmitting the disease is unknown. An older child or adult who denies cat contact may have had a brief encounter as long as 1 month prior to the recognition of lymphadenopathy.

Pathologists usually report findings as "compatible with" or "suggestive of" CSD because lymph node changes are not diagnostic. The basic pathology is the formation of a granuloma. There are three stages of change in lymph nodes: an enlargement with hypertrophy of the germinal centers and a thickening of the cortex; the formation of granulomas with invasion of lymphocytes and epithelial cells; and fusion of the granulomas with central necrosis and infiltration with neutrophils. All may be present simultaneously, but regression occurs usually before pus formation. Pus may be loculated.

CLINICAL PRESENTATION

About 3 to 5 days after an intimate exposure to a cat, usually immature, an inoculation site appears and progresses through stages similar to chickenpox lesions. First, a pink or red macule becomes papular and later forms a vesicle filled with sterile, opaque liquid. On breaking, a brief crust phase may be observed, which is much shorter than that of chickenpox. These changes, which usually last 1 to 3 days, often pass unnoticed, but the remaining papule, a few millimeters to 1 cm in diameter, may be present for weeks. A remaining macule may be observed for as long as 2 to 3 months.

In most patients, the illness is mild with generalized aching, malaise, anorexia, and rarely nausea and abdominal pain. About 40% of patients are afebrile. Only about 10% have temperatures above 102°F.

Although virtually all patients have lymphadenopathy, the extent of involvement and clinical course are highly variable. It may be concurrent with recognition of the papule, but because of the location or size of the lymph node, it may be undetected for 1 month or more. It may increase in size for several weeks and then regress over a period of 2 or more months. In approximately 12% of cases, the involved lymph node proceeds to suppuration.

Lymphadenopathy in CSD is usually single. When regional, usually only two nodes are enlarged; three nodes are

Table 207-1. Location of Lymphadenopathy Among 1200 Patients with Cat-Scratch Disease

LOCATION	NUMBER	PERCENT
Total upper extremity	610	46.1
Axillary	586	
Epitrochlear	24	
Total neck and jaw	340	26.1
Cervical	191	
Submandibular	149	
Total groin	228	17.5
Inguinal	143	
Femoral	85	
Preauricular	87	6.6
Postauricular	2	
Clavicular	31	2.3
Chest	4	

Note: The number of patients totals 1302; some had more than one location.

occasionally enlarged, and four or more are rarely enlarged. The location of involved lymph nodes among my first 1200 patients with CSD is shown in Table 207-1.

Generalized lymphadenopathy has been reported but is unlikely unless an immune deficiency is present.

An accurate measurement is essential at the initial examination to detect the progression or regression of lymphadenopathy. Because enlarged lymph nodes are sometimes ovoid rather than round, two planes, horizontal and vertical, should be measured. A convenient way to assure accuracy is the use of calipers. Those used in electrocardiographic interpretation are readily available.

The most unusual manifestation of CSD is the oculoglandular form (of Parinaud) that is manifested by a granuloma of the conjunctiva, preauricular lymphadenopathy, no purulent discharge from the eye, and a surprising lack of local discomfort. The prognosis is excellent. Recently, neuroretinitis has been recognized as a complication of CSD in variable locations of the United States. Other rarely encountered manifestations include erythema nodosum, thrombocytopenia, erythema marginatum, and an osteolytic lesion, which has been reported in only a few patients. Encephalopathy accompanying CSD is abrupt and severe in onset; convulsions are often the first sign. This form of encephalopathy has a better prognosis than most other types of encephalitis.

DIFFERENTIAL DIAGNOSIS

A helpful aid in the diagnosis of CSD is the *Rule of Five*, as shown in the display entitled "Diagnosis of Cat-Scratch Disease."

Some authorities believe that other causes of lymphadenopathy should be eliminated before making a diagnosis

Diagnosis of Cat-Scratch Disease: *The Rule of Five*

Lymphadenopathy, single (mostly) or regional (sometimes)	1.0
Intimate exposure to a cat (usually immature)	2.0
Inoculation site	2.0
Positive skin test	2.0

Note: Five points strongly suggest cat-scratch disease; seven points indicate a definite diagnosis.

of CSD. The differential diagnosis, however, is usually apparent. For example, infectious mononucleosis may begin as a single enlarged lymph node, almost always in the neck, but acute tonsillopharyngitis distinguishes it from CSD. The Kawasaki syndrome is characterized by lymphadenopathy, but confusion with CSD is highly unlikely because of its other features.

A mycobacterial infection causes more difficulty in differential diagnosis. Lymphadenopathy caused by *Mycobacterium tuberculosis,* which is usually regarded as a bilateral infection of the lymph nodes of the neck, can be diagnosed readily in most patients. On the other hand, with atypical mycobacteria, single-node lymphadenopathy in the neck is characteristic.

A malignant disease involving the lymph nodes may present as a single node or regional lymphadenitis. In children, especially, other nodes usually become involved quickly (see also Chap. 84, "Neck Masses," and Chap. 127, "Lymphadenopathy").

WORK-UP

The diagnosis of CSD presents little difficulty in most patients. All have lymphadenopathy, usually single, sometimes regional, and rarely bilateral; therefore, the diagnosis primarily depends on determining the cause of lymph node enlargement or excluding other causes of lymphadenopathy.

A history of handling a cat, usually an immature one that is not ill, is almost essential in the diagnosis. Finding the inoculation site may clinch the diagnosis. Locating the entry site of the organism that causes CSD is the most neglected feature in the examination. When it is not apparent, a history from the patient or his or her family will often reveal a lesion remembered as a "bump" or pimple at the time or just before lymphadenopathy was recognized.

Laboratory work is not helpful, although there may be an elevation of the white blood cell count and occasionally an eosinophilia. The sedimentation rate may be elevated, but not consistently.

Skin Test

The skin test need not be performed in most patients; however, it can be invaluable in complicated cases. When the physician is unwilling to observe a patient with lymphadenopathy, and to avoid embarking on a complicated diagnostic evaluation and treatment such as lymph node removal, the test can be the means of preventing unnecessary surgery and antibiotics. It may thus be argued that the benefit of the skin test, in preventing anguish among patients and their families with regard to the cause of undiagnosed lymphadenopathy, far outweighs its vague danger, as yet undiscovered or even defined.

The test uses a crude substance made from pus aspirated from a fluctuant node of a patient with the disease. If the test is applied more than 1 week after the enlargement of the involved node, all patients should have a positive result. There may be an occasional false-positive reaction, but I believe that many such patients have had an inapparent infection in childhood.

A reaction to the test in the form of a wheal may be immediate in a few patients. An anaphylactic reaction has not been reported.

TREATMENT

Treatment is usually symptomatic and is aimed at protection of the involved lymph node. Isolation of the patient is not indicated.

While controlled studies on the use of antibiotics in the treatment of CSD have never been made, there is recent evidence that the use of gentamicin has been highly effective in rarely seen systemic CSD. The causative organism may also be sensitive to third-generation cephalosporins and sulfa compounds. Because the disease is self-limited and rarely severe, antibiotic treatment is recommended only for the unusual patient who is severely ill. However, one recent retrospective study reported that trimethoprim-sulfamethoxazole effectively treated uncomplicated cases of CSD and prevented nodes from suppuration or drainage.

A limitation of activity is advised to prevent trauma to enlarged lymph nodes. Analgesics and bed rest are indicated for the minority of patients who have a fever. Normal activity may be continued by most patients during the weeks to a few months required for the complete regression of lymphadenopathy.

Aspiration is indicated in patients who have suppuration of lymph nodes. This should be done with a 16- or 18-gauge needle after ethyl chloride has been sprayed over the puncture site. The skin is usually too thin to permit the injection of a local anesthetic. Unless there is considerable pain, a delay of aspiration until suppuration is marked may prevent repeated aspiration.

Surgical removal of involved lymph nodes is not justified except rarely when diagnosis is in doubt and a delay might hinder the treatment of a malignancy. Moreover, an incision of suppurant lymph nodes is not recommended because aspiration is nearly always successful and is less likely to result in chronic drainage.

The patient and his or her family are almost always interested in the care of the involved cat. Because these animals are not ill and the length of time during which they may transmit disease is unknown, I do not recommend the removal of the cat.

ANNOTATED BIBLIOGRAPHY

Carithers HA: Cat scratch disease: An overview based on a study of 1,200 patients. Am J Dis Child 139:1124–1133, 1985. (Extended study.)

Carithers HA: Cat scratch disease associated with an osteolytic lesion. Am J Dis Child 137:968–970, 1983. (Describes in detail this unusual manifestation.)

Carithers HA: Oculoglandular disease of Parinaud, manifestations of cat scratch disease. Am J Dis Child 132:1195–1200, 1978. (Describes this most common unusual manifestation.)

Carithers HA: Treatment of cat scratch disease. In Gellis SS, Kagan BM: Current Pediatric Therapy, 13th ed. Philadelphia, WB Saunders, 1990. (Discusses use of antibiotics and other means of treatment.)

Carithers HS, Margileth AM: Cat scratch disease. Acute encephalopathy and other neurological manifestations. Am J Dis Child 145:98–101, 1991. (A review of all known cases.)

Collipp, PJ: Cat scratch disease: Therapy with trimethoprim-sulfamethoxazole. Am J Dis Child 146: 397–399, 1992. (In this uncontrolled series of 71 children with cat scratch disease, trimethoprim-sulfamethoxazole was quite effective. Of the 30 children who were treated with cephalosporins and other antibiotics, 7 had nodes that suppurated and drained, in contrast with none from the TMP–SMZ-treated group.)

Margileth AM: Cat scratch disease: Non-bacterial regional lymphadenitis. Pediatrics 42:803–818, 1968. (Excellent reference.)

Margileth AM, Wear DJ, Hadfield TL et al: Cat scratch disease: Bacteria in skin at primary inoculation site. JAMA 252:928–931, 1984. (Important advance in understanding the disease.)

208

Common Intestinal Parasites

Stephen J. Lerman

Because of increasing worldwide travel, immigration from tropical areas, and attendance by young children in day-care centers, pediatricians in the United States confront new trends in parasitic disease. This chapter deals with the four intestinal parasites that the pediatrician will most commonly encounter: *Giardia lamblia, Enterobius vermicularis, Trichuris trichiura, and Ascaris lumbricoides.* Common stool protozoa that are not pathogenic and therefore should not be treated are listed in Table 208-1.

GIARDIA LAMBLIA

This flagellated protozoan has emerged in recent years as the most common intestinal parasite in the United States.

For example, 14% of 916 children who had stool examinations at one large New England health maintenance organization (Harvard Community Health Plan) from August 1, 1990, to January 31, 1991, were positive for *Giardia lamblia.* This figure is higher than that for any other stool parasite. Infection can be transmitted by contaminated mountain streams, municipal water supplies, and food, and person-to-person by the direct fecal–oral route in day-care, institutional, household, and homosexual settings. Day-care centers appear to play an important role in maintaining endemic *Giardia* transmission in the community.

Pathophysiology

The active trophozoite form of *G. lamblia* resides in the upper part of the small intestine of man. Encystation occurs as liquid feces become dehydrated in transit down the colon. Excretion of cysts may continue for months or years. Cysts are resistant to the levels of chlorine usually used for municipal water purification. However, cysts can be killed by treating water with iodine or by boiling it.

The cyst is the infective stage of the parasite. When ingested, it excysts, and two trophozoites emerge that attach themselves to the surface of the small intestine and multiply there. Symptoms usually appear 1 to 3 weeks after infection, but the incubation period is sometimes longer.

Giardia may induce malabsorption either by damaging the microvillae of the small intestine or by adhering to the epithelial surface and interfering mechanically with absorption of nutrients.

Patients with decreased gastric acidity or secretory IgA deficiency have more severe infections.

Clinical Presentation

Diarrhea is the most frequent symptom. It may be acute and self-limited, protracted, or intermittent. Stools are usually loose and foul-smelling; sometimes they are watery or greasy. They rarely contain mucus or blood. Anorexia, abdominal cramps, bloating, flatulence, and weight loss are common. Children may also develop a severe spruelike syndrome with abdominal distention; malabsorption of fat, lactose, iron, folic acid, and vitamins A and B_{12}; and growth retardation. The concentration of IgE is normal, and eosinophilia is rare. As many as 76% of infected individuals are asymptomatic.

Differential Diagnosis

In the extensive differential diagnosis of infectious and noninfectious causes of diarrhea, features favoring giardiasis include an appropriate epidemiologic setting (e.g., day-care center), duration of greater than 1 week, and the smelly, greasy nature of the stools.

Table 208-1. Nonpathogenic Intestinal Protozoa

Blastocystis hominis
Chilomastix mesnili
Endolimax nana
Entamoeba coli
Entamoeba hartmanni
Iodoamoeba beutschlii
Trichomonas hominis

Diagnosis

At least three separate stools collected over the period of a week should be examined for *G. lamblia* cysts and trophozoites. The frequency of positive stool examinations in various studies ranges from 50% to over 90%. If giardiasis is still suspected after multiple negative stool examinations, duodenal contents should be sampled by intubation and aspiration, or through the use of a string that is coiled inside a weighted gelatin capsule (Entero-Test and Entero-Test Pediatric, H.D.C. Corporation, San Jose, CA). Biopsy of the small intestine may provide the only positive result in a small proportion of infected patients.

Management

The author recommends treatment not only of symptomatic but also of asymptomatic infection. Some authorities do not endorse treating asymptomatic infection. Effective therapy stops diarrhea in a few days in symptomatic patients and, in currently asymptomatic children, terminates prolonged cyst excretion, reducing the risk of spreading infection to others, and prevents the possible later appearance of symptoms. Quinacrine (Atabrine) is the drug of choice, and metronidazole (Flagyl) and furazolidone (Furoxone) are alternatives. None of the three agents, however, is ideal for the treatment of giardiasis in children.

Quinacrine is over 90% effective and inexpensive. The adult dose is 100 mg three times a day, and the pediatric dose is 6 mg/kg/day in three divided doses for 5 days. There are two impediments to the use of quinacrine in children: it is available only as an unscored tablet corresponding to the adult dose, and it is bitter-tasting. Some pharmacists may be willing to pulverize the tablets and dispense measured individual doses in glycine envelopes or in gelatin capsules. The bitter taste of quinacrine can be disguised by giving it with jam, honey, chocolate syrup, apple sauce, or ice cream.

Frequent side effects include dizziness, headache, vomiting, and diarrhea. Quinacrine is excreted into the urine, turning it deep yellow, and can be deposited in the skin, causing a yellowish discoloration that is fluorescent when exposed to ultraviolet light. This discoloration is noticeable in about 5% of children 1 to 2 weeks after initiation of therapy and persists for 2 weeks to 4 months. Quinacrine

can cause severe exacerbations in patients with psoriasis, transient toxic psychosis, and, rarely, exfoliative dermatitis. Prolonged high-dose therapy with quinacrine has caused rare instances of retinopathy, similar to that associated with chloroquine. Quinacrine is contraindicated in patients who are receiving primaquine for malaria prophylaxis because concurrent administration of the two drugs results in markedly elevated concentrations of primaquine and greatly enhances its toxicity.

Metronidazole, like quinacrine, is over 90% effective. However, it is more expensive than quinacrine. Although metronidazole is not approved for the treatment of giardiasis by the U.S. Food and Drug Administration, it is widely used for this indication. The commonly recommended dose is 250 mg three times a day for adults and 15 mg/kg/day in three divided doses for children for 5 days. It is supplied as an unscored tablet corresponding to the adult dose. However, a pharmacist can prepare a liquid suspension of metronidazole following directions available from the pharmaceutical company (G.D. Searle & Co.). Nausea, headache, and an unpleasant metallic taste in the mouth occur frequently. Less common adverse effects include vomiting, diarrhea, stomatitis, sensory neuropathy, dark urine, a disulfiramlike reaction with alcohol, and reversible neutropenia. Use during pregnancy is not recommended. In addition, there is concern about its carcinogenic potential, based on the occurrence of tumors in experimental animals fed metronidazole and mutagenesis in bacteria exposed to the urine of humans taking recommended doses of the drug.

Furazolidone is only about 80% effective and is the most expensive of the three drugs used for giardiasis. However, it has a major advantage for pediatric prescribing in that it is available as a flavored liquid (50 mg/15 ml) as well as a scored tablet (100 mg). The recommended adult dose of furazolidone is 100 mg four times a day and the pediatric dose is 6 mg/kg/day in four divided doses for 7 to 10 days. Nausea and vomiting are frequent adverse effects. Like metronidazole, furazolidone turns the urine dark and can cause a disulfiramlike reaction with alcohol. It also can cause red blood cell hemolysis and anemia in individuals with G6PD deficiency and in young infants. Furazolidone is a monoamine oxidase inhibitor, and caution is required when it is co-administered with other monoamine oxidase inhibitors, sympathomimetic amines, and tyramine-containing foods. Furazolidone caused tumors in experimental animals, raising concern about its carcinogenic potential.

ENTEROBIUS VERMICULARIS

Generally known as the pinworm because the tail of the adult female is pointed or pin-shaped, *Enterobius vermicularis* is the commonest parasitic nematode in the United States. Spread within families, day-care groups, and institutionalized populations occurs readily and without regard to socioeconomic status or level of hygiene.

Pathophysiology

Enterobius vermicularis is a white threadlike worm 1 cm in length that lives in the lumen of the colon and rectum. At night, the pregnant female lays her fertilized eggs on the perianal skin and dies. Pruritus results from an allergic response to the worm proteins. The eggs embryonate and become infective within a few hours. Scratching leads to direct anus–finger–mouth transmission with autoinfection and the opportunity for passage to others. In addition, the eggs survive on clothing, on bedding, and in house dust for about 2 weeks. The eggs hatch into larvae in the small intestine, and when they have matured, the adult worms migrate to the colon. The cycle from ingested egg to adult worm takes 4 to 6 weeks.

Clinical Presentation

The principal symptom is perianal itching, which can be intense and result in excoriation. In girls, an adult worm may occasionally move from the anal to the vaginal area and cause perivaginal itching. The majority of infected children, however, have no symptoms. *Enterobius vermicularis* is not a tissue parasite and is not associated with eosinophilia or elevated serum IgE levels.

Differential Diagnosis

The most common source of confusion is "pinworm neurosis," a fantasy of infestation leading to rectal itching that may develop in uninfected contacts of a case, or in patients who have been successfully treated.

Diagnosis

Pinworms can be seen with the naked eye, although they can easily be confused with bits of white thread or toilet paper. Diagnosis is usually made by pressing transparent adhesive tape (Scotch tape swab or pinworm paddle) repeatedly against the perianal skin immediately after the child wakes up in the morning, before the child bathes or defecates, and examining it microscopically for adherent eggs. A single test detects about 50% of infections, three tests detect 90%, and five tests detect 99%. Eggs are rarely seen in conventional stool examinations.

Management

The drug of choice is either pyrantel pamoate (Antiminth) or mebendazole (Vermox). A single dose of either agent cures over 90% of pinworm infections. To destroy worms that have hatched from eggs after the first treatment, a second dose is advised 2 weeks after the initial dose. Because of the high rate of infection in families and other close groups and the frequency with which infection is asymptom-atic, I recommend simultaneous treatment of all family or group members. Recurrence, frequently introduced from outside the family or group, is common and can be treated the same way as the original infection.

Pyrantel pamoate is supplied as an oral suspension (50 mg/ml) and can be given without regard to meals. The individual dose for both children and adults is 11 mg/kg body weight to a maximum of 1 g. This corresponds to a simplified dose regimen of 1 ml of pyrantel pamoate per 10 lb of body weight or 1 tsp per 50 lb of body weight to a maximum of 4 tsp. Although usually well tolerated, pyrantel pamoate can occasionally cause gastrointestinal disturbance, headache, dizziness, rash, or fever.

Mebendazole is supplied as a 100-mg tablet, and the individual dose, a single tablet, is the same for both children and adults because very little is systemically absorbed. This results in a clear-cut cost advantage for mebendazole in adolescents and adults, while a treatment course of pyrantel pamoate is less expensive for children. Diarrhea and abdominal pain are occasional side effects. Mebendazole should not be given to children less than 2 years of age or to pregnant women.

Parents need to understand that pinworm infestation is not due to a failure of personal cleanliness. Sheets, pajamas, and underclothes should be changed at the time of treatment and washed in hot water and detergent. Customary hygienic practices, such as washing hands after defecating and before eating or preparing food, should be observed. However, excessively stringent sanitary measures, such as sterilizing sheets and clothing, daily cleaning of each room in the house, twice-a-day showers, and frequent nail brushing, should be avoided; they are useless and only serve to heighten guilt and anxiety.

TRICHURIS TRICHIURA

Known as whipworm because of the whiplike shape of the adult worm, *Trichuris trichiura* is common in young children in the rural southeastern United States and among immigrants from the tropics where the infection rate may be as high as 80%.

Pathophysiology

The adult worms are 3 to 5 cm in length and live attached to the wall of the large intestine. The adult females produce several thousand eggs per day and live 1.5 to 2 years. Eggs leave the body in the feces and are deposited in soil, where they must embryonate before becoming infectious. Under favorable soil conditions of shade, warmth, and moisture, the eggs embryonate in 2 to 4 weeks. The embryonated eggs are picked up on the hands of young children who play in the contaminated soil, or they can be found on the surface of fruits and vegetables fertilized with human feces. When ingested, the infective eggs hatch in the upper duodenum;

the larvae mature in the small intestine and then migrate to the colon. Adult female worms begin to lay eggs about 90 days after the embryonated eggs are ingested.

Clinical Presentation

Most children with whipworm infection tolerate it without symptoms. Some have subtle periumbilical pain and mild diarrhea. In association with heavy worm burdens, children may have prolonged watery diarrhea with copious mucus, and sometimes blood, tenesmus, right lower quadrant tenderness, and occasionally rectal prolapse. Whipworm infection does not elicit eosinophilia.

Anemia is often found in children with whipworm infection, but these children often suffer from multiple parasitic infections (including hookworm) and malnutrition. The whipworm itself probably does not cause significant blood loss.

Differential Diagnosis

If severe or prolonged diarrhea occurs in association with whipworm infection, particularly if symptoms do not respond to therapy for trichuriasis, other bacterial or parasitic (e.g., *Entamoeba histolytica, G. lamblia*) causes should be sought.

Diagnosis

Characteristic eggs are readily identified in a stool sample. On sigmoidoscopic examination, adult worms can be seen attached to the wall of the colon.

Management

With the availability of safe and effective drug therapy for whipworm, even asymptomatic infections should be treated. Mebendazole (Vermox) 100 mg b.i.d. for 3 days in both children and adults is the treatment of choice. Its cure rate is 70% to 96%, and it reduces egg counts by 90% to 99%. As noted above, mebendazole causes occasional diarrhea and abdominal pain and should be avoided in children less than 2 years of age and in pregnant women.

ASCARIS LUMBRICOIDES

Ascaris lumbricoides is known as the giant intestinal roundworm because it can grow to a length of more than 30 cm. It is endemic among young children in some rural communities in the southeastern United States and is common among immigrants from tropical areas with poor sanitation and where human feces are used for fertilizer. An estimated one billion people have ascariasis worldwide; in some parts of Africa, 95% of the population is infected. Enormous egg output by the worms and resistance of the eggs to a variety of environmental conditions facilitate the spread of infection.

Pathophysiology

Ascaris lumbricoides lives in the upper small intestine. Each female produces approximately 200,000 eggs per day over a life span of about 1 year. The eggs are passed in the feces in an unembryonated, noninfective state. They can survive extreme cold and drying for a considerable period of time and are also resistant to chemical disinfectants. Under optimal conditions of warm, moist soil, eggs embryonate in about 3 weeks and can then remain infective for months. When embryonated eggs are ingested, either by the hands of young children who play in contaminated soil or on fecally contaminated fruits and vegetables, the larvae hatch, penetrate the wall of the small intestine, and pass through the circulation to the lungs. They break out of the blood vessels into the alveoli and pass up the trachea and are swallowed. When they reach the small intestine again, they develop into adult worms. The elapsed time from ingestion of eggs to production of eggs by adults is 2 months.

Clinical Presentation

Heavy *Ascaris* infections can aggravate nutritional deficiency. The worm secretes an antitrypsin and competes for proteins that the host ingests. Infection may also induce malabsorption of fats and carbohydrates.

The majority of people have no symptoms or only vague abdominal discomfort. They may become aware of infection only through stool examination for another reason, or when they pass a live worm in the stool or from the mouth or nose. During the intestinal phase of ascariasis, the eosinophil count is normal or only slightly elevated. In 2 cases per 1000 infected children, a tangled bolus of worms obstructs the lumen of the small intestine, causing vomiting, abdominal pain, and distention. Even less frequently, a worm obstructs the biliary tract, penetrates the liver, or perforates the intestine. Fever, certain drugs, or general anesthetic agents can excite adult worms and stimulate their migration.

During migration of larvae to the lung, with heavy infection, the highly allergenic antigens of *A. lumbricoides* can cause *Löffler's syndrome* (fever, respiratory symptoms, transient pulmonary infiltrates, and marked eosinophilia).

Differential Diagnosis

The dog and cat roundworms *Toxocara canis* and *Toxocara cati,* respectively, whose immature larvae migrate more widely in young children (liver, central nervous system, eye, and lung) than does *A. lumbricoides,* may cause Löffler's syndrome as one aspect of visceral larval migrans. The etiologic diagnosis of Löffler's syndrome requires serologic testing.

Diagnosis

Even with a light infection, there is no difficulty identifying eggs in stool samples because they have a distinctive appearance and are present in large numbers.

Management

Either pyrantel pamoate (Antiminth) or mebendazole (Vermox) is the drug of choice for uncomplicated intestinal infection, and both are highly effective. There is no specific drug therapy for the migrating larvae causing Löffler's syndrome. For intestinal obstruction, piperazine is the preferred drug, and most cases can be managed without surgery.

Pyrantel pamoate is given as a single dose of 11 mg/kg of body weight to a maximum of 1 g for both children and adults. It is supplied as an oral suspension (50 mg/ml), and this corresponds to a simplified dose regimen of 1 ml of pyrantel pamoate per 10 lb of body weight, or 1 tsp per 50 lb to a maximum of 4 tsp. Occasionally, pyrantel pamoate causes gastrointestinal disturbance, headache, dizziness, rash, or fever.

The dose of mebendazole is a single 100-mg tablet b.i.d. for 3 days for both children and adults. Compared to single-dose therapy with pyrantel pamoate, the longer course with mebendazole is a disadvantage in terms of both cost and convenience. Ascariasis and trichuriasis frequently coexist in the same patient, and with mebendazole, treatment can be directed at both infections. Occasional side effects include diarrhea and abdominal pain. Mebendazole should not be given to children less than 2 years of age or to pregnant women.

ANNOTATED BIBLIOGRAPHY

Bartlett AV, Moore M, Gary GW, Starko KM, Erben JJ, Meredith BA: Diarrheal illness among infants and toddlers in day care centers. I. Epidemiology and pathogens. II. Comparison with day care homes and households. J Pediatr 107(4):495, 503, 1985. (One of several studies showing the high rate of *Giardia* infection in toddlers in day-care centers, the frequency of asymptomatic infection, and the common occurrence of transmission to the child's family.)

Craft JC: *Giardia* and giardiasis in childhood. Pediatr Infect Dis 1(3):196, 1982. (Comprehensive review.)

Drugs for parasitic infections. Med Lett Drugs Ther 34(865):17, 1992. (Authoritative recommendations on drugs and doses.)

Katz M, Despommier DD, Gwadz R: Parasitic Diseases, 2nd ed. New York, Springer-Verlag, 1989. (Clinically oriented textbook with outstanding photographs and life-cycle drawings.)

Lerman SJ, Walker RA: Treatment of giardiasis. Literature review and recommendations. Clin Pediatr 21(7):409, 1982. (Critical evaluation of the three drugs used to treat giardiasis.)

Miller RA, Minshew BH: *Blastocystis hominis:* An organism in search of a disease. Rev Infect Dis 10(5):930, 1988. (Concludes that "*B. hominis* is rarely, if ever, a human pathogen, and treatment directed at the eradication of *B. hominis* is not indicated".)

Schantz PM, Glickman LT: Toxocaral visceral larva migrans. N Engl J Med 298(8):436, 1978. (Comprehensive review.)

Senay H, MacPherson D: *Blastocystis hominis:* Epidemiology and natural history. J Infect Dis 162:987, 1990. (Concludes that *B. hominis* is most likely a commensal organism.)

24

MISCELLANEOUS SUBJECTS AND CONDITIONS

209

Preventive Measures for Third-World Travel

Kenneth M. Boyer

Pediatricians are often asked about appropriate health precautions and official requirements for children traveling with their families from the United States to developing countries. The physician need not be an ultimate authority on such issues but ought to be prepared to provide sensible advice. Authoritative sources of information include *Health Information for International Travel,* published annually by the Centers for Disease Control (CDC); the *Report of the Committee on Infectious Diseases* (the "Red Book"), published biennially or triennially by the American Academy of Pediatrics; and the *Morbidity and Mortality Weekly Report* (MMWR), published by the CDC. The CDC also provides a Disease Information Hotline for general information and updated recommendations (404-639-1610) as well as a Malaria Hotline regarding malaria prophylaxis (404-332-4599). A subscription to Travel Health Information Service, a for-profit company (1-800-755-2301), may prove useful to those who frequently counsel international travelers. Information is updated weekly and is available either in a print format or in IBM-PC–compatible software. Uncertainties regarding official requirements or current risks can usually be resolved by communication with the particular country's consulate or embassy, or with medical authorities at the family's destination. A number of university medical centers in the United States maintain "travelers clinics" that are authorized to provide specialized vaccines (e.g., yellow fever) and can also serve as a source of information.

Conditions in many countries resemble those of a century or more ago in the United States—before the development and near universal use of childhood vaccination, before the introduction of reliable systems for water purification and sewage disposal, before the establishment of regulatory agencies for food and medicine quality, before the widespread availability of emergency medical services, before virtually every home had a refrigerator, stove, and flush toilet, and before the elimination of at least some important vectors of disease (such as body lice and malaria-transmitting mosquitoes).

Key considerations in providing advice to a family include the ages of children traveling, the destination country, the expected duration of stay, and the living conditions. Obviously, an exclusively breast-fed infant visiting well-to-do relatives in a major city for a week would have risks quite different from those of a weaned toddler staying for 2 years in a remote village with marginal food, water, and sanitation, especially if the destination country were in the midst of a cholera epidemic. Preexisting medical conditions must be taken into account in planning. For example, the absence of reliable refrigeration at the destination would make management of insulin-dependent diabetes mellitus impossible. The family of a child with asthma would be well advised to be self-sufficient in managing an attack before venturing away from ready access to emergency services. Insurance companies should be contacted before leaving to ascertain extent of coverage during the trip. If inadequate, coverage can often be extended to include international travel for a nominal fee. In general, plans for a trip should be made well enough in advance so that all appropriate interventions can be made before leaving and timed so that they are effective. Specific recommendations for preventive measures are given in Table 209-1.

Table 209-1. Recommendations for Prophylaxis of Children Traveling from the United States to Endemic Developing Countries, According to Length of Stay

	LENGTH OF TRAVEL		
PREVENTIVE MEASURES	Brief (<2 wk)	Intermediate (2 wk to 3 mo)	Long-term Residential (>3 mo)
Routine immunizations			
Review and update	+	+	+
Accelerated primary DTP	+	+	+
Accelerated primary OPV	+	+	+
Accelerated primary measles	±	+	+
Specialized immunizations			
Yellow fever*	+	+	+
Typhoid fever	±	±	+
Hepatitis B	−	±	+
Meningococcus	−	±	+
Japanese encephalitis	−	±	+
Rabies	−	−	+
Cholera	−	−	−
ISG for hepatitis A	±	+	+
Chemoprophylaxis for malaria	+	+	+

*An International Certificate of Yellow Fever Vaccination is REQUIRED for entry into 15 equatorial African countries (see *Health Information for International Travel* for specifics) and one in South America (French Guiana). For other endemic areas, yellow fever vaccine is recommended but not mandatory.

+ = recommended; ± = consider; − = not recommended; DTP = diphtheria and tetanus toxoids with pertussis vaccine; OPV = oral, attenuated poliovirus vaccine containing poliovirus types 1, 2, and 3; ISG = immune serum globulin. (Adapted from the Report of the Committee on Infectious Diseases, 22nd ed, p 65. Elk Grove Village, IL, American Academy of Pediatrics, 1991.)

IMMUNIZATIONS

Routine

The common vaccine-preventable pediatric infections remain prevalent in developing countries. Thus, a pediatrician's first priority for patients traveling to the Third World is to make sure all age-appropriate vaccinations recommended in the United States have been given. This includes both primary series and boosters. In children who have not received full primary series, accelerated schedules are recommended.

DTP. Diphtheria–tetanus–pertussis immunizations can be initiated as early as 4 weeks of age. Intervals between doses in a primary series can be shortened to 6 weeks, thus ensuring completion of the primary series by age 14 weeks. The normal 18-month booster may be given as early as age 12 months.

OPV. Like DTP immunization, trivalent oral polio vaccine can be initiated as early as 4 weeks of age. Intervals between doses can be shortened to 6 weeks. Although not recommended in the United States, a third dose should be included as part of the primary series, or as an extra dose if the infant is between 6 and 14 months old.

HbCV. *Haemophilus influenzae* type b conjugate vaccine should be initiated at the recommended age of 2 months.

For infant travelers, there is a potential advantage for the PRP-OMP (Pedvax HIB, MSD) conjugate vaccine, based on its rapid stimulation of protective levels of antibody with one or two injections. The second dose may be given as soon as 6 weeks after the first. The recommended age for booster vaccination with PRP-OMP is 12 months.

MMR. Measles–mumps–rubella vaccine administration should also be accelerated, although it is the measles component that is by far the most important. MMR may be given at age 12 months. For younger babies, monovalent measles vaccine should be administered between 6 and 11 months of age, with a dose of MMR given subsequently at age 15 months. The Edmonston–Zagreb measles vaccine, available in many developing countries but not in the United States, is a monovalent immunogen superior to the Moraten strain used routinely in the U.S. It should be recalled that simultaneous or prior administration of immune serum globulin (ISG) (for hepatitis A prophylaxis) will inactivate measles vaccine (as well as mumps and rubella) and thus result in primary vaccine failure.

Specialized

With the global eradication of smallpox, only one vaccination—for yellow fever—remains as a mandatory requirement for entry to a select list of tropical countries. However, a number of other specialized immunizations are prudent to consider, particularly for children who will have long-term stays. The following guidelines apply to vaccinations against diseases known to be endemic in the destination country or countries.

Yellow Fever. Yellow fever vaccine is a live attenuated vaccine given subcutaneously. A single dose (0.5 ml, all ages) confers immunity. The lower age limit for vaccination is 9 months. Although not all countries in the yellow fever belt mandate immunization, vaccination is recommended for all individuals entering rural endemic areas. This vaccine can be given only at authorized vaccination centers in the United States. Simultaneous administration of cholera vaccine is not recommended because lower antibody levels are achieved. Other live attenuated vaccines and ISG can be administered concurrently without interference. Booster doses are indicated after 10 years.

Typhoid Fever. Although not required for entry into any country, typhoid immunization is prudent for families with long-term residential stays and, depending on the living circumstances to be encountered, also for short stays in endemic areas of Africa, Asia, and South America. Two typhoid vaccines are now available—the conventional inactivated vaccine and a newly licensed oral attenuated vaccine, Ty21a. Inactivated vaccine has 70% to 95% efficacy, but febrile responses after vaccination are common. Ty21a has comparable efficacy but far fewer side effects. Unfortunately, efficacy studies with Ty21a have not been done in children <6 years of age. Thus, this new vaccine is recommended only for children ≥6 years of age. For the inactivated vaccine, two doses (0.5 ml for children ≥ age 10 years, 0.25 ml for ages <10) are given at 4-week intervals. Ty21a is taken as one enteric-coated capsule every other day for a total of four doses. Booster doses are indicated after 5 years. A liquid form of Ty21a, with superior immunizing properties, is nearing FDA licensure.

Hepatitis B. Recombinant hepatitis B vaccine is recommended for long-term residential travelers to endemic regions of Africa, Asia, Eastern Europe, Arctic areas of North America, and South America. Because venereal and perinatal transmissions are the dominant mechanisms of acquiring hepatitis B virus (HBV) in these areas, children are at generally lower risk than adults. However, the vaccine is very safe and is increasingly being incorporated into routine pediatric health maintenance in the United States. Doses differ for the two available recombinant hepatitis B vaccines (Recombivax HB, MSD, and Engerix-B, SKF), but they yield equivalent antibody responses. A primary series generally consists of three intramuscular doses of vaccine given over a period of 6 months (see Chap. 14 for recommendations by age, vaccine manufacturer, and schedule). An accelerated four-dose schedule has been FDA-approved for one vaccine (Eugerix-B) involving doses at 0, 1, and 2 months, with a booster at 6 to 12 months. Administration

of the first three doses before departure is likely to provide short-term protection; the booster will provide prolonged immunity.

Meningococcus. Tetravalent meningococcal polysaccharide vaccine is recommended for travelers to the "meningitis belt" of equatorial Africa. The vaccine confers immunity against serogroups A, C, Y, and W135. Its highest efficacy is against serogroup A, the most important of the infecting serogroups in this region. The dose is 0.5 ml subcutaneously. Boosters are unnecessary if primary immunization is given at ≥ age 2.

Japanese Encephalitis. Japanese encephalitis vaccine is recommended for travelers to certain areas of China and Southeast Asia where this important arbovirus is endemic. The inactivated vaccine is unavailable in the United States, however. Thus, long-term visitors are advised to obtain the vaccination at their destination.

Rabies. Rabies preexposure immunization is a reasonable consideration for children who will have long-term residence in areas where dog rabies remains highly prevalent. In these countries, rabies immune globulin may be relatively unavailable or unstandardized, and human diploid cell vaccine (with its advantages of infrequent side effects and high immunogenicity) may be unavailable as well. Preexposure immunization may avoid these potential difficulties associated with emergency postexposure management. Regimens for preexposure prophylaxis include three-dose series of human diploid cell vaccine administered intramuscularly (1.0 ml per dose, days 0, 7, and 28) or subcutaneously (0.1 ml per dose, same schedule).

Cholera. Although the vaccine is still available, cholera vaccination is no longer required for entry to any country or territory. With its marginal efficacy, cholera vaccine is considered much less valuable than avoidance of potentially contaminated water and food.

ISG. Standard immune serum globulin, either as a single intramuscular dose for short-term travel or as repetitive doses for residential stays, is recommended for prevention of hepatitis A. Dosages are 0.02 ml/kg for intermediate stays (between 2 weeks and 3 months) and 0.06 ml/kg given every 5 months for long-term residence (>3 months). Because immune globulin manufactured in the United States is unlikely to harbor IgG antibodies to yellow fever virus or *Salmonella typhi*, the only vaccination with which one must be concerned about interference is measles.

MALARIA

Malaria is endemic in most of the tropical and subtropical Third World. Repeated exposure of long-term residents in endemic countries results in complete or partial immunity. Travelers without previous exposure to malaria are not only susceptible to the disease but are more likely to manifest its

Table 209-2. Recommended Drugs for Prophylaxis and Presumptive Treatment of Malaria in Children

DRUG	USE	DOSE
Choroquine phosphate (Aralen®)	Chemoprophylaxis (all ages)	5 mg/kg base (= 8.3 mg/kg salt) once/week, up to adult dose (300 mg base)
Mefloquine (Lariam®)	Chemoprophylaxis (areas of chloroquine-resistant *P. falciparum;* wt >15 kg)	15–19 kg: ¼ tab (=62 mg salt)/wk 20–30 kg: ½ tab (=125 mg salt)/wk 31–45 kg: ¾ tab (=188 mg salt)/wk >45 kg: 1 tab (=250 mg salt)/wk
Doxycycline	Chemoprophylaxis (areas of chloroquine-resistant *P. falciparum;* age >8 yr)	2 mg/kg once/day, up to adult dose (100 mg)
Pyrimethamine/ sulfadoxine (Fansidar®)	Temporary presumptive treatment (when medical evaluation is unavailable, given as a single dose)	5–10 kg: ½ tab (=12/250 mg pyr/sulfa) 11–20 kg: 1 tab (=25/500 mg pyr/sulfa) 21–30 kg: 1½ tab (=38/750 mg pyr/sulfa) 31–45 kg: 2 tab (=50/1000 mg pyr/sulfa) >45 kg: 3 tab (=75/1500 mg pyr/sulfa)

Adapted from Centers for Disease Control: Health Information for International Travel. Washington, DC, U.S. Government Printing Office, 1991, p. 100.

more severe and life-threatening consequences. Current estimates of malaria risk, according to destination, are available in *Health Information for International Travel*. Within a given country, risk is further enhanced in rural areas (e.g., an African game park) and with outdoor exposure at dusk and during evening hours when mosquitoes are most active (e.g., overnight camping on a safari). With potential mosquito exposure, judicious use of mosquito repellents, such as N, N-diethylmetatoluamide (DEET), and mosquito nets when sleeping is recommended.

Chemoprophylaxis

If malaria exposure during travel is possible, chemoprophylaxis should be undertaken (Table 209-2). The key consideration is whether chloroquine-resistant *Plasmodium falciparum* infections occur at the destination. This problem of drug resistance has become a major therapeutic and prophylactic issue in the past decade. Chloroquine is the only prophylactic medication that can safely be administered to children of all ages. Thus, if exposure to resistant *P. falciparum* is possible, travel by young children should be discouraged. Mefloquine and doxycycline provide effective prophylaxis against resistant *P. falciparum* in older children and adults.

The other key consideration in malaria chemoprophylaxis is timing of initiation and discontinuation of medications. Chloroquine and mefloquine need to be initiated 1 to

2 weeks prior to departure and *must be continued* for 4 weeks after leaving the endemic area. Doxycycline must also be continued for 4 weeks after leaving an area of endemicity, but it can be started 1 to 2 days prior to departure.

Treatment

In endemic areas, unexplained symptoms of fever, persistent headache, muscle aches, or vomiting are suggestive of malaria. Prompt medical evaluation and examination of blood for malaria parasites are essential. Families who use chloroquine prophylaxis should carry age-appropriate treatment doses of pyrimethamine/sulfadoxine (Fansidar). If medical evaluation is unavailable, a single dose of Fansidar should be taken promptly in the event of a febrile illness. Families should be aware that such self-treatment is only a temporary measure and that medical evaluation should still be sought.

TRAVELER'S DIARRHEA

Limitations in water quality and food sanitation in many Third-World countries make traveler's diarrhea an important risk. Most cases are caused by enterotoxigenic *Escherichia coli,* but *Salmonella, Shigella, Campylobacter, Giardia, Entamoeba histolytica,* and *Vibrio cholerae* are other possible etiologies of enteric infection.

Prophylaxis

The CDC recommendation to "boil it, cook it, peel it, or forget it" should be kept in mind as the most effective means of prevention. Implementation of this simple admonition is often difficult, primarily because hidden sources of ingestion of fecally contaminated water can easily be overlooked. For example, ice should be avoided, teeth should be brushed without the use of tap water, and only canned or bottled *carbonated* beverages should be drunk. Raw meat, raw seafoods, and raw fruits and vegetables are especially risky foods. For infants, the safest food and water source is breast-feeding. Infant formula prepared from commercial powder and boiled water is the safest alternative.

A number of seemingly logical preventive medications may actually be harmful. For example, the antiperistaltic agents diphenoxylate hydrochloride (Lomotil) and loperamide (Imodium) have no preventive efficacy and can actually increase the severity of infections caused by invasive enteric pathogens. Bismuth subsalicylate (Pepto-Bismol), taken in large quantities, has some preventive efficacy but is impractical. Antimicrobial prophylaxis is effective; data have demonstrated the efficacy of trimethoprim-sulfamethoxazole (Bactrim, Septra), doxycycline, ciprofloxacin (Cipro), and norfloxacin (Noroxin). With the exception of trimethoprim-sulfamethoxazole, all of these medications have contraindications or age limitations for pediatric use. Thus, prophylactic use for children is not generally recommended.

Treatment

Although prophylactic use is not recommended, early therapeutic use of trimethoprim-sulfamethoxazole is recommended for children (or parents) who develop traveler's diarrhea. A dose of 10 mg/kg/day of the trimethoprim component (with 50 mg/kg/day sulfamethoxazole), divided b.i.d., is effective. The adult treatment dose is 160 mg trimethoprim with 800 mg sulfamethoxazole once daily. If dehydration develops, oral rehydration is the most important aspect in treating traveler's diarrhea in children. The World Health Organization Oral Rehydration Solution (ORS) is recommended. It can be purchased at stores and pharmacies in almost all developing countries and is supplied as packets designed to be added to a liter of boiled water. It consists of a fixed combination of sodium chloride, sodium citrate, potassium chloride, and glucose. ORS should be offered ad lib and will correct most mild to moderate dehydration. Persistent vomiting, bloody diarrhea, high fever, and severe dehydration require medical attention.

ANNOTATED BIBLIOGRAPHY

Centers for Disease Control: Health Information for International Travel. Washington, DC, U.S. Government Printing Office, 1991. (Authoritative annual summary of current recommendations and requirements.)

Kozicki M, Steffen R, Schar M: "Boil it, cook it, peel it or forget it": Does this rule prevent traveler's diarrhea? Int J Epidemiol 14:169–172, 1985. (Shows that it lowers the odds.)

La Russa PS: Infections associated with international travel. In Nelson JD (ed): Current Therapy in Pediatric Infectious Disease—2. Toronto, BC Dekker, 1988. (Good, brief summary for planning an international trip.)

Peter G, Lepow ML, McCracken GH, Phillips CF: Report of the Committee on Infectious Diseases, 22nd ed. Elk Grove Village, IL, American Academy of Pediatrics, 1991. (Authoritative source of immunization requirements and recommendations for children, with short summaries of essential information on the most important infectious disease hazards to international travelers.)

Rodriguez WJ: Traveler's diarrhea. In Nelson JD: Current Therapy in Pediatric Infectious Disease—2. Toronto, BC Dekker, 1988. (Good, brief summary of prophylactic and therapeutic measures.)

210

Chronic Illness

Paula Kienberger Jaudes

A chronic illness may be defined as a physical disorder that continues for 3 months or more, requires hospitalization for at least 1 month, or is expected at the time of diagnosis to last for more than 3 months.

Approximately 10% of all individuals under 21 years of age in the United States have a chronic illness or disability. For more than two million children, chronic conditions cause some degree of limitation of their daily activities. These conditions include arthritis, asthma, autism, central nervous system (CNS) injury, cerebral palsy, chronic renal failure, cleft lip and palate, congenital heart disease, cystic fibrosis, diabetes mellitus, Down syndrome, hearing impairment, hemophilia, leukemia, mental retardation, muscular dystrophy, neural tube defects, phenylketonuria, sickle cell disease, seizure disorders, and visual impairment. Asthma is the most common of these conditions.

A pediatrician in practice will manage between 200 and 300 chronically ill children per year. Because of measures such as vaccinations and effective antibiotic treatment, which have resulted in decreased morbidity from acute illnesses and an increase in the survival rate of children with chronic illness, chronic disease has both increased and become more evident in medical practice. Parents, physicians, educators, and society are also more aware of chronic disease.

The Vanderbilt Institute for Public Policy Studies has examined the issues concerning the care of chronically ill children and has identified three principles related to public policy concerning such children. These principles are also applicable to the care of these children: "(1) Children with chronic illnesses and their families have special needs which merit attention, beyond that provided to the health needs of able-bodied children. (2) Families have the central role in caring for their own members, and the goal of policy [care] should be to enable families to carry out their responsibilities to nurture their children and encourage their most effective development. (3) Policy [care] should encourage professional services of a highly ethical nature. Key elements include truth-telling, confidentiality, maintenance of dignity and respect for family preference, professionals' recognition of their own effectiveness, and emphasis on collaboration." (Hutchins, 1985)

The impact of chronic illness on children and their families is similar regardless of the specific type of illness. Issues that need to be addressed in all cases of chronic disease include the effects of the illness on the child's growth and development; the parents' emotional reactions to the child's illness; the impact of the illness on siblings, parents, and the functioning of the family; worry about the future; and the choice and comprehension of the appropriate treatment. Discussion of these issues and the role of the pediatrician in the care of these children now follows.

THE CHILD

The goals of all therapeutic interventions on behalf of a child with a chronic illness should be to minimize the biologic manifestations, complications, and progression of the illness and to enable the child to function as independently as possible. The care of the chronically ill child is directed not at a cure, which may be unattainable, but at optimal achievable function. Children with chronic illnesses should be regarded as children with special needs and not as special children.

The effect of a specific chronic disease on the development of the child is determined by the nature of the illness, its severity, the limitations that it imposes, the experience of pain, the treatment modalities, isolation and separation from others, and the visibility of the illness. The developmental problems faced by a 1-year-old are different from those of a school-aged child or an adolescent. A visible deformity (e.g., cerebral palsy) may have an impact different from that of an invisible illness (e.g., asthma). Children with an invisible chronic illness may have stress and adaptive problems, because although they appear normal, they have limits and restrictions caused by illness. Thus, the children cannot always behave like their peers. At each stage of development, a child must accomplish certain tasks of cognition and social and emotional development in order to advance to the next stage. Chronic illness can interfere with the child's development by delaying or interrupting these sequences.

The main purpose in any therapeutic plan is to regard the child as a whole person, not only considering medical care but also devoting attention to psychosocial function. Psychosocial adjustment is adequate for most chronically ill children and adolescents. Adjustment not only refers to the ability to adapt to the medical problem but also indicates that an individual is free from disabling psychiatric or social abnormalities. Treatment strategies should be aimed at promoting adjustment.

Maladjustment to a chronic illness was previously considered to be caused by the nature and severity of that disability. It is now apparent from population surveys that, compared to their healthy peers, children with chronic illnesses are generally at increased risk of experiencing significant psychological or social problems. Children who have a poor functional status have more difficulty in making a good psychological adjustment. The degree of psychological adjustment seems to bear little relationship to traditional measures of morbidity, such as the number of days in the hospital. Among children within a medical diagnostic category, there is a great variability in adjustment; therefore, the medical diagnosis may provide little information, or may even be misleading, regarding the psychological and social well-being of the patient. Personality attributes that can be regarded as assets, such as intelligence, diminish the likelihood of psychosocial problems, whereas liabilities such as low intelligence or unattractiveness serve to increase the probability of maladjustment. The most important factors in adjustment involve how the family functions with the child and how together they can adapt to the child's illness and its demands.

THE FAMILY

A common characteristic of children with chronic illnesses is their potential to disrupt the life of the family. Research on families with a chronically ill child has focused on the psychopathology of the family members, with little awareness of the positive aspects of the way in which the families adapt. Research has also been performed on how families function within specific diagnostic categories as opposed to generic problems faced by families who have a child with a chronic disease.

Both mothers and fathers experience successive or simultaneous reactions after learning of the diagnosis of a chronic illness in their child. These reactions may include shock, anger, resentment, self-blame, denial, sadness, and acceptance. During this process of grieving and reattachment, parents may stop at any one of these stages and may need help to complete this process.

Mothers, who are usually the primary care-givers, vary greatly in their response to their child's illness. Most research has focused on maternal response. Their response is likely to depend on the mother's own developmental history and on her relationship with her own parents. The relationship to her chronically ill child may range from rejection to overprotectiveness to adapting well. The reactions of fathers have been less well studied. Fathers are usually not the primary care-givers, but they are usually psychologically involved with the chronically ill child.

Studies on the incidence of divorce in families of chronically ill children have failed to show a consistent increase in the divorce rate. This topic is controversial and has only minimally been studied; the divorce rate may be elevated in families of children with certain diseases. However, parents of chronically ill children seem to have more marital stress than that experienced by families without chronically ill children.

The effects on growth and development of siblings of chronically ill children are varied. Problems for siblings can include fear of catching the disease, guilt, resentment of the burden inflicted, jealousy at attention to the affected child, a real or imagined fear of stigmatization, and problems at school. Factors that may affect the adjustment of siblings include the severity of the illness and the sex, birth order, and age of the affected sibling.

SERVICES NEEDED

Children with chronic illnesses and their families need medical, educational, financial, and advocacy services.

Medical

The child with a chronic illness needs general pediatric care and, in many cases, subspecialty care. The pediatrician provides ongoing health care to the child and family, whereas the subspecialist provides technological expertise in the treatment of the particular disease or deformity. The generalist and the subspecialist complement each other's role in meeting the medical needs of the child and family.

Educational

The patient and the family need to understand the medical aspects of the chronic illness because they must live with the illness. It is important for them to be educated and to educate themselves, so that they can make appropriate choices concerning schooling, housing, financial matters, equipment, and medical care. The parents may also need this information for the purpose of advocacy.

In 1975, the Educational Act (PL 94-142) for All Handicapped Children was signed; it became fully effective in 1978. The major assumptions from which the law was developed are that all children have the right to education, and that all children, no matter how profoundly handicapped they may be, are able to learn. The law mandates that the states provide appropriate free education for all handicapped children in minimally restrictive environments, with the concurrence of the parents. All states are mandated to implement educational programs for handicapped children 3 years of age and older. In some states, education is available for these children starting at birth.

Specifically, the law states that a public school must make a multidisciplinary assessment of each child, on the basis of which an individual educational plan (IEP) will be formulated. According to the IEP, the child is then placed in an environment that will enhance his or her development. The child's educational progress is monitored according to the IEP. The parents participate in all major decisions, and they have the right to appeal placement decisions. The IEP is based on information about the child's illness, developmental status, capacity for daily functioning, and perceived academic potential.

The physician, who is usually the first person to identify children with chronic diseases, will refer a child needing services to the local school district. For physicians, becoming involved in the education of their patients may be a new role. The school forms must be filled out, with information provided about the specific services that will be needed for the child. The physician may, in some cases, have to be the child's advocate to obtain these services from the school system. The physician may also have to educate the school professionals about the illness, and he or she should be prepared to be active in helping to plan the best educational program for the child.

In 1986, Congress passed PL 99-457, Amendments of The Education of the Handicapped Act, which took effect in August 1989. This law requires each state to establish a comprehensive system to provide *early intervention* to disabled infants from birth until their third birthday. Its purpose is to foster better cooperation between health care and special education professionals and to strengthen the role of the family. The development of an individual family service plan (IFSP) for the child and family is mandated. During the first 4 years of the law's implementation, a system is to be established that will identify, evaluate, and provide services to handicapped infants. The pediatrician's role during this time is to work with the state in the planning stages and to advocate for services for handicapped children from birth to age 3.

Finally, the community must be educated to the needs of the chronically ill child. The community should understand the nature of chronic illness and should respond by removing barriers, both by providing access for handicapped persons and by breaking down stereotyped views of the chronically ill.

Financial

Chronic disease can place major financial stress on a family. Expenses arise not only for direct health care but also for home care, transportation, extra telephone bills, loss of time from work, special diets, counseling, and so forth.

The extent to which these expenses are reimbursable—and some never are—depends on the parents' insurance coverage, income, state of residence, and the child's specific medical condition. Private insurance frequently does not cover primary health care, counseling, or home health care.

The pediatrician can advise a family that needs financial help to investigate the availability of funding from Medicaid (Title XIX funds), crippled children's services (Title V), supplemental social security income programs, disease-oriented voluntary associations, or special state programs. The possible public funding sources differ among states and have different eligibility requirements. A resource for the pediatrician could be a nurse/social worker who works for the state agency that handles funding for children with chronic diseases, or a pediatric social worker at a medical center.

Advocacy

Parents and physicians may need to join in being advocates for the chronically ill child to assure that the child's medical, psychosocial, behavioral, and educational needs are being met. In many cases, the community, government, and society have to be educated and motivated to action to meet these needs. Examples of advocacy include the provision of handicapped-accessible sidewalks, ensuring that the child is in the appropriate classroom, or petitioning the state for funding of in-home care of a child rather than having the child in a hospital.

Specific Services

The child or family may have other specific needs that depend on the type of chronic illness. For example, a child or family under stress may have psychological difficulties and may need counseling. This counseling may be provided by a physician, psychologist, or social worker.

The child may require treatment by one or more health care professionals, such as a speech therapist, physical therapist, occupational therapist, vocational therapist, or infant development specialist. Equipment may be needed that could range from simple bracing to an electric wheelchair or a computerized communication board. The home may have to be modified so that the activities of daily living are optimized and so that space can be allocated for equipment. The child and family may need help with transportation to and from therapy and medical facilities. The necessary service can sometimes consist of the provision of bus fare or access to specialized vans.

Social service assistance may help the family in coping with medical, educational, financial, and psychological problems. Legal assistance may be needed in advocacy for the child. An example is ensuring that a child is not denied medical benefits because he or she is poor or in poor housing facilities.

Home care rather than hospitalization may be preferable for some children whose chronic illness has high technology needs. With home care, the chronically ill child may have as normal a life as possible with his or her family and may thus maximize growth and development. High technology may include a ventilator, a phrenic nerve pacer, hyperalimentation, or respiratory treatment. Several requirements should be met for home care to be successful. These requirements include a family willing to care for the child, a flexible, well-thought-out plan of care with a designated coordinator, a backup plan for emergencies, a mechanism for providing social and emotional support for the child and family, and appropriate alternative respite care.

ROLE OF THE PEDIATRICIAN

The general pediatrician assumes the primary care for the chronically ill child. The often complex medical problems are dealt with by the generalist in collaboration with subspecialists. Ideally, this teamwork prevents fragmentation of medical care. However, the chronically ill child and the family have needs beyond purely medical ones. The pediatrician, as the primary care provider, is in a position to also recognize problems of adjustment and development.

The pediatrician, together with the family, helps with the case management of the health care of the whole child. Case management includes the management of medical care, the continuity of care, the coordination of comprehensive services, and the support of the family. The parents have the primary responsibility for the care of their child. The pediatrician can lend his or her knowledge, support, medical expertise, coordination of services, and advocacy to the parents in their efforts to meet the various needs in support of their chronically ill child.

ANNOTATED BIBLIOGRAPHY

Blum RW (ed): Chronic Illness and Disabilities in Childhood and Adolescence. Orlando, Grune & Stratton, 1984. (Many medical disease chapters; emphasizes the adolescent.)

Haggerty RJ (ed): Chronic disease in children. Pediatr Clin North Am 31: Feb, 1984. (Excellent overall review of problems.)

Hobbs N, Perrin JM (eds): Issues in the Care of Children with Chronic Illness. San Francisco, Jossey-Bass, 1985. (Defines and examines the opportunities available to families who have a child with a chronic illness.)

Hobbs N, Perrin JM, Ireys HT: Chronically Ill Children and Their Families. San Francisco, Jossey-Bass, 1985. (Findings from a study of public policies affecting chronically ill children and their families.)

Hutchins V: Chronic illness: Old and new perspectives. Presented at New Directions in Care of Children with Chronic Illness, sponsored by the United Hospital Fund of New York, New York, May 1985. (Keynote address.)

Jaudes PK: The medical care of children with complex home health care needs: An overview for caretakers. In Hochstadt NJ, Yost DM (eds): The medically Complex Child. The Transition to Home Care, pp 29–60. New York, Harwood Academic Publishers, 1991. (Home care resource book on children with chronic illness.)

Sabbeth BF, Leventhal JM: Marital adjustment to chronic childhood illness: A critique of the literature. Pediatrics 73:762, 1984. (Controversial topic; good review.)

Stein REK (ed): Caring for Children with Chronic Illness. Issues and Strategies. New York, Springer, 1989. (Framework for considering the range of issues and dilemmas posed by chronic illness.)

211

Colic

Marc Weissbluth

Colic in infants is characterized by spells or paroxysmal attacks of crying, irritability, or fussiness occurring in the evening hours in babies who are clinically healthy. Unfortunately, there is disagreement among researchers and practitioners on almost every clinical feature of colic because there are no objective diagnostic criteria. Thus, data regarding infantile colic have been obtained almost exclusively by a reliance on reports from parents. Obviously, parental anxiety, fatigue, and preconceptions may influence their descriptions of their infants' behavior.

PRESENTATION

Illingworth defined colic as "violent rhythmical, screaming attacks which did not stop when the infants were picked up, and for which no cause, such as underfeeding, could be found." Wessel diagnosed a colicky infant as "one who, otherwise healthy and well-fed, had paroxysms of irritability, fussing or crying lasting for a total of more than 3 hours a day and occurring on more than 3 days in one week . . . and that the paroxysms continued to recur for more than 3 weeks." These pediatricians studied ~150 infants. Their combined results showed that the attacks do not usually occur during the first few days but are present in about 80% of affected infants by 2 weeks of age. All affected infants have the onset of their spells by 3 weeks of age. About 80% of colicky infants begin their spells between 5 P.M. and 8 P.M., and their spells usually end by midnight. An additional 12% of infants experience their spells later in the evening, starting between 7 P.M. and 10 P.M. and ending by 2 A.M. At 2 months of age, about 50% of colicky infants no longer have these crying spells, and by 3 months of age, an additional 30% of infants are free of colic. By about 4 months of age, an additional 10%, or 90% of all previously colicky infants, are free of symptoms. The average duration of the colic spell lasts almost 4 hours. The onset of colic in premature infants is usually delayed and starts near the expected date of delivery regardless of the gestational age at birth.

Some pediatricians view the colicky crying spells as qualitatively different from normal infant crying, and they use specific clinical features as diagnostic criteria. For example, colicky infants are diagnosed as such only if they are observed to draw up their legs onto their abdomen or only if they exhibit inconsolability. Most practitioners, however, would agree that crying with the legs drawn up onto the abdomen is not a pathognomonic sign of colic.

Inconsolability means that the infant does not become quiet with conventional soothing techniques and may be defined differently by different pediatricians. A pediatrician with a background in temperament research or psychophysiology might describe inconsolability as a within-the-child trait, but another pediatrician with a psychodynamic perspective might consider inconsolability from an interactional viewpoint and might focus on maternal anxiety as the major contributing factor.

Other pediatricians view colicky crying spells not as qualitatively different from normal crying but differing from normal infant crying only in intensity, duration, or persistence. Data from several studies tend to support this viewpoint because there are no measurable discontinuities in crying behavior between infants who do and do not have colic. For example, for the upper 25% of crying duration in normal babies at age 6 weeks, the mean duration is 3.5 hours, which is close to the mean duration of colicky crying spells (3.7–3.9 hours). The documented natural history of infant crying regarding its onset, time of occurrence, and cessation parallels that of colic and lends support to the notion that colic represents only an extreme form of normally occurring infant behaviors. Thus, colic and unexplained crying in infants may reflect normal developmental or maturational processes that occur during the first few months. The delayed onset in prematures also supports the view that colic is time-locked to postconceptual age.

During colic spells, the infant is often described as hypertonic because the entire body is stiffened, the fists are tightly clenched, and the legs are flexed rigidly over the abdomen. The babies sometimes have uncoordinated jerky movements of their limbs described as batting or flapping of the arms or kicking the legs. At other times the movements are described as writhing, twisting, or turning. These movements are not present at other times, and these babies have normal neurologic examinations. Air swallowing occurs during these agitated movements and during the crying spells, and this swallowed air is probably the explanation for the gassiness that is another feature of colicky infants. There is no evidence to suggest that the gassiness in colicky infants is caused by primary gastrointestinal pathology. There is also no strong evidence associating colic with the method of feeding or food allergy.

Another feature of some, but not all, colicky infants is stimulus sensitivity; they appear to be either easily startled or easily awakened. Frequent awakenings at night often occur in these infants. A bothersome feature of colicky infants in general is extreme daytime wakefulness manifested by brief naps or no naps.

DIFFERENTIAL DIAGNOSIS

Most pediatric texts include in their list of possible causes of colic or in their differential diagnosis of colic every organ system or disease known to cause pain or gassiness in infants. When a condition is diagnosed, such as cow's milk protein allergy, then the child has pain or discomfort from that problem, not colic. The term *infantile colic* is usually used when there is no diagnosable medical or surgical problem. If the infant is clinically well on repeated physical examinations and the presentation fits the usual description of colic, then there are only a few alternative diagnostic possibilities. Problems relating to feeding are often mentioned because the gassiness suggests gastrointestinal cramps or pain. Feeding problems are rarely discovered, and these can easily be detected by a careful history and repeated weight measurements. Urinary tract infections tend to cause crying and irritability at any time, and the pain does not occur with the evening periodicity of colic. Children with urinary tract infections do not usually gain weight well, or they may develop fever.

The progressive quality over time of increasingly severe pain, increasing weakness, or increasing listlessness that commonly occurs with organic diseases is notably absent in colicky infants. They appear completely healthy when they are not having their characteristic evening spells.

WORK-UP

A careful history and physical examination are usually sufficient to establish the diagnosis of infantile colic. The physical examination, or repeated examinations, should be considered as a sufficient diagnostic test. Laboratory tests or radiographic examinations, sometimes including hospitalization, are usually unnecessary if the child is gaining weight normally and has a normal physical examination. Tests such as blood counts or urine cultures are sometimes performed on the infant to create the impression of professional thoroughness in order to reduce *parental* anxiety. Under the guise of a laboratory work-up, the physician hopes to better convince the family (and sometimes himself or herself) that there is no organic disease. Thus, after winning their trust and confidence, the pediatrician can better support the parents as they wait out the 3 or 4 months of colic. However, one potential problem of doing laboratory tests with the intent of reducing parental anxiety, rather than based on clinical suspicions, is that a somewhat abnormal result may occur. Obviously, the slightly abnormal test result does not necessarily signify pathology. Nevertheless, one abnormal test could lead to further unneeded tests in a fruitless search to eliminate some uncommon or obscure condition. Another disadvantage in performing laboratory tests is that the performance of the tests themselves or hospitalizing the infant might reinforce the parents' belief that something must be medically wrong with their child. After all, they may think, why else would the doctor do these tests if he or she did not truly suspect something might be wrong with my baby? With this attitude, the discovery of a few normal results might only cause parents to request additional tests, studies, or consultations.

On the other hand, if the physician does not perform tests, this might lead to heightened anxiety or parental dissatisfaction based on a perception of a lack of thoroughness, and it may cause the parents to change pediatricians. There is enormous variability among families and pediatricians in how they handle the stresses caused by a colicky infant. Sensitivity to this variability of how the parents are affected and how the pediatrician is affected should encourage a highly individualized approach to working up and treating an infant who might have colic.

MANAGEMENT

The major principle of management is not exactly *what* the physician recommends but *how* he or she does it. The physician should take the parents' complaint *seriously*, and should perform a *thorough* examination. When the physician suspects colic, a thorough examination is diagnostic and also therapeutic because the thoroughness itself reassures the parents that their child is healthy and is being looked after by someone who really cares. This situation is analogous to carefully examining the child with fever even when a common cold is suspected. The physician should be patient, sympathetically supportive, and appropriately tentative when offering advice regarding remedies of questionable value, such as herbal teas or hot water bottles. The way in which the physician presents these therapies is important, because overly encouraging home remedies or formula switching may only heighten parental anxiety when each of these items might eventually fail.

If the physician spends extra time in the office or on the phone expressing optimism regarding the health of the child and emphasizing that this stressful period will soon end, this will help the parents maintain their morale. Their increased optimism from the physician's reassurance might reduce parental anxiety and might also cause them to handle their baby in a calmer fashion and thus actually reduce the crying. The major error in management is to trivialize the parents' complaint, because colic is known to be a transitory condition with no known morbidity or complications.

Parents must be explicitly told that they are not causing the crying. Self-doubt, feelings of inadequate parenting skills, and failure to nurse well are topics that should be openly discussed, because parents blame themselves for the infant crying.

TREATMENT

The three major methods of reducing infant crying are (1) rhythmic rocking motions using swings, cradles, springs on crib casters, automobile rides, rocking chairs, or parents' arms; (2) encouraging sucking at the breast, bottle, pacifier, wrist, fist, or thumb; and (3) swaddling, bundling, or cuddling. These methods should be encouraged whenever the infant needs to be soothed, and parents need to be told explicitly that the young infant will not become "spoiled" from all this attention. In other words, the child will not learn a crying habit or always expect to be picked up when the parents behave this way during the first 6 weeks.

In order to alleviate unnecessary guilt and prevent misdirected therapies focused on parental psychological factors, parents should be informed that there is no good scientific evidence to suggest that their inexperience, anxiety, or parenting practices are directly causing the colic. Parents should also be told that treatments with sedatives, hypnotics, antiflatulents, antacids, antihistamines, alcohol, or gripe water are no better than a placebo. Antispasmodics are commonly used, but only dicyclomine hydrochloride has been shown to be an effective drug to reduce crying; however, it is no longer used because of questions regarding its safety. Placebo effects commonly occur during the first few weeks after an initial brief period of fussiness subsides, shortly after about 6 weeks of age when the peak of unexplained fussiness or crying is passed, and after 3 to 4 months of age when all unexplained crying or fussiness disappears.

During the first month or so, it is important for the parents to learn to accept and love their baby despite his or her crying. To maintain their morale, they need to have time away from their baby by hiring help, even for short periods of time. The pediatrician can help the parents cultivate a watchful waiting attitude until the colic passes. Parents can learn to become sensitive to subtle shifts in their baby's behavior so that they can begin to modify their care-giving behaviors as the colic begins to subside.

After about 6 weeks of age, for some mild colicky babies, when the baby begins to exhibit specific social smiling, the baby might benefit from less attention when overly tired. The soothing parental efforts might be so socially pleasurable to the child that he or she fights sleep to enjoy the parents' company. The end result is fatigue-driven fussiness. However, for severe colicky babies, because they are so irregular regarding sleep/wake transitions, it is difficult for parents to distinguish between colicky crying and fatigue-driven crying until about 3 to 4 months of age. At this age, for all colicky babies, the evening crying spells have diminished, and most parents should now be encouraged to give their child less attention when they think that the child is tired and needs to sleep. After 3 to 4 months, most parents are better able to differentiate the child's *need* to sleep from his or her *desire* to play.

The failure of parents to shift their parenting strategies after about 3 to 4 months of age, in response to the increasing social maturity of the child, often causes severe postcolic sleep problems. Letting the child "cry it out" probably helps no one when the child is under several weeks of age. However, letting the child "learn to sleep" after 3 to 4 months helps produce a calmer, less fussy baby. Parents should be told that they should allow their child to learn the self-soothing skill of falling asleep unassisted, and they should be reassured that they are not hurting their child.

Learning to be alone to develop self-soothing skills is a developmental healthy habit for the child, and pediatricians can guide parents' behavior, which helps or hinders its evolution (see also Chap. 30, "Sleep Disturbances").

ANNOTATED BIBLIOGRAPHY

Brazelton TB: Crying in infancy. Pediatrics 29:579–588, 1962. (Naturalistic study of infant crying based on parents' reports.)

Illingworth RS: Infantile colic revisited. Arch Dis Child 60:981–985, 1985. (Update from his classic 1954 article and a review of current therapeutic ideas.)

Illingworth RS: Three months' colic. Arch Dis Child 29:167–174, 1954. (Comprehensive review of the literature and a clinical study comparing colicky and noncolicky babies.)

Rebelsky F, Black R: Crying in infancy. J Genet Psychol 121:49–57, 1972. (Infant crying study based on tape recordings.)

Weissbluth M: Crybabies. New York, Berkley, 1989. (Data-based guide for parents and professionals describing how colic relates to normal crying, temperament, and sleep disturbances.)

Weissbluth M: Healthy Sleep Habits, Happy Child. New York, Fawcett Columbine, 1987. (Detailed discussion on postcolic sleep problems.)

Weissbluth M, Christoffel KK, Davis AT: Treatment of infantile colic with dicyclomine hydrochloride. J Pediatr 104:951–955, 1984. (Randomized, placebo-controlled, double-blind study regarding colic, temperament, and sleep.)

Wessel MA, Cobb JC, Jackson EB, Harris GS, Detwiller AC: Paroxysmal fussing in infancy sometimes called "colic." Pediatrics 14:421–434, 1954. (Comprehensive description of the clinical features of colic.)

212

Breath-Holding Spells

Peter T. Heydemann

Breath-holding spells constitute a distinct variety of syncope in early childhood and are the most dramatic benign episodes of childhood. They consist typically of a sudden upset to the child followed by a period of unconsciousness and perhaps convulsive movement. There are *cyanotic* and *pallid* subtypes, both of which have their highest incidence in the first 2 years of life and are uncommon after the age of 6 years. Such spells have been estimated to occur in nearly 1% of children, and mild variations occur in up to 5% of young children. Recurrences of spells are common.

The term "breath-holding spell" is well entrenched in American medical literature but is somewhat misleading. In cyanotic spells, the term breath-holding inappropriately suggests a willful component to the episode; it would be more correct for it to be called "prolonged expiratory apnea." In the pallid type of spell, breath-holding is a minimal feature of the episode, and the term "pallid anoxic seizure" or "reflex anoxic seizure" would be more appropriate.

PATHOPHYSIOLOGY

The pathophysiologies of the cyanotic and pallid types of spells differ. Cyanotic spells occur during episodes in which the child cries and then suddenly holds his breath in expiration. During crying, the pCO_2 is lowered, thus causing cerebral vasoconstriction and diminished cerebral perfusion. The diminished perfusion is aggravated by the child's Valsalva maneuver, which decreases cardiac stroke volume and may cause reflex bradycardia. As breath-holding continues, progressive hypoxia ensues and the child loses consciousness. A seizure may result if the hypoxia or ischemia is severe. As breathing resumes during the seizure, cerebral hypoxia improves, the seizure ends, and consciousness is restored.

Most children with pallid spells have abnormally active vagal reflexes that produce severe bradycardia with decreased cardiac output and cerebral perfusion. A sudden scare or mild physical trauma induces reflex vagal cardiac slowing. The ensuing loss of postural tone and consciousness is equivalent to fainting. If diminished cerebral perfusion lasts more than a few seconds, a generalized seizure follows. At that point, the heart rate improves and awareness resumes. The neural circuitry of this presumed limbic-vagal pathway is poorly delineated.

CLINICAL PRESENTATION

The physician is usually presented with the history that a small child has had a spell consisting of a sudden brief interruption of normal behavior and consciousness. Cyanotic breath-holding spells are the most common. Nearly all spells are preceded by crying, which is brought on most frequently by anger; sudden pain, surprise, and fear are the other usual precipitants. Vigorous crying is interrupted within 1 to 2 minutes by the sudden quiet of breath-holding in expiration. The initial reddish facial flush of crying turns into cyanosis, which is most prominent on the face. After a few seconds of cyanosis, the child becomes limp. At this point, the spell may resolve or develop into a true anoxic seizure with tonic (opisthotonic) or tonic-clonic movements. As with all convulsions, incontinence may accompany the event, and a postictal state lasting minutes to several hours may follow.

Pallid breath-holding spells typically are preceded by sudden pain, mild head trauma, or an emotional "startle." The child lets out a quick cry or whimper, becomes quite pale, and loses consciousness and postural tone. If the pulse is monitored, severe bradycardia is noted, with a transient rate as low as 15 beats per minute. Asystole up to 50 seconds has been reported. When the limpness lasts more than a few seconds or the child's head is elevated, a generalized convulsion, which typically lasts less than a minute, may

occur and may be followed by a postictal state. The child's color returns at the end of the unconsciousness. If the child should begin to rise (or be carried head up) too quickly, the sequence to unconsciousness may recur.

DIFFERENTIAL DIAGNOSIS

Breath-holding spells are one cause of recurrent seizures. Diagnostic difficulties occur in separating such spells from epilepsy and febrile seizures. In the small group of children with congenital cardiac disease, it is important to distinguish *tet* spells (as seen in tetralogy of Fallot).

Epileptic seizures rarely are provoked by emotional or external stimuli. Although small children with epilepsy may suddenly fall and have a seizure, it is important to note if the child was frightened by the fall or sustained an injury immediately before the spell.

When a brief, uncomplicated generalized seizure occurs during a febrile illness, the physician usually diagnoses a febrile convulsion. Febrile illnesses probably also reduce the seizure threshold for other types of convulsions, including those from breath-holding spells. In the infant with cyanotic heart disease (especially tetralogy of Fallot), paroxysmal attacks of dyspnea and increased cyanosis may occur as a result of spasm of the right ventricular outflow tract and diminished pulmonary circulation. The onset of a *tet* spell may be spontaneous or may be brought on by crying, feeding, or straining at bowel movement. The spell may cause marked hypoxia and convulsions. It resolves over minutes to hours and should be treated acutely by putting the infant in the knee–chest position, giving O_2, and injecting morphine and bicarbonate. Correct diagnosis and prompt treatment are critical (see Chap. 194).

WORK-UP

A careful history is the cornerstone of the diagnosis. As with the evaluation of any paroxysmal event, it is important to elicit the details that preceded the spell (e.g., environmental occurrences, child's actions, or parental actions), the sequence of events during the spell, and the nature of the postspell behavior. A mild trauma, fright, or frustration precedes all breath-holding spells. In the cyanotic type, crying is prominent, in contrast to the brief whimper heard in the pallid variety. In the cyanotic type, the cyanosis occurs prior to the seizure, whereas the occasional cyanosis of epilepsy occurs later in the seizure. In the pallid type, a child has often fallen to the ground and then stands or is carried over an adult's shoulder. In minor cyanotic or pallid spells, the child simply becomes limp, but more severe spells include typical tonic-clonic (generalized) convulsions.

The standard physical and neurologic examinations are not generally helpful. Most children appear perfectly healthy, although lethargy may be present immediately after the spell. The physician should check factors that predispose to syncope, such as pallor, pulse, blood pressure, fever, and hydration state. With regard to the differential diagnosis of other causes of seizures, the physician should look for signs of neurocutaneous diseases (e.g., hypopigmented macules, shagreen patches, café-au-lait spots, other nevi); he should also examine optic fundi, palpate the fontanel, measure the head circumference, and evaluate for hepatosplenomegaly.

Laboratory testing may be avoided when a clear picture has emerged from the history and physical examinations. When necessary, blood may be drawn for CBC and simple chemistries (e.g., sodium, BUN, glucose, calcium) to rule out anemia and metabolic causes of seizures. An EEG is a helpful adjunctive test in evaluating for epilepsy; however, the history is more important, and it must be remembered that up to 3% of normal children may have epileptiform abnormalities on EEG. If an EGG is obtained during a breath-holding attack, a high voltage slowing is noted during the hypoxic–ischemic phase. In rare instances (in the differential diagnosis of epilepsy), a CT or MRI scan of the brain is indicated when there are abnormal neurologic findings, an atypical history, or a focal EEG abnormality. Some experienced physicians will perform an evocative test under ECG monitoring as part of the physical examination: firm, gentle ocular compression evokes bradycardia in most children with pallid spells, and a complete spell with convulsion may follow. A good history, however, generally provides an accurate enough diagnosis to avoid the ocular compression test.

MANAGEMENT

Cyanotic breath-holding spells are best managed by counseling the care-giver to avoid preventable frustrations and confrontations with the child. In this manner, the crying that precedes the spell will be avoided. The child should adhere to nap and bedtime routines. If a potential tantrum begins, the care-giver should walk out of sight in an effort to interrupt the child's focus on secondary gain from the care-giver. For the care-giver who wants to keep the child in view, care should be taken to avoid reinforcement of the child's behavior. If a cyanotic spell with seizure occurs, routine seizure advice should be heeded: Keep the child horizontal with the head turned toward the side to avoid pooling of saliva in the posterior pharynx.

Pallid spells should also be managed by attempting to avoid situations that produce sudden frights or minor physical trauma. When the fright or trauma occurs, the child should be kept supine in an effort to prevent exacerbating the cerebral ischemia. This is an effective treatment in many cases. Thus, the susceptible child should not be comforted in the standard parental hug position with the child's head upright at the parent's shoulder. Children who have frequent pallid spells may be treated effectively with vagolytic agents; however, the need for such treatment is rare, and there is no widely established regimen. Atropine sulfate

0.01 mg/kg/dose or hyoscyamine (Levsin solution or elixir) may be used b.i.d. to q.i.d.

PATIENT EDUCATION

The aforementioned counseling measures are important in treating breath-holding spells. In addition, it is imperative to reassure parents that the spells are benign, that they do not predispose to epilepsy, and that they resolve typically in early childhood.

ANNOTATED BIBLIOGRAPHY

DiMario F, Chee C, Berman P: Pallid breath-holding spells: Evaluation of the autonomic nervous system. Clin Pediatr 29:17–24, 1990. (Demonstrates mild autonomic differences between pallid breath-holders and controls.)

Gordon N: Breath-holding spells. Dev Med Child Neurol 29:811–814, 1987. (Brief, well-written review of the subject.)

Laxdal T, Gomez MR, Reiher J: Cyanotic and pallid syncopal attacks in children (breath-holding spells). Dev Med Child Neurol 11:755–763, 1969. (Descriptive retrospective series of 150 children with prolonged follow-up results.)

Lombroso CT, Lerman P: Breathholding spells (cyanotic and pallid infantile syncope). Pediatrics 39:563–581, 1967. (Large prospective and retrospective study including incidence figures, descriptive findings, and case reports; includes use of the ocular compression test with ECG and EEG monitoring.)

McGee JP, Saidel DH: Individual behavior therapy. In Harrison S, Noshpitz J (eds): Basic Handbook of Child Psychiatry, Vol 3, Chap 5, pp 98–99. New York, Basic Books, 1979. (Gives a brief discussion of behavior modification techniques as applied to tantrums.)

McWilliam RC, Stephenson JBP: Atropine treatment of reflex anoxic seizures. Arch Dis Child 59:473–485, 1984. (Documents success of anticholinergic therapy in pallid spells.)

213

Home Medical Care

Edward S. Gross

In recent years there has been an enormous surge of interest in home care for patients with illnesses previously thought to require hospitalization. Much of this is, in effect, the transfer of modalities of care that were developed in pediatric hospitals. A major impetus for this shift is an appreciation of the therapeutic milieu, which permits a child to feel nurtured and hopeful and leads to more rapid recovery from acute illness or better survival in a chronic condition. Being at home often is the best means of providing this therapeutic requirement.

Another important influence has been the cost of care. Both private and public third-party payers in the United States have placed limitations on the extent of reimbursement for hospital services based on diagnosis-related groups (DRGs). These efforts have been felt especially in the care of adults and have stimulated advances in home care for adults. Pediatric home care has been enriched by these advances, though not all of them are readily transferable to the particular care needs of children.

MODALITIES CURRENTLY AVAILABLE IN THE HOME SETTING

Infusion Therapy

The widespread use of the heparin lock has made intravenous therapy at home easy and liberating. Nursing agencies are widely available to support this modality. Home administration of fluids or medications is generally begun and supervised by specialist nurses; when a patient is hospitalized, it is useful to begin teaching the family how to manage the fluids and heparin flush. Patients fitted with heparin locks may often go about routine activities, including school attendance, while maintaining a therapy schedule. School nurses are often willing to assist in this effort, permitting administration of medications in school.

Peripheral vein catheters for long-term intravenous fluid administration have improved substantially in recent years and now are often left in place without change for weeks.

Respiratory Therapy

Chest physical therapy (CPT) is usually mastered by the parents (or even siblings) of children with chronic lung problems such as cystic fibrosis (CF) and bronchopulmonary dysplasia (BPD). With exacerbations, however, it is often helpful to have a respiratory therapist provide some of the treatments in order to assure that optimal intensity is given, as well as to refresh the family's knowledge and skills. These services are widely available.

Home administration of oxygen has long been available, largely because of the prevalence of chronic pulmonary disease in adults. The growing numbers of neonatal intensive care unit graduates with bronchopulmonary dysplasia have made pediatric home oxygen much more common in recent years. Support for this and related illnesses includes ongoing pulmonary function testing, oximetry, and monitoring devices for apnea and arrhythmias. Children on monitors may, of course, need intervention; hence, parent training in resuscitation techniques is an integral component of home cardiac or pulmonary monitoring.

Nutritional Services

Feeding through gastrostomy or nasogastric tubes has also long been available as a home therapy. More recently, total parenteral nutrition (TPN) with use of a pump and central venous access has become more widely available for home use, chiefly in the management of primary gastrointestinal problems or chemotherapy causing these problems. Central venous access can be obtained through the traditional, direct surgical approach to large central vessels or through the use of long catheters placed through peripheral veins. The latter have won wide acceptance in recent years because of their lack of reactivity and easier placement.

Rehabilitative Services

Programs designed to support rehabilitative programs after neurologic or orthopedic injury have become available from several agencies. Services of the rehabilitative hospital are offered without its environment, which can be daunting and discouraging to parents and can delay their becoming proficient in taking care of their child's needs. Neuropsychological assessment and physical and occupational therapy evaluations done at home are successfully performed by some suppliers of these services in the stability of the home setting.

Phototherapy

Equipment for performing phototherapy ranges from conventional light-boxes, used with the infant wearing eye patches and minimal clothing, to the "Wallaby," a fiberoptic mat placed next to the infant's skin and connected by fiberoptic cable to a light source, permitting the patient to be clothed, fed, and handled while still receiving therapy. Home phototherapy has provided a welcome solution to the conflict between a longer stay (and greater expense) in the hospital for an otherwise discharge-ready mother and the forced separation from a baby receiving phototherapy as an inpatient. If an infant requires close surveillance and if exchange transfusion is a real possibility, the home setting may not be best because of the time required for readmission, blood matching, and so on. Because most phototherapy occurs under low-risk conditions, most of it can be done at home (see also Chap. 195).

A sample protocol for home phototherapy is listed in Table 213-1. This, as well as the other guidelines that follow, assumes the 24-hour availability of a responsible person or agency if problems arise.

GUIDELINES FOR TRANSFER TO ACUTE HOME CARE

In determining when a patient should be considered for the Acute Home Care program, the physician should consider the following points. Since every patient is unique, these are not intended to serve as rigid criteria.

a. *Patient's overall condition.* The most important consideration is the *state of improvement of the patient* in

Table 213-1. Home Phototherapy Guidelines

	BILIRUBIN TREATMENT THRESHOLDS	
Age	*Bili (Indirect) for Home RX*	*Inpatient RX Only*
Term/Normal Risk Infant		
<24 hrs	10–14	15 or more
24–72 hrs	15–19	More than 19.0

At least once every 24 hours, evaluate jaundice, hydration and feeding status; repeat bilirubin (review blood type and Coombs', reticulocyte count, hemoglobin).

Increased Risk Group		
<24 hrs	NA	5 or more (NICU above 10)
24–48 hrs	5–9	10–14 (NICU if 15 or more)
48–72 hrs	10–14	15 or more
>72 hrs	15–19	Above 19

NICU = neonatal intensive care unit.

Home phototherapy is excluded if: feeding adequacy questionable; poor care-giving skills; questionable home situation; reticulocyte count 10% or more; Rh incompatibility.

Increased risk group if: birth weight was below 2500 g; hemolysis is present (positive Coombs'— ABO only); sepsis present.

relation to the condition on admission; if the patient presented for the first time today, would his or her overall condition (other than the need for continuing medication or fluids) require hospitalization? Could the care be managed at home?

b. *Fever.* Fever during the previous 24 hours ≥38.9°C (102.0°F) is a *relative* contraindication to transfer to home care. The source and significance of the fever should be acknowledged and discussed if transfer is contemplated.

c. *Hydration and fluid and electrolyte management.* A patient to be transferred home should be in good fluid balance and should have stable fluid and electrolyte requirements (i.e., the patient's clinical hydration and electrolyte status should require revision of fluid orders no more often than every 24 hours).

d. *Respiratory status.* Patients who require oxygen or who are having episodes of respiratory distress are not good candidates for home care transfer. Those who have established diagnoses of heart or chronic respiratory disease (e.g., BPD, CF) with supplemental oxygen requirements are exceptions. Their families may be accustomed to oxygen administration or may need to learn to give it.

One measure of respiratory status is respiratory rate at rest in room air. A resting rate approaching the normal range for age is a useful indication of the absence of distress. An alternative measurement of respiratory status, if available, is oximetry: O_2 saturation of 94% or more at rest in room air is evidence of adequately compensated respiratory function.

e. *Family capability and willingness.* Parents must appear competent to undertake home care. Parents should agree to the program and should sign the care

request. Staff and supports must be in place to manage the patient at home.

f. *Consultations with hospital staff.* House-staff physicians caring for the patient are often aware of issues not otherwise apparent and should be included in discussions of whether the patient is ready for transfer to home care.

Hospital house-staff physicians usually wish to be advised of patient outcome. A copy of the home care visits from the patient record can be sent to the house officer who cared for the patient.

g. *Age of the patient.* Guidelines usually apply only to children over 6 weeks of age. Newborns with these conditions require additional consultation by the appropriate subspecialist.

SPECIFIC ILLNESSES: TREATMENT PATTERNS

Acute Infectious Diseases

A number of acute infectious diseases requiring hospitalization can be expected to have a long convalescent course in an otherwise stable patient. Some of these conditions include osteomyelitis, septic arthritis, bacteremia, deep-tissue cellulitis (especially facial or buccal cellulitis and pre-septal or periorbital cellulitis), and bacterial meningitis. At our institution, in collaboration with the hospitals to which we send our ill patients, we have developed guidelines that permit much shorter hospital stays than in the past (see sample protocols at the end of this chapter). Patients whose illness appears to be following a predictable pattern are permitted to go home on intravenous medications as soon as they have turned a clinical corner toward recovery. The care of patients in this group involves daily assessments by a skilled nurse practitioner who provides case management, 24-hour availability for parental concerns, and coordination of care with the pediatrician and IV nursing service. It is not required that the patient be afebrile or fully convalescent; however, the child must be able to tolerate oral fluids and able to maintain the intravenous connection (usually with a heparin lock).

Management of meningitis in the home setting has been the most controversial of these illnesses. Additional experience must be gained before this debate is settled. However, advances in antibiotic technology may create newer issues that supplant the current concerns. If, for example, the cerebrospinal fluid (CSF) can reliably be sterilized in only a few days, and patients have not yet recovered from the effects of localized brain swelling, then the need for supportive care may continue beyond the need for antimicrobial therapy. Under these circumstances, the focus of attention will be the patient's ability to tolerate supports at home (rather than to be given critically necessary antibiotic doses on schedule).

Patients receiving intravenous medications need a schedule of regular contact with a skilled clinician for evaluation of recovery, review of the overall condition, a search for complications of disease or therapy, and planning for necessary rehabilitative steps, such as resumption of activities. Some programs provide ongoing assessments in conjunction with delivery and administration of medications. In other programs, the physician is expected to plan for and provide these services, some of which can be obtained through skilled nurses, such as the Visiting Nurse Association.

Cystic Fibrosis

Patients with cystic fibrosis have had their lives lengthened and enhanced by a cycle of health interventions in addition to daily care. One component of this cycle is the periodic "clean-out" performed when a deterioration of the patient's clinical condition occurs or is anticipated. The care in the hospital usually entails intravenous antibiotics and, often, intensive chest physical therapy and inhalation therapy, along with individual measures needed by a particular patient. The hospital has traditionally been the setting for this care, but in recent years many CF programs have shifted the bulk of routine "clean-outs" to the home setting. In many communities the Cystic Fibrosis Foundation has become a vendor of these services. Receiving care at home greatly reduces the interruptions in a patient's and family's lives, and the concomitant feelings of isolation and inferiority (see also Chap. 171).

Chemotherapy

Chemotherapy patients profit greatly from home modalities, which may include infusion pumps for management of chronic pain as well as parenteral nutrition and chemotherapy. Drug interactions can be problematic; it is helpful

for the family to have access to a knowledgeable pharmacist. Here, as with AIDS and other chronic life-threatening illnesses, a physician should be available to the family at all times to assess unusual events or reactions and to institute changes or hospitalization if needed. The primary care physician or team manages the care of these patients, who are continually moving between home and hospital, clinic and office. Their sense of despair and overwhelming illness can, to some extent, be offset by providing as much care as possible at home.

Technology-Dependent

Technology-dependent children have a variety of deficits requiring long-term ventilator use or tracheostomies with oxygen. They have generally been cared for in hospitals, but recent studies have demonstrated the cost-effectiveness of home care. The experience of home care for infants on nasal-prong oxygen for bronchopulmonary dysplasia has been excellent, as has been the experience of home care for technology-dependent children.

CONCERNS FOR THE PEDIATRICIAN

Insurance programs often have confusing limitations on home care based on the concept of home care as part of a convalescent process rather than as treatment or chronic care. It is therefore essential to be quite clear with insurance representatives about the plans and focus of a course of home care.

If infusion therapy is planned, it is essential to arrange for the inevitable failure of venous access. It is also desirable to have a backup for the home IV nurse. If a cut-down is needed to maintain venous access, who will do it? Where will it be done? In caring for active toddlers, it is often difficult to maintain venous access, and sometimes parents are less able than hospital personnel to restrain a child.

A patient undergoing care at home as an alternative to hospitalization is dependent upon the primary care physician for supervision and management. A suitable coverage arrangement is necessary when the primary physician is unavailable; the covering colleague should be ready to see a home care patient with the understanding that the home care patient is the equivalent of a hospitalized one and may need prompt intervention, more so than most ambulatory problems. It is also necessary to be more sensitive to questions and concerns voiced by the families of home care patients, who may be reluctant to take so much of a physician's time and attention. Parents may need to be encouraged to communicate concerns rather than to "tough it out" and risk serious consequences.

FRONTIERS OF HOME CARE

Computers and communications are expected to have an important impact on the ability to deliver care to patients at home in the near future. Measurements, such as pulmonary function tests and temperature, can be stored and compared, and appropriate warnings can be sent to the physician. Computer-based record systems permit central coordination of complex care, as, for example, in managing premature infants at home. Intake and output, cumulative drug doses, apnea and bradycardia, and so on, are easily stored on a computer and improve the effectiveness of the home as a care setting. Data from monitoring and tests can be fed to a central record whose clinician users will be able to review a patient's recent and past record in detail, from any location with a phone line, and make well-informed decisions.

Telephone devices permitting rapid and direct access to a central "nursing station" extend the notion of "home as hospital." These devices are already in use in some locations.

Antibiotic technology will also change home care in the future. Already, many illnesses that required parenteral antibiotics can be managed with drugs that achieve parenteral-like levels on oral administration (e.g., amoxicillin-clavulanate, trimethoprim-sulfamethoxazole). Rapid sterilization of body fluids with rapidly diffusing drugs has already been demonstrated with ceftriaxone in treating meningitis. This and similarly aggressive drugs can be expected to shorten the antibiotic-infusion component of hospitalizations for many acute infections and will lessen the need for home intravenous therapy.

Can patients recovering from surgery, such as uncomplicated appendectomy, be sent home from the recovery room with suitable monitors to send needed information to the surgeon? Will the physician of the next decade make rounds using a monitor screen and telephone? It is clear that many exciting innovations that will allow children and adults to recover from illness at home are on the horizon.

ANNOTATED BIBLIOGRAPHY

Committee on Infectious Diseases, American Academy of Pediatrics: Treatment of bacterial meningitis. Pediatrics 81:904–907, 1988. (Policy statement concerning the current overall approach to treatment, setting, and concerns in the management of common bacterial meningitis in children; home care for meningitis is advocated only in very carefully defined circumstances.)

Fields A, Rosenblatt A, Pollack M, Kaufman J: Home care cost-effectiveness for respiratory technology–dependent children. Am J Dis Child 145:729–733, 1991. (Demonstration of cost savings produced by home care [compared to hospital care] for children with a range of chronic illnesses who require a chronic respirator or tracheostomy plus oxygen support; discussion of Health Care Finance Agency and Medicaid coverage for home care.)

Peter G (ed): Q & A. Outpatient management of bacterial meningitis. Pediatr Infect Dis J 8:258–60, 1989. (Two authorities offer slightly differing approaches to patient selection for out-of-hospital management for the postacute days of treatment of bacterial meningitis in children.)

Rosenfeld W, Twist P, Concepcion L: A new device for phototherapy. Pediatr Res 25:272A, 1989. (First published description of the fiberoptic mat device for phototherapy.)

Schoumacher R: Saving money with home care. Am J Dis Child 145:725, 1991. (Editorial comment on the achievements and prospects in home care of respiratory technology–dependent children; discussion of drawbacks and needed studies related to home care, particularly for prolonged periods.)

Home Care Guidelines for Select Infectious Diseases

BACTERIAL MENINGITIS (*Haemophilus,* meningococcal, pneumococcal)

1. Irritability: Patient is tolerant of handling by parent, as necessary for care at home. Patient is able to be fed by parent.
2. Mental status: Patient is generally alert with no severe changes in level of irritability or alertness.
   An evolving neurological abnormality (e.g., changing or unstable motor loss or cranial nerve palsy) requires caution until fully evaluated or stable.
3. Overall "toxicity," lack of interaction, and poor responsiveness: improved from admission, nearly absent.
4. SIADH: if present and unresolved, fluids ordered for home infusion should reflect appropriate restriction, and measurement of sodium (daily) and urinary specific gravity (most voids) is needed.
5. Vomiting: Volume and frequency not sufficient to require changes in IV fluid replacement more often than once every 24 hours.
6. Bacteriology: Causative organism sensitive to antibiotics selected for use in home program.
7. Rifampin prophylaxis: In cases of *Haemophilus* or meningococcal meningitis, rifampin prophylaxis for appropriate contacts, including those who will care for the child at home, should be in progress or completed before child transfers to home setting.
8. Usual duration of therapy in uncomplicated cases is 10 days for *Haemophilus* and pneumococcal disease, 7 days for meningococcal; in unusual circumstances, therapy may be prolonged (see also Chap. 153).

PNEUMONIA

1. Respiratory status: Improvement from admission; no oxygen requirement (except in patients with established chronic disease requiring oxygen for home maintenance); no need for suctioning; no bouts of distress or cyanosis.

2. Respiratory physical therapy can usually be continued at home by parents or, if necessary, by home care providers (vendors).
3. Duration of therapy based on severity of illness and rate of recovery; usually 7–10 days overall, part of course may be PO (see also Chap. 169).

CELLULITIS (DEEP TISSUE, OTHER THAN PERIORBITAL OR BUCCAL)

1. Fever: Follow guidelines of clinician.
2. Overall "toxicity," lack of interaction, and poor responsiveness: improved from admission, nearly absent.
3. Usual course of therapy is 7–10 days. Oral antibiotics may be used after a definite clinical response has been observed on IV therapy; however, it is important to be sure that the PO doses provide blood levels comparable to those of IV.

PERIORBITAL AND BUCCAL CELLULITIS

1. Fever, hydration: Follow "routine" guidelines.
2. Overall "toxicity" improved from admission.
3. If lumbar puncture was performed during initial evaluation and CSF culture is negative, treat for 7–10 days, according to cellulitis protocol. If positive or if no LP was done, treat patient as for meningitis, for 10–14 days.
4. Patient established on, and responsive to, medications with appropriate penetration for parameningeal focus, such as parenteral ampicillin or ceftriaxone; parenteral or PO chloramphenicol in meningitis doses.

Discuss with infectious disease (ID) service if any doubt regarding appropriateness or duration of therapy (see also Chap. 95).

BACTEREMIA, CULTURE POSITIVE

1. Fever: Follow "routine"guidelines.
2. No clinical evidence or meningitis, pericarditis, septic arthritis, or osteomyelitis.
3. Patient established on, and responsive to, medications with appropriate penetration for proven bacteremia, such as parenteral ampicillin or ceftriaxone; parenteral or PO chloramphenicol; doses appropriate for bacteremia.
4. Usual course of therapy: For Haemophilus influenzae, pneumococcus or meningococcus: 7–10 days. P.O. therapy possible, depending on organism. Consult with infectious disease service for duration of treatment of other organisms.

Discuss with ID service if any doubt regarding choice or duration of therapy (see also Chap. 198).

OSTEOMYELITIS

1. Patient has completed appropriate initial evaluation in hospital: Surgical evaluation, biopsy, debridement as indicated.
2. Patient established on, and responsive to, appropriate antibiotic therapy. No increasing pain, joint limitation, or other suggestions of clinical failure of therapy.
3. Consult with orthopedist service to ascertain that there is no requirement for continued hospitalization on surgical grounds, such as additional biopsy, additional sites of infection to be evaluated, bony abnormalities, debridement, or chronic foci.
4. Orthopedic physician contacted, agrees with management plans, and is available for backup.
5. Usual course of therapy is 4 weeks, part of which may be PO Switching to PO medication is often done after a week or more of IV therapy, but it is essential to assure that the PO medication and dose provide adequate blood levels. This may be predicted from available references. Consult with ID service if there is any doubt.
6. Chronic and recurrent osteomyelitis are special circumstances requiring consultation with infectious disease service to design therapeutic plan.

Note: The sedimentation rate, usually used to follow progress in patients with osteomyelitis and septic arthritis, usually does not improve in the first week of therapy. A rising sedimentation rate implies treatment failure or complications and requires reevaluation by the orthopedic specialist and possible readmission.

SEPTIC ARTHRITIS

1. Patient has completed appropriate initial evaluation in hospital: Surgical evaluation, joint immobilization, aspiration, and drainage as indicated.
2. Patient established on, and responsive to, appropriate antibiotic therapy. No increasing pain, joint limitation, or other suggestions of clinical failure of therapy.
3. Consult with orthopedist service to ascertain that there is no requirement for continued hospitalization on surgical grounds, such as continuing need for joint drainage procedures or further measures to secure immobilization.
4. Orthopedic physician contacted, agrees with management plans, and is available for backup.
5. Usual course of therapy is three weeks, part of which may be PO Switching to PO medication is often done after a week or more of IV therapy, but it is essential to assure that the PO medication and dose provide adequate blood levels. Consult with ID service if there is any doubt.

See note on sedimentation rate under Osteomyelitis.

214

Perioperative Management of Ambulatory Pediatric Surgical Patients

Victor C. Baum and
Corrie T.M. Anderson

There are approximately three million operations each year on pediatric patients. Economic, psychological, and infectious disease factors have led to the increase in the number of pediatric patients having outpatient surgery in the last decade. Currently, up to 60% of pediatric operations are performed as outpatient procedures. This chapter focuses on several specific issues that may face the primary care physician whose patient is to be scheduled for elective outpatient surgery.

Retention of secretions, the production of which is increased with an upper respiratory infection (URI), is likely to occur in the presence of a weak cough, predisposing the patient to airway plugging and atelectasis. It is generally assumed that avoiding endotracheal intubation of the airway will decrease the frequency of untoward events.

The differences between children and adults in chest wall compliance and functional residual capacity (on a surface area basis) predispose infants more than adults to the risks of developing hypoxemia under general anesthesia. In addition, the composition of the diaphragm and intercostal muscles differs between children and adults. These muscles in children have less type 1 slow-twitch muscle than do adults, meaning that they cannot sustain the increased work of breathing as well as can adults.

THE PATIENT WITH AN UPPER RESPIRATORY INFECTION

Upper respiratory infections (URIs) are very common in the pediatric population. Often, elective cases are canceled if a patient has, or has recently had, symptoms of a URI. Several studies have demonstrated an increased risk of cough, laryngospasm, pneumonia, atelectasis, and hypoxemia when surgery is performed in these patients. Multiple cancellations due to the high incidence of URI can wreak havoc with surgical schedules but, more important, can create scheduling problems for families and emotional problems for children. Thus, several studies have tried to define appropriate criteria to distinguish between a URI and a chronic or other noninfectious condition. At least two studies have shown that children with a URI who have general anesthesia but are not intubated (e.g., for tympanostomy

tubes) have no increased morbidity. Although they may have an increased incidence of mild arterial desaturation (O_2 saturation <95%) on arrival in the recovery room, they have no increase in major hypoxemic events (O_2 saturation <85%).

Differentiating infections from noninfectious causes of URI-like symptoms may be difficult. One set of widely quoted criteria is that of Tait and Knight. Symptoms identified in this study as qualifying as a URI included any combination of two symptoms from the following list, except as noted in #8.

1. Sore or scratchy throat
2. Sneezing
3. Rhinorrhea
4. Congestion
5. Malaise
6. Nonproductive cough
7. Fever less than 101°F
8. Combinations of 1 & 5, 2 & 3, 3 & 6, or 4 & 6 required one additional symptom from #1 to #7 for diagnosis of a URI.

The history and physical examination are most helpful in ruling in or ruling out a URI. Other family members may have symptoms or may have just gotten over symptoms. An afebrile child with a clear discharge most likely has allergic rhinitis and has no increased anesthetic risk. The presence of grunting, flaring, or accessory muscle use suggests the presence of lower respiratory tract involvement. Wheezing from whatever cause is reason to cancel an elective operation. Laboratory data such as pulmonary function tests, arterial blood gas analysis, and oximetry are not predictive and are not practical as screening modalities.

Several questions need to be addressed if a diagnosis of respiratory tract infection is made. "Is this elective surgery?" If it is not elective, then every effort should be made to improve the patient's clinical condition prior to surgery. This may include chest physiotherapy, bronchodilator therapy, humidified oxygen, and so forth. If the surgery can be performed without having to intubate the patient, the surgery may proceed, because this method of airway control does not appear to carry the same risk of airway irritation. If the anesthetic cannot be performed without intubation, or if a regional anesthetic technique cannot be used, then one must be prepared for the possibility of major airway obstruction occurring during the perioperative period. From this follows the second question: "What is the understanding of the patient, surgeon, and parent of the risks?" These risks should be discussed frankly so the family is not caught by surprise. If the child will require endotracheal intubation for an elective case that can be delayed, then it should be postponed. Studies indicate that the optimal timing of the surgery is a minimum of 6 weeks after the disappearance of lower tract symptoms and 2 to 4 weeks after the last upper tract symptoms have abated. This allows for a safe surgery when optimal pulmonary conditions are likely to be present, because airway ciliary cells have been repaired and the tendency for bronchoconstriction has passed.

Communication between the parent, pediatrician, anesthesiologist, and surgeon will help to facilitate the best care for the patient. If there are any concerns, they should be addressed as soon as possible (e.g., the anesthesiologist should be called in advance). This will allow optimal preoperative care and will prevent unexpected last-minute cancellations.

THE PRETERM INFANT

In general, younger children are at a higher risk of morbidity and mortality during the perioperative period. With advances in medical technology, the survival rate of preterm infants continues to increase. The major questions surrounding the care of these premature infants address adequate pain control, risks of respiratory compromise, and possible postoperative apnea.

Pain is a highly subjective and extremely variable phenomenon. Preverbal children, especially newborns, are at a severe disadvantage because of their inability to communicate the extent of their suffering. Attitudes among physicians, nurses, and lay personnel based on misconceptions about addiction, safety, and the postulated immature physiological system of the preterm infant have acted as barriers to the delivery of adequate pain control to the preverbal child. Anatomical, biochemical, physiological, and behavioral aspects of the preterm infant indicate the existence of an intact neurophysiological system capable of responding to nociceptive (painful) stimuli. Additionally, preterm infants demonstrate metabolic catabolism if not treated with optimal anesthesia, which can be harmful to a developing newborn.

Another barrier to adequate pain relief in newborns is the erroneous belief that they do not remember the pain and thus it will have no effect on them. Current evidence suggests that the basic reactive components of the emotion of fear are present at birth and are activated by nociceptive stimuli. Thus, adequate pain control during the perioperative period is imperative for the newborn.

Prematurity is accompanied by undeveloped lung parenchyma and an immature respiratory control system. These children are at greater risk for developing bronchopulmonary dysplasia (BPD), pulmonary infections, and respiratory control problems. These infants have numerous clinical problems because of their disease. Their response to hypoxia is depressed, their neurologic control of breathing is abnormal, and their response to ventilatory stress (i.e., infection or anesthesia) is limited.

There is a difference between adults and infants in the control of ventilation. The differences in both the neural control and the mechanics of the respiratory system influence the response to anesthesia and the recovery from an-

esthesia. Preterm infants, as well as some term infants, are subject to episodes of periodic breathing and apnea. Premature infants have an increased risk of apnea after general anesthesia. In addition, there are frequent postoperative hypoxic episodes that go unnoticed in the recovery room and during transport. Postoperative apnea has even been noted in a full-term infant. Premature infants have been found to tolerate the work of breathing poorly because of the incomplete development and growth of their skeletal muscles. It does not appear from the most recent studies that the presence of preoperative apnea or the absence of apnea in the premature infant reliably predicts the postoperative risk of apnea. In addition, preoperative pneumocardiographic studies are unable to foretell future apneic episodes.

An infant with a history of BPD or a preterm infant undergoing surgery should have a careful history and physical examination. A history of long-term intubation or oxygen requirement or a history of apnea should alert the physician to possible postoperative problems. The respiratory pattern should be noted on physical examination. If the infant has labored breathing, the stress of surgery and anesthetic agents may place him or her at more risk. In the case of an infant with BPD, a recent chest x-ray, hematocrit, and arterial blood gas should be obtained. A PaO_2 less than 88 is indicative of pulmonary disease. The recommendations for transfusion vary with each institution, surgeon, and anesthesiologist. The hematocrit at which the infant is to be transfused should be discussed with all concerned individuals prior to surgery. Diuretics, bronchodilators, and supplemental oxygen therapy may be beneficial. The medications the patient is taking will help direct preoperative laboratory studies ordered.

Apnea is clearly the major risk to young ex-premature infants who are at home and return for a minor surgical procedure. There have been no definitive studies to determine the exact age at which the risk of apnea is abolished. Practice varies between institutions. The most conservative recommendations are that premature infants should have elective surgery delayed until they are greater than 60 weeks postconception. Term infants should have elective surgery delayed until they are 44 weeks postconception. For nonelective surgery, if the above criteria are not met, infants should be monitored with an apnea monitor for 12 to 18 hours postoperation. If apneic episodes occur, monitoring should continue for at least 12 hours after the last apneic episode. Fatigue of the respiratory musculature is also a potential contributor to the respiratory depression seen in premature infants. The option of regional anesthesia without supplemental intravenous agents such as midazolam or ketamine appears to offer a safe alternative for the premature infant and the infant with BPD.

Postoperatively, the infant with BPD should be given supplemental oxygen therapy and should be monitored with pulse oximetry. Intraoperative use of a local anesthetic can obviate the need for opiates and thus limit the child's exposure to their side effects. Diuretics and bronchodilator therapy should be given when warranted.

PREOPERATIVE FASTING

A major potential risk of anesthesia is aspiration of gastric contents into the lungs. This risk is related to both gastric pH (pH <2.5) and gastric volume (>0.4 ml/kg). The usual approach has been a prolonged period of fasting, typically 4 hours in newborns and young infants, 6 hours in children under 3 years of age, and 8 hours in children 3 years of age and older. It was assumed that this would assure an empty stomach at the time of induction of anesthesia. Unfortunately, it also meant that those children typically began surgery with a fluid deficit, were irritable because they were hungry or thirsty, and occasionally had surgery canceled because of inadvertent feeding during the period of fasting. Fortunately for all concerned, several recent studies in children have shown that a fast of only 2 hours after *clear* liquids is all that is needed. In fact, gastric volumes were lower in these children than they were in children with a protracted fast. This 2-hour period is just for clear liquids and does not apply to children needing emergency surgery. The child who has had solid food 2 hours before surgery will still find surgery delayed or canceled.

PREOPERATIVE TESTS

Until recently, a preoperative hematocrit and urinalysis were required of all surgical patients, and additional tests were required of many patients. Recent work has resulted in a significant modification of these requirements, based on conclusions that routine random testing:

a. cannot be demonstrated to improve postoperative morbidity, mortality, or length of hospital stay
b. does not result in the discovery of significant abnormalities that would not have been uncovered by the history and physical examination
c. results in pursuing and treating borderline and false-positive laboratory abnormalities
d. results in abnormal test results not pursued, posing a medicolegal risk
e. results in operating room delays when borderline or false-positive results become available shortly before surgery
f. most often would not affect conduction of a safe anesthetic, even if a positive laboratory finding were noted

These findings have been documented in pediatric and adult patients. Although specific requirements may vary in individual hospitals, more and more centers are discon-

tinuing mandatory preoperative hematocrits and urinalyses for routine surgery in otherwise healthy pediatric ambulatory patients. UCLA Medical Center, for example, does not require a urinalysis for any ambulatory pediatric patients and does not require a hematocrit for boys or premenarcheal girls. These recommendations have been instituted, in part, by noting that patients, even without chronic anemia, tolerate low hematocrits much better than was previously thought, making the previous recommendation of a minimum hematocrit of 30% invalid. Healthy adults, for instance, do not raise their cardiac output dramatically until their hemoglobin is less than 7 g/dl or their hematocrit is below 21%. The inutility of routine preoperative chest x-rays has been known for several years, and they are therefore not routinely required now.

These guidelines apply only to healthy children scheduled for routine ambulatory surgery. Children with an underlying disease should be evaluated and have appropriate preoperative testing as dictated by their disease. Similarly, pediatric patients scheduled for "same-day admission" surgery might require a hematocrit if the planned surgery is major and might result in significant blood loss.

ANNOTATED BIBLIOGRAPHY

Anand KJS, Sippell WG, Aynsley-Green A: Randomized trial of fentanyl anaesthesia in preterm babies undergoing surgery: Effects on the stress response. Lancet i:243–248, 1987. (One of a series evaluating the perioperative stress response in young infants.)

Cohen MM, Cameron CB: Should you cancel the operation when a child has an upper respiratory infection? Anesth Analg 72:282–288, 1991. (Study [using a large data base] documenting increased risk of perioperative respiratory complications in children with URIs.)

Cote CJ: NPO after midnight for children—A reappraisal. Anesthesiology 75:589–592, 1990. (Well-referenced editorial reviewing the lack of need for a prolonged preoperative fast.)

Dalens B, Hasnasoui A: Caudal anesthesia in pediatric surgery: Success rate and adverse effects in 750 consecutive patients. Anesth Analg 68:83–89, 1989. (Report on regional anesthesia in pediatrics; regional anesthesia is being used more and more as the primary anesthetic or in conjunction with general anesthesia.)

Kurth CD, Spitzer AR, Broennle AM, Downes JJ: Post-operative apnea in pre-term infants. Anesthesiology 66:483–488, 1987. (Study documenting the incidence and period of risk of postoperative apnea in preterm infants.)

Tait AR, Knight PR: The effects of general anesthesia on upper respiratory tract infections in children. Anesthesiology 67:930–935, 1987. (Frequently referenced paper evaluating general anesthesia risks in children with URIs.)

Zeltzer LK, Anderson CTM, Schechter NL: Pediatric pain: Current status and new directions. Curr Probl Pediatr 20:409–486, 1990. (Discussion of issues, including postoperative pain management, in children.)

Appendix A

TRANSFER OF DRUGS AND OTHER CHEMICALS INTO HUMAN BREAST MILK*

Robert A. Dershewitz

Table 1. Drugs That Are Contraindicated During Breast-Feeding

DRUG	REPORTED SIGN OR SYMTPOM IN INFANT OR EFFECT ON LACTATION
Bromocriptine	Supresses lactation
Cocaine	Cocaine intoxication
Cyclophosphamide	Possible immune suppression; unknown effect on growth or association with carcinogenesis; neutropenia
Cyclosporine	Possible immune suppression; unknown effect on growth or association with carcinogenesis
Doxorubicin	Possible immune suppression; unknown effect on growth or association with carcinogenesis
Ergotamine	Vomiting, diarrhea, convulsions (doses used in migraine medications)
Lithium	⅓ to ½ therapeutic blood concentration in infants
Methotrexate	Possible immune suppression; unknown effect on growth or association with carcinogenesis; neutropenia
Phencyclidine (PCP)	Potent hallucinogen
Phenindione	Anticoagulant; increased prothrombin and partial thromboplastin time in 1 infant (not used in USA)

Table 2. Drugs of Abuse That Are Contraindicated During Breast-Feeding

DRUG	EFFECT
Amphetamine	Irritability, poor sleep pattern
Cocaine	Cocaine intoxication
Heroin	
Marijuana	Only one report in literature; no effect mentioned
Nicotine (smoking)	Shock, vomiting, diarrhea, rapid heart rate, restlessness; decreased milk production
Phencyclidine	Potent hallucinogen

*Adapted from Pediatrics 84:924–931, 1989. Reprinted with permission from the American Academy of Pediatrics.

Table 3.   Radiopharmaceuticals That Require Temporary Cessation of Breast-Feeding*

DRUG	RECOMMENDED ALTERATION IN BREAST-FEEDING PATTERN
Gallium-67 (^{67}Ga)	Radioactivity in milk present for 2 wk
Indium-111 (^{111}In)	Small amount present at 20 h
Iodine-125 (^{125}I)	Risk of thyroid cancer; radioactivity in milk present for 12 d
Iodine-131 (^{131}I)	Radioactivity in milk present 2–14 d depending on study
Radioactive sodium	Radioactivity in milk present 96 h
Technetium-99m (^{99m}TC), ^{99m}Tc macroaggregates, ^{99m}TcO$_4$	Radioactivity in milk present 15 h to 3 d

*Consult nuclear medicine physician before performing diagnostic study so that a radionuclide with the shortest excretion time in breast milk can be used. Before study, the mother should pump her breast and store enough milk in freezer for feeding the infant; after study, the mother should pump her breast to maintain milk production but discard all milk pumped for the required time that radioactivity is present in milk.

Table 4.   Drugs Whose Effect on Nursing Infants Is Unknown but May Be of Concern

DRUG	EFFECT
Psychotropic drugs	Special concern when given to nursing mothers for long periods of time
Antianxiety	
Diazepam	None
Lorazepam	None
Prazepam	None
Quazepam	None
Antidepressant	
Amitriptyline	None
Amoxapine	None
Desipramine	None
Dothiepin	None
Doxepin	None
Imipramine	None
Trazodone	None
Trazodone	None
Antipsychotic	
Chlorpromazine	Galactorrhea in adult; drowsiness and lethargy in infant
Chlorprothixene	None
Haloperidol	None
Mesoridazine	None
Chloramphenicol	Possible idiosyncratic bone marrow suppression
Metoclopramide K	None described; potent central nervous system drug
Metronidazole	In vitro mutagen; may discontinue breast-feeding 12–24 h to allow excretion of dose when single-dose therapy given to mother
Tinidazole	See Metronidazole

Table 5.   Drugs That Have Caused Significant Effects on Some Nursing Infants and Should Be Given to Nursing Mothers With Caution

DRUG	EFFECT
Aspirin (salicylates)	Metabolic acidosis (dose related); may affect platelet function; rash
Clemastine	Drowsiness, irritability, refusal to feed, high-pitched cry, neck stiffness (1 case)
Phenobarbitol	Sedation; infantile spasms after weaning from milk containing phenobarbitol, methemoglobinemia (1 case)
Primidone	Sedation, feeding problems
Salicylazosulfapyridine (sulfasalazine)	Bloody diarrhea in 1 infant

Table 6.   Maternal Medication Usually Compatible With Breast-Feeding*

DRUG	REPORTED SIGN OR SYMPTOM IN INFANT OR EFFECT ON LACTATION
Anesthetics, Sedatives	
Alcohol	Drowsiness, diaphoresis, deep sleep, weakness, decrease in linear growth, abnormal weight gain; maternal ingestion of 1 g/kg daily decreases milk ejection reflex
Barbituate	See Table 5
Bromide	Rash, weakness, absence of cry with maternal intake of 5.4 g/d
Chloral hydrate	Sleepiness
Chloroform	None
Halothane	None
Lidocaine	None
Magnesium sulfate	None
Methyprylon	Drowsiness
Secobarbital	None
Thiopental	None
Anticoagulants	
Bishydroxcoumarin	None
Warfarin	None
Antiepileptics	
Carbamazepine	None
Ethosuximide	None; drug appears in infant serum
Phenobarbital	See Table 5
Phenytoin	Methemoglobinemia (1 case)
Primidone	See Table 5
Thiopental	None
Valporic acid	None
Antihistamines, decongestants, and bronchodilators	
Dexbrompheniramine maleate with *d*-isoephedrine	Crying, poor sleep patterns, irritability
Dyphylline	None
Iodides	May affect thyroid activity; see Miscellaneous, iodine
Pseudoephedrine	None
Terbutaline	None
Theophylline	Irritability
Triprolidine	None
Antihypertensive and cardiovascular drugs	
Acebutolol	None
Atenolol	None
Captopril	None
Digoxin	None
Diltiazem	None
Disopyramide	None
Hydralazine	None
Labetalol	None
Lidocaine	None
Methyldopa	None
Metoprolol	None
Mexiletine	None
Minoxidil	None
Nadolol	None
Oxprenolol	None
Procainamide	None
Propranolol	None
Quinidine	None
Timolol	None
Verapamil	None
Antiinfective drugs (all antibiotics transfer into breast milk in limited amounts)	
Acyclovir	None
Amoxicillin	None

(continued)

Table 6. Maternal Medication Usually Compatible With Breast-Feeding* (*continued*)

DRUG	REPORTED SIGN OR SYMPTOM IN INFANT OR EFFECT ON LACTATION
Antiinfective drugs, *continued*	
Aztreonam	None
Cefadroxil	None
Cefazolin	None
Cefotaxime	None
Cefoxitin	None
Ceftazidine	None
Ceftriaxone	None
Chloroquine	None
Clindamycin	None
Cycloserine	None
Dapsone	None; sulfonamide detected in infant's urine
Erythromycin	None
Ethambutol	None
Hydroxychloroquine	None
Isoniazid	None; acetyl metabolite also secreted; ? hepatoxicity
Kanamycin	None
Moxalactam	None
Nalidixic acid	Hemolysis in infant with glucose-6-phosphate deficiency (G-6-PD)
Nitrofurantoin	Hemolysis in infant with G-6-PD
Pyrimethamine	None
Quinine	None
Rifampin	None
Salicylazosulfapyridine (sulfasalazine)	See Table 5
Streptomycin	None
Sulbactam	None
Sulfapyridine	Caution in infant with jaundice or G-6-PD, and in ill, stressed, or premature infant. Appears in infant's urine.
Sulfisoxazole	Caution in infant with jaundice or G-6-PD, and in ill, stressed, or premature infant. Appears in infant's urine.
Tetracycline	None; negligible absorption by infant
Ticarcillin	None
Trimethoprim/sulfamethoxazole	None
Antithyroid drugs	
Carbimazole	Goiter
Methimazole (active metabolite of carbimazole)	None
Propylthiouracil	None
Thiouracil	None mentioned; drug not used in USA
Cathartics	
Cascara	None
Danthron	Increased bowel activity
Senna	None
Diagnostic agents	
Iodine	Goiter; see Miscellaneous, iodine
Iopanoic acid	None
Metrizamide	None
Diuretic agents	
Bendroflumethiazide	Suppresses lactation
Chlorothiazide, hydrochlorothiazide	None
Chlorthalidone	Excreted slowly
Spironolactone	None
Hormones	
^{3}H-norethynodrel	None
19-norsteroids	None
Clogestone	None

(continued)

Table 6. Maternal Medication Usually Compatible With Breast-Feeding* (*continued*)

DRUG	REPORTED SIGN OR SYMPTOM IN INFANT OR EFFECT ON LACTATION
Hormones, *continued*	
Contraceptive pill with estrogen/progesterone	Rare breast enlargement; decrease in milk production and protein content (not confirmed in several studies)
Estradiol	Withdrawal, vaginal bleeding
Medroxyprogesterone	None
Prednisolone	None
Prednisone	None
Progesterone	None
Muscle relaxants	
Baclofen	None
Methocarbamol	None
Narcotics, nonnarcotic analgesics, anti-inflammatory agents	
Acetaminophen	None
Butorphanol	None
Codeine	None
Dipyrone	None
Flufenamic acid	None
Gold salts	None
Hydroxychloroquine	None
Ibuprofen	None
Indomethacin	Seizure (1 case)
Mefenamic acid	None
Methadone	None if mother receiving $\leq$ 20 mg/24 h
Morphine	None
Nefopam	None
Phenylbutazone	None
Piroxicam	None
Prednisolone, prednisone	None
Propoxyphene	None
Salicylates	See Table 5
Suprofen	None
Tolmetin	None
Stimulants	
Caffeine	Irritability, poor sleep pattern, excreted slowly; no effect with usual amount of caffeine beverages
Vitamins	
B₁ (thiamin)	None
B₆ (pyridoxine)	None
B₁₂	None
D	None; follow infant's serum calcium if mother receives pharmacologic doses
Folic acid	None
K₁	None
Riboflavin	None
Miscellaneous	
Acetazolamide	None
Atropine, scopolamine	None
Cimetidine	None
Cisapride	None
Cisplatin	Not found in milk
Domperidone	None
Iodine (povidone-iodine/vaginal douche)	Elevated iodine levels in breast milk, odor of iodine on infant's skin
Metoclopramide	See Table 4
Noscapine	None
Pyridostigmine	None
Tolbutamide	? Jaundice

*Drugs listed have been reported in the literature as having the effects listed or effect. The word "none" means that no observable change was seen in the nursing infant while the mother was ingesting the compound. It is emphasized that most of the literature concerns single case reports or small series of infants.

Table 7.   Food and Environmental Agents and Their Effect on Breast-Feeding

AGENT	REPORTED SIGN OR SYMPTOM IN INFANT OR EFFECT ON LACTATION
Aflatoxin	None
Aspartame	Caution if mother or infant has phenylketonuria
Bromide (photographic laboratory)	Potential absorption and bromide transfer into milk; see Table 6, Anesthetics, sedatives
Cadmium	None reported
Chlordane	None reported
Chocolate (theobromine)	Irritability or increased bowel activity if excess amounts (16 oz/d consumed by mother)
DDT, benzenehexachlorides, dieldrin, aldrin, hepatachlorepoxide	None
Fava beans	Hemolysis in patient with glucose-6-phosphate deficiency (G-6-PD)
Fluorides	None
Hexachlorobenzene	Skin rash, diarrhea, vomiting, dark urine, neurotoxicity, death
Hexachlorophene	None; possible contamination of milk from nipple washing
Lead	Possible neurotoxicity
Methyl mercury, mercury	May affect neurodevelopment
Monosodium glutamate (MSG)	None
Polychlorinated biphenyls and polybrominated biphenyls	Lack of endurance, hypotonia, sullen expressionless facies
Tetrachlorethylene-cleaning fluid (perchloroethylene)	Obstructive jaundice, dark urine
Vegetarian diet	Signs of B_{12} deficiency; see Chap. 15

Appendix B

AGE-APPROPRIATE TOYS

Lucinda Lee Katz

There are many video games, educational tapes, and family entertainment resources, including the computer, that are wonderful and invaluable. This appendix does not deal with technology as a resource.

BIRTH TO 24 MONTHS

Activities that encourage adult–child interaction

Activities that encourage large body movement—reaching, rolling, pulling

Activities that encourage batting, retrieving, mouthing, tracking, watching

Activities that encourage listening, sound making, turn taking

Activities that encourage problem solving, making relationships between ideas, people, places, and objects

Crib toys: peekaboo, crib gyms, rattles, key rings, teethers, busy boxes, mobiles, track and watch, flip fingers, small balls

Stuffed toys: teddy bears, monkeys, and other stuffed animals

Music boxes: Jack-in-the-box, mobiles, merry-go-music, animal wind-up music boxes

Rolling toys: water floating toys, Nerf and small rubber balls, flutter-balls, larger balls, plastic see-through toys

Pop-up toys: pop-up animals, Jack-in-the-ball, Jack-in-the-box

Blocks: soft blocks, unit blocks

Push and pull toys: corn poppers, vacuum cleaners, lawn bubbler, clatter-pillar

Pounding toys: pots and pans, peg pounders, hammer boards

Puzzles: large 2- to 10-piece puzzles

Housekeeping toys: telephones, cash registers, dress-up clothes, dolls

2 TO 5 YEARS

Activities that encourage problem solving

Activities that encourage fantasy play

Activities that encourage child-to-child and adult-to-child interactions

Activities that encourage multiple skill levels (e.g., scribbling an order for lunch, pretend making the food, serving the food to friend)

Activities that encourage observations of cause and effect, logic and order, strategy skills

Blocks; dress-up clothes; water play; sand play; wheel toys; superhero figures; small construction toys; Legos; books; pencils, paper, scissors, crayons, markers; dolls; stuffed animals; transformers; puzzles (10–300 pieces); simple board games; simple card games; simple group games; items for pretend play; paints; small collections of cars, animals, fantasy figures

5 TO 12 YEARS

Activities that encourage problem solving, strategy building, and multidimensional thinking

Activities that encourage child–group, child–child, child–adult interactions

Activities that encourage independence

Activities that encourage team, club, group activities

Board games; card games; group games that encourage rituals, rules, and specific roles; collections of baseball cards, stickers, stuffed animals, porcelain animal families, dolls, books, hats, cars; athletics; books; science and math activities; computers; bike riding; skateboards; swimming; skating; instruments; hobbies

12 YEARS TO ADULTHOOD

Activities that encourage depth and breadth of subject matter

Activities that encourage skill acquisition, problem solving, and multidimensional thinking

Activities that encourage more involvement with larger community

Activities that encourage friendship patterns, group activities, developing individual roles

Community service projects; clubs; international and national travel; long and short planned trips; tutoring; sports activities; intergenerational projects; apprenticeship in adult roles or hobbies and interest areas

Appendix C

AGE-APPROPRIATE BOOKS

Lucinda Lee Katz and Franny Billingsley

The books listed in this Appendix are not exhaustive. A more extensive guide to selecting books for children is *Choosing Books for Children: A Commonsense Guide*, by Betsy Hearne (Delacorte Press, New York, 1990). The following books are examples of age-appropriate books that we recommend.

BIRTH TO 18 MONTHS

Soft books (cloth and bath books) that infants can participate with—touch, crumple, chew, and so forth. Big simple shapes, bold primary colors, animal noises, and everyday objects with clear and simple pictures should be the focus. Try to avoid long texts and cartoon figures. Older baby can participate with "peekaboo" books such as Eric Hill's lift-the-flap *Where's Spot* series, or books that focus on touch and other senses, such as *Pat the Bunny*.

Board books should be simple and clear with objects to identify easily recognizable. Examples of two authors are Helen Oxenbury's big board book series *Clap Hands, Tickle, Tickle All Fall Down*, and *Say Goodnight* and Fiona Pragoff's beautifully photographed series that includes *Growing* and *Colors*.

Lyrical language books expose the child to the music of our language, such as nursery rhymes, song books, and poem books. The books should have bright illustrations or photographs, such as Aliki's *Hush Little Baby*, Bruce McMillan's *Mary Had a Little Lamb*, and Bruce Degen's *Jamberry*.

Story books that encourage making relationships with people, places, ideas, and objects, such as Ruth Bornstein's *Little Gorilla* and Eric Carle's *The Very Hungry Caterpillar*.

18 MONTHS TO 3 YEARS

Nursery rhymes, picture books with a short story line or repetition of an idea, cumulative folktales, choral-response stories and songs, simple poems, finger-plays, conversational books, goodnight books. Books in this category should have a short story line, with clear and simple illustrations that emphasize the beauty of language. Books should be sturdy so that young children can handle the books and feel some ownership of the book.

Books to encourage listening, singing, talking, and repetition, such as Margaret Mahy's *17 Kings and 42 Elephants*, Bill Martin Jr.'s *Barn Dance!*, and Charlotte Pomerantz's *The Piggy in the Puddle*.

Books that encourage building from simple ideas to more complex relationships of people, places, ideas, and objects. Examples include *A House Is a House for Me*, by Mary Ann Hoberman, and Ezra Jack Keat's *The Snowy Day*.

Books that encourage repetition of ideas, words, and sentence building, such as *The Napping House*, by Audrey and Don Wood, and Michael Rosen and Helen Oxenbury's *We're Going on a Bear Hunt*.

3 TO 5 YEARS

Books in this category should have a simple story line with clear illustrations, although the plot should be more complicated and the characters more detailed. Simple chapter books can be introduced at this age. Reading aloud is pleasurable for a child this age.

Books that encourage reading aloud, storytelling, and story dramatization. These might include Barbara Cooney's *Miss Rumphius*, Debra Frasier's *On the Day You Were Born*, and *The Pig's Picnic*, by Keiko Kasza.

ABC and counting books, and books that encourage picture, word, and idea identification and recognition, such as *Animalia*, by Graeme Base, Sally Gridley's *Knock, Knock! Who's There?*, and *Annie and the Wild Animals*, by Jan Brett.

Fairy tales, simple hero tales, and stories with animals as the main characters, such as Steven Kellogg's *Paul Bunyan* and *Wild Robin*, by Susan Jeffers.

Books that encourage building a story line with beginning, middle, and end, such as *The Wolf's Chicken Stew*, by Keiko Kasza.

Books that encourage story and sequence building, rhythm and repetition, logic and order. Examples include *Ox-Cart Man*, by Donald Hall, and Nancy White Carlstrum's *Jesse Bear, What Will You Wear?*

5 TO 8 YEARS

A child this age is beginning to independently select books to read. However, being read to is still extremely important, although the books for read-aloud can be more complex and at a higher level of character and plot development. Listening skills can far exceed reading ability.

Books that encourage oral expression, reading aloud, and storytelling. These include Virginia Hamilton's folktales, such as *In the Beginning: Creation Stories from Around the World*, and Julius Lester's *How Many Spots Does a Leopard Have?*

Chapter books, family adventure, and fantasy stories are excellent read-aloud books.

Complex stories with detailed pictures are especially popular.

Books that share an interest of the child. Some examples are:

Mystery and ghost stories (John Bellairs, Alvin Schwartz)

Poetry (Shel Silverstein, Jack Prelutsky)

Adventure (Lynne Reid Banks, Sid Fleischman, Joan Aiken)

Humor (Roald Dahl, Daniel Pinkwater, James Howe, Lois Lowry)

Fantasy (Diana Wynne Jones, Natalie Babbitt, Lloyd Alexander)

Family life, family tension (Patricia MacLachlan, Katherine Paterson, Zilpha Keatly Synder, Beverly Cleary)

Animal stories (Marguerite Henry, Jim Kjelgaard, Arnold Lobel, Else Minarik, E.B. White)

Sports (Matt Christopher, John Tunis)

Ethnic groups (Virginia Hamilton, Laurence Yep, Mildred Taylor, Bette Bao Lord)

Science fiction (William Sleator)

Nonfiction stories (science, nature, technology, animals, plants, space, and weather)

Games, riddle-joke-nonsense books

Magazines

Comic books

9 TO 12 YEARS

Books for this age group should be well written and should fall into categories of interest to that child. Favorites include mysteries, adventure, fantasy, sports, relationships with family and friends, information, documentation and research on special topics, and good literature. Children enjoy stories about peers and situations in which they might find themselves. Many books focus on issues such as separation and being separated from parents or friends. Another popular theme is "feeling like an outsider."

12 YEARS TO ADULTHOOD

Any books that are well written and encourage pleasure, enjoyment, and the interest of the young adult are recommended. Many books written for adults are in this category. Books that help build self-esteem; books that focus on current interests, emotional-social-psychological issues, suspense and mysteries, personal problems, family relationships, gender relationships, imagination, hobbies, diaries, biographies, and travel; and content-specific books are especially worthwhile.

Resource books should be made available, such as encyclopedias, dictionaries, atlases, almanacs, thesaurus.

Appendix D

CHILD DEVELOPMENT RESOURCES FOR PARENTS

Lucinda Lee Katz and Thomas J. Hathaway

INFANCY

Ames LB: Questions Parents Ask. New York, Delta, 1988. (Offers sensible solutions to common parenting problems—infancy through early schooling.)

Brazelton TB: Infants and Mothers. New York, Delacorte, 1969. (Profiles three different types of temperaments in infants, giving parents a sense of the wide range of infant dispositions.)

Caplan F: The First Twelve Months of Life. New York, Bantam, 1978. (Details developmental characteristics of infants month by month.)

Dunn J: Distress and Comfort. Cambridge, MA, Harvard University Press, 1977. (First in the series The Developing Child, edited by Jerome Bruner, Michael Cole, and Barbara Lloyd; provides good introduction to theories of attachment and separation in the first months of life.)

Eisenberg A, Murkoff H, Hathaway S: What to Expect the First Year. New York, Workman Publishing, 1989. (Includes thorough information on the first year of parenting and addresses common child care issues such as colic, sleep and eating patterns, nursing, and weaning.)

Greenspan S: The First Feelings. New York, Penguin/Viking, 1985. (Focuses on the parent–infant dyad and the importance of establishing healthy interaction from the beginning.)

Kaye K: The Mental and Social Life of Babies. Chicago, University of Chicago Press, 1982. (Author describes the development of the parent–infant interaction, progressing from the child as an apprentice to the child as an adult.)

Leach P: Babyhood. New York, Alfred A. Knopf, 1983. (Developmental approach to the first 2 years of life; presents stages of emotional, physical, and intellectual growth of infants.)

Mahler M: The Psychological Birth of the Human Infant. New York, Basic Books, 1975. (Describes the process of separation/individuation that culminates in the psychological birth of a human infant; traces the symbiotic union through ego identity.)

PRESCHOOL

Brazelton TB: Toddlers and Parents. New York, Dell, 1976. (Profiles of families illuminating the universal struggle for independence and self-mastery by children between the ages of 1 and 3 years.)

Caplan T de F: The Early Childhood Years: Two to Six. New York, GP Putnam, 1983. (Practical information about raising children between the ages of 2 and 6 years; includes health care, toilet training, major areas of growth and development, extensive reading lists.)

Fraiberg S: The Magic Years. New York, Scribner, 1959. (Describes the wonder of childhood and the development of imagination.)

Kagan J: The Second Year. Cambridge, MA, Harvard University Press, 1981. (Provides information on the emotional and cognitive changes in the second year of life, such as the child's recognition of standards of behavior and of his or her own ability to meet those standards.)

SCHOOL AGE

Best R: We've All Got Scars. Indiana University Press, 1984. (Concentrates on the "informal curriculum" that the schools teach versus the academic one. In this "informal curriculum," the boys and girls are seen to learn patterns of behavior and socialization skills that are passed to them depending on their gender. Also discussed is their experiences of an informal sex education from their peers. Interesting insights for all those interested in the socialization and schooling of children.)

Clarke-Stewart A, Koch J: Children: Development Through Adolescence. New York, Wiley, 1983.

Kagan J: The Nature of the Child. New York, Basic Books, 1984. (In challenging many long-held views of human development, the author argues that early experience does not shape our lives forever; rather, humans have the potential for changing and continually transforming their own experiences.)

Kelley M: The Mother's Almanac II: Your Child from Six to Twelve. New York, Doubleday, 1989. (Uses the mother's perspective to understand the demands and challenges of parenting the 6- to 12-year-old on topics such as independence, family dynamics, and family traditions.)

ADOLESCENCE

Elkind D: All Grown Up and No Place to Go. New York, Addison-Wesley, 1984. (Book for parents; uses research, case studies, and personal experiences to communicate the situation that today's teenagers face. The book speaks to the "me" generation of parents, giving advice about supporting and raising the adolescent in the computer age.)

Faber A, Mazlish E: How to Talk So Kids Will Listen and Listen So Kids Will Talk. New York, Avon Books, 1982. (Addresses the relationship between parent and child regarding feelings. The exercises and cartoons give parents practical and useful information on discipline, cooperation, and autonomy.)

Group for the Advancement of Psychiatry: Normal Adolescence. New York, Scribner, 1968. (Compiles the research and perceptions of a group of psychiatrists, psychologists, and an anthropologist who came together in this informative book about adolescents. They discuss adolescence in terms of biologic, cultural, and psychological development. The authors believe that adolescence can be positive and that its conflicts and resolution can be a constructive force in our society.)

Kaplan L: Adolescence: The Farewell to Childhood. New York, Simon and Schuster, 1984. (Author treats the adolescent period with respect, showing it to be a phase that is profoundly complicated. Within the historical context of philosophy, psychology, and literature, the author draws a vivid series of contrasts that characterize the adolescent. She shows us how it is a time of life that has both an ending and a frightening, exciting beginning.)

Steinberg L, Levine A: You and Your Adolescent: A Parent's Guide for Ages 10–20. New York, Harper Collins Publishers, 1990. (Focuses on the basics of parenting adolescents on topics such as family communication, problem solving, physical and psychological development, and the social world of adolescents.)

CHILD CARE–PARENT CARE

Bettelheim B: Dialogues with Mothers. New York, The Free Press of Glencoe, 1962. (This is not a book that gives answers; it helps parents to learn to ask questions of themselves about the type of child they wish to have. By helping parents understand their own expectations in bringing up a child, it enhances the family's chances of being emotionally healthy.)

Christophersen ER: The Baby Owner's Manual. Shawnee Mission, KA, Overland Press, 1984. (What to expect and how to survive the first 30 days of having a baby. This illustrated book also provides expectant parents with practical, basic information to help them in their daily routine, both before childbirth and during the first month of the baby's life.)

Ferber R: Solve Your Child's Sleep Problems. New York, Simon & Schuster, 1988. (Guides parents on how to handle sleep problems in children aged 1–6; topics such as sleeping patterns, bed-wetting, night terrors, insomnia, and so forth, are addressed.)

Fraiberg S: Every Child's Birthright: In Defense of Mothering. New York, Bantam, 1977. (Concerned with the love affair that exists between parents and their children. Discusses the treatment that a human infant needs and is entitled to receive from his or her care-givers. This treatment is seen to be related to the bond that forms between the care-giver and the infant, and the value that our society puts on the act of mothering.)

Kanter CN: And Baby Makes Three: Your Feelings and Needs as New Parents. Minneapolis, Winston Press, 1983. (Book about parenting that focuses not only on the care of the infant but also on the feelings of the new parent. The author is a psychiatric social worker, and her clear style of writing, interwoven with developmental theory, makes this a good book for parents.)

Kitzinger S: Your Baby, Your Way. New York, Pantheon Books, 1987. (Addresses typical concerns about pregnancy and birthing; topics include emotional, physical, nutritional, and psychological issues on having a child.)

Leach P: Your Baby and Child: From Birth to Age Five. New York, Alfred A. Knopf, 1984. (Developmental approach to the first 5 years of life. Covers the psychological, social, and physical development of the child. The author includes many topics such as feeding, play, and interaction, and emphasizes reading and responding to the child's needs rather than rigidly following rules or generalizations about children.)

McBride AB: The Growth and Development of Mothers. New York, Harper & Row, 1975. (Looks at the process of becoming a mother. Written by a professor of psychiatric nursing who is also a mother of two, this book combines personal experience, case studies, and theoretical analysis in an attempt to explain the challenging, ever-changing experience of motherhood.)

Rakowitz E, Rubin GS: Living With Your New Baby. New York, Franklin Watts, 1978. (Provides practical information to help couples deal with the emotional and physiologic changes that occur during the first 3 months after childbirth. It gives a view of prenatal occurrences, including choosing a pediatrician and preparing the home, as well as advice about the legal aspects of parenthood and single parenting.)

Samuels M, Samuels N. The Well Baby Book. New York, Simon and Schuster, 1991. (Comprehensive manual for parenting including such topics as the working mother, sibling relationships, single parenting, developmental landmarks, television viewing, and common illnesses.)

Spock B: Baby and Child Care. New York, Pocket, 1975. (Best-seller in the child care field for over 30 years. It is an informative, practical book that gives advice on the psychological and physical care of infants and children. The author covers a wide array of subjects, including childbirth, fathering, nutrition, choosing day care, and single-family homes.)

Stoppard M: Day by Day Baby Care. New York, Ballantine Books, 1983. (Covers every aspect of child care, from birth through age 3. It has easily accessible organization and full illustrations. The author is a physician, a medical educator, and a mother of two herself. This book is an extremely usable and valuable resource for new parents or professionals working with infants.)

CHILD DEVELOPMENT AND INFANT MENTAL HEALTH

The Developing Child Series. Cambridge, MA, Harvard University Press (applies to all references in this section.)

Bower TGR: The Perceptual World of the Child. 1977 (Traces key elements in the development of perception in the child, concluding that the human perceptual system remains fairly constant throughout life but that our interpretation of the perceptual data changes with growth.)

Clarke-Stewart A: Daycare. 1982 (Practical book based on research exploring the effects of day care on young children. The author presents information on U.S. society and its need for day care, the history of day care, the types of day care currently used, the effects of day care, and hints for parents on making practical day-care decisions.)

deVillier PA, deVillier JG: Early Language. 1979 (Gives a summary of work in the area of early language development, tracing development in the sequence that it appears in the infant. Little information on theories of language development is offered.)

Dunn J: Distress and Comfort. 1977 (Good introduction on the theories of attachment/separation in the first months of life, including a cross-cultural view of attachment and distress, and the long-term consequences of the care-givers' method of handling early distress.)

Farnham-Diggory S: Learning Disabilities. 1978 (Gives definitions and descriptions of learning disabilities. It provides a historical review, describes brain functions, gives statistics and case studies, compares learning disabilities with hyperactivity, and examines the information processing approach to disabilities.)

Garvey C: Children's Talk. 1984 (The major discussions in this book bring together information from several bodies of research that discuss the child's attempt to use language in a social context.)

Garvey C: Play. 1977 (Not an introductory book: this well-written volume covers the definition of play, play in connection with elements in the child's environment, and learning to play. The reader is advised to have prior experience before reading this book.)

Goodnow J: Children's Drawing. 1977 (Examines research on children's drawing, looking at drawing as a reflection of cognitive development rather than of emotional development.)

Greenfield PM: Mind and Media: The Effects of Television, Video, Games and Computers. 1984 (Using information from an array of disciplines, this book summarizes what television, video games, and computers can and should do. This book shows us that although the media can be effective tools, they are not a substitute for teaching.)

Kempe CH, Kempe RS: Child Abuse. 1978 (Focuses on the nature and treatment of child abuse and describes the organization of programs that treat child abuse. This book is useful to all those who come into contact with children.)

Macfarlane A: The Psychology of Childbirth. 1977 (Discusses life before birth, psychosocial factors in pregnancy, variations during delivery, the beginning of life, the capabilities of the newborn, research on early bonding, and other issues. This is a good introduction to research on early socialization.)

Parke RD: Fathers. 1981 (Describes new research on the history of fathering, the role of the father, the expectant father, the relationship between father and infant, the role of fathers in socialization and intellectual development, and the issues of job sharing, divorce, and career families.)

Rubin Z: Children's Friendships. 1980 (Describes the development of friendships, beginning with a historical summary and then tracing the development of friendship from the first year through the changes that accompany growing up. The author discusses such issues as what it means to be a friend, what it means to lose a friend, children's division into same-sex friendship groups, and friendship patterns across different ages and cultures.)

Schaffer R: Mothering. 1977 (Describes mothering from various perspectives: (1) the traditional, (2) the writers of practical handbooks for parents, and (3) the last 10 years of research. A good introductory book.)

Stern D: The First Relationship: Infant and Mother. 1977 (Describes the social interaction of the parent–infant dyad during the first 6 months of life. It shows in detail how the interactive nature of the relationship is critically dependent on input and participation from both the parent and the infant. A fascinating and new way to look at infants and their parents.)

COMBINING CAREER AND FAMILY

Brazelton TB: Working Parents. 1986.

Curley J, Ladar S, Siegler A et al: The Balancing Act. Chicago, Review Press, 1975. (Composed of the essays of five young professional women who have become mothers for the first time. They are all committed to their work and to their children. They describe their experiences, their successes, and failures at balancing their careers and their home life. An interesting, honest, and helpful account for parents and would-be parents in this career-oriented age.)

Curley J, Ladar S, Siegler A et al: The Balancing Act II. Chicago, Review Press, 1981.

Grossman C: Infant care guide for new mothers who are considering returning to a job before the baby is toddler. In The Robert Hamilton Wallace Infant Care Program, Evanston Hospital, 1984.

BREAST-FEEDING

Ewy D, Ewy R: Preparation for Breast-feeding. New York, Dolphin Books, 1975. (Fully explains breast-feeding in a step-by-step coverage of how to prepare and what to expect in the months prior to birth; comprehensive for parents.)

Kitzinger S: Breastfeeding Your Baby. New York: Alfred A. Knopf, 1989. (Reassures parents on how to approach breast-feeding; step-by-step approach with clear illustrations and photographs.)

La Leche League: The Womanly Art of Breast-feeding. Franklin Park, IL, La Leche League, 1981. (Fully illustrated, complete manual to breast-feeding based on research and vast practical experience. Written by a worldwide organization that is considered one of the world's foremost authorities on breast-feeding.)

Pryor K: Nursing Your Baby. New York, Pocket, 1972. (Describes the psychological as well as the physical adjustments that a mother must make in order to breast-feed her infant. Gives helpful information, complete with photographs, on day-to-day management of nursing; also reviews current knowledge in the field from a wide variety of disciplines.)

PREPARING THE CHILD FOR HOSPITALIZATION

Elliott I: Hospital Roadmap: A Book to Help Explain the Hospital Experience to Young Children. Cambridge, MA, Resources for Children in Hospitals, 1984. (For parents and early school-age children; clearly written in simple, straightforward language; covers common hospital experiences and feelings.)

Hautzig D: A Visit to Sesame Street Hospital. New York, Random House, 1985. (For preschool and early school-age children. Sesame Street characters go on a brief tour of the hospital. Style, content, and depth most appropriate for younger children.)

Hogan P: The Hospital Scares Me. Milwaukee, Raintree, 1980. (For preschool and early school-age children. The story of a young boy's hospital experience, including hospital procedures and his feelings during hospitalization. Attractively illustrated.)

Howe J: The Hospital Book. New York, Crown, 1981. (For older school-age children. Detailed coverage of common hospital procedures, personnel, tests, and experiences. Slightly dated black and white photographs.)

Richter E: The Teenage Hospital Experience. You Can Handle It! New York, Coward, 1982. (Interviews with teenagers regarding the hospital experience, common feelings, reactions, and how to cope with these. Also includes interviews with medical and nursing professionals. Dated language and photographs.)

Rogers I: Going to the Hospital. New York, Putnam, 1988. (For preschool and early school-age children. Well-written and illustrated. Style, content, and depth most appropriate for younger children.)

Appendix E

A CORE LIST OF OFFICE EMERGENCY EQUIPMENT*

Robert A. Dershewitz

The office is not a proxy emergency room and cannot be expected to be as well equipped or as proficient in dealing with emergencies. However, because true emergencies sometimes occur or present themselves in an office, this setting must be prepared to initiate appropriate emergency care. Basic or minimal equipment and medications need to be available to respond to a wide, though realistic, array of emergencies—at least until emergency medical services arrive. It is suggested that all equipment be stored in a portable unit such as a tool cart.

AIRWAY/BREATHING EQUIPMENT

Portable oxygen tank with flow meter, tubing, and oxygen masks (pediatric and adult sizes)

Self-inflating bag–valve ventilation device with oxygen reservoir (adult and child sizes)

Ventilation masks (newborn, infant, child, and adult sizes)

Portable suction machine with suction catheters

Suction bulb and/or DeLee catheter

Desirable, But Not Necessary

Pediatric laryngoscope and blades (sizes 0–3)

Endotracheal tubes (sizes 3.0–8.0 [uncuffed through 6; cuffed 6–8])

Stylettes for endotracheal tubes

Oropharyngeal airways (sizes 0–5)

CPR resuscitation board

Tincture of benzoin

Magill forceps

EQUIPMENT TO SUPPORT CIRCULATION

IV fluids
> ½–1 liter bag of normal saline
> ½–1 liter bag of normal saline in 5% dextrose

Infusion set

IV butterfly needles 18–25 gauge

IV catheters 18–22 gauge

IV pole

Intraosseous infusion needles (16 or 18 gauge)

Armboard

Tourniquet

Tape, alcohol pads

Sphygmomanometer with infant-, child-, and adult-sized cuffs

4×4 sponges

2×2 sponges

Syringes (10 ml, 3 ml, 1 ml)

DRUGS

It is highly recommended to have a list of emergency drugs along with a quick guide for easy use where the drugs are stored.

Epinephrine (diluted 1:10,000 for intravenous, endotracheal, or intraosseous use; 1:1000 for subcutaneous use)

Atropine

---

*For a more complete listing of emergency drugs and dosages, as well as a discussion on office emergencies, the reader is referred to the article by Sapien and Hodge in *Pediatric Annals* 19:659–667, 1990.

Sodium bicarbonate

Lidocaine

Dextrose

Insulin

Ipecac

Activated charcoal

Diazepam

Corticosteroids for IV and P.O. use

Narcan

Diphenhydramine

Parenteral antibiotics (e.g., ampicillin, ceftriaxone)

Sterile eye irrigation

Aminophylline

TRAUMA

C-spine stabilization equipment (hard cervical collars or sandbags with tape)

Splinting materials

Wound dressing

Index

Page numbers followed by *f* indicate figures; those followed by *t* indicate tabular material.

Abdominal pain
  acute, 396–400
    from appendicitis, 397
    character of, 397
    differential diagnosis of, 397–399
    from ectopic pregnancy, 397
    management of, 400
    from obstruction with strangulation, 397
    referral in, 400
    visceral vs. parietal, 397
    work-up for, 399–400
  in pelvic inflammatory disease, 471–472
  recurrent, 400–404
    definition of, 400
    gastroenterology referral for, 404
    hospitalization for, 404
    in irritable bowel syndrome, 401
    laboratory tests in, 402, 402t
    management of, 403–404
    organic causes of, 402–403, 403f
    presentation of, 401
    from stress, 401, 402
    work-up for, 401
ABR. *See* Auditory brain stem response, 299
Abrasions
  cleansing of, 540
  dressings for, 539
  referral for, 540
Abscess(es)
  brain, 703
  cold, 673
Absences
  school
    parental cause, 162–163
    truancy, 163
Absence seizures, 581, 582, 585–586
  myoclonic
    in epilepsy syndromes, 583
Abuse. *See* Child abuse; Sexual abuse;
    Substance abuse
Accident prevention. *See* Injury prevention
Acetaminophen (N-acetylpara-aminophenol)
  clinical presentation of, 645
  clinical uses of
    for fever, 669
    for analgesia, 678
  poisoning from, 645–646
    evaluation of, 645–646
    oral N-acetylcysteine for, 646
    Rumack-Mathew nomogram in, 646f
  hepatotoxicity in, 645
  vs. toxic hepatitis, 645
Achilles tendonitis, 518
Acidemia
  metabolic
    in salicylate poisoning, 644
Acidic compound ingestions
  clinical presentation of, 655
  pathophysiology of, 655
  prevention of, 656–657
  treatment of
    nutrition following, 656
    steroids in, 656
    surgical, 656
  work-up for
    esophagoscopy in, 655–656
    history and physical examination in, 655
Acne, 279–282
  clinical presentation of, 279
    lesions in, 279–280
    scars from, 280
  differential diagnosis of, 281
  pathophysiology of, 279
  treatment of, 281–282
    antibiotics, systemic, 282

dermabrasion in, 282
  keratolytics in, 281–282
  topicals in, 281, 282
  types of
    acne vulgaris, 279–280
    conglobata, 280
    drug-induced, 281
    fulminans, 280
    gram-negative folliculitis, 281
    infantile, 280
    neonatorum, 280
    occlusion-induced, 280–281
    occupational, 281
  work-up for, 281
Acne keloidalis, 253
Acoustic reflectometry
  acoustic otoscope in, 301
  in otitis media with effusion, 296
  vs. typanometry, 301
Acquired immunodeficiency syndrome (AIDS)
  in children, 200–204
    AIDS dementia in, 202
    CDC classification of, 201
    clinical manifestations of HIV infection in,
      201–202, 210t
    differential diagnosis of, 202
    laboratory test for, 203
    pathophysiology of, 201
    transmission to, 200–201
    treatment and management of, 203
    vs. adult HIV infection, 201t
    work-up for, 202–203
Acrocyanosis. *See* Cyanosis
Acrodermatitis enteropathica
  vs. atopic dermatitis, 237
  vs. diaper rash, 241
Acrodermatitis of childhood
  papular, 264
Acromioclavicular joint
  injury to, 527
Acropustulosis of infancy, 249
Activity
  suppression of
    in development, 38
Acute abdomen, 397
Acute care regimens, 99
Acyanotic lesion(s)
  neonatal, 210–211, 212t
    anomalous origin of left coronary
      artery, 210
    aortic stenosis, 209, 211
    arteriovenous malformations, 210
    atrial septal defect, 210
    coarctation of the aorta, 209
    from diabetic mother, 211
    endocardial cushion defect, 209
    hypoplastic left heart, 210
    patent ductus arteriosus, 209, 211
    peripheral pulmonic stenosis, 209
    Pompe's disease, 211
    vascular rings, pulmonary slings, 211
    ventricular septal defect, 210, 211
Acyclovir
  for acute herpetic gingivostomatitis, 321
  for herpes virus, 739, 739t
Adenoidectomy
  for otitis media with effusion, 297
ADHD. *See* Attention deficit hyperactivity
    disorder
Adhesive agents
  contact dermatitis from, 243
Adjustment disorder
  rebelliousness vs., 173

Adolescence
  pregnancy in, 54, 165–169
  sexually transmitted diseases in, 54, 732,
    735–736
  street drug usage in, 54, 175–178
  suicide in, 142–143
  truancy in, 163
Adoption
  of foster child, 119
Adrenarche
  in sexual development, 348
Advocacy
  for chronic illness, 773
Advocacy role
  of physician
    in child abuse and neglect, 93
    for foster child, 118, 119
    for safety, 89
Affective disorder(s)
  manic depression, 120
  rebelliousness vs., 173
β-agonists
  for anaphylaxis, 189
  for chronic asthma, 186–187
    oral or inhalation
AIDS. *See* Acquired immunodeficiency
    syndrome
Air conduction
  in hearing, 298, 299, 299f
Air pollution
  indoor
    formaldehyde in, 81
    nitrogen dioxide in, 81
    tobacco smoke in, 80–82
    wood stove and fireplace smoke in, 81
  outdoor
    Clean Air Act of 1970 and, 81–82
    ozone in, 81, 82
    pollutants in, 81
Airway
  inflammatory illness of, 609–612
    airway obstruction from, 609
    croup, 610–612
    supraglottitis, 609–610
    tracheitis, bacterial, 612
  obstruction of
    in cystic fibrosis, 627, 628–629
    from foreign body aspiration, 607–609
    in inflammatory illness, 609
Akinetic seizures
  syncope vs., 695
Alar. *See* Daminozide
Albright's syndrome, 273
Alcohol
  in breast milk, 18
  fetal exposure to
    birth defects from, 16
    fetal alcohol syndrome from, 18
    effect on newborn, 18
Alcohol intoxication, 660–662. *See also*
    Substance abuse
  from benzyl alcohol, 662
  blood levels in, 661, 661t
  from ethanol
    blood level/clinical syndrome in, 661, 661t
    pathophysiology of, 660–661
    in small children, 660
    treatment of, 661
  from ethylene alcohol, 662
  from isopropyl alcohol
    pathophysiology of, 661–662
    toxicity of, 661–662
    treatment of, 661–662
  from methanol
    pathophysiology of, 661
    signs and symptoms of, 661

ISBN 0-397-51196-5

90000

9 780397 511969